HUMAN PHYSIOLOGY AND MECHANISMS OF DISEASE

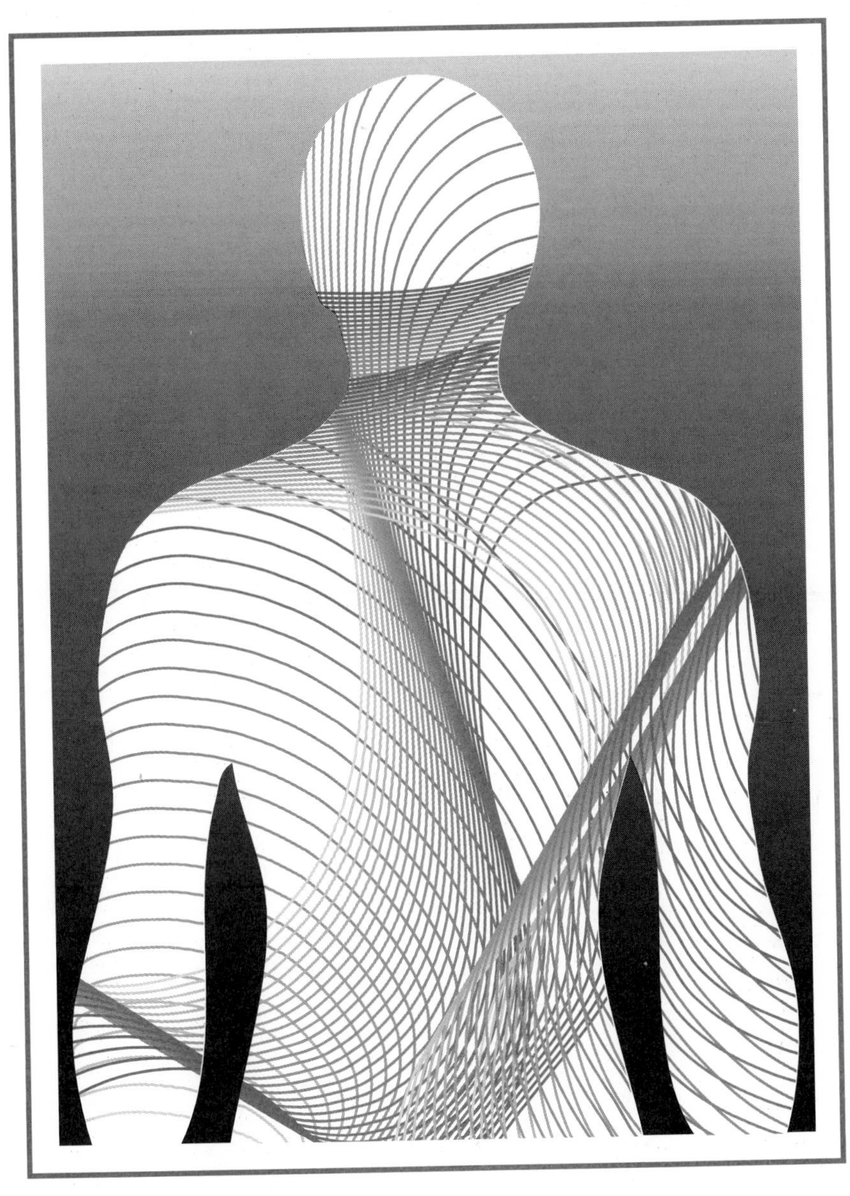

fifth edition

HUMAN PHYSIOLOGY AND MECHANISMS OF DISEASE

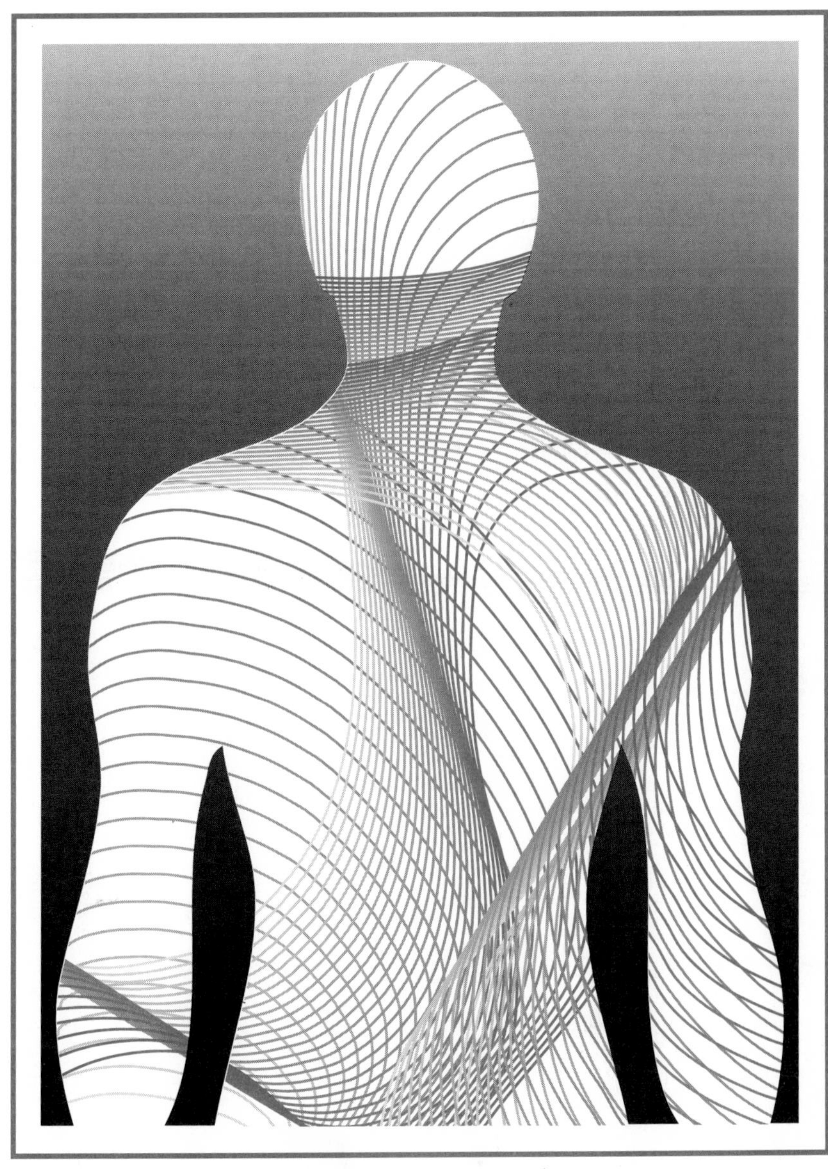

ARTHUR C. GUYTON, M.D.
Professor of Physiology and Biophysics
Department of Physiology and Biophysics
University of Mississippi Medical Center
Jackson, Mississippi

W.B. SAUNDERS COMPANY
Harcourt Brace Jovanovich, Inc.
Philadelphia
London Toronto Montreal Sydney Tokyo

fifth edition

W. B. SAUNDERS COMPANY
Harcourt Brace Jovanovich Inc.

The Curtis Center
Independence Square West
Philadelphia, Pennsylvania 19106

Library of Congress Cataloging-in-Publication Data

Guyton, Arthur C.
Human physiology and mechanisms of disease / Arthur C. Guyton. — 5th ed.
p. cm.
Includes bibliographical references and index.
ISBN 0-7216-3961-5
1. Human physiology. 2. Physiology, Pathological. I. Title.
[DNLM: 1. Disease. 2. Physiology. QT 104 G992b]
QP34.5.G87 1992
612—dc20
DNLM/DLC
for Library of Congress 91-36020
CIP

Editor: Martin J. Wonsiewicz
Designer: Ellen Bodner-Zanolle
Production Manager: Peter Faber
Manuscript Editor: Wynette Kommer
Illustration Specialist: Cecilia Roberts
Indexer: Nancy Matthews

Listed here is the latest translated edition of this book together with the language of the translation and the publisher. 9/26/89, Portuguese, Editora Guanabara, S.A.A., Rio de Janeiro, Brazil

Bahasa Malaysia (3rd Edition) — Universiti Sains Malaysia, Minden, Malaysia

Greek (3rd Edition) — C. G. Listsas, Athens, Greece

Portuguese (2nd Edition) — DISCO CBS Industria e Comercio Ltd., Rio de Janeiro, Brazil

Spanish (2nd Edition) — Nueva Editorial Interamerica S.A.

Indonesian (3rd Edition) — EGC Medical Publishers, Jakarta, Indonesia

Portions of this book, including both text and illustrations, have appeared previously in the *Textbook of Medical Physiology* by Arthur C. Guyton, published by W. B. Saunders, 1991.

Human Physiology and Mechanisms of Disease ISBN 0-7216-3961-5

Printed in the United States of America

Last digit is the print number: 9 8 7 6 5 4 3 2 1

Preface

This textbook, entitled Human Physiology and Mechanisms of Disease, is written for those students who do not have the time to study one of the more formidable books and yet require much more than the usual college introduction to the physiology of the human body. These include medical students, dental students, pharmacy students, other paramedical students in all fields, and upper level biology students. In general, the types of material presented are threefold: first, the basic fundamental principles of life itself, beginning with the physical, chemical, and molecular laws of cellular function; second, the important concepts and principles necessary for understanding the overall integrated function of the human body; and, third, multiple illustrative examples of how physiological function can become abnormal in human disease conditions.

This is the fifth edition of this text. The changes from the fourth edition have been many, including update of the physiological understanding of virtually every functional area of the body. However, the most extensive changes have come in two special areas: First is the fundamental molecular mechanisms of physiology, a field that is advancing exceedingly rapidly. Fortunately, newer knowledge in this area simplifies many of the explanations for which only speculation could be given previously. The second major area of change has been in the higher functions of the nervous system. Research on nervous mechanisms has always been difficult, so that new fundamental principles of nervous function have been very slow to develop. Yet, within the past decade, especially with the advancing knowledge of neuronal molecular physiology, many of the deeper levels of nervous function are at last beginning to fall in place.

I hope especially that this text can convey to the student that our bodies are among the most complex and yet logical and beautiful of all functional mechanisms. I hope, too, that he or she will understand that each individual living cell carries within its nucleus all the genetic information required to create an entire human being; yet, this same genetic pool serves as almost 100,000 separate intracellular control systems that regulate the chemical reactions within the cells. And, finally, I hope that all students will recognize, as a special example, the majesty of the human brain as a powerful computer having capabilities that all the electronic computers in the world cannot at present achieve.

I could go on detailing the miracles of the human body. That, indeed, is the purpose of this entire text. The success of the book will be measured by the degree of excitement that it leaves with the student for further study in the field of physiology or for a lifetime of physiological thinking.

A small but important portion of this text presents not only knowledge that has come from basic experiments in animals but also knowledge that has come from human experiments, especially unplanned experiments caused by disease. For instance, a major share of our knowledge of the regulation of blood glucose and of the mechanisms of carbohydrate metabolism has come from study of diabetes mellitus, a disease that alters these physiological functions profoundly and that is widespread among the human population. Likewise, literally thousands of human "experiments" proceed each day in the fields of high blood pressure, congestive heart failure, gastrointestinal disturbances, respiratory diseases, and so forth. The physiology of each of these abnormalities is discussed briefly, partly because study of the diseases themselves can be enlightening but even more, because they give important insights into basic physiological concepts.

Finally, I would like to thank many others who have contributed to the development of this text. For the illustrations in the text I am especially indebted to Ms. Tomiko Mita, Mr. Michael Schenk, Ms. Tina Burnham, and Ms. Dianne Fleming, and for excellent secretarial services I owe my gratitude to Mrs. Ivadelle Osberg Heidke, Ms. Gwendolyn Robbins, and Mrs. Nancy Kimmel. I also extend my appreciation to the staff of the W. B. Saunders Company for its continued excellence in all publication matters, with appreciation especially to Martin J. Wonsiewicz, Senior Editor; Ellen Bodner-Zanolle, Designer; Peter Faber, Production Manager; Wynette Kommer, Manuscript Editor; and Cecilia Roberts, Illustration Specialist, whose editorial and technical help have been invaluable.

ARTHUR C. GUYTON, M.D.

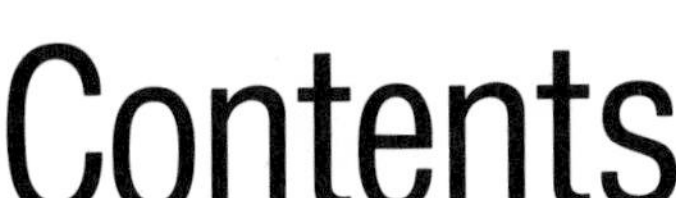

Contents

I

Introduction to Physiology: The Cell and General Physiology

1 Functional Organization of the Human Body and Control of the "Internal Environment"

2 The Cell and Its Function

3 Genetic Control of Protein Synthesis, Cell Function, and Cell Reproduction

4 Transport Through the Cell Membrane

1

Functional Organization of the Human Body and Control of the "Internal Environment"

In human physiology, we are concerned with the specific characteristics and mechanisms of the human body that make it a living being. The very fact that we remain alive is almost beyond our own control, for hunger makes us seek food and fear makes us seek refuge. Sensations of cold make us provide warmth, and other forces cause us to seek fellowship and to reproduce. Thus, the human being is actually an automaton, and the fact that we are sensing, feeling, and knowledgeable beings is part of this automatic sequence of life; these special attributes allow us to exist under widely varying conditions that otherwise would make life impossible.

CELLS AS THE LIVING UNITS OF THE BODY

The basic living unit of the body is the cell, and each organ is an aggregate of many different cells held together by intercellular supporting structures. Each type of cell is specially adapted to perform one particular function. For instance, the red blood cells, 25 trillion in all, transport oxygen from the lungs to the tissues. Although this type of cell is perhaps the most abundant, there are perhaps another 75 trillion cells. The entire body, then, contains about 100 trillion cells.

Although the many cells of the body often differ markedly from each other, all of them have certain basic characteristics that are alike. For instance, in all cells oxygen combines with carbohydrate, fat, or protein to release the energy required for cell function. Furthermore, the general mechanisms for changing nutrients into energy are basically the same in all cells, and all the cells also deliver the end-products of their chemical reactions into the surrounding fluids.

Almost all cells also have the ability to reproduce, and whenever cells of a particular type are destroyed from one cause or another, the remaining cells of this type often regenerate new cells until the appropriate number is replenished.

THE EXTRACELLULAR FLUID—THE INTERNAL ENVIRONMENT

About 56 per cent of the adult human body is fluid. Although most of this fluid is inside the cells and is called *intracellular fluid,* about one third is in the spaces outside the cells and is called *extracellular fluid.* This extracellular fluid is in constant motion throughout the body. It is rapidly transported in the circulating blood and then mixed between the blood and the tissue fluids by diffusion through the capillary walls. In the extracellular fluid are the ions and nutrients needed by the cells for maintenance of cellular life. Therefore, all cells live in essentially the same environment, the extracellular fluid, for which reason the extracellular fluid is called the *internal environment* of the body, or the *milieu intérieur,* a term introduced over a hundred years ago by the great 19th century French physiologist Claude Bernard.

Cells are capable of living, growing, and performing their special functions so long as the proper concentrations of oxygen, glucose, different ions, amino acids, fatty substances, and other constituents are available in this internal environment.

Differences Between Extracellular and Intracellular Fluids. The extracellular fluid contains large amounts of *sodium, chloride,* and *bicarbonate ions,* plus nutrients for the cells, such as *oxygen, glucose, fatty acids,* and *amino acids.* It also contains carbon dioxide that is being transported from the cells to the lungs to be excreted and other cellular products that are being transported to the kidneys for excretion.

The intracellular fluid differs significantly from the extracellular fluid; particularly, it contains large amounts of *potassium, magnesium,* and *phosphate ions* instead of the sodium and chloride ions found in the extracellular fluid. Special mechanisms for transporting ions through the cell membranes maintain these differences. These mechanisms are discussed in Chapter 4.

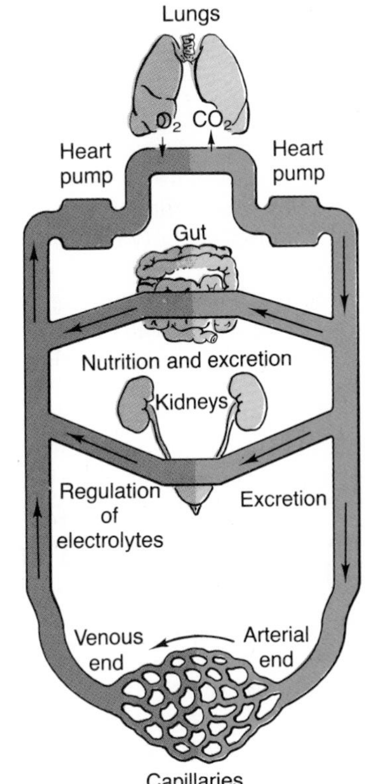

Figure 1–1. General organization of the circulatory system.

"HOMEOSTATIC" MECHANISMS OF THE MAJOR FUNCTIONAL SYSTEMS

Homeostasis

The term *homeostasis* is used by physiologists to mean *maintenance of static, or constant, conditions in the internal environment.* Essentially all the organs and tissues of the body perform functions that help maintain these constant conditions. For instance, the lungs provide oxygen to the extracellular fluid to replenish continually the oxygen that is being used by the cells, the kidneys maintain constant ion concentrations, and the gastrointestinal system provides nutrients. A large segment of this text is concerned with the manner in which each organ or tissue contributes to homeostasis. To begin this discussion, the different functional systems of the body and their homeostatic mechanisms are outlined briefly.

The Extracellular Fluid Transport System —The Circulatory System

Extracellular fluid is transported through all parts of the body in two different stages. The first stage entails movement of blood around and around the circulatory system, and the second, movement of fluid between the blood capillaries and the cells. Figure 1–1 illustrates the overall circulation of blood. All the blood in the circulation traverses the entire circuit of the circulation an average of once each minute at rest and as many as six times each minute when a person becomes extremely active.

As blood passes through the capillaries, continual exchange of extracellular fluid occurs between the plasma portion of the blood and the interstitial fluid that fills the spaces between the cells, the *intercellular spaces.* This process is illustrated in Figure 1–2. Note that the capillaries are porous so that large amounts of fluid and its dissolved constituents can *diffuse* back and forth between the blood and the tissue spaces, as illustrated by the arrows. This process of diffusion is caused by kinetic motion of the molecules in both the plasma and the interstitial fluid. That is, the fluid and dissolved molecules are continually moving and bouncing in all directions within the fluid itself and also through the pores and through the tissue spaces. Almost no cell is located more than 25 to 50 micrometers from a capillary, which insures diffusion of almost any substance from the capillary to the cell within a few seconds. Thus, the extracellular fluid everywhere in the body, both that of the plasma and that in interstitial spaces, is continually being mixed, thereby maintaining almost complete homogeneity.

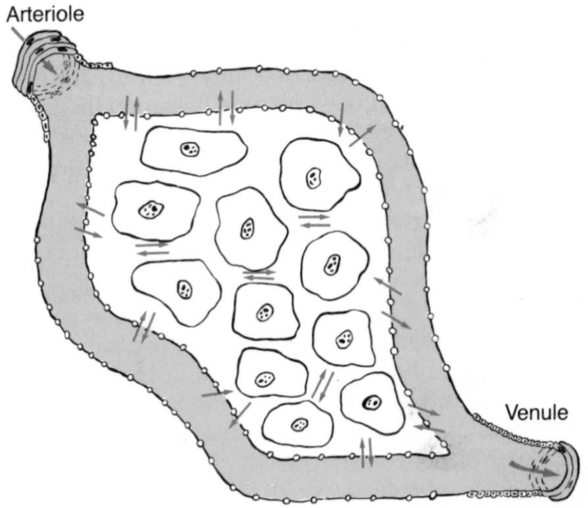

Figure 1–2. Diffusion of fluids through the capillary walls and through the interstitial spaces.

Origin of Nutrients in the Extracellular Fluid

The Respiratory System. Figure 1–1 shows that each time the blood passes through the body it also flows through the lungs. The blood picks up oxygen in the alveoli, thus acquiring the *oxygen* needed by the cells. The membrane between the alveoli and the lumen of the pulmonary capillaries is only 0.4 to 2.0 micrometers in thickness, and oxygen diffuses through this membrane into the blood in exactly the same manner that water and ions diffuse through the tissue capillaries.

The Gastrointestinal Tract. A large portion of the blood pumped by the heart passes also through the walls of the gastrointestinal organs. Here different dissolved nutrients, including *carbohydrates, fatty acids, amino acids,* and others, are absorbed into the extracellular fluid.

The Liver and Other Organs That Perform Primarily Metabolic Functions. Not all substances absorbed from the gastrointestinal tract can be used in their absorbed form by the cells. The liver changes the chemical compositions of many of these to more usable forms, and other tissues of the body—the fat cells, the gastrointestinal mucosa, the kidneys, and the endocrine glands—help modify the absorbed substances or store them until they are needed at a later time.

The Musculoskeletal System. Sometimes the question is asked: How does the musculoskeletal system fit into the homeostatic functions of the body? The answer to this is obvious and simple: Were it not for this system, the body could not move to the appropriate place at the appropriate time to obtain the foods required for nutrition. The musculoskeletal system also provides motility for protection against adverse surroundings, without which the entire body, and along with it all the homeostatic mechanisms, could be destroyed instantaneously.

Removal of Metabolic End-Products

Removal of Carbon Dioxide by the Lungs. At the same time that blood picks up oxygen in the lungs, *carbon dioxide* is released from the blood into the alveoli, and the respiratory movement of air into and out of the alveoli carries the carbon dioxide to the atmosphere. Carbon dioxide is the most abundant of all the end-products of metabolism.

The Kidneys. Passage of the blood through the kidneys removes most substances from the plasma that are not needed by the cells. These substances include especially different end-products of cellular metabolism and excesses of ions and water that might have accumulated in the extracellular fluid. The kidneys perform their function by, first, filtering large quantities of plasma through the glomeruli into the tubules and then reabsorbing into the blood those substances needed by the body, such as glucose, amino acids, appropriate amounts of water, and many of the ions. However, most of the substances not needed by the body, especially the metabolic end-products such as urea, are poorly reabsorbed and, instead, pass on through the renal tubules into the urine.

Regulation of Body Functions

The Nervous System. The nervous system is composed of three major parts: the *sensory portion,* the *central nervous system* (or *integrative portion*), and the *motor portion.* Sensory receptors detect the state of the body or the state of the surroundings. For instance, receptors present everywhere in the skin apprise one every time an object touches that person at any point. The eyes are sensory organs that give one a visual image of the surrounding area. The ears also are sensory organs. The central nervous system is composed of the brain and spinal cord. The brain can store information, generate thoughts, create ambition, and determine reactions the body performs in response to the sensations. Appropriate signals are then transmitted through the motor portion of the nervous system to carry out the person's desires.

A large segment of the nervous system is called the *autonomic system.* It operates at a subconscious level and controls many functions of the internal organs, including the action of the heart, the movements of the gastrointestinal tract, and the secretion by different glands.

The Hormonal System of Regulation. Located in the body are eight major endocrine glands that secrete chemical substances, the *hormones.* Hormones are transported in the extracellular fluid to all parts of the body to help regulate cellular function. For instance, thyroid hormone increases the rates of most chemical reactions in all cells. In this way thyroid hormone helps to set the tempo of bodily activity. Insulin controls glucose metabolism, adrenocortical hormones control ion and protein metabolism, and parathyroid hormone controls bone metabolism. Thus, the hormones are a system of regulation that complements the nervous system. The nervous system, in general, regulates mainly muscular and secretory activities of the body, whereas the hormonal system regulates mainly the metabolic functions.

Reproduction

Reproduction sometimes is not considered to be a homeostatic function. However, reproduction does help maintain static conditions by generating new beings to take the place of ones that are dying. This perhaps sounds like a permissive usage of the term homeostasis, but it does illustrate that, in the final analysis, essentially all structures of the body are so organized that they help maintain the automaticity and the continuity of life.

THE CONTROL SYSTEMS OF THE BODY

The human body has literally thousands of control systems in it. The most intricate of all these are the genetic control systems that operate in all cells to control intracellular function and all extracellular functions as well. This subject is discussed in Chapter 3. Many other control systems operate within the organs to control functions of the individual parts of the organs; others operate throughout the entire body to control the interrelationships between the organs. For instance, the respiratory system, operating in association with the nervous system, regulates the concentration of carbon dioxide in the extracellular fluid. The liver and the pancreas regulate the concentration of glucose in the extracellular fluid. The kidneys regulate the concentrations of hydrogen, sodium, potassium, phosphate, and other ions in the extracellular fluid.

Examples of Control Mechanisms

Regulation of Oxygen and Carbon Dioxide Concentrations in the Extracellular Fluid. Because oxygen is one of the major substances required for chemical reactions in the cells, it is fortunate that the body has a special control mechanism to maintain an almost exact and constant oxygen concentration in the extracellular fluid. This mechanism depends principally on the chemical characteristics of *hemoglobin,* which is present in all the red blood cells. Hemoglobin combines with oxygen as the blood passes through the lungs. Then, as the blood passes through the tissue capillaries, the hemoglobin will not release oxygen into the tissue fluid if too much oxygen is already there, but if the oxygen concentration is too little, sufficient oxygen will be released to re-establish an adequate tissue oxygen concentration. Thus, the regulation of oxygen concentration in the tissues is vested principally in the chemical characteristics of hemoglobin itself. This regulation is called the *oxygen-buffering function of hemoglobin.*

Carbon dioxide concentration in the extracellular fluid is regulated in quite a different way. Carbon dioxide is one of the major end-products of the oxidative reactions in cells. If all the carbon dioxide formed in the cells were to continue to accumulate in the tissue fluids, the mass action of the carbon dioxide itself would soon halt all the energy-giving reactions of the cells. Fortunately, a nervous mechanism controls the expiration of carbon dioxide through the lungs and in this way maintains a constant and reasonable concentration of carbon dioxide in the extracellular fluid. That is, a high carbon dioxide concentration *excites the respiratory center,* causing the person to breathe rapidly and deeply. This increases the expiration of carbon dioxide and therefore increases its removal from the blood and the extracellular fluid, and the process continues until the concentration returns to normal.

Regulation of Arterial Pressure. Several different systems contribute to the regulation of arterial pressure. One of these, the *baroreceptor system,* is a very simple and excellent example of a control mechanism. In the walls of most of the great arteries of the upper body, especially in the bifurcation region of the carotids and the arch of the aorta, are many nerve receptors, called *baroreceptors,* which are stimulated by stretch of the arterial wall. When the arterial pressure becomes great, these baroreceptors are stimulated excessively, and impulses are transmitted to the medulla of the brain. Here the impulses inhibit the *vasomotor center,* which in turn decreases the number of impulses transmitted through the sympathetic nervous system to the heart and blood vessels. Lack of these impulses causes diminished pumping activity by the heart and increased ease of blood flow through the peripheral vessels, both of which lower the arterial pressure back toward normal. Conversely, a fall in arterial pressure relaxes the stretch receptors, allowing the vasomotor center to become more active than usual and thereby causing the arterial pressure to rise back toward normal.

Normal Ranges of Important Extracellular Fluid Constituents

Table 1–1 lists the more important constituents and physical characteristics of extracellular fluid, along with their normal values, normal ranges, and

Table 1–1 SOME IMPORTANT CONSTITUENTS AND PHYSICAL CHARACTERISTICS OF THE EXTRACELLULAR FLUID, THE NORMAL RANGE OF CONTROL, AND THE APPROXIMATE NONLETHAL LIMITS

	Normal Value	Normal Range	Approximate Nonlethal Limits	Units
Oxygen	40	35–45	10–1000	mm Hg
Carbon dioxide	40	35–45	5–80	mm Hg
Sodium ion	142	138–146	115–175	mmol/L
Potassium ion	4.2	3.8–5.0	1.5–9.0	mmol/L
Calcium ion	1.2	1.0–1.4	0.5–2.0	mmol/L
Chloride ion	108	103–112	70–130	mmol/L
Bicarbonate ion	28	24–32	8–45	mmol/L
Glucose	85	75–95	20–1500	mg/dl
Body temperature	98.4 (37.0)	98–98.8 (37.0)	65–110 (18.3–43.3)	F° (C°)
Acid-base	7.4	7.3–7.5	6.9–8.0	pH

maximum limits for short periods of time without causing death. Note especially the narrowness of the normal range for each one of these. Values outside these ranges are usually the cause of or the result of illness.

Even more important are the limits beyond which abnormalities can cause death. For instance, an increase in the body temperature of only 10° to 12°F (6° to 7°C) above normal can often lead to a vicious circle of increasing cellular metabolism that literally destroys the cells. Note also the very narrow range for the acid-base balance of the body, with a normal pH value of 7.4 and lethal values only about 0.5 on either side of the normal value. Another especially important factor is potassium ion, for whenever its concentration falls to less than one third normal, the person is likely to be paralyzed because of inability of the nerves to carry nerve signals, and if ever it rises to two or more times normal, the heart muscle is likely to be depressed severely. Also, when the calcium ion concentration falls below about one half normal, the person is likely to experience tetanic contraction of muscles throughout the body because of spontaneous generation of nerve impulses in the peripheral nerves. When the glucose concentration falls below one half normal, the person frequently develops extreme mental irritability and sometimes even convulsions.

Thus, consideration of these examples should give one an extreme appreciation of the value and even necessity of the vast numbers of control systems that keep the body operating in health; in absence of any one of these controls, serious illness or death can result.

Characteristics of Control Systems—Negative Feedback Nature of Most Control Systems

Most control systems of the body act by a process of *negative feedback,* which can be explained by analyzing the regulation of carbon dioxide concentration. A high concentration of carbon dioxide in the extracellular fluid causes increased pulmonary ventilation, and this in turn causes decreased carbon dioxide concentration because the lungs then excrete greater amounts of carbon dioxide out of the body. In other words, the high concentration causes a decreased concentration, which is *negative* to the initiating stimulus. Conversely, if the carbon dioxide concentration falls too low, this causes a feedback increase in the concentration. This response also is negative to the initiating stimulus.

Therefore, in general, if some factor becomes excessive or too little, a control system initiates *negative feedback,* which consists of a series of changes that return the factor toward a certain mean value, thus maintaining homeostasis.

"Gain" of a Control System. The degree of effectiveness with which a control system maintains constant conditions is determined by the *gain* of the negative feedback. For instance, let us assume that a large volume of blood is transfused into a person whose baroreceptor pressure control system is not functioning, and the arterial pressure rises from the normal level of 100 mm Hg up to 175 mm Hg. Then, assume the same volume of blood is injected into the same person when the baroreceptor system is functioning, and this time the pressure rises only 25 mm Hg. Thus, the feedback control system has caused a "correction" of −50 mm Hg; that is, from 175 mm Hg to 125 mm Hg. Yet, there still remains an increase in pressure of +25 mm Hg, called the "error," which means that the control system is not 100 per cent effective in preventing change. The gain of the system is then calculated by the following formula:

$$\text{Gain} = \frac{\text{Correction}}{\text{Error}}$$

Thus, in the previous example, the correction is −50 mm Hg, and the error still persisting is +25 mm Hg. Therefore, the gain of the person's baroreceptor system for control of arterial pressure is −50 divided by +25, or −2. That is, an extraneous factor that tends to increase or decrease the arterial pressure does so only one third as much as would occur if this control system were not present.

The gains of some other physiological control systems are much greater than that of the baroreceptor system. For instance, the gain of the system controlling body temperature is approximately −33. Therefore, one can see that the temperature control system is much more effective than the acute pressure control system.

SUMMARY—AUTOMATICITY OF THE BODY

The purpose of this chapter has been to point out, first, the overall organization of the body and, second, the means by which the different parts of the body operate in harmony. To summarize, the body is actually a *social order of about 100 trillion cells* organized into different functional structures, some of which are called *organs.* Each functional structure provides its share in the maintenance of homeostatic conditions in the extracellular fluid, which is called the *internal environment.* As long as normal conditions are maintained in the internal environment, the cells of the body continue to live and function properly. Thus, each cell benefits from homeostasis, and in turn each cell contributes its share toward the maintenance of homeostasis. This reciprocal interplay provides continuous automaticity of the body until one or more functional systems lose their ability to contribute their share of function. When this happens, all the cells of the body suffer. Extreme dysfunction leads to death, whereas moderate dysfunction leads to sickness.

REFERENCES

Adolph, E. F.: Physiological integrations in action. Physiologist, 25:(Suppl.) 1, 1982.

Bernard, C.: Lectures on the Phenomena of Life Common to Animals and Plants. Springfield, Ill., Charles C Thomas, 1974.

Bryant, P. J., and Simpson, P.: Intrinsic and extrinsic control of growth in developing organs. Q. Rev. Biol., 59:387, 1984.

Burattini, R., and Borgdorff, P.: Closed-loop baroreflex control of total peripheral resistance in the cat: Identification of gains by aid of a model. Cardiovasc. Res., 18:715, 1984.

Cannon, W. B.: The Wisdom of the Body. New York, W. W. Norton & Co., 1932.

Frisancho, A. R.: Human Adaptation. St. Louis, C. V. Mosby Co., 1979.

Gann, D. S., et al.: Neural interaction in control of adrenocorticotropin. Fed. Proc., 44:161, 1985.

Guyton, A. C., et al.: Dynamics and Control of the Body Fluids. Philadelphia, W. B. Saunders Co., 1975.

Klevecz, R. R., et al.: Cellular clocks and oscillators. Int. Rev. Cytol., 86: 97, 1984.

Randall, J. E.: Microcomputers and Physiological Simulation. 2d ed. New York, Raven Press, 1987.

Thompson, R. F.: The neurobiology of learning and memory. Science, 233:941, 1986.

Yates, F. E. (ed.): Self-Organizing Systems. New York, Plenum Publishing Corp., 1987.

QUESTIONS

1. Approximately how may cells are there in the body?
2. Explain what is meant by the "internal environment."
3. Explain the differences between the extracellular and intracellular fluids.
4. What is the meaning of the word *homeostasis*?
5. What role does the circulatory system play in homeostasis?
6. Explain what is meant by diffusion.
7. What is the role of the kidneys in homeostasis?
8. What are the three major portions of the nervous system?
9. Explain the importance of *negative feedback* as the basis for most control mechanisms.
10. If the arterial blood pressure suddenly becomes 80 mm Hg too high, but one of the pressure-controlling mechanisms then returns the pressure to a level that is only 10 mm Hg too high, what is the gain of that control mechanism?

2

The Cell and Its Function

Each of the 75 to 100 trillion cells in the human being is a living structure that can survive indefinitely and, in most instances, can even reproduce itself, provided its surrounding fluids contain appropriate nutrients. A typical cell, as seen by the light microscope, is illustrated in Figure 2–1. Its two major parts are the *nucleus* and the *cytoplasm.* The nucleus is separated from the cytoplasm by a *nuclear membrane,* and the cytoplasm is separated from the surrounding fluids by a *cell membrane.*

The different substances that make up the cell are collectively called *protoplasm.* Protoplasm is composed mainly of five basic substances: water, electrolytes, proteins, lipids, and carbohydrates.

PHYSICAL STRUCTURE OF THE CELL

The cell is not merely a bag of fluid, enzymes, and chemicals; it also contains highly organized physical structures, many of which are called *organelles,* and the physical nature of each of these is equally as important to the function of the cell as the cell's chemical constituents. For instance, without one of the organelles, the *mitochondria,* more than 95 per cent of the energy supply of the cell would cease immediately. Some principal organelles or structures of the cell are illustrated in Figure 2–2, including the *cell membrane, nuclear membrane, endoplasmic reticulum, Golgi apparatus, mitochondria, lysosomes,* and *centrioles.*

The Membranous Structures of the Cell

Essentially all organelles of the cell are lined by membranes composed primarily of lipids and proteins. These membranes include the *cell membrane,* the *nuclear membrane,* the *membrane of the endoplasmic reticulum,* and the *membranes of the mitochondria, lysosomes,* and *Golgi apparatus,* as well as still others. The lipids of the membranes provide a barrier that prevents free movement of water and water-soluble substances from one cell compartment to the other. The protein molecules in the membrane, on the other hand, often penetrate all the way through the membrane, thus interrupting the continuity of the lipid barrier, and therefore provide pathways for passage of specific substances through the membrane.

The Cell Membrane

The Lipid Barrier of the Cell Membrane. Figure 2–3 illustrates the cell membrane. Its basic structure is a *lipid bilayer,* which is a thin film of lipids only 2 molecules thick that is continuous over the entire cell surface. Interspersed in this lipid film are large globular protein molecules.

The lipid bilayer is composed almost entirely of phospholipids and cholesterol. One part of the phospholipid and the cholesterol molecules is soluble in water, that is, *hydrophilic,* whereas the other part is soluble only in fats, that is, *hydrophobic.* The phosphate radical of the phospholipid is hydrophilic, and the fatty acid radicals are hydrophobic. The cholesterol has a hydroxyl radical that is water soluble and a steroid nucleus that is fat soluble. Because the hydrophobic portions of both these molecules are repelled by water but are mutually attracted to each other, they have a natural tendency to line up, as illustrated in Figure 2–3, the fatty portions occupying the center of the membrane and the hydrophilic portions projecting to the two surfaces in contact with the surrounding water.

The membrane lipid bilayer is a major barrier impermeable to the usual water-soluble substances, such

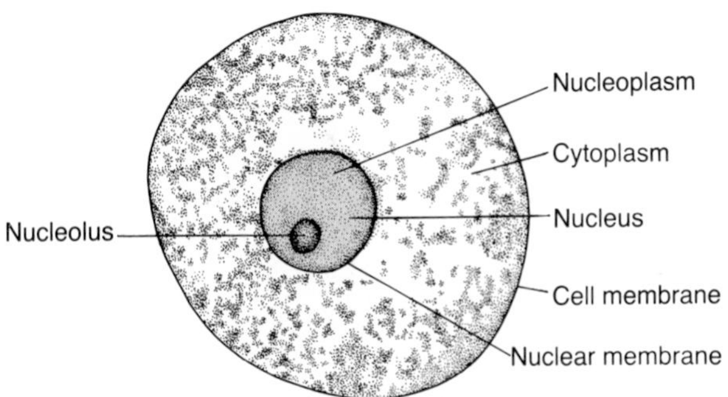

Figure 2–1. Structure of the cell as seen with the light microscope.

as ions, glucose, urea, and others. On the other hand, fat-soluble substances, such as oxygen, carbon dioxide, and alcohol, can penetrate this portion of the membrane with ease.

A special feature of the lipid bilayer is that it is a *fluid* and not a solid. Therefore, portions of the membrane can literally flow from one point to another along the surface of the membrane. Proteins or other substances dissolved in or floating in the lipid bilayer tend to diffuse to all areas of the cell membrane.

The Cell Membrane Proteins. Figure 2–3 illustrates globular masses floating in the lipid bilayer. These are membrane proteins, most of which are *glycoproteins.* Two types of proteins occur: the *integral proteins* that protrude all the way through the membrane and the *peripheral proteins* that are attached only to the surface of the membrane and do not penetrate.

Many of the integral proteins provide structural *channels* (or *pores*) through which water-soluble substances, especially the ions, can diffuse between the extracellular and intracellular fluid. However, these proteins have selective properties that cause preferential diffusion of some substances more than others. Others of the integral proteins act as *carrier proteins* for transporting substances in the direction opposite to their natural direction of diffusion, which is called "active transport."

The peripheral proteins occur either entirely or almost entirely on the inside of the membrane, and they are normally attached to one of the integral proteins. These proteins function almost entirely as enzymes that catalyze a multitude of different chemical reactions essential to the cell's function.

The Membrane Carbohydrates—The Cell "Glycocalyx." The membrane carbohydrates occur almost invariably in combination with proteins and lipids in the form of *glycoproteins* and *glycolipids.* In fact, most of the integral proteins are glycoproteins, and about one tenth of the lipid molecules are glycoli-

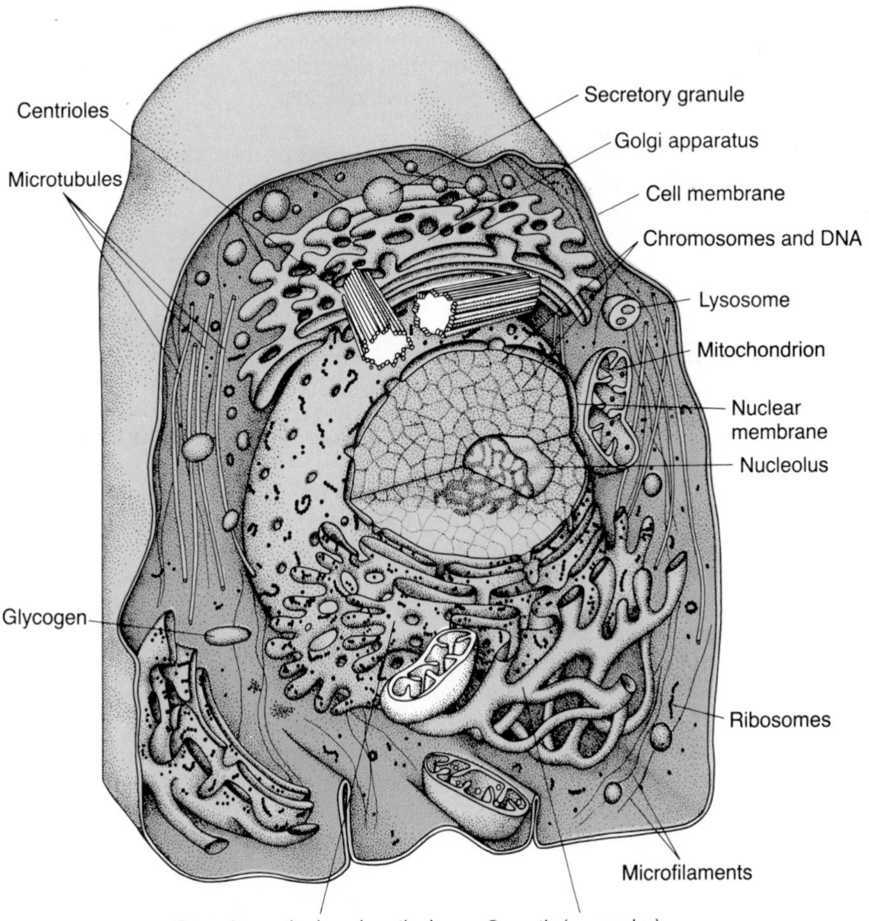

Figure 2–2. Reconstruction of a typical cell, showing the internal organelles in the cytoplasm and in the nucleus.

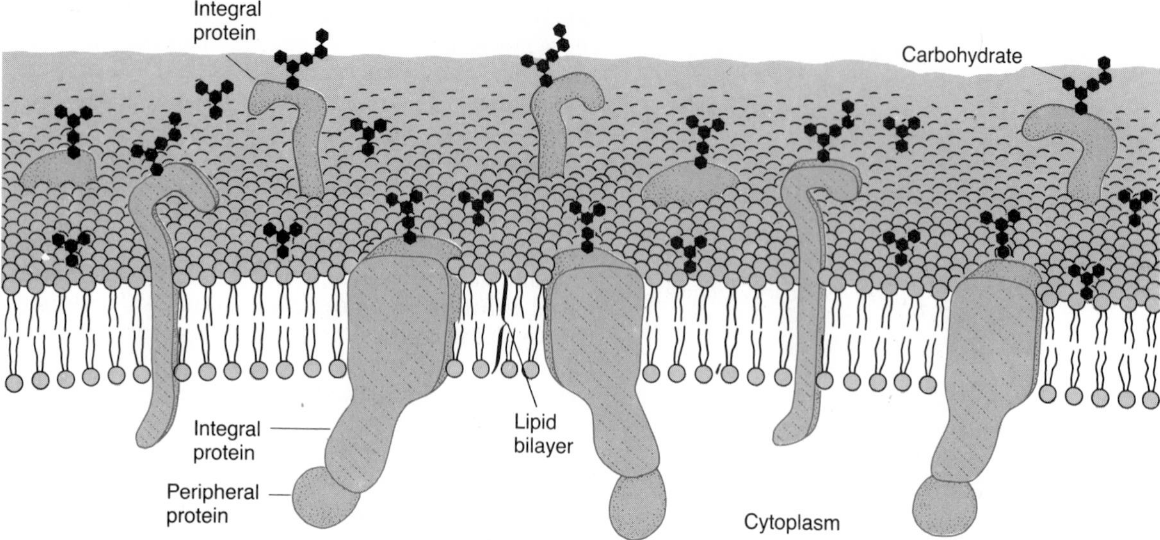

Figure 2-3. Structure of the cell membrane, showing that it is composed mainly from a lipid bilayer but with large numbers of protein molecules protruding through the layer. Also, carbohydrate moieties are attached to the protein molecules on the outside of the membrane and additional protein molecules are attached on the inside. (From Lodish and Rothman: The assembly of cell membranes. *Sci. Am., 240:*48, 1979. ©1979 by Scientific American, Inc. All rights reserved.)

pids. The "glyco" portions of these molecules almost invariably protrude to the outside of the cell, dangling outward from the cell surface. Many other carbohydrate compounds, called *proteoglycans,* which are mainly carbohydrate substances bound together by small protein cores, are often loosely attached to the outer surface of the cell as well. Thus, the entire surface of the cell often has a loose carbohydrate coat called the *glycocalyx.*

The carbohydrate moieties attached to the outer surface of the cell have several important functions: (1) Many of them are negatively charged, which gives most cells an overall negative surface charge that repels other negative objects. (2) The glycocalyx of some cells attaches to the glycocalyx of other cells, thus attaching the cells to each other as well. (3) Many of the carbohydrates act as *receptor substances* for binding hormones like insulin and in doing so activate attached integral proteins that in turn also activate a cascade of intracellular enzymes. (4) Some enter into immune reactions, as we discuss in Chapter 25.

The Cytoplasm and Its Organelles

The cytoplasm is filled with both minute and large dispersed particles and organelles, ranging in size from a few nanometers to many micrometers. The clear fluid portion of the cytoplasm in which the particles are dispersed is called *cytosol;* this contains mainly dissolved proteins, electrolytes, glucose, and minute quantities of lipid compounds.

Dispersed in the cytoplasm are neutral fat globules, glycogen granules, ribosomes, secretory granules, and five especially important organelles: the *endoplasmic reticulum,* the *Golgi apparatus,* the *mitochondria,* the *lysosomes,* and the *peroxisomes.*

The Endoplasmic Reticulum

Figure 2-2 illustrates in the cytoplasm a network of tubular and flat vesicular structures called the *endoplasmic reticulum.* The tubules and vesicles all interconnect with each other. Also, their walls are constructed of lipid bilayer membranes containing large amounts of proteins, similar to the cell membrane. The total surface area of this structure in some cells — the liver cells, for instance — can be as much as 30 to 40 times as great as the cell membrane area.

The detailed structure of a small portion of endoplasmic reticulum is illustrated in Figure 2-4. The space inside the tubules and vesicles is filled with *endoplasmic matrix,* a fluid medium that is different from the fluid outside the endoplasmic reticulum.

Substances formed in some parts of the cell enter the space of the endoplasmic reticulum and are then conducted to other parts of the cell. Also, the vast surface area of the reticulum and multiple enzyme systems attached to its membranes provide the ma-

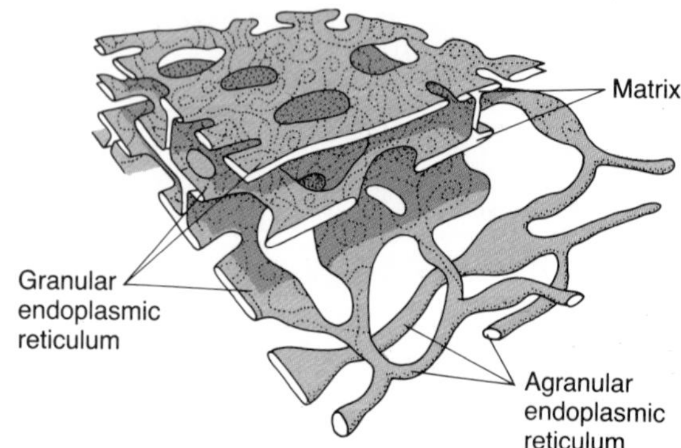

Figure 2-4. Structure of the endoplasmic reticulum. (Modified from De Robertis, Saez, and De Robertis: Cell Biology. 6th ed. Philadelphia, W. B. Saunders Company, 1975.)

chinery for a major share of the metabolic functions of the cell.

Ribosomes and the Granular Endoplasmic Reticulum. Attached to the outer surfaces of many parts of the endoplasmic reticulum are large numbers of small granular particles called *ribosomes.* Where these are present, the reticulum is frequently called the *granular endoplasmic reticulum.* The ribosomes are composed of a mixture of ribonucleic acid (RNA) and proteins, and they function in the synthesis of protein in the cells, as discussed later in this and the following chapter.

The Agranular Endoplasmic Reticulum. Part of the endoplasmic reticulum has no attached ribosomes. This part is called the *agranular,* or *smooth, endoplasmic reticulum.* The agranular reticulum functions in the synthesis of lipid substances and in many other enzymatic processes of the cell.

Golgi Apparatus

The Golgi apparatus, illustrated in Figure 2–5, is closely related to the endoplasmic reticulum. It has membranes similar to those of the agranular endoplasmic reticulum. It is usually composed of four or more stacked layers of thin, flat enclosed vesicles lying near the nucleus. This apparatus is very prominent in secretory cells.

The Golgi apparatus functions in association with the endoplasmic reticulum. As illustrated in Figure 2–5, small "transport vesicles," also called endoplasmic reticulum vesicles or simply *ER vesicles,* continually pinch off from the endoplasmic reticulum and shortly thereafter fuse with the Golgi apparatus. In this way, substances are transported from the endoplasmic reticulum to the Golgi apparatus. The transported substances are then processed in the Golgi apparatus to form *lysosomes, secretory vesicles,* or other cytoplasmic components.

The Lysosomes

Lysosomes are vesicular organelles formed by the Golgi apparatus that then become dispersed throughout the cytoplasm. The lysosomes provide an intracellular digestive system that allows the cell to digest and thereby remove unwanted substances and structures, such as bacteria. The lysosome, illustrated in Figure 2–2, is quite different from one cell to another, but it is usually 250 to 750 nanometers in diameter. It is surrounded by a typical lipid bilayer membrane and is filled with large numbers of small granules, which are protein aggregates of hydrolytic (digestive) enzymes. A hydrolytic enzyme is capable of splitting an organic compound into two or more parts by combining hydrogen from a water molecule with part of the compound and by combining the hydroxyl portion of the water molecule with the other part of the compound. For instance, protein is hydrolyzed to form amino acids, and glycogen is hydrolyzed to form glucose. More than 50 different *acid hydrolases* have been found in lysosomes, and the principal substances that they digest are proteins, nucleic acids, mucopolysaccharides, lipids, and glycogen.

Ordinarily, the membrane surrounding the lysosome prevents the enclosed hydrolytic enzymes from coming in contact with other substances in the cell. However, many different conditions of the cell will break the membranes of some of the lysosomes, allowing release of the enzymes. These enzymes then split the organic substances with which they come in contact into small, highly diffusible substances, such as amino acids and glucose. Some of the more specific functions of lysosomes are discussed later in the chapter.

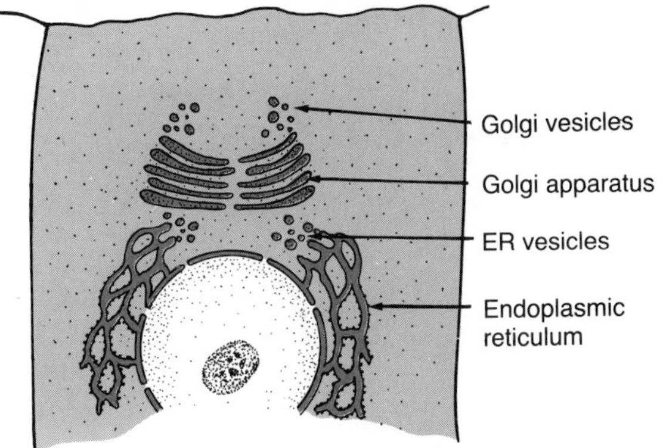

Figure 2–5. A typical Golgi apparatus and its relationship to the endoplasmic reticulum and the nucleus.

The Mitochondria

The mitochondria are called the "powerhouses" of the cell. Without them, the cells would be unable to extract significant amounts of energy from the nutrients and oxygen, and as a consequence essentially all cellular functions would cease. As illustrated in the cell of Figure 2–2, these organelles are present in essentially all portions of the cytoplasm, but the total number per cell varies from less than a hundred up to several thousand, depending on the amount of energy required by each cell.

The basic structure of the mitochondrion is illustrated in Figure 2–6, which shows it to be composed mainly of two lipid bilayer–protein membranes: an *outer membrane* and an *inner membrane.* Many infoldings of the inner membrane form *shelves* onto which oxidative enzymes are attached. In addition, the inner cavity of the mitochondrion is filled with a *matrix* containing large quantities of dissolved enzymes that are necessary for extracting energy from nutrients. These enzymes operate in association with the oxidative enzymes on the shelves to cause oxidation of the nutrients, thereby forming carbon dioxide and water. The liberated energy is used to synthesize a high-energy substance called *adenosine triphosphate (ATP).* ATP is then transported out of the mitochondrion, and it diffuses throughout the cell to release its energy wherever it is needed for performing cellular

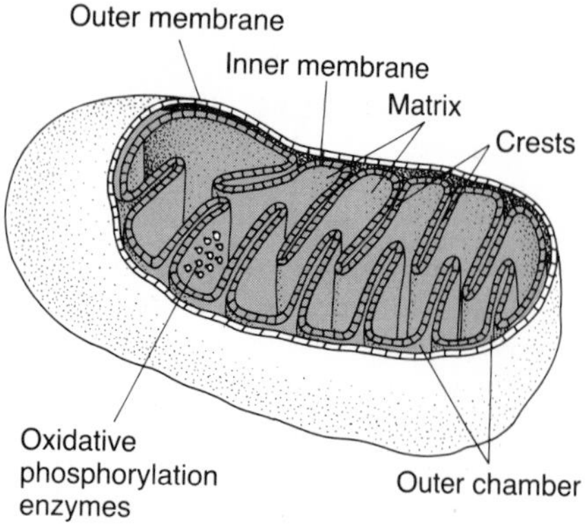

Figure 2-6. Structure of a mitochondrion. (Modified from De Robertis, Saez, and De Robertis: Cell Biology. 6th ed. Philadelphia, W. B. Saunders Company, 1975.)

functions. The details of ATP formation by the mitochondrion are given in Chapter 45, and some of the important functions of ATP in the cell are introduced later in this chapter.

Mitochondria are self-replicative, which means that one mitochondrion can form a second one, a third one, and so on, whenever there is need in the cell for increased amounts of ATP.

Other Cytoplasmic Structures and Organelles

Throughout this text we learn that there are literally hundreds of different types of cells, and each of these has special unique structures. For instance, some of the cells are rigid. This is usually achieved by the presence in the cytoplasmic compartment of large numbers of filamentous or tubular structures composed of fibrillar proteins. Also, some of the tubular structures, called *microtubules,* can actually transport substances from one part of a cell to another, thus providing an intracellular circulatory system. Also, it is structures composed of microtubules that form the rigid structures of (a) cilia that protrude from certain cell surfaces and move fluids along the surfaces, (b) the tail of the sperm that beats rhythmically and propels the sperm through the genital tract of the female, and (c) the mitotic apparatus that plays an essential role in cell division.

Fibrillar proteins also form the contractile apparatus of muscle cells, which we shall discuss in great detail in Chapter 6.

Finally, one of the important functions of many cells is to secrete special substances. All such substances are formed by the endoplasmic reticulum–Golgi apparatus system and are released from the Golgi apparatus into the cytoplasm inside storage vesicles called *secretory vesicles* or *secretory granules.* Then, at a later time, these are expelled through the cell membrane, as we shall discuss later in this chapter.

The Nucleus

The nucleus is the control center of the cell. Briefly, the nucleus contains large quantities of *DNA,* which we have called *genes* for many years. The genes determine the characteristics of the protein enzymes of the cytoplasm and in this way control cytoplasmic activities. They also control reproduction; the genes first reproduce themselves, and after this the cell splits by a special process called *mitosis* to form two daughter cells, each of which receives one of the two sets of genes. All these activities of the nucleus are considered in detail in the following chapter.

The appearance of the nucleus under the microscope does not give much of a clue to the mechanisms by which it performs its control activities. Figure 2-7 illustrates the light microscopic appearance of the interphase nucleus (period between cell divisions), showing darkly staining *chromatin material* throughout the nucleoplasm. During cell division, called *mitosis,* the chromatin material becomes readily identifiable as the highly structured *chromosomes,* which can be seen easily with the light microscope.

The Nuclear Envelope

The nuclear envelope is frequently called the *nuclear membrane.* However, it is actually two separate membranes, one inside the other. The outer membrane is continuous with the endoplasmic reticulum, and the space between the two nuclear membranes is also continuous with the compartment inside the endoplasmic reticulum.

The nuclear envelope is penetrated by several thousand *nuclear pores* large enough to allow some molecules up to 44,000 molecular weight to pass through with relative ease and molecules with molecular weight less than 15,000 to pass extremely rapidly.

Nucleoli

The nuclei of most cells contain one or more lightly staining structures called nucleoli. The nucleolus, unlike most of the organelles that we have discussed,

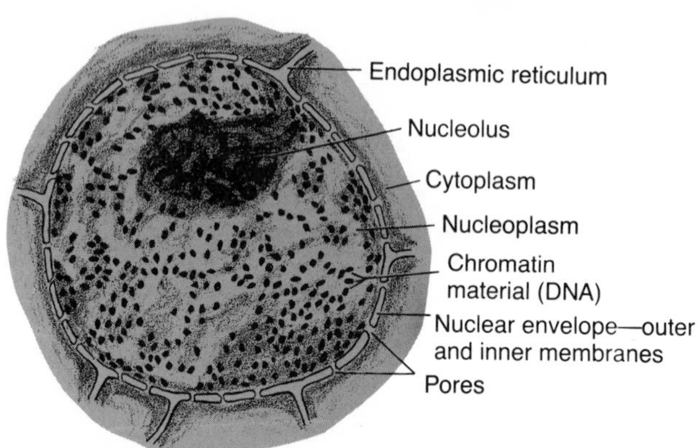

Figure 2-7. Structure of the nucleus.

does not have a limiting membrane. Instead, it is simply a structure that contains a large amount of *RNA* and proteins. The nucleolus becomes considerably enlarged when a cell is actively synthesizing proteins. The genes of five separate chromosome pairs synthesize the RNA and then store it in the nucleolus, beginning with a loose fibrillar RNA that later condenses with the proteins to form granular "subunits" of ribosomes. These in turn are transported through the nuclear membrane pores into the cytoplasm, where they assemble together to form the "mature" ribosomes that play an essential role for the formation of proteins, either in the cytosol or in association with the endoplasmic reticulum, as we discuss more fully in the following chapter.

FUNCTIONAL SYSTEMS OF THE CELL

In the remainder of this chapter, we will discuss several representative functional systems of the cell that make it a living organism.

Ingestion by the Cell—Endocytosis

If a cell is to live and grow, it must obtain nutrients and other substances from the surrounding fluids. Most substances pass through the cell membrane by *diffusion* and *active transport,* which are considered in detail in Chapter 4. However, large particles enter the cell by a specialized function of the cell membrane called *endocytosis.* The two principal forms of endocytosis are *pinocytosis* and *phagocytosis.* Pinocytosis means the ingestion of extremely small vesicles containing extracellular fluid. Phagocytosis means ingestion of large particles, such as bacteria, cells, or portions of degenerating tissue.

Pinocytosis. Pinocytosis occurs continually at the cell membranes of most cells but especially rapidly in some cells. For instance, it occurs so rapidly in macrophages that about 3 per cent of the total macrophage membrane is engulfed in the form of vesicles each minute. Even so, the pinocytic vesicles are so small, usually only 100 to 200 nanometers in diameter, that most of them can be seen only with the electron microscope.

Pinocytosis is the only means by which some very large macromolecules, such as most protein molecules, can enter cells. In fact, the rate at which pinocytic vesicles form usually is enhanced when such macromolecules attach to the cell membrane.

Figure 2-8 illustrates the successive steps of pinocytosis, showing three molecules of protein attaching to the membrane. These molecules usually attach to *receptors* on the surface of the membrane that are specific for the types of proteins that are to be absorbed. The receptors generally are concentrated in small pits in the cell membrane, called *coated pits.* On the inside of the cell membrane beneath these pits is a latticework of a fibrillar protein called *clathrin* as well as additional contractile filaments of *actin* and *myosin.* Once the protein molecules have bound with the receptors, the surface properties of the membrane change in such a way that the entire pit invaginates inward and the contractile proteins cause its borders to close over the attached proteins as well as over a small amount of extracellular fluid. Immediately thereafter, the invaginated portion of the membrane breaks away from the surface of the cell, forming a *pinocytic vesicle.*

What causes the cell membrane to go through the necessary contortions for forming pinocytic vesicles remains mainly a mystery. However, this process requires energy from within the cell; this is supplied by ATP, a high energy substance that is discussed later in the chapter. Also, it requires the presence of calcium ions in the extracellular fluid, which probably react with the contractile filaments beneath the coated pits to provide the force for pinching the vesicles away from the cell membrane.

Phagocytosis. Phagocytosis occurs in much the same way as pinocytosis except that it involves large particles rather than molecules. Only certain cells have the capability of phagocytosis, most notably the tissue macrophages and some of the white blood cells.

Phagocytosis is initiated when proteins or large polysaccharides on the surface of the particle that is to be phagocytized—such as a bacterium, a dead cell, or other tissue debris—bind with receptors on the sur-

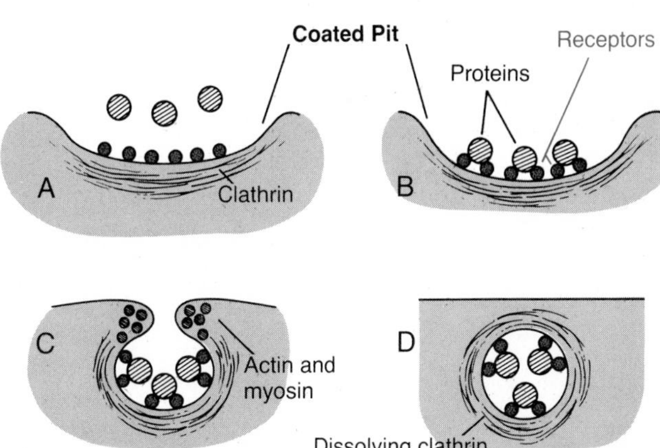

Figure 2-8. Mechanism of pinocytosis.

face of the phagocyte. In the case of bacteria, these usually are attached to specific antibodies, and the antibodies in turn attach to the phagocyte receptors. This intermediation of antibodies is called *opsonization,* which is discussed in Chapters 24 and 25.

Phagocytosis occurs in the following steps:

1. The cell membrane receptors attach to the surface ligands of the particle.
2. The edges of the membrane around the points of attachment evaginate outward within a fraction of a second to surround the particle; then, progressively more and more membrane receptors attach to the particle ligands, all this occurring suddenly in a zipperlike fashion, completely surrounding the particle.
3. Actin and other contractile fibrils in the cytoplasm surround the engulfed particle and contract around its outer edge, pushing the object further to the interior.
4. The contractile proteins then pinch the *phagocytic vesicle* off, leaving it in the cell interior in the same way that pinocytic vesicles are formed.

Digestion of Foreign Substances in the Cell—Function of the Lysosomes

Almost immediately after a pinocytic or phagocytic vesicle appears inside a cell, one or more lysosomes become attached to the vesicle and empty their acid hydrolases into the vesicle, as illustrated in Figure 2-9. Thus, a *digestive vesicle* is formed in which the hydrolases begin hydrolyzing the proteins, glycogen, nucleic acids, mucopolysaccharides, and other substances in the vesicle. The products of digestion are small molecules of amino acids, glucose, phosphates, and so forth that can then diffuse through the membrane of the vesicle into the cytoplasm. What is left of the digestive vesicle, called the *residual body,* represents the undigestible substances. In most instances this is finally excreted through the cell membrane by a process called *exocytosis,* which is essentially the opposite of endocytosis.

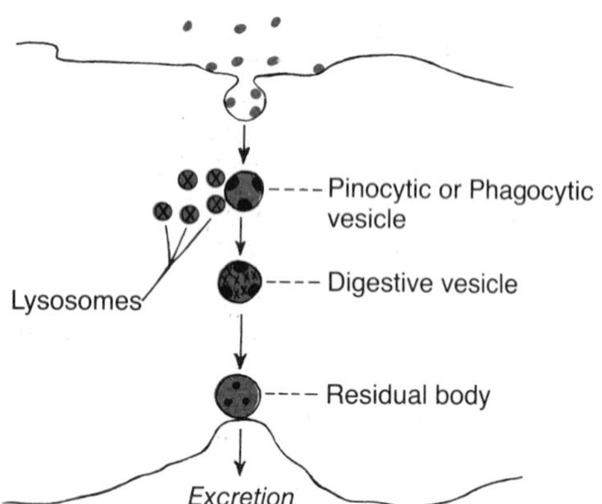

Figure 2-9. Digestion of substances in pinocytic vesicles by enzymes derived from lysosomes.

Thus, the lysosomes may be called the *digestive organs* of the cells.

The lysosomes also contain bactericidal agents that can kill phagocytized bacteria before they can cause cellular damage. These agents include *lysozyme* that dissolves the bacterial cell membrane, *lysoferrin* that binds iron and other metals that are essential for bacterial growth, and acid at a pH of about 5.0 that activates the hydrolases and also inactivates some of the bacterial metabolic systems.

Synthesis and Formation of Cellular Structures by the Endoplasmic Reticulum and the Golgi Apparatus

The extensiveness of the endoplasmic reticulum and the Golgi apparatus, especially in secretory cells, has already been emphasized. These two structures are formed primarily of lipid bilayer membranes, and their walls are literally loaded with protein enzymes that catalyze the synthesis of many of the substances required by the cell.

In general, most of the synthesis begins in the endoplasmic reticulum, but most of the products that are formed are then passed on to the Golgi apparatus, where they are further processed prior to release into the cytoplasm. But, first, let us note the specific products that are synthesized in the specific portions of the endoplasmic reticulum and the Golgi apparatus.

Formation of Proteins by the Granular Endoplasmic Reticulum. The granular endoplasmic reticulum is characterized by the presence of large numbers of ribosomes attached to the outer surfaces of the reticulum membrane. As we shall discuss in the following chapter, protein molecules are synthesized within the structures of the ribosomes. Furthermore, the ribosomes extrude many of the synthesized protein molecules not into the cytosol but instead through the endoplasmic reticulum wall into the endoplasmic matrix.

Almost as rapidly as the protein molecules enter the endoplasmic matrix, enzymes in the endoplasmic reticulum wall cause rapid changes in these molecules. First, almost all of them are immediately conjugated with carbohydrate moieties to form *glycoproteins.* Therefore, essentially all the endoplasmic proteins are glycoproteins, in contrast to the proteins that are formed by the ribosomes in the cytosol, which are mainly free proteins. Second, the proteins are cross-linked and folded to form more compact molecules.

Synthesis of Lipids by the Endoplasmic Reticulum, Especially by the Smooth Endoplasmic Reticulum. The endoplasmic reticulum also synthesizes lipids, especially phospholipids and cholesterol. These are rapidly incorporated into the lipid bilayer of the endoplasmic reticulum itself, thus causing the endoplasmic reticulum to grow continually. This occurs mainly in the smooth portion of the endoplasmic reticulum.

To keep the endoplasmic reticulum from growing

beyond the limits of the cell, however, small vesicles called *endoplasmic reticulum vesicles*, or *transport vesicles*, continually break away from the smooth reticulum; most of these vesicles migrate rapidly to the Golgi apparatus.

Synthetic Functions of the Golgi Apparatus. Although the major function of the Golgi apparatus is to process substances already formed in the endoplasmic reticulum, it also has the capability of synthesizing certain carbohydrates that cannot be formed in the endoplasmic reticulum. This is especially true of sialic acid and galactose. In addition, the Golgi apparatus can cause the formation of very large saccharide polymers bound with only small amounts of protein; the most important of these are hyaluronic acid and chondroitin sulfate. A few of the many functions of hyaluronic acid and chondroitin sulfate in the body are as follows: (1) They are the major components of proteoglycans secreted in mucus and other glandular secretions. (2) They are the major components of the ground substance in the interstitial spaces, acting as a filler between collagen fibers and cells. (3) They are principal components of the organic matrix in both cartilage and bone.

Processing of Endoplasmic Secretions by the Golgi Apparatus—Formation of Vesicles. Figure 2–10 summarizes the major functions of the endoplasmic reticulum and Golgi apparatus. As substances are formed in the endoplasmic reticulum, especially the proteins, they are transported through the reticular tubules toward the portions of the smooth endoplasmic reticulum that lie nearest the Golgi apparatus. At this point, small transport vesicles of smooth endoplasmic reticulum continually break away and diffuse to the *deeper layers* of the Golgi apparatus. Inside these vesicles are the synthesized proteins and other products. These vesicles instantly fuse with the Golgi apparatus and empty their contained substances into the vesicular spaces of the Golgi apparatus. Here, additional carbohydrate moieties are added to the secretions. Also, a most important function of the Golgi apparatus is to compact the endoplasmic reticular secretions into highly concentrated packets. As the secretions pass toward the outermost layers of the Golgi apparatus, the compaction and processing proceed; finally, both small and large vesicles continually break away from the Golgi apparatus, carrying with them the compacted secretory substances, and they then diffuse throughout the cell.

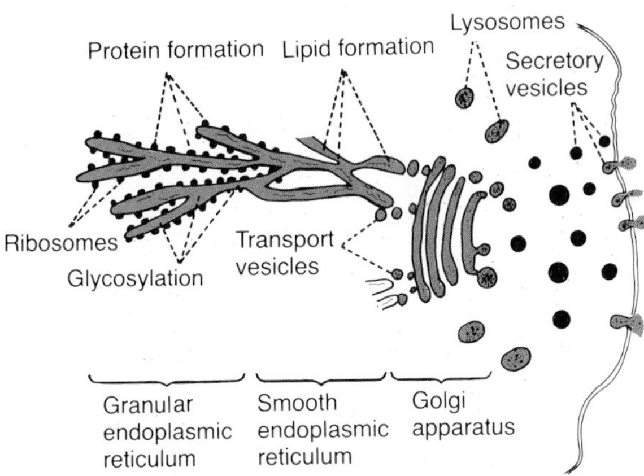

Figure 2–10. Formation of proteins, lipids, and cellular vesicles by the endoplasmic reticulum and Golgi apparatus.

To give one an idea of the timing of these processes: When a glandular cell is bathed in radioactive amino acids, newly formed radioactive protein molecules can be detected in the granular endoplasmic reticulum within 3 to 5 minutes. Within 20 minutes, the newly formed proteins are present in the Golgi apparatus, and within 1 or 2 hours, radioactive proteins are secreted from the surface of the cell.

Types of Vesicles Formed by the Golgi Apparatus—Secretory Vesicles and Lysosomes. In a highly secretory cell, the vesicles that are formed by the Golgi apparatus are mainly *secretory vesicles*, containing especially the protein substances that are to be secreted through the surface of the cell. These vesicles diffuse to the cell membrane and then fuse with it and empty their substances to the exterior by a mechanism called *exocytosis*, which is essentially the opposite of endocytosis. Exocytosis, in most cases, is stimulated by entry of calcium ions into the cell; the calcium ions interact with the vesicular membrane, in some way not understood, to cause its fusion with the cell membrane.

On the other hand, some of the vesicles are destined for intracellular use. For instance, specialized portions of the Golgi apparatus form the *lysosomes* that have already been discussed.

Use of Intracellular Vesicles to Replenish Cellular Membranes. Many of the vesicles finally fuse with the cell membrane or with the membranes of other intracellular structures, such as the mitochondria and even the endoplasmic reticulum itself. This obviously increases the expanse of these membranes and thereby replenishes these membranes as they themselves are destroyed. For instance, the cell membrane loses much of its substance every time it forms a phagocytic or pinocytic vesicle, and it is vesicles from the Golgi apparatus that continually replenish the cell membrane.

Thus, in summary, the membranous system of the endoplasmic reticulum and the Golgi apparatus represents a highly metabolic organ capable of forming both new cellular structures and secretory substances to be extruded from the cell.

Extraction of Energy from Nutrients—Function of the Mitochondria

The principal substances from which cells extract energy are oxygen and one or more of the foodstuffs—carbohydrates, fats, and proteins. In the human body, essentially all carbohydrates are converted into *glucose* before they reach the cell, the proteins are converted into *amino acids*, and the fats are converted into *fatty acids*. Figure 2–11 shows oxygen and the

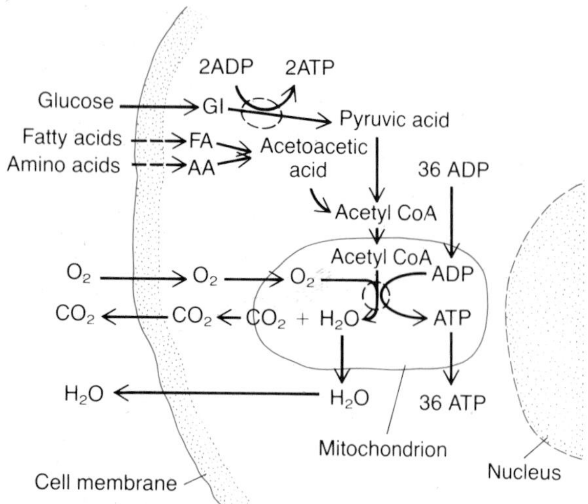

Figure 2-11. Formation of adenosine triphosphate (ATP) in the cell, showing that most of the ATP is formed in the mitochondria.

foodstuffs—glucose, fatty acids, and amino acids—all entering the cell. Inside the cell, the foodstuffs react chemically with the oxygen under the influence of various enzymes that control their rates of reactions and channel the energy that is released in the proper direction.

Almost all these oxidative reactions occur inside the mitochondria, and the energy that is released is used to form mainly *ATP*. Then, the ATP, not the original foodstuffs themselves, is used throughout the cell to energize almost all the intracellular metabolic reactions.

Functional Characteristics of ATP

The formula for ATP is:

NH_2 — Adenine — $CH_2—O—P—O\sim P—O\sim P—O^-$ (each P bearing $=O$ and O^-) — Phosphate — Ribose (OH OH)

Adenosine triphosphate

ATP is a nucleotide composed of the nitrogenous base *adenine,* the pentose sugar *ribose,* and three *phosphate radicals.* The last two phosphate radicals are connected with the remainder of the molecule by so-called *high-energy phosphate bonds,* which are represented by the symbol ~. Each of these bonds contains about 12,000 calories of energy per mole of ATP under the physical conditions of the body (7300 calories under standard conditions), which is much greater than the energy stored in the average chemical bond of other organic compounds, thus giving rise to the term "high-energy" bond. Furthermore, the high-energy phosphate bond is very labile so that it can be split instantly on demand whenever energy is required to promote other cellular reactions.

When ATP releases its energy, a phosphoric acid radical is split away, and *adenosine diphosphate (ADP)* is formed. Then, energy derived from the cellular nutrients causes the ADP and phosphoric acid to recombine to form new ATP, the entire process continuing over and over again. For these reasons, ATP has been called the *energy currency* of the cell, for it can be spent and remade again and again, usually having a turnover time of only a few minutes at most.

Chemical Processes in the Formation of ATP—Role of the Mitochondria. On entry into the cells, glucose is subjected to enzymes in the cytoplasm that convert it into *pyruvic acid* (a process called *glycolysis*). A small amount of ADP is changed into ATP by energy released during this conversion, but this amount accounts for less than 5 per cent of the overall energy metabolism of the cell.

By far the major portion of the ATP formed in the cell is formed in the mitochondria. The pyruvic and fatty acids and most of the amino acids are all converted into the compound *acetyl-CoA* in the matrix of the mitochondrion. This substance, in turn, is acted upon by another series of enzymes in the mitochondrion matrix, undergoing dissolution in a sequence of chemical reactions called the *citric acid cycle,* or *Krebs cycle.* These chemical reactions are explained in detail in Chapter 45.

In the citric acid cycle, acetyl-CoA is split into its component parts, *hydrogen atoms* and *carbon dioxide.* The carbon dioxide, in turn, diffuses out of the mitochondria and eventually out of the cell.

The hydrogen atoms, on the other hand, are very highly reactive, and they eventually combine with oxygen that has diffused into the mitochondria. This releases a tremendous amount of energy, which is used by the mitochondria to convert large amounts of ADP to ATP. The processes of these reactions are very complex, requiring the participation of large numbers of protein enzymes that are integral parts of the mitochondrial *membranous shelves* that protrude into the mitochondrial matrix. The initial event is removal of an electron from the hydrogen atom, thus converting it to a hydrogen ion. The terminal event is movement of these ions through large globular proteins called *ATP synthetase* that protrude like knobs through the membranes of the mitochondrial shelves. ATP synthetase is an enzyme that uses the energy from the movement of the hydrogen ions to cause the conversion of ADP to ATP, while at the same time the hydrogen ions combine with oxygen to form water. Finally, the newly formed ATP is transported out of the mitochondria into all parts of the cytoplasm and

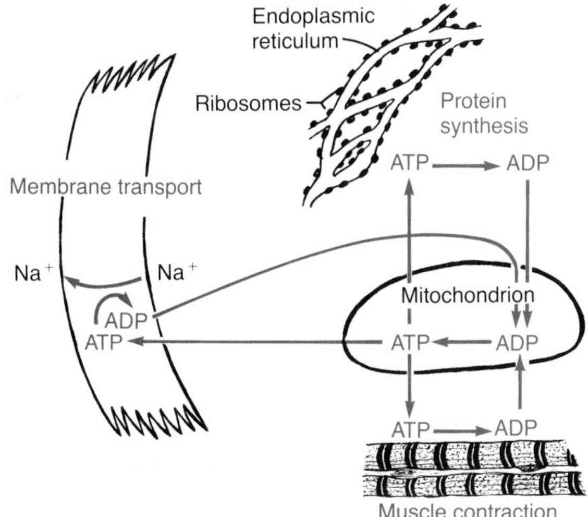

Figure 2-12. Use of adenosine triphosphate to provide energy for three major cellular functions: (1) membrane transport, (2) protein synthesis, and (3) muscle contraction.

nucleoplasm, where its energy is used to energize the functions of the cell.

This overall process for the formation of ATP is called the *chemiosmotic mechanism* of ATP formation. The chemical and physical details of this mechanism are presented in Chapter 45.

Uses of ATP for Cellular Function. ATP is used to promote three major categories of cellular functions: (1) *membrane transport,* (2) *synthesis of chemical compounds* throughout the cell, and (3) *mechanical work.* These three different uses of ATP are illustrated by examples in Figure 2-12: (1) to supply energy for the transport of sodium through the cell membrane, (2) to promote protein synthesis by the ribosomes, and (3) to supply the energy needed during muscle contraction.

In addition to membrane transport of sodium, energy from ATP is required either directly or indirectly for transport of potassium ions, calcium ions, magnesium ions, phosphate ions, chloride ions, urate ions, hydrogen ions, and still many other ions and various organic substances. Membrane transport is so important to cellular function that some cells, the renal tubular cells for instance, use as much as 80 per cent of the ATP formed in the cells for this purpose alone.

In addition to synthesizing proteins, cells also synthesize phospholipids, cholesterol, purines, pyrimidines, and a great host of other substances. Synthesis of almost any chemical compound requires energy. Indeed, some cells use as much as 75 per cent of all the ATP formed in the cell simply to synthesize new chemical compounds; this is particularly true during the growth phase of cells.

The final major use of ATP is to supply energy for special cells to perform mechanical work. We see in Chapter 6 that each contraction of a muscle fiber requires expenditure of tremendous quantities of ATP. Other cells perform mechanical work in additional ways, especially by *ciliary* and *ameboid motion,* which are described later in this chapter. The source of energy for all these types of mechanical work is ATP.

In summary, therefore, ATP is always available to release its energy rapidly and almost explosively wherever in the cell it is needed. To replace the ATP used by the cell, other much slower chemical reactions break down carbohydrates, fats, and proteins, and use the energy derived from these to form new ATP. Over 95 per cent of this ATP is formed in the mitochondria, which accounts for the name given to the mitochondria, the "powerhouses" of the cell.

Ameboid Locomotion of Cells

By far the most important type of cell movement that occurs in the body is that of the specialized muscle cells in skeletal, cardiac, and smooth muscle, which constitute almost 50 per cent of the entire body mass. The specialized functions of these cells are discussed in Chapters 6 through 9. However, two other types of movement occur in other cells, *ameboid locomotion* and *ciliary movement.*

Ameboid locomotion means movement of an entire cell in relation to its surroundings, such as the movement of white blood cells through tissues. Typically, ameboid locomotion begins with protrusion of a *pseudopodium* from one end of the cell. The pseudopodium projects far out away from the cell body and then attaches to the new tissue area, and finally the remainder of the cell moves toward the pseudopodium. Figure 2-13 illustrates this process, showing an elongated cell, the right-hand end of which is a protruding pseudopodium. The membrane of this end of the cell is continually moving forward, and the membrane at the left-hand end of the cell is continually following along as the cell moves.

Mechanism of Ameboid Locomotion. Figure 2-13 illustrates the general principle of ameboid motion. Basically, it results from continual exocytosis that forms new cell membrane at the leading edge of the pseudopodium and continual endocytosis of the membrane in mid and rear portions of the cell. Also, one other effect is essential for forward movement of the cell. This effect is attachment of the pseudopodium to the surrounding tissues so that it becomes fixed in its leading position, while the remainder of the cell body is pulled forward toward the point of attachment. This attachment is effected by receptor

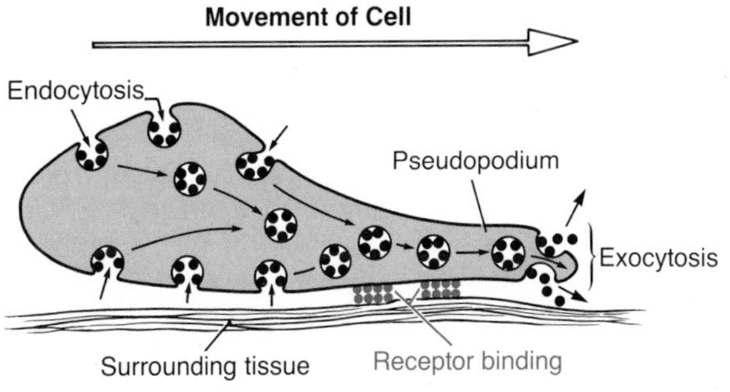

Figure 2-13. Ameboid motion by a cell.

proteins that line the insides of the exocytotic vesicles. When the vesicles become part of the pseudopodial membrane, they open so that their insides evert to the outside and the receptors now protrude to the outside and contact ligands in the surrounding tissues. An especially important ligand is a protein called *fibrinectin*, which is bound to the collagen fibers of the tissue.

At the opposite end of the cell, the endocytotic activity pulls the receptors away from their ligands to form endocytotic vesicles. Then, inside the cell, these vesicles stream toward the pseudopodial end of the cell, where they are used to form still new membrane for the pseudopodium.

One of the unknowns in the process of ameboid motion is the source of the energy that causes the vesicular streaming from the endocytotic end of the cell toward the tip of the pseudopodium. Part of this might result from contraction of actin and myosin filaments in the ectoplasm of the cell, contracting the cell at its rear end and literally pushing the vesicles and cytoplasm toward the pseudopodial end.

Control of Ameboid Locomotion—"Chemotaxis." The most important factor that usually initiates ameboid locomotion is the process called *chemotaxis.* This results from the appearance of certain chemical substances in the tissues. The chemical substance that causes chemotaxis to occur is called a *chemotactic substance.* Most cells that exhibit ameboid locomotion move toward the source of the chemotactic substance—that is, from an area of lower concentration toward an area of higher concentration—which is called *positive chemotaxis.* However, some cells move away from the source, which is called *negative chemotaxis.*

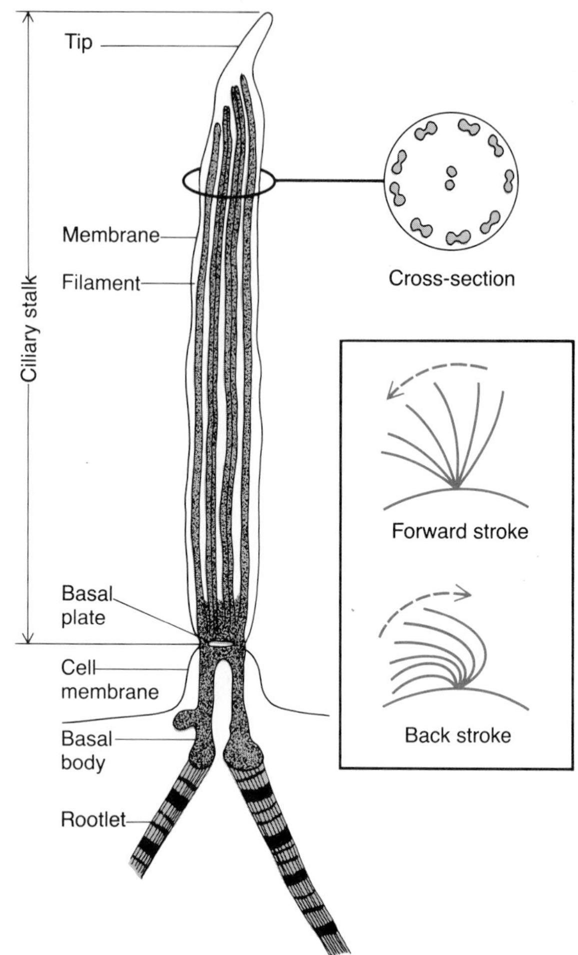

Figure 2–14. Structure and function of the cilium. (Modified from Satir: Cilia. *Sci. Am., 204:*108, 1961. ©1961 by Scientific American, Inc. All rights reserved.)

Cilia and Ciliary Movements

A second type of cellular motion, *ciliary movement,* is a whiplike movement of cilia on the surfaces of cells. This occurs in only two places in the human body: on the inside surfaces of the respiratory airways and on the inside surfaces of the uterine tubes (fallopian tubes) of the reproductive tract. In the nasal cavity and lower respiratory airways, the whiplike motion of the cilia causes a layer of mucus to move at a rate of about 1 cm/min toward the pharynx, in this way continually clearing these passageways of mucus and any particles that have become entrapped in the mucus. In the uterine tubes, the cilia cause slow movement of fluid from the ostium of the uterine tube toward the uterine cavity; it is this movement of fluid that transports the ovum from the ovary to the uterus.

As illustrated in Figure 2–14, a cilium has the appearance of a sharp-pointed curved hair that projects 2 to 4 micrometers from the surface of the cell. Many cilia project from each single cell—for instance, as many as 200 cilia on the surface of each epithelial cell in the respiratory tract. The cilium is covered by an outcropping of the cell membrane, and it is supported by 11 microtubules, consisting of 9 double tubules located around the periphery of the cilium, and 2 single tubules down the center, as shown in the cross-section illustrated in the figure. Each cilium is an outgrowth of a structure that lies immediately beneath the cell membrane, called the *basal body* of the cilium.

The *flagellum of a sperm* is also similar to a cilium; in fact, it has much the same type of structure and same type of contractile mechanism. However, the flagellum is much longer and moves in quasisinusoidal waves instead of with whiplike movements.

In the inset of Figure 2–14, movement of the cilium is illustrated. The cilium moves forward with a sudden rapid stroke, 10 to 20 times per second, bending sharply where it projects from the surface of the cell. Then it moves backward very slowly in a whiplike manner. The rapid forward movement pushes the fluid lying adjacent to the cell in the direction that the cilium moves; then the slow whiplike movement in the other direction has almost no effect on the fluid. As a result, fluid is continually propelled in the direction of the fast forward stroke. Since most ciliated cells have large numbers of cilia on their surfaces, and since all the cilia are oriented in the same direction, this is a very effective means for moving fluids from one part of the surface to another.

Mechanism of Ciliary Movement. Although all aspects of ciliary movement are not yet clear, we do know the following: First, the nine double tubules and the two single tubules are all linked to each other by a complex of protein cross-linkages; this total complex of tubules and cross-linkages is called the *axoneme.* Second, even after removal of the membrane and destruction of other elements of the cilium besides the axoneme, the cilium can still beat under appropriate conditions. Third, there are two necessary conditions for continued beating of the axoneme after removal of the other structures of the cilium: (1) the presence of ATP and (2) appropriate ionic conditions, including especially appropriate concentrations of magnesium and calcium. Fourth, during forward motion of the cilium, the tubules on the front edge of the cilium slide outward toward the tip of the cilium while the tubules on the back edge remain in place. Fifth, three protein arms, composed of the protein *dynein* that has ATPase activity, project from each set of peripheral tubules toward the next set.

Given this basic information, it has been postulated that the release of energy from ATP in contact with the ATPase dynein arms causes the arms to "crawl" along the surface of the adjacent pair of tubules. If the front tubules crawl outward while the back tubules remain stationary, this obviously will cause bending.

The way in which cilium contraction is controlled is not understood. However, the cilia of some genetically abnormal cells do not have the two central single tubules, and these cilia fail to beat at all. Therefore, it is presumed that some signal, perhaps an electrochemical signal, is transmitted along these two tubules to activate the dynein arms.

REFERENCES

Bershadsky, A. D., and Vasiliev, J. M.: Cytoskeleton. New York, Plenum Publishing Corp., 1988.

Bettger, W. J., and McKeehan, W. L.: Mechanisms of cellular nutrition. Physiol. Rev., 66:1, 1986.

Bohr, D. F.: Cell membrane in hypertension. News Physiol. Sci., 4:85, 1989.

Cereijido, M., et al.: Tight junction: Barrier between higher organisms and environment. New Physiol. Sci., 4:72, 1989.

Chien, S. (ed.): Molecular Biology in Physiology. New York, Raven Press, 1988.

DeMello, W. C. (ed.): Cell-to-Cell Communication. New York, Plenum Publishing Corp., 1987.

DeRobertis, E. D. P., and DeRobertis, E. M. F., Jr.: Cell and Molecular Biology. 8th ed. Philadelphia, Lea & Febiger, 1987.

Fawcett, D. W.: Bloom & Fawcett: A Textbook of Histology. 11th ed. Philadelphia, W. B. Saunders Co., 1986.

Fawcett, D. W.: The Cell. 2nd ed. Philadelphia, W. B. Saunders Co., 1981.

Holtzman, E.: Lysosomes, New York, Plenum Publishing Corp., 1989.

Hubbard, A. L., et al.: Biogenesis of endogenous plasma membrane proteins in epithelian cells. Annu. Rev. Physiol., 51:755, 1989.

Kudlow, J. E., et al. (eds.): Biology of Growth Factors. New York, Plenum Publishing Corp., 1988.

Lane, M. D., et al.: The mitochondrion updated. Science, 234:526, 1986.

Lemasters, J. J., et al. (eds.): Integration of Mitochondrial Function. New York, Plenum Publishing Corp., 1988.

Sowers, A. E. (ed.): Cell Fusion. New York, Plenum Publishing Corp., 1987.

Thomas, K. A.: Fibroblast growth factors. FASEB J., 1:434, 1987.

van der Laarse, W. J., et al.: Energetics at the single cell level. News Physiol. Sci., 4:91, 1989.

QUESTIONS

1. Name the membranous structures of the cell.
2. Discuss the chemical and physical characteristics of the cell membrane.
3. What are the roles of cell membrane proteins and carbohydrates?
4. Describe the endoplasmic reticulum and its synthesis functions.
5. How does the role of the Golgi apparatus differ from that of the endoplasmic reticulum?
6. How are the lysosomes formed, and what are the principal constituents of the lysosomes?
7. What is the structure of the mitochondria, and what is the special significance of the enzymes located in the mitochondrial shelves?
8. What are the characteristics of the nuclear pores?
9. Explain the mechanisms of pinocytosis and phagocytosis.
10. Describe the digestive vesicle and the events that take place in it.
11. Trace the synthesis of proteins by the granular endoplasmic reticulum, their transport to the Golgi apparatus, the formation of secretory vesicles, and final extrusion of secretory proteins through the cell surface.
12. What are some of the special substances and organelles formed by the Golgi apparatus?
13. Explain the special characteristics of the chemical substance adenosine triphosphate that allow it to function as "energy currency" in a cell.
14. Explain briefly the role of the mitochondrion in the formation of ATP.
15. What are the uses of ATP in the cell?
16. Describe ameboid and ciliary motions and their mechanisms.

3

Genetic Control of Protein Synthesis, Cell Function, and Cell Reproduction

Virtually everyone knows that the genes control heredity from parents to children, but most persons do not realize that the same genes control the reproduction of and the day-by-day function of all cells. The genes control cell function by determining what substances will be synthesized within the cell — what structures, what enzymes, what chemicals.

Figure 3–1 illustrates the general schema of genetic control. Each gene, which is a nucleic acid called *deoxyribonucleic acid (DNA),* automatically controls the formation of another nucleic acid, *ribonucleic acid (RNA),* which spreads throughout the cell and controls the formation of a specific protein. Some proteins are *structural proteins,* which, in association with various lipids and carbohydrates, form the structures of the various organelles that are discussed in Chapter 2. By far the majority of the proteins are *enzymes* that catalyze the different chemical reactions in the cells. For instance, enzymes promote all the oxidative reactions that supply energy to the cell, and they promote the synthesis of various chemicals, such as lipids, glycogen, adenosine triphosphate (ATP), and so on.

For the formation of each cellular protein, there is usually only a single gene pair in each cell. It is estimated that cells of the human being have over 100,000 such gene pairs, which means that as many as 100,000 different proteins are formed in different cells, though not all of these in the same cell, for reasons that we discuss later in the chapter.

The Genes

Large numbers of genes attached end on end are contained in extremely long, double-stranded helical molecules of *DNA* having molecular weights measured in the billions. A very short segment of such a molecule is illustrated in Figure 3–2. This molecule is composed of several simple chemical compounds arranged in a regular pattern explained in the following few paragraphs.

The Basic Building Blocks of DNA. Figure 3–3 illustrates the basic chemical compounds involved in the formation of DNA. These include (1) *phosphoric acid,* (2) a sugar called *deoxyribose,* and (3) four nitrogenous *bases* (two purines, *adenine* and *guanine,* and two pyrimidines, *thymine* and *cytosine*). The phosphoric acid and deoxyribose form the two helical strands that are the backbone of the DNA molecule, and the bases lie between the two strands and connect them.

The Nucleotides. The first stage in the formation of DNA is the combination of one molecule of phosphoric acid, one molecule of deoxyribose, and one of the four bases to form a nucleotide. Four separate nucleotides are thus formed, one for each of the four bases: *deoxyadenylic, deoxythymidylic, deoxyguanylic,* and *deoxycytidylic acids.* Figure 3–4 illustrates the chemical structure of adenylic acid, and Figure 3–5 illustrates simple symbols for all the four basic nucleotides that form DNA.

Organization of the Nucleotides to Form DNA. Figure 3–6 illustrates the manner in which multiple numbers of nucleotides are bound together to form DNA. Note that these are combined in such a way that phosphoric acid and deoxyribose alternate with each other in the two separate strands, and these strands are held together by loose bonds between the purine and pyrimidine bases. But note carefully that

1. The purine base *adenine* always bonds with the pyrimidine base *thymine* and
2. The purine base *guanine* always bonds with the pyrimidine base *cytosine.*

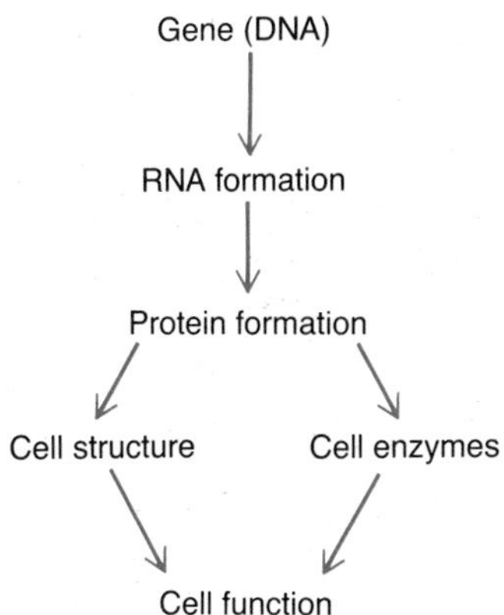

Figure 3-1. General schema by which the genes control cell function.

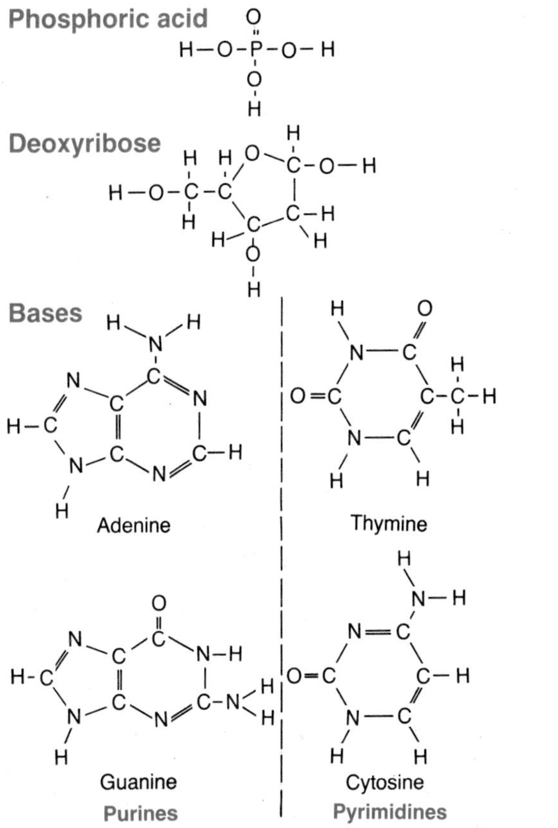

Thus, in Figure 3-6 the sequence of complementary pairs of bases is CG, CG, GC, TA, CG, TA, GC, AT, and AT. However, the bases are bound together by very loose *hydrogen bonding,* represented in the figure by dashed lines. Because of the looseness of these bonds, the two strands can pull apart with ease, and they do so many times during the course of their function in the cell.

Now, to put the DNA of Figure 3-6 into its proper physical perspective, one needs merely to pick up the two ends and twist them into a helix. Ten pairs of nucleotides are present in each full turn of the helix in the DNA molecule, as is illustrated in Figure 3-2.

The Genetic Code

The importance of DNA lies in its ability to control the formation of other substances in the cell. It does this by means of the so-called *genetic code.* When the two strands of a DNA molecule are split apart, this exposes the purine and pyrimidine bases projecting to the side of each strand. It is these projecting bases that form the code.

The genetic code consists of successive "triplets" of bases—that is, each group of three successive bases is a code word. The successive triplets eventually control the sequence of amino acids in a protein molecule during its synthesis in the cell. Note in Figure 3-6 that each of the two strands of the DNA molecule carries its own genetic code. For instance, the top strand, reading from left to right, has the genetic code GGC, AGA, CTT, the triplets being separated from each other by the arrows. As we follow this genetic code through Figures 3-7 and 3-8, we see that these three respective triplets are responsible for successive placement of the three amino acids *proline, serine,* and *glutamic acid* in a molecule of protein.

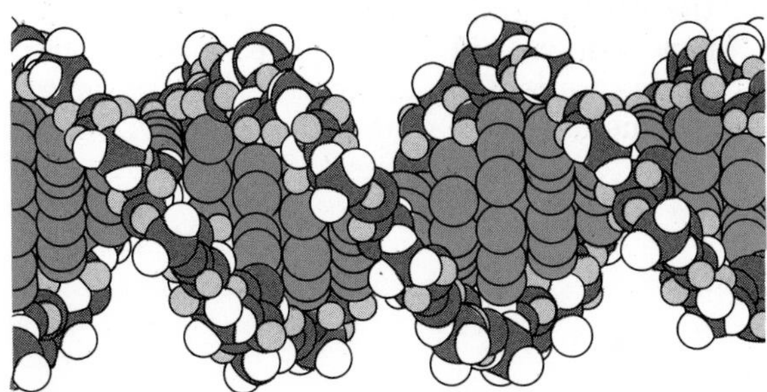

Figure 3-2. The helical, double-stranded structure of the gene. The outside strands are composed of phosphoric acid and the sugar deoxyribose. The internal molecules connecting the two strands of the helix are purine and pyrimidine bases; these determine the "code" of the gene.

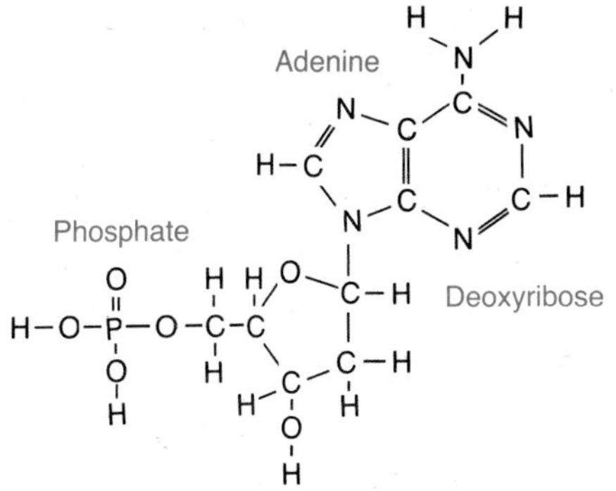

Phosphoric acid

Deoxyribose

Bases

Adenine

Thymine

Guanine

Cytosine

Purines

Pyrimidines

Figure 3-3. The basic building blocks of deoxyribonucleic acid (DNA).

RNA—THE PROCESS OF TRANSCRIPTION

Because almost all DNA is located in the nucleus of the cell and yet most of the functions of the cell are

Adenine

Phosphate

Deoxyribose

Figure 3-4. Deoxyadenylic acid, one of the nucleotides that make up DNA.

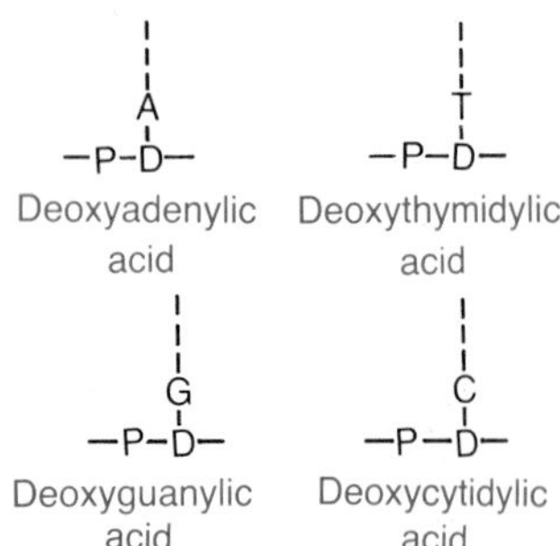

Figure 3-5. Combinations of the basic building blocks of DNA to form nucleotides. (*P*, phosphoric acid; *D*, deoxyribose.) The four nucleotide bases are *A*, adenine; *T*, thymine; *G*, guanine; and *C*, cytosine. These four different types of nucleotides make up DNA.

carried out in the cytoplasm, some means must be available for the genes of the nucleus to control the chemical reactions of the cytoplasm. This is achieved through the intermediary of another type of nucleic acid, *RNA*, the formation of which is controlled by the DNA of the nucleus. In this process the code is transferred to the RNA, which is called *transcription.* The RNA then diffuses from the nucleus through the nuclear pores into the cytoplasmic compartment, where it controls protein synthesis.

Synthesis of RNA

During synthesis of RNA, the two strands of the DNA molecule separate temporarily; one of these strands is then used as a template for synthesis of the RNA molecules. The code triplets in the DNA cause the formation of *complementary* code triplets (called *codons*) in the RNA; these codons in turn control the sequence of amino acids in a protein to be synthesized later in the cytoplasm. When one strand of DNA is used in this manner to cause the formation of RNA, the opposite strand remains inactive. Each DNA strand in each chromosome is such a large molecule that it carries the code for an average of about 4000 genes.

The Basic Building Blocks of RNA. The basic building blocks of RNA are almost the same as those of DNA except for two differences. First, the sugar deoxyribose is not used in the formation of RNA. In its place is another sugar of very slightly different composition, *ribose.* Second, thymine is replaced by another pyrimidine, *uracil.*

Formation of RNA Nucleotides. The basic building blocks of RNA first form nucleotides exactly as previously described for the synthesis of DNA. Here again, four separate nucleotides are used in the formation of RNA. These nucleotides contain the bases *adenine, guanine, cytosine,* and *uracil.* Note that these are the same as the bases in DNA except for one of them; the uracil replaces the thymine in DNA.

Activation of the Nucleotides. The next step in the synthesis of RNA is activation of the nucleotides. This occurs by addition to each nucleotide of two phosphate radicals to form triphosphates. These last two phosphates are combined with the nucleotide by *high-energy phosphate bonds* derived from the ATP of the cell.

The result of this activation process is that large quantities of energy are made available to each of the nucleotides, and this energy is used in promoting the subsequent chemical reactions that eventuate in the formation of the RNA chain.

Assembly of the RNA Molecule from Activated Nucleotides Using the DNA Strand as a Template — The Process of "Transcription"

Assembly of the RNA molecule is accomplished in the manner illustrated in Figure 3-7 under the influence of the enzyme *RNA polymerase.* This is a very large enzyme that has many functional properties necessary for the formation of the RNA molecule, the most important of which are the following:

1. In the DNA strand immediately ahead of the initial gene is a sequence of nucleotides called the *promoter.* The RNA polymerase has an appropriate complementary structure that recognizes this promoter and becomes attached to it. This is the essential step in initiating the formation of the RNA molecule.
2. Once the RNA polymerase attaches to the promoter, it causes unwinding of about two turns of the DNA helix and separation of the unwound portions of the two strands.
3. Then the polymerase moves along the DNA strand and begins forming the RNA molecule by binding complementary RNA nucleotides with the DNA strand.
4. Next the successive RNA nucleotides bind successively with each other to form an RNA strand.
5. When the RNA polymerase reaches the end of the gene or sequence of genes, it encounters a new sequence of DNA nucleotides called the *chain-terminating sequence;* this causes the polymerase to break away from the DNA strand,

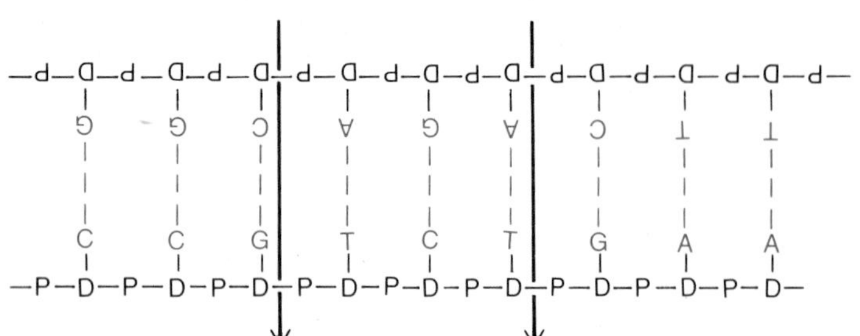

Figure 3-6. Arrangement of deoxyribose nucleotides in DNA.

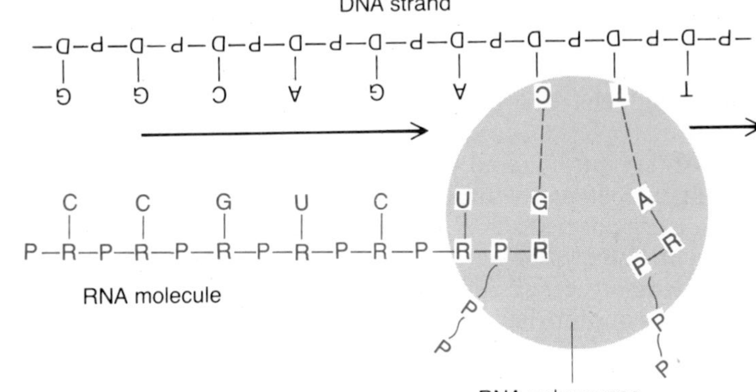

Figure 3-7. Combination of ribose nucleotides with a strand of DNA to form a molecule of ribonucleic acid (RNA) that carries the DNA code from the gene to the cytoplasm. The RNA polymerase moves along the DNA strand and builds the RNA molecule.

and at the same time the RNA strand is released into the nucleoplasm.

It should be remembered that there are four different types of DNA bases and also four different types of RNA nucleotide bases. Furthermore, these always combine with each other in specific combinations. Therefore, the code that is present in the DNA strand is transmitted in *complementary* form to the RNA molecule in the following combinations:

DNA base	*RNA base*
guanine	cytosine
cytosine	guanine
adenine	uracil
thymine	adenine

There are three separate types of RNA, each of which plays an independent and entirely different role in protein formation. These are

1. *Messenger RNA,* which carries the genetic code to the cytoplasm for controlling the formation of the proteins;
2. *Transfer RNA,* which transports activated amino acids to the ribosomes to be used in assembling the protein molecules; and
3. *Ribosomal RNA,* which, along with about 75 different proteins, forms the *ribosomes,* the physical and chemical structures on which protein molecules are actually assembled.

Messenger RNA—The "Codons"

Messenger RNA molecules are composed of several hundred to several thousand nucleotides in single strands, and they contain *codons* that are exactly complementary to the code triplets of the genes. Figure 3-8 illustrates a small segment of a molecule of messenger RNA. Its codons are CCG, UCU, and GAA. These are the codons for the amino acids proline, serine, and glutamic acid. The transcription of these codons from the DNA molecule is demonstrated in Figure 3-7.

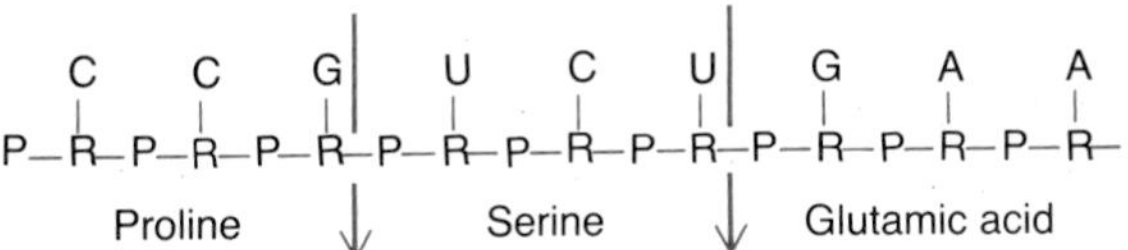

Figure 3-8. Portion of a ribonucleic acid molecule, showing three "code" words, CCG, UCU, and GAA, which represent the three amino acids *proline, serine,* and *glutamic acid.*

RNA Codons for the Different Amino Acids. Table 3-1 gives the RNA codons for the 20 common amino acids found in protein molecules. Note that most of the amino acids are represented by more than one codon; also, one codon represents the signal "start manufacturing a protein molecule," and three codons represent "stop manufacturing a protein molecule." In Table 3-1, these two types of codons are designated CI for "chain-initiating" and CT for "chain-terminating."

Transfer RNA—The "Anticodons"

Another type of RNA that plays an essential role in protein synthesis is called *transfer RNA* because it

Table 3-1 RNA CODONS FOR THE DIFFERENT AMINO ACIDS AND FOR START AND STOP

Amino Acid	RNA Codons					
Alanine	GCU	GCC	GCA	GCG		
Arginine	CGU	CGC	CGA	CGG	AGA	AGG
Asparagine	AAU	AAC				
Aspartic acid	GAU	GAC				
Cysteine	UGU	UGC				
Glutamic acid	GAA	GAG				
Glutamine	CAA	CAG				
Glycine	GGU	GGC	GGA	GGG		
Histidine	CAU	CAC				
Isoleucine	AUU	AUC	AUA			
Leucine	CUU	CUC	CUA	CUG	UUA	UUG
Lysine	AAA	AAG				
Methionine	AUG					
Phenylalanine	UUU	UUC				
Proline	CCU	CCC	CCA	CCG		
Serine	UCU	UCC	UCA	UCG	AGC	AGU
Threonine	ACU	ACC	ACA	ACG		
Tryptophan	UGG					
Tyrosine	UAU	UAC				
Valine	GUU	GUC	GUA	GUG		
Start (CI)	AUG					
Stop (CT)	UAA	UAG	UGA			

transfers amino acid molecules to the messenger RNA strand as the protein is synthesized. Each type of transfer RNA combines specifically with one of the 20 amino acids that are to be incorporated into proteins. The transfer RNA then acts as a *carrier* to transport its specific type of amino acid to the ribosomes, where protein molecules are forming. In the ribosomes, each specific type of transfer RNA recognizes a particular codon on the messenger RNA, as is described subsequently, and thereby delivers the appropriate amino acid to the appropriate place in the chain of the newly forming protein molecule.

Transfer RNA, containing only about 80 nucleotides, is a relatively small molecule in comparison with messenger RNA. It is a folded chain of nucleotides with a cloverleaf appearance similar to that illustrated in Figure 3–9.

Since the function of transfer RNA is to cause attachment of a specific amino acid to a forming protein chain, it is essential that each type of transfer RNA bind with only one type of amino acid as well as have specificity for a particular codon in the messenger RNA. The specific code in the transfer RNA that allows it to recognize a specific codon is again a triplet of nucleotide bases and is called an *anticodon.* This is located approximately in the middle of the transfer RNA molecule (at the bottom of the cloverleaf configuration illustrated in Figure 3–9). During formation of a protein molecule, the anticodon bases combine loosely by hydrogen bonding with the codon bases of the messenger RNA. In this way the respective amino acids are lined up one after another along the messenger RNA chain, thus establishing the appropriate sequence of amino acids in the protein molecule.

Ribosomal RNA

The third type of RNA in the cell is ribosomal RNA; it constitutes about 60 per cent of the *ribosome.* The remainder of the ribosome is protein, containing about 75 different types of proteins that are both structural proteins and enzymes needed in the manufacture of protein molecules.

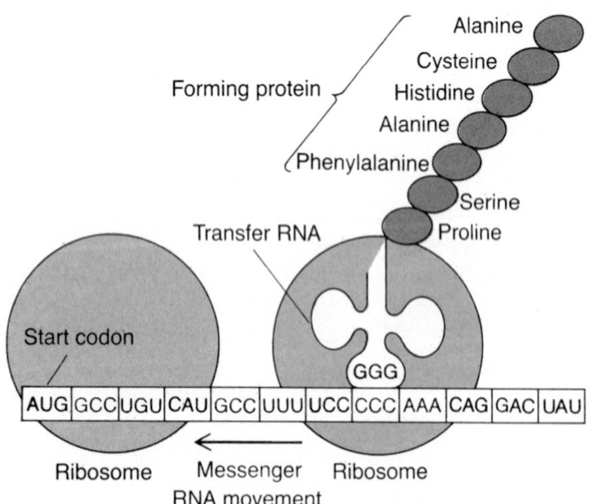

Figure 3–9. Mechanism by which a protein molecule is formed in ribosomes in association with messenger RNA and transfer RNA.

The ribosome is the physical structure in the cytoplasm on which protein molecules are actually synthesized. However, it always functions in association with both the other types of RNA as well: transfer RNA transports amino acids to the ribosome for incorporation into the developing protein molecule, whereas messenger RNA provides the information necessary for sequencing the amino acids in proper order for each specific type of protein to be manufactured.

The ribosomes of nucleated cells are composed of two physical subunits, called the *small subunit,* containing 1 RNA molecule and 33 proteins, and the *large subunit,* containing 3 RNAs and more than 40 proteins. Although we have only partial knowledge of the mechanism of protein manufacture in the ribosome, it is known that messenger RNA and transfer RNA first complex with the small subunit. Then the large subunit provides most of the enzymes that promote peptide linkages between the successive amino acids. Thus, the ribosome acts as a manufacturing plant in which the protein molecules are formed.

Formation of Proteins on the Ribosomes —The Process of "Translation"

When a molecule of messenger RNA comes in contact with a ribosome, it travels along the ribosome, beginning at a predetermined end of the RNA molecule specified by an appropriate sequence of RNA bases. Then, as illustrated in Figure 3–9, while the messenger RNA travels along the ribosome, a protein molecule is formed—a process called *translation.* Thus, the ribosome reads the code of the messenger RNA in much the same way that a tape is "read" as it passes through the playback head of a tape recorder. Then, when a "stop" (or "chain-terminating") codon slips past the ribosome, the end of a protein molecule is signaled, and the protein molecule is freed into the cytoplasm.

Attachment of Ribosomes to the Endoplasmic Reticulum. In the previous chapter it was noted that many ribosomes become attached to the endoplasmic reticulum. This does not occur until the ribosomes begin to form the protein molecules. It occurs because the initial ends of some protein molecules have amino acid sequences that immediately attach to specific receptor sites on the endoplasmic reticulum; this causes these molecules to penetrate the reticulum wall and enter the endoplasmic reticulum matrix. This occurs while the protein molecule is still being formed by the ribosome, which pulls the ribosome against the endoplasmic reticulum, thereby giving the "granular" appearance to the reticulum.

Figure 3–10 shows the functional relationship of messenger RNA to the ribosomes and also the manner in which the ribosomes attach to the membrane of the

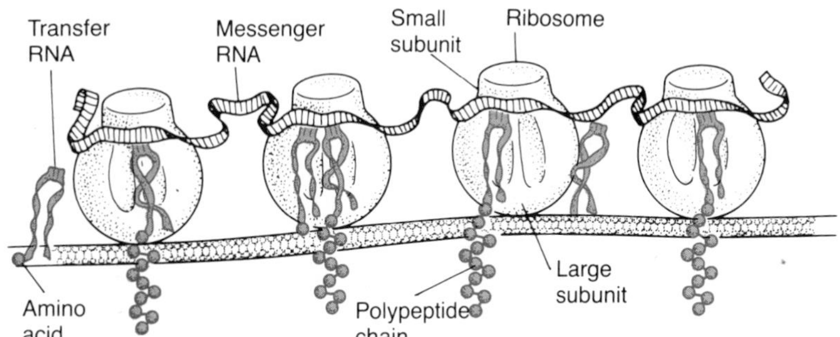

Figure 3-10. An artist's concept of the physical structure of the ribosomes as well as their functional relationship to messenger RNA, transfer RNA, and the endoplasmic reticulum during the formation of protein molecules. (From Bloom and Fawcett: A Textbook of Histology. 10th ed. Philadelphia, W. B. Saunders Company, 1975.)

endoplasmic reticulum. Note the process of translation occurring in several ribosomes at the same time in response to the same strand of messenger RNA. And note also the newly forming polypeptide chains passing through the endoplasmic reticulum membrane into the endoplasmic matrix.

Yet, it should be noted that except in glandular cells that form large amounts of protein-containing secretory vesicles, the other proteins formed by the ribosomes are released directly into the cytosol. These are the enzymes and internal structural proteins of the cell.

Peptide Linkage. The successive amino acids in the protein chain combine with each other according to the following typical chemical reaction:

$$R-\overset{\overset{NH_2}{|}}{C}-\overset{\overset{O}{\|}}{C}-OH + H-\overset{\overset{H}{|}}{N}-\overset{\overset{R}{|}}{C}-COOH \longrightarrow$$

$$R-\overset{\overset{NH_2}{|}}{C}-\overset{\overset{O}{\|}}{C}-\overset{\overset{H}{|}}{N}-\overset{\overset{R}{|}}{C}-COOH + H_2O$$

In this chemical reaction, a hydroxyl radical is removed from the COOH portion of one amino acid, while a hydrogen of the NH_2 portion of the other amino acid is removed. These combine to form water, and the two reactive sites left on the two successive amino acids bond with each other, resulting in a single molecule. This process is called *peptide linkage.*

For each peptide linkage formed during the manufacture of a protein molecule in the ribosome, a very large amount of energy is consumed, requiring the breakdown of four molecules of ATP. Thus, protein synthesis is one of the most energy-consuming of all the life processes of the cell.

Synthesis of Other Substances in the Cell

Many thousands of protein enzymes formed in the manner just described control essentially all the other chemical reactions that take place in cells. These enzymes promote synthesis of lipids, glycogen, purines, pyrimidines, and hundreds of other substances. We discuss many of these synthetic processes in relation to carbohydrate, lipid, and protein metabolism in Chapters 45 and 46. It is by means of all these different substances that the many functions of the cells are performed.

CONTROL OF GENETIC FUNCTION AND BIOCHEMICAL ACTIVITY IN CELLS

There are basically two different methods by which the biochemical activities in the cell are controlled. One of these is called *genetic regulation,* in which the activities of the genes themselves are controlled, and the other is called *enzyme regulation,* in which the levels of activity of the enzymes within the cell are controlled.

Genetic Regulation

The Operon of the Prokaryote and Its Control of Biochemical Synthesis—Function of the "Promoter." Formation of all the enzymes needed for a specific synthetic process is usually controlled by a sequence of genes located in series one after the other on the same chromosomal DNA strand. This area of the DNA strand is called an *operon,* and the genes responsible for forming the respective enzymes are called *structural genes.* In Figure 3-11, three respective structural genes are illustrated in an operon, and it is shown that they control the formation of three respective enzymes used in a particular biochemical synthetic process.

Now note in the figure the shaded areas on the DNA strand. These areas are called the *promoter.* This is a series of nucleotides that has specific affinity for RNA polymerase, as already discussed. The polymerase must bind with this promoter before it can begin traveling along the DNA strand to synthesize RNA. Therefore, the promoter is the essential element in activating the operon.

Control of the Operon by a "Repressor Protein"—The "Repressor Operator." Also note in Figure 3-11 an additional band of nucleotides lying in the middle of the promoter. This area is called a *repressor operator* because a "regulatory" protein can bind here and prevent attachment of RNA polymerase to the promoter, thereby blocking transcription of the genes. Such a regulatory protein is called a *repressor protein.* Various nonprotein substances in the cell, such as some of the cell metabolites, can bind

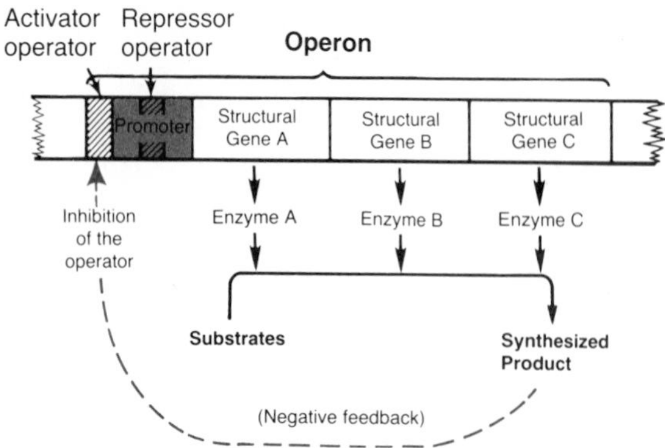

Figure 3-11. Function of the operon to control biosynthesis. Note that the synthesized product exerts a negative feedback to inhibit function of the operon, in this way automatically controlling the concentration of the product itself.

with the repressor protein to change its state. A substance that causes it to change so that it will bind with the operator and stop transcription is called a *repressor substance* or *inhibitor substance.* On the other hand, a substance that changes the repressor protein so that it will break its bond with the operator is called an *activator substance* or *inducer substance* because it activates, or induces, the transcription process by removing the repressor protein.

To illustrate the control of gene transcription by a repressor protein, let us give an example. The saccharide lactose usually is not available to *E. coli* cells as a food substrate. Therefore, the bacterium normally will not synthesize the required enzymes for metabolic breakdown of lactose. However, when lactose does become available, it induces a change in a repressor protein, causing it to break away from a repressor operator on the operon that transcribes for the necessary metabolic enzymes. Therefore, the operon becomes derepressed, and within a few minutes the appropriate enzymes are present in the bacterium to cause breakdown of the lactose.

Control of the Operon by an "Activator Protein"—The "Activator Operator." Now note in Figure 3-11 another operator, called the *activator operator,* that lies adjacent to but ahead of the promoter. When a regulatory protein binds to this operator, it helps attract the RNA polymerase to the promoter, in this way activating the operon. Therefore, a regulatory protein of this type is called an *activator protein.* The operon can be activated or inhibited through the activator operator in ways exactly opposite to the control of the repressor operator.

Negative Feedback Control of the Operon. Finally, note in Figure 3-11 that the presence of a critical amount of a synthesized product in the cell can cause negative feedback inhibition of the operon that is responsible for its synthesis. It can do this either by causing a regulatory repressor protein to bind at the repressor operator or by causing a regulatory activator protein to break its bond with the activator operator. In either case, the operon becomes inhibited. Therefore, once the required synthesized product has become abundant enough, the operon becomes dormant. On the other hand, when the synthesized product becomes degraded in the cell and its concentration falls, the operon once again becomes active. In this way, the concentration of the product is automatically controlled.

Other Mechanisms for Control of Transcription by the Operon. Variations in the basic mechanism for control of the operon have been discovered with rapidity in the last several years. Without giving details, let us list some of these:

1. An operon is frequently controlled by a *regulatory gene* located elsewhere in the genetic complex of the nucleus. That is, the regulatory gene causes the formation of a regulatory protein that in turn acts either as an activator or as a repressor substance to control the operon.
2. Occasionally, many different operons are controlled at the same time by the same regulatory protein. In some instances, the same regulatory protein functions as an activator for one operon and as a repressor for another operon. When multiple operons are controlled simultaneously in this manner, all the operons that function together are called a *regulon.*
3. In eukaryotes, the nuclear DNA is packaged in specific structural units, the *chromosomes.* And within each chromosome, the DNA is wound around small proteins called *histones,* which in turn are compacted tightly together by still other proteins. As long as the DNA is in this compacted state, it cannot function to form RNA. However, multiple control mechanisms are beginning to be discovered that can cause selected areas of the chromosomes to become decompacted one part at a time so that RNA transcription can occur.

Because there are as many as 100,000 different genes in each human cell, the large number of different ways in which genetic activity can be controlled is not surprising. The genetic control systems are especially important for controlling the intracellular concentrations of amino acids, amino acid derivatives, and the intermediate substrates of carbohydrate, lipid, and protein metabolism.

Control of Enzyme Activity

In addition to control of the genetic regulatory system, some of the intracellular enzymes themselves can be directly controlled by intracellular inhibitors or activators. This, therefore, represents a second category of mechanisms by which cellular biochemical functions can be controlled.

Enzyme Inhibition. When their concentrations become too great, some of the chemical substances formed in the cell have a direct feedback effect in inhibiting the respective enzyme systems that synthesize them. Almost always the synthesized product acts on the first enzyme in a sequence, rather than on the subsequent enzymes, usually binding directly with the enzyme and causing an allosteric conformational change that inactivates it. One can readily recognize the importance of inactivating this first enzyme: It prevents buildup of intermediary products that will not be used.

This process of enzyme inhibition is another example of negative feedback control; it is responsible for controlling the intracellular concentrations of some of the amino acids, purines, pyrimidines, vitamins, and other substances.

Enzyme Activation. Enzymes either that are normally inactive or that have been inactivated by some inhibitor substance often can be activated. An example of this is the action of cyclic adenosine monophosphate (cAMP) in causing glycogen to split and release glucose molecules to form high-energy ATP. When most of the ATP has been depleted in a cell, a considerable amount of cAMP begins to be formed as a breakdown product of the ATP; this cAMP immediately activates the glycogen-splitting enzyme phosphorylase, liberating glucose molecules that are rapidly metabolized and their energy used for replenishment of the ATP stores. Thus, in this case the cAMP acts as an enzyme activator and thereby helps control intracellular ATP concentration.

In summary, there are two principal methods by which the cells control proper proportions and proper quantities of different cellular constituents: (1) the mechanism of genetic regulation and (2) the mechanism of enzyme regulation. The genes can be either activated or inhibited, and, likewise, the enzyme systems can be either activated or inhibited. Most often, these regulatory mechanisms function as feedback control systems that continually monitor the cell's biochemical composition and make corrections as needed. But, on occasion, substances from without the cell (especially some of the hormones that will be discussed later in this text) also control the intracellular biochemical reactions by activating or inhibiting one or more of the intracellular control systems.

CELL REPRODUCTION

Cell reproduction is another example of the pervading, ubiquitous role that the DNA-genetic system plays in all life processes. The genes and their regulatory mechanisms determine the growth characteristics of the cells and also when or whether these cells divide to form new cells. In this way, the all-important genetic system controls each stage in the development of the human being from the single-cell fertilized ovum to the whole functioning body. Thus, if there is any central theme to life, it is the DNA-genetic system.

The Life Cycle of the Cell. The life cycle of a cell is the period of time from cell reproduction to reproduction. When mammalian cells are not inhibited and are reproducing as rapidly as they can, this life cycle lasts for 10 to 30 hours. It is terminated by a series of distinct physical events called *mitosis* that cause division of the cell into two new daughter cells. The events of mitosis are illustrated in Figure 3–12 and are described later. The actual stage of mitosis, however, lasts for only about 30 minutes, so that more than 95 per cent of the life cycle even of rapidly reproducing cells is represented by the interval between mitosis, called *interphase*. In fact, except in special conditions of rapid cellular reproduction, inhibitory factors almost always slow or stop the uninhibited life cycle of the cell. Therefore, different cells of the body have life cycle periods that vary from as little as 10 hours for stimulated bone marrow cells to an entire lifetime of the human body for nerve and striated muscle cells.

Replication of the DNA, the Initial Step in Cell Reproduction

As is true of almost all other important events in the cell, reproduction begins in the nucleus itself. The first step is *replication (duplication) of all DNA in the chromosomes.* Only after this has occurred can mitosis take place.

The DNA begins to be duplicated some 5 to 10 hours before mitosis, and this is completed in 4 to 8 hours. The DNA is duplicated only once, so that the net result is two exact *replicates* of all DNA. These

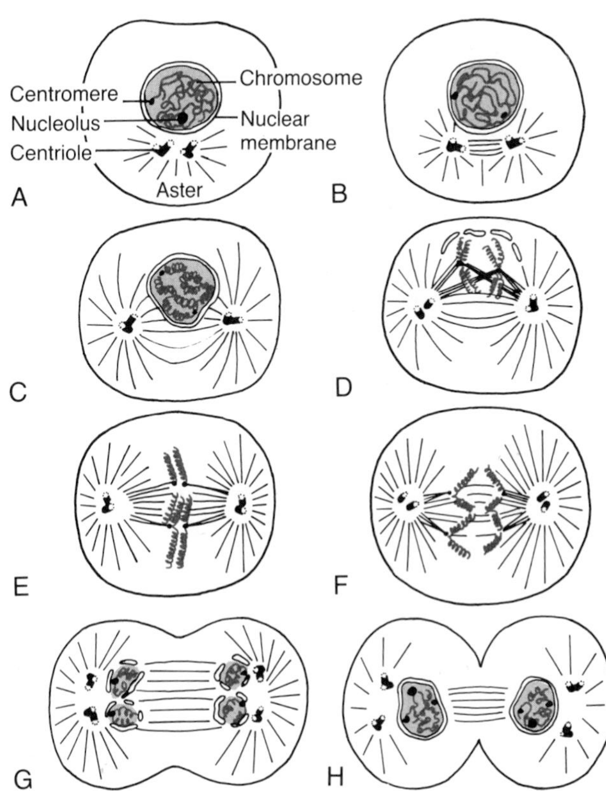

Figure 3–12. Stages in the reproduction of the cell. *A, B,* and *C,* prophase; *D,* prometaphase; *E,* metaphase; *F,* anaphase; *G* and *H,* telophase. (Redrawn from Mazia: How cells divide. *Sci. Am., 205*:102, 1961. © by Scientific American, Inc. All rights reserved.)

replicates, in turn, become the DNA in the two new daughter cells that will be formed at mitosis. Following replication of the DNA, there is another period of 1 to 2 hours before mitosis begins abruptly. However, even during this period, preliminary changes are already beginning to take place that will lead to the mitotic process.

Chemical and Physical Events of DNA Replication. DNA is replicated in much the same way that RNA is transcribed by DNA except for a few important differences:

1. Both strands of the DNA in each chromosome are replicated, not simply one of them.
2. Both entire strands of the DNA helix are replicated from end to end rather than small portions of them, as occurs in the transcription of RNA by the genes.
3. The principal enzymes for replicating DNA are a complex of several enzymes called *DNA polymerase,* which is comparable to RNA polymerase. It attaches to and moves along the DNA template strand, while another enzyme, *DNA ligase,* causes bonding of the successive nucleotides to each other, using high-energy phosphate bonds to energize these attachments.
4. Each newly formed strand of DNA remains attached by loose hydrogen bonding to the original DNA strand that is used as its template. Therefore, two new DNA helixes are formed that are exact duplicates of each other and that are still coiled together.
5. Because the DNA helixes in each chromosome are about 6 centimeters in length and have millions of turns in each helix, it would be impossible for the two newly formed DNA helixes to uncoil from each other were it not for some special mechanism. This is achieved by enzymes that periodically cut each helix along its entire length, rotate each segment enough to cause separation, and then resplice the helix. Thus, the two new helixes become uncoiled.

DNA Repair and DNA "Proofreading." During the hour or so between DNA replication and the beginning of mitosis, there is a period of very active repair and "proofreading" of the DNA strands. That is, wherever inappropriate DNA nucleotides have been matched up with the nucleotides of the original template strand, special enzymes cut out the defective areas and replace these with the appropriate complementary nucleotides. This is achieved by the same DNA polymerases and DNA ligase that are used in the process of replication. This repair process is referred to as *DNA proofreading.*

Because of repair and proofreading, the transcription process almost never makes a mistake. But when a mistake is made, this is called a *mutation;* it in turn will cause the formation of some abnormal protein in the cell, often leading to abnormal cellular function and sometimes even to death.

The Chromosomes and Their Replication

The DNA helixes of the nucleus are packaged in chromosomes. The human cell contains 46 chromosomes arranged in 23 pairs. Most of the genes in the two chromosomes of each pair are identical or almost identical with each other, so that it is usually stated that the different genes also exist in pairs, although occasionally this is not the case.

Aside from the DNA in the chromosome, there is also a large amount of protein, composed mainly of many small molecules of electropositively charged *histones.* The histones are organized into vast numbers of small, bobbin-like cores. Successive segments of each DNA helix are coiled sequentially around one core after another. Then, during mitosis the successive cores are packed one against the other, thus allowing the tremendously long DNA molecule, having a linear length of 6 centimeters and a molecular weight of about 60 billion, to be packaged in a coiled and folded arrangement of the *mitotic chromosome* that is only a few micrometers in length, 1/10,000 the stretched-out length of the DNA itself.

Replication of the chromosomes in their entirety follows during the next few minutes after replication of the DNA helixes; the new DNA helixes collect new protein molecules as needed. At this stage, the two newly formed chromosomes are called *chromatids.* They remain temporarily attached to each other (until the time for mitosis) at a point called the *centromere* located near the center of each of the chromatids.

Mitosis

The actual process by which the cell splits into two new cells is called *mitosis.* Once each chromosome has been replicated to form the two chromatids, mitosis follows automatically within an hour or two.

The Mitotic Apparatus. One of the first events of mitosis takes place in the cytoplasm, occurring during the latter part of interphase and the early part of prophase, in or around the small structures called *centrioles.* As illustrated in Figure 3–12, two pairs of centrioles lie close to each other near one pole of the nucleus. (These centrioles, like the DNA and chromosomes, had also been replicated during interphase, usually shortly before the replication of the DNA.) Each centriole is a small cylindrical body about 0.4 micrometer long and about 0.15 micrometer in diameter, consisting mainly of nine parallel tubular structures arranged in the form of a cylinder. The two centrioles of each pair lie at right angles to each other.

Shortly before mitosis is to take place, the two pairs of centrioles begin to move apart from each other. This is caused by successive polymerization of protein microtubules growing between the respective centriole pairs and actually pushing them apart. At the same time, other microtubules grow radially away from each of the centriole pairs, forming a spiny star, called the *aster,* in each end of the cell. Some of the spines penetrate the nucleus and play a role in separating the two sets of chromatids during mitosis. The complex of microtubules connecting the two centriole pairs is called the *spindle,* and the entire set of microtubules plus the two pairs of centrioles is called the *mitotic apparatus.*

Prophase. The first stage of mitosis, called *prophase,* is shown in Figure 3–12A, B, and C. While the spindle is forming, the chromosomes of the nucleus, which in interphase consist of loosely coiled strands, become condensed into well-defined chromosomes.

Prometaphase. During this stage (Fig. 3–12D), the nuclear envelope fragments. At the same time, a new set of microtubules begins to extend outward from a small condensed portion of each chromatid called the *kinetochore,* located on the outside of the centromere, where the two chromatids are attached to each other. These new microtubules, in turn, either become attached to or interact with the microtubules from the two asters of the mitotic apparatus, with one chromatid connecting to the aster at one pole of the cell and the other chromatid connecting to the opposite aster.

Metaphase. During metaphase (Fig. 3–12E), the two asters of the mitotic apparatus are pushed farther apart by additional growth of the mitotic spindle. Simultaneously the chromatids are pulled tightly by the attached microtubules to the very center of the cell, lining up to form the *equatorial plate* of the mitotic spindle.

Anaphase. During this phase (Fig. 3–12F), the two chromatids of each chromosome are pulled apart at the centromere. Exactly how the microtubular system causes this is not known, except that it is known that the microtubules contain *actin* in addition to tubulin; actin is one of the contractile proteins of muscle. Therefore, it has been presumed that the microtubules might contract or that the chromosomal tubules might interact in a sliding way with the microtubules of the aster to cause the pulling force. Regardless of the mechanism, all 46 pairs of chromatids are separated, forming two separate sets of 46 *daughter chromosomes.* One of these sets is pulled toward one mitotic aster and the other toward the other aster at the two respective poles of the dividing cell.

Telophase. In telophase (Fig. 3–12G and H), the two sets of daughter chromosomes are now pulled completely apart. Then the mitotic apparatus dissolutes, and a new nuclear membrane develops around each set of chromosomes, this membrane being formed from portions of the endoplasmic reticulum that are already present in the cytoplasm. Shortly thereafter, the cell pinches in two midway between the two nuclei. This is caused by a contractile ring of *microfilaments* composed of *actin* and probably *myosin,* the two contractile proteins of muscle, forming at the juncture of the newly developing cells and pinching them off from each other.

Control of Cell Growth and Reproduction

We all know that certain cells grow and reproduce all the time, such as the blood-forming cells of the bone marrow, the germinal layers of the skin, and the epithelium of the gut. However, many other cells, such as smooth muscle cells, may not reproduce for many years. A few cells, such as the neurons and most striated muscle cells, reproduce only in the fetus and do not reproduce during the entire postnatal life of the person.

In certain tissues, an insufficiency of some types of cells causes these to grow and reproduce very rapidly until appropriate numbers of them are again available. For instance, seven eighths of the liver can be removed surgically, and the cells of the remaining one eighth will grow and divide until the liver mass returns almost to normal. The same occurs for almost all glandular cells, cells of the bone marrow, subcutaneous tissue, intestinal epithelium, and almost any other tissue except highly differentiated cells, such as nerve and muscle cells.

We know very little about the mechanisms that maintain proper numbers of the different types of cells in the body. However, experiments have shown at least three ways in which growth can be controlled. First, growth is often controlled by *growth factors* that come from other parts of the body. Some of these circulate in the blood, but others originate in adjacent tissues. For instance, the epithelial cells of some glands, such as the pancreas, will fail to grow without a growth factor from the sublying connective tissue of the gland. Second, most normal cells will stop growing when they have run out of space for growth. This occurs when cells are grown in tissue culture; the cells grow until they contact a solid object and then growth stops. Third, cells grown in tissue culture often stop growing when minute amounts of their own secretions are allowed to collect in the culture medium. This, too, could provide a means for negative feedback control of growth.

CANCER

Cancer is caused in all or almost all instances by *mutation* or *abnormal activation* of cellular genes that control cell growth and cell mitosis. The abnormal genes are called *oncogenes.*

Only a minute fraction of the cells that mutate in the body ever lead to cancer. There are several reasons for this. First, most mutated cells have less survival capability than normal cells and therefore simply die. Second, only a few of the mutated cells that do survive lose the normal feedback controls that prevent excessive growth. Third, those cells that are potentially cancerous are often, if not usually, destroyed by the body's immune system before they grow into a cancer.

But what is it that causes the altered genes? When one realizes that many trillions of new cells are formed each year in the human being, this question should probably better be asked in the following form: Why is it that we do not develop literally millions or billions of mutant cancerous cells? The answer is the incredible precision with which DNA chromosomal strands are replicated in each cell before mitosis takes place and also because the "proofreading" process cuts and repairs any abnormal DNA strand before the mitotic process is allowed to proceed. Yet, despite all these precautions, probably one newly formed cell in every few million still has significant mutant characteristics.

Thus, chance alone is all that is required for mutations to take place, so we may suppose that a very large number of cancers are merely the result of an unlucky occurrence.

Yet, the probability of mutations can be increased manyfold when a person is exposed to certain chemical, physical, or biological factors. Some of these are the following:

1. It is well known that *ionizing radiation,* such as x-rays, gamma rays, and particle radiations from radioactive substances, and even ultraviolet light can predispose to cancer. Ions formed in tissue cells under the influence of such radiation are highly reactive and can rupture DNA strands, thus causing many mutations.
2. *Chemical substances* of certain types also have a high propensity for causing mutations. Historically, it was long ago discovered that various aniline dye derivatives are very likely to cause cancer, so that workers in chemical plants producing such substances, if unprotected, have a special predisposition to cancer. Chemical substances that can cause mutation are called *carcinogens.* The carcinogens that cause by far the greatest number of deaths in our present-day society are those in cigarette smoke. These cause about one quarter of all cancer deaths.
3. *Physical irritants* can also lead to cancer, such as continued abrasion of the linings of the intestinal tract by some types of food.
4. In many families there is a strong *hereditary tendency to cancer.* In those families, it is presumed that one or more of the genes that predispose to cancer are already mutated in the inherited genome.
5. In experimental animals, certain types of viruses can cause some kinds of cancer, including leukemia.

Invasive Characteristic of the Cancer Cell. The three major differences between the cancer cell and the normal cell are (1) The cancer cell does not respect usual cellular growth limits; the reason for this is that the cells presumably do not require the growth factors that are necessary to cause growth of normal cells. (2) Cancer cells are far less adhesive to each other than are normal cells. Therefore, they have a tendency to wander through the tissues, to enter the blood stream, and to be transported all through the body, where they form nidi for numerous new cancerous growths. (3) Some cancers also produce *angiogenic factors* that cause many new blood vessels to grow into the cancer, thus supplying the nutrients required for cancer growth.

Why Do Cancer Cells Kill? The answer to this question is usually very simple. Cancer tissue competes with normal tissues for nutrients. Because cancer cells continue to proliferate indefinitely, their number multiplying day by day, one can readily understand that the cancer cells will soon demand essentially all the nutrition available to the body. As a result, the normal tissues gradually suffer nutritive death.

REFERENCES

Bradshaw, R. A., and Prentis, S.: Oncogenes and Growth Factors. New York, Elsevier Science Publishing Co., 1987.

Echols, H.: Multiple DNA-protein interactions governing high-precision DNA transactions. Science, 233:1050, 1986.

Fox, J. L.: Contemplating the human genome. BioScience, 37:457, 1987.

Macara, I. G.: Oncogenes and cellular signal transduction. Physiol. Rev., 69:797, 1989.

Marx, J. L.: Zipping up DNA binding proteins. Science, 240:1732, 1988.

Nora, J. J., and Fraser, F. C.: Medical Genetics: Principles and Practice. 3rd ed. Philadelphia, Lea & Febiger, 1989.

Schleif, R.: DNA looping. Science, 240:127, 1988.

Schlesinger, D. H. (ed.): Macromolecular Sequencing and Synthesis: Selected Methods and Applications. New York, Alan R. Liss, Inc., 1988.

Scriver, C. R., et al. (eds.): The Metabolic Basis of Inherited Disease. 6th ed. New York, McGraw-Hill Book Co., 1989.

Thomas, K. A.: Fibroblast growth factors. FASEB J., 1:434, 1987.

Thompson, M. W., et al.: Genetics in Medicine. 5th ed. Philadelphia, W. B. Saunders Co., 1989.

Varmus, H. E.: Oncogenes and transcriptional control. Science, 238:1337, 1987.

Weiss, L., et al.: Interactions of cancer cells with the microvasculature during metastasis. FASEB J., 2:12, 1988.

QUESTIONS

1. What is a gene?
2. Give the overall schema by which genes control cellular function and reproduction.
3. What are the building blocks of DNA?
4. Explain the genetic code and how it is transferred from DNA to RNA and then to the formation of proteins.
5. What are the different types of RNA, and what are their specific functions?
6. How do the building blocks of RNA differ from those of DNA?
7. What is meant by the anticodons of transfer RNA and how do they function in relation to the codons of messenger RNA?
8. Explain the role of ribosomes in the formation of protein.
9. What is the role of peptide linkages in the formation of

proteins, and how much energy is expended in the formation of each peptide linkage?
10. Explain the genetic regulation mechanism for regulating synthetic function in a cell.
11. What is meant by an "operon"?
12. How do repressor substances and activator substances function in the regulation of cell activity?
13. Explain the difference between genetic regulation and enzyme regulation.
14. During cell reproduction, how is the replication of DNA different from the transcription process for the formation of RNA?
15. Explain the mechanism of DNA "proofreading."
16. Explain the formation of the mitotic apparatus as well as its functions during mitosis.
17. Describe the stages of mitosis.
18. What are some of the factors that control cell growth?
19. How do cancer cells differ from normal cells, and what prevents the formation of literally thousands of cancers in all persons?

4

Transport Through the Cell Membrane

The fluid inside the cells of the body, called *intracellular fluid,* is very different from that outside the cells, called *extracellular fluid.* The extracellular fluid includes both the *interstitial fluid* that circulates in the spaces between the cells and also the fluid of the *blood plasma* that mixes freely with the interstitial fluid through the capillary walls. It is the extracellular fluid that supplies the cells with nutrients and other substances needed for cellular function. But before the cell can utilize these substances, they must also be transported through the cell membrane.

Figure 4–1 gives the approximate compositions of the *extracellular fluid,* which lies outside the cell membranes, and the *intracellular fluid,* inside the cells. Note that the extracellular fluid contains large quantities of *sodium* but only small quantities of *potassium.* Exactly the opposite is true of the intracellular fluid. Also, the extracellular fluid contains large quantities of chloride, whereas the intracellular fluid contains very little. But the concentrations of phosphates, essentially all of which are organic metabolic intermediates, and proteins in the intracellular fluid are considerably greater than in the extracellular fluid. These many differences are extremely important to the life of the cell. The purpose of this chapter is to explain how these differences are brought about by the transport mechanisms of the cell membranes.

The Lipid Barrier and the Transport Proteins of the Cell Membrane

The structure of the cell membrane is discussed in Chapter 2 and shown in Figure 2–3. It consists almost entirely of a *lipid bilayer,* with large numbers of protein molecules floating in the lipid, many penetrating all the way through, as illustrated in Figure 4–2.

The lipid bilayer is not miscible with either the extracellular fluid or the intracellular fluid. Therefore, it constitutes a barrier for the movement of most water molecules and water-soluble substances between the extracellular and intracellular fluid compartments. However, as illustrated by the lefthand arrow of Figure 4–2, a few substances can penetrate this bilayer and can either enter the cell or leave it, passing directly through the lipid substance itself.

The protein molecules, on the other hand, have entirely different transport properties. Their molecular structures interrupt the continuity of the lipid bilayer and therefore constitute an alternate pathway through the cell membrane. Most of these penetrating proteins, therefore, are *transport proteins.* Different proteins function differently. Some have watery spaces all the way through the molecule and allow free movement of certain ions or molecules; these are called *channel proteins.* Others, called *carrier proteins,* bind with substances that are to be transported, and conformational changes in the protein molecules then move the substances through the interstices of the molecules to the other side of the membrane. Both the channel proteins and the carrier proteins can be highly selective in the type or types of molecules or ions that are allowed to cross the membrane.

Diffusion Versus Active Transport. Transport through the cell membrane, either directly through the lipid bilayer or through the proteins, occurs by one of two basic processes, *diffusion* (which is also called "passive transport") or *active transport.* Although there are many different variations of these two basic mechanisms, as we see later in this chapter, diffusion means random molecular movement of substances molecule by molecule either through intermolecular spaces in the membrane or in combination with a carrier protein. The energy that causes diffusion is the energy of the normal kinetic motion of matter. By contrast, active transport means movement of ions or other substances across the membrane in combina-

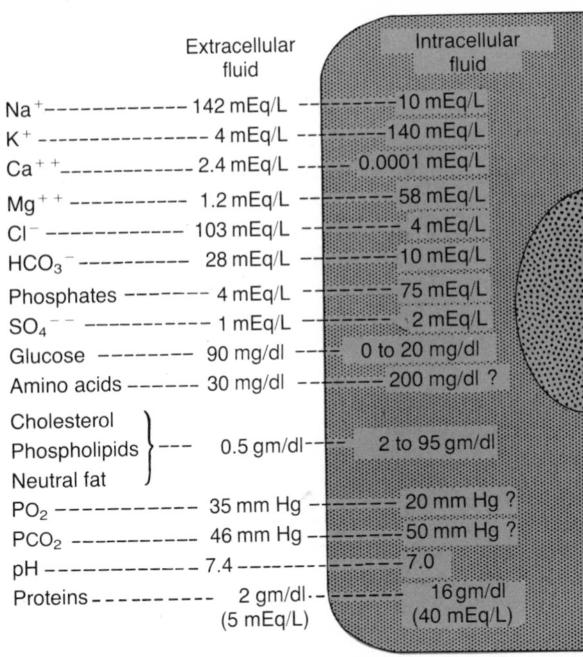

Figure 4-1. Chemical compositions of extracellular and intracellular fluids.

tion with a carrier protein but additionally *against an energy gradient,* such as from a low concentration state to a high concentration state, a process that requires an additional source of energy besides kinetic energy to cause the movement. Let us explain in more detail the basic physics and physical chemistry of these two separate processes.

DIFFUSION

All molecules and ions in the body fluids, including both water molecules and dissolved substances, are in constant motion, each particle moving its own separate way. Motion of these particles is what physicists call heat—the greater the motion, the higher the temperature—and motion never ceases under any conditions except at absolute zero temperature. When a moving molecule, A, approaches a stationary molecule, B, the electrostatic and internuclear forces

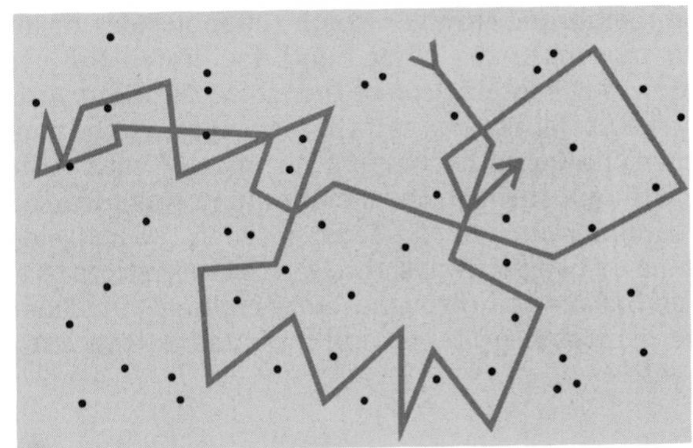

Figure 4-3. Diffusion of a fluid molecule during a billionth of a second.

of molecule A repel molecule B, transferring some of the energy of motion to molecule B. Consequently, molecule B gains kinetic energy of motion, while molecule A slows down, losing some of its kinetic energy. Thus, as shown in Figure 4-3, a single molecule in solution bounces among the other molecules first in one direction, then another, then another, and so forth, bouncing randomly billions of times each second.

This continual movement of molecules among each other in liquids, or in gases, is called *diffusion.* Ions diffuse in exactly the same manner as whole molecules, and even suspended colloid particles diffuse in a similar manner except that they diffuse far less rapidly than molecular substances because of their very large sizes.

Diffusion Through the Cell Membrane

Diffusion through the cell membrane is divided into two separate subtypes called *simple diffusion* and *facilitated diffusion.* Simple diffusion means the molecular kinetic movement of molecules or ions through a membrane opening or intermolecular spaces without the necessity of binding with carrier proteins in the membrane. The rate of diffusion is determined by the amount of substance available, by the velocity of kinetic motion, and by the number of openings in the

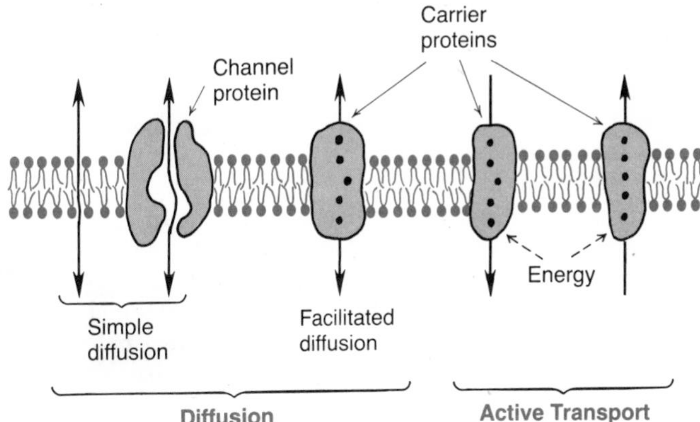

Figure 4-2. Transport pathways through the cell membrane, and the basic mechanisms of transport.

cell membrane through which the molecules or ions can move. On the other hand, facilitated diffusion requires the interaction of the molecule or ion with a carrier protein that aids its passage through the membrane, probably by binding chemically with it and shuttling it through the membrane in this form.

Simple diffusion can occur through the cell membrane by two pathways: through the interstices of the lipid bilayer and through watery channels in some of the transport proteins, as illustrated to the left in Figure 4-2.

Simple Diffusion Through the Lipid Bilayer

Diffusion of Lipid-Soluble Substances. In experimental studies, the lipids of cells have been separated from the proteins and then reconstituted as artificial membranes consisting of a lipid bilayer but without any transport proteins. Using such an artificial membrane, the transport properties of the lipid bilayer by itself have been determined.

One of the most important factors that determines how rapidly a substance will move through the lipid bilayer is the *lipid solubility* of the substance. For instance, the lipid solubilities of oxygen, nitrogen, carbon dioxide, and alcohols are very high, so that all these can dissolve directly in the lipid bilayer and diffuse through the cell membrane in exactly the same manner that diffusion occurs in a watery solution. For obvious reasons, the rate of diffusion of these substances through the membrane is directly proportional to their lipid solubility. Especially large quantities of oxygen can be transported in this way; therefore, oxygen is delivered to the interior of the cell almost as though the cell membrane did not exist.

Transport of Water and Other Lipid-Insoluble Molecules. Even though water is highly insoluble in the membrane lipids, nevertheless it penetrates the cell membrane very readily, much of it passing directly through the lipid bilayer and still more passing through protein channels. The rapidity with which water molecules can penetrate the cell membrane is astounding. As an example, the total amount of water that diffuses in each direction through the red cell membrane during each second is approximately 100 times as great as the volume of the red cell itself.

The reason for the large amount of diffusion of water through the lipid bilayer is still not certain, but it is believed that water molecules are small enough and their kinetic energy great enough that they can simply penetrate like bullets through the lipid portion of the membrane before the "hydrophobic" character of the lipids can stop them.

Other lipid-insoluble molecules also can pass through the lipid bilayer in the same way as water molecules if they are small enough. However, as they become larger, their penetration falls off extremely rapidly. For instance, the diameter of the urea molecule is only 20 per cent greater than that of water. Yet its penetration through the cell membrane is about a thousand times less than that of water. Even so, remembering the astonishing rate of water penetration, this amount of penetration still allows rapid transport of urea through the cell membrane.

Failure of Ions to Diffuse Through the Lipid Bilayer. Even though water and other very small uncharged molecules diffuse easily through the lipid bilayer, ions—even small ones, such as hydrogen ions, sodium ions, potassium ions, and so forth—penetrate the lipid bilayer about one million times less rapidly than does water. Therefore, any significant transport of these through the cell membrane must occur through channels in the proteins, as we discuss shortly.

The reason for the impenetrability of the lipid bilayer to ions is the electrical charge of the ions; this impedes ionic movement in two separate ways: (1) The electrical charge of these ions causes multiple molecules of water to become bonded to the ions, forming so-called *hydrated ions.* This greatly increases the sizes of ions, which alone impedes penetration of the lipid bilayer. (2) Even more important, the electrical charge of the ion also interacts with the charges of the lipid bilayer in the following way. It will be recalled that each half of the bilayer is composed of "polar" lipids that have an excess of negative charge facing toward the surfaces of the membrane. Therefore, when a charged ion tries to penetrate either the negative or the positive electrical barrier, it is instantaneously repulsed.

Table 4-1 gives the relative permeabilities of the lipid bilayer to a number of different molecules or ions of different diameters. Note especially the *extremely poor permeance of the ions* because of their electrical charges and the *poor permeance of glucose* because of its molecular diameter. Note also that glycerol penetrates the membrane almost as easily as urea even though its diameter is almost twice as great. The reason for this is a slight degree of lipid solubility.

Simple Diffusion Through Protein Channels and "Gating" of These Channels

Many of the protein channels provide watery pathways through the interstices of the protein molecules. Therefore, substances can diffuse directly through these channels from one side of the membrane to the other. However, the protein channels are distinguished by two important characteristics: (1) They

Table 4-1 RELATIONSHIP OF EFFECTIVE DIAMETERS OF DIFFERENT SUBSTANCES TO THEIR LIPID BILAYER PERMEABILITIES

Substance	Diameter (nm)	Relative Permeability
Water molecule	0.3	1.0
Urea molecule	0.36	0.0006
Hydrated chloride ion	0.386	0.00000001
Hydrated potassium ion	0.396	0.0000000006
Hydrated sodium ion	0.512	0.0000000002
Glycerol	0.62	0.0006
Glucose	0.86	0.000009

are often selectively permeable to certain substances. (2) Many of the channels can be opened or closed by *gates.*

Selective Permeability of Different Protein Channels. Most, but not all, protein channels are highly selective for the transport of one or more specific ions or molecules. This results from the characteristics of the channel itself, such as its diameter, its shape, and the nature of the electrical charges along its inside surfaces. To give an example, one of the most important sets of protein channels, the so-called *sodium channels,* calculate to be only 0.3 by 0.5 nanometer in size, but more important, the inner surfaces of these channels are *strongly negatively charged,* as illustrated by the negative signs inside the channel proteins in the top panel of Figure 4–4. These strong negative charges are postulated to pull sodium ions more than they pull other physiologically important ions into the channels because of the smaller ionic diameter of the dehydrated sodium ions than of the others. Once in the channel, the sodium ions then diffuse in either direction according to the usual laws of diffusion. Thus, the sodium channel is specifically selective for the passage of sodium ions.

On the other hand, another set of protein channels is selective for potassium transport, illustrated in the lower panel of Figure 4–4. These channels calculate to be slightly smaller than the sodium channels, only 0.3 by 0.3 nanometer, but *they are not negatively charged.* Therefore, no strong attractive force is pulling ions into the channels, and the ions are not pulled away from the water molecules that hydrate them. The hydrated form of the potassium ion is considerably smaller than the hydrated form of sodium because the sodium ion has one whole orbital set of electrons less than the potassium ion, which allows

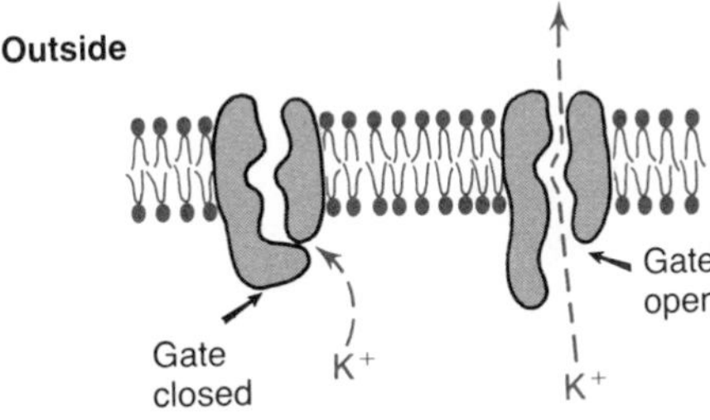

Figure 4–4. Transport of sodium and potassium ions through protein channels. Also shown are conformational changes of the channel protein molecules that open or close the "gates" guarding the channels.

the sodium nucleus to attract far more water molecules than can the potassium. Therefore, the smaller hydrated potassium ions can pass easily through this smaller channel, whereas sodium ions are mainly rejected, thus once again providing selective permeability for a specific ion.

Gating of Protein Channels. Gating of protein channels provides a means for controlling the permeability of the channels. This is illustrated in both the upper and the lower panels of Figure 4–4 for the sodium and the potassium ion. It is believed that the gates are actual gatelike extensions of the transport protein molecule, which can close over the opening of the channel or can be lifted away from the opening by a conformational change in the shape of the protein molecule itself. In the case of the sodium channels, this gate opens and closes on the outer surface of the cell membrane, whereas for the potassium channels it opens and closes on the inner surface.

The opening and closing of gates are controlled in two principal ways:

1. *Voltage gating.* In this instance, the molecular conformation of the gate responds to the electrical potential across the cell membrane. For instance, when there is a strong negative charge on the inside of the cell membrane, the sodium gates remain tightly closed; on the other hand, when the negative charge is lost, the gates open. This is the basic cause of action potentials in nerves that in turn are responsible for nerve signals. These events are discussed in the following chapter.
2. *Ligand gating.* Some protein channel gates are opened by the binding of another molecule with the protein; this causes a conformational change in the protein molecule that opens or closes the gate. This is called *ligand gating,* and the substance that binds is the *ligand.* One of the most important instances of ligand gating is the effect of acetylcholine on the so-called *acetylcholine channel.* This opens the gate of this channel, providing a pore about 0.65 nanometer in diameter that allows all molecules and positive ions smaller than this diameter to pass through. This gate is exceedingly important in the transmission of signals from one nerve cell to another and from nerve cells to muscle cells.

The Open-State, Closed-State of Gated Channels. Figure 4–5 illustrates an especially interesting characteristic of voltage-gated channels. This figure shows two recordings of electrical current flowing through a single sodium channel when there was an approximately 25 millivolt potential gradient across the membrane. Note that the channel conducts current either all or none. That is, the gate of the channel snaps open and then snaps closed, each snapping event occurring within a few millionths of a second. This illustrates the rapidity with which conformational changes can occur in the shape of the protein molecular gates. At one voltage potential the channel may remain closed all the time or almost all the time, whereas at another voltage level it may remain open either all or most of the time. However, at in-between voltages, the gates tend to snap open and closed intermittently, as illustrated in the upper recording, giving an average current flow somewhere between the minimum and the maximum.

The Patch-Clamp Method for Recording Ion Current Flow Through Single Channels. One might wonder how it is technically possible to record ion current flow through single channels, as shown in Figure 4–5A. This has been achieved by using the "patch-clamp" method illustrated in Figure 4–5B. Very simply, a micropipette, having a tip diameter of only 1 or 2 micrometers, is abutted against the outside of a cell membrane. Then suction is applied inside the pipette to pull the membrane slightly into the tip of the pipette. This creates a seal where the edges of the pipette touch the cell membrane. The result is a minute "patch" at the tip of the pipette through which current flow can be recorded.

Alternatively, as shown to the right in Figure 4–5B, the small cell membrane patch at the end of the pipette can be torn away from the cell. The pipette with its sealed patch is then inserted into a free solution. This allows the concentration of the ions both inside the micropipette and in the outside solution to be altered as desired. Also, the voltage between the two sides of the membrane can be set at will—that is, "clamped" to a given voltage.

Fortunately, it has been possible to make such patches small enough that one often finds only a single channel protein in the membrane patch that is being studied. By varying the concentrations of different ions and the voltage across the membrane, one can determine the transport characteristics of the channel as well as its gating properties.

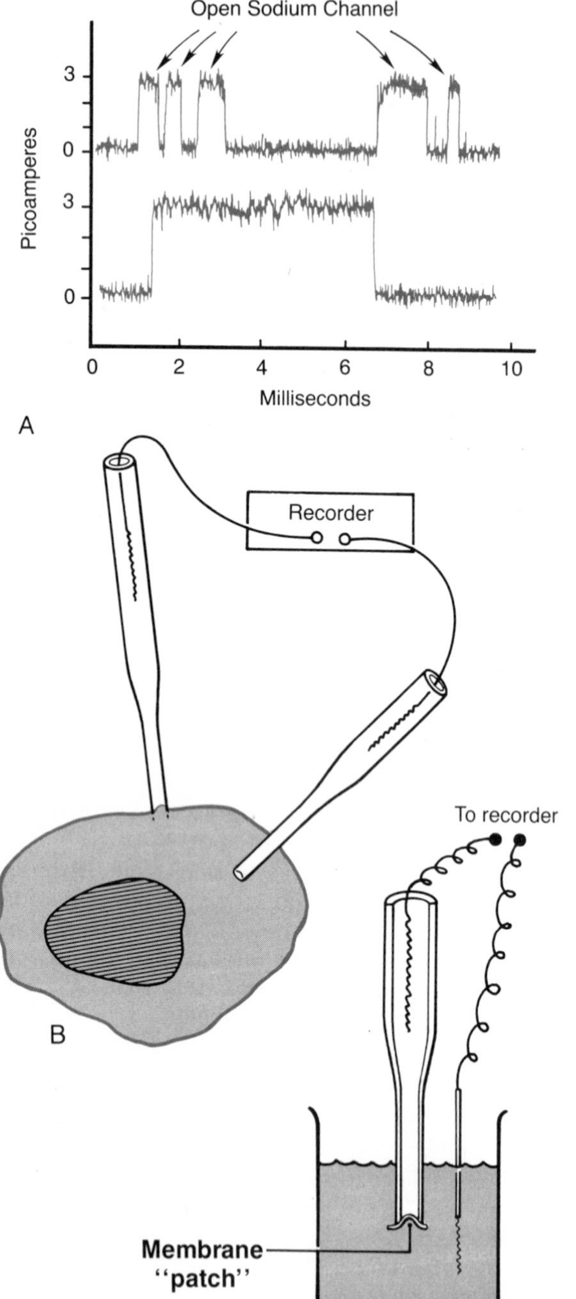

Figure 4–5. *A,* Record of current flow through a single voltage-gated sodium channel, demonstrating the all-or-none principle for opening of the channel. *B,* The "patch-clamp" method for recording current flow through a single protein channel. To the left, recording is performed from a "patch" of a living cell membrane. To the right, recording is from a membrane patch that has been torn away from the cell.

Facilitated Diffusion

Facilitated diffusion is also called *carrier-mediated diffusion* because a substance transported in this manner usually cannot pass through the membrane without a specific carrier protein helping it. That is, the carrier *facilitates* the diffusion of the substance to the other side.

Facilitated diffusion differs from simple diffusion through an open channel in the following very important way: Although the rate of diffusion through an open channel increases proportionately with the concentration of the diffusing substance, in facilitated diffusion the rate of diffusion approaches a maximum, called V_{max}, as the concentration of the substance increases.

What is it that limits the rate of facilitated diffusion? A probable answer is that the molecule to be transported enters the protein channel and becomes bound. Then in a fraction of a second a conformational change occurs in the carrier protein, so that the channel now opens to the opposite side of the membrane. Obviously, the rate at which molecules can be transported by this mechanism can never be greater than the rate at which the carrier protein molecule can undergo conformational change back and forth between its two states.

Among the most important substances that cross cell membranes by facilitated diffusion are *glucose* and most of the *amino acids.* In the case of glucose, the carrier molecule is known to have a molecular weight of about 45,000; it can also transport several other monosaccharides that have structures similar to that of glucose, including mannose, galactose, xylose, and arabinose. Also, insulin can increase the rate of facilitated diffusion of glucose as much as 10-fold to 20-

fold. This is the principal mechanism by which insulin controls glucose use in the body, as we discuss in Chapter 52.

Factors That Affect Net Rate of Diffusion

By now it is evident that many different substances can diffuse either through the lipid bilayer of the cell membrane or through protein channels. However, please understand clearly that substances that diffuse in one direction can also diffuse in the opposite direction. Usually, what is important to the cell is not the total substance diffusing in both directions but the difference between these two, which is the *net rate of diffusion* in one direction. The factors that affect this are (1) the permeability of the membrane, (2) the area of the membrane, (3) the difference in concentration of the diffusing substance between the two sides of the membrane, (4) the pressure difference across the membrane, and (5) in the case of ions, the electrical potential difference between the two sides of the membrane.

Permeability of the Membrane. The permeability of a membrane for a given substance is expressed as the *net* rate of diffusion of the substance through each unit area of the membrane for a unit concentration difference (when there are no electrical or pressure differences). The different factors that affect cell membrane permeability are (1) thickness of the membrane, (2) lipid solubility of the substance diffusing through the membrane, (3) number of protein channels through which the substance can pass, (4) temperature, and (5) molecular weight of the diffusing substance.

Finally, to determine the total effect on diffusion we must consider the area of the membrane as well. When permeability is multiplied by area, this gives the diffusion coefficient. That is:

$$D = P \times A$$

where D is the diffusion coefficient, P is the permeability, and A is the total area.

Effect of a Concentration Difference. Figure 4-6A illustrates a cell membrane with a substance in high concentration on the outside and low concentration on the inside. The rate at which the substance diffuses *inward* is proportional to the concentration of molecules on the *outside,* for this concentration determines how many molecules strike the outside of the channels each second. On the other hand, the rate at which molecules diffuse *outward* is proportional to their concentration *inside* the membrane. Obviously, therefore, the rate of net diffusion into the cell is proportional to the concentration on the outside *minus* the concentration on the inside, or

$$\text{Net diffusion} \propto D(C_o - C_i)$$

in which C_o is the concentration on the outside, C_i is the concentration on the inside, and D is the diffusion coefficient of the membrane for the substance.

A

Outside Membrane Inside

C_o Ci

B

C

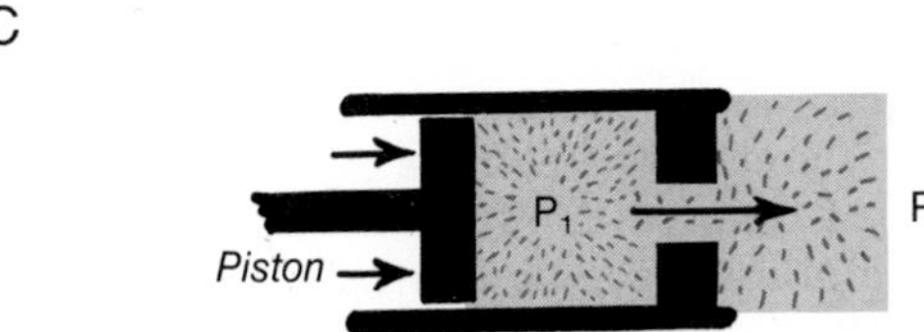

Figure 4-6. Effect of *(A)* concentration difference, *(B)* electrical difference, and *(C)* pressure difference on net diffusion of molecules and ions through a cell membrane.

Effect of an Electrical Potential on the Diffusion of Ions. If an electrical potential is applied across the membrane, as shown in Figure 4-6B, because of their electrical charges ions will move through the membrane even though no concentration difference exists to cause their movement. Thus, in the left panel of the figure, the concentrations of negative ions are exactly the same on both sides of the membrane, but a positive charge has been applied to the right side of the membrane and a negative charge to the left, creating an electrical gradient across the membrane. The positive charge attracts the negative ions, whereas the negative charge repels them. Therefore, net diffusion occurs from left to right. After much time, large quantities of negative ions will have moved to the right, creating the condition illustrated in the right panel of Figure 4-6B, in which a concentration difference of the same ions has developed in the direction opposite to the electrical potential difference. Obviously, the concentration difference is now tending to move the ions to the left, while the electrical difference is tending to move them to the right. When the concentration difference rises high enough, the two effects exactly balance each other. At normal body temperature (37°C), the electrical difference that will exactly balance a given concentration difference of *univalent* ions, such as sodium (Na^+), potassium (K^+), or chloride (Cl^-), can be determined from the following formula, called the *Nernst equation:*

$$\text{EMF (in millivolts)} = \pm 61 \log \frac{C_1}{C_2}$$

in which EMF is the electromotive force (voltage) between side 1 and side 2 of the membrane, C_1 is the concentration on side 1, and C_2 is the concentration on side 2. The polarity of the voltage on side 1 in the above equation is + for negative ions and − for positive ions. This relationship is extremely important in understanding the transmission of nerve impulses, for which reason it is discussed in even greater detail in the next chapter.

Effect of a Pressure Difference. At times, considerable pressure difference develops between the two sides of a membrane. This occurs, for instance, at the capillary membrane, which has a pressure approximately 20 mm Hg greater inside the capillary than outside. Pressure actually means the sum of all the forces of the different molecules striking a unit surface area at a given instant. Therefore, when the pressure is higher on one side of a membrane than on the other, this means that the sum of all the forces of the molecules striking the channels on that side of the membrane is greater than on the other side. This can result either from greater numbers of molecules striking the membrane per second or from greater kinetic energy of the average molecule striking the membrane. In either event, increased amounts of energy are available to cause net movement of molecules from the high pressure side toward the low pressure side. This effect is illustrated in Figure 4–6C, which shows a piston developing high pressure on one side of a cell membrane, thereby causing net diffusion through the membrane to the other side.

Osmosis Across Selectively Permeable Membranes—Net Diffusion of Water

By far the most abundant substance to diffuse through the cell membrane is water. It should be recalled that enough water ordinarily diffuses in each direction through the red cell membrane per second to equal about *100 times the volume of the cell itself.* Yet, *normally,* the amount that diffuses in the two directions is so precisely balanced that not even the slightest *net* movement of water occurs. Therefore, the volume of the cell remains constant. However, under certain conditions, a *concentration difference for water* can develop across a membrane, just as concentration differences for other substances can also occur. When this happens, net movement of water does occur across the cell membrane, causing the cell either to swell or to shrink, depending on the direction of the net movement. This process of net movement of water caused by a concentration difference of water is called *osmosis.*

To give an example of osmosis, let us assume the conditions shown in Figure 4–7, with pure water on one side of the cell membrane and a solution of sodium chloride on the other side. Referring back to Table 4–1, we see that water molecules pass through the cell

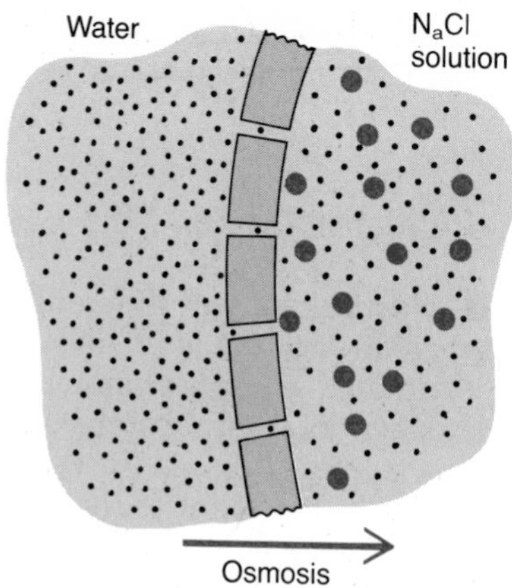

Figure 4–7. Osmosis at a cell membrane when a sodium chloride solution is placed on one side of the membrane and water on the other side.

membrane with ease, whereas sodium and chloride ions pass through only with extreme difficulty. Therefore, sodium chloride solution is actually a mixture of permeant water molecules and nonpermeant sodium and chloride ions, and the membrane is said to be *selectively permeable* (or "semipermeable") to water but not to sodium and chloride ions. Yet the presence of the sodium and chloride has displaced some of the water molecules and therefore has reduced the concentration of water molecules to less than that of pure water. As a result, in the example of Figure 4–7, more water molecules strike the channels on the left side, where there is pure water, than on the right side, where the water concentration has been reduced. Thus, net movement of water occurs from left to right—that is, osmosis occurs from the pure water into the sodium chloride solution.

Osmotic Pressure

If in Figure 4–7 pressure were applied to the sodium chloride solution, osmosis of water into this solution would be slowed, stopped, or even reversed. The amount of pressure required exactly to stop osmosis is called the *osmotic pressure* of the sodium chloride solution.

The principle of a pressure difference opposing osmosis is illustrated in Figure 4–8, which shows a selectively permeable membrane separating two columns of fluid, one containing water and the other containing a solution of water and any solute that will not penetrate the membrane. Osmosis of water from chamber B into chamber A causes the levels of the fluid columns to become farther and farther apart, until eventually a pressure difference is developed that is great enough to oppose the osmotic effect. The pressure difference across the membrane at this point is the osmotic pressure of the solution containing the nondiffusible solute.

Importance of Numbers of Osmotic Particles in Determining Osmotic Pressure. The osmotic pressure exerted by particles in a solution, whether they be molecules or ions, is determined by the *numbers* of particles per unit volume of fluid and not the

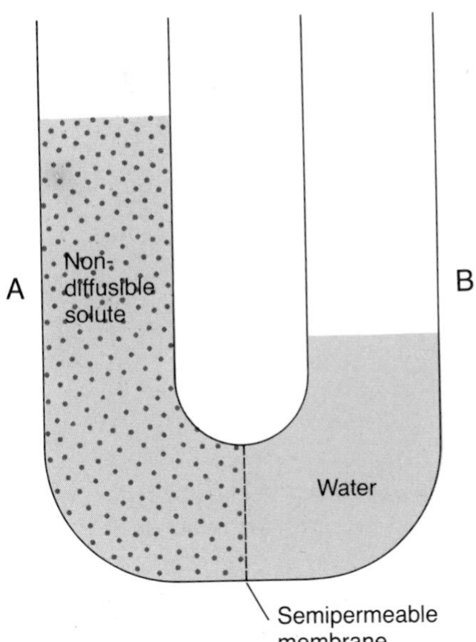

Figure 4-8. Demonstration of osmotic pressure on the two sides of a semipermeable membrane.

mass of the particles. The reason for this is that each particle in a solution, regardless of its mass, exerts, on the average, the same amount of pressure against the membrane. That is, all particles are bouncing among each other with, on the average, equal energy. If some particles have greater kinetic energy of movement than others, their impact with the low-energy particles will impart part of their energy to these, thus decreasing the energy level of the high-energy particles, while increasing the energy level of others until the energy level of all of them, averaged over a period of time, is the same. Therefore, the large particles, which have greater mass (m) than the small particles, move at lower velocities (v), while the small particles move at higher velocities in such a way that their average kinetic energies (k), determined by the equation

$$k = \frac{mv^2}{2},$$

become equal to each other. Therefore, on the average, the kinetic energy of each molecule or ion that strikes a membrane is approximately the same regardless of its molecular size. Consequently, the factor that determines the osmotic pressure of a solution is the concentration of the solution in terms of numbers of particles and not in terms of mass of the solute.

"Osmolality"—the Osmole. Because the amount of osmotic pressure exerted by a solute is proportional to the concentration of the solute in numbers of molecules or ions, expressing the solute concentration in terms of mass is of no value in determining osmotic pressure. To express the concentration in terms of numbers of particles, the unit called the *osmole* is used in place of grams.

One osmole is the number of molecules in 1 gram molecular weight of undissociated solute. Thus, 180 grams of glucose, which is 1 gram molecular weight of glucose, is equal to 1 osmole of glucose because glucose does not dissociate. On the other hand, if the solute dissociates into two ions, 1 gram molecular weight of the solute equals 2 osmoles because the number of osmotically active particles is now twice as great as is the case in the undissociated solute. Therefore, 1 gram molecular weight of sodium chloride, 58.5 grams, is equal to 2 osmoles.

A solution that has *1 osmole of solute dissolved in each kilogram of water* is said to have an *osmolality of 1 osmole per kilogram,* and a solution that has 1/1000 osmole dissolved per kilogram has an osmolality of 1 milliosmole per kilogram. The normal osmolality of the extracellular and intracellular fluids is about 300 milliosmoles per kilogram.

Relationship of Osmolality to Osmotic Pressure. At normal body temperature, 37°C, a concentration of 1 osmole per liter will cause *19,300 mm Hg* osmotic pressure in the solution. Likewise, 1 milliosmole per liter concentration is equivalent to *19.3 mm Hg* osmotic pressure. Multiplying this value times the 300 milliosmolar concentration of the body fluids gives a total calculated osmotic pressure of these fluids of 5790 mm Hg. The measured value for this, however, averages only about 5500 mm Hg. The reason for this difference is that many of the ions in the body fluids, such as the sodium and the chloride ions, are highly attracted to each other; consequently, they cannot move totally unrestrained in the fluids and create their full osmotic potential.

ACTIVE TRANSPORT

From the discussion thus far, it is evident that *no substances can diffuse against an "electrochemical gradient,"* which is the sum of all the diffusion forces acting at the membrane—the forces caused by concentration difference, electrical difference, and pressure difference. That is, it is often said that substances cannot diffuse "uphill."

Yet, at times a large concentration of a substance is required in the intracellular fluid even though the extracellular fluid contains only a minute concentration. This is true, for instance, for potassium ions. Conversely, it is important to keep the concentrations of other ions very low inside the cell even though their concentrations in the extracellular fluid are very great. This is especially true for sodium ions. Obviously, neither of these two effects could occur by the process of simple diffusion, for simple diffusion tends always to equilibrate the concentrations on the two sides of the membrane. Instead, some energy source must cause movement of potassium ions "uphill" to the inside of cells and cause movement of sodium ions also "uphill" but in this instance to the outside of the cell. When a cell membrane moves molecules or ions uphill against a concentration gradient (or uphill against an electrical or pressure gradient), the process is called *active transport.*

Among the different substances that are actively transported through cell membranes are sodium ions, potassium ions, calcium ions, iron ions, hydrogen ions, chloride ions, iodide ions, urate ions, several different sugars, and most of the amino acids.

Primary Active Transport and Secondary Active Transport. Active transport is divided into two types according to the source of the energy used to cause the transport. These are called *primary active transport* and *secondary active transport.* In primary active transport, the energy is derived directly from the breakdown of adenosine triphosphate (ATP) or some other high-energy phosphate compound. In secondary active transport, the energy is derived secondarily from ionic concentration gradients that have been created in the first place by primary active transport. In both instances, transport depends on *carrier proteins* that penetrate through the membrane, the same as is true for facilitated diffusion. However, in active transport, the carrier protein functions differently from the carrier in facilitated diffusion, for in active transport it imparts energy to the transported substance to move it against an electrochemical gradient. Let us give some examples of primary active transport and secondary active transport and explain their principles of function more fully.

Primary Active Transport — The Sodium-Potassium "Pump"

Among the substances that are transported by primary active transport are sodium, potassium, calcium, hydrogen, chloride, and a few other ions. However, not all of these substances are transported by the membranes of all cells. Furthermore, some of the pumps function at intracellular membranes rather than (or in addition to) the surface membrane of the cell, such as at the membrane of the muscle sarcoplasmic reticulum or at one of the two membranes of the mitochondria. Nevertheless, they all operate by essentially the same basic mechanism.

The active transport mechanism that has been studied in greatest detail is the *sodium-potassium pump,* a transport process that pumps sodium ions outward through the cell membrane and at the same time pumps potassium ions from the outside to the inside. This pump is present in all cells of the body, and it is responsible for maintaining the sodium and potassium concentration differences across the cell membrane as well as for establishing a negative electrical potential inside the cells. Indeed, we see in the next chapter that this pump is the basis of nerve function to transmit nerve signals throughout the nervous system.

Figure 4–9 illustrates the basic components of the Na^+-K^+ pump. The *carrier protein* is a complex of two separate globular proteins, a larger one with a molecular weight of about 100,000 and a smaller one with a molecular weight of 55,000. Although the function of the smaller protein is not known, the larger protein has three specific features that are important for function of the pump:

1. It has three *receptor sites for binding sodium ions* on the portion of the protein that protrudes to the interior of the cell.

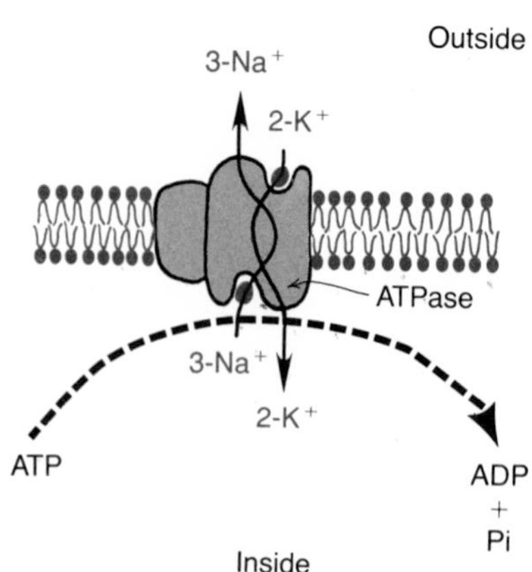

Figure 4–9. The postulated mechanism of the sodium-potassium pump.

2. It has two *receptor sites for potassium ions* on the outside.
3. The inside portion of this protein adjacent to or near the sodium binding sites has ATPase activity.

Now to put the pump into perspective: When three sodium ions bind on the inside of the carrier protein and two potassium ions on the outside, the ATPase function of the protein becomes activated. This then cleaves one molecule of ATP, splitting it to adenosine diphosphate (ADP) and liberating a high-energy phosphate bond of energy. This energy is then believed to cause a conformational change in the protein carrier molecule, extruding the sodium ions to the outside and the potassium ions to the inside. Unfortunately, the precise mechanism of the conformational change of the carrier is still to be discovered.

The Calcium Pump

Another very important primary active transport mechanism is the calcium pump. Calcium ions are normally maintained at extremely low concentration in the intracellular cytosol, at a concentration about 10,000 times less than that in the extracellular fluid. This is achieved by two calcium pumps. One is in the cell membrane and pumps calcium to the outside of the cell. The other pumps calcium ions into one or more of the internal vesicular organelles of the cell, such as into the sarcoplasmic reticulum of muscle cells and into the mitochondria in all cells. In both instances, the carrier protein penetrates the membrane from side to side and also serves as an ATPase having the same capability to cleave ATP as the ATPase sodium carrier protein. The difference is that this protein has a binding site for calcium instead of sodium.

Saturation of Active Transport

Active transport saturates in exactly the same way that facilitated diffusion saturates. The saturation is caused by limitation of the rates at which the chemical reactions of binding, release, and carrier conformational changes can occur.

Energetics of Active Transport

The amount of energy required to transport a substance actively through a membrane (aside from energy lost as heat in the chemical reactions) is determined by the degree that the substance is concentrated during transport. Compared with the energy required to concentrate a substance tenfold, to concentrate it hundredfold requires twice as much energy and to concentrate it thousandfold requires three times as much. In other words, the energy required is proportional to the *logarithm* of the degree that the substance is concentrated, as expressed by the following formula:

$$\text{Energy (in calories per osmole)} = 1400 \log \frac{C_1}{C_2}$$

That is, in terms of calories, the amount of energy required to concentrate 1 osmole of substance tenfold is about 1400 calories, or hundredfold, 2800 calories. One can see that the energy expenditure for concentrating substances in cells or for removing substances from cells against a concentration gradient can be tremendous. Some cells, such as those lining the renal tubules, as well as many glandular cells, expend as much as 90 per cent of their energy for this purpose alone.

Secondary Active Transport—Co-Transport and Counter-Transport

When sodium ions are transported out of cells by primary active transport, a very large concentration gradient of sodium usually develops—very high concentration outside the cell and very low concentration inside. This gradient represents a storehouse of energy because the excess sodium outside the cell membrane is always attempting to diffuse to the interior. Under the appropriate conditions, this diffusion energy of sodium can literally pull other substances along with the sodium through the cell membrane. This phenomenon is called *co-transport;* it is one form of secondary active transport.

For sodium to pull another substance along with it, a coupling mechanism is required. This is achieved by means of still another carrier protein in the cell membrane. The carrier in this instance serves as an attachment point for both the sodium ion and the substance to be co-transported. Once they both are attached, a conformational change occurs in the carrier protein, and the energy gradient of the sodium ion causes both the sodium ion and the other substance to be transported together to the interior of the cell.

In *counter-transport,* sodium ions again attempt to diffuse to the interior of the cell because of their large concentration gradient. However, this time, the substance to be transported is on the inside of the cell and must be transported to the outside. Therefore, the sodium ion binds to the carrier protein where it projects through the exterior surface of the membrane, while the substance to be counter-transported binds to the interior projection of the carrier protein. Once both have bound, a conformational change occurs again, with the energy of the sodium ion moving to the interior causing the other substance to move to the exterior.

Sodium Co-Transport of Glucose and Amino Acids. Glucose and many amino acids are transported into most cells against very large concentration gradients; the mechanism of this is entirely by the co-transport mechanism illustrated in Figure 4-10. Note that the transport carrier protein has two binding sites on its exterior side, one for sodium and one for glucose. Also, the concentration of sodium ions is very high on the outside and very low inside, which provides the energy for the transport. A special property of the transport protein is that the conformational change to allow sodium movement to the interior will not occur until a glucose molecule also attaches. But when they are both attached, the conformational change takes place automatically, and both the sodium and the glucose are transported to the inside of the cell at the same time. Hence, this is a *sodium-glucose co-transport* mechanism.

Sodium co-transport of the amino acids occurs in the same manner as for glucose except that it uses a different set of transport proteins. Five separate *amino acid transport proteins* have been identified, each of which is responsible for transporting one subset of amino acids with specific molecular characteristics.

Sodium co-transport of glucose and amino acids occurs especially in the epithelial cells of the intestinal tract and renal tubules to aid in the absorption of these substances into the blood, as we discuss in later chapters.

Sodium Counter-Transport of Calcium and Hydrogen Ions. Two especially important counter-transport mechanisms are *sodium-calcium counter-transport* and *sodium-hydrogen counter-transport.* Calcium counter-transport occurs in all or almost all cell membranes, with sodium ions moving to the interior and calcium ions to the exterior, both bound to the same transport protein in a counter-transport mode. This is in addition to primary active transport of calcium that occurs in some cells.

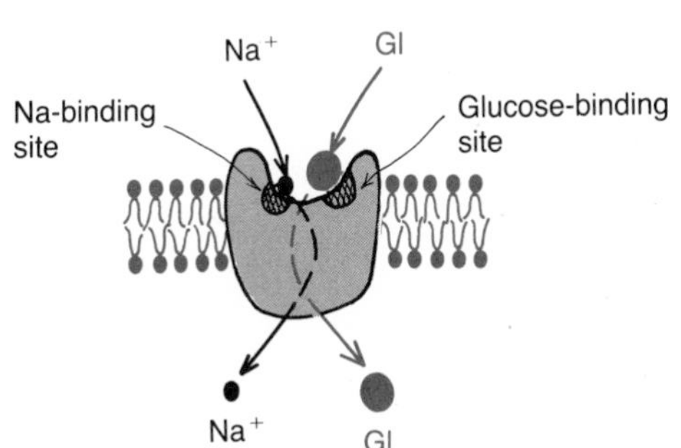

Figure 4-10. A postulated mechanism for sodium co-transport of glucose.

Sodium-hydrogen counter-transport occurs in several tissues. An especially important example is in the proximal tubules of the kidneys, where sodium ions move from the lumen of the tubule to the interior of the tubular cells, while hydrogen ions are counter-transported into the lumen. This mechanism is a key to hydrogen ion control in the body fluids.

REFERENCES

Biggio, G., and Costa, E. (eds.): Chloride Channels and Their Modulation by Neurotransmitters and Drugs. New York, Raven Press, 1988.

Bretag, A. H.: Muscle chloride channels. Physiol. Rev., 67:618, 1987.

Chasis, J. A., and Shohet, S. B.: Red cell biochemical anatomy and membrane properties. Annu. Rev. Physiol., 49:237, 1987.

Dinno, M. A., and Armstrong, W. M. (eds.): Membrane Biophysics III: Biological Transport. New York, Alan R. Liss, Inc., 1988.

Forgac, M.: Structure and function of vacuolar class of ATP-driven proton pumps. Physiol. Rev., 69:765, 1989.

Haas, M.: Properties and diversity of Na-K-Cl cotransporters. Annu. Rev. Physiol., 51:443, 1989.

Hidalgo, C. (ed.): Physical Properties of Biological Membranes and Their Functional Implications. New York, Plenum Publishing Corp., 1988.

Hoffmann, E. K., and Simonsen, L. O.: Membrane mechanisms in volume and pH regulation in vertebrate cells. Physiol. Rev., 69:315, 1989.

Kim, C. H., and Tedeschi, H. (eds.): Advances in Membrane Biochemistry and Bioenergetics. New York, Plenum Publishing Corp., 1987.

Latorre, R., et al.: Varieties of calcium-activated potassium channels. Annu. Rev. Physiol., 51:385, 1989.

Lauger, P.: Dynamics of ion transport systems in membranes. Physiol. Rev., 67:1296, 1987.

Narahashi, T.: Ion Channels. New York, Plenum Publishing Corp., 1988.

Petersen, O. H., and Petersen, C. C. H.: The patch-clamp technique: Recording ionic currents through single pores in the cell membrane. News Physiol. Sci., 1:5, 1986.

Reuter, H.: Modulation of ion channels by phosphorylation and second messengers. News Physiol. Sci., 2:168, 1987.

Schatzmann, H. J.: The calcium pump of the surface membrane and of the sarcoplasmic reticulum. Annu. Rev. Physiol., 51:473, 1989.

Stein, W. D. (ed.): The Ion Pumps: Structure, Function, and Regulation. New York, Alan R. Liss, Inc., 1988.

Trimmer, J. S., and Agnew, W. S.: Molecular diversity of voltage-sensitive Na channels. Annu. Rev. Physiol., 51:401, 1989.

Verner, K., and Schatz, G.: Protein translocation across membranes. Science, 241:1307, 1988.

Welsh, M. J.: Electrolyte transport by airway epithelia. Physiol. Rev., 67:1143, 1987.

QUESTIONS

1. What are the principal differences between the composition of extracellular fluid and that of intracellular fluid?
2. Describe the transport properties of the cell membrane lipid barrier. What substances penetrate this barrier with ease, and why?
3. Describe the characteristics of the transport proteins.
4. Explain the mechanism of diffusion. Also explain the difference between simple diffusion and facilitated diffusion.
5. What are some of the substances that are transported through the cell membrane by simple diffusion?
6. What are some of the substances transported through the cell membrane by facilitated diffusion? Why do both facilitated diffusion and active transport "saturate"—that is, why do each of these reach a maximum rate at which they can transport substances?
7. How do ions pass through the cell membrane? Explain what is meant by *gating* of protein transport channels. Also explain *voltage gating* and *ligand gating.*
8. Explain how each of the following factors affects net diffusion through the cell membrane: (a) permeability of the membrane, (b) concentration difference across the membrane, (c) electrical potential difference across the membrane, and (d) pressure difference across the membrane.
9. Give the Nernst equation. If the concentration of sodium ions is ten times as great inside a membrane as outside and only sodium ions can pass through the membrane, what is the electrical potential across the membrane?
10. Explain the mechanisms of osmosis and osmotic pressure.
11. Why is osmotic pressure determined by the molar concentration of a solution rather than by its mass concentration of the dissolved solute?
12. Give the numerical relationship between osmolality of a solution and its osmotic pressure.
13. In what way does active transport differ from facilitated diffusion?
14. Describe the mechanism of the sodium-potassium "pump."
15. What substances are transported by the mechanism of active transport in different cells of the body?
16. How much energy is required to concentrate 1 osmol of a substance 10-fold? To concentrate it 1000-fold?
17. Explain the mechanism of sodium co-transport. What important substances are normally transported by the mechanism of co-transport in many cells of the body?

Nerve and Muscle

5

Membrane Potentials and Action Potentials

Electrical potentials exist across the membranes of essentially all cells of the body, and some cells, such as nerve and muscle cells, are "excitable"—that is, capable of self-generation of electrochemical impulses at their membranes and, in most instances, employment of these impulses to transmit signals along the membranes. In still other types of cells, such as glandular cells, macrophages, and ciliated cells, other types of changes in membrane potentials probably play significant roles in controlling many of the cell's functions.

BASIC PHYSICS OF MEMBRANE POTENTIALS

Membrane Potentials Caused by Diffusion

Figure 5-1A and B illustrates a nerve fiber when there is no active transport of either sodium or potassium ions. In Figure 5-1A, the potassium concentration is very great inside the membrane, whereas that outside is very low. Let us also assume that the membrane in this instance is very permeable to the potassium ions but not to any other ions. Because of the large potassium concentration gradient from the inside toward the outside, there is a strong tendency for potassium ions to diffuse outward. As they do so, they carry positive charges to the outside, thus creating a state of electropositivity outside the membrane and electronegativity on the inside because of the negative anions that remain behind, which do not diffuse outward along with the potassium. This new potential difference repels the positively charged potassium ions in a backward direction from the outside to the inside. Within a millisecond or so, the potential change becomes great enough to block further net diffusion of potassium ions to the exterior despite the high potassium ion concentration gradient. In the normal large mammalian nerve fiber, the potential difference required is about 94 millivolts (mV), with negativity inside the fiber membrane.

Figure 5-1B illustrates the same phenomenon as that in Figure 5-1A but this time with a high concentration of sodium ions outside the membrane and a low sodium concentration inside. These ions are also positively charged, and this time the membrane is highly permeable to the sodium ions but impermeable to all other ions. Diffusion of the sodium ions to the inside creates a membrane potential now of opposite polarity, with negativity outside and positivity inside. Again, the membrane potential rises high enough within milliseconds to block further net diffusion of the sodium ions to the inside; however, this time, for the large mammalian nerve fiber, the potential is about 61 mV and with positivity inside the fiber.

Thus, in both parts of Figure 5-1 we see that a concentration difference of ions across a selectively permeable membrane can, under appropriate conditions, cause the creation of a membrane potential. In later sections of this chapter, we see that many of the rapid changes in membrane potentials observed during the course of nerve and muscle impulse transmission result from the occurrence of rapidly changing diffusion potentials of this nature.

Relationship of the Diffusion Potential to the Concentration Difference—the Nernst Equation. The potential level across the membrane that will exactly prevent net diffusion of an ion in either direction through the membrane is called the *Nernst potential* for that ion. The magnitude of this potential is determined by the *ratio* of the ion concentrations on the two sides of the membrane—the greater this ratio, the greater the tendency for the ions to diffuse in one direction, and therefore the greater the Nernst potential. The following equation, called the *Nernst equation,* can be used to calculate the Nernst potential for any univalent ion at normal body temperature of 37°C:

$$\text{EMF (mV)} = \pm 61 \log \frac{\text{Conc. inside}}{\text{Conc. outside}}.$$

When using this formula, the sign of the potential is positive (+) when the ion under consideration is a negative ion and negative (−) when it is a positive ion.

Thus, when the concentration of a positive ion (potassium ions, for instance) on the inside is ten times that on the outside, the log of 10 is 1, so that the Nernst potential calculates to be −61 mV inside the membrane.

Measuring the Membrane Potential

The method for measuring the membrane potential is simple in theory but often very difficult in practice because of the small sizes of many of the fibers. Figure 5–2 illustrates a small pipette, filled with a very strong electrolyte solution (KCl), that is impaled through the cell membrane to the interior of the fiber. Then another electrode, called the "indifferent electrode," is placed in the interstitial fluids, and the potential difference between the inside and outside of the fiber is measured using an appropriate voltmeter. This is a highly sophisticated electronic apparatus that is capable of measuring very small voltages despite extremely high resistance to electrical flow through the tip of the micropipette, which has a diameter usually less than 1 micrometer and a resistance often as great as a billion ohms. For recording rapid *changes* in the membrane potential during the transmission of nerve impulses, the microelectrode is connected to an oscilloscope, as explained later in the chapter.

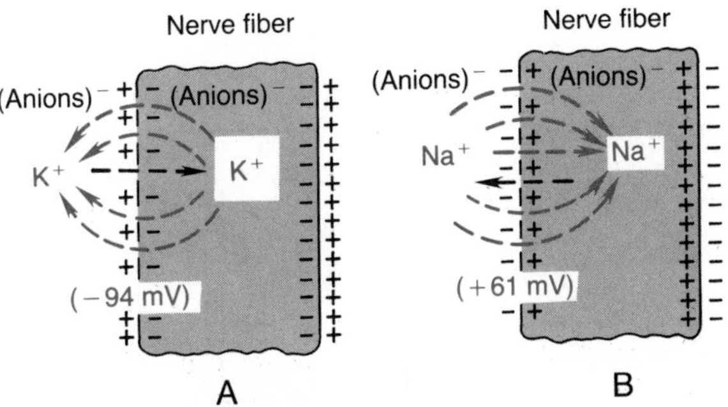

Figure 5–1. *A,* Establishment of a diffusion potential across a cell membrane, caused by potassium ions diffusing from inside the cell to the outside through a membrane that is selectively permeable only to potassium. *B,* Establishment of a diffusion potential when the membrane is permeable only to sodium ions. Note that the internal membrane potential is negative when potassium ions diffuse and positive when sodium ions diffuse because of opposite concentration gradients of these two ions.

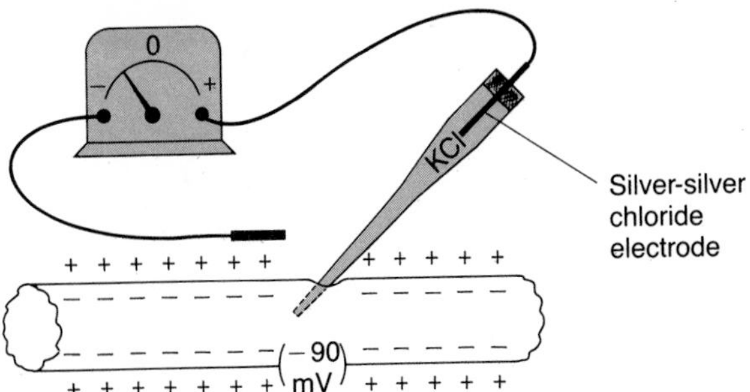

Figure 5–2. Measurement of the membrane potential of the nerve fiber using a microelectrode.

THE RESTING MEMBRANE POTENTIAL OF NERVES

The membrane potential of large nerve fibers when they are not transmitting nerve signals is about −90 mV. That is, the potential *inside the fiber* is 90 mV more negative than the potential in the interstitial fluid on the outside of the fiber. In the next few paragraphs, we explain all the factors that determine the level of this potential, but before doing so we must describe the transport properties of the resting nerve membrane for sodium and potassium.

Active Transport of Sodium and Potassium Ions through the Membrane—the Sodium-Potassium Pump. First, let us recall from the discussions of the previous chapter that all cell membranes of the body have a powerful sodium-potassium pump and that, as illustrated in Figure 5–3, this continually pumps sodium to the outside of the fiber and potassium to the inside. Further, let us remember that more positive charges are pumped to the outside than to the inside (three Na^+ ions to the outside for each two K^+ ions to the inside), leaving a net deficit of positive ions on the inside; this is the same as causing a negative charge inside the cell membrane.

This sodium-potassium pump also causes the tremendous concentration gradients for sodium and potassium across the resting nerve membrane. These gradients are the following:

Na^+ (outside):	142 mEq/L
Na^+ (inside):	14 mEq/L
K^+ (outside):	4 mEq/L
K^+ (inside):	140 mEq/L

The ratios of these two respective ions from the inside to the outside are

$$Na^+_{inside}/Na^+_{outside} = 0.1$$
$$K^+_{inside}/K^+_{outside} = 35.0$$

Leakage of Potassium and Sodium Through the Nerve Membrane. To the right in Figure 5–3 is

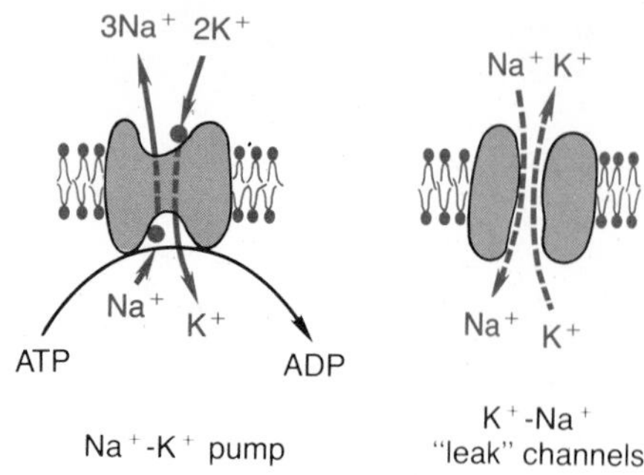

Figure 5-3. The functional characteristics of the Na^+-K^+ pump and also of the potassium-sodium "leak" channels.

illustrated a channel protein in the cell membrane, through which potassium and sodium ions can leak, called a *potassium-sodium "leak" channel.* There are actually multiple different proteins of this type with different leak characteristics. However, the emphasis is on potassium leakage because, on the average, the channels are far more permeable to potassium than to sodium, normally about 100 times as permeable. We see later that this differential in permeability is exceedingly important in determining the level of the normal resting membrane potential.

Origin of the Normal Resting Membrane Potential

Figure 5-4 illustrates the important factors in the establishment of the normal resting membrane potential of −90 mV. These are as follows:

Contribution of the Potassium Diffusion Potential. In Figure 5-4A, we make the assumption that the only movement of ions through the membrane is the diffusion of potassium ions, as illustrated by the open channels between the potassium inside the membrane and the outside. Because of the high ratio of potassium ions inside to outside, 35 to 1, the Nernst potential corresponding to this ratio is −94 mV, since the logarithm of 35 is 1.54, and this times −61 mV is −94 mV. Therefore, if potassium ions were the only factor causing the resting potential, this resting potential would also be equal to −94 mV, as illustrated in the figure.

Contribution of Sodium Diffusion Through the Nerve Membrane. Figure 5-4B illustrates the addition of very slight permeability of the nerve membrane to sodium ions, caused by the minute diffusion of the sodium ions through the K^+-Na^+ leak channels. The ratio of sodium ions from inside to outside the membrane is 0.1, and this gives a calculated Nernst potential for the inside of the membrane of +61 mV. But also shown in Figure 5-4B is the Nernst potential for potassium diffusion of −94 mV. How do these interact with each other, and what will be the summated potential? Intuitively, one can see that if the membrane is highly permeable to potassium but only very slightly permeable to sodium, it is logical that the diffusion of potassium will contribute far more to the membrane potential than will the diffusion of sodium. In the normal nerve fiber, the permeability of the membrane to potassium is about 100 times as great as to sodium, so that the net result is an approximate internal membrane potential of −86 mV, as shown to the right in the figure.

Contribution of the Na^+-K^+ Pump. Finally, in Figure 5-4C an additional contribution of the Na^+-K^+ pump is illustrated. In this figure, there is continuous pumping of three sodium ions to the outside for each two potassium ions pumped to the inside of the membrane. The fact that more sodium ions are being pumped to the outside than potassium to the inside causes a continual loss of positive charges from inside the membrane; this creates an additional degree of negativity (about −4 mV additional) on the inside beyond that which can be accounted for by

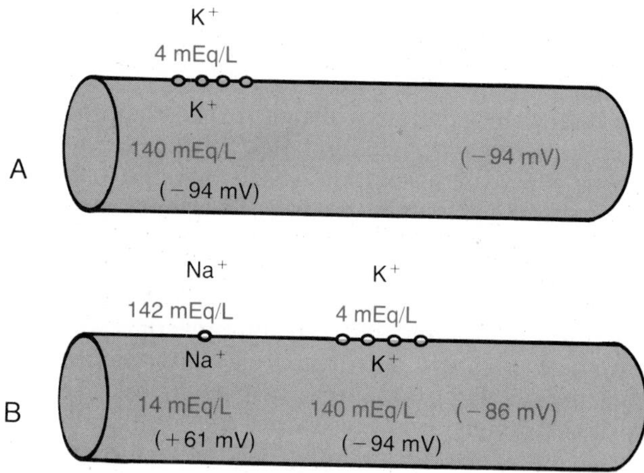

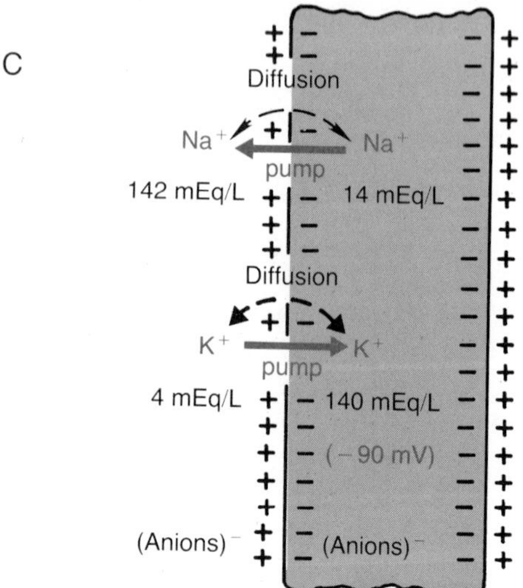

Figure 5-4. Establishment of resting membrane potentials in nerve fibers under three separate conditions: *A*, when the membrane potential is caused entirely by potassium diffusion alone; *B*, when the membrane potential is caused by diffusion of both sodium and potassium ions; and *C*, when the membrane potential is caused by diffusion of both sodium and potassium ions plus pumping of both these ions by the Na^+-K^+ pump.

diffusion alone. Therefore, as illustrated in Figure 5–4C, the net membrane potential with all these factors operative at the same time is −90 mV.

In summary, the diffusion potentials alone caused by potassium and sodium diffusion would give a membrane potential of approximately −86 mV, almost all of this being determined by potassium diffusion. Then, an additional −4 mV is contributed to the membrane potential by the electrogenic Na^+-K^+ pump, giving a net resting membrane potential of −90 mV.

The resting membrane potential in large skeletal muscle fibers is approximately the same as that in large nerve fibers, also −90 mV. However, in both small nerve fibers and small muscle fibers—smooth muscle, for instance—as well as in many of the neurons of the central nervous system, the membrane potential is often as little as −40 to −60 mV instead of −90 mV.

THE NERVE ACTION POTENTIAL

Nerve signals are transmitted by *action potentials,* which are rapid changes in the membrane potential. Each action potential begins with a sudden change from the normal resting negative potential to a positive membrane potential and then ends with an almost equally rapid change back again to the negative potential. To conduct a nerve signal, the action potential moves along the nerve fiber until it comes to the fiber's end. The upper panel of Figure 5–5 shows the disturbances that occur at the membrane during the action potential, with transfer of positive charges to the interior of the fiber at its onset and return of positive charges to the exterior at its end. The lower panel illustrates graphically the successive changes in the membrane potential over a few 10,000ths of a second, illustrating the explosive onset of the action potential and the almost equally as rapid recovery.

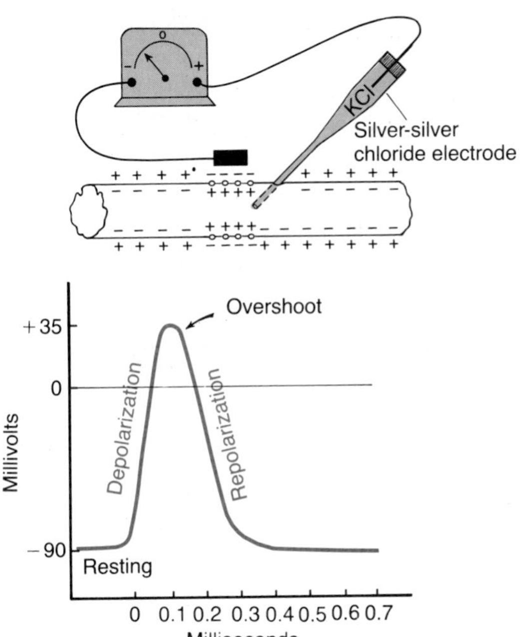

Figure 5–5. A typical action potential recorded by the method illustrated in the upper panel of the figure.

The successive stages of the action potential are as follows:

Resting Stage. This is the resting membrane potential before the action potential occurs. The membrane is said to be "polarized" during this stage because of the very large negative membrane potential that is present.

Depolarization Stage. At this time, the membrane suddenly becomes very permeable to sodium ions, allowing tremendous numbers of sodium ions to flow to the interior of the axon. The normal "polarized" state of −90 mV is lost, with the potential rising rapidly in the positive direction. This is called *depolarization.* In large nerve fibers, the membrane potential actually "overshoots" beyond the zero level and becomes somewhat positive, but in some smaller fibers as well as many central nervous system neurons, the potential merely approaches the zero level and does not overshoot to the positive state.

Repolarization Stage. Within a few 10,000ths of a second after the membrane becomes highly permeable to sodium ions, the sodium channels begin to close, and the potassium channels open more than normally. Then, rapid diffusion of potassium ions to the exterior re-establishes the normal negative resting membrane potential. This is called *repolarization* of the membrane.

To explain more fully the factors that cause both the depolarization and the repolarization processes, we need now to describe the special characteristics of yet two other types of transport channels through the nerve membrane: the voltage-gated sodium and potassium channels.

The Voltage-Gated Sodium and Potassium Channels

The necessary actor in causing both depolarization and repolarization of the nerve membrane during the action potential is the *voltage-gated sodium channel.* However, the *voltage-gated potassium channel* plays an important role in increasing the rapidity of repolarization of the membrane. *These two voltage-gated channels are in addition to the Na^+-K^+ pump and also in addition to the Na^+-K^+ leak channels.*

The Voltage-Gated Sodium Channel—"Activation" and "Inactivation" of the Channel

The upper panel of Figure 5–6 illustrates the voltage-gated sodium channel in three separate states. This channel has two *gates,* one near the outside of the channel called the *activation gate* and another near the inside called the *inactivation gate.* To the left is shown the state of these two gates in the normal resting membrane when the membrane potential is −90 mV. In this state, the activation gate is closed, which

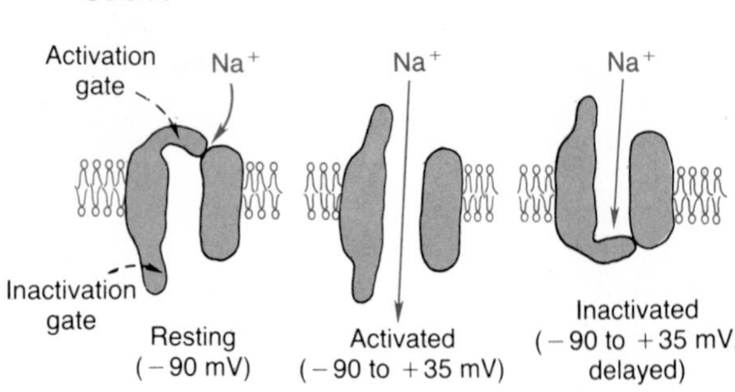

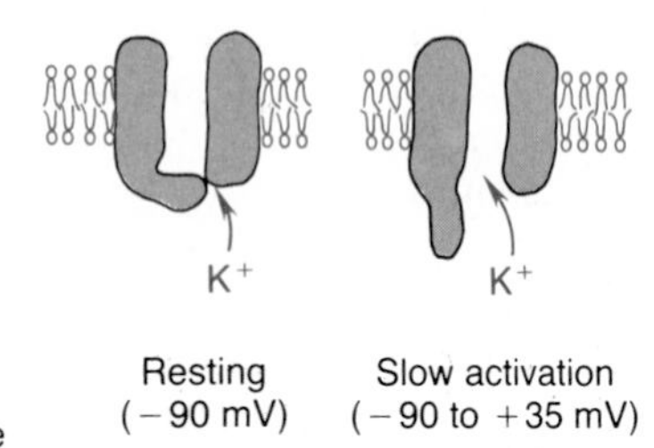

Figure 5-6. Characteristics of the voltage-gated sodium and potassium channels, showing both activation and inactivation of the sodium channels but activation of the potassium channels only when the membrane potential is changed from the normal resting negative value to a positive value.

prevents any entry of sodium ions to the interior of the fiber through these sodium channels. On the other hand, the inactivation gate is open and does not at this time constitute any barrier to the movement of the sodium ions.

Activation of the Sodium Channel. When the membrane potential becomes less negative than during the resting state, rising from −90 mV toward zero, it finally reaches a voltage, usually somewhere between −70 and −50 mV, that causes a sudden conformational change in the activation gate, flipping it to the open position. This is called the *activated state;* during this state, sodium ions can literally pour inward through the channel, increasing the sodium permeability of the membrane as much as 500-fold to 5000-fold.

Inactivation of the Sodium Channel. To the far right in the upper panel of Figure 5-6 is illustrated a third state of the sodium channel. The same increase in voltage that opens the activation gate also closes the inactivation gate. However, closure of the inactivation gate occurs a few 10,000ths of a second after the activation gate opens. That is, the conformational change that flips the inactivation gate to the closed state is a slower process, whereas the conformational change that opens the activation gate is a very rapid process. Therefore, after the sodium channel has remained open for a few 10,000ths of a second, it closes, and sodium ions can no longer pour to the inside of the membrane. At this point the membrane potential begins to recover back toward the resting membrane state, which is the repolarization process.

A very important characteristic of the sodium channel inactivation process is that *the inactivation gate will not reopen again until the membrane potential returns nearly to the original resting membrane potential level.* Therefore, it is not possible for the sodium channels to open again without the nerve fiber first repolarizing.

The Voltage-Gated Potassium Channels and Their Activation

The lower panel of Figure 5-6 illustrates the voltage-gated potassium channel in two separate states: during the resting state and toward the end of the action potential. During the resting state, the gate of the potassium channel is closed, as illustrated to the left in the figure, and potassium ions are prevented from passing through this channel to the exterior. When the membrane potential rises from −90 mV toward zero, this voltage change causes a slow conformational opening of the gate and allows increased potassium diffusion outward through the channel. However, because of slowness of opening of these potassium channels, they normally do not open until the sodium channels are beginning to become inactivated and therefore are closing. Thus, the decrease in sodium entry to the cell and simultaneous increase in potassium exit from the cell greatly speeds the repolarization process, leading within a few 10,000ths of a second to full recovery of the resting membrane potential.

Summary of the Events That Cause the Action Potential

Figure 5-7 illustrates in summary form the sequential events that occur during and shortly after the action potential. These are as follows:

At the bottom of the figure are shown the changes in membrane conductances for sodium and potassium ions. During the resting state, before the action potential begins, the conductance for potassium ions is shown to be 50 to 100 times as great as the conductance for sodium ions. This is caused by much greater leakage of potassium ions than sodium ions through the leak channels. However, at the onset of the action potential, the sodium channels instantaneously become activated and allow an up to 5000-fold increase in sodium conductance. Then the inactivation process closes the sodium channels within another few fractions of a millisecond. The onset of the action potential also causes voltage gating of the potassium channels, causing them to begin opening a fraction of a millisecond after the sodium channels open. And at the end of the action potential, the return of the membrane potential to the negative state causes the potassium channels to close back to their original status, but again only after a short delay.

In the middle portion of Figure 5-7 is shown the ratio of sodium conductance to potassium conduct-

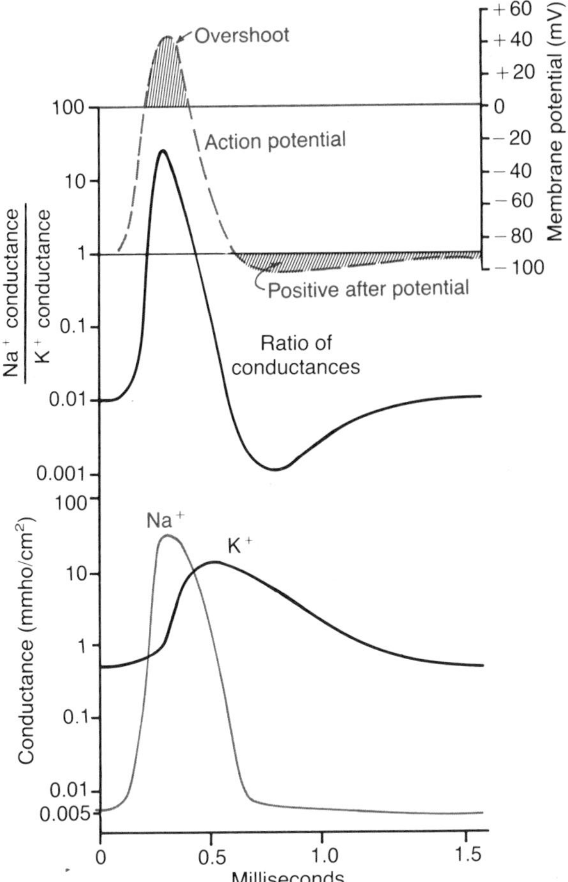

Figure 5–7. Changes in sodium and potassium conductances during the course of the action potential. Note that sodium conductance increases several thousandfold during the early stages of the action potential, whereas potassium conductance increases only about 30-fold during the latter stages of the action potential and for a short period thereafter. (Curves constructed from data in Hodgkin and Huxley papers but transposed from squid axon to apply to the membrane potentials of large mammalian nerve fibers.)

ance at each instant during the action potential, and above this is shown the action potential itself. During the early portion of the action potential, this ratio increases more than 1000-fold. Therefore, far more sodium ions now flow to the interior of the fiber than do potassium ions to the exterior. This is what causes the membrane potential to become positive. Then the sodium channels begin to become inactivated, and at the same time the potassium channels open, so that the ratio of conductance now shifts far in favor of high potassium conductance but low sodium conductance. This allows extremely rapid loss of potassium ions to the exterior, while essentially no sodium ions flow to the interior. Consequently, the action potential quickly returns to its baseline level.

Roles of Other Ions During the Action Potential

Thus far, we have considered only the roles of sodium and potassium ions in the generation of the action potential. However, at least two other types of ions must be considered. These are as follows:

The Impermeant Negatively Charged Ions (Anions) Inside the Axon. Inside the axon are many negatively charged ions that cannot go through the membrane channels. These include protein molecules, many organic phosphate compounds, sulfate compounds, and so forth. Because these cannot leave the interior of the axon, any deficit of positive ions inside the membrane leaves an excess of the impermeant negative ions. Therefore, these impermeant negative ions are responsible for the negative charge inside the fiber when there is a deficit of the positively charged potassium and sodium ions.

Calcium Ions. The cell membranes of almost all, if not all, cells of the body have a calcium pump similar to the sodium pump. Like the sodium pump, this device pumps calcium ions from the interior to the exterior of the cell membrane (or into the endoplasmic reticulum), creating a calcium ion gradient of about 10,000-fold, leaving an internal concentration of calcium ions of about 10^{-7} molar in contrast to an external concentration of about 10^{-3} molar.

In addition, there are also voltage-gated calcium channels. These channels are very slow to become activated, requiring 10 to 20 times as long for activation as the sodium channels.

Calcium channels are very numerous in both cardiac muscle and smooth muscle. In fact, in some types of smooth muscle, the fast sodium channels are hardly present at all, so the action potentials then are caused almost entirely by activation of the slow calcium channels.

Initiation of the Action Potential

Up to this point, we have explained the action potential itself but not what initiates the action potential. The answer to this is really quite simple:

A Positive Feedback Opens the Sodium Channels. First, as long as the membrane of the nerve fiber remains totally undisturbed, no action potential occurs in the normal nerve. However, if any event at all causes enough initial rise in the membrane potential from −90 mV up toward the zero level, the rising voltage itself will cause many voltage-gated sodium channels to begin opening. This allows rapid inflow of sodium ions, which causes still further rise of the membrane potential, thus opening still more voltage-gated sodium channels and more streaming of sodium ions to the interior of the fiber. Obviously, this process is a positive-feedback vicious circle that, once the feedback is strong enough, will continue until all the voltage-gated sodium channels have become totally activated (opened). Then, within another fraction of a millisecond, the rising membrane potential causes beginning inactivation of the sodium channels as well as opening of potassium channels, and the action potential soon terminates.

Threshold for Initiation of the Action Potential. An action potential will not occur until the initial rise in membrane potential is great enough to create the vicious circle described in the last paragraph. Usually, a sudden rise in membrane potential of 15 to 30 mV is required. Therefore, a sudden increase in the membrane potential in a large nerve fiber of from −90 mV up to about −65 mV will usually cause the explosive development of the action potential. This level of −65 mV, therefore, is said to be the *threshold* for stimulation.

PROPAGATION OF THE ACTION POTENTIAL

In the preceding paragraphs we have discussed the action potential as it occurs at one spot on the membrane. However, an action potential elicited at any one point on an excitable membrane usually excites adjacent portions of the membrane, resulting in propagation of the action potential. The mechanism of this is illustrated in Figure 5–8. Figure 5–8A shows a normal resting nerve fiber, and Figure 5–8B shows a nerve fiber that has been excited in its midportion —that is, the midportion has suddenly developed increased permeability to sodium. The arrows illustrate a "local circuit" of current flow between the depolarized areas of the membrane and the adjacent resting membrane areas; positive electrical charges carried by the inward diffusing sodium ions flow not only inward through the depolarized membrane but also for several millimeters along the core of the axon. These positive charges increase the voltage for a distance of 1 to 3 millimeters inside large fibers to above the threshold voltage value for initiating an action potential. Therefore, the sodium channels in these new areas immediately activate, and, as illustrated in Figure 5–8C and D, the explosive action potential spreads. Then these newly depolarized areas cause additional local circuits of current flow still farther along the membrane, causing progressively more and more depolarization. Thus, the depolarization process travels along the entire extent of the fiber. The transmission of the depolarization process along a nerve or muscle fiber is called a *nerve* or *muscle impulse.*

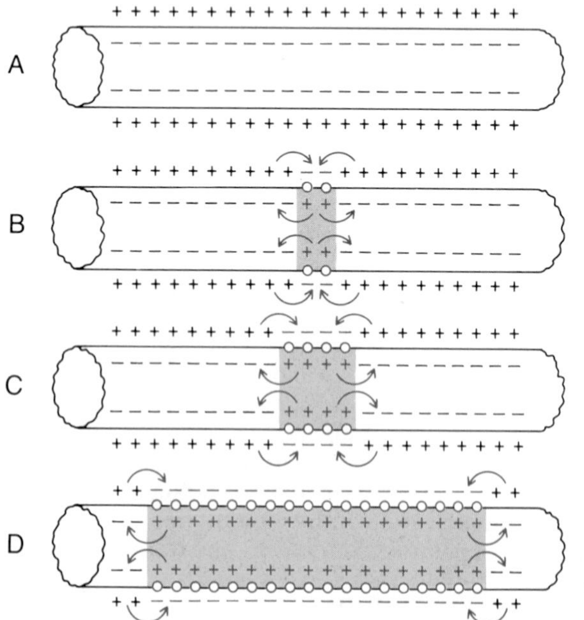

Figure 5–8. Propagation of action potentials in both directions along a conductive fiber.

Direction of Propagation. It is obvious, as illustrated in Figure 5–8, that an excitable membrane has no single direction of propagation, but that the action potential can travel in both directions away from the stimulus—and even along all branches of a nerve fiber—until the entire membrane has become depolarized.

The All-or-Nothing Principle. It is equally obvious that, once an action potential has been elicited at any point on the membrane of a normal fiber, the depolarization process will travel over the entire membrane if conditions are right, or it might not travel at all if conditions are not right. This is called the all-or-nothing principle.

RE-ESTABLISHING SODIUM AND POTASSIUM IONIC GRADIENTS AFTER ACTION POTENTIALS—IMPORTANCE OF ENERGY METABOLISM

Transmission of each impulse along the nerve fiber reduces infinitesimally the concentration differences of sodium and potassium between the inside and outside of the membrane because of diffusion of sodium ions to the inside during depolarization and diffusion of potassium ions to the outside during repolarization. For a single action potential, this effect is so minute that it cannot be measured. Indeed, 100,000 to 50,000,000 impulses can be transmitted by nerve fibers, the number depending on the size of the fiber and several other factors, before the concentration differences have run down to the point that action potential conduction ceases. Yet, even so, with time it becomes necessary to re-establish the sodium and potassium membrane concentration differences. This is achieved by the action of the Na^+-K^+ pump in exactly the same way as that described earlier in the chapter for original establishment of the resting potential. That is, the sodium ions that have diffused to the interior of the cell during the action potentials and the potassium ions that have diffused to the exterior are returned to their original state by the Na^+-K^+ pump. Since this pump requires energy for operation, this process of "recharging" the nerve fiber is an active metabolic one, using energy derived from the adenosine triphosphate energy system of the cell.

PLATEAU IN SOME ACTION POTENTIALS

In some instances, the excitable membrane does not repolarize immediately after depolarization, but,

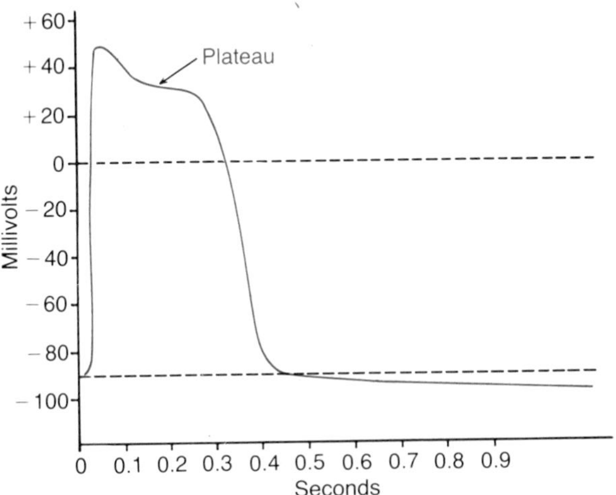

Figure 5-9. An action potential from a Purkinje fiber of the heart, showing a "plateau."

instead, the potential remains on a plateau near the peak of the spike for many milliseconds before repolarization begins. Such a plateau is illustrated in Figure 5-9; one can readily see that the plateau greatly prolongs the period of depolarization. This type of action potential occurs in heart muscle fibers, where the plateau lasts for as long as two to three tenths of a second and causes each contraction of the heart muscle also to last for this same period of time.

The cause of the plateau is a combination of several different factors. First, in heart muscle, two separate types of channels enter into the depolarization process: (1) the usual voltage-activated sodium channels, called *fast channels,* and (2) the voltage-activated calcium channels, which are slow to be activated and therefore are called *slow channels*—these channels allow diffusion mainly of calcium ions but of some sodium ions as well. Activation of the fast channels causes the spike portion of the action potential, whereas the slow but prolonged activation of the slow channels is mainly responsible for the plateau portion of the action potential.

A second factor partly responsible for the plateau is that the voltage-gated potassium channels are slow to be activated in some instances, often not opening until the very end of the plateau. This, too, delays the return of the membrane potential toward the resting value.

RHYTHMICITY OF CERTAIN EXCITABLE TISSUES—REPETITIVE DISCHARGE

Repetitive self-induced discharges, or *rhythmicity,* occur normally in the heart, in most smooth muscle, and in many of the neurons of the central nervous system. It is these rhythmical discharges that cause the heart rhythm, that cause peristalsis, and that cause such neuronal events as the rhythmical control of breathing.

Also, all other excitable tissues can discharge repetitively if the threshold for stimulation is reduced low enough. For instance, even nerve fibers and skeletal muscle fibers, which normally are highly stable, discharge repetitively when they are placed in a solution containing the drug veratrine or when the calcium ion concentration falls below a critical value.

The Re-excitation Process Necessary for Rhythmicity. For rhythmicity to occur, the membrane, even in its natural state, must already be permeable enough to sodium ions (or to calcium and sodium ions through the slow calcium channels) to allow automatic membrane depolarization. Thus, Figure 5-10 shows that the "resting" membrane potential is only −60 to −70 mV. This is not enough negative voltage to keep the sodium and calcium channels closed. That is, (1) sodium and calcium ions flow inward, (2) this further increases the membrane permeability, (3) still more ions flow inward, (4) the permeability increases more, and so forth, thus eliciting the regenerative process of sodium and calcium channel openings until an action potential is generated. Then, at the end of the action potential, the membrane repolarizes. But shortly thereafter, the depolarization process begins again, and a new action potential occurs spontaneously. This cycle continues again and again and causes self-induced rhythmical excitation of the excitable tissue.

Yet, why does the membrane not depolarize immediately after it has become repolarized rather than delaying for nearly a second before the onset of the next action potential? The answer to this is that toward the end of all action potentials, and continuing for a short period thereafter, the membrane becomes excessively permeable to potassium. The excessive outflow of potassium ions carries tremendous numbers of positive charges to the outside of the membrane, creating inside the fiber considerably more negativity than would otherwise occur for a short period after the preceding action potential is over, thus drawing the membrane potential nearer to the potassium Nernst potential. This is a state called *hyperpolarization,* which is illustrated in Figure 5-10. As long as this state exists, re-excitation will not occur; but gradually the excess potassium conductance (and the state of hyperpolarization) disappears, as shown in the figure, thereby allowing the membrane potential to increase until it reaches the *threshold* for excitation; then suddenly a new action potential results, the process occurring again and again.

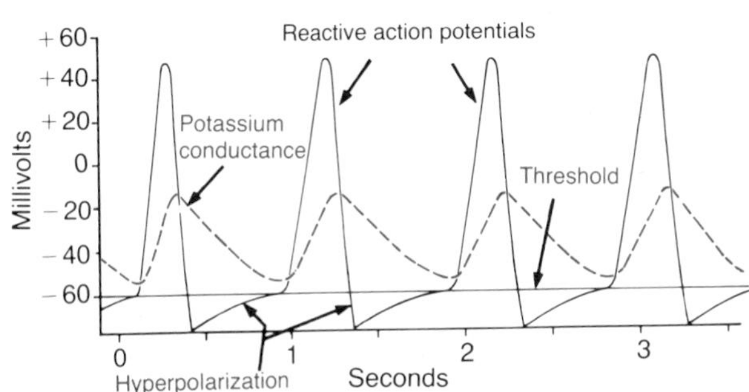

Figure 5-10. Rhythmic action potentials similar to those recorded in the rhythmical control center of the heart. Note their relationship to potassium conductance and to the state of hyperpolarization.

SPECIAL ASPECTS OF SIGNAL TRANSMISSION IN NERVE TRUNKS

Myelinated and Unmyelinated Nerve Fibers. A typical nerve trunk comprises a few very large nerve fibers that occupy most of the cross-sectional area and many more small fibers lying between the large ones. The large fibers are *myelinated* and the small ones are *unmyelinated.* The average nerve trunk contains about twice as many unmyelinated fibers as myelinated fibers.

Figure 5–11 illustrates a typical myelinated fiber. The central core of the fiber is the *axon,* and the membrane of the axon is the actual *conductive membrane.* The axon is filled in its center with *axoplasm,* which is a viscid intracellular fluid. Surrounding the axon is a *myelin sheath* that is often thicker than the axon itself, and about once every 1 to 3 millimeters along the length of the axon the myelin sheath is interrupted by a *node of Ranvier.*

The myelin sheath is deposited around the axon by Schwann cells in the following manner: The membrane of a Schwann cell first envelops the axon. Then the cell rotates around the axon many times, laying down multiple layers of cellular membrane containing the lipid substance *sphingomyelin.* This substance is an excellent insulator that decreases the ion flow through the membrane approximately 5000-fold. However, at the juncture between each two successive Schwann cells along the axon, a small, uninsulated area remains, only 2 to 3 *micro*meters in length, where ions can still flow with ease between the extracellular fluid and the axon. This area is the node of Ranvier.

"Saltatory" Conduction in Myelinated Fibers from Node to Node. Even though ions cannot flow significantly through the thick myelin sheaths of myelinated nerves, they can flow with considerable ease through the nodes of Ranvier. Therefore, action potentials can occur *only at the nodes.* Yet, the action potentials are conducted from node to node, as illustrated in Figure 5–12; this is called *saltatory conduction.* That is, electrical current flows through the surrounding extracellular fluids and also through the axoplasm from node to node, exciting successive nodes one after another. Thus, the nerve impulse jumps down the fiber, which is the origin of the term "saltatory."

Saltatory conduction is of value for two reasons. First, by causing the depolarization process to jump long intervals along the axis of the nerve fiber, this mechanism increases the velocity of nerve transmission in myelinated fibers as much as 5-fold to 50-fold. Second, saltatory conduction conserves energy for the axon, for only the nodes depolarize, allowing perhaps a hundred times smaller loss of ions than would otherwise be necessary and therefore requiring little extra metabolism for re-establishing the sodium and potas-

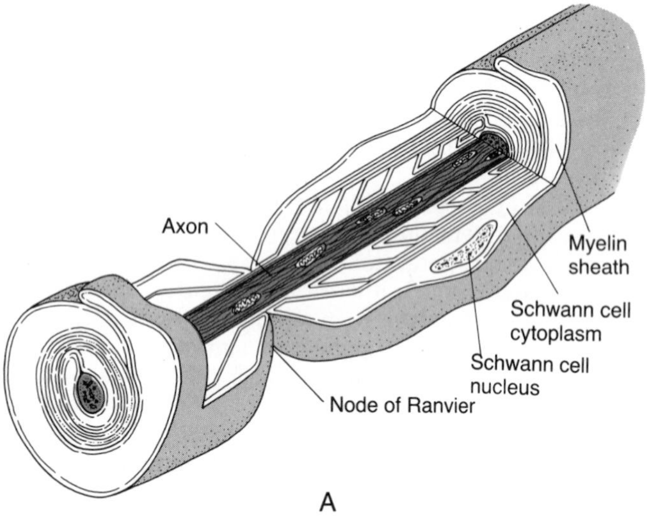

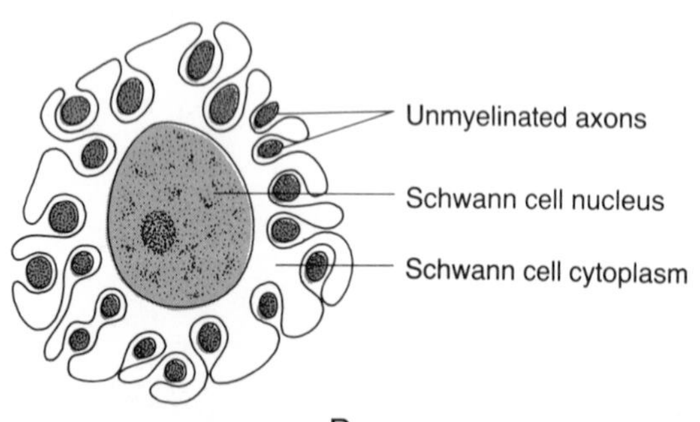

Figure 5–11. Function of the Schwann cell to insulate nerve fibers. *A,* The wrapping of a Schwann cell membrane around a large axon to form the myelin sheath of the myelinated nerve fiber. (Modified from Leeson and Leeson: Histology. Philadelphia, W. B. Saunders Company, 1979.) *B,* Evagination of the membrane and cytoplasm of a Schwann cell around multiple unmyelinated nerve fibers.

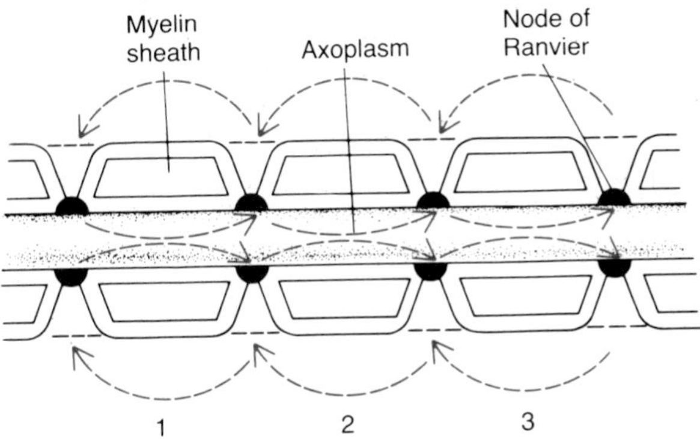

Figure 5-12. Saltatory conduction along a myelinated axon.

sium concentration differences across the membrane after a series of nerve impulses.

Velocity of Conduction in Nerve Fibers

The velocity of conduction in nerve fibers varies from as little as 0.5 m/sec in very small unmyelinated fibers to as high as 100 m/sec (the length of a football field in 1 second) in very large myelinated fibers. The velocity increases approximately with the fiber diameter.

EXCITATION—THE PROCESS OF ELICITING THE ACTION POTENTIAL

Basically, any factor that causes sodium ions to begin to diffuse inward through the membrane in sufficient numbers will set off the automatic, regenerative opening of the sodium channels. This can result from (1) simple *mechanical* disturbance of the membrane, (2) *chemical* effects on the membrane, or (3) passage of *electricity* through the membrane. All these are used at different points in the body to elicit nerve or muscle action potentials: mechanical pressure to excite sensory nerve endings in the skin, chemical neurotransmitters to transmit signals from one neuron to the next in the brain, and electrical current to transmit signals between muscle cells in the heart and intestine. For the purpose of understanding the excitation process, let us discuss briefly the principles of electrical stimulation.

Excitation of a Nerve Fiber by a Negatively Charged Metal Electrode. The usual means for exciting a nerve or muscle in the experimental laboratory is to apply electricity at the nerve or muscle surface through two small electrodes, one of which is negatively charged and the other positively charged. When this is done, one finds that the excitable membrane becomes stimulated at the negative electrode.

The cause of this effect is the following: Remember that the action potential is initiated by the opening of voltage-gated sodium channels. Furthermore, these channels are opened by a decrease in the electrical voltage across the membrane. The negative current from the negative electrode reduces the voltage immediately outside the membrane, drawing this voltage nearer to the voltage of the negative membrane potential inside the fiber. This decreases the electrical voltage across the membrane and allows activation of the sodium channels, thus resulting in an action potential.

RECORDING MEMBRANE POTENTIALS AND ACTION POTENTIALS

The Cathode Ray Oscilloscope. Earlier in this chapter we noted that the membrane potential changes occur very rapidly throughout the course of an action potential. Indeed, most of the action potential complex of large nerve fibers takes place in less than 1/1000 second. In some figures of this chapter an electrical meter has been shown recording these potential changes. However, it must be understood that any meter capable of recording them must be capable of responding extremely rapidly. For practical purposes, the only common type of meter that is capable of responding accurately to the very rapid membrane potential changes is the cathode ray oscilloscope.

Figure 5-13 illustrates the basic components of a cathode ray oscilloscope. The cathode ray tube itself is composed basically of an *electron gun* and a *fluorescent surface* against which electrons are fired. Where the electrons hit the surface, the fluorescent material glows. If the electron beam is moved across the surface, the spot of glowing light also moves and draws a fluorescent line on the screen.

In addition to the electron gun and fluorescent surface, the cathode ray tube is provided with two sets of electrically charged plates, one set positioned on either side of the electron beam and the other set positioned above and below. Appropriate electronic control circuits change the voltage on these plates so that the electron beam can be bent up or down in response

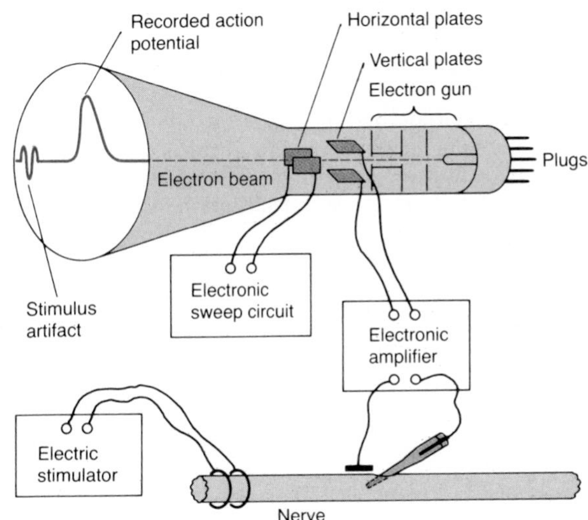

Figure 5-13. The cathode ray oscilloscope for recording transient action potentials.

to electrical signals coming from recording electrodes on nerves. The beam of electrons is also swept horizontally across the screen at a constant rate. This gives the record illustrated on the face of the cathode ray tube, giving a time base horizontally and the voltage changes at the nerve electrodes vertically. Note at the left end of the record a small *stimulus artifact* caused by the electrical stimulus used to elicit the action potential. Then farther to the right is the recorded action potential itself.

Recording the Monophasic Action Potential. Throughout this chapter, "monophasic" action potentials have been shown in the different diagrams. To record these, a micropipette electrode, illustrated earlier in the chapter in Figure 5–2, is inserted into the interior of the fiber. Then, as the action potential spreads down the fiber, the changes in the potential inside the fiber are recorded, as illustrated in several different figures earlier in the chapter.

REFERENCES

Auerbach, A., and Sachs, F.: Patch clamp studies of single ionic channels. Annu. Rev. Biophys. Bioeng., 13:269, 1984.

Byrne, J. H., and Schultz, S. G.: An Introduction to Membrane Transport and Bioelectricity. New York, Raven Press, 1988.

Clausen, T.: Regulation of active Na^+-K^+ transport in skeletal muscle. Physiol. Rev., 66:542, 1986.

DeWeer, P., et al.: Voltage dependence of the Na-K pump. Annu. Rev. Physiol., 50:225, 1988.

Grinnell, A. D., et al. (eds.): Calcium and Ion Channel Modulation. New York, Plenum Publishing Corp., 1988.

Hodgkin, A. L.: The Conduction of the Nervous Impulse. Springfield, Ill., Charles C Thomas, 1963.

Hodgkin, A. L., and Huxley, A. F.: Movement of sodium and potassium ions during nervous activity. Cold Spr. Harb. Symp. Quant. Biol., 17:43, 1952.

Hodgkin, A. L., and Huxley, A. F.: Quantitative description of membrane current and its application to conduction and excitation in nerve. J. Physiol. (Lond.), 117:500, 1952.

Miller, R. J.: Multiple calcium channels and neuronal function. Science, 235:46, 1987.

Narahashi, T.: Ion Channels. New York, Plenum Publishing Corp., 1988.

Reuter, H.: Modulation of ion channels by phosphorylation and second messengers. News Physiol. Sci., 2:168, 1987.

Ross, W. N.: Changes in intracellular calcium during neuron activity. Annu. Rev. Physiol., 51:491, 1989.

Shepherd, G. M.: Neurobiology. New York, Oxford University Press, 1987.

Skene, J. H. P.: Axonal growth-associated proteins. Annu. Rev. Neurosci., 12:127, 1989.

Trimmer, J. A., and Agnew, W. S.: Molecular diversity of voltage-sensitive Na channels. Annu. Rev. Physiol., 51:401, 1989.

QUESTIONS

1. What is meant by a membrane potential?
2. Explain how membrane potentials can be caused by diffusion of ions through a membrane.
3. Calculate the Nernst potentials for sodium and potassium for the normal nerve, using the concentration values given in the text.
4. Explain why the sodium-potassium pump is called an electrogenic pump.
5. Describe the method for measuring the membrane potential.
6. Why is the normal resting membrane potential nearly equal to the Nernst potential for potassium?
7. Explain the events that occur during the depolarization and repolarization stages of the action potential.
8. Describe the voltage-gated sodium and potassium channels. What is meant by *activation* of the sodium channel, and what is meant by *inactivation* of this channel?
9. Approximately how much does the sodium conductance increase during the early part of the action potential?
10. Explain how action potentials are initiated. What is meant by the *threshold* for initiation of the action potential?
11. Explain the means by which action potentials are propagated along the nerve fiber.
12. What is meant by the term *all-or-nothing principle*?
13. Why must a nerve fiber be recharged after nerve impulses have been transmitted? Approximately how many nerve impulses can be transmitted before the nerve fiber will "run-down"?
14. What causes increased heat production in nerve fibers?
15. Explain what causes a plateau in some action potentials. In what tissues is one likely to find such action potentials?
16. Describe the re-excitation process that occurs in some tissues, such as the heart and some smooth-muscle organs, that causes repetitive discharge. What is the difference between a *myelinated* and an *unmyelinated* nerve fiber, and how does saltatory conduction occur in myelinated fibers?
17. Explain the different methods by which nerve fibers can be excited.
18. Describe the use of the oscilloscope for recording action potentials.

6

Contraction of Skeletal Muscle

Approximately 40 per cent of the body is skeletal muscle, and almost another 10 per cent is smooth and cardiac muscle. Many of the same principles of contraction apply to all these different types of muscle, but in the present chapter the function of skeletal muscle is considered mainly; the specialized functions of smooth muscle are discussed in Chapter 7 and of cardiac muscle in Chapter 8.

PHYSIOLOGICAL ANATOMY OF SKELETAL MUSCLE

The Skeletal Muscle Fiber

Figure 6-1 illustrates the organization of skeletal muscle, showing that all skeletal muscles are made of numerous fibers ranging between 10 and 80 micrometers in diameter. In most muscles the fibers extend the entire length of the muscle; and, except for about 2 per cent of the fibers, each is innervated by only one nerve ending, located near the middle of the fiber.

The Sarcolemma. The sarcolemma is the cell membrane of the muscle fiber. However, the sarcolemma consists of a true cell membrane, called the *plasma membrane,* and an outer coat made up of a thin layer of polysaccharide material containing numerous thin collagen fibrils. At the end of the muscle fiber, this surface layer of the sarcolemma fuses with a tendon fiber, and the tendon fibers in turn collect into bundles to form the muscle tendons and thence insert into the bones.

Myofibrils; Actin and Myosin Filaments. Each muscle fiber contains several hundred to several thousand *myofibrils,* which are illustrated by the many small open dots in the cross-sectional view of Figure 6-1C. Each myofibril (Figure 6-1D and E) in turn has, lying side-by-side, about 1500 *myosin filaments* and 3000 *actin filaments,* which are large polymerized protein molecules that are responsible for muscle contraction. These can be seen in longitudinal view in the electron micrograph of Figure 6-2 and are represented diagrammatically in Figure 6-1, parts E through L. The thick filaments in the diagrams are *myosin,* and the thin filaments are *actin.*

Note that the myosin and actin filaments partially interdigitate and thus cause the myofibrils to have alternate light and dark bands. The light bands contain only actin filaments and are called *I bands* because they are *isotropic* to polarized light. The dark bands contain the myosin filaments as well as the ends of the actin filaments where they overlap the myosin and are called *A bands* because they are *anisotropic* to polarized light. Note also the small projections from the sides of the myosin filaments. These are called *cross-bridges.* They protrude from the surfaces of the myosin filaments along the entire extent of the filament except in the very center. It is the interaction between these cross-bridges and the actin filaments that causes contraction.

Figure 6-1E also shows that the ends of the actin filaments are attached to a so-called *Z disc.* From this disc, these filaments extend in both directions to interdigitate with the myosin filaments. The Z disc, which itself is composed of filamentous proteins different from the actin and myosin filaments, passes from myofibril to myofibril, attaching the myofibrils to each other all the way across the muscle fiber. Therefore, the entire muscle fiber has light and dark bands, as do the individual myofibrils. These bands give skeletal and cardiac muscle their "striated" appearance.

The portion of a myofibril (or of the whole muscle fiber) that lies between two successive Z discs is called a *sarcomere.* When the muscle fiber is at its normal,

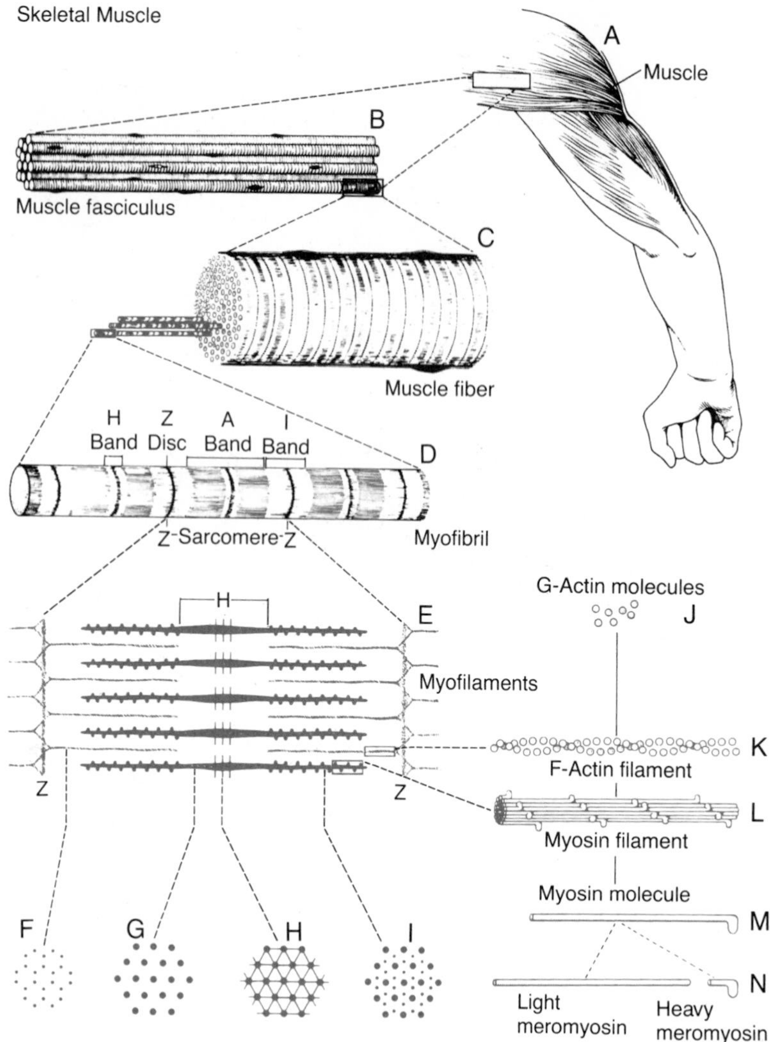

Figure 6–1. Organization of skeletal muscle, from the gross to the molecular level. *F, G, H,* and *I* are cross-sections at the levels indicated. (Drawing by Sylvia Colard Keene. Modified from Fawcett: Bloom and Fawcett: A Textbook of Histology. Philadelphia, W. B. Saunders Company, 1986.)

fully stretched resting length, the length of the sarcomere is about 2 micrometers. At this length, the actin filaments completely overlap the myosin filaments and are just beginning to overlap each other. We see later that at this length the sarcomere also is capable of generating its greatest force of contraction.

The Sarcoplasm. The mofibrils are suspended inside the muscle fiber in a matrix called *sarcoplasm,* which is composed of usual intracellular constituents. The fluid of the sarcoplasm contains large quantities of potassium, magnesium, phosphate, and protein enzymes. Also present are tremendous numbers of *mitochondria* that lie between and parallel to the myofibrils, which is indicative of the great need of the contracting myofibrils for large amounts of adenosine triphosphate (ATP) formed by the mitochondria.

The Sarcoplasmic Reticulum. Also in the sarcoplasm is an extensive endoplasmic reticulum, which in the muscle fiber is called the *sarcoplasmic reticulum.* This reticulum has a special organization that is extremely important in the control of muscle contraction, which is discussed later in the chapter. The electron micrograph of Figure 6–3 illustrates the arrangement of this sarcoplasmic reticulum and shows how extensive it can be.

MOLECULAR MECHANISM OF MUSCLE CONTRACTION

Sliding Mechanism of Contraction. Figure 6–4 illustrates the basic mechanism of muscle contraction. It shows the relaxed state of a sarcomere (above) and the contracted state (below). In the relaxed state, the ends of the actin filaments derived from two successive Z discs barely begin to overlap each other, while at the same time completely overlapping the myosin filaments. On the other hand, in the contracted state these actin filaments have been pulled inward among the myosin filaments, so that they now overlap each other to a major extent. Also, the Z discs have been pulled by the actin filaments up to the ends of the myosin filaments. Thus, muscle contraction occurs by a *sliding filament mechanism.*

But what causes the actin filaments to slide inward among the myosin filaments? This is caused by mechanical forces generated by the interaction of the cross-bridges of the myosin filaments with the actin filaments, as we discuss in the following sections. Under resting conditions, these forces are inhibited, but when an action potential travels over the muscle

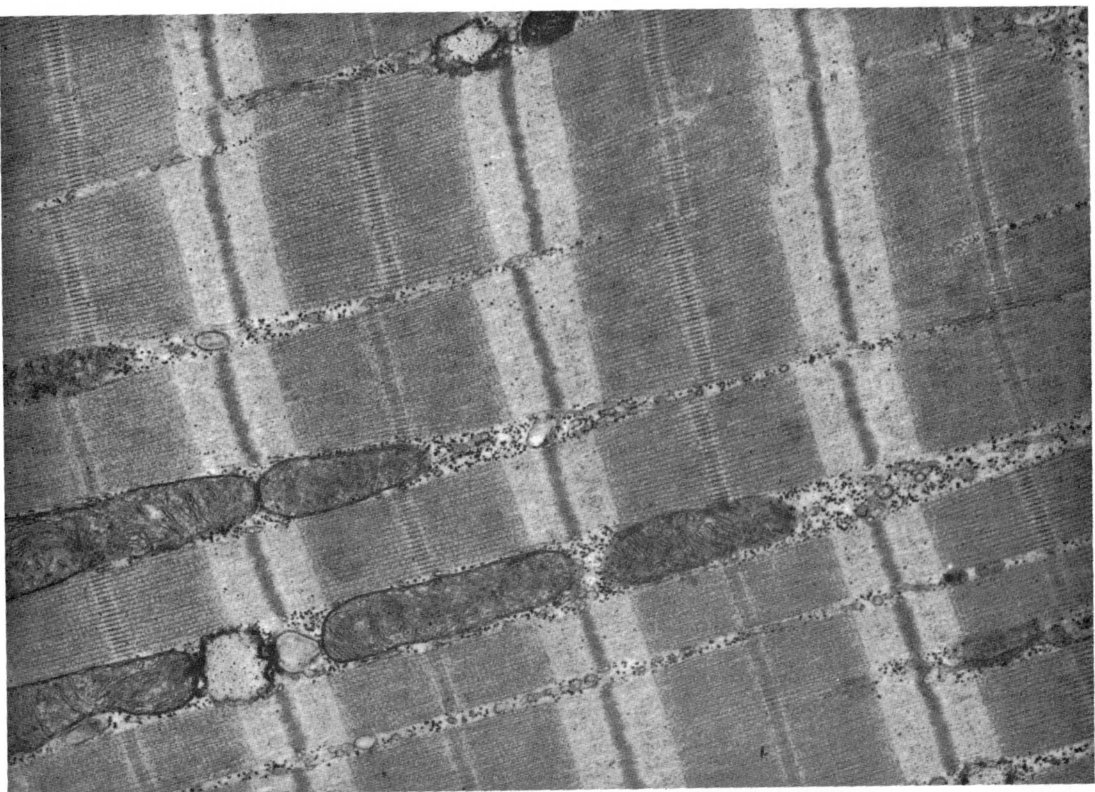

Figure 6-2. Electron micrograph of muscle myofibrils, showing the detailed organization of actin and myosin filaments. Note the mitochondria lying between the myofibrils. (From Fawcett: The Cell. Philadelphia, W. B. Saunders Company, 1981.)

fiber membrane, this causes the release of large quantities of calcium ions into the sarcoplasm surrounding the myofibrils. These calcium ions in turn activate the forces between the filaments, and contraction begins, but energy is also needed for the contractile process to proceed. This energy is derived from the high-energy bonds of ATP, which is degraded to adenosine diphosphate (ADP) to liberate the energy required.

In the next few sections, we describe what is known about the details of the molecular processes of contraction. To begin this discussion, however, we must first characterize in detail the myosin and actin filaments.

Molecular Characteristics of the Contractile Filaments

The Myosin Filament. The myosin filament is composed of multiple myosin molecules, each having a molecular weight of about 480,000. Figure 6-5A illustrates an individual molecule; section B illus-

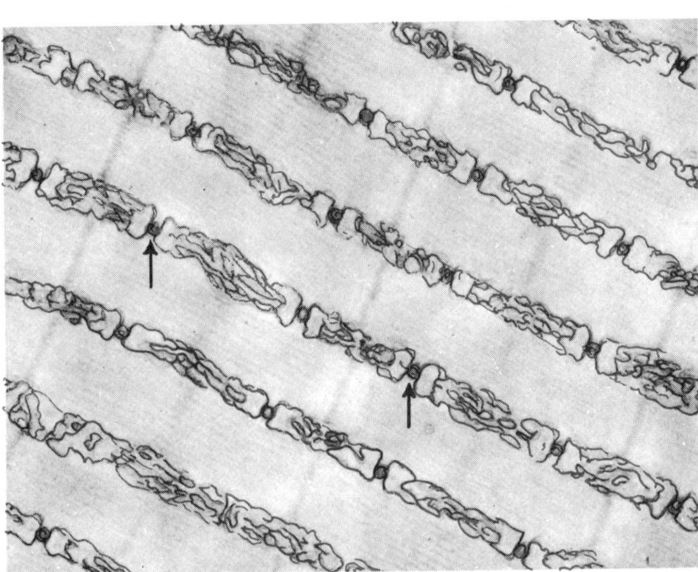

Figure 6-3. Sarcoplasmic reticulum surrounding the myofibrils, showing the longitudinal system paralleling the myofibrils. Also shown in cross-section are the T tubules (arrows) that lead to the exterior of the fiber membrane and that contain extracellular fluid. (From Fawcett: The Cell. Philadelphia, W. B. Saunders Company, 1981.)

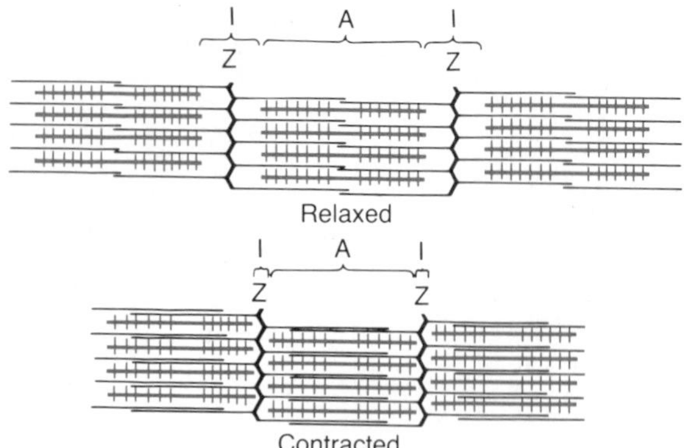

Figure 6-4. The relaxed and contracted states of a myofibril, showing sliding of the actin filaments (black) into the spaces between the myosin filaments (red).

trates the organization of the molecules to form a myosin filament as well as its interaction on one side with the ends of two actin filaments.

The *myosin molecule* is composed of six polypeptide chains: two *heavy chains* each with a molecular weight of about 200,000 and four *light chains* with molecular weights of about 20,000 each. The two heavy chains wrap spirally around each other to form a double helix. However, one end of each of these chains is folded into a globular protein mass called the myosin *head.* Thus, there are two free heads lying side by side at one end of the double helix myosin molecule; the elongated portion of the coiled helix is called the *tail.* The four light chains are also parts of the myosin heads, two to each head. These light chains help control the function of the head during the process of muscle contraction.

The *myosin filament* is made up of 200 or more individual myosin molecules. The central portion of

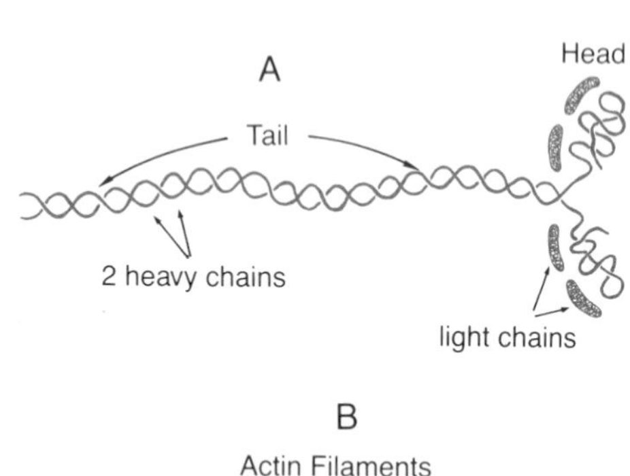

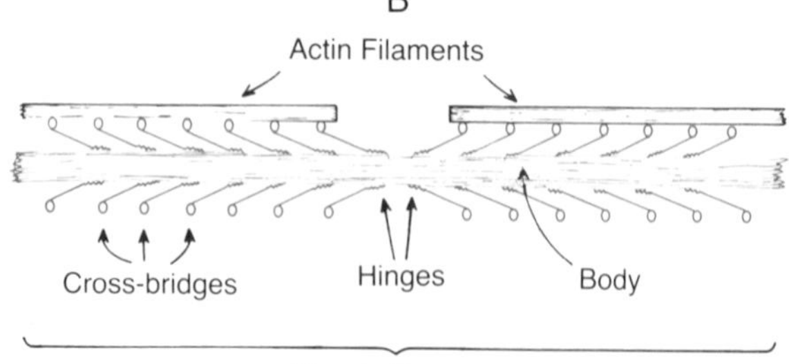

Figure 6-5. *A,* The myosin molecule. *B,* Combination of many myosin molecules to form a myosin filament. Also shown are the cross-bridges and the interaction between the heads of the cross-bridges and adjacent actin filaments.

one of these filaments is illustrated in Figure 6-5B, showing the tails of the myosin molecules bundled together to form the *body* of the filament, while many heads of the molecules hang outward to the sides of the body. Also, part of the helix portion of each myosin molecule extends to the side along with the head, thus providing an *arm* that extends the head outward from the body, as shown in the figure. The protruding arms and heads together are called *cross-bridges.* Each cross-bridge is believed to be flexible at two points called *hinges,* one where the arm leaves the body of the myosin filament and the other where the two heads attach to the arm. The hinged arms allow the heads either to be extended far outward from the body of the myosin filament or to be brought close to the body. The hinged heads are believed to participate in the actual contraction process.

The total length of each myosin filament is very uniform, almost exactly 1.6 micrometers. However, note that there are no cross-bridge heads in the very center of the myosin filament because the hinged arms extend toward both ends of the myosin filament away from the center; therefore, in the center there are only tails of the myosin molecules and no heads.

ATPase Activity of the Myosin Head. Another feature of the myosin head that is essential for muscle contraction is that it functions as an ATPase enzyme. As we see later, this property allows the head to cleave ATP and to use the energy derived from the ATP's high-energy phosphate bond to energize the contraction process.

The Actin Filament. The actin filament is also complex. It is composed of three different protein components: *actin, tropomyosin,* and *troponin.*

The backbone of the actin filament is a double-stranded F-actin protein molecule, illustrated by the two lighter-colored strands in Figure 6-6. The two strands are wound in a helix in the same manner as the myosin molecule.

Each strand of the double F-actin helix is composed of polymerized G-actin molecules, each having a molecular weight of about 42,000. There are approximately 13 of these molecules in each revolution of each strand of helix. Attached to each one of the G-actin molecules is one molecule of ADP. It is believed that these ADP molecules are the active sites on the actin filaments with which the cross-bridges of the myosin filaments interact to cause muscle contraction.

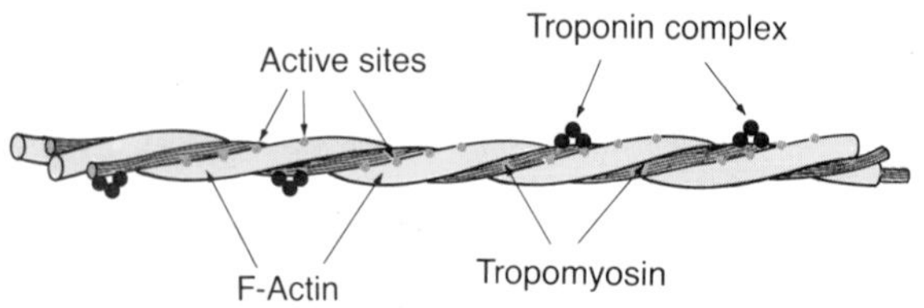

Figure 6-6. The actin filament, composed of two helical strands of F-actin and tropomyosin molecules that fit loosely in the grooves between the actin strands. Attached to one end of each tropomyosin molecule is a troponin complex that initiates contraction.

Each actin filament is approximately 1 micrometer long. The bases of the actin filaments are inserted strongly into the Z discs, while the other ends protrude in both directions into the adjacent sarcomeres to lie in the spaces between the myosin molecules, as illustrated in Figure 6–4.

Tropomyosin Molecules. The actin filament also contains another protein, *tropomyosin.* Each molecule of tropomyosin has a molecular weight of 70,000 and a length of 40 nanometers. These molecules are connected loosely with the F-actin strands, wrapped spirally around the sides of the F-actin helix. In the resting state, the tropomyosin molecules are believed to lie on top of the active sites of the actin strands, so that attraction cannot occur between the actin and myosin filaments to cause contraction.

Troponin and Its Role in Muscle Contraction. Attached near one end of each tropomyosin molecule is still another protein molecule called *troponin.* This is actually a complex of three loosely bound protein subunits, each of which plays a specific role in the control of muscular contraction. One of the subunits (troponin I) has a strong affinity for actin, another (troponin T) for tropomyosin, and a third (troponin C) for calcium ions. This complex is believed to attach the tropomyosin to the actin. The strong affinity of the troponin for calcium ions is believed to initiate the contraction process, as is explained in the following section.

Interaction of Myosin, Actin Filaments, and Calcium Ions to Cause Contraction

Inhibition of the Actin Filament by the Troponin-Tropomyosin Complex; Activation by Calcium Ions. A pure actin filament without the presence of the troponin-tropomyosin complex binds strongly with myosin molecules in the presence of magnesium ions and ATP, both of which are normally abundant in the myofibril. However, if the troponin-tropomyosin complex is added to the actin filament, this binding does not take place. Therefore, it is believed that the active sites on the normal actin filament of the relaxed muscle are inhibited or actually physically covered by the troponin-tropomyosin complex. Consequently, the sites cannot attach to the myosin filaments to cause contraction. Before contraction can take place, the inhibitory effect of the troponin-tropomyosin complex must itself be inhibited.

Now, let us discuss the role of the calcium ions. In the presence of large amounts of calcium ions, the inhibitory effect of the troponin-tropomyosin on the actin filaments is itself inhibited. The mechanism of this is not known, but one suggestion is the following: When calcium ions combine with troponin C, the troponin complex supposedly undergoes a conformational change that in some way tugs on the tropomyosin molecule and moves it deeper into the groove between the two actin strands. This "uncovers" the active sites of the actin, thus allowing contraction to proceed. Although this is a hypothetical mechanism, nevertheless it does emphasize that the normal relationship between the tropomyosin-troponin complex and actin is altered by calcium ions, producing a new condition that leads to contraction.

Interaction Between the "Activated" Actin Filament and the Myosin Cross-Bridges — The "Walk-Along" Theory of Contraction. As soon as the actin filament becomes activated by the calcium ions, the heads of the cross-bridges from the myosin filaments immediately become attracted to the active sites of the actin filament, and this in some way causes contraction to occur. Although the precise manner by which this interaction between the cross-bridges and the actin causes contraction is still unknown, a suggested hypothesis for which considerable evidence exists is the "walk-along" theory (or *"ratchet" theory) of contraction.*

Figure 6–7 illustrates the postulated walk-along mechanism for contraction. This figure shows the heads of two cross-bridges attaching to and disengaging from the active sites of an actin filament. It is postulated that when the head attaches to an active site, this attachment simultaneously causes profound changes in the intramolecular forces between the head and arm of the cross-bridge. The new alignment of forces causes the head to tilt toward the arm and to drag the actin filament along with it. This tilt of the head is called the *power stroke.* Then, immediately after tilting, the head automatically breaks away from the attach site. Next, the head returns to its normal perpendicular direction. In this position it combines with a new active site farther down along the actin filament; then, the head tilts again to cause a new power stroke, and the actin filament moves another step. Thus, the heads of the cross-bridges bend back and forth and step by step walk along the actin filament, pulling the ends of the actin filaments toward the center of the myosin filament.

Each one of the cross-bridges is believed to operate independently of all others, each attaching and pulling in a continuous but random cycle. Therefore, the greater the number of cross-bridges in contact with the actin filament at any given time, the greater, theoretically, is the force of contraction.

ATP as the Source of Energy for Contraction — Chemical Events in the Motion of the Myosin Heads. When a muscle contracts against a load, work is performed and energy is required. Large amounts of

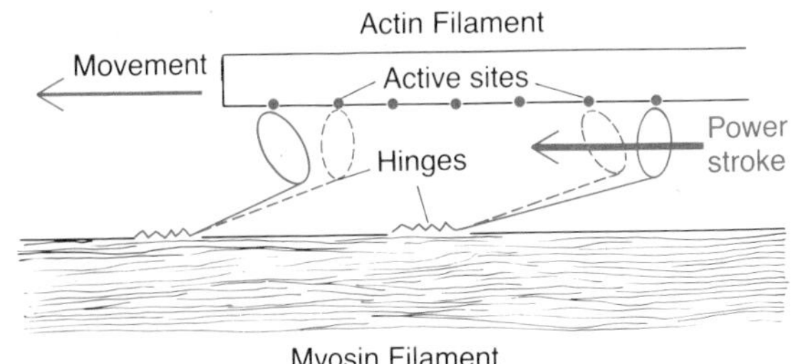

Figure 6–7. The "walk-along" mechanism for contraction of the muscle.

ATP are cleaved to form ADP during the contraction process. Furthermore, the greater the amount of work performed by the muscle, the greater the amount of ATP that is cleaved. Although it is still not known exactly how ATP is used to provide the energy for contraction, the following is a sequence of events that has been suggested as the means by which this occurs:

1. Before contraction begins, the heads of the cross-bridges bind with ATP. The ATPase activity of the myosin head immediately cleaves the ATP but leaves the cleavage products, ADP plus Pi, bound to the head. In this state, the conformation of the head is such that it extends perpendicularly toward the actin filament but is not yet attached to the actin.
2. Next, when the inhibitory effect of the troponin-tropomyosin complex is itself inhibited by calcium ions, active sites on the actin filament are uncovered, and the myosin heads do then bind with these, as illustrated in Figure 6–7.
3. The bond between the head of the cross-bridge and the active site of the actin filament causes a conformational change in the head, prompting the head to tilt toward the arm of the cross-bridge. This provides the *power stroke* for pulling the actin filament. The energy that activates the power stroke is the energy already stored, like a "cocked" spring, by the conformational change in the head when the ATP molecule had been cleaved.
4. Once the head of the cross-bridge is tilted, this allows release of the ADP and Pi that were previously attached to the head; at the site of release of the ADP, a new molecule of ATP binds. This binding in turn causes detachment of the head from the actin.
5. After the head has detached from the actin, the new molecule of ATP is also cleaved, and the energy again "cocks" the head back to its perpendicular condition ready to begin a new power stroke cycle.

Thus, the process proceeds again and again until the actin filament pulls the Z membrane up against the ends of the myosin filaments or until the load on the muscle becomes too great for further pulling to occur.

Degree of Actin and Myosin Filament Overlap—Effect on Tension Developed by the Contracting Muscle

Figure 6–8 illustrates the effect of sarcomere length and of myosin-actin filament overlap on the active tension developed by a contracting muscle fiber. To the right are illustrated different degrees of overlap of the myosin and actin filaments at different sarcomere lengths. At point D on the diagram, the actin filament has pulled all the way out to the end of the myosin filament with no overlap at all. At this

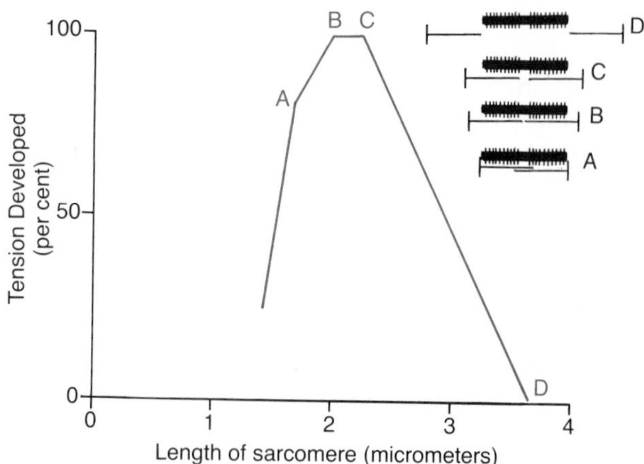

Figure 6–8. Length-tension diagram for a single sarcomere, illustrating maximum strength of contraction when the sarcomere is 2.0 to 2.2 micrometers in length. At the upper right are shown the relative positions of the actin and myosin filaments at different sarcomere lengths from point A to point D. (Modified from Gordon, Huxley, and Julian: The length-tension diagram of single vertebrate striated muscle fibers. *J. Physiol., 171*:28P, 1964.)

point, the tension developed by the activated muscle is zero. Then, as the sarcomere shortens and the actin filament begins to overlap the myosin filament, the tension increases progressively until the sarcomere length decreases to about 2.2 micrometers. At this point, the actin filament has already overlapped all the cross-bridges of the myosin filament but has not yet reached the center of the myosin filament. Upon further shortening, the sarcomere maintains full tension until point B at a sarcomere length of approximately 2.0 micrometers. At this point, the ends of the two actin filaments begin to overlap each other, in addition to overlapping the myosin filaments. As the sarcomere length falls from 2 micrometers down to about 1.65 micrometers, at point A, the strength of contraction decreases. At this point the two Z discs of the sarcomere abut the ends of the myosin filaments. Then, as contraction proceeds to still shorter sarcomere lengths, the ends of the myosin filaments are actually crumpled, and as illustrated in the figure, the strength of contraction also decreases precipitously.

This diagram illustrates that maximum contraction occurs when there is maximum overlap between the actin filaments and the cross-bridges of the myosin filaments, and it supports the idea that the greater the number of cross-bridges pulling the actin filaments, the greater the strength of contraction.

INITIATION OF MUSCLE CONTRACTION: EXCITATION-CONTRACTION COUPLING

Initiation of contraction in skeletal muscle begins with action potentials in the muscle fibers. These elicit electrical currents that spread to the interior of the fiber, where they cause release of calcium ions from the sarcoplasmic reticulum. It is the calcium ions that in turn initiate the chemical events of the contractile process. This overall process for controlling muscle contraction is called *excitation-contraction coupling.*

The Muscle Action Potential

Almost everything discussed in Chapter 5 regarding initiation and conduction of action potentials in nerve fibers applies equally well to skeletal muscle fibers, except for quantitative differences. Some of the quantitative aspects of muscle potentials are the following:

1. Resting membrane potential: Approximately −80 to −90 millivolts in skeletal fibers—the same as in large myelinated nerve fibers.
2. Duration of action potential: 1 to 5 milliseconds in skeletal muscle—about five times as long as in large myelinated nerves.
3. Velocity of conduction: 3 to 5 meters per second—about 1/18 the velocity of conduction in the large myelinated nerve fibers that excite skeletal muscle.

Excitation of Skeletal Muscle Fibers by Nerves. In normal function of the body, skeletal muscle fibers are excited by large myelinated nerve fibers. These attach to the skeletal muscle fibers at the neuromuscular junction, which will be discussed in detail in the following chapter. Except for 2 per cent of the muscle fibers, there is only one neuromuscular junction to each muscle fiber; this junction is located near the middle of the fiber. Therefore, the action potential spreads from the middle of the fiber toward its two ends. This dual direction of spreading from the center is important because it allows nearly coincident contraction of all sarcomeres of the muscles so that they can all contract together rather than separately.

Spread of the Action Potential to the Interior of the Muscle Fiber by Way of the Transverse Tubule System

The skeletal muscle fiber is so large that action potentials spreading along its surface membrane cause almost no current flow deep within the fiber. Yet, to cause contraction, electrical currents must penetrate to the vicinity of all the separate myofibrils. This is achieved by transmission of the action potentials along *transverse tubules* (T tubules) that penetrate all the way through the muscle fiber from one side to the other. The T tubule action potentials in turn cause the sarcoplasmic reticulum to release calcium ions in the immediate vicinity of all the myofibrils, and these calcium ions then cause contraction. This overall process is called *excitation-contraction* coupling. Now, let us describe this in much greater detail.

The Transverse Tubule–Sarcoplasmic Reticulum System

Figure 6–9 illustrates several myofibrils surrounded by the transverse tubule–sarcoplasmic reticulum system. The transverse tubules are very small and run transverse to the myofibrils. They begin at the cell membrane and penetrate all the way from one side of the muscle fiber to the opposite side. Not shown in the figure is the fact that these tubules branch among themselves so that they form entire *planes* of T tubules interlacing among all the separate myofibrils. Also, it should be noted that *where the T tubules originate from the cell membrane they are open to the exterior.* Therefore, they communicate with the fluid surrounding the muscle fiber and contain extracellular fluid in their lumens. In other words, the T tubules are internal extensions of the cell membrane. Therefore, when an action potential spreads over a muscle fiber membrane, it spreads along the T tubules to the deep interior of the muscle fiber as well. The action potential currents surrounding these transverse tubules then elicit the muscle contraction.

Figure 6–9 shows the *sarcoplasmic reticulum* as well, shown in red. This is composed of two major parts: (1) long *longitudinal tubules* that run parallel to the myofibrils and terminate in (2) large chambers called *terminal cisternae* that abut the transverse tubules.

Release of Calcium Ions by the Sarcoplasmic Reticulum

One of the special features of the sarcoplasmic reticulum is that it contains calcium ions in very high concentration, and many of these ions are released when the adjacent T tubule is excited.

Figure 6–10 shows that the action potential of the T tubule causes current flow through the tips of the cisternae that abut the T tubule. At these points, each cisterna projects *junctional feet* that attach to the membrane of the T tubule, presumably facilitating passage of some signal from the T tubule to the cisterna. Possibly this signal is electical current of the action potential itself. However, there are also reasons to believe that it could be some chemical or mechanical signal. Whatever the signal, it causes rapid opening of large numbers of calcium channels through the membranes of the cisternae and their attached longitudinal tubules of the sarcoplasmic reticulum. These channels remain open for a few milliseconds; during this time the calcium ions responsible for muscle contraction are released into the sarcoplasm surrounding the myofibrils.

The calcium ions that are thus released from the sarcoplasmic reticulum diffuse to the adjacent myofibrils, where they bind strongly with troponin C, as discussed earlier in the chapter, and this in turn elicits the muscle contraction.

The Calcium Pump for Removing Calcium Ions from the Sarcoplasmic Fluid. Once the calcium ions have been released from the sarcoplasmic tubules and have diffused to the myofibrils, muscle contraction will continue as long as the calcium ions remain in high concentration in the sarcoplasmic

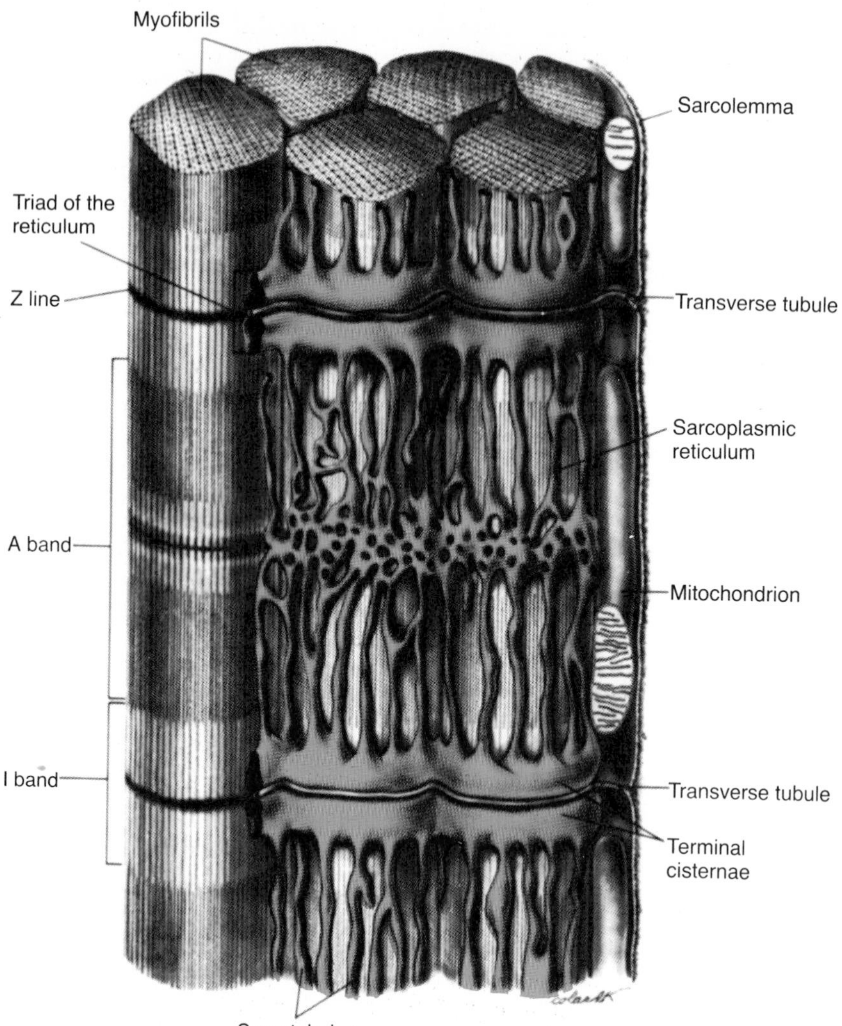

Figure 6–9. The transverse tubule–sarcoplasmic reticulum system. Note the *longitudinal tubules* that terminate in large *cisternae.* The cisternae in turn abut the transverse tubules. Note also that the transverse tubules communicate with the outside of the cell membrane. This illustration was drawn from frog muscle, which has one transverse tubule per sarcomere, located at the Z line. A similar arrangement is found in mammalian heart muscle, but mammalian skeletal muscle has two transverse tubules per sarcomere, located at the A-I junctions. (From Fawcett: Bloom and Fawcett: A Textbook of Histology. Philadelphia, W. B. Saunders Company, 1986. Modified after Peachey: *J. Cell Biol., 25:*209, 1965. Drawn by Sylvia Colard Keene.)

fluid. However, a continually active calcium pump located in the walls of the sarcoplasmic reticulum pumps calcium ions out of the sarcoplasmic fluid back into the sarcoplasmic tubules. This pump can concentrate the calcium ions about 10,000-fold inside the sarcoplasmic reticulum. In addition, inside the reticulum is a protein called *calsequestrin* that can bind over 40 times as much calcium as that in the ionic state, thus providing another 40-fold increase in the storage of calcium. Thus, this massive transfer of calcium into

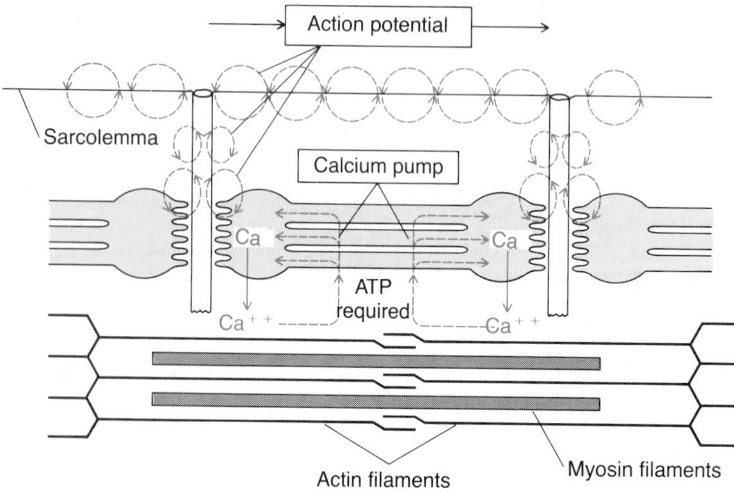

Figure 6–10. Excitation-contraction coupling in the muscle, showing an action potential that causes release of calcium ions from the sarcoplasmic reticulum and then reuptake of the calcium ions by a calcium pump.

the sarcoplasmic reticulum causes virtual total depletion of calcium ions in the fluid of the myofibrils. Therefore, except immediately after an action potential, the calcium ion concentration in the myofibrils is kept at an extremely low level.

The Excitatory "Pulse" of Calcium Ions. The normal concentration (less than 10^{-7} molar) of calcium ions in the cytosol that bathes the myofibrils is too little to elicit contraction. Therefore, in the resting state, the troponin-tropomyosin complex keeps the actin filaments inhibited and maintains a relaxed state of the muscle.

On the other hand, full excitation of the T tubule–sarcoplasmic reticulum system causes enough release of calcium ions to increase the concentration in the myofibrillar fluid to as high as 2×10^{-4} molar concentration, which is about ten times the level required to cause maximum muscle contraction (about 2×10^{-5} molar). Immediately thereafter, the calcium pump depletes the calcium ions again. The total duration of this calcium "pulse" in the usual skeletal muscle fiber lasts about 1/20 second, though it may last several times as long as this in some skeletal muscle fibers and be several times shorter in others (in heart muscle, the calcium pulse lasts for as long as 1/3 second because of the long duration of the cardiac action potential). It is during this calcium pulse that muscle contraction occurs. If the contraction is to continue without interruption for longer intervals, a series of such pulses must be initiated by a continuous series of repetitive action potentials, as discussed later in the chapter.

EFFICIENCY OF MUSCLE CONTRACTION

The efficiency of an engine or a motor is calculated as the percentage of energy input that is converted into muscle work instead of heat. The percentage of the input energy to the muscle (the chemical energy in the nutrients) that can be converted into muscle work is less than 20 to 25 per cent, the remainder becoming heat. The reason for this low efficiency is that about half of the energy in the foodstuffs is lost during the formation of ATP, and even then only 40 to 45 per cent of the energy in the ATP itself can later be converted into work. Also, maximum efficiency can be realized only when the muscle contracts at a moderate velocity. If the muscle contracts very slowly or without any movement at all, large amounts of *maintenance heat* are released during the process of contraction even though little or no work is being performed, thereby decreasing the efficiency. On the other hand, if contraction is too rapid, large proportions of the energy are used to overcome the viscous friction within the muscle itself, and this, too, reduces the efficiency of contraction. Ordinarily, maximum efficiency is developed when the velocity of contraction is about 30 per cent of maximum.

CHARACTERISTICS OF A SINGLE MUSCLE TWITCH

Many features of muscle contraction can be especially well demonstrated by eliciting single *muscle twitches*. This can be accomplished by instantaneously exciting the nerve to a muscle or by passing a short electrical stimulus through the muscle itself, giving rise to a single, sudden contraction lasting for a fraction of a second.

Isometric Versus Isotonic Contraction. Muscle contraction is said to be *isometric* when the muscle does not shorten during contraction and *isotonic* when it shortens with the tension on the muscle remaining constant.

There are several basic differences between isometric and isotonic contractions. First, isometric contraction does not require much sliding of myofibrils among each other. Second, in isotonic contraction a load is moved, which involves the phenomena of inertia. That is, the weight or other type of object being moved must first be accelerated, and once a velocity has been attained the load has momentum that causes it to continue moving even after the contraction is over. Therefore, an isotonic contraction is likely to last considerably longer than an isometric contraction of the same muscle. Third, isotonic contraction entails the performance of external work. Therefore, a greater amount of energy is used by the muscle.

Muscles can contract both isometrically and isotonically in the body, but most contractions are actually a mixture of the two. When standing, a person tenses the quadriceps muscles to tighten the knee joints and to keep the legs stiff. This is isometric contraction. On the other hand, when a person lifts a weight using the biceps, this is mainly an isotonic contraction. Finally, contractions of leg muscles during running are a mixture of isometric and isotonic contractions—isometric mainly to keep the limbs stiff when the legs hit the ground and isotonic mainly to move the limbs.

Characteristics of Isometric Twitches Recorded from Different Muscles. The body has many different sizes of skeletal muscles—from the very small stapedius muscle of only a few millimeters length and a millimeter or so in diameter up to the very large quadriceps muscle. Furthermore, the fibers may be as small as 10 microns in diameter or as large as 80 microns. And, finally, the energetics of muscle contraction vary considerably from one muscle to another. These different physical and chemical characteristics often manifest themselves in the form of different speeds of contraction: some muscles contract rapidly while others contract slowly.

Fast Versus Slow Muscle. Figure 6–11 illustrates isometric contractions of three different types of skeletal muscles: an ocular muscle, which has a duration of contraction of less than 1/40 second; the gastrocnemius muscle, which has a duration of contraction of about 1/15 second; and the soleus muscle, which has a duration of contraction of about 1/5 sec-

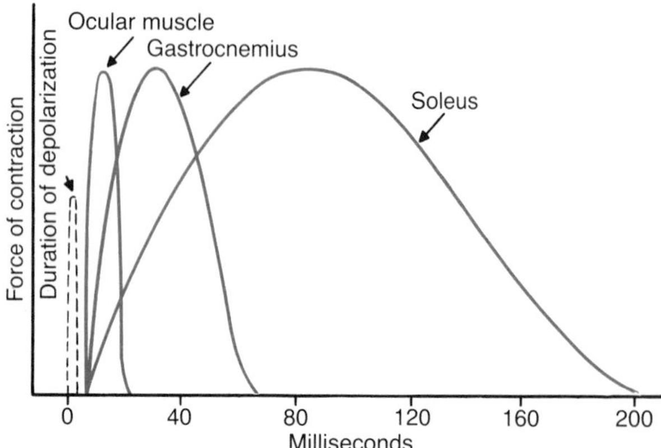

Figure 6-11. Duration of isometric contractions of different types of mammalian muscles, showing also a latent period between the action potential and muscle contraction.

ond. It is interesting that these durations of contractions are adapted to the function of each of the respective muscles, for ocular movements must be extremely rapid to maintain fixation of the eyes upon specific objects, the gastrocnemius muscle must contract moderately rapidly to provide sufficient velocity of limb movement for running and jumping, while the soleus muscle is concerned principally with slow reactions for continual support of the body against gravity.

As we shall discuss more fully in Chapter 57 on sports physiology, every muscle of the body is composed of a mixture of so-called *fast* and *slow* muscle fibers, with still other fibers graduated between these two extremes. The muscles that react very rapidly usually are composed mainly of the fast fibers, which are much larger and contain a much more extensive sarcoplasmic reticulum than found in the slow fibers.

MECHANICS OF SKELETAL MUSCLE CONTRACTION

The Motor Unit

Each motor nerve fiber that leaves the spinal cord usually innervates many different muscle fibers, the number depending on the type of muscle. All the muscle fibers innervated by a single motor nerve fiber are called a *motor unit.* In general, small muscles that react rapidly and whose control is exact have few muscle fibers in each motor unit (as few as two to three in some of the laryngeal muscles) and have a large number of nerve fibers going to each muscle. On the other hand, the large muscles that do not require a very fine degree of control, such as the gastrocnemius muscle, may have several hundred muscle fibers in a motor unit. An average figure for all the muscles of the body can be considered to be about 150 muscle fibers to the motor unit.

Summation of Muscle Contraction

Summation means the adding together of individual muscle twitches to make strong and concerted muscle movements. In general, summation occurs in two different ways: (1) by increasing the number of motor units contracting simultaneously, and (2) by increasing the rapidity of contraction of individual motor units. These are called, respectively, *multiple motor unit summation* and *frequency summation.*

Frequency Summation and Tetanization. When a muscle is stimulated at progressively greater frequencies, its degree of contraction becomes progressively greater, which is *frequency* summation. This is illustrated in Figure 6-12. Also, at the higher frequencies of stimulation the successive contractions fuse together and cannot be distinguished one from the other. This state is called *tetanization,* and the lowest frequency at which it occurs is called the *critical frequency.*

Tetanization results partly from the viscous properties of the muscle and partly from the nature of the contractile process itself. The muscle fibers are filled with sarcoplasm, which is a viscous fluid, and the fibers are encased in fasciae and muscle sheaths that have a viscous resistance to change in length. Therefore, these viscous factors play a role in causing the successive contractions to fuse with each other.

But in addition to the viscous property of muscle, the activation process itself lasts for a definite period of time, and successive pulsatile states of activation of the muscle fiber can occur so rapidly that they fuse into a long continual state of activation; that is, the level of free calcium ions in the myofibrils remains continuously above the level required for full activation of the contractile process, thus providing an uninterrupted stimulus for maintenance of contraction. Once the critical frequency for tetanization is reached, further increase in rate of stimulation increases the force of contraction only a few more per cent, as shown in Figure 6-12.

Maximum Strength of Contraction. The maximum strength of tetanic contraction of a muscle operating at a normal muscle length is about 3.5 kilograms per square centimeter of muscle, or 50 pounds per square inch. Since a quadriceps muscle can at times

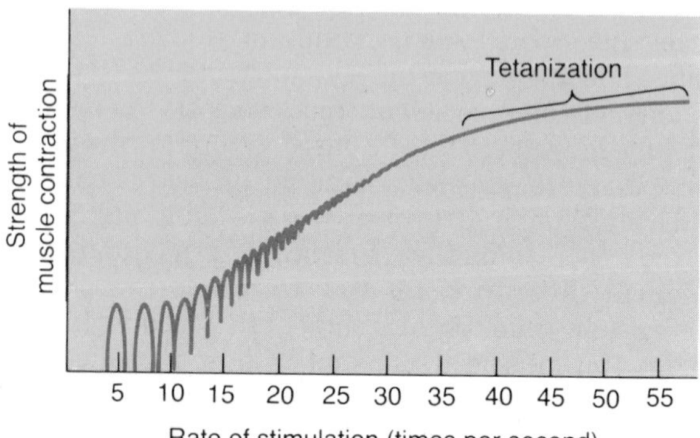

Figure 6-12. Frequency summation and tetanization.

have as much as 16 square inches of muscle belly, as much as 800 pounds of tension may at times be applied to the patellar tendon. One can readily understand, therefore, how it is possible for muscles sometimes to pull their tendons out of the insertions in bones.

MUSCLE FATIGUE

Prolonged and strong contraction of a muscle leads to the well-known state of muscle fatigue. Studies in athletes have shown that muscle fatigue increases in almost direct proportion to the rate of depletion of muscle glycogen. Therefore, most fatigue probably results simply from inability of the contractile and metabolic processes of the muscle fibers to continue supplying the same work output. However, experiments have also shown that transmission of the nerve signal through the neuromuscular junction can occasionally diminish following prolonged muscle activity, thus further diminishing muscle contraction.

Interruption of blood flow through a contracting muscle leads to almost complete muscle fatigue within a minute or more because of the obvious loss of nutrient supply—especially loss of oxygen.

REMODELING OF MUSCLE TO MATCH FUNCTION

All the muscles of the body are continually being remodeled to match the functions that are required of them. Their diameters are altered, their lengths are altered, their strengths are altered, their vascular supplies are altered, and even the types of muscle fibers are altered at least to a slight extent. This remodeling process is often quite rapid, within a few weeks. Indeed, experiments have shown that even normally the muscle contractile proteins can be totally replaced once every 2 weeks.

Muscle Hypertrophy and Muscle Atrophy

When the total mass of a muscle enlarges, this is called *muscle hypertrophy.* When it decreases, the process is called *muscle atrophy.*

Virtually all muscle hypertrophy results from hypertrophy of the individual muscle fibers, which is called simply *fiber hypertrophy.* This usually occurs in response to contraction of a muscle at maximal or almost maximal force. Hypertrophy occurs to a much greater extent when the muscle is simultaneously stretched during the contractile process. Only a few such strong contractions each day are required to cause almost maximum hypertrophy within 6 to 10 weeks.

Unfortunately, the manner in which forceful contraction leads to hypertrophy is not known. Yet it is known that the rate of synthesis of muscle contractile proteins is far greater during developing hypertrophy than their rate of decay, leading to progressively greater numbers of both actin and myosin filaments in the myofibrils. In turn, the myofibrils themselves split within each muscle fiber to form new myofibrils. Thus, it is mainly this great increase in numbers of additional myofibrils that causes muscle fibers to hypertrophy.

Along with the increasing numbers of myofibrils, the enzyme systems that provide energy also increase. This is especially true of the enzymes for glycolysis, allowing a rapid supply of energy during short-term forceful muscle contraction.

When a muscle remains unused for long periods of time, the rate of decay of the contractile proteins as well as the numbers of myofibrils occurs more rapidly than the rate of replacement. Therefore, muscle atrophy occurs.

Effects of Muscle Denervation

When a muscle loses its nerve supply, it no longer receives the contractile signals that are required to maintain normal muscle size. Therefore, atrophy begins almost immediately. After about 2 months, degenerative changes also begin to appear in the muscle fibers themselves. If the nerve supply grows back to the muscle, full return of function will usually occur up to about 3 months, but from that time onward the capability of functional return becomes less and less, with no return of function after 1 to 2 years. In the final stage of denervation atrophy, most of the muscle fibers are completely destroyed and replaced by fibrous and fatty tissue.

REFERENCES

Clausen, T.: Regulation of active Na^+-K^+ transport in skeletal muscle. Physiol. Rev., 66:542, 1986.

Gowitzke, B. A., et al.: Scientific Bases of Human Movement. Baltimore, Williams & Wilkins, 1988.

Haynes, D. H., and Mandveno, A.: Computer modeling of Ca^{2+}–Mg^{2+}–ATPase of sarcoplasmic reticulum. Physiol. Rev., 67:244, 1987.

Huxley, A. F.: Muscular Contraction. Annu. Rev. Physiol., 50:1, 1988.

Huxley, A. F., and Gordon, A. M.: Striation patterns in active and passive shortening of muscle. Nature (Lond.), 193:280, 1962.

Huxley, H. E., and Faruqi, A. R.: Time-resolved x-ray diffraction studies on vertebrate striated muscle. Annu. Rev. Biophys. Bioeng., 12:381, 1983.

Laufer, R., et al.: Regulation of acetylcholine receptor biosynthesis during motor endplate morphogenesis. News Physiol. Sci., 4:5, 1989.

Oho, S. J.: Electromyography: Neuromuscular Transmission Studies. Baltimore, Williams & Wilkins, 1988.

Rios, E., and Pizarro, G.: Voltage sensors and calcium channels of excitation-contraction coupling. News Physiol. Sci., 3:223, 1988.

Rowland, L. P., et al. (eds.): Molecular Genetics in Diseases of Brain, Nerve, and Muscle. New York, Oxford University Press, 1989.

Soderberg, G. L.: Kinesiology. Baltimore, Williams & Wilkins, 1986.

Steinbach, J. H.: Structural and functional diversity in vertebrate skeletal muscle nicotinic acetylcholine receptors. Annu. Rev. Physiol., 51:353, 1989.

Sugi, H., and Pollack, G. H. (eds.): Molecular Mechanism of Muscle Contraction. New York, Plenum Publishing Corp., 1988.

Vergara, J., and Asotra, K.: The chemical transmission mechanism of excitation-contraction coupling in skeletal muscle. News Physiol. Sci., 2:182, 1987.

QUESTIONS

1. Describe the component parts of a skeletal muscle fiber, beginning with the fiber itself; then describe the nature of the myofibrils and the organization of myosin and actin filaments in the myofibrils.
2. How are the actin and myosin filaments organized within each sarcomere of the skeletal muscle fiber?
3. Describe the manner in which the sarcolemma attaches to the tendons.
4. Explain the manner in which the actin and myosin filaments interdigitate with each other to cause contraction.
5. How do multiple myosin molecules combine with each other to form the myosin filament?
6. Describe the cross-bridges of the myosin filaments and their component parts.
7. Describe the manner in which the actin molecules are combined together to form the actin filament.
8. Explain the relationship of tropomyosin and troponin to the actin filament.
9. Explain the manner in which the myosin and actin filaments interact with each other to cause contraction by the "walk-along" mechanism.
10. Give the postulated steps for the mechanism by which ATP is used as an energy source to cause the power stroke of the myosin heads.
11. Explain why the strength of contraction of a skeletal muscle fiber is determined by the degree of overlap of the actin and myosin filaments. Also, what is the relationship between sarcomere length and strength of contraction?
12. Describe the organization of the sarcoplasmic reticulum in the skeletal muscle fiber, and also explain the relationship of the transverse tubules to this sarcoplasmic reticulum.
13. How does the muscle action potential travel to the interior of the skeletal muscle fiber?
14. Explain how the "pulse" of calcium ions in the sarcoplasm occurs and how the calcium ions disappear during each skeletal muscle twitch.
15. Explain the postulated mechanism by which calcium ions cause muscle contraction.
16. What is meant by efficiency of muscle contraction? Approximately how efficient is the contraction of most skeletal muscle?
17. Explain the difference between *isometric* and *isotonic* muscle contractions.
18. Explain how muscle contraction summates as a result of *multiple motor unit summation* and *wave summation.*
19. What is meant by *tetanization* during muscle contraction, and what causes this?
20. If a muscle has 10 square centimeters of cross-sectional area, what will be its approximate maximal strength of contraction?
21. What factors can lead to muscle fatigue?
22. What type of muscle contraction leads to muscle hypertrophy, and what are the changes in the muscle itself?
23. What factors can lead to muscle atrophy? Following denervation, how long can a muscle fiber remain alive while awaiting a nerve fiber to reinnervate it?

7

Neuromuscular Transmission; Function of Smooth Muscle

TRANSMISSION OF IMPULSES FROM NERVES TO SKELETAL MUSCLE FIBERS: THE NEUROMUSCULAR JUNCTION

The skeletal muscle fibers are innervated by large, myelinated nerve fibers that originate in the large motoneurons of the anterior horns of the spinal cord. Each nerve fiber normally branches many times and stimulates from three to several hundred skeletal muscle fibers. The nerve ending makes a junction, called the *neuromuscular junction,* with the muscle fiber near the fiber's midpoint, and the action potential in the fiber travels in both directions toward the muscle fiber ends. With the exception of about 2 per cent of the muscle fibers, there is only one such junction per muscle fiber.

Physiological Anatomy of the Neuromuscular Junction — The "Motor End-Plate." Figure 7–1, parts A and B, illustrates the neuromuscular junction between a large, myelinated nerve fiber and a skeletal muscle fiber. The nerve fiber branches at its end to form a complex of branching nerve *terminals,* which invaginate into the muscle fiber but lie entirely outside the muscle fiber plasma membrane. The entire structure is called the *motor end-plate.* It is covered by one or more Schwann cells that insulate it from the surrounding fluids.

Figure 7–1C shows an electron micrographic sketch of the junction between a single-branch axon terminal and the muscle fiber membrane. The invagination of the membrane is called the *synaptic gutter* or *synaptic trough,* and the space between the terminal and the fiber membrane is called the *synaptic cleft.* The synaptic cleft is 20 to 30 nanometers wide and is occupied by a basal lamina, which is a thin layer of spongy reticular fibers through which diffuses extracellular fluid. At the bottom of the gutter are numerous smaller *folds* of the muscle membrane called *subneural clefts,* which greatly increase the surface area at which the synaptic transmitter can act.

In the axon terminal are many mitochondria that supply energy mainly for synthesis of the excitatory transmitter *acetylcholine* that, in turn, excites the muscle fiber. The acetylcholine is synthesized in the cytoplasm of the terminal but is rapidly absorbed into many small synaptic vesicles, approximately 300,000 of which are normally in the terminals of a single end-plate. Attached to the matrix of the basal lamina are large quantities of the enzyme *acetylcholinesterase,* which is capable of destroying acetylcholine, to be explained in further detail.

Secretion of Acetylcholine by the Nerve Terminals

When a nerve impulse reaches the neuromuscular junction, about 300 vesicles of acetylcholine are released from the terminals into the synaptic trough. Figure 7–2 illustrates some of the details of this mechanism, showing an expanded view of a synaptic trough with the neural membrane above and the muscle membrane and its subneural clefts below.

On the inside surface of the neural membrane are linear *dense bars,* shown in cross-section in Figure 7–2. To each side of each dense bar are protein particles that penetrate the membrane, believed to be voltage-gated calcium channels. When the action potential spreads over the terminal, these channels open and allow large quantities of calcium to diffuse to the interior of the terminal. The calcium ions in turn exert an attractive influence on the acetylcholine ves-

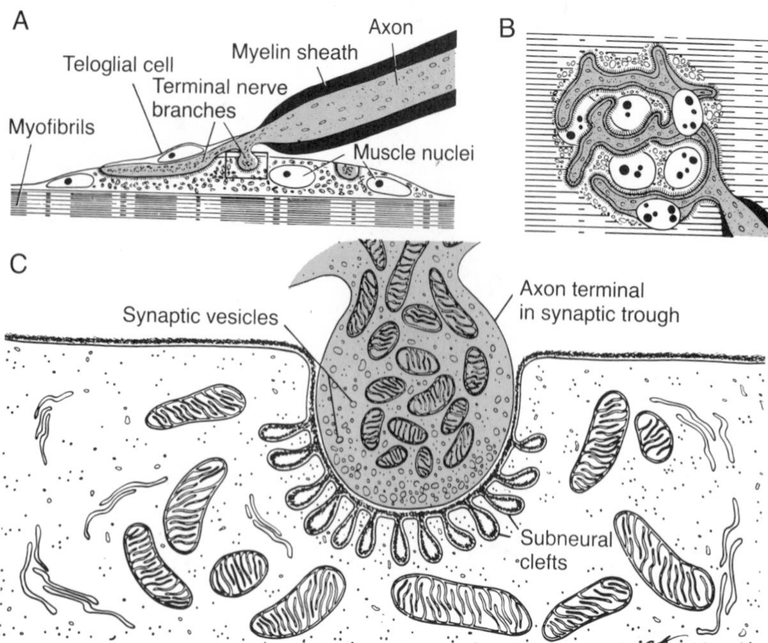

Figure 7-1. Different views of the motor end-plate. *A*, Longitudinal section through the end-plate. *B*, Surface view of the end-plate. *C*, Electron micrographic appearance of the contact point between one of the axon terminals and the muscle fiber membrane, representing the rectangular area shown in *A*. (From Fawcett, as modified from R. Couteaux: Bloom and Fawcett: A Textbook of Histology. Philadelphia, W. B. Saunders Company, 1986.)

icles, drawing them to the neural membrane adjacent to the dense bars. Some of the vesicles fuse with the neural membrane and empty their acetylcholine into the synaptic trough by the process of exocytosis.

Although some of the aforementioned details are still speculative, it is known that the effective stimulus for causing acetylcholine release from the vesicles is entry of calcium ions. Furthermore, the vesicles are emptied through the membrane adjacent to the dense bars.

Effect of Acetylcholine to Open Acetylcholine-Gated Ion Channels. Figure 7-2 shows many acetylcholine receptors in the muscle membrane; these are actually acetylcholine-gated ion channels, located almost entirely near the mouths of the subneural clefts lying immediately below the dense bar areas, where the acetylcholine vesicles empty into the synaptic trough.

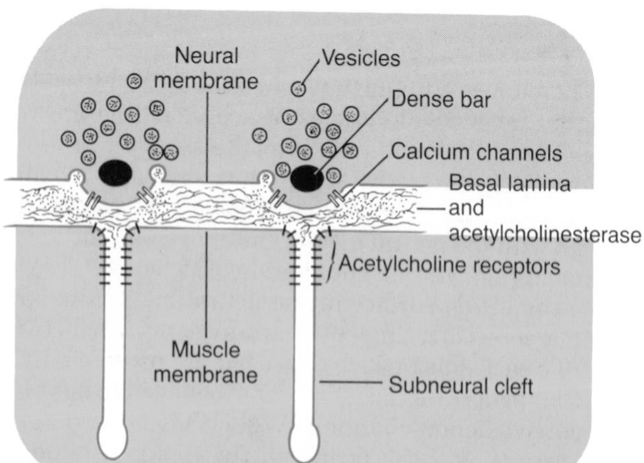

Figure 7-2. Release of acetylcholine from synaptic vesicles at the neural membrane of the neuromuscular junction. Note the close proximity of the release sites to the acetylcholine receptors at the mouths of the subneural clefts.

Each receptor is a large protein complex having a total molecular weight of 275,000. The complex is composed of five subunit proteins, which penetrate all the way through the membrane lying side by side in a circle to form a tubular channel. The channel remains constricted until acetylcholine attaches to one of the subunits. This causes a conformational change that opens the channel, as illustrated in Figure 7-3; the channel in the upper figure has a constricted point, while the bottom one has been opened by attachment of an acetylcholine molecule.

The acetylcholine channel has a diameter when open of about 0.65 nanometer, which is large enough to allow all the important positive ions—sodium (Na^+), potassium (K^+), and calcium (Ca^{++})—to move easily through the opening. On the other hand, negative ions, such as chloride ions, do not pass through because of strong negative charges in the mouth of the channel that repel the negative chloride ions.

However, in practice, far more sodium ions flow through the acetylcholine channels than any other ions for two reasons. First, there are only two positive ions in great enough concentration to matter greatly: sodium ions in the extracellular fluid and potassium ions in the intracellular fluid. Second, the very negative potential on the inside of the muscle membrane, −80 to −90 mV, pulls the positively charged sodium ions to the inside of the fiber, while at the same time preventing the efflux of the potassium ions when they attempt to pass outward.

Therefore, as illustrated in the lower panel of Figure 7-3, the net effect of opening the acetylcholine-gated channels is to allow large numbers of sodium ions to pour to the inside of the fiber, carrying with them large numbers of positive charges. This creates a local potential inside the fiber called the *end-plate potential* of as much as 50 to 75 mV, which initiates an action potential at the muscle membrane and thus causes muscle contraction.

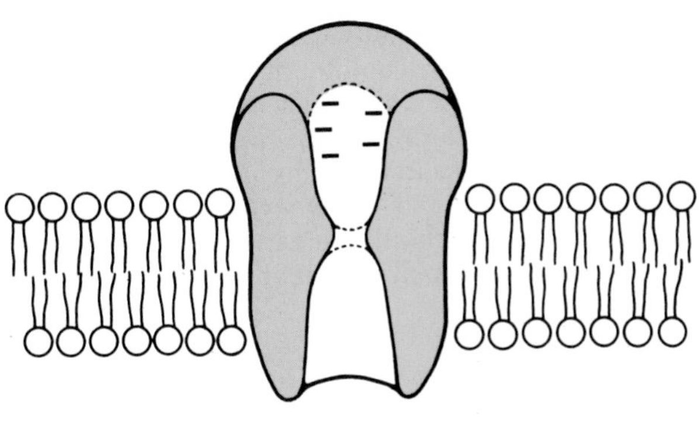

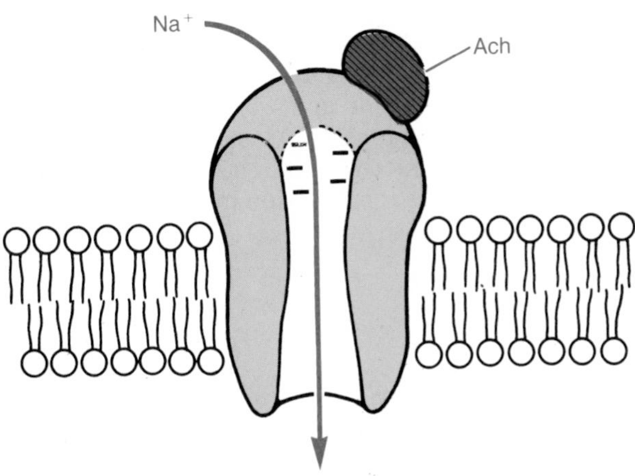

Figure 7-3. The *acetylcholine channel:* Above, while in the closed state. Below, after acetylcholine has become attached and a conformational change has opened the channel, allowing excess sodium to enter the muscle fiber and excite contraction. Note the negative charges at the channel mouth that prevent passage of negative ions.

Destruction of the Released Acetylcholine by Acetylcholinesterase. The acetylcholine, once released into the synaptic trough, continues to activate the acetylcholine receptors as long as it persists in the trough. However, it is rapidly destroyed by the enzyme *acetylcholinesterase* that is attached mainly to the *basal lamina,* a spongy layer of fine connective tissue that fills the synaptic trough between the presynaptic terminal and the postsynaptic muscle membrane.

Yet, the very short period of time that the acetylcholine remains in the synaptic trough—a few milliseconds at most—is almost always sufficient to excite the muscle fiber. Then the rapid removal of the acetylcholine prevents muscle re-excitation after the fiber has recovered from the first action potential.

Molecular Biology of Acetylcholine Formation and Release

Because the neuromuscular junction is large enough to be easily studied, it is one of the few synapses of the nervous system at which most of the details of chemical transmission have been worked out. The formation and release of acetylcholine at this junction occurs in the following stages:

1. Very small vesicles are formed by the Golgi apparatus in the cell body of the motoneuron in the spinal cord. These vesicles are then transported by "streaming" of the axoplasm through the core of the axon from the central cell body to the neuromuscular junction at the tips of the nerve fibers. About 300,000 of these small vesicles collect in the nerve terminals of a single end-plate.
2. Acetylcholine is synthesized in the cytosol of the terminal nerve fibers but is then transported through the membranes of the vesicles to their interior, where it is stored in highly concentrated form, with about 10,000 molecules of acetylcholine in each vesicle.
3. When an action potential arrives at the nerve terminal, this opens many calcium channels in the membrane of the terminal because this terminal has an abundance of voltage-gated calcium channels. As a result, the calcium ion concentration in the terminal increases about 100-fold, which in turn increases the rate of fusion of the acetylcholine vesicles with the terminal membrane about 10,000-fold. As each vesicle fuses, its outer surface ruptures through the cell membrane, thus causing *exocytosis* of acetylcholine into the synaptic cleft. Usually about 200 to 300 vesicles rupture with each action potential. The acetylcholine is then split by acetylcholinesterase into acetate ion and choline, and the choline is actively reabsorbed back into the neural terminal to be reused in forming new acetylcholine. This entire sequence of events occurs in 5 to 10 milliseconds.
4. After each vesicle has released its acetylcholine, the membrane of the vesicle becomes part of the cell membrane. However, the number of vesicles available in the nerve ending is sufficient to allow transmission of only a few thousand nerve impulses. Therefore, for continued function of the neuromuscular junction, the vesicles need to be retrieved from the nerve membrane. Retrieval is achieved by the process of *endocytosis.* Within a few seconds after the action potential is over, "coated pits" appear on the surface of the terminal nerve membrane, caused by contractile proteins of the cytosol, especially the protein *cathrin,* attaching underneath the membrane in the areas of the original vesicles. Within about 20 seconds, the proteins contract and cause the pits to break away to the interior of the membrane, thus forming new vesicles. Within another few seconds, acetylcholine is transported to the interior of these vesicles, and they are then ready for a new cycle of acetylcholine release.

Drugs That Affect Transmission at the Neuromuscular Junction

Drugs That Stimulate the Muscle Fiber by Acetylcholine-like Action. Many different compounds, including *methacholine, carbachol,* and *nicotine,* have the same effect on the muscle fiber as does acetylcholine. The difference between these drugs and acetylcholine is that they are not destroyed by cholinesterase or are destroyed very slowly, so that when once applied to the muscle fiber the action persists for many minutes to several hours.

Drugs That Block Transmission at the Neuromuscular Junction. A group of drugs, known as the *curariform drugs,* can prevent passage of impulses from the end-plate into the muscle. Thus, D-tubocurarine affects the membrane by competing with acetylcholine for the receptor sites of the membrane, so that the acetylcholine cannot increase the permeability of the acetylcholine channels sufficiently to initiate a depolarization wave.

Drugs That Stimulate the Neuromuscular Junction by Inactivating Acetylcholinesterase. Three particularly well-known drugs, *neostigmine, physostigmine,* and *diisopropyl fluorophosphate,* inactivate acetylcholinesterase so that the cholinesterase normally in the synapses will not hydrolyze the acetylcholine released at the end-plate. As a result, acetylcholine increases in quantity with successive nerve impulses so that extreme amounts of acetylcholine can accumulate and then repetitively stimulate the muscle fiber. This causes *muscular spasm* when even a few nerve impulses reach the muscle; this can cause death due to laryngeal spasm, which smothers the person.

Diisopropyl fluorophosphate, which has military potential as a very powerful "nerve" gas, actually inactivates acetylcholinesterase for weeks, which makes this a particularly lethal drug.

Myasthenia Gravis

The disease *myasthenia gravis,* which occurs in about one of every 20,000 persons, causes the person to become paralyzed because of inability of the neuromuscular junctions to transmit signals from the nerve fibers to the muscle fibers. Pathologically, antibodies that attack the acetylcholine-gated transport proteins have been demonstrated in the blood of most of these patients. Therefore, it is believed that myasthenia gravis is an autoimmune disease in which patients have developed antibodies against their own acetylcholine-activated ion channels.

Regardless of the cause, the end-plate potentials developed in the muscle fibers are too weak to stimulate the muscle fibers adequately. If the disease is intense enough, the patient dies of paralysis—in particular, of paralysis of the respiratory muscles. However, the disease can usually be ameliorated with several different drugs, as follows:

Treatment with Drugs. When a patient with myasthenia gravis is treated with a drug, such as neostigmine, that is capable of inactivating acetylcholinesterase, the acetylcholine secreted by the end-plate is not destroyed immediately. If a sequence of nerve impulses arrives at the end-plate, the quantity of acetylcholine present at the membrane increases progressively until finally the end-plate potential caused by the acetylcholine rises above threshold value for stimulating the muscle fiber. Thus, it is sometimes possible, by diminishing the quantity of acetylcholinesterase in the muscles of a patient with myasthenia gravis, to allow even the inadequate quantities of acetylcholine secreted at the end-plates to effect almost normal muscular activity.

SMOOTH MUSCLE AND ITS CONTRACTION

In the previous chapter and the first part of this chapter, the discussion has been concerned with skeletal muscle. We now turn to smooth muscle, which is composed of far smaller fibers—usually 2 to 5 micrometers in diameter and only 20 to 500 micrometers in length—in contrast to the skeletal muscle fibers that are as much as 20 times as large (in diameter) and thousands of times as long. Nevertheless, many of the principles of contraction apply to smooth muscle the same as to skeletal muscle. Most important, essentially the same attractive forces between myosin and actin filaments cause contraction in smooth muscle as in skeletal muscle.

Types of Smooth Muscle

The smooth muscle of each organ is distinctive from that of most other organs. Yet, for the sake of simplicity, smooth muscle can generally be divided into two major types, which are illustrated in Figure 7–4: *multiunit smooth muscle* and *single-unit smooth muscle.*

Multiunit Smooth Muscle. This type of smooth muscle is composed of discrete smooth muscle fibers. Each fiber operates entirely independently of the others and is often innervated by a single nerve ending, as occurs for skeletal muscle fibers. Furthermore, the outer surfaces of these fibers, like those of skeletal muscle fibers, are covered by a thin layer of "basement

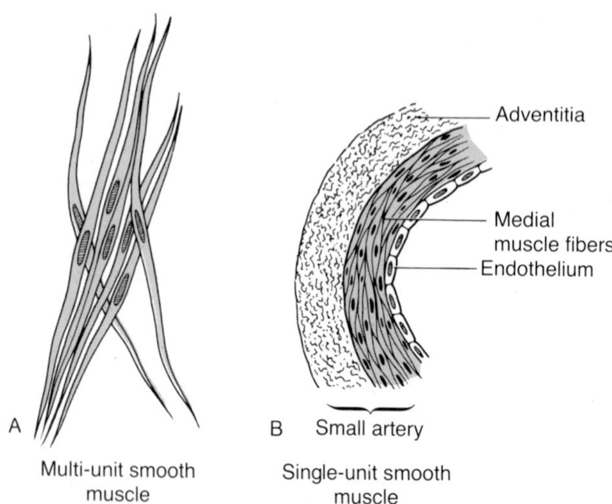

Figure 7–4. Multiunit and single-unit smooth muscle.

membrane-like" substance, a mixture of fine collagen and glycoprotein fibrillae that helps insulate the separate fibers from each other.

The most important characteristic of multiunit smooth muscle fibers is that their control is exerted mainly by nerve signals. This is in contrast to a major share of the control of visceral smooth muscle by nonnervous stimuli.

Some examples of multiunit smooth muscle found in the body are the smooth muscle fibers of the ciliary muscle of the eye, the iris of the eye, the nictitating membrane that covers the eyes in some lower animals, and the piloerector muscles that cause erection of the hairs when stimulated by the sympathetic nervous system.

Single-Unit Smooth Muscle. The term "single-unit" is confusing because it does not mean single muscle fibers. Instead, it means a whole mass of hundreds to millions of muscle fibers that contract together as a single unit. The fibers are usually aggregated into sheets or bundles, and their cell membranes are adherent to each other at multiple points so that force generated in one muscle fiber can be transmitted to the next. In addition, the cell membranes are joined by many *gap junctions* through which ions can flow freely from one cell to the next so that action potentials travel from one fiber to the next and cause the muscle fibers all to contract together. This type of smooth muscle is also known as *syncytial smooth muscle* because of its interconnections among fibers. Because such muscle is found in the walls of most viscera of the body—including the gut, the bile ducts, the ureters, the uterus, and many blood vessels—it is also often called *visceral smooth muscle.*

The Contractile Process in Smooth Muscle

The Chemical Basis for Smooth Muscle Contraction

Smooth muscle contains both *actin* and *myosin filaments,* having chemical characteristics similar to but not exactly the same as those of the actin and myosin filaments in skeletal muscle. Chemical studies have shown that actin and myosin filaments derived from smooth muscle interact with each other in much the same way that this occurs for actin and myosin derived from skeletal muscle. Furthermore, the contractile process is activated by calcium ions, and adenosine triphosphate (ATP) is degraded to adenosine diphosphate (ADP) to provide the energy for contraction.

On the other hand, there are major differences between the physical organization of smooth muscle and that of skeletal muscle, as well as differences in excitation-contraction coupling, control of the contractile process by calcium ions, duration of contraction, and amount of energy required for the contractile process.

The Physical Basis for Smooth Muscle Contraction

Smooth muscle does not have the same striated arrangement of the actin and myosin filaments as that found in skeletal muscle. Recent special electron micrographic techniques suggest the physical organization illustrated in Figure 7-5. This shows large numbers of actin filaments attached to so-called *dense bodies.* Some of these bodies are attached to the cell membrane. Others are dispersed inside the cell and are held in place by a scaffold of structural proteins linking one dense body to another. Note in Figure 7-5 that some of the membrane-dense bodies of adjacent cells are also bonded together by intercellular protein bridges. It is mainly through these bonds that the force of contraction is transmitted from one cell to the next.

Interspersed among the many actin filaments in the muscle fiber are a few myosin filaments. These have a diameter over two times as great as that of the actin filaments.

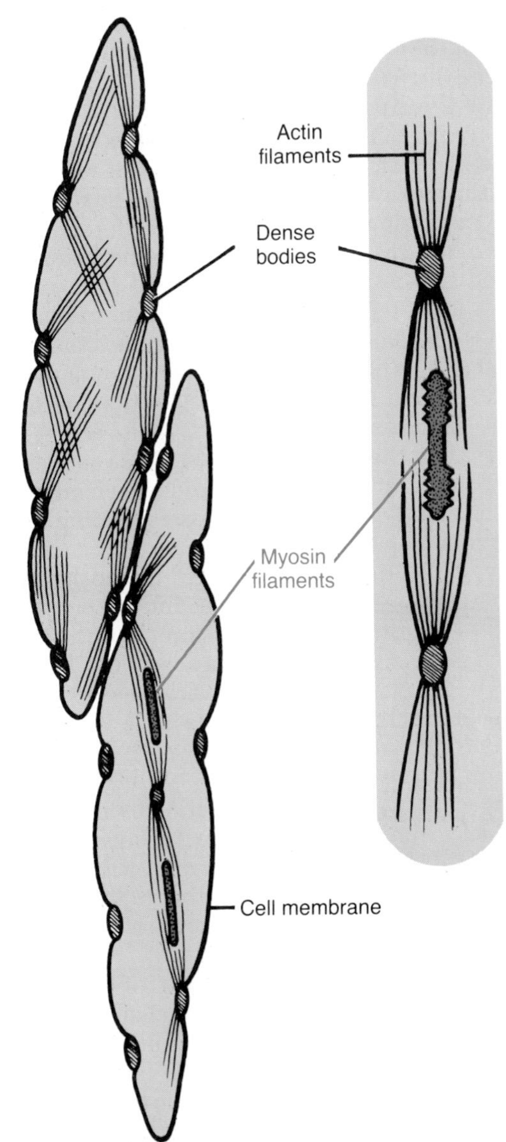

Figure 7-5. Physical structure of smooth muscle. The upper lefthand fiber shows actin filaments radiating from "dense bodies." The lower fiber in the righthand insert demonstrates the relationship of myosin filaments to the actin filaments.

To the right in Figure 7–5 is the postulated structure of individual contractile units within smooth muscle cells, showing large numbers of actin filaments radiating from two dense bodies; these filaments overlap a single myosin filament located midway between the dense bodies. Obviously, this contractile unit is similar to the contractile unit of skeletal muscle but without the regularity of the skeletal muscle structure; in fact, the dense bodies of smooth muscle serve the same role as the Z discs in skeletal muscle.

Comparison of Smooth Muscle Contraction with Skeletal Muscle Contraction

Although most skeletal muscle contracts rapidly, most smooth muscle contraction provides prolonged tonic contraction, often lasting hours or even days. Therefore, it is to be expected that both the physical and the chemical characteristics of smooth muscle versus skeletal muscle contraction would differ. The following are some of the differences:

Slow Cycling of the Cross-Bridges. The rapidity of cycling of the cross-bridges in smooth muscle—that is, their attachment to actin, then release from the actin, and attachment again for the next cycle—is much, much slower in smooth muscle than in skeletal muscle, in fact as little as 1/10 to 1/300 the frequency in skeletal muscle. Yet, the *fraction of time* that the cross-bridges remain attached to the actin filaments, which is the major factor that determines the force of contraction, is believed to be very greatly increased in smooth muscle. A possible reason for the slow cycling is that the cross-bridge heads have far less ATPase activity than that in skeletal muscle, so that degradation of the ATP that energizes the movements of the heads is greatly reduced, with corresponding slowing of the rate of cycling.

Energy Required to Sustain Smooth Muscle Contraction. Only 1/10 to 1/300 as much energy is required to sustain the same tension of contraction in smooth muscle as in skeletal muscle. This, too, is believed to result because of the very slow attachment cycling of the cross-bridges and because only one molecule of ATP is required for each cycle regardless of its duration.

This economy of energy utilization by smooth muscle is exceedingly important to the overall energy economy of the body because organs, such as the intestines, the urinary bladder, the gallbladder, and other viscera must maintain tonic muscle contraction on a daily basis.

Slowness of Onset of Contraction and Relaxation of Smooth Muscle. A typical smooth muscle tissue begins to contract 50 to 100 milliseconds after it is excited, reaches full contraction about ½ second later, and then declines in contractile force in another 1 to 2 seconds, giving a total contraction time of 1 to 3 seconds. This is about 30 times as long as a single contraction of an average skeletal muscle. However, because of the many different types of smooth muscle, contraction of some types can be as short as 0.2 second or as long as 30 seconds.

The slow onset of contraction in smooth muscle as well as the prolonged contraction is probably caused by the slowness of attachment and detachment of the cross-bridges. In addition, the initiation of contraction in response to calcium ions, called the excitation-contraction coupling mechanism, is much slower than in skeletal muscle, as we discuss later.

Force of Muscle Contraction. Despite the relatively few myosin filaments in smooth muscle and despite the slow cycling time of the cross-bridges, the maximum force of contraction of smooth muscle is often even greater than that of skeletal muscle—as great as 4 to 6 kg/cm^2 cross-sectional area for smooth muscle in comparison with 3 to 4 kg for skeletal muscle. This great force of attraction is postulated to result from the prolonged period of attachment of the myosin cross-bridges to the actin filaments.

Percentage Shortening of Smooth Muscle During Contraction. A characteristic of smooth muscle that is different from skeletal muscle is its ability to shorten a far greater percentage of its length than can skeletal muscle while still maintaining almost full force of contraction. Skeletal muscle has a useful distance of contraction of only about one third its stretched length, whereas smooth muscle can often contract quite effectively more than two thirds its stretched length. This allows smooth muscle to perform especially important functions in the hollow viscera, allowing the gut, the bladder, the blood vessels, and other internal bodily structures to change their lumen diameters from very large down to almost zero.

The "Latch" Mechanism for Prolonged Holding Contractions of Smooth Muscle. Once smooth muscle has developed full contraction, the degree of activation of the muscle can usually be reduced to far less than the initial level and yet the muscle will still maintain its full strength of contraction. Furthermore, the energy consumed to maintain contraction is often minuscule, sometimes as little as 1/300 the energy required for comparable skeletal muscle continuous contraction. This is called the "latch" mechanism. This same effect occurs to a slight extent in skeletal muscle but to an extent many times less than that in smooth muscle.

The importance of the latch mechanism is that it can maintain prolonged tonic contraction in smooth muscle for hours and hours with very little use of energy. Also, very little excitatory signal is required from nerve fibers or hormonal sources.

The cause of the latch phenomenon is undoubtedly related to the prolonged attachment of the myosin cross-bridges to the actin filaments.

Stress-Relaxation of Smooth Muscle. Another important characteristic of smooth muscle, especially of the visceral type of smooth muscle in many hollow organs, is its ability to return nearly to its original *force* of contraction seconds or minutes after it has been elongated or shortened. For example, a sudden increase in volume of fluid in the urinary bladder causes an immediate large increase in pressure in the bladder. However, during the next 15 seconds to a minute or so, despite continued stretch of the bladder wall, the pressure returns almost exactly back to the original level. Then, when the volume is increased by another step, the same effect occurs again. When the volume is suddenly decreased, the pressure falls very low at first but then returns in another few seconds or minutes back to the original level. This phenomenon is called *stress-relaxation.* Its obvious importance is that it allows a hollow organ to maintain approximately the same amount of pressure inside its lumen regardless of length of the muscle fibers.

Regulation of Contraction by Calcium Ions

As is true for skeletal muscle, the initiating event in most smooth muscle contraction is an increase in intracellular calcium ions. This increase can be caused by nerve stimulation of the smooth muscle fiber, hormonal stimulation, stretch of the fiber, or even changes in the chemical environment of the fiber.

Yet, *smooth muscle does not contain troponin,* the regulatory protein that is activated by calcium ions to cause skeletal muscle contraction. Instead, smooth muscle contraction is activated by an entirely different mechanism, as follows:

Combination of Calcium Ions with "Calmodulin"—Activation of Myosin Kinase and Phosphorylation of the Myosin Head. In place of troponin, smooth muscle cells contain large quantities of another regulatory protein called *calmodulin.* Although this protein is similar to troponin in that it reacts with four calcium ions, it is different in the manner in which it initiates the contraction. Calmodulin does this by activating the myosin cross-bridges. This activation and subsequent contraction occurs in the following sequence:

1. The calcium ions bind with calmodulin.
2. The calmodulin-calcium combination then joins with and activates myosin kinase, a phosphorylating enzyme.
3. One of the light chains of each myosin head, called the *regulatory chain,* becomes phosphorylated in response to the myosin kinase. When this chain is not phosphorylated, the attachment-detachment cycling of the head will not occur. But, when the regulatory chain is phosphorylated, the head has the capability of binding with the actin filament and proceeding through the entire cycling process, thus causing muscle contraction.

Cessation of Contraction—Role of "Myosin Phosphatase." When the calcium ion concentration falls below a critical level, the aforementioned processes all automatically reverse except for the phosphorylation of the myosin head. Reversal of this requires another enzyme, *myosin phosphatase,* which splits the phosphate from the regulatory light chain. Then, the cycling stops and the contraction ceases. The time required for relaxation of muscle contraction, therefore, is determined to a great extent by the amount of active myosin phosphatase in the cell.

NEURAL AND HORMONAL CONTROL OF SMOOTH MUSCLE CONTRACTION

Although skeletal muscle is activated exclusively by the nervous system, smooth muscle can be stimulated to contract by multiple types of signals: by nervous signals, by hormonal stimulation, and in several other ways. The principal reason for the difference is that the smooth muscle membrane contains many different types of receptor proteins that can initiate the contractile process. Still other receptor proteins inhibit smooth muscle contraction, which is another difference from skeletal muscle. Therefore, in this section, we discuss, first, neural control of smooth muscle contraction, followed by hormonal control and other means of control.

Neuromuscular Junctions of Smooth Muscle

Physiological Anatomy of Smooth Muscle Neuromuscular Junctions. Neuromuscular junctions of the type found on skeletal muscle fibers do not occur in smooth muscle. Instead, the *autonomic nerve fibers* that innervate smooth muscle generally branch diffusely on top of a sheet of muscle fibers, as illustrated in Figure 7–6. In most instances, these fibers do not make direct contact with the smooth muscle fibers at all but instead form so-called *diffuse junctions* that secrete their transmitter substance into the interstitial fluid from a few nanometers to a few microns away from the muscle cells; the transmitter substance then diffuses to the cells. Furthermore, where there are many layers of muscle cells, the nerve fibers often innervate only the outer layer, and the muscle excitation then travels from this outer layer to

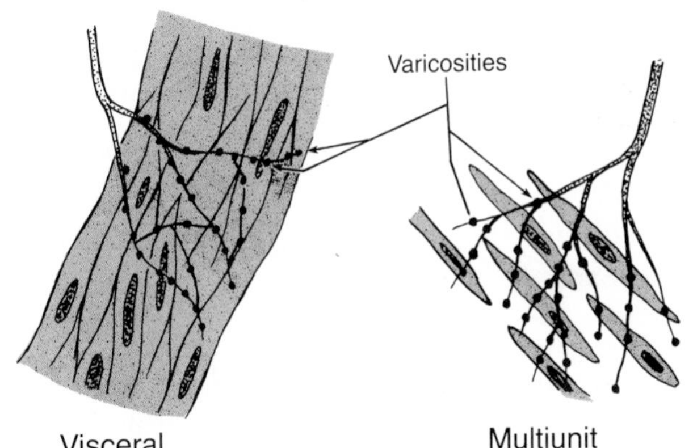

Figure 7–6. Innervation of smooth muscle.

the inner layers by action potential conduction in the muscle mass or by subsequent diffusion of the transmitter substance.

The axons innervating smooth muscle fibers also do not have typical branching end-feet of the type in the motor end-plate on skeletal muscle fibers. Instead, most of the fine terminal axons have multiple *varicosities* distributed along their axes. In the varicosities are vesicles similar to those in the skeletal muscle end-plate containing transmitter substance. However, in contrast to the vesicles of skeletal muscle junctions that contain only acetylcholine, the vesicles of some autonomic nerve fiber endings contain *acetylcholine* while others contain *norepinephrine.*

In a few instances, particularly in the multiunit type of smooth muscle, the varicosities lie directly on the muscle fiber membrane with a separation from this membrane of as little as 20 to 30 nanometers—the same width as the synaptic cleft that occurs in the skeletal muscle junction. These *contact junctions* function in much the same way as the skeletal muscle neuromuscular junction, and the latent period of contraction of these smooth muscle fibers is considerably shorter than of fibers stimulated by the diffuse junctions.

Excitatory and Inhibitory Transmitter Substances at the Smooth Muscle Neuromuscular Junction. Two different transmitter substances known to be secreted by the autonomic nerves innervating smooth muscle are *acetylcholine* and *norepinephrine.* Acetylcholine is an excitatory transmitter substance for smooth muscle fibers in some organs but an inhibitory transmitter for smooth muscle in other organs. When acetylcholine excites a muscle fiber, norepinephrine ordinarily inhibits it. Conversely, when acetylcholine inhibits a fiber, norepinephrine usually excites it.

Both acetylcholine and norepinephrine excite or inhibit smooth muscle by first binding with a *receptor protein* on the surface of the muscle cell membrane. This receptor in turn controls the opening or closing of ion channels or controls some other means for activating or inhibiting the smooth muscle fiber. Furthermore, some of the receptor proteins are *excitatory receptors,* whereas others are *inhibitory receptors.* Thus, it is the type of receptor that determines whether the smooth muscle will be inhibited or excited and also determines which of the two transmitters, acetylcholine or norepinephrine, will be effective in causing the excitation or inhibition.

Membrane Potentials and Action Potentials in Smooth Muscle

In the normal resting state, the membrane potential of smooth muscle is usually about −50 to −60 mV, or about 30 mV less negative than in skeletal muscle. Action potentials occur in single-unit smooth muscle in the same way that they occur in skeletal muscle. However, action potentials do not normally occur in many if not most multiunit types of smooth muscle, as is discussed in a subsequent section.

The action potentials of visceral smooth muscle occur in two different forms: (1) spike potentials and (2) action potentials with plateaus.

Spike Potentials. Typical spike action potentials, such as those seen in skeletal muscle, occur in most types of single-unit smooth muscle. The duration of this type of action potential is 10 to 50 milliseconds, as illustrated in Figure 7–7A and B. Such action potentials can be elicited in many ways, such as by electrical stimulation, by the action of hormones on the smooth muscle, by the action of transmitter substances from nerve fibers, or as a result of spontaneous generation in the muscle fiber itself.

Action Potentials with Plateaus. Figure 7–7C illustrates an action potential with a plateau. The onset of this action potential is similar to that of the typical spike potential. However, instead of rapid repolarization of the muscle fiber membrane, the repolarization is delayed for several hundred to several thousand milliseconds. The importance of the plateau is that it can account for the prolonged periods of contraction that occur in some types of smooth muscle, such as the ureter, the uterus under some condi-

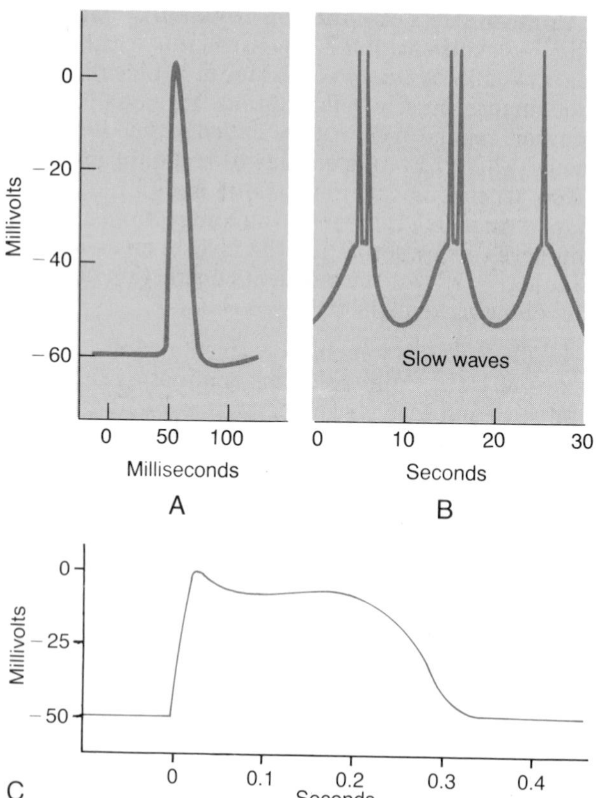

Figure 7–7. *A,* Typical smooth muscle action potential (spike potential) elicited by an external stimulus. *B,* Repetitive spike potentials elicited by slow rhythmical electrical waves that occur spontaneously in the smooth muscle of the intestinal wall. *C,* An action potential with a plateau recorded from a smooth muscle fiber of the uterus.

tions, and some types of vascular smooth muscle. (Also, this is the type of action potential seen in cardiac muscle fibers that have a prolonged period of contraction, as we discuss in the next two chapters.)

Importance of Calcium Channels in Generating the Smooth Muscle Action Potential. The smooth muscle cell membrane has far more voltage-gated calcium channels than does skeletal muscle but very few voltage-gated sodium channels. Therefore, sodium participates very little in the generation of the action potential in most smooth muscle. Instead, flow of calcium ions through the membrane to the interior of the fiber is mainly responsible for the action potential. This occurs in the same self-regenerative way as occurs for the sodium channels in nerve fibers and in skeletal muscle fibers. However, calcium channels open many times more slowly than do sodium channels. This accounts in large measure for the slow action potentials of smooth muscle fibers.

Another important feature of calcium entry into the cells during the action potential is that this same calcium acts directly on the smooth muscle contractile mechanism to cause contraction. Thus, the calcium performs two tasks at once.

Slow Wave Potentials in Single-Unit Smooth Muscle and Spontaneous Generation of Action Potentials. Some smooth muscle is self-excitatory. That is, action potentials arise within the smooth muscle itself without an extrinsic stimulus. This is often associated with a basic *slow wave rhythm* of the membrane potential. A typical slow wave of this type in the visceral smooth muscle of the gut is illustrated in Figure 7–7B. The slow wave (the sinusoidal wave at the bottom of Figure 7–7B) is not an action potential. It is not a self-regenerative process that spreads progressively over the membranes of the muscle fibers. Instead, it is a local property of the smooth muscle fibers that make up the muscle mass.

The cause of the slow wave rhythm is unknown; one suggestion is that the slow waves are caused by waxing and waning of the pumping of sodium ions outward through the muscle fiber membrane; the membrane potential becomes more negative when sodium is pumped rapidly and less negative when the sodium pump becomes less active. Another suggestion is that the conductances of the ion channels increase and decrease rhythmically.

The importance of the slow waves lies in the fact that they can initiate action potentials. The slow waves themselves cannot cause muscle contraction, but when the potential of the slow wave rises above the level of approximately −35 mV (the approximate threshold for eliciting action potentials in most visceral smooth muscle), an action potential develops and spreads over the muscle mass, and then contraction does occur. Figure 7–7B illustrates this effect, showing that at each peak of the slow wave, one or more action potentials occur. This effect can obviously promote a series of rhythmical contractions of the smooth muscle mass. Therefore, the slow waves are frequently called *pacemaker waves.* In Chapter 42, we see that this type of activity controls the rhythmical contractions of the gut.

Excitation of *Visceral Smooth Muscle* by Stretch. When visceral (single-unit) smooth muscle is stretched sufficiently, spontaneous action potentials are usually generated. These result from a combination of the normal slow wave potentials plus a decrease in the negativity of the membrane potential caused by the stretch itself. This response to stretch allows a hollow organ that is excessively stretched to contract automatically and therefore to resist the stretch. For instance, when the gut is overstretched by intestinal contents, a local automatic contraction often sets up a peristaltic wave that moves the contents away from the excessively stretched intestine.

Depolarization of *Multiunit Smooth Muscle* Without Action Potentials. The smooth muscle fibers of multiunit smooth muscle normally contract mainly in response to nerve stimuli. However, action potentials most often do not develop. The reason for this is that the fibers are too small to generate an action potential. Yet, even without an action potential in the multiunit smooth muscle fibers, the local depolarization, called the "junctional potential," caused by the nerve transmitter substance itself spreads by direct electrical conduction over the entire fiber and is all that is needed to cause the muscle contraction.

Smooth Muscle Contraction Without Action Potentials—Effect of Local Tissue Factors and Hormones

Probably half or more of all smooth muscle contraction is initiated not by action potentials but by stimulatory factors acting directly on the smooth muscle contractile machinery. The two types of nonnervous and nonaction potential stimulating factors most often involved are (1) local tissue factors and (2) various hormones.

Smooth Muscle Contraction in Response to Local Tissue Factors. In Chapter 13, we discuss the control of contraction of the arterioles, meta-arterioles, and precapillary sphincters. The smaller of these vessels have little or no nervous supply. Yet, the smooth muscle is highly contractile, responding rapidly to changes in local conditions in the surrounding interstitial fluid. In this way, a powerful local feedback control system controls the blood flow to the local tissue area. Some of the specific control factors are as follows:

1. Lack of oxygen in the local tissues causes smooth muscle relaxation and therefore vasodilatation.
2. Excess carbon dioxide also causes vasodilatation.
3. Increased hydrogen ion concentration also causes vasodilatation.

Such factors as adenosine, lactic acid, increased potassium ions, diminished calcium ion concentration, and decreased body temperature also cause local vasodilatation.

Effects of Hormones on Smooth Muscle Contraction. Most of the circulating hormones in the body affect smooth muscle contraction at least to some degree, and some have very profound effects. Some of the more important blood-borne hormones that affect contraction are *norepinephrine, epinephrine, acetylcholine, angiotensin, vasopressin, oxytocin, serotonin,* and *histamine.*

A hormone causes contraction of smooth muscle when the muscle cell membrane contains *excitatory receptors* for the respective hormone. However, the hormone causes inhibition instead of contraction if the membrane contains *inhibitory receptors* rather than excitatory receptors.

Smooth Muscle Excitation or Inhibition Caused by Hormones or Local Tissue Factors. Some hormone receptors in the smooth muscle membrane open sodium or calcium ion channels and depolarize the membrane the same as following nerve stimulation. Occasionally, but not always, action potentials result, or rhythmical action potentials that are already occurring may be enhanced. However, in many instances depolarization occurs without action potentials; nevertheless, even this depolarization is associated with calcium ion entry into the cell that promotes contraction.

Activation of other membrane receptors inhibits contraction. This is achieved by closing sodium and calcium channels to prevent the entry of these positive ions or by opening potassium channels to allow positive potassium ions to flow to the exterior, in both instances increasing the degree of negativity inside the muscle cell, a state called *hyperpolarization.*

Source of Calcium Ions That Cause Contraction

Although the contractile process in smooth muscle, as in skeletal muscle, is activated by calcium ions, the source of the calcium ions differs at least partly in smooth muscle; the difference is that the sarcoplasmic reticulum, from which virtually all the calcium ions are derived in skeletal muscle contraction, is often only rudimentary in most smooth muscle. Instead, in many types of smooth muscle, almost all the calcium ions that cause contraction enter the muscle cell from the extracellular fluid at the time of the action potential. There is a reasonably high concentration of calcium ions in the extracellular fluid, greater than 10^{-3} molar in comparison with less than 10^{-7} molar in the cell sarcoplasm, and as was pointed out earlier, the smooth muscle action potential is caused mainly by influx of calcium ions into the muscle fiber. Because the smooth muscle fibers are extremely small (in contrast to the sizes of the skeletal muscle fibers), these calcium ions can diffuse to all parts of the smooth muscle and elicit the contractile process.

Role of the Sarcoplasmic Reticulum. Some smooth muscle contains a moderately developed sarcoplasmic reticulum, and some of the sarcoplasmic tubules lie near the cell membrane. Small invaginations of the external cell membrane, called *caveoli,* penetrate into the cell and abut the surfaces of these sarcoplasmic tubules. The caveoli are believed to represent a rudimentary analog of the T tubule system of skeletal muscle. When an action potential is transmitted into the caveoli invaginations, this seems to excite calcium ion release from the sarcoplasmic tubules, in the same way that action potentials in skeletal muscle T tubules also cause release of calcium ions.

In general, the more extensive the sarcoplasmic reticulum in the smooth muscle fiber, the more rapidly it contracts, presumably because calcium entry through the cell membrane is much slower than internal release of calcium ions from the sarcoplasmic reticulum.

The Calcium Pump. To cause relaxation of the smooth muscle contractile elements, it is necessary to remove the calcium ions. This removal is achieved by calcium pumps that pump the calcium ions out of the smooth muscle fiber back into the extracellular fluid or pump the calcium ions into the sarcoplasmic reticulum. However, these pumps are very slow-acting in comparison with the fast-acting sarcoplasmic reticulum pump in skeletal muscle. Therefore, the duration of smooth muscle contraction is often in the order of seconds rather than hundredths to tenths of a second, as occurs for skeletal muscle.

REFERENCES

Campbell, J. H., and Campbell, G. R.: Endothelial cell influences on vascular smooth muscle phenotype. Annu. Rev. Physiol., 48:295, 1986.

Furchgott, R. F.: The role of endothelium in the responses of vascular smooth muscle to drugs. Annu. Rev. Pharmacol. Toxicol., 24:175, 1984.

Gabella, G.: Structural apparatus for force transmission in smooth muscle. Physiol. Rev., 64:455, 1984.

Hai, C. M., and Murphy, R. A.: Ca^{2+}, crossbridge phosphorylation, and contraction. Annu. Rev. Physiol., 51:285, 1989.

Hirst, G. D. S., and Edwards, F. R.: Sympathetic neuroeffector transmission in arteries and arterioles. Physiol. Rev., 69:546, 1989.

Kamm, K. E., and Stull, J. T.: Regulation of smooth muscle contractile elements by second messengers. Annu. Rev. Physiol., 51:299, 1989.

Kito, S., et al. (eds.): Neuroreceptors and Signal Transduction. New York, Plenum Publishing Corp., 1988.

Murphy, R. A.: Muscle cells of hollow organs. News Physiol. Sci., 3:124, 1988.

Paul, R. J.: Smooth muscle energetics. Annu. Rev. Physiol., 51:331, 1989.

Rosenthal, W., et al.: Control of voltage-dependent Ca^{2+} channels by G protein-coupled receptors. FASEB J., 2:2784, 1988.

Rowland, L. P., et al. (eds.): Molecular Genetics in Diseases of Brain, Nerve, and Muscle. New York, Oxford University Press, 1989.

Seidel, C. L., and Schildmeyer, L. A.: Vascular smooth muscle adaptation to increased load. Annu. Rev. Physiol., 49:489, 1987.

van Breemen, C., and Saida, K.: Cellular mechanisms regulating $[Ca^{2+}]$ smooth muscle. Annu. Rev. Physiol., 51:315, 1989.

Vanhoutte, P. M.: Calcium-entry blockers, vascular smooth muscle and systemic hypertension. Am. J. Cardiol., 55:17B, 1985.

QUESTIONS

1. Describe the anatomy of a neuromuscular junction.
2. Explain how acetylcholine is secreted by the axon terminals, how it is destroyed by acetylcholine, and how it excites the muscle fiber.
3. What are the characteristics of acetylcholine-gated channels?
4. Approximately what is the voltage of the end-plate potential, and how does it excite the muscle membrane? Describe the disease *myasthenia gravis,* its cause, and its treatment.
5. What are the differences between *multiunit smooth muscle* and *visceral smooth muscle*?
6. How does smooth muscle contraction differ chemically from that of skeletal muscle? How does smooth muscle contraction differ physically from that of skeletal muscle contraction?
7. What are the interrelationships of actin and myosin fibrils during smooth muscle contraction? How do the action potential of smooth muscle differ from those of skeletal muscle?
8. What is the role of calcium ions in the generation of the smooth muscle action potential?
9. Explain how slow waves cause rhythmical contraction in some smooth muscle masses.
10. What is the difference between the manner in which calcium ions cause contraction of smooth muscle and the manner in which they cause contraction of skeletal muscle?
11. Explain the differences between neuromuscular junctions of smooth muscle and those of skeletal muscle.
12. Why does nervous stimulation of some smooth muscle cause excitation while it causes inhibition of other smooth muscle?
13. Explain how local tissue factors and hormones can cause smooth muscle contraction or inhibition without eliciting action potentials.
14. What causes tone in smooth muscle, and what is the importance of tone in the function of organs?

The Heart

8

Heart Muscle; The Heart as a Pump

With this chapter we begin discussion of the heart and circulatory system. The heart, illustrated in Figure 8-1, is actually two separate pumps: a *right heart* that pumps the blood through the lungs and a *left heart* that pumps the blood through the peripheral organs. In turn, each of these two separate hearts is a pulsatile two-chamber pump composed of an *atrium* and a *ventricle.* The atrium functions principally as a blood reservoir and as an entryway to the ventricle, but it also pumps weakly to help move the blood into the ventricle. The ventricle in turn supplies the main force that propels the blood through either the pulmonary or the peripheral circulation.

Special mechanisms in the heart maintain cardiac rhythmicity and transmit action potentials throughout the heart muscle to cause the heart's rhythmical beat. This rhythmical control system is explained in the following chapter. In the present chapter, we explain how the heart operates as a pump, beginning with the special features of heart muscle itself.

PHYSIOLOGY OF CARDIAC MUSCLE

Physiological Anatomy of Cardiac Muscle

Figure 8-2 illustrates a typical histological picture of cardiac muscle, showing the cardiac muscle fibers arranged in a latticework, the fibers dividing, then recombining, and then spreading again. One notes immediately from this figure that cardiac muscle is *striated* in the same manner as typical skeletal muscle. Furthermore, cardiac muscle has typical myofibrils that contain *actin* and *myosin filaments* almost identical to those found in skeletal muscle, and these filaments interdigitate and slide along each other during the process of contraction in the same manner as occurs in skeletal muscle. (See Chapter 6.)

Cardiac Muscle as a Syncytium. The angulated dark areas crossing the cardiac muscle fibers in Figure 8-2 are called *intercalated discs;* they are actually cell membranes that separate individual cardiac muscle cells from each other. That is, cardiac muscle fibers are made up of many individual cells connected in series with each other. Yet electrical resistance through the intercalated disc is only 1/400 the resistance through the outside membrane of the cardiac muscle fiber because the cell membranes fuse with each other and form very permeable "communicating" junctions (gap junctions) that allow relatively free diffusion of ions. Therefore, from a functional point of view, ions move with ease along the axes of the cardiac muscle fibers, so that action potentials travel from one cardiac muscle cell to another, past the intercalated discs, with only slight hindrance. Therefore, cardiac muscle is a *syncytium* of many heart muscle cells, in which the cardiac cells are so interconnected that when one of these cells becomes excited, the action potential spreads to all of them, spreading from cell to cell and spreading throughout the latticework interconnections.

The heart is composed of two separate syncytiums: the *atrial syncytium* that constitutes the walls of the two atria and the *ventricular syncytium* that constitutes the walls of the two ventricles. The atria are separated from the ventricles by fibrous tissue that surrounds the valvular openings between the atria and ventricles. Normally, action potentials can be conducted from the atrial syncytium into the ventricular syncytium only by way of a specialized conductive system, the *A-V bundle,* which is discussed in detail in the following chapter. This division of the muscle mass of the heart into two separate functional syncytiums allows the atria to contract a short time ahead of ventricular contraction, which is important for the effectiveness of heart pumping.

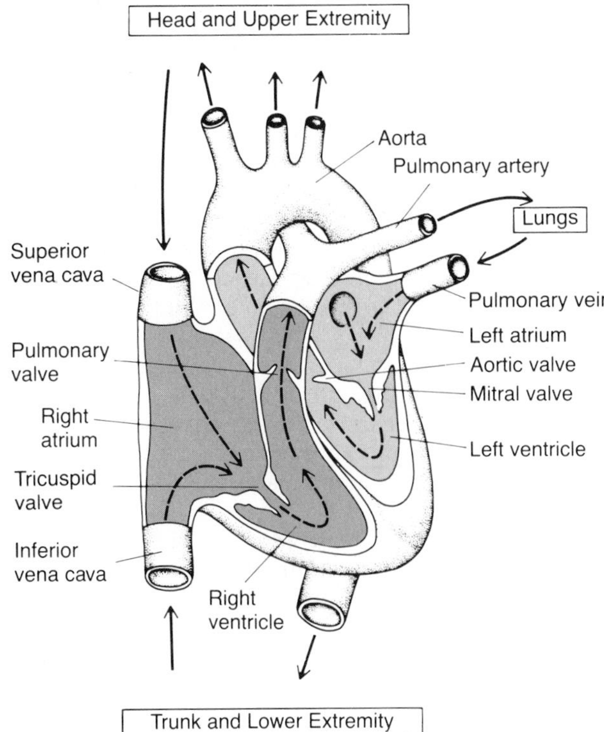

Figure 8-1. Structure of the heart and course of blood flow through the heart chambers.

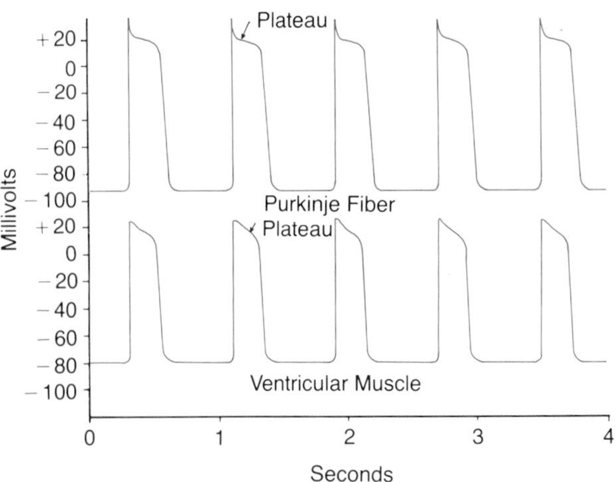

Figure 8-3. Rhythmic action potentials from a Purkinje fiber and from a ventricular muscle fiber, recorded by means of microelectrodes.

Action Potentials in Cardiac Muscle

The *resting membrane potential* of normal cardiac muscle is approximately −85 to −95 millivolts (mV) and approximately −90 to −100 mV in the specialized conductive fibers, the Purkinje fibers, which are discussed in the following chapter.

The *action potential* recorded in ventricular muscle, shown by the bottom record of Figure 8-3, is 105 mV, which means that the membrane potential rises from its normally very negative value to a slightly positive value of about +20 mV. Then, after the initial *spike,* the membrane remains depolarized for about 0.2 second in atrial muscle and about 0.3 second in ventricular muscle, exhibiting a *plateau* as illustrated in Figure 8-3, followed at the end of the plateau by abrupt repolarization. The presence of this plateau in the action potential causes muscle contraction to last 3 to 15 times as long in cardiac muscle as in skeletal muscle.

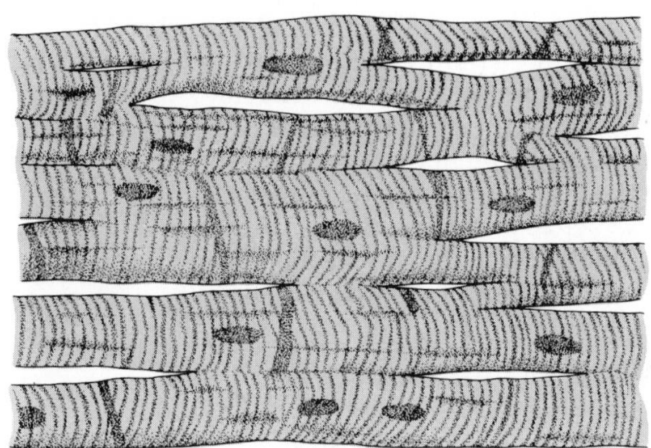

Figure 8-2. The "syncytial," interconnecting nature of cardiac muscle.

At least one major difference between the membrane properties of cardiac and skeletal muscle accounts for the prolonged action potential and the plateau in cardiac muscle. That is, the action potential of skeletal muscle is caused almost entirely by sudden opening of large numbers of so-called *fast sodium channels* that allow tremendous numbers of sodium ions to enter the skeletal muscle fiber. These channels are called "fast" channels because they remain open for only a few 10,000ths of a second and then abruptly close. At the end of this closure, the process of repolarization occurs, and the action potential is over within another 10,000th of a second or so. In cardiac muscle, on the other hand, the action potential is caused by the opening of two types of channels: (1) the same *fast sodium channels* as those in skeletal muscle and (2) another entire population of so-called *slow calcium channels,* also called *calcium-sodium channels.* This second population of channels differs from the fast sodium channels in being slower to open, but, more importantly, they remain open for several tenths of a second. During this time, large amounts of both calcium and sodium ions flow through these channels to the interior of the cardiac muscle fiber, and this maintains a prolonged period of depolarization, causing the plateau in the action potential. Furthermore, the calcium ions that enter the muscle during this action potential play an important role in helping excite the muscle contractile process, which is another difference between cardiac muscle and skeletal muscle, as we discuss later in this chapter.

Velocity of Conduction in Cardiac Muscle. The velocity of conduction of the action potential in both atrial and ventricular muscle fibers is about 0.3 to 0.5 meter per second, or about 1/250 the velocity in very large nerve fibers and about 1/10 the velocity in skeletal muscle fibers. The velocity of conduction in the specialized conductive system varies from 0.02

to 4 meters per second in different parts of the system, as is explained in the following chapter.

Refractory Period of Cardiac Muscle. Cardiac muscle, like all excitable tissue, is refractory to restimulation during the action potential. Therefore, the refractory period of the heart is the interval of time during which a normal cardiac impulse cannot re-excite an already excited area of cardiac muscle. The normal refractory period of the ventricle is 0.25 to 0.3 second, which is approximately the duration of the action potential. There is an additional *relative refractory period* of about 0.05 second during which the muscle is more difficult than normal to excite but nevertheless can be excited.

The refractory period of atrial muscle is much shorter than that for the ventricles (about 0.15 second), and the relative refractory period is another 0.03 second. Therefore, the rhythmical rate of contraction of the atria can be much faster than that of the ventricles.

Excitation-Contraction Coupling — Function of Calcium Ions and of the T Tubules

As is true for skeletal muscle, when an action potential passes over the cardiac muscle membrane, the action potential also spreads to the interior of the cardiac muscle fiber along the membranes of penetrating T tubules. The T tubule action potentials in turn act on the membranes of the longitudinal sarcoplasmic tubules to cause instantaneous release of very large quantities of calcium ions into the muscle sarcoplasm from the sarcoplasmic reticulum. In another few thousandths of a second, these calcium ions diffuse into the myofibrils and catalyze the chemical reactions that promote sliding of the actin and myosin filaments along each other; this in turn produces the muscle contraction.

Thus far, this mechanism of excitation-contraction coupling is the same as that for skeletal muscle, but there is a second effect that is quite different. In addition to the calcium ions released into the sarcoplasm from the cisternae of the sarcoplasmic reticulum, large quantities of extra calcium ions also diffuse into the sarcoplasm from the T tubules at the time of the action potential. Indeed, without this extra calcium from the T tubules, the strength of cardiac muscle contraction would be considerably reduced because the sarcoplasmic reticulum of cardiac muscle is less well developed than that of skeletal muscle and does not store enough calcium to provide full contraction. The T tubules of cardiac muscle have a diameter 5 times as great as that of the skeletal muscle tubules and a volume 25 times as great; also, inside the T tubules is a large quantity of mucopolysaccharides that are electronegatively charged and bind an abundant extra store of calcium ions, keeping this always available for diffusion to the interior of the cardiac muscle fiber when the T tubule action potential occurs.

The strength of contraction of cardiac muscle depends to a great extent on the concentration of calcium ions in the extracellular fluids. The reason for this is that the ends of the T tubules open directly to the outside of the cardiac muscle fibers, allowing the same extracellular fluid that is in the cardiac muscle interstitium to percolate through the T tubules as well. Consequently, the quantity of calcium ions in the T tubule system as well as the availability of calcium ions to cause cardiac muscle contraction depends directly on the extracellular fluid calcium ion concentration.

By way of contrast, the strength of skeletal muscle contraction is hardly affected by the extracellular fluid calcium concentration because its contraction is caused almost entirely by calcium ions released from the sarcoplasmic reticulum inside the skeletal muscle fiber itself.

At the end of the plateau of the action potential, the influx of calcium ions to the interior of the muscle fiber is suddenly cut off, and the calcium ions in the sarcoplasm are rapidly pumped back into both the sarcoplasmic reticulum and the T tubules. As a result, the contraction ceases until a new action potential occurs.

Duration of Contraction. Cardiac muscle begins to contract a few milliseconds after the action potential begins and continues to contract for a few milliseconds after the action potential ends. Therefore, the duration of contraction of cardiac muscle is mainly a function of the duration of the action potential — about 0.2 second in atrial muscle and 0.3 second in ventricular muscle.

THE CARDIAC CYCLE

The period from the beginning of one heartbeat to the beginning of the next is called the *cardiac cycle.* Each cycle is initiated by spontaneous generation of an action potential in the sinus node, as is explained in the following chapter. This node is located in the superior lateral wall of the right atrium near the opening of the superior vena cava, and the action potential travels rapidly through both atria and thence through the A-V bundle into the ventricles. However, because of a special arrangement of the conducting system from the atria into the ventricles, there is a delay of more than 1/10 second between passage of the cardiac impulse from the atria into the ventricles. This allows the atria to contract ahead of the ventricles, thereby pumping blood into the ventricles prior to the very strong ventricular contraction. Thus, the atria act as *primer pumps* for the ventricles, and the ventricles then provide the major source of power for moving blood through the vascular system.

Systole and Diastole

The cardiac cycle consists of a period of relaxation called *diastole,* during which the heart fills with blood, followed by a period of contraction called *systole.*

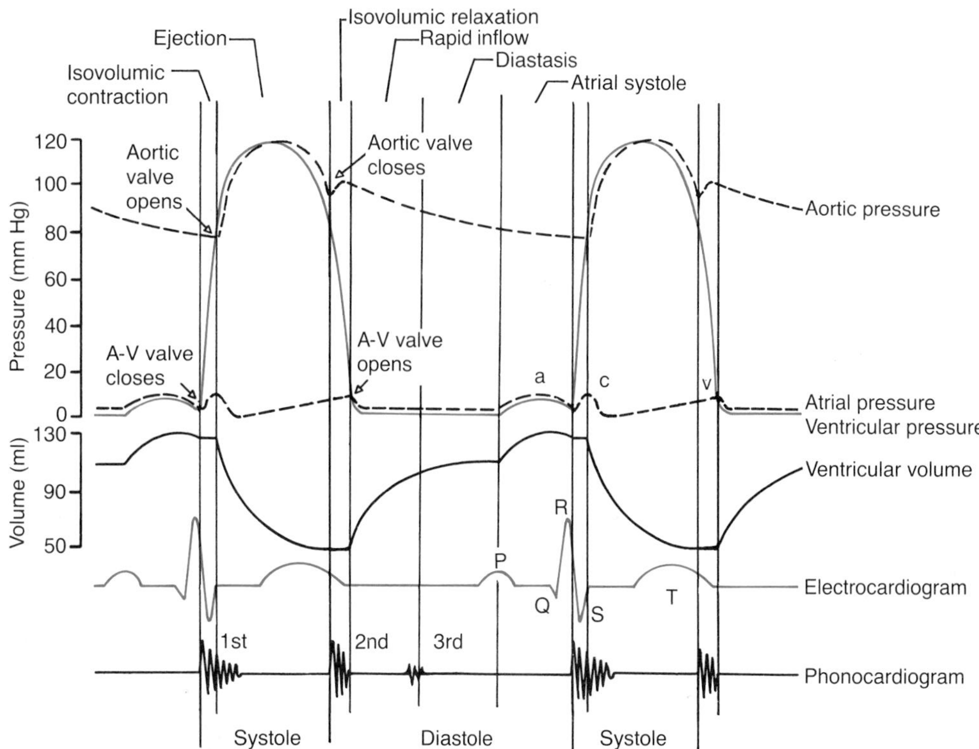

Figure 8-4. The events of the cardiac cycle, showing changes in left atrial pressure, left ventricular pressure, aortic pressure, ventricular volume, the electrocardiogram, and the phonocardiogram.

Figure 8-4 illustrates the different events during the cardiac cycle. The top three curves show the pressure changes in the aorta, the left ventricle, and the left atrium, respectively. The fourth curve depicts the changes in ventricular volume, the fifth the electrocardiogram, and the sixth a phonocardiogram, which is a recording of the sounds produced by the heart—mainly by the heart valves—as it pumps. It is especially important that the reader study in detail the diagram of this figure and understand the causes of all the events illustrated. These are explained as follows:

Relationship of the Electrocardiogram to the Cardiac Cycle

The electrocardiogram in Figure 8-4 shows the *P, Q, R, S,* and *T waves,* which will be discussed in Chapter 10. These are electrical voltages generated by the heart and recorded by the electrocardiograph from the surface of the body. The *P wave* is caused by the *spread of depolarization* through the atria, and this is followed by atrial contraction, which causes a slight rise in the atrial pressure curve immediately after the P wave. Approximately 0.16 second after the onset of the P wave, the *QRS waves* appear as a result of depolarization of the ventricles, which initiates contraction of the ventricles and causes the ventricular pressure to begin rising, as also illustrated in the figure. Therefore, the QRS complex begins slightly before the onset of ventricular systole.

Finally, one observes the *ventricular T wave* in the electrocardiogram. This represents the stage of repolarization of the ventricles, at which time the ventricular muscle fibers begin to relax. Therefore, the T wave occurs slightly prior to the end of ventricular contraction.

Function of the Atria as Pumps. Blood normally flows continuously from the great veins into the atria; approximately 75 per cent of blood flows directly through the atria into the ventricles even before the atria contract. Then, atrial contraction usually causes an additional 25 per cent filling of the ventricles. Therefore, the atria simply function as primer pumps that increase the ventricular pumping effectiveness as much as 25 per cent. Yet, the heart can continue to operate quite satisfactorily under normal resting conditions even without this extra 25 per cent effectiveness because it normally has the capability of pumping 300 to 400 per cent more blood than is required by the body anyway. Therefore, when the atria fail to function, the difference is unlikely to be noticed unless a person exercises; then acute signs of heart failure occasionally develop, especially shortness of breath.

Function of the Ventricles as Pumps

Filling of the Ventricles. During ventricular systole, large amounts of blood accumulate in the atria because of the closed A-V valves. Therefore, just as soon as systole is over and the ventricular pressures fall again to their low diastolic values, the high pressures in the atria immediately push the A-V valves open and allow blood to flow rapidly into the ventricles, as shown by the rise of the *ventricular volume* *curve* in Figure 8–4. This is called the *period of rapid filling of the ventricles.*

The period of rapid filling lasts approximately the first third of diastole. During the middle third of diastole only a small amount of blood normally flows into the ventricles; this is blood that continues to empty into the atria from the veins and passes on through the atria directly into the ventricles.

During the latter third of diastole, the atria contract and give an additional thrust to the inflow of blood into the ventricles; this accounts for approximately 25 per cent of the filling of the ventricles during each heart cycle.

Emptying of the Ventricles During Systole. ***Period of Isovolumic (Isometric) Contraction.*** Immediately after ventricular contraction begins, the ventricular pressure abruptly rises, as shown in Figure 8–4, causing the A-V valves to close. Then an additional 0.02 to 0.03 second is required for the ventricle to build up sufficient pressure to push the semilunar (aortic and pulmonary) valves open against the pressures in the aorta and pulmonary artery. Therefore, during this period of time, contraction is occurring in the ventricles, but there is no emptying.

Period of Ejection. When the left ventricular pressure rises slightly above 80 mm Hg (and the right ventricular pressure slightly above 8 mm Hg), the ventricular pressures now push the semilunar valves open. Immediately, blood begins to pour out of the ventricles, with about 70 per cent of the emptying occurring during the first third of the period of ejection and the remaining 30 per cent during the next two thirds. Therefore, the first third is called the *period of rapid ejection* and the last two thirds the *period of slow ejection.*

Period of Isovolumic (Isometric) Relaxation. At the end of systole, ventricular relaxation begins suddenly, allowing the intraventricular pressures to fall rapidly. The elevated pressures in the distended large arteries immediately push blood back toward the ventricles, which snaps the aortic and pulmonary valves closed. For another 0.03 to 0.06 second, the ventricular muscle continues to relax, even though the ventricular volume does not change, giving rise to the period of *isovolumic* or *isometric relaxation.* During this period, the intraventricular pressures fall rapidly back to their very low diastolic levels. Then the A-V valves open to begin a new cycle of ventricular pumping.

End-Diastolic Volume, End-Systolic Volume, and Stroke Volume Output. During diastole, filling of the ventricles normally increases the volume of each ventricle to about 110 to 120 milliliters (ml). This volume is known as the *end-diastolic volume.* Then, as the ventricles empty during systole, the volume decreases about 70 ml, which is called the *stroke volume output.* The remaining volume in each ventricle, about 40 to 50 ml, is called the *end-systolic volume.* The fraction of the end-diastolic volume that is ejected is called the *ejection fraction*—usually equal to about 60 per cent.

When the heart contracts strongly, the end-systolic volume can fall to as little as 10 to 20 ml. On the other hand, when large amounts of blood flow into the ventricles during diastole, their end-diastolic volumes can become as great as 150 to 180 ml in the normal heart. And by both increasing the end-diastolic volume and decreasing the end-systolic volume, the stroke volume output can at times be increased to about double normal.

Function of the Valves

The Atrioventricular Valves. The *A-V valves* (the *tricuspid* and the *mitral* valves) prevent backflow of blood from the ventricles to the atria during systole, and the *semilunar valves* (the *aortic* and *pulmonary* valves) prevent backflow from the aorta and pulmonary arteries into the ventricles during diastole. All these valves, which are illustrated in Figure 8–5, close and open *passively.* That is, they close when a backward pressure gradient pushes blood backward, and they open when a forward pressure gradient forces blood in the forward direction. For obvious anatomical reasons, the thin, filmy A-V valves require almost no backflow to cause closure, whereas the much heavier semilunar valves require rather strong backflow for a few milliseconds.

Function of the Papillary Muscles. Figure 8–5 also illustrates the papillary muscles that attach to the vanes of the A-V valves by the *chordae tendineae.* The papillary muscles contract when the ventricular walls contract, but, contrary to what might be expected, they *do not* help the valves to close. Instead, they pull the vanes of the valves inward toward the ventricles to prevent their bulging too far backward toward the atria during ventricular contraction. If a chorda tendinea becomes ruptured or if one of the papillary muscles becomes paralyzed, the valve bulges far backward, sometimes so far that it leaks severely and results in severe or even lethal cardiac incapacity.

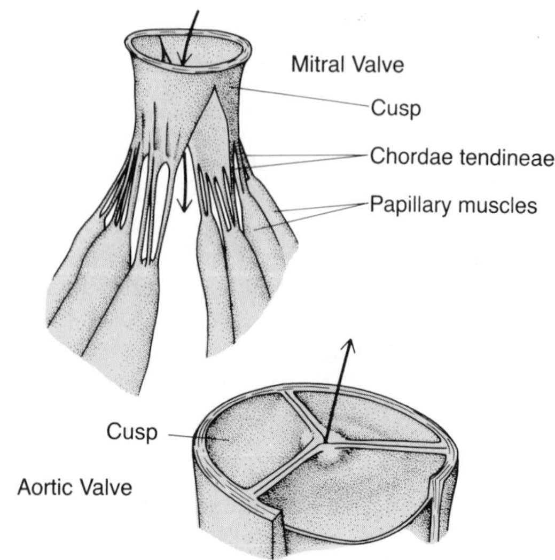

Figure 8–5. Mitral and aortic valves.

The Aortic and Pulmonary Valves. There are differences between the operation of the aortic and pulmonary valves and that of the A-V valves. First, the high pressures in the arteries at the end of systole cause the semilunar valves to snap to the closed position in comparison with a much softer closure of the A-V valves. Second, because of smaller openings, the velocity of blood ejection through the aortic and pulmonary valves is far greater than that through the much larger A-V valves. Also, because of the rapid closure and rapid ejection, the edges of the semilunar valves are subjected to much greater mechanical abrasion than are the A-V valves, which also are supported by the chordae tendineae. It is obvious from the anatomy of the aortic and pulmonary valves, as illustrated in Figure 8–5, that they are well adapted to withstand this extra physical trauma.

The Aortic Pressure Curve

When the left ventricle contracts, the ventricular pressure rises rapidly until the aortic valve opens. Then the pressure in the ventricle rises much less thereafter, as illustrated in Figure 8–4, because blood immediately flows out of the ventricle into the aorta.

The entry of blood into the arteries causes the walls of these arteries to stretch and the pressure to rise. Then, at the end of systole, after the left ventricle stops ejecting blood and the aortic valve closes, the elastic recoil of the arteries maintains a high pressure in the arteries even during diastole.

After the aortic valve has closed, pressure in the aorta falls slowly throughout diastole because blood stored in the distended elastic arteries flows continuously through the peripheral vessels back to the veins. Before the ventricle contracts again, the aortic pressure usually falls to approximately 80 mm Hg (diastolic pressure), which is two thirds the maximal pressure of 120 mm Hg (systolic pressure) occurring in the aorta during ventricular contraction.

The pressure curve in the pulmonary artery is similar to that in the aorta except that the pressures are only about one sixth as great.

Relationship of the Heart Sounds to Heart Pumping

When listening to the heart with a stethoscope, one does not hear the opening of the valves, for this is a relatively slowly developing process that makes no noise. However, when the valves close, the vanes of the valves and the surrounding fluids vibrate under the influence of the sudden pressure differentials that develop, giving off sound that travels in all directions through the chest.

When the ventricles first contract, one hears a sound that is caused by closure of the A-V valves. The vibration is low in pitch and relatively long continued and is known as the *first heart sound.* When the aortic and pulmonary valves close, one hears a relatively rapid snap, for these valves close extremely rapidly, and the surroundings vibrate for only a short period of time. This sound is known as the *second heart sound.*

The Chemical Energy for Cardiac Contraction: Oxygen Utilization by the Heart

Heart muscle, like skeletal muscle, uses chemical energy to provide the work of contraction. This energy is derived mainly from oxidative metabolism of fatty acids and to a lesser extent of other nutrients, especially lactate and glucose. Therefore, the rate of oxygen consumption by the heart is an excellent measure of the chemical energy liberated while the heart performs its work. The different reactions that liberate this energy are discussed in Chapters 45 and 46.

Experimental studies on isolated hearts have shown that the oxygen consumption of the heart, and therefore the chemical energy expended during contraction, is directly related to the *work output* of the heart, which in turn is determined mainly by the amount of blood pumped and the arterial pressure level at which it is pumped.

REGULATION OF HEART PUMPING

When a person is at rest, the heart pumps only 4 to 6 liters of blood each minute. However, during severe exercise, the heart may be required to pump as much as four to seven times this amount.

The two basic means by which the volume pumped by the heart is regulated are (1) intrinsic cardiac regulation of pumping in response to changes in volume of blood flowing into the heart and (2) control of the heart by the autonomic nervous system.

Intrinsic Regulation of Heart Pumping—The Frank-Starling Mechanism

In Chapter 17 we see that the amount of blood pumped by the heart each minute is determined by the rate of blood flow into the heart from the veins, which is called *venous return.* That is, each peripheral tissue of the body controls its own blood flow, and the total of all the local blood flows through all the peripheral tissues returns by way of the veins to the right atrium. The heart in turn automatically pumps this incoming blood on into the systemic arteries, so that it can flow around the circuit again.

This intrinsic ability of the heart to adapt to changing volumes of inflowing blood is called the *Frank-Starling mechanism of the heart,* in honor of Frank and Starling, two great physiologists of nearly a century ago. Basically, the Frank-Starling mechanism means that the greater the heart is filled during diastole, the greater will be the quantity of blood pumped into the aorta. Or another way to express this is: *Within physiological limits, the heart pumps all the blood that comes to it without allowing excessive damming of blood in the veins.*

What Is the Explanation of the Frank-Starling Mechanism? When an extra amount of blood flows into the ventricles, the cardiac muscle itself is stretched to a greater length. This in turn causes the muscle to contract with increased force because the actin and myosin filaments are then brought to a more nearly optimal degree of interdigitation for force generation. Therefore, the ventricle, because of its increased pumping, automatically pumps the extra blood into the arteries. This ability of stretched muscle, up to an optimal length, to contract with increased force is characteristic of all striated muscle, as explained in Chapter 6, not simply of cardiac muscle.

Ventricular Function Curves

One of the best ways to express the functional ability of the ventricles to pump blood is by ventricular function curves, as shown in Figure 8-6. This figure illustrates a type of ventricular function curve called the *ventricular output curve.* The two curves represent function of the two ventricles of the human heart based on data extrapolated from lower animals. As each atrial pressure rises, the respective ventricular volume output per minute also increases.

Thus, ventricular function curves are another way of expressing the Frank-Starling mechanism of the heart. That is, as the ventricles fill to higher atrial pressures, the ventricular volume and strength of cardiac contraction increase, causing the heart to pump increased quantities of blood into the arteries.

Control of the Heart by the Sympathetic and Parasympathetic Nerves

The pumping effectiveness of the heart is highly controlled by the *sympathetic* and *parasympathetic* (vagus) nerves, which abundantly supply the heart, as illustrated in Figure 8-7. The amount of blood pumped by the heart each minute, the *cardiac output,*

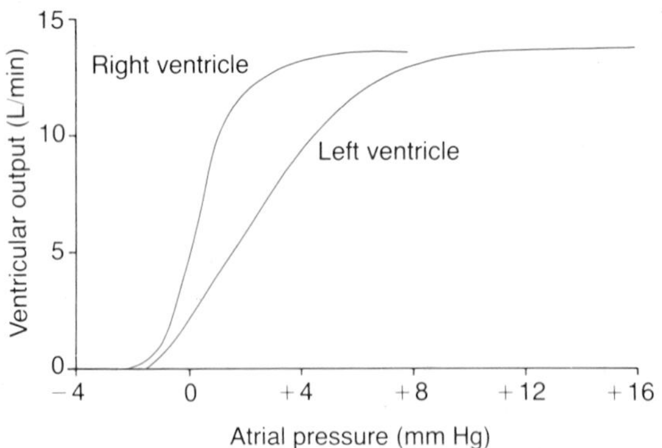

Figure 8-6. Approximate normal right and left ventricular output curves for the human heart, as extrapolated from data obtained in dogs.

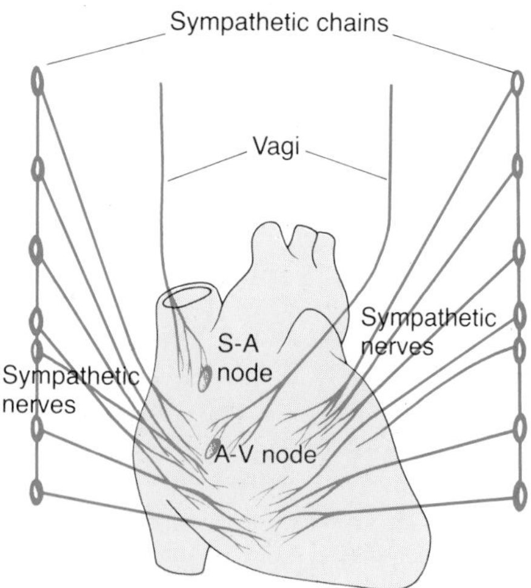

Figure 8-7. The cardiac nerves.

can often be increased several hundred per cent by sympathetic stimulation. By contrast, it can be decreased to as low as zero or almost zero by vagal (parasympathetic) stimulation.

Excitation of the Heart by the Sympathetic Nerves. Strong sympathetic stimulation can increase the heart rate in the human to as high as 200 and rarely even 250 beats per minute in young people. Also, sympathetic stimulation increases the force with which the heart muscle contracts, therefore also increasing the volume of blood pumped as well as increasing the ejection pressure. Thus, sympathetic stimulation can often increase the cardiac output as much as twofold to threefold.

Parasympathetic (Vagal) Stimulation of the Heart. Strong vagal stimulation of the heart can actually stop the heart beat for a few seconds, but then the heart usually "escapes" and beats at a rate of 20 to 30 beats per minute thereafter. In addition, strong parasympathetic stimulation decreases the strength of heart contraction by as much as 20 to 30 per cent. This is not a great decrease because the vagal fibers are distributed mainly to the atria and not much to the ventricles, where the power contraction of the heart occurs. Nevertheless, the great decrease in heart rate combined with a slight decrease in heart contraction can decrease ventricular pumping as much as 50 or more per cent — especially so when the heart is working under great workload.

Effect of Sympathetic or Parasympathetic Stimulation on the Cardiac Function Curve. Figure 8-8 illustrates four separate cardiac function curves. These are much the same as the ventricular function curves of Figure 8-6 except that they represent function of the entire heart rather than of a single ventricle; they show the relationship between the right atrial pressure at the input of the heart and cardiac output into the aorta.

The curves of Figure 8-8 demonstrate that at any given right atrial pressure, the cardiac output increases with increasing sympathetic stimulation and decreases with increasing parasympathetic stimula-

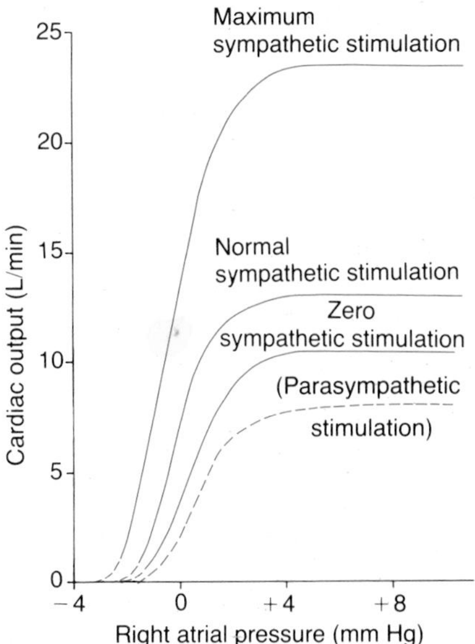

Figure 8–8. Effect on the cardiac output curve of different degrees of sympathetic and parasympathetic stimulation.

tion. It should be remembered that the changes in output caused by nerve stimulation are brought about by both *changes in heart rate* and *changes in contractile strength of the heart,* because both of these affect cardiac output.

EFFECT OF POTASSIUM AND CALCIUM IONS ON HEART FUNCTION

In the discussion of membrane potentials in Chapter 5, it was pointed out that potassium ions have a marked effect on membrane potentials and action potentials, and in Chapter 6 it was noted that calcium ions play an especially important role in initiating the muscle contractile process. Therefore, it is to be expected that the concentrations of these two ions in the extracellular fluids will have important effects on cardiac pumping.

Effect of Potassium Ions. Excess potassium in the extracellular fluids causes the heart to become extremely dilated and flaccid and slows the heart rate. Very large quantities can also block conduction of the cardiac impulse from the atria to the ventricles through the A-V bundle. Elevation of potassium concentration to only 9 to 12 mEq/liter—two to three times the normal value—can cause such weakness of the heart and abnormal rhythm that this can cause death.

These effects are caused partially by the fact that a high potassium concentration in the extracellular fluids causes a decreased resting membrane potential in the cardiac muscle fibers, as explained in Chapter 5. As the membrane potential decreases, the intensity of the action potential also decreases, which makes the contraction of the heart progressively weaker.

Effect of Calcium Ions. An excess of calcium ions causes effects almost exactly opposite of those of potassium ions, causing the heart to go into spastic contraction. This is caused by the direct effect of calcium ions in exciting the cardiac contractile process, as explained earlier in the chapter. Conversely, a deficiency of calcium ions causes cardiac flaccidity, similar to the effect of potassium. However, because the calcium ion levels in the blood are normally regulated within narrow ranges, it is rare that these cardiac effects of abnormal calcium concentrations are of clinical concern.

REFERENCES

Cooper, G., IV: Cardiocyte adaptation to chronically altered load. Annu. Rev. Physiol., 49:501, 1987.

Cowley, A. W., Jr., and Guyton, A. C.: Heart rate as a determinant of cardiac output in dogs with arteriovenous fistula. Am. J. Cardiol., 28:321, 1971.

Ellis, D.: Na-Ca exchange in cardiac tissue. Adv. Myocardiol., 5:295, 1985.

FitzGerald, P. G.: Gap junction heterogeneity in liver, heart, and lens. News Physiol. Sci., 3:206, 1988.

Fozzard, H. A., et al.: The Heart and Cardiovascular System: Scientific Foundations. New York, Raven Press, 1986.

Guyton, A. C.: Determination of cardiac output by equating venous return curves with cardiac response curves. Physiol. Rev., 35:123, 1955.

Guyton, A. C., et al.: Circulatory Physiology: Cardiac Output and Its Regulation. 2nd ed. Philadelphia, W. B. Saunders Co., 1973.

Hurst, J. W., et al.: The Heart. New York, McGraw-Hill Book Co., 1990.

Morgan, H. E., et al.: Biochemical mechanisms of cardiac hypertrophy. Annu. Rev. Physiol., 49:533, 1987.

Nozawa, T., et al.: Relation between oxygen consumption and pressure-volume area of in situ dog heart. Am. J. Physiol., 253:H31, 1987.

Roegg, J. C.: Dependence of cardiac contractility on myofibrillar calcium sensitivity. News Physiol. Sci., 2:179, 1987.

Starling, E. H.: The Linacre Lecture on the Law of the Heart. London, Longmans Green & Co., 1918.

Suga, H., et al.: Prospective prediction of O_2 consumption from pressure-volume area in dog hearts. Am. J. Physiol., 252:H1258, 1987.

Swynghedauw, B.: Developmental and functional adaptation of contractile proteins in cardiac and skeletal muscles. Physiol. Rev., 66:710, 1986.

Winegrad, S.: Calcium release from cardiac sarcoplasmic reticulum. Annu. Rev. Physiol., 44:451, 1982.

QUESTIONS

1. Describe the differences between cardiac muscle and skeletal muscle.
2. What is meant by the *atrial cardiac muscle syncytium* and the *ventricular cardiac muscle syncytium*?
3. How do action potentials of cardiac muscle differ from those in skeletal muscle?
4. How does excitation-contraction coupling in cardiac muscle differ from that in skeletal muscle? Explain especially the importance of calcium ions in the T tubules.
5. Explain what is meant by *systole* and *diastole.*
6. Give the relationships of the waves in the electrocardiogram to the periods of systole and diastole.

7. Explain the role of the atria as "primer" pumps.
8. Describe the different stages of filling of the ventricles during diastole.
9. Describe the stages of ventricular emptying during the pumping cycle.
10. What are meant by *end-diastolic volume, end-systolic volume,* and *stroke volume output*?
11. Explain the function of the valves, pointing out especially the differences in anatomy and function of the A-V valves versus the semilunar valves (aortic and pulmonary valves).
12. Describe the successive stages of the aortic pressure curve and explain the causes of its features.
13. Give the relationship of the heart sounds to the systolic and diastolic periods of the cardiac cycle.
14. Explain the mechanism and importance of the Frank-Starling law of the heart.
15. What is the effect on cardiac output of changing the arterial pressure load?
16. Describe the ventricular function curves for the right and left heart.
17. What is the approximate range of control of heart rate by the parasympathetic and sympathetic nerves?
18. How much can parasympathetic and sympathetic nerve stimulation of the heart change the contractile strength of the heart?
19. Describe the effects of cardiac debility and cardiac hypertrophy on overall heart function as represented by cardiac output curves.
20. What are the respective effects of excess potassium ions and excess calcium ions on heart function?
21. Explain the effect of changes in body temperature on heart rate and heart contraction.

9

Rhythmical Excitation of the Heart

The heart is endowed with a specialized system (1) for generating rhythmical impulses to cause rhythmical contraction of the heart muscle and (2) for conducting these impulses rapidly throughout the heart. When this system functions normally, the atria contract about one sixth of a second ahead of ventricular contraction, which allows extra filling of the ventricles before they pump the blood through the lungs and peripheral circulation.

Unfortunately, though, this rhythmical and conduction system of the heart is very susceptible to damage by heart disease, especially by ischemia of the heart tissues resulting from poor coronary blood flow. The consequence is often a very bizarre heart rhythm, even to the extent of causing death.

THE SPECIALIZED EXCITATORY AND CONDUCTIVE SYSTEM OF THE HEART

Figure 9–1 illustrates the specialized excitatory and conductive system of the heart that controls cardiac contractions. The figure shows (A) the *sinus node* (also called *sinoatrial* or *S-A node*), in which the normal rhythmical impulse is generated; (B) the *internodal pathways* that conduct the impulse from the sinus node to the A-V node; (C) the *A-V node* (also called *atrioventricular node*), in which the impulse from the atria is delayed before passing into the ventricles; (D) the *A-V bundle,* which conducts the impulse from the atria into the ventricles; and (E) the *left* and *right bundles of Purkinje fibers,* which conduct the cardiac impulse to all parts of the ventricles.

The Sinus Node

The sinus node is a small, flattened, ellipsoid strip of specialized muscle approximately 3 millimeters wide, 15 millimeters long, and 1 millimeter thick; it is located in the superior lateral wall of the right atrium immediately below and lateral to the opening of the superior vena cava. The fibers of this node have almost no contractile filaments and are each 3 to 5 micrometers in diameter, in contrast to a diameter of 10 to 15 micrometers for the surrounding atrial muscle fibers. However, the sinus fibers are continuous with the atrial fibers, so that any action potential that begins in the sinus node spreads immediately into the atria.

Automatic Rhythmicity of the Sinus Fibers

Many cardiac fibers have the capability of *self-excitation,* a process that can cause automatic rhythmical contraction. This is especially true of the fibers of the sinus node. For this reason, the sinus node ordinarily controls the rate of beat of the entire heart, as is discussed in detail later in this chapter.

Mechanism of Sinus Nodal Rhythmicity. Figure 9–2 illustrates action potentials recorded from a sinus nodal fiber for three heart beats and, by comparison, a single ventricular muscle fiber action potential, shown to the right. Note that the potential of the sinus nodal fiber between discharges has a negativity of only −55 to −60 millivolts (mV) in comparison with −85 to −90 mV for the ventricular fiber. The cause of this reduced negativity is that the cell membranes of the sinus fibers are naturally leaky to sodium ions.

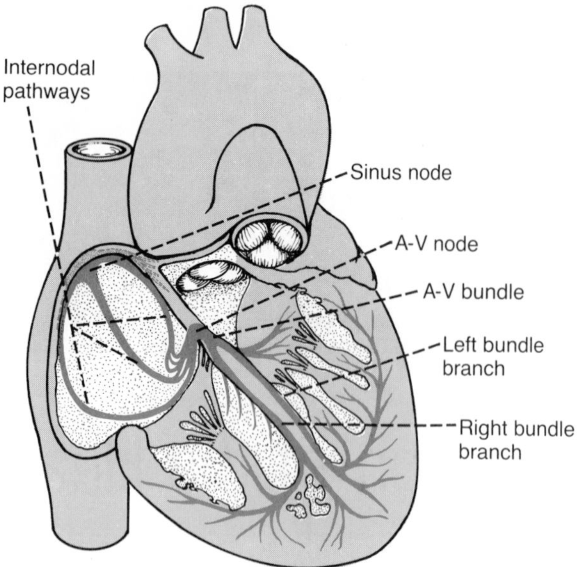

Figure 9-1. The sinus node and the Purkinje system of the heart, showing also the A-V node, the atrial internodal pathways, and the ventricular bundle branches.

Before attempting to explain the rhythmicity of the sinus nodal fibers, first recall from the discussions of Chapters 5 and 8 that in cardiac muscle three different types of membrane ion channels play important roles in causing the voltage changes of the action potential. These are (1) the *fast sodium channels,* (2) the *slow calcium-sodium channels,* and (3) the *potassium channels.* The opening of the fast sodium channels for a few 10,000ths of a second is responsible for the very rapid spikelike onset of the action potential observed in ventricular muscle because of rapid influx of positive sodium ions to the interior of the fiber. Then the plateau of the ventricular action potential is caused primarily by slower opening of the slow calcium-sodium channels, which lasts for a few tenths of a second. Finally, increased opening of the potassium channels and diffusion of large amounts of positive potassium ions out of the fiber return the membrane potential to its resting level.

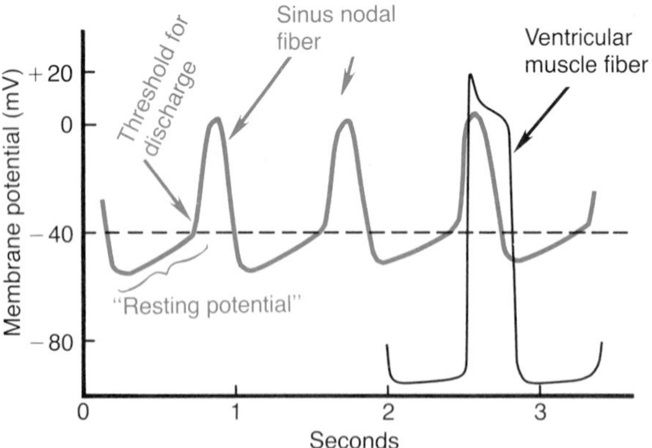

Figure 9-2. Rhythmical discharge of a sinus nodal fiber and comparison of the sinus nodal action potential with that of a ventricular muscle fiber.

But there is a difference in the function of these channels in the sinus nodal fiber because of the much lesser negativity of the "resting" potential—only −55 mV. At this level of negativity, the fast sodium channels have mainly become "inactivated," which means that they have become blocked. The cause of this is that any time the membrane potential remains less negative than about −60 mV for more than a few milliseconds, the inactivation gates on the inside of the cell membrane that close these channels become closed and remain so. Therefore, only the slow calcium-sodium channels can open (that is, can become "activated") and thereby cause the action potential. Therefore, the action potential is slower to develop than that of the ventricular muscle and also recovers slowly as well, rather than the abrupt recovery that occurs for the ventricular fiber.

Self-Excitation of Sinus Nodal Fibers. Sodium ions naturally tend to leak to the interior of the sinus nodal fibers through multiple membrane channels, and this influx of positive charges also causes a rising membrane potential. Thus, as illustrated in Figure 9-2, the "resting" potential gradually rises between each two heart beats. When it reaches a *threshold voltage* of about −40 mV, the calcium-sodium channels become activated, leading to very rapid entry of both calcium and sodium ions, thus causing the action potential. Therefore, basically, the inherent leakiness of the sinus nodal fibers to sodium ions causes their self-excitation.

Why does this leakiness to sodium ions not cause the sinus nodal fibers to remain depolarized all the time? The answer is, first, the calcium-sodium channels become inactivated (that is, they close) within about 100 to 150 milliseconds after opening, and second, at about the same time greatly increased numbers of potassium channels open. Therefore, now the influx of calcium and sodium ions through the calcium-sodium channels ceases while large quantities of positive potassium ions diffuse *out* of the fiber, thus terminating the action potential. Furthermore, the potassium channels remain open for another few tenths of a second, carrying a great excess of positive potassium charges out of the cell, which temporarily causes considerable excess negativity inside the fiber; this is called *hyperpolarization.* This hyperpolarization initially carries the "resting" membrane potential down to about −55 to −60 mV at the termination of the action potential.

Last, we must explain why the state of hyperpolarization also is not maintained forever. The reason is that during the next few tenths of a second after the action potential is over, progressively more and more of the potassium channels begin to close. Now the inward-leaking sodium ions once again overbalance the outward flux of potassium ions, which causes the "resting" potential to drift upward, finally reaching the threshold level for discharge at a potential of about −40 mV. Then the entire process begins again: self-excitation, recovery from the action potential, hyperpolarization after the action potential is over, upward drift of the "resting" potential, then re-excitation still again to elicit another cycle. This process continues indefinitely throughout the life of the person.

Internodal Pathways and Transmission of the Cardiac Impulse Through the Atria

The ends of the sinus nodal fibers fuse with the surrounding atrial muscle fibers, and action potentials originating in the sinus node travel outward into these fibers. In this way, the action potential spreads through the entire atrial muscle mass and eventually also to the A-V node. The velocity of conduction in the atrial muscle is approximately 0.3 m/sec. However, conduction is somewhat more rapid — about 1 m/sec — in several small bundles of atrial muscle fibers. One of these passes through the anterior walls of the atria to the left atrium, and three others curve through the atrial walls and terminate in the A-V node, also conducting the cardiac impulse at a rapid velocity. These three small bundles, illustrated in Figure 9–1, are called *internodal pathways.* The cause of the more rapid velocity of conduction in these bundles is the presence of a number of specialized conduction fibers mixed with the atrial muscle. These fibers are similar to the very rapidly conducting Purkinje fibers of the ventricles, which are discussed subsequently.

The A-V Node and Delay in Impulse Conduction

Fortunately, the conductive system is organized so that the cardiac impulse will not travel from the atria into the ventricles too rapidly; this allows time for the atria to empty their contents into the ventricles before ventricular contraction begins. It is primarily the A-V node and its associated conductive fibers that delay this transmission from the atria into the ventricles.

The A-V node is located in the posterior septal wall of the right atrium immediately behind the tricuspid valve, as illustrated in Figure 9–1. Figure 9–3 shows the different parts of this node and its connections with the atrial internodal pathway fibers and the A-V bundle. The figure also shows the approximate intervals of time in fractions of a second between the genesis of the cardiac impulse in the sinus node and its appearance at different points in the A-V nodal system. Note that the impulse, after traveling through the internodal pathway, reaches the A-V node approximately 0.03 second after its origin in the sinus node. Then there is a further delay of 0.09 second in the A-V node itself before the impulse enters the *penetrating portion of the A-V bundle.* A final delay of another 0.04 second occurs mainly in this penetrating A-V bundle, which is composed of multiple small fascicles passing through the fibrous tissue separating the atria from the ventricles.

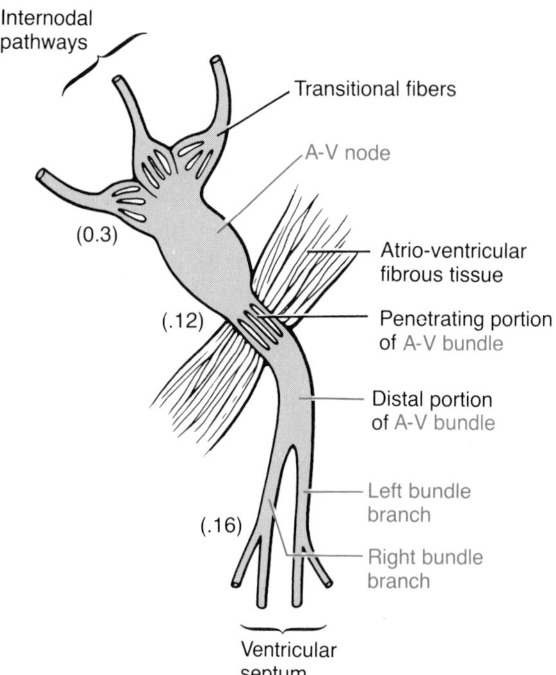

Figure 9–3. Organization of the A-V node. The numbers represent the interval of time from the origin of the impulse in the sinus node. The values have been extrapolated to the human being.

Thus, the total delay in the A-V nodal and A-V bundle system is approximately 0.13 second. About a quarter of this time lapse occurs in the *transitional fibers,* which are very small fibers that connect the fibers of the atrial internodal pathways with the A-V node (see Fig. 9–3). The velocity of conduction in these fibers is as little as 0.02 to 0.05 m/sec (about 1/12 that in normal cardiac muscle), which greatly delays entrance of the impulse into the A-V node. After entering the node proper, the velocity of conduction in the nodal fibers is still quite low, only 0.05 m/sec, about one eighth the conduction velocity in normal cardiac muscle. This low velocity of conduction is also approximately true for the penetrating portion of the A-V bundle.

Cause of the Slow Conduction. The cause of the extremely slow conduction in the transitional as well as the nodal and penetrating A-V bundle fibers is partly that their sizes are considerably smaller than the sizes of the normal atrial muscle fibers. However, most of the slow conduction is probably caused by two other factors. First, all these fibers have resting membrane potentials that are much less negative than the normal resting potential of other cardiac muscle. Second, very few gap junctions connect the successive fibers in the pathway, so that there is great resistance to the conduction of excitatory ions from one fiber to the next. Thus, with both low voltage to drive the ions and great resistance to the movement of the ions, it is easy to see why each succeeding fiber is slow to be excited.

Transmission in the Purkinje System

The *Purkinje fibers* lead from the A-V node through the A-V bundle into the ventricles. Except for the initial portion of these fibers where they penetrate the atrioventricular fibrous barrier, they have functional characteristics quite the opposite of those of the A-V nodal fibers; they are very large fibers, even larger than the normal ventricular muscle fibers, and they transmit action potentials at a velocity of 1.5 to 4.0 m/sec, a velocity about 6 times that in the usual cardiac muscle and 150 times that in some transitional fibers of the A-V node. This allows almost immediate transmission of the cardiac impulse throughout the entire ventricular system.

The very rapid transmission of action potentials by Purkinje fibers is believed to be caused by increased permeability of the gap junctions at the intercalated discs between the successive cardiac cells that make up the Purkinje fibers. At these discs, ions are transmitted easily from one cell to the next, thus enhancing the velocity of transmission.

Distribution of the Purkinje Fibers in the Ventricles. After penetrating through the atrioventricular fibrous tissue, the distal portion of the A-V bundle passes downward in the ventricular septum for 5 to 15 millimeters toward the apex of the heart, as shown in Figures 9–1 and 9–3. Then the bundle divides into the *left* and *right bundle branches* that lie beneath the endocardium of the two respective sides of the septum. Each branch spreads downward to the apex of the ventricle, dividing into smaller branches that course around each ventricular chamber and back toward the base of the heart. The terminal Purkinje fibers penetrate about one third of the way into the muscle mass and then become continuous with the cardiac muscle fibers.

From the time that the cardiac impulse first enters the bundle branches until it reaches the terminations of the Purkinje fibers, the total time that elapses averages only 0.03 second; therefore, once the cardiac impulse enters the Purkinje system, it spreads almost immediately to the entire endocardial surface of the ventricular muscle.

Transmission of the Cardiac Impulse in the Ventricular Muscle

Once the impulse has reached the ends of the Purkinje fibers, it is then transmitted through the ventricular muscle mass by the ventricular muscle fibers themselves. The velocity of transmission is now only 0.3 to 0.5 m/sec, one sixth that in the Purkinje fibers.

The cardiac muscle wraps around the heart in a double spiral with fibrous septa between the spiraling layers; therefore, the cardiac impulse does not necessarily travel directly outward toward the surface of the heart but instead angulates toward the surface along the directions of the spirals. Because of this, transmission from the endocardial surface to the epicardial surface of the ventricle requires as much as another 0.03 second, approximately equal to the time required for transmission through the entire Purkinje system. Thus, the total time for transmission of the cardiac impulse from the initial bundle branches leaving the A-V bundle to the last of the ventricular muscle fibers in the normal heart is about 0.06 second.

Summary of the Spread of the Cardiac Impulse Through the Heart

Figure 9–4 illustrates in summary form the transmission of the cardiac impulse through the human heart. The numbers on the figure represent the intervals of time in hundredths of a second that lapse between the origin of the cardiac impulse in the sinus node and its appearance at each respective point in the heart. Note that the impulse spreads at moderate velocity through the atria but is delayed more than 0.1 second in the A-V nodal region before appearing in the ventricular septal A-V bundle. Once it has passed through this bundle, it spreads rapidly through the Purkinje fibers to the entire endocardial surfaces of the ventricles. Then the impulse once again spreads more slowly through the ventricular muscle to the epicardial surfaces.

It is extremely important that the reader learn in detail the course of the cardiac impulse through the heart and the times of its appearance in each separate part of the heart, for a quantitative knowledge of this process is essential to the understanding of electro-

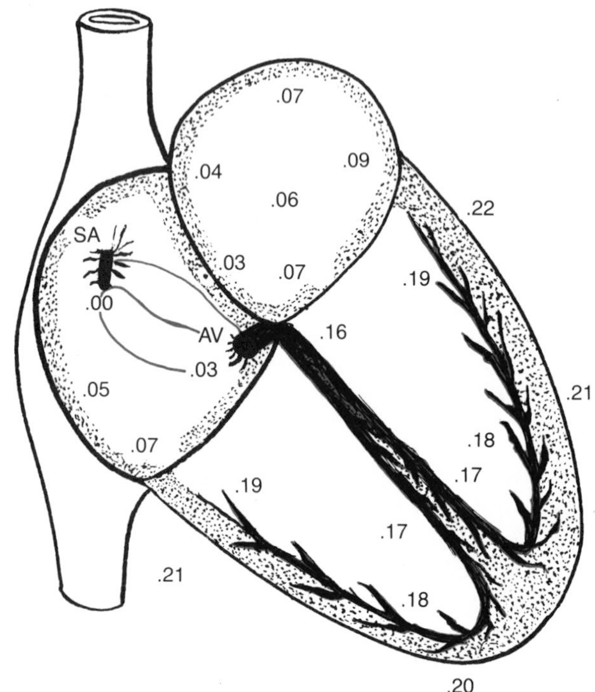

Figure 9–4. Transmission of the cardiac impulse through the heart, showing the time of appearance (in fractions of a second) of the impulse in different parts of the heart.

cardiography, which is discussed in the following chapter.

CONTROL OF EXCITATION AND CONDUCTION IN THE HEART

The Sinus Node as the Pacemaker of the Heart

In the previous discussion of the genesis and transmission of the cardiac impulse through the heart, we have noted that the impulse normally arises in the sinus node. However, this often is not the case under abnormal conditions, for other parts of the heart can exhibit rhythmic contraction in the same way that the sinus nodal fibers can; this is particularly true of the A-V nodal and Purkinje fibers.

The A-V nodal fibers, when not stimulated from some outside source, discharge at an intrinsic rhythmic rate of 40 to 60 times per minute, and the Purkinje fibers discharge at a rate of somewhere between 15 and 40 times per minute. These rates are in contrast to the normal rate of the sinus node of 70 to 80 times per minute.

Therefore, the question that we must ask is: Why does the sinus node control the heart's rhythmicity rather than the A-V node or the Purkinje fibers? The answer to this derives from the fact that the discharge rate of the sinus node is considerably greater than that of either the A-V node or the Purkinje fibers. Each time the sinus node discharges, its impulse is conducted into both the A-V node and the Purkinje fibers, discharging their excitable membranes. Then these tissues as well as the sinus node recover from the action potential and become hyperpolarized. But the sinus node loses its hyperpolarization much more rapidly than does either of the other two and emits a new impulse before either one of them can reach its own threshold for self-excitation. The new impulse again discharges both the A-V node and Purkinje fibers. This process continues on and on, the sinus node always exciting these other potentially self-excitatory tissues before self-excitation can actually occur.

Thus, the sinus node controls the beat of the heart because its rate of rhythmic discharge is greater than that of any other part of the heart. Therefore, the sinus node is the normal *pacemaker* of the heart.

Abnormal Pacemakers—the Ectopic Pacemaker. Occasionally some other part of the heart develops a rhythmic discharge rate that is more rapid than that of the sinus node. For instance, this often occurs in the A-V node or in the Purkinje fibers. In either of these cases, the pacemaker of the heart shifts from the sinus node to the A-V node or to the excitable Purkinje fibers. Under more rare conditions, a point in the atrial or ventricular muscle develops excessive excitability and becomes the pacemaker.

A pacemaker elsewhere than the sinus node is called an *ectopic pacemaker.* Obviously, an ectopic pacemaker causes an abnormal sequence of contraction of the different parts of the heart.

Control of Heart Rhythmicity and Conduction by the Sympathetic and Parasympathetic Nerves

The heart is supplied with both sympathetic and parasympathetic nerves, as illustrated in Figure 8–7 of the previous chapter. The parasympathetic nerves (the vagi) are distributed mainly to the sinus and A-V nodes, to a lesser extent to the muscle of the two atria, and even less to the ventricular muscle. The sympathetic nerves, on the other hand, are distributed to all parts of the heart, with a strong representation to the ventricular muscle as well as to all the other areas.

Effect of Parasympathetic (Vagal) Stimulation on Cardiac Rhythm and Conduction—Ventricular Escape. Stimulation of the parasympathetic nerves to the heart (the vagi) causes the hormone *acetylcholine* to be released at the vagal endings. This hormone has two major effects on the heart. First, it decreases the rate of rhythm of the sinus node, and, second, it decreases the excitability of the A-V junctional fibers between the atrial musculature and the A-V node, thereby slowing transmission of the cardiac impulse into the ventricles. Very strong stimulation of the vagi can completely stop the rhythmic contraction of the sinus node or completely block transmission of the cardiac impulse through the A-V junction. In either case, rhythmic impulses are no longer transmitted into the ventricles. The ventricles stop beating for 4 to 10 seconds, but then some point in the Purkinje fibers, usually in the ventricular septal portion of the A-V bundle, develops a rhythm of its own and causes ventricular contraction at a rate of 15 to 40 beats per minute. This phenomenon is called *ventricular escape.*

Mechanism of the Vagal Effects. The acetylcholine released at the vagal nerve endings greatly increases the permeability of the fiber membranes to potassium, which allows rapid leakage of potassium to the exterior. This causes increased negativity inside the fibers, an effect called *hyperpolarization,* which makes excitable tissue much less excitable, as was explained in Chapter 5.

Effect of Sympathetic Stimulation on Cardiac Rhythm and Conduction. Sympathetic stimulation causes essentially the opposite effects on the heart to those caused by vagal stimulation as follows: First, it increases the rate of sinus nodal discharge. Second, it increases the rate of conduction as well as the level of excitability in all portions of the heart. Third, it increases greatly the force of contraction of all the cardiac musculature, both atrial and ventricular, as discussed in the previous chapter.

In short, sympathetic stimulation increases the overall activity of the heart. Maximal stimulation can almost triple the rate of heartbeat and can increase the strength of heart contraction as much as twofold.

Mechanism of the Sympathetic Effect. Stimulation of the sympathetic nerves releases the hormone *norepinephrine* at the sympathetic nerve endings. The precise mechanism by which this hormone acts on cardiac muscle fibers is still somewhat doubtful, but the present belief is that it increases the permeability of the fiber membrane to sodium and calcium. In the sinus node, an increase of sodium permeability causes a more positive resting potential and an increased rate of upward drift of the membrane potential to the threshold level for self-excitation, both of which obviously accelerate the onset of self-excitation and therefore increase the heart rate.

In the A-V node, increased sodium permeability makes it easier for the action potential to excite the succeeding portion of the conducting fiber, thereby decreasing the conduction time from the atria to the ventricles.

The increase in permeability to calcium ions is at least partially responsible for the increase in contractile strength of the cardiac muscle under the influence of sympathetic stimulation because calcium ions play a powerful role in exciting the contractile process of the myofibrils.

REFERENCES

Ellis, D.: Na-Ca exchange in cardiac tissues. Adv. Myocardiol., 5:295, 1985.

Fozzard, H. A., et al.: The Heart and Cardiovascular System: Scientific Foundations. New York, Raven Press, 1986.

Gravanis, M. B. (ed.): Cardiovascular Pathophysiology. New York, McGraw-Hill Book Co., 1987.

Guyton, A. C., and Satterfield, J.: Factors concerned in electrical defibrillation of the heart, particularly through the unopened chest. Am. J. Physiol., 167:81, 1951.

Josephson, M. E., and Singh, B. N.: Use of calcium antagonists in ventricular dysfunction. Am. J. Cardiol., 55:81B, 1985.

Latorre, R., et al.: K^+ channels gated by voltage and ions. Annu. Rev. Physiol., 46:485, 1984.

Mazzanti, M., and DeFelice, L. J.: K channel kinetics during the spontaneous heart beat in embryonic chick ventricle cells. Biophys. J., 54:1139, 1988.

Mazzanti, M., and DeFelice, L. J.: Na channel kinetics during the spontaneous heart beat in embryonic chick ventricle cells. Biophys. J., 52:95, 1987.

Mazzanti, M., and DeFelice, L. J.: Regulation of the Na-conducting Ca channel during the cardiac action potential. Biophys. J., 51:115, 1987.

Meijler, F. L., and Janse, M. J.: Morphology and electrophysiology of the mammalian atrioventricular node. Physiol. Rev., 68:608, 1988.

Reuter, H.: Ion channels in cardiac cell membranes. Annu. Rev. Physiol., 44:473, 1984.

Sheridan, J. D., and Atkinson, M. M.: Physiological roles of permeable junctions: Some possibilities. Annu. Rev. Physiol., 47:337, 1985.

QUESTIONS

1. Describe the special excitatory and conductive system of the heart.
2. What is the mechanism of S-A nodal rhythmicity?
3. What causes the delay in transmission at the A-V node? And, what is the importance of this delay for cardiac function?
4. Describe the Purkinje system for rapid conduction of the cardiac impulse to all parts of the ventricles.
5. Why is it important that all parts of the ventricles receive the cardiac impulse simultaneously?
6. Why does the S-A node normally function as the pacemaker of the heart?
7. Under what conditions can other areas of the heart besides the S-A node become the pacemaker of the heart?
8. What are the effects of parasympathetic (vagal) stimulation on cardiac rhythmicity and conduction of the cardiac impulse through the conductive system of the heart?
9. What are the effects of sympathetic stimulation on cardiac rhythm, cardiac conduction, and cardiac contractile strength?

10

The Electrocardiogram and Electrocardiographic Interpretation of Heart Abnormalities

As the cardiac impulse passes through the heart, electrical currents spread into the tissues surrounding the heart, and a small proportion of these spreads all the way to the surface of the body. If electrodes are placed on the skin on opposite sides of the heart, electrical potentials generated by these currents can be recorded; the recording is known as an *electrocardiogram.* A normal electrocardiogram for two beats of the heart is illustrated in Figure 10–1.

CHARACTERISTICS OF THE NORMAL ELECTROCARDIOGRAM

The normal electrocardiogram (Fig. 10–1) is composed of a P wave, a "QRS complex," and a T wave. The QRS complex is often three separate waves, the Q wave, the R wave, and the S wave.

The P wave is caused by electrical potentials generated as the atria depolarize prior to their contraction. The QRS complex is caused by potentials generated when the ventricles depolarize prior to their contraction, that is, as the depolarization wave spreads through the ventricles. Therefore, both the P wave and the components of the QRS complex are *depolarization waves.*

The T wave is caused by potentials generated as the ventricles recover from the state of depolarization. This process occurs in ventricular muscle 0.25 to 0.35 second after depolarization, and this wave is known as a *repolarization wave.*

Thus, the electrocardiogram is composed of both depolarization and repolarization waves. The principles of depolarization and repolarization are discussed in Chapter 5. However, the distinction between depolarization waves and repolarization waves is so important in electrocardiography that further clarification is needed, as follows:

Depolarization Waves Versus Repolarization Waves

Figure 10–2 illustrates a muscle fiber in four different stages of depolarization and repolarization. During the process of depolarization the normal negative potential inside the fiber is lost and the membrane potential actually reverses; that is, it becomes slightly positive inside and negative outside.

In Figure 10–2A, the process of depolarization, illustrated by the red positive charges inside and negative charges outside, is traveling from left to right, and the first half of the fiber has already depolarized, while the remaining half is still polarized. This causes the meter to record positively. To the right of the muscle fiber is illustrated a record of the potential between the electrodes as recorded by a high-speed recording meter at this particular stage of depolarization.

In Figure 10–2B, depolarization has extended over the entire muscle fiber, and the recording to the right has returned to the zero baseline because both electrodes are now in areas of equal negativity. The completed wave is a *depolarization wave* because it results from spread of depolarization along the entire extent of the muscle fiber.

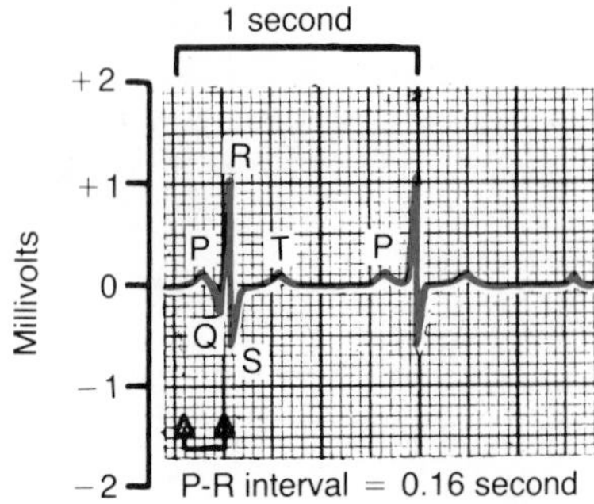

Figure 10–1. The normal electrocardiogram.

Figure 10–2C illustrates the repolarization process in the muscle fiber, which has proceeded halfway along the fiber from left to right. At this point, the left electrode is in an area of positivity, while the right electrode is in an area of negativity. This is opposite to the polarity in Figure 10–2A. Consequently, the recording, as illustrated to the right, becomes negative.

In Figure 10–2D, the muscle fiber has completely repolarized, and both electrodes are now in areas of positivity, so that no potential is recorded between them. Thus, in the recording to the right, the potential returns once more to the zero level. This completed negative wave is a *repolarization wave* because it results from spread of the repolarization process over the muscle fiber.

Relationship of the Monophasic Action Potential of Cardiac Muscle to the QRS and T Waves. The monophasic action potential of ventricular muscle, which was discussed in the preceding chapter, normally lasts between 0.25 and 0.35 second. The top part of Figure 10–3 illustrates a monophasic action potential recorded from a microelectrode inserted into the inside of a single ventricular muscle fiber. The upsweep of this action potential is caused by *depolarization,* and the return of the potential to the baseline is caused by *repolarization.*

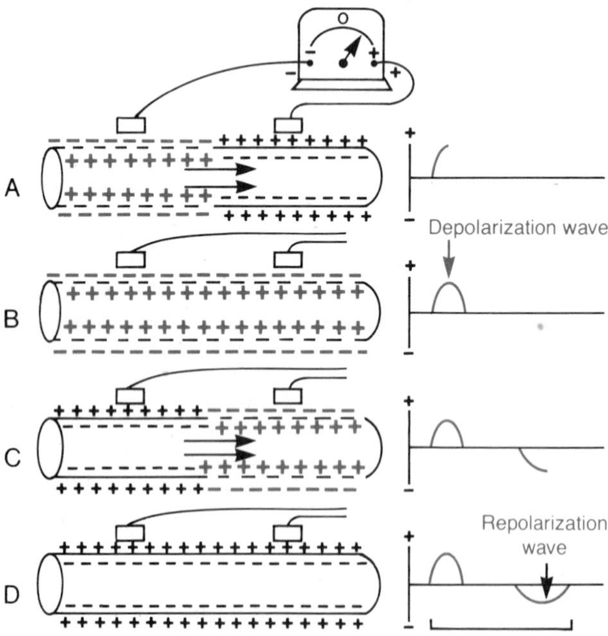

Figure 10–2. Recording the *depolarization wave* and the *repolarization wave* from a cardiac muscle fiber.

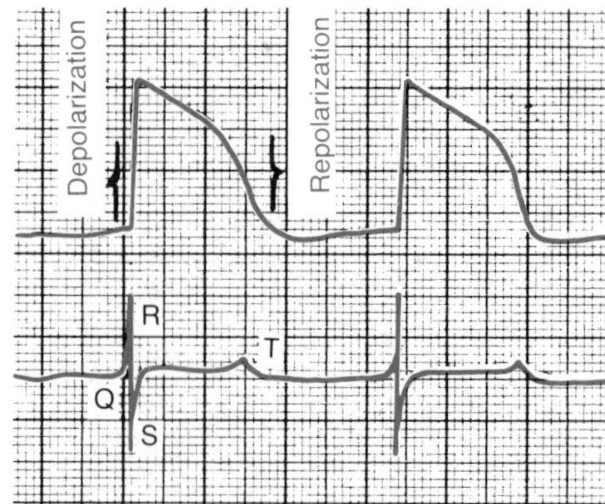

Figure 10–3. *Above:* Monophasic action potential from a ventricular muscle fiber during normal cardiac function, showing rapid depolarization and then repolarization occurring slowly during the plateau stage but very rapidly toward the end. *Below:* Electrocardiogram recorded simultaneously.

Note below in the figure the simultaneous recording of the electrocardiogram from this same ventricle, which shows the QRS wave appearing at the beginning of the monophasic action potential and the T wave appearing at the end. Note especially that *no potential at all is recorded in the electrocardiogram when the ventricular muscle is either completely polarized or completely depolarized.*

Relationship of Atrial and Ventricular Contraction to the Waves of the Electrocardiogram

Before contraction of muscle can occur, depolarization must spread through the muscle to initiate the chemical processes of contraction. Therefore, the P wave occurs immediately before the *beginning of contraction of the atria,* and the QRS wave occurs immediately before the *beginning of contraction of the ventricles.* The ventricles remain contracted until a few milliseconds after repolarization has occurred, that is, until after the end of the T wave.

The ventricular repolarization wave is the T wave of the normal electrocardiogram. Ordinarily, ventricular muscle begins to repolarize in some fibers approximately 0.20 second after the beginning of the depolarization wave but in many others not until as long as 0.35 second. Thus, the process of repolarization extends over a long period of time, about 0.15 second. For this reason, the T wave in the normal electrocardiogram is often a prolonged wave, but the voltage of the T wave is considerably less than the voltage of the QRS complex, partly because of its prolonged length.

The atria repolarize approximately 0.15 to 0.20 second after the P wave. However, this occurs just at the moment that the QRS wave is being recorded in the electrocardiogram. Therefore, the atrial repolarization wave, known as the *atrial T wave,* is usually totally obscured by the much larger QRS wave. For this reason, an atrial T wave is rarely observed in the electrocardiogram.

Voltage and Time Calibration of the Electrocardiogram

All recordings of electrocardiograms are made with appropriate calibration lines on the recording paper. Either these calibration lines are already ruled on the paper, as is the case when a pen recorder is used, or they are recorded on the paper at the same time that the electrocardiogram is recorded, which is the case with the photographic types of electrocardiographs.

As illustrated in Figure 10–1, the horizontal calibration lines are arranged so that 10 small divisions upward or downward in the standard electrocardiogram represent 1 millivolt (mV) with positivity in the upward direction and negativity in the downward direction.

The vertical lines on the electrocardiogram are time calibration lines. Each inch in the horizontal direction is 1 second, and each inch in turn is usually broken into five segments by dark vertical lines; the intervals between these lines represent 0.20 second.

Normal Voltages in the Electrocardiogram. The voltages of the waves in the normal electrocardiogram depend on the manner in which the electrodes are applied to the surface of the body. When one electrode is placed directly over the heart and the second electrode is placed elsewhere on the body, the voltage of the QRS complex may be as great as 3 to 4 mV. Even this voltage is very small in comparison with the monophasic action potential of 110 mV recorded directly at the heart muscle membrane. When electrocardiograms are recorded from electrodes on the two arms or on one arm and one leg, the voltage of the QRS complex usually is approximately 1 mV from the top of the R wave to the bottom of the S wave; the voltage of the P wave, between 0.1 and 0.3 mV; and that of the T wave, between 0.2 and 0.3 mV.

The P-Q or P-R Interval. The duration of time between the beginning of the P wave and the beginning of the QRS wave is the interval between the beginning of contraction of the atrium and the beginning of contraction of the ventricle. This period of time is called the P-Q interval. The normal P-Q interval is approximately 0.16 second. This interval is sometimes also called the P-R interval because the Q wave is frequently absent.

The Q-T Interval. Contraction of the ventricle lasts almost from the beginning of the Q wave to the end of the T wave. This interval of time is called the Q-T interval and ordinarily is approximately 0.35 second.

The Rate of the Heart as Determined from Electrocardiograms. The rate of heartbeat can be determined easily from electrocardiograms because the time interval between two successive beats is the reciprocal of the heart rate. If the interval between two beats as determined from the time calibration lines is 1 second, the heart rate is 60 beats per minute. The normal interval between two successive QRS complexes is approximately 0.83 second. This is a heart rate of 60/0.83 times per minute, or 72 beats per minute.

METHODS FOR RECORDING ELECTROCARDIOGRAMS—THE PEN RECORDER

The electrical currents generated by the cardiac muscle during each beat of the heart sometimes change potentials and polarity in less than 0.01 second. Therefore, it is essential that any apparatus for recording electrocardiograms be capable of responding rapidly to these changes in electrical potentials.

Most modern clinical electrocardiographic apparatus employ a direct pen writing recorder that writes the electrocardiogram directly on a moving sheet of paper. The pen is often a thin tube connected at one end to an inkwell, and its recording end is connected to a powerful electromagnet system that is capable of moving the pen back and forth at high speed. As the paper moves forward, the pen records the electrocardiogram. The movement of the pen in turn is controlled by means of appropriate electronic amplifiers connected to electrocardiographic electrodes on the patient.

Other pen recording systems use special paper that does not require ink in the recording stylus. One such paper turns black when electrical current flows from the tip of the stylus through the paper to an electrode at its back. This leaves a black line everywhere on the paper that the stylus touches.

Flow of Electrical Currents Around the Heart in the Chest

Figure 10–4 illustrates the ventricular muscle lying within the chest. Even the lungs, though mostly filled with air, conduct electricity to a surprising extent, and fluids of the other tissues surrounding the heart conduct electricity even more easily. Therefore, the heart is actually suspended in a conductive medium. When one portion of the ventricles becomes electronegative with respect to the remainder, electrical current flows from the depolarized area to the polarized area in large circuitous routes, as noted in the figure.

It should be recalled from the discussion of the Purkinje system in Chapter 9 that the cardiac impulse first arrives in the ventricles in the septum and shortly thereafter reaches the endocardial surfaces of the remainder of the ventricles, as shown by the colored areas and the negative signs in Figure 10–4. This provides electronegativity on the insides of the ventricles and electropositivity on the outer walls of the

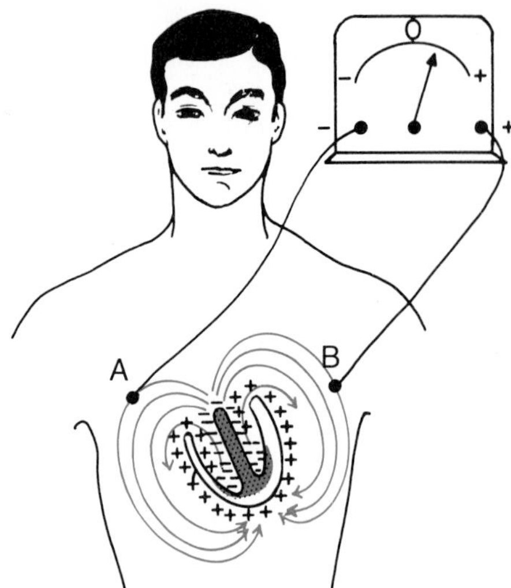

Figure 10-4. Flow of current in the chest around a partially depolarized heart.

ventricles, and current flows through the fluids surrounding the ventricles along elliptical paths, as illustrated in the figure. If one algebraically averages all the lines of current flow (the elliptical lines), one finds that the average current flow, *in the negative to positive direction,* is from the base of the heart toward the apex. During most of the remainder of the depolarization process, the current continues to flow in this direction as the depolarization spreads from the endocardial surface outward through the ventricular muscle. However, immediately before the depolarization has completed its course through the ventricles, the direction of current flow reverses for about 1/100 second, flowing then from the apex toward the base because the very last part of the heart to become depolarized is the outer walls of the ventricles near the base of the heart.

Thus, in the normal heart current flows primarily in the direction from the base toward the apex during almost the entire cycle of depolarization except at the very end. Therefore, if a meter is connected to the surface of the body, as shown in Figure 10-4, the electrode nearer the base will be negative, whereas the electrode nearer the apex will be positive, and the recording meter will show a positive recording in the electrocardiogram.

ELECTROCARDIOGRAPHIC LEADS

The Three Bipolar Limb Leads

Figure 10-5 illustrates electrical connections between the limbs and the electrocardiograph for recording electrocardiograms from the so-called standard bipolar limb leads. The term "bipolar" means that the electrocardiogram is recorded from two electrodes on the body, in this case on the limbs. Thus, a "lead" is not a single wire connecting from the body but a combination of two wires and their electrodes to make a complete circuit with the electrocardiograph. The electrocardiograph in each instance is illustrated by mechanical meters in the diagram, though the actual electrocardiograph is a high-speed recording meter with a moving paper.

Lead I. In recording limb lead I, the *negative terminal of the electrocardiograph is connected to the right arm* and the *positive terminal to the left arm.* Therefore, when the point on the chest where the right arm connects to the chest is electronegative with respect to the point where the left arm connects, the electrocardiograph records positively—that is, above the zero voltage line in the electrocardiogram. When the opposite is true, the electrocardiograph records below the line.

Lead II. In recording limb lead II, the *negative terminal of the electrocardiograph is connected to the right arm* and the *positive terminal to the left leg.* Therefore, when the right arm is negative with respect to the left leg, the electrocardiograph records positively.

Lead III. In recording limb lead III, the *negative terminal of the electrocardiograph is connected to the left arm* and the *positive terminal to the left leg.* This means that the electrocardiograph records positively when the left arm is negative with respect to the left leg.

Normal Electrocardiograms Recorded from the Three Standard Bipolar Limb Leads. Figure 10-6 illustrates recordings of the electrocardiogram in leads I, II, and III. It is obvious from this figure that

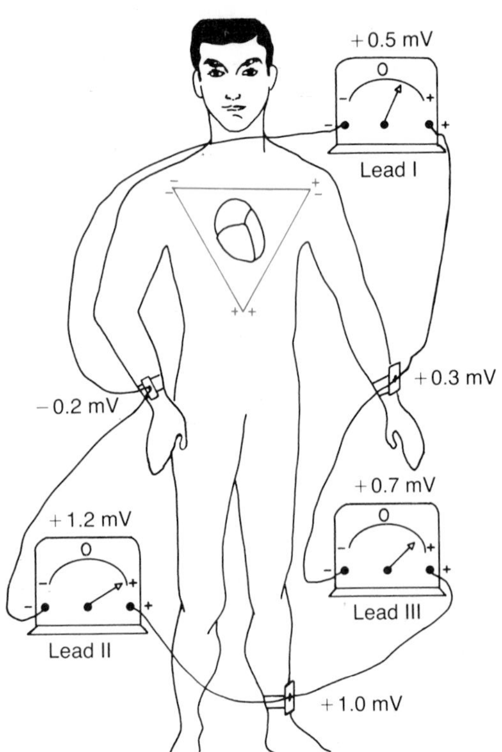

Figure 10-5. Conventional arrangement of electrodes for recording the standard electrocardiographic leads. Einthoven's triangle is superimposed on the chest.

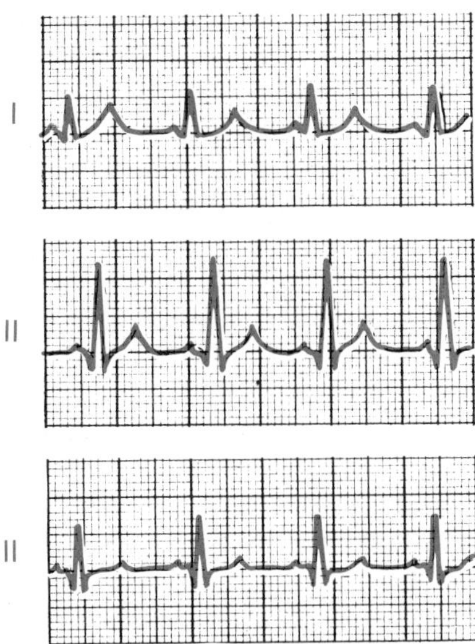

Figure 10-6. Normal electrocardiograms recorded from the three standard electrocardiographic leads.

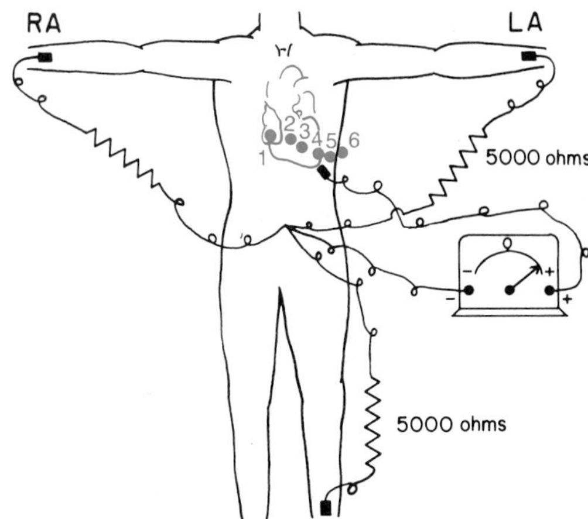

Figure 10-7. Connections of the body with the electrocardiograph for recording chest leads.

the electrocardiograms in these three leads are very similar to each other, for they all record positive *P* waves and positive *T* waves, and the major portion of the QRS complex is also positive in each electrocardiogram.

Because the recordings from all the bipolar limb leads are similar to each other, it does not matter greatly which lead is recorded when one wishes to diagnose the different cardiac arrhythmias, for diagnosis of arrhythmias depends mainly on the time relationships between the different waves of the cardiac cycle. On the other hand, when one wishes to diagnose damage in the ventricular or atrial muscle or in the conducting system, it does matter greatly which leads are recorded, for abnormalities of the cardiac muscle change the patterns of the electrocardiograms markedly in some leads and yet may not affect other leads.

Chest Leads (Precordial Leads)

Often electrocardiograms are recorded with an electrode placed on the anterior surface of the chest over the heart at one of the six separate red points in Figure 10-7. This electrode is connected to the positive terminal of the electrocardiograph, while the negative electrode, called the *indifferent electrode,* is normally connected through electrical resistances to the right arm, left arm, and left leg all at the same time, as also shown in the figure. Usually six different standard chest leads are recorded from the anterior chest wall, the chest electrode being placed respectively at the six points illustrated in the diagram. The different recordings are known as leads V_1, V_2, V_3, V_4, V_5, and V_6.

Figure 10-8 illustrates the electrocardiograms of the normal heart as recorded from these six standard chest leads. Because the heart surfaces are close to the chest wall, each chest lead records mainly the electrical potential of the cardiac musculature immediately beneath the electrode. Therefore, relatively minute abnormalities in the ventricles, particularly in the anterior ventricular wall, frequently cause marked changes in the electrocardiograms recorded from chest leads.

ELECTROCARDIOGRAPHIC INTERPRETATION OF CARDIAC ARRHYTHMIAS

The rhythmicity of the heart and its normal control were discussed in Chapter 9. The major purpose of the present section is to describe the electrocardiograms recorded in a few conditions known clinically as "cardiac arrhythmias."

ATRIOVENTRICULAR BLOCK

The only means by which impulses can ordinarily pass from the atria into the ventricles is through the *A-V bundle,* which is also known as the *bundle of His.* Different conditions that can either decrease the rate of conduction of the impulse through this bundle or totally block the impulse are:

1. *Ischemia of the A-V bundle fibers.*
2. *Compression of the A-V bundle* by scar tissue or by calcified portions of the heart.

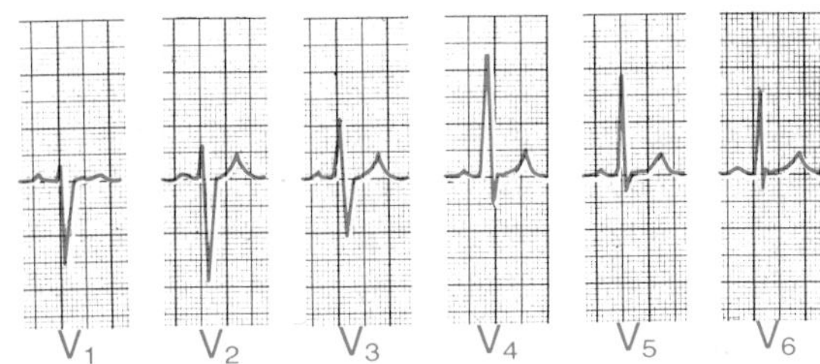

Figure 10-8. Normal electrocardiograms recorded from the six standard chest leads.

3. *Inflammation of the A-V bundle or fibers of the A-V junction.*
4. *Extreme stimulation of the heart by the vagi.*

Incomplete Heart Block. When conduction through the A-V junction is prolonged from a normal value of 0.16 second to as great as 0.25 to 0.50 second, the action potentials traveling through the A-V bundle fibers are sometimes strong enough to pass on into the A-V node and at other times are not strong enough. Often the impulse passes into the ventricles on one heart beat and fails to pass on the next one or two beats, thus alternating between conduction and nonconduction. In this instance, the atria beat many times without a corresponding beat of the ventricles, and it is said that there are "dropped beats" of the ventricles. This condition is called *incomplete heart block.*

Figure 10–9 illustrates P-R intervals as long as 0.30 second, and it also illustrates one dropped beat as a result of failure of conduction from the atria to the ventricles.

At times every other beat of the ventricles is dropped, so that a 2:1 rhythm develops in the heart, with the atria beating twice for every single beat of the ventricles. Sometimes other rhythms, such as 3:2 or 3:1, also develop.

Complete Atrioventricular Block. When the condition causing poor conduction in the A-V bundle becomes extremely severe, complete block of the impulse from the atria into the ventricles occurs. In this instance the P waves become completely dissociated from the QRS-T complexes, as illustrated in Figure 10–10. Note that the rate of rhythm of the atria in this electrocardiogram is approximately 100 beats per minute, while the rate of ventricular beat is less than 40 per minute. Furthermore, there is no relationship whatsoever between the rhythm of the atria and that of the ventricles, for the ventricles have "escaped" from control by the atria, and they are beating at their own natural rate.

Stokes-Adams Syndrome — Ventricular Escape. In some patients with atrioventricular block, total block comes and goes — that is, impulses are conducted from the atria into the ventricles for a period of time, and then suddenly no impulses at all are transmitted. This condition occurs particularly in hearts with borderline coronary ischemia.

Immediately after A-V conduction is first blocked, the ventricles stop contracting entirely for about 5 to 10 seconds. Then some part of the Purkinje system beyond the block, usually in the A-V bundle itself, begins discharging rhythmically at a rate of 15 to 40 times per minute and acting as the pacemaker of the ventricles. This is called *ventricular escape.* Because the brain cannot remain active for more than 3 to 5 seconds without blood supply, patients usually faint between block of conduction and "escape" of the ventricles. These periodic fainting spells are known as the Stokes-Adams syndrome.

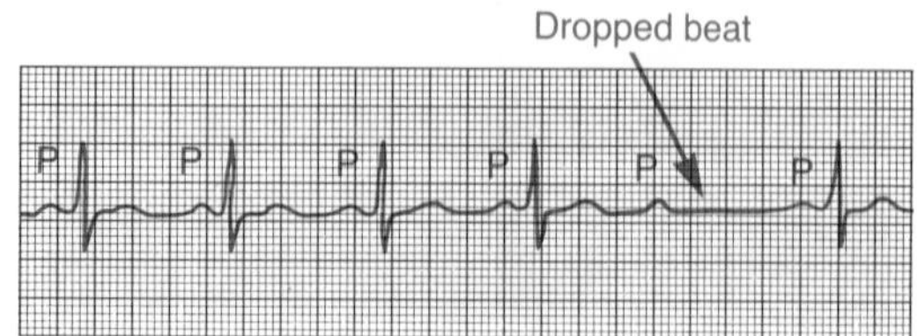

Figure 10–9. Second-degree incomplete atrioventricular block (lead V_3).

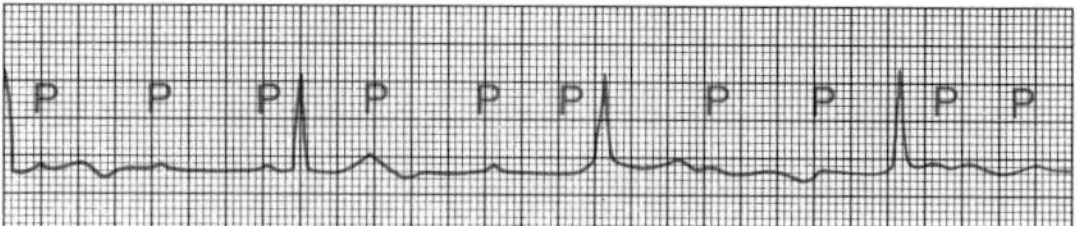

Figure 10–10. Complete atrioventricular block (lead II).

Premature Contractions

A premature contraction is a contraction of the heart prior to the time when normal contraction would have been expected. This condition is also frequently called *premature beat* or *extrasystole.*

Most premature contractions result from *ectopic foci* in the heart, which emit abnormal impulses at odd times during the cardiac rhythm. The possible causes of ectopic foci are (1) local areas of ischemia; (2) small calcified plaques at different points in the heart, which press against the adjacent cardiac muscle so that some of the fibers are irritated, and (3) toxic irritation of the A-V node, Purkinje system, or myocardium caused by drugs, nicotine, or caffeine, and so forth.

Atrial Premature Contraction. Figure 10–11 illustrates an electrocardiogram showing a single atrial premature contraction (premature beat). This is caused by irritation at some point in the atrium leading to generation of a spurious action potential at an abnormal time in the cardiac cycle. As a result, the interval between the preceding beat and the premature beat is shortened. Also, the interval between the premature beat and the next succeeding beat is slightly prolonged. The reason is that the premature beat originated in the atrium at some distance from the S-A node, and the impulse of the premature beat had to travel through a short distance of atrial muscle before it discharged the S-A node. Consequently, the S-A node discharged late in the cycle and made the succeeding heartbeat also late in appearing.

Premature Ventricular Contractions. The electrocardiogram of Figure 10–12 illustrates a series

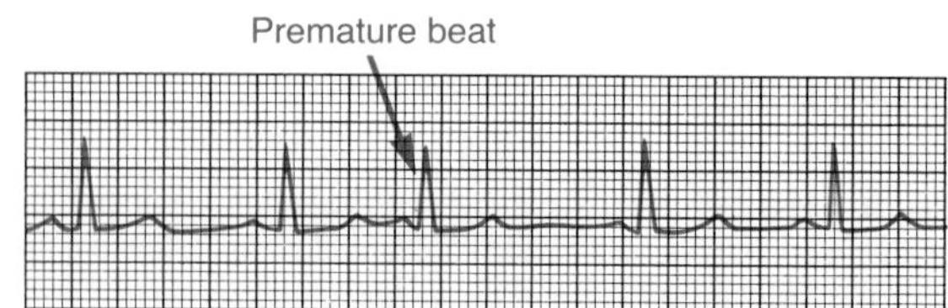

Figure 10–11. Atrial premature contraction (lead I).

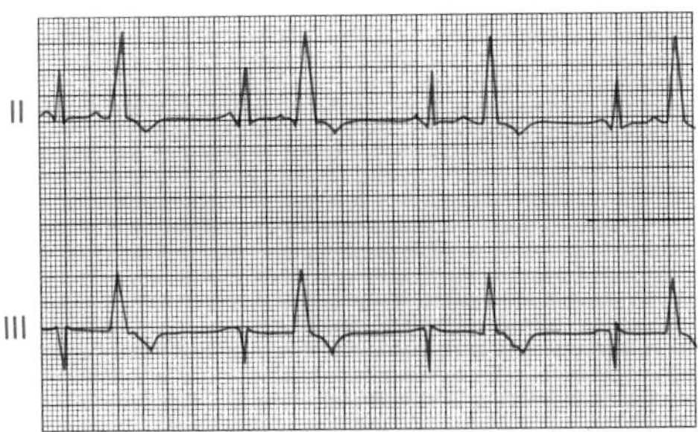

Figure 10-12. Premature ventricular contractions (PVCs) illustrated by the large abnormal QRS-T complexes (leads II and III).

of premature ventricular contractions (called PVCs) alternating with normal beats. These, too, are caused by an irritable focus in the heart, but this time occurring in the ventricles. Premature ventricular contractions cause several special effects in the electrocardiogram, as follows: First, the QRS complex is usually considerably prolonged. The reason is that the impulse is conducted mainly through the muscle of the ventricles rather than through the Purkinje system.

Second, the QRS complex has a very high voltage, for the following reason: When the normal impulse passes through the heart, it passes through both ventricles approximately simultaneously; consequently, the depolarization waves of the two sides of the heart partially neutralize each other. However, when a premature ventricular contraction occurs, the impulse travels in only one direction, so that there is no such neutralization effect.

Third, following almost all premature ventricular contractions, the T wave has a potential opposite to that of the QRS complex because the *slow conduction of the impulse* through the cardiac muscle causes the area first depolarized to repolarize first as well. As a result, the direction of the potential in the heart during repolarization is opposite to that during depolarization. This is not true of the normal T wave.

Some premature ventricular contractions result from simple factors such as cigarettes, coffee, lack of sleep, various mild toxic states, and even emotional irritability. On the other hand, a large share of ventricular premature beats result from some actual pathological condition of the heart. For instance, many ventricular premature beats occur following coronary thrombosis because of stray impulses originating around the borders of the infarcted area of the heart.

Paroxysmal Tachycardia

The term *tachycardia* means rapid rate of heart beat. Abnormalities in any portion of the heart, including the atria, the Purkinje system, and the ventricles, can sometimes cause rapid rhythmic discharge of impulses which then spread through the heart, thus "pacing" the heart at a rapid rate of contraction.

Atrial Paroxysmal Tachycardia. Figure 10-13 illustrates a sudden increase in rate of heart beat from approximately 95 beats per minute to approximately 150 beats per minute. Close analysis of the electrocardiogram shows that an inverted P wave occurs before each of the QRS-T complexes during the paroxysm of rapid heart beat, though this P wave is partially superimposed on the normal T wave of the preceding beat. This indicates that the origin of this particular paroxysmal tachycardia is in the atrium, but because the P wave is abnormal, the origin is not near the S-A node.

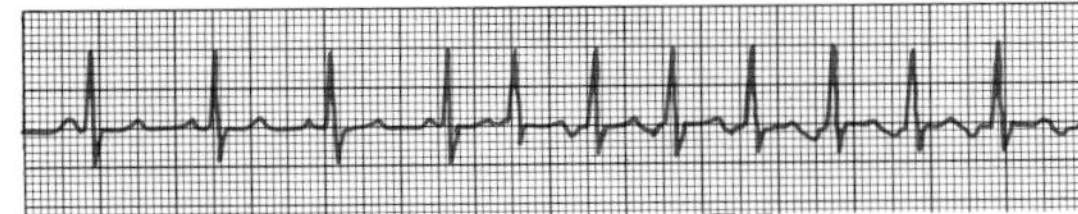

Figure 10-13. Atrial paroxysmal tachycardia—onset in middle of record (lead I).

Ventricular Paroxysmal Tachycardia. Figure 10-14 illustrates a typical short paroxysm of ventricular tachycardia. The electrocardiogram of ventricular paroxysmal tachycardia has the appearance of a series of ventricular premature beats occurring one after another without any normal beats interspersed.

Ventricular paroxysmal tachycardia is usually a serious condition for two reasons. First, this type of tachycardia usually does not occur unless considerable damage is present in the ventricles. Second, ventricular tachycardia predisposes to ventricular fibrillation, which is almost invariably fatal, as we shall discuss in the following sections.

VENTRICULAR FIBRILLATION

The most serious of all cardiac arrhythmias is *ventricular fibrillation,* which, if not treated instantly, is almost invariably fatal.

Ventricular fibrillation results from cardiac impulses that have gone berserk within the ventricular muscle mass, stimulating first one portion of the ventricular muscle, then another portion, then another, and eventually feeding back onto itself to re-excite the same ventricular muscle over and over again—never stopping. When this happens, many small portions of the ventricular muscle will be contracting at the same time, while equally as many other portions will be relaxing. Thus, there is never a coordinate contraction of all of the heart muscle at once, which is required for a pumping cycle of the heart. Therefore, despite massive flow of stimulatory signals throughout the ventricles, the ventricular chamber neither enlarges nor contracts but remains in partial contrac-

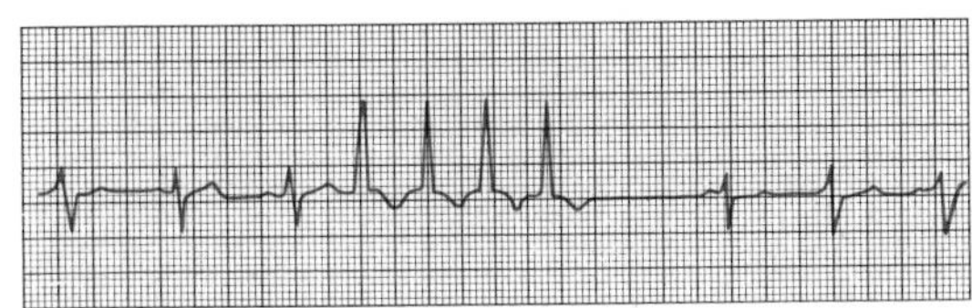

Figure 10-14. Ventricular paroxysmal tachycardia (lead III).

tion, pumping either no blood at all or negligible amounts. Therefore, after fibrillation begins, unconsciousness occurs within 4 to 5 seconds for lack of blood flow to the brain, and irretrievable death of the tissues occurs throughout the body within a few minutes.

Multiple factors can spark the beginning of ventricular fibrillation—with a normal heart beat one second and a second later the ventricles in fibrillation. Especially likely to initiate fibrillation are (1) sudden electrical shock of the heart or (2) ischemia of the heart muscle, its specialized conducting system, or both. In either instance, an instantaneous pattern of re-entry signals can be established, so that the contractile impulses travel around and around through the heart muscle. This phenomenon is also frequently called a *circus movement.*

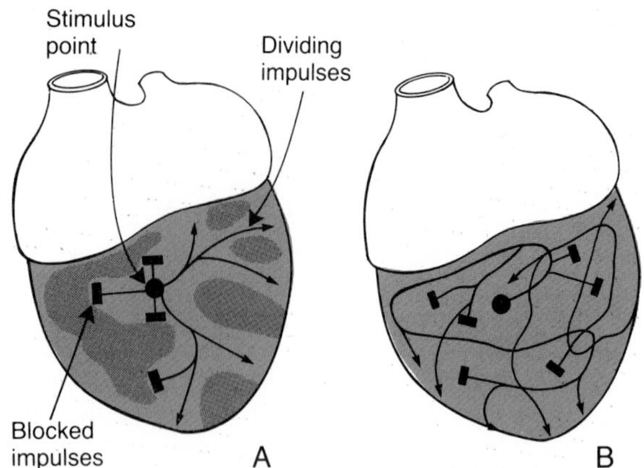

Figure 10-16. *A,* Initiation of fibrillation in a heart when patches of refractory musculature are present. *B,* Continued propagation of *fibrillatory impulses* in the fibrillating ventricle.

The Phenomenon of "Re-Entry"—Circus Movements as the Basis for Ventricular Fibrillation

When the *normal* cardiac impulse has traveled through the entire extent of the ventricles, it then has no place else to go because all of the ventricular muscle is at that time refractory and cannot conduct the impulse further. Therefore, that impulse dies, and the heart awaits a new signal to begin in the sinus node.

However, under some circumstances this normal sequence of events does not occur. Therefore, let us explain more fully the background conditions that can initiate re-entry and lead to the circus movements of ventricular fibrillation.

Figure 10-15 illustrates several small cardiac muscle strips cut in the form of circles. If such a strip is stimulated at the 12 o'clock position *so that the impulse travels in only one direction,* the impulse spreads progressively around the circle until it returns to the 12 o'clock position. If the originally stimulated muscle fibers are still in a refractory state, the impulse then dies out, for refractory muscle cannot transmit a second impulse. However, three different conditions can cause this impulse to continue to travel around the circle, that is, to cause "re-entry" of the impulse into muscle that has already been excited.

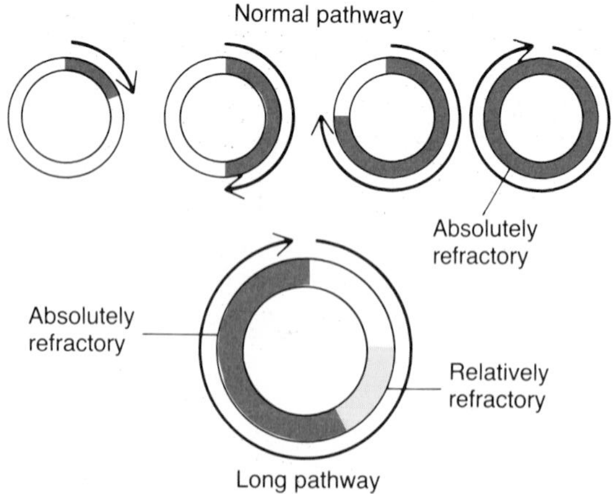

Figure 10-15. The circus movement, showing annihilation of the impulse in the short pathway and continued propagation of the impulse in the long pathway.

First, if the *length of the pathway around the circle is long,* by the time the impulse returns to the 12 o'clock position the originally stimulated muscle will no longer be refractory, and the impulse will continue around the circle again and again.

Second, if the length of the pathway remains constant but the *velocity of conduction becomes decreased* enough, an increased interval of time will elapse before the impulse returns to the 12 o'clock position. By this time the originally stimulated muscle might be out of the refractory state, and the impulse can continue around the circle again and again.

Third, *the refractory period of the muscle might become greatly shortened.* In this case, the impulse could also continue around and around the circle.

All three of these conditions occur in different pathological states of the human heart.

The "Chain Reaction" Mechanism of Fibrillation

In ventricular fibrillation one sees many separate and small contractile waves spreading at the same time in different directions over the cardiac muscle. Obviously, then, the re-entrant impulses in fibrillation are not simply a single impulse moving in a circle as illustrated in Figure 10-15. Instead, they have degenerated into a series of multiple wave fronts that have the appearance of a "chain reaction." One of the best ways to explain this process in fibrillation is to describe the initiation of fibrillation by electric shock caused by 60-cycle alternating electrical current.

Fibrillation Caused by 60-Cycle Alternating Current. At a central point in the ventricles of heart A in Figure 10-16, a 60-cycle electrical stimulus is applied through a stimulating electrode. The first cycle of the electrical stimulus causes a depolarization wave to spread in all directions, leaving all the muscle beneath the electrode in a refractory state. After about 0.25 second, this muscle begins to come out of the refractory state. However, some portions of the muscle come out of refractoriness prior to other portions. This state of events is depicted in heart A by many light patches, which represent excitable cardiac muscle, and dark patches, which represent still refractory muscle. New stimuli from the electrode can now cause impulses to travel in certain directions through the heart but not in all directions. Thus, in heart A certain impulses travel for short distances until they reach refractory areas of the heart and then are blocked. Other impulses, however, pass between the refractory areas and continue to travel in the excitable patches of muscle. Now, several events transpire in rapid succession, all occurring simultaneously and eventuating in a state of fibrillation. These are as follows:

First, block of the impulses in some directions but successful transmission in other directions creates one of the necessary conditions for a re-entrant signal to develop—that is, *transmission of some of the depolarization waves around the heart in only one direction.* As a result, these waves do not run into waves traveling in the opposite direction and therefore do not annihilate themselves on the opposite side of the heart but can continue around and around the ventricles.

Second, the rapid stimulation of the heart causes two changes in the cardiac muscle itself, both of which predispose to circus movement: (1) the *velocity of conduction through the heart becomes decreased,* which allows a longer time interval for the impulses to travel around the heart. (2) The *refractory period of the muscle becomes shortened,* allowing re-entry of the impulse into previously excited heart muscle within a much shorter period of time than normally.

Third, one of the most important features of fibrillation is the *division of impulses,* as illustrated in heart A. When a depolarization wave reaches a refractory area in the heart, it travels to both sides around the area. Thus, a single impulse becomes two impulses. Then when each of these reaches another refractory area it, too, divides to form still two more impulses. In this way many different new wave fronts are continually being formed in the heart by a progressive *chain reaction* until, finally, there are many small depolarization waves traveling in many different directions at the same time.

Heart B in Figure 10–16 illustrates the final state that develops in fibrillation. Here one can see many impulses traveling in all directions, some dividing and increasing the number of impulses, while others are blocked entirely by refractory areas.

The Electrocardiogram in Ventricular Fibrillation

In ventricular fibrillation the electrocardiogram is extremely bizarre, as seen in Figure 10–17, and ordinarily shows no tendency toward a regular rhythm of any type. In the early phases of ventricular fibrillation, relatively large masses of muscle contract simultaneously, and this causes strong, though irregular, waves in the electrocardiogram. However, after only a few seconds the coarse contractions of the ventricles disappear, and the electrocardiogram changes into a new pattern of low-voltage, very irregular waves. Thus, no repetitive electrocardiographic pattern can be ascribed to ventricular fibrillation except that the electrical potentials constantly and spasmodically change because the currents in the heart flow first in one direction, then in another, and rarely repeat any specific cycle.

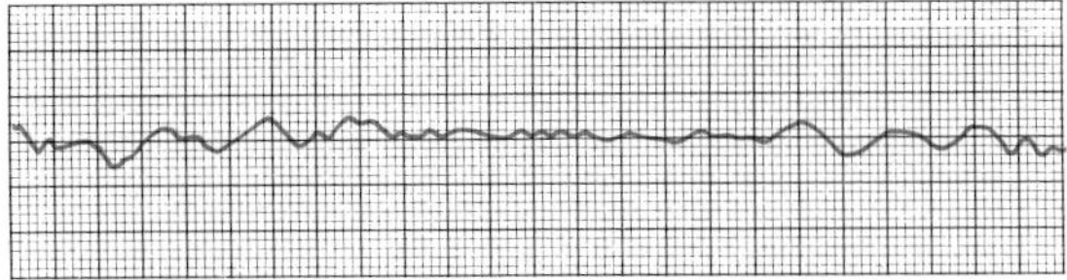

Figure 10–17. Ventricular fibrillation (lead II).

The voltages of the waves in the electrocardiogram in ventricular fibrillation are usually about 0.5 mV when ventricular fibrillation first begins, but these decay rapidly so that after 20 to 30 seconds they are usually only 0.2 to 0.3 mV.

Electroshock Defibrillation of the Ventricles

Although a weak alternating current almost invariably throws the ventricles into fibrillation, a very strong electrical current passed through the ventricles for a short interval of time can stop fibrillation by throwing all the ventricular muscle into refractoriness simultaneously. This is accomplished by passing intense current—several thousand volts for a small fraction of a second—through electrodes placed on the chest, as illustrated in Figure 10–18. The current penetrates most of the fibers of the ventricles, thus stimulating essentially all parts of the ventricles simultaneously and causing them to become refractory. All impulses stop, and the heart then remains quiescent for 3 to 5 seconds, after which it begins to beat again, usually with the sinus node or some other part of the heart becoming the pacemaker.

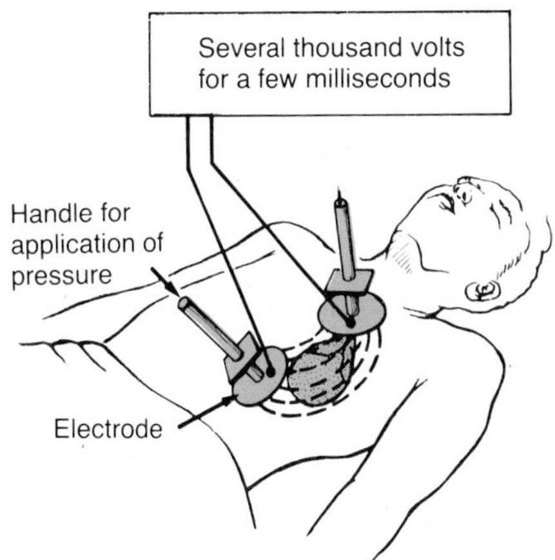

Figure 10–18. Application of electrical current to the chest to stop ventricular fibrillation.

ATRIAL FIBRILLATION

Remember that, except for the connection through the A-V bundle, the atrial muscle mass is entirely separated from the ventricular muscle mass, and they are insulated from each other by fibrous tissue. Therefore, ventricular fibrillation often occurs entirely independently of atrial fibrillation. Likewise, fibrillation often occurs in the atria independently of ventricular fibrillation and is called *atrial fibrillation.*

The mechanism of atrial fibrillation is identical with that of ventricular fibrillation except that the process occurs in the atrial muscle mass instead of the ventricular mass. A very frequent cause of atrial fibrillation is atrial enlargement resulting from heart valve lesions that prevent the atria from emptying adequately into the ventricles or resulting from ventricular failure with excess damming of blood in the atria. The dilated atrial walls provide the ideal conditions of a long conductive pathway as well as slow conduction, both of which predispose to atrial fibrillation.

Pumping Characteristics of the Atria During Atrial Fibrillation. For the same reasons that the ventricles will not pump blood during ventricular fibrillation, neither do the atria pump blood in atrial fibrillation. Therefore, the atria become useless as primer pumps for the ventricles. Even so, blood flows passively through the atria into the ventricles, and the efficiency of ventricular pumping is decreased only 20 to 30 per cent. Therefore, in contrast to the lethality of ventricular fibrillation, a person can live for months or even years with atrial fibrillation, though at a reduced efficiency of overall heart pumping.

The Electrocardiogram in Atrial Fibrillation. Figure 10–19 illustrates the electrocardiogram during atrial fibrillation. Numerous small depolarization waves spread in all directions through the atria during atrial fibrillation. Because the waves are weak and because many of them are of opposite polarity at any given time, they usually almost completely neutralize each other. Therefore, in the electrocardiogram one can see no P waves from the atria but instead only a fine, high-frequency, very low voltage wavy record. On the other hand, the QRS-T complexes are completely normal unless there is some pathology of the ventricles, but their timing is very irregular for the following reasons:

Irregularity of the Ventricular Rhythm During Atrial Fibrillation. When the atria are fibrillating, impulses arrive at the A-V node rapidly but also irregularly. Because the A-V node will not pass a second impulse for approximately 0.35 second after a previous one, at least 0.35 second must elapse between one ventricular contraction and the next, and an additional but variable interval of 0 to 0.6 second occurs before one of the irregular fibrillatory impulses happens to arrive at the A-V node. Thus, the interval between successive ventricular contractions varies from a minimum of about 0.35 second to a maximum of about 0.95 second, causing a very irregular heartbeat.

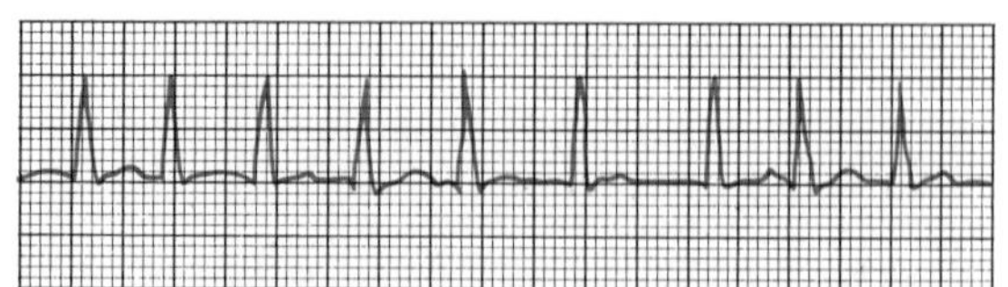

Figure 10–19. Atrial fibrillation (lead I).

CARDIAC ARREST

A final serious abnormality of the cardiac rhythmicity-conduction system is cardiac arrest. This results from cessation of all rhythmic impulses of the heart. That is, no spontaneous rhythm at all remains.

Cardiac arrest is especially likely to occur during deep anesthesia when patients often develop severe hypoxia because of inadequate respiration. The hypoxia prevents the muscle fibers and conductive fibers from maintaining normal electrolyte concentration differentials across their membranes, and their excitability may be so affected that the automatic rhythmicity disappears.

Following temporary cardiac arrest, cardiopulmonary resuscitation is usually quite successful in re-establishing a normal heart rhythm. However, in some patients, severe myocardial disease leads to permanent or semipermanent cardiac arrest, which obviously will cause death. In many cases, however, rhythmical electrical impulses from an implanted electronic cardiac pacemaker have been used successfully to keep patients alive for many years.

ELECTROCARDIOGRAPHIC INTERPRETATION IN NONARRHYTHMICAL CARDIAC ABNORMALITIES

From the discussion in Chapter 9 of impulse transmission through the heart, it is obvious that many changes in this transmission can cause not only altered heart rhythms but also altered shapes of the waves in the electrocardiogram. For this reason, most serious abnormalities of the heart can be detected by analyzing the contours of the different waves in the different electrocardiographic leads. The purpose of the present section is to present several representative electrocardiograms when the muscle of the heart, especially of the ventricles, contracts abnormally.

The Mean Electrical Axis of the Ventricles

It was shown in Figure 10–4 that during most of the cycle of ventricular depolarization, the polarity of the electrical potential is from the base of the ventricle toward the apex — that is, the base of the ventricle is negative, and the apex is positive. This preponderant direction of potential during depolarization is called the *mean electrical axis of the ventricles.* The mean electrical axis of the normal ventricles is 59 degrees (zero degrees is toward the left side of the heart, and the axis is measured clockwise from this direction). However, in certain pathological conditions of the heart, the direction of the potential is changed markedly — sometimes even to opposite poles of the heart.

Hypertrophy of One Ventricle

When one ventricle becomes greatly hypertrophied, the principal direction of the electrical potential in the heart during depolarization — that is, the axis of the heart — shifts toward the hypertrophied ventricle for two reasons. First, far greater quantity of muscle exists on the hypertrophied side of the heart than on the other side, and this allows excess generation of electrical current on that side. Second, more time is required for the depolarization wave to travel through the hypertrophied ventricle than through the normal ventricle. Consequently, the normal ventricle becomes depolarized (negative) considerably in advance of the hypertrophied ventricle, and this causes a strong potential from the normal side of the heart toward the hypertrophied side. Thus the axis deviates toward the hypertrophied ventricle.

Left Axis Deviation Resulting from Hypertrophy of the Left Ventricle. Figure 10-20 illustrates the three standard leads of an electrocardiogram in which the potential is strongly positive in lead I and strongly negative in lead III. This means that the major axis of the potential in the heart is mainly in the direction of lead I, which is from right arm toward left arm; and the potential is opposite to the direction of lead III, which is from left arm toward left leg. That is, the axis of the heart points upward toward the left shoulder. This is called *left axis deviation* because it is to the left of the normal axis of the heart, which points downward and only slightly to the left in the chest.

The electrocardiogram of Figure 10-20 is typical of that resulting from increased muscular mass of the left ventricle. In this instance the axis deviation was caused by *high blood pressure,* which caused the left ventricle to hypertrophy in order to pump blood against the elevated systemic arterial pressure. However, a similar picture of left axis deviation occurs when the left ventricle hypertrophies as a result of aortic valvular stenosis, aortic valvular regurgitation, or any of a number of congenital heart conditions in which the left ventricle enlarges while the right side of the heart remains relatively normal in size.

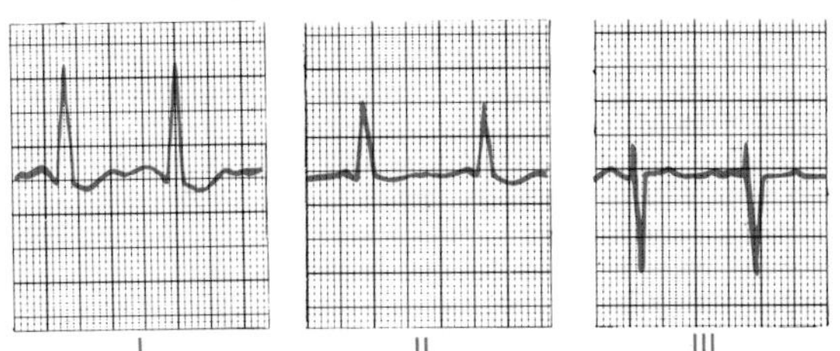

Figure 10-20. Left axis deviation in hypertensive heart disease. Note the slightly prolonged QRS complex as well.

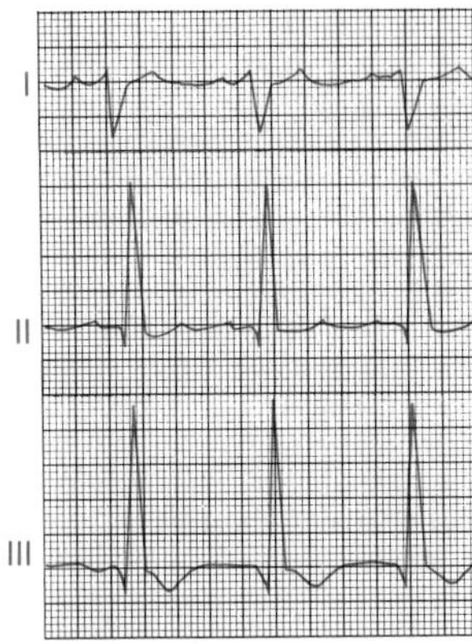

Figure 10-21. Right axis deviation due to right bundle branch block. Note the greatly prolonged QRS complex.

Right axis deviation occurs when the right ventricle enlarges. That is, the potential in lead I then becomes negative while that in lead III becomes strongly positive.

Bundle Branch Block

Ordinarily, the two lateral walls of the ventricles depolarize at almost the same time, because both the left and right bundle branches transmit the cardiac impulse to the endocardial surfaces of the two ventricular walls at almost the same instant. As a result, the potentials from the walls of the two ventricles almost exactly neutralize each other. However, if one of the major bundle branches is blocked, depolarization of the two ventricles does not occur simultaneously, and the depolarization potentials do not neutralize each other. As a result, axis deviation occurs, as follows:

Right or Left Bundle Branch Block. When the right bundle branch is blocked, the left ventricle depolarizes far more rapidly than the right ventricle (because the normal left bundle still conducts a rapid signal to the left ventricle), so that the left becomes electronegative while the right remains electroposi-

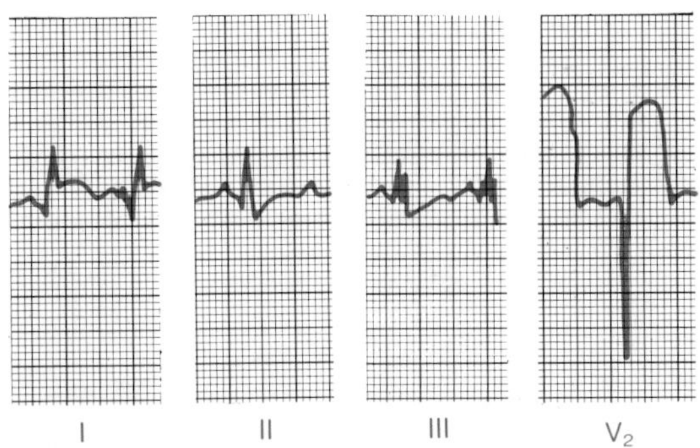

Figure 10-22. Current of injury in acute anterior wall infarction. Note the intense current of injury in lead V_2.

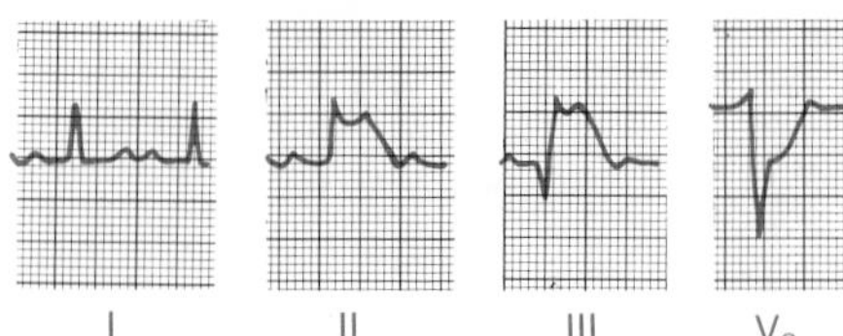

Figure 10–23. Current of injury in acute posterior wall, apical infarction.

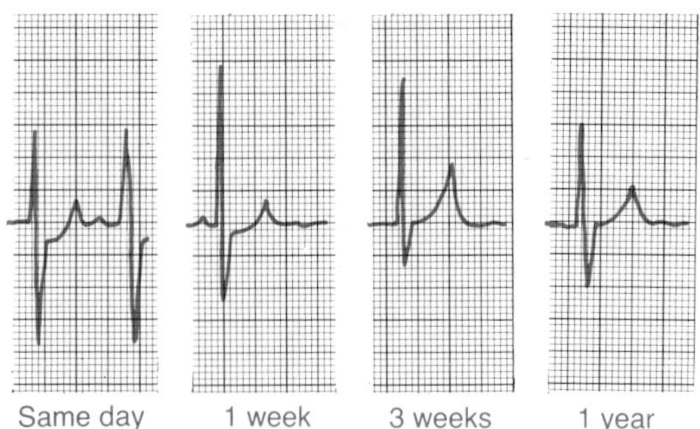

Figure 10–24. Recovery of the myocardium following moderate posterior wall infarction, illustrating disappearance of the current of injury (lead V_3).

tive. Therefore, a very strong potential develops with its negative end toward the left ventricle and its positive end toward the right ventricle. In other words, intense right axis deviation occurs because the positive end of the axis is to the right of the normal downward direction.

Right axis deviation (denoted especially by the very negative QRS in lead I) caused by right bundle branch block is illustrated in Figure 10–21, which also shows a prolonged QRS complex due to blocked conduction.

Left bundle branch block causes the opposite effect, namely, left axis deviation but also prolonged QRS complex.

Current of Injury

Many different cardiac abnormalities, especially those that damage the heart muscle itself, cause part of the heart to remain *depolarized all the time.* When this occurs, current flows between the pathologically depolarized and the normally polarized areas. This is called a *current of injury.* The most common cause of a current of injury is *ischemia of the muscle caused by coronary occlusion.*

Effect of Current Injury on the QRS Complex — The S-T Segment Shift. It will be recalled that in the normal heart no electrical current flows from the heart either when the heart is totally polarized during the T-P interval or when the heart is totally depolarized during the S-T interval. Therefore, in the normal electrocardiogram, both the T-P and the S-T intervals record on the same voltage level. However, when there is a current of injury, the heart cannot completely repolarize during the T-P interval. For this reason, the voltage level of the T-P interval is different from that of the S-T interval. This effect is called the *S-T segment shift,* which unfortunately is a misnomer because the abnormality is actually a T-P segment shift.

Current of Injury Caused by Acute Anterior Wall Infarction. Figure 10–22 illustrates the electrocardiogram in the three standard leads and in one chest lead recorded from a patient with acute anterior wall cardiac infarction caused by coronary thrombosis. (*Infarction* means loss of coronary blood flow.) The most important diagnostic feature of this electrocardiogram is the current of injury *in the chest lead* (V_2 lead) as denoted by the S-T segment shift (the broad wave at the top of the record following the QRS complex).

Posterior Wall Infarction. Figure 10–23 illustrates the three standard leads and one chest lead from a patient with posterior wall infarction. The major diagnostic feature of this electrocardiogram is the S-T segment shift in the chest lead (V_2 lead) and in leads II and III.

Recovery from Coronary Thrombosis. Figure 10–24 illustrates the chest lead from a patient with posterior wall infarction, showing the change in this chest lead from the day of the attack to 1 week later, then 3 weeks later, and finally 1 year later. From this electrocardiogram it can be seen that a slight current of injury (S-T segment shift) is present immediately after the acute attack, but after approximately 1 week the current of injury has diminished considerably and after 3 weeks it is completely gone. After that, the electrocardiogram changes slightly during the following year because of progressive repair of the damaged muscle.

REFERENCES

Chung, E. K.: Principles of Cardiac Arrhythmias. 4th ed. Baltimore, Williams & Wilkins, 1988.

Guyton, A. C., and Crowell, J. W.: A stereovectorcardiograph. J. Lab. Clin. Med., 40:726, 1952.

Hurst, J. W., et al. (eds.): The Heart. 7th ed. New York, McGraw-Hill Book Co., 1990.

Johnson, R., and Swartz, M. H.: A Simplified Approach to Electrocardiography. Philadelphia, W. B. Saunders Co., 1986.

Josephson, M. E.: Clinical Cardiac Electrophysiology: Techniques and Interpretations. 2nd Ed. Philadelphia, Lea & Febiger, 1989.

Kennedy, H. L.: Ambulatory Electrocardiography and Its Technology. 2nd ed. Philadelphia, Lea & Febiger, 1989.

Laiken, N., et al.: Interpretation of Electrocardiograms: A Self-Instructional Approach. 2nd ed. New York, Raven Press, 1988.

Marriott, H. J. L., and Conover, M. B.: Advanced Concepts in Arrhythmias. 2nd ed. St. Louis, C. V. Mosby Co., 1989.

Marriott, H. J. L., and Wagner, G.: Practical Electrocardiography. 8th ed. Baltimore, Williams & Wilkins, 1988.

Morganroth, J.: Ambulatory Holter electrocardiography: Choice of technologies and clinical uses. Ann. Intern. Med., 102:73, 1985.

Saksena, S., and Goldschlager, N. F. (ed.): Electrical Therapy for Cardiac Arrhythmias. Philadelphia, W. B. Saunders Co., 1989.

Stein, E.: Interpretation of Arrhythmias: A Self-Study Program. Philadelphia, Lea & Febiger, 1988.

QUESTIONS

1. Explain what is meant by a *depolarization wave* and by a *repolarization wave* in the electrocardiogram. Which of the normal electrocardiographic waves are depolarization and which are repolarization waves?
2. At what point in the monophasic action potential of ventricular cardiac muscle does the QRS wave occur? At what point does the T wave occur?
3. Explain the voltage and time calibration marks on the electrocardiogram.
4. What is the significance of the *P-Q interval*?
5. Draw a diagram of the heart showing the flow of current around the ventricles when they are approximately half depolarized.
6. Explain the connections of the electrodes to the body for recording the three standard limb leads.
7. Explain how the electrocardiographic chest leads are recorded.
8. What are the characteristics of the electrocardiogram in *incomplete heart block* and *complete heart block*?
9. Describe the characteristics of the electrocardiogram when either *atrial* or *ventricular premature contractions* occur. Explain the differences between the electrocardiographic patterns.
10. Describe the electrocardiogram in *atrial paroxysmal tachycardia.*
11. Explain the mechanism of the circus movement.
12. What happens to the heart in ventricular fibrillation?
13. Explain the "chain reaction" mechanism of fibrillation as well as the means by which 60-cycle alternating current elicits ventricular fibrillation.
14. Why is very strong electric shock to the heart capable of causing defibrillation, whereas weak electric shock is a very common cause of fibrillation?
15. Describe the electrocardiographic pattern in *atrial fibrillation* and in *ventricular fibrillation.* Explain the irregular timing of the heart beat in atrial fibrillation.
16. What conditions can cause cardiac arrest?
17. What is meant by the mean electrical axis of the ventricles?
18. Explain why the electrical axis deviates to the left in both *hypertrophy* of the left ventricle and *left bundle branch block.*
19. What is the cause of *current of injury* in the electrocardiogram? How can it be used to determine the locus of a myocardial infarct in the heart?

IV

The Circulation

11

Overview of the Circulation; Medical Physics of Pressure, Flow, Resistance, and Vascular Compliance

The function of the circulation, illustrated in Figure 11–1, is to service the needs of the tissues—to transport nutrients to the tissues, to transport waste products away, to conduct hormones from one part of the body to another, and in general to maintain an appropriate environment in all the tissue fluids for optimal survival and function of the cells.

The circulation is divided into the *systemic circulation* and the *pulmonary circulation.* Because the systemic circulation supplies all the tissues of the body except the lungs with blood flow, it is also frequently called the *peripheral circulation.*

The Functional Parts of the Circulation. Before attempting to discuss the details of function in the circulation, it is important to understand the overall role of each of its parts, as follows:

The function of the *arteries* is to transport blood *under high pressure* to the tissues. For this reason, the arteries have strong vascular walls, and blood flows rapidly in the arteries.

The *arterioles* are the last small branches of the arterial system, and they act as *control valves* through which blood is released into the capillaries. The arteriole has a strong muscular wall that is capable of closing the arteriole completely or of allowing it to be dilated severalfold, thus having the capability of vastly altering blood flow to the capillaries in response to the needs of the tissues.

The function of the *capillaries* is to exchange fluid, nutrients, electrolytes, hormones, and other substances between the blood and the interstitial fluid. For this role, the capillary walls are very thin and are permeable to small molecular substances.

The *venules* collect blood from the capillaries; they gradually coalesce into progressively larger veins.

The *veins* function as conduits for transport of blood from the tissues back to the heart, but, equally important, they serve as a major reservoir of blood. Because the pressure in the venous system is very low, the venous walls are thin. Even so, they are muscular, and this allows them to contract or expand and thereby act as a reservoir for extra blood, either a small or a large amount, depending on the needs of the body.

Volumes of Blood in the Different Parts of the Circulation. By far the greater proportion of the blood in the circulation is contained in the systemic veins. Figure 11–1 shows this, illustrating that approximately 84 per cent of the entire blood volume of the body is in the systemic circulation, with 64 per cent in the veins, 13 per cent in the arteries, and 7 per cent in the systemic arterioles and capillaries. The heart contains 7 per cent of the blood and the pulmonary vessels 9 per cent. Most surprising is the very low blood volume in the capillaries of the systemic circulation. Yet, it is here that the most important function of the systemic circulation occurs, diffusion of substances back and forth between the blood and the tissues. This function is so important that it is discussed in detail in Chapter 13.

Pressures in the Various Portions of the Circulation. Because the heart pumps blood continually into the aorta, the pressure in the aorta is obviously high, averaging approximately 100 mm Hg. Also, because the pumping by the heart is pulsatile, the arterial pressure fluctuates between a *systolic level* of

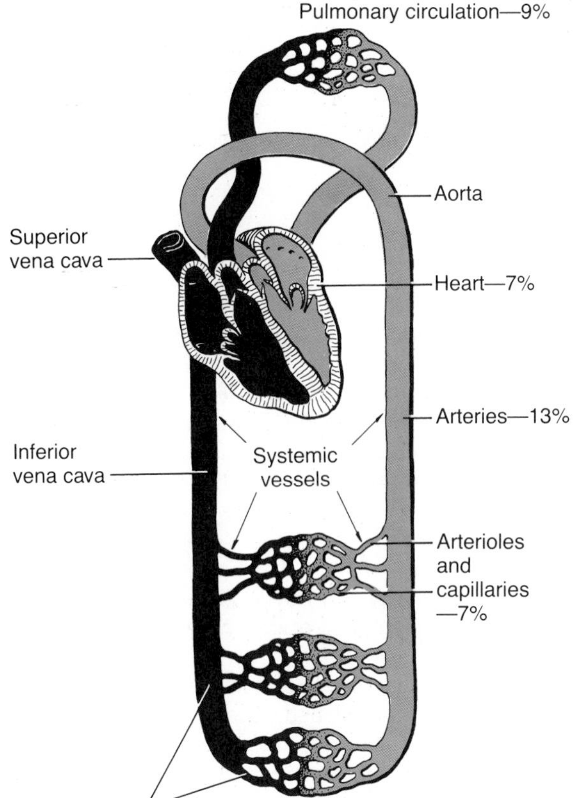

Figure 11-1. Distribution of blood volume in the different portions of the circulatory system.

120 mm Hg and a *diastolic level* of 80 mm Hg, as illustrated in Figure 11-2. As the blood flows through the systemic circulation, its pressure falls progressively to approximately 0 mm Hg by the time it reaches the termination of the venae cavae in the right atrium.

The pressure in the systemic capillaries varies from as high as 35 mm Hg near the arteriolar ends to as low as 10 mm Hg near their venous ends, but the average "functional" capillary pressure in most vascular beds is about 17 mm Hg, a pressure low enough that very little of the plasma leaks out of the porous capillaries even though nutrients can diffuse easily to the tissue cells.

Note to the far right in Figure 11-2 the respective pressures in the different parts of the pulmonary circulation. In the pulmonary arteries, the pressure is pulsatile, just as in the aorta, but the pressure level is far less, at a systolic arterial pressure of about 25 mm Hg and a diastolic pressure of 8 mm Hg, with a mean pulmonary arterial pressure of only 16 mm Hg. The pulmonary capillary pressure averages only 7 mm Hg. Yet, the total blood flow through the lungs each minute is the same as that through the systemic circulation. The low pressures of the pulmonary system are in accord with the needs of the lungs, for all that is required is to expose the blood in the pulmonary capillaries to the oxygen and other gases in the pulmonary alveoli.

THE BASIC THEORY OF CIRCULATORY FUNCTION

Although the details of circulatory function are often complex, three basic principles underlie all functions of the system. These are as follows:

The Blood Flow to Each Tissue of the Body Is Almost Always Precisely Controlled in Relation to the Tissue Needs. When tissues are active, they need much more blood flow than when at rest, occasionally as much as 20 to 30 times the resting level. Yet, the heart normally cannot increase its cardiac output more than four to seven times. Therefore, it is not possible simply to increase the blood flow everywhere in the body when a particular tissue demands increased flow. Instead, the microvessels of each tissue continuously monitor the tissue needs, such as the availability of nutrition and the accumulation of tissue waste products, and these in turn control the local blood flow very precisely to the level

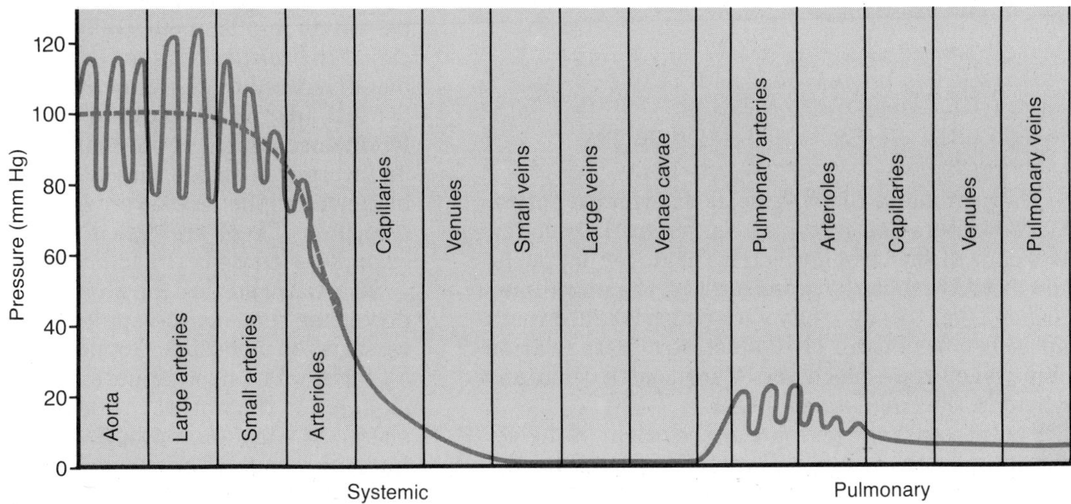

Figure 11-2. Blood pressures in the different portions of the circulatory system.

required for the tissue activity. Also, nervous control of the circulation provides additional specific attributes to tissue blood flow control.

The Cardiac Output Is Controlled Mainly by the Local Tissue Flow. When blood flows through a tissue, it immediately returns by way of the veins to the heart. Fortunately, the heart responds to this increased inflow of blood by pumping almost all of it immediately back into the arteries from whence it came. In this sense, the heart acts as an automaton, responding to the demands of the tissues. Unfortunately, though, the heart is not perfect in its response. Therefore, it often needs help in the form of special nerve signals to make it pump the required amounts of blood flow.

In General, the Arterial Pressure Is Controlled Independently of Either Local Blood Flow Control or Cardiac Output Control. The circulatory system is provided with a very extensive system for controlling the arterial pressure. For instance, if at any time the pressure falls significantly below its normal mean level of about 100 mm Hg, a barrage of nervous reflexes within seconds elicits a series of circulatory changes to raise the pressure back to normal, including increased force of heart pumping, contraction of the large venous reservoirs to provide more blood for the heart, and generalized constriction of most of the arterioles throughout the body, so that more blood will accumulate in the arterial tree. Then, over more prolonged periods of time, hours and days, the kidneys play an additional major role in pressure control both by secreting pressure-controlling hormones and by regulating the blood volume.

The importance of pressure control is that it prevents changes in blood flow in one area of the body from significantly affecting flow elsewhere in the body because the common pressure head for both areas is not allowed to change greatly.

Thus, in summary the needs of the local tissues are served by the circulation. In the remainder of this chapter, we begin to discuss the basic details of the management of blood flow and the control of cardiac output and arterial pressure.

INTERRELATIONSHIPS AMONG PRESSURE, FLOW, AND RESISTANCE

Flow through a blood vessel is determined entirely by two factors: (1) the *pressure difference* between the two ends of the vessel, which is the force that pushes the blood through the vessel, and (2) the impediment to blood flow through the vessel, which is called vascular *resistance.* Figure 11-3 illustrates these relationships, showing a blood vessel segment located anywhere in the circulatory system.

P_1 represents the pressure at the origin of the vessel; at the other end the pressure is P_2. The flow through the vessel can be calculated by the following formula, which is called *Ohm's law:*

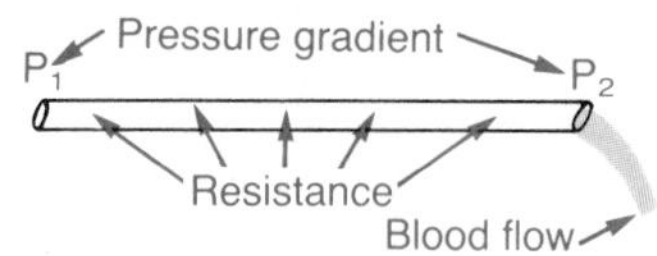

Figure 11-3. Relationships among pressure, resistance, and blood flow.

$$Q = \frac{\Delta P}{R} \quad (1)$$

in which Q is blood flow, ΔP is the pressure difference ($P_1 - P_2$) between the two ends of the vessel, and R is the resistance. This formula states, in effect, that the blood flow is directly proportional to the pressure difference but inversely proportional to the resistance.

It should be noted especially that it is the *difference* in pressure between the two ends of the vessel, not the absolute pressure in the vessel, that determines the rate of flow. For instance, if the pressure at both ends of the segment were 100 mm Hg and yet no difference existed between the two ends, there would be no flow despite the presence of 100 mm Hg pressure.

Ohm's law expresses the most important of all the relationships that the reader needs to understand to comprehend the hemodynamics of the circulation. Because of the extreme importance of this formula, the reader should also become familiar with its other two algebraic forms:

$$\Delta P = Q \times R \quad (2)$$

$$R = \frac{\Delta P}{Q} \quad (3)$$

Blood Flow

Blood flow means simply the quantity of blood that passes a given point in the circulation in a given period of time. Ordinarily, blood flow is expressed in *milliliters* or *liters per minute,* but it can be expressed in milliliters per second or in any other unit of flow.

The overall blood flow in the circulation of an adult person at rest is about 5000 ml per minute. This is called the *cardiac output* because it is the amount of blood pumped by the heart in a unit period of time.

Methods for Measuring Blood Flow. Many different mechanical or mechanoelectrical devices can be inserted in series with a blood vessel or in some instances applied to the outside of the vessel to measure flow. These are called simply *flowmeters.* One example of these is the following:

The Ultrasonic Doppler Flowmeter. A type of flowmeter that can be applied to the outside of the vessel is the ultrasonic Doppler flowmeter, illustrated in Figure 11-4. A minute piezoelectric crystal is mounted in the wall of the device. This crystal, when energized with an appropriate electronic apparatus, transmits sound at a frequency of several million cycles per second downstream along the flowing blood. A portion of the sound is reflected by the flow-

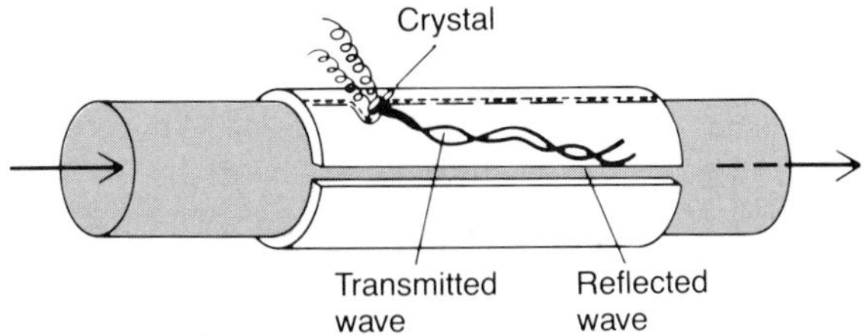

Figure 11-4. An ultrasonic Doppler flowmeter.

ing red blood cells, so that reflected sound waves travel backward from the blood toward the crystal. However, these reflected waves have a lower frequency than the transmitted wave because the red cells are moving away from the transmitter crystal. This is called the Doppler effect. (It is the same effect that one experiences when a train approaches and passes by while blowing its whistle. Once the whistle has passed by the person, the pitch of the sound from the whistle suddenly becomes much lower than when the train is approaching.) The transmitted wave is intermittently cut off, and the reflected wave is received back onto the crystal, then amplified greatly by the electronic apparatus. Another portion of the apparatus determines the frequency difference between the transmitted wave and the reflected wave, thus also determining the velocity of blood flow.

Obviously, the ultrasonic Doppler flowmeter is capable of recording very rapid, pulsatile changes in flow as well as steady flow.

Blood Pressure

The Standard Units of Pressure. Blood pressure is almost always measured in *millimeters of mercury (mm Hg)* because the mercury manometer has been used since antiquity as the standard reference for measuring blood pressure. Actually, blood pressure means the *force exerted by the blood against any unit area of the vessel wall.* When one says that the pressure in a vessel is 50 mm Hg, this means that the force exerted is sufficient to push a column of mercury up to a level 50 mm high. If the pressure is 100 mm Hg, it will push the column of mercury up to 100 millimeters.

Occasionally, pressure is measured in *centimeters of water.* A pressure of 10 centimeters of water means a pressure sufficient to raise a column of water to a height of 10 cm. *One millimeter of mercury equals 1.36 centimeter of water* because the specific gravity of mercury is 13.6 times that of water, and 1 centimeter is 10 times as great as 1 millimeter. Dividing 13.6 by 10, we derive the factor 1.36.

High-Fidelity Methods for Measuring Blood Pressure. Unfortunately, the mercury in the mercury manometer has so much *inertia* that it cannot rise and fall rapidly. For this reason the mercury manometer, though excellent for recording steady pressures, cannot respond to pressure changes that occur more rapidly than approximately one cycle every 2 to 3 seconds. Whenever it is desired to record rapidly changing pressures, some other type of pressure recorder is needed. Figure 11-5 demonstrates the basic principles of three electronic pressure *transducers* commonly used for converting pressure into electrical signals and then recording the pressure on a high-speed electrical recorder. Each of these transducers employs a very thin and highly stretched metal membrane that forms one wall of the fluid chamber. The fluid chamber in turn is connected through a needle or catheter with the vessel in which the pressure is to be measured. Pressure variations in the vessel cause changes of pressure in the chamber beneath the membrane. When the pressure is high, the membrane bulges outward slightly, and when low, it returns toward its resting position.

In Figure 11-5A, a simple metal plate is placed a few thousandths of an inch above the membrane. When the membrane bulges outward, the *capacitance* between the plate and membrane increases, and this change in capacitance can be recorded by an appropriate electronic system.

In Figure 11-5B, a small iron slug rests on the membrane, and this can be displaced upward into a coil. Movement of the iron changes the *inductance* of the coil, and this, too, can be recorded electronically.

Finally, in Figure 11-5C, a very thin, stretched resistance wire is connected to the membrane. When this wire is greatly stretched, its resistance increases, and when less stretched, the resistance decreases. These changes also can be recorded by means of an electronic system.

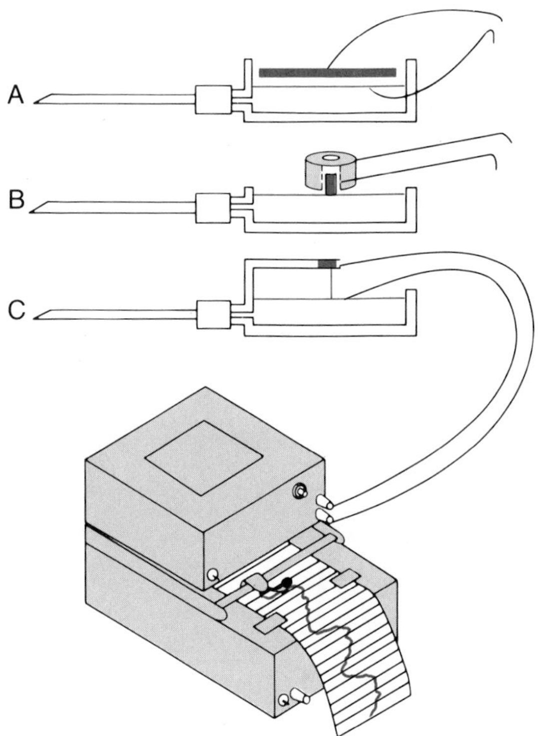

Figure 11-5. Principles of three different types of electronic transducers for recording rapidly changing blood pressures.

With some of these high-fidelity types of recording systems, pressure cycles up to 500 cycles per second have been recorded accurately.

Resistance to Blood Flow

Units of Resistance. Resistance is the impediment to blood flow in a vessel, but it cannot be measured by any direct means. Instead, resistance must be calculated from measurements of blood flow and pressure difference in the vessel. If the pressure difference between two points in a vessel is 1 mm Hg and the flow is 1 ml/sec, the resistance is said to be 1 *peripheral resistance unit,* usually abbreviated *PRU.*

Total Peripheral Resistance and Total Pulmonary Resistance. The rate of blood flow through the circulatory system when a person is at rest is close to 100 ml/sec, and the pressure difference from the systemic arteries to the systemic veins is about 100 mm Hg. Therefore, in round figures the resistance of the entire systemic circulation, called the *total peripheral resistance,* is approximately 100/100 or 1 PRU. In some conditions in which all the blood vessels throughout the body become strongly constricted, the total peripheral resistance rises to as high as 4 PRU, and when the vessels become greatly dilated, it can fall to as little as 0.2 PRU.

In the pulmonary system, the mean arterial pressure averages 16 mm Hg, and the mean left atrial pressure averages 2 mm Hg, giving a net pressure difference of 14 mm. Therefore, in round figures the *total pulmonary resistance* at rest calculates to be about 0.14 PRU.

Vessel Diameter Has a Tremendous Effect on Resistance — Poiseuille's Law

Observe in Figure 11-6A that increasing the diameter of a blood vessel from a diameter of 1 to a diameter four times as great increases the blood flow from 1 milliliter per minute to 256 milliliters per minute, an extreme increase in flow for a relatively small increase

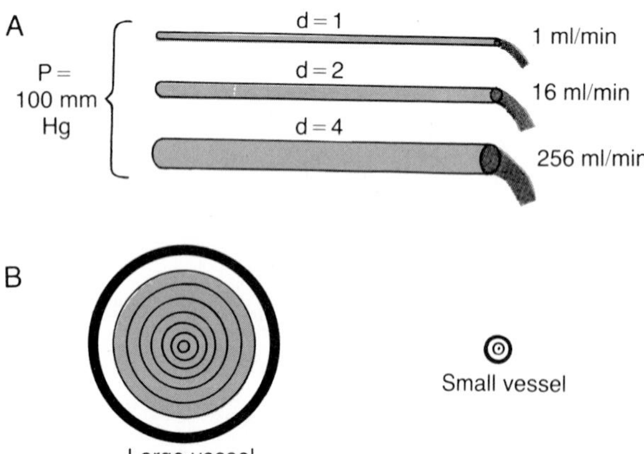

Figure 11-6. *A,* Demonstration of the effect of vessel diameter on blood flow. *B,* Concentric rings of blood flowing at different velocities; the farther away from the vessel wall, the faster the flow.

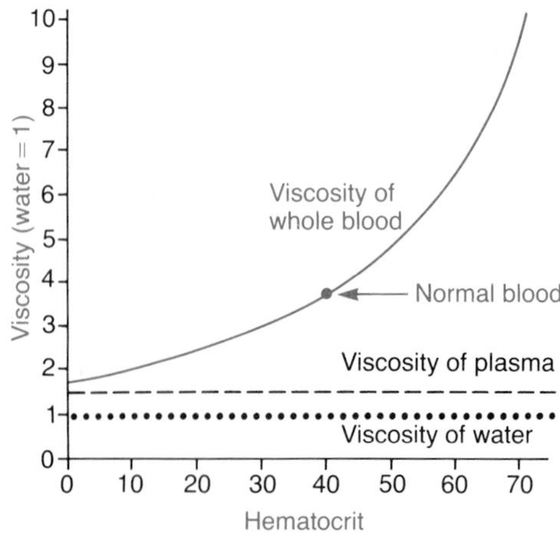

Figure 11-7. Effect of hematocrit on viscosity.

in diameter. Poiseuille discovered that this increase in flow is proportional to the fourth power of the diameter; that is $4 \times 4 \times 4 \times 4$ is equal to 256. Thus, the larger vessel has very little resistance while the smaller vessel has 256 times as much resistance. The reason for this is that most of the resistance occurs near the wall of the vessel where the blood drags against the endothelium. Therefore, in larger vessels vastly more blood can flow in the vessel middle, far away from the wall where the resistance becomes very little.

The importance of this fourth power relationship between resistance and vessel diameter is that the resistance of the body's small arterioles is tremendous while the resistance of the aorta and other large arteries is almost nothing. Consequently, the flow of blood in each tissue is controlled almost entirely by changes in the diameters of the arterioles, not by changes in the diameters of the larger arteries.

Effect of Blood Hematocrit and Viscosity on Vascular Resistance and Blood Flow

Another very important factor in vascular resistance is the viscosity of the blood. The greater the viscosity, the less the flow in a vessel if all other factors are constant. Furthermore, the viscosity of normal blood is about three times as great as the viscosity of water.

But what is it that makes the blood so viscous? It is mainly the large numbers of suspended red cells in the blood, each of which exerts frictional drag against adjacent cells and against the wall of the blood vessel. The per cent of cells in the blood is called the *hematocrit.* Thus, if a person has a hematocrit of 40, 40 per cent of the blood volume is cells, and the remainder is plasma. The hematocrit of normal men averages about 42, whereas that of normal women averages about 38.

The viscosity of blood increases drastically as the hematocrit increases, as illustrated in Figure 11-7. If we consider the viscosity of whole blood at normal hematocrit to be about 3, this means that the resistance for blood flow is about three times the resistance for water flow, and three times as much pressure is required to force whole blood as to force water through the same tube. Note that when the hematocrit rises to 60 or 70, which it often does in polycythemia, the blood viscosity can become as great as ten times that of water, and its flow through blood vessels is greatly retarded.

VASCULAR COMPLIANCE (OR CAPACITANCE)

Usually in hemodynamic studies it is much more important to know the *total quantity of blood* that can be stored in a given portion of the circulation for each mm Hg pressure rise than to know the distensibility of the individual vessels. This value is called the *compliance* or *capacitance* of the respective vascular bed. That is,

$$\text{Vascular compliance} = \frac{\text{Increase in volume}}{\text{Increase in pressure}} \quad (4)$$

Compliance and distensibility are quite different. A highly distensible vessel that has a very slight volume may have far less compliance than a much less distensible vessel that has a very large volume, for *compliance is equal to distensibility × volume.*

The compliance of a vein is about 24 times that of its corresponding artery because it is about 8 times as distensible and it has a volume about three times as great ($8 \times 3 = 24$).

Volume-Pressure Curves of the Arterial and Venous Circulations

A convenient method for expressing the compliance—that is, the relationship of pressure to volume in a vessel or in a large portion of the circulation—is the so-called *volume-pressure curve* (also frequently called the *pressure-volume curve*). The two solid curves of Figure 11–8 represent, respectively, the volume-pressure curves of the normal arterial and venous systems, showing that when the arterial system, including the larger arteries, small arteries, and arterioles, is filled with approximately 750 ml of blood, the mean arterial pressure is 100 mm Hg, but when filled with only 500 milliliters, the pressure falls to zero.

In the entire venous system, on the other hand, the volume of blood normally is about 2500 milliliters, and tremendous changes in this volume are required to change the venous pressure only a few millimeters of mercury because of the very great venous compliance.

Effect of Sympathetic Stimulation or Sympathetic Inhibition on the Volume-Pressure Relationships of the Arterial and Venous Systems. Also shown in Figure 11–8 are the effects of sympathetic stimulation and sympathetic inhibition on the volume-pressure curves. It is evident that the increase in vascular smooth muscle tone caused by sympathetic stimulation increases the pressure at each volume of the arteries or veins, whereas sympathetic inhibition decreases the pressure at each volume. Obviously, control of the vessels in this manner by the sympathetics is a valuable means for diminishing the dimensions of one segment of the circulation, thus transferring blood to other segments. For instance, an increase in vascular tone throughout the systemic circulation often causes large volumes of blood to shift into the heart, which is a major way in which pumping by the heart is increased.

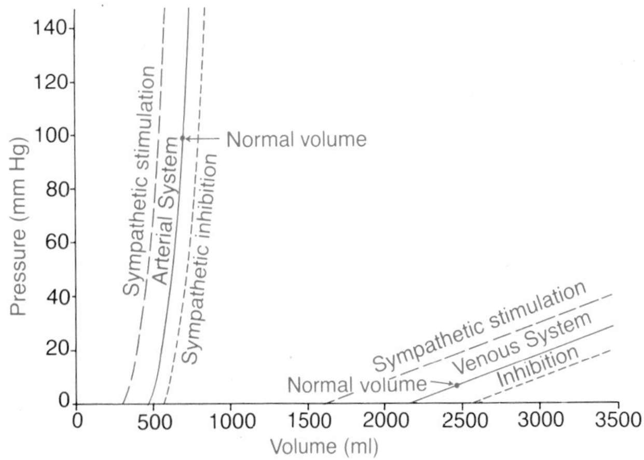

Figure 11–8. Volume-pressure curves of the systemic arterial and venous systems, showing also the effects of sympathetic stimulation and sympathetic inhibition.

Sympathetic control of vascular capacity is also especially important during hemorrhage. Enhancement of the sympathetic tone of the vessels, especially of the veins, reduces the dimensions of the circulatory system, and the circulation continues to operate almost normally even when as much as 25 per cent of the total blood volume has been lost.

Importance of the Tremendous Venous Compliance

The very large compliance of the venous system allows most of the extra blood of the circulation to be stored in the veins. By constricting the veins even a slight amount, this forces extra blood into the heart and thereby causes the heart to pump greatly increased volumes of blood throughout the circulation, called the *cardiac output*. For instance, stimulation of the veins by the sympathetic nerves can translocate large amounts of extra blood into the heart within seconds and in this way increase the cardiac output severalfold almost immediately. We shall see later that this is especially important in such conditions as exercise.

Therefore, the veins play a special role both in storing extra blood and in rapid control of cardiac output.

REFERENCES

See references for Chapter 12.

QUESTIONS

1. State approximately the quantities of blood in the different parts of the circulation.
2. Trace the change in the pressure as the blood flows from the arteries to the arterioles, the capillaries, the venules, and the veins in the systemic circulation.
3. What are the specific characteristics of the arterioles and small arteries that make these the main controllers of blood flow through local tissue areas?
4. State Ohm's law in all of its three different hemodynamic forms.
5. What are the usual units used in expressing blood flow?
6. Explain the function of the ultrasonic Doppler flowmeter.
7. Give the standard units for expressing blood pressure.
8. What are the relative advantages of the mercury manometer versus the high-fidelity methods for measuring blood pressure?
9. State the standard units for expressing resistance to blood flow.
10. How does one determine the resistance to blood flow?
11. What is the quantitative relationship between vascular diameter and vascular resistance?
12. How does sympathetic stimulation affect vascular resistance and tissue blood flow?
13. How much more compliant is the systemic venous system than the systemic arterial system?

12

Special Functions of the Systemic Circulation—Arteries, Veins, and Capillaries

THE ARTERIAL PRESSURE PULSATIONS

With each beat of the heart a new surge of blood fills the arteries. Were it not for the distensibility of the arterial system, blood flow through the tissues would occur only during cardiac systole, and no blood flow at all would occur during diastole. Fortunately, the combination of distensibility of the arteries and their resistance reduces the pressure pulsations almost to zero by the time the blood reaches the capillaries; therefore, tissue blood flow is hardly affected by the pulsatile nature of heart pumping.

A typical record of the *pressure pulsations* at the root of the aorta is illustrated in Figure 12–1. In the normal young adult, the pressure at the height of each pulse, the *systolic pressure,* is about 120 mm Hg and at its lowest point, the *diastolic pressure,* is about 80 mm Hg. The difference between these two pressures, about 40 mm Hg, is called the *pulse pressure.*

Two major factors affect the pulse pressure: (1) the *stroke volume output* of the heart and (2) the *compliance (total distensibility)* of the arterial tree.

In general, the greater the stroke volume output, the greater the amount of blood that must be accommodated in the arterial tree with each heart beat, and, therefore, the greater the pressure rise and fall during systole and diastole, thus causing a greater pulse pressure.

On the other hand, the less the compliance of the arterial system, the greater the rise in pressure for a given stroke volume of blood pumped into the arteries. For instance, the pulse pressure sometimes rises to as much as two times normal in old age because the arteries become hardened with *arteriosclerosis* and therefore are noncompliant.

In effect, then, the pulse pressure is determined approximately by the *ratio of stroke volume output to compliance of the arterial tree.* Therefore, any condition of the circulation that affects either of these two factors will also affect the pulse pressure.

Transmission of Pressure Pulses to the Peripheral Arteries

When the heart ejects blood into the aorta during systole, at first only the proximal portion of the aorta becomes distended because the inertia of the blood prevents sudden movement all the way to the periphery. However, the rising pressure in the central aorta rapidly overcomes this inertia and the wave front of distension spreads farther and farther along the aorta, as illustrated in Figure 12–2. This is called *transmission of the pressure pulse* in the arteries.

Damping of the Pressure Pulses in the Smaller Arteries, Arterioles, and Capillaries. Figure 12–3 shows typical changes in the contours of the pressure pulse as the pulse travels into the peripheral vessels. Note especially in the three lower curves that the intensity of pulsation becomes progressively less in the smaller arteries, the arterioles, and especially the capillaries. In fact, only when the aortic pulsations are extremely large or when the arterioles are greatly dilated can pulsations be observed at all in the capillaries.

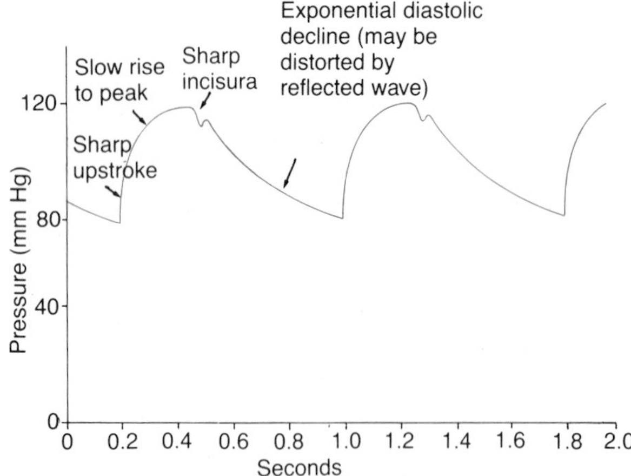

Figure 12-1. A normal pressure pulse contour recorded from the ascending *aorta.* (From Opdyke: *Fed. Proc., 11*:734, 1952.)

This progressive diminishment of the pulsations in the periphery is called *damping* of the pressure pulses. The cause of this is twofold: (1) the resistance to blood movement in the vessels and (2) the compliance of the vessels. The resistance damps the pulsations because a small amount of blood must flow forward at the pulse wave front to distend the next segment of the vessel; the greater the resistance, the more difficult it is for this to occur. The compliance damps the pulsations because the more compliant a vessel, the more the quantity of blood flow at the pulse wave front must be to cause the rise in pressure.

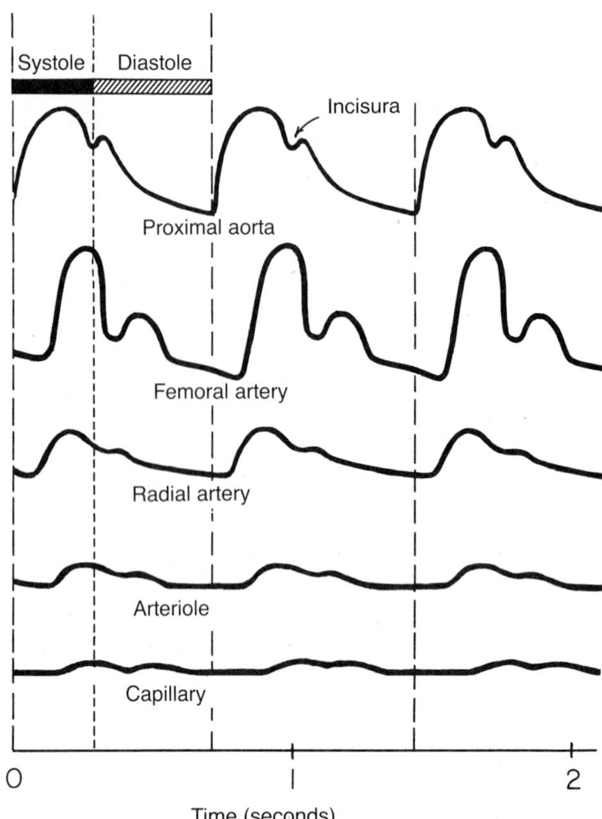

Figure 12-3. Changes in the pulse pressure contour as the pulse wave travels toward the smaller vessels.

The Auscultatory Method for Measuring Systolic and Diastolic Pressures

Obviously, it is impossible to use the various pressure recorders that require needle insertion into an artery for making routine pressure measurements in human patients, although they are used on occasion when special studies are necessary. Instead, the clinician determines systolic and diastolic pressures by indirect means, usually by the auscultatory method.

Figure 12-4 illustrates the auscultatory method for determining systolic and diastolic arterial pressures. A stethoscope is placed over the antecubital artery, while a blood pressure cuff is inflated around the upper arm. As long as the cuff presses against the arm with so little pressure that the artery remains distended with blood, no sounds whatsoever are heard by the stethoscope, despite the fact that the blood within the artery is pulsating. When the cuff pressure is great enough to close the artery during part of the arterial

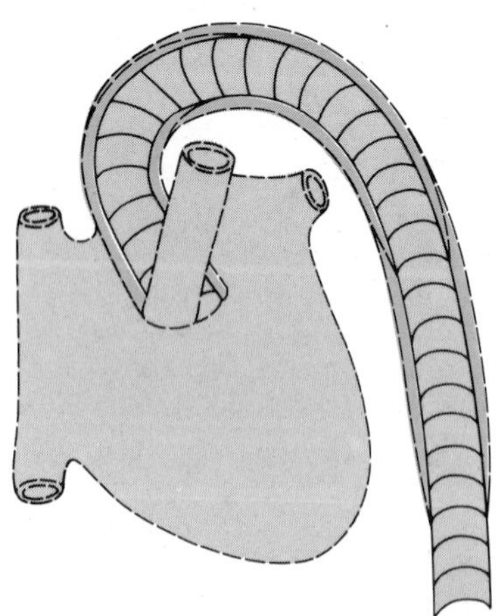

Figure 12-2. Progressive stages in the transmission of the pressure pulse along the aorta.

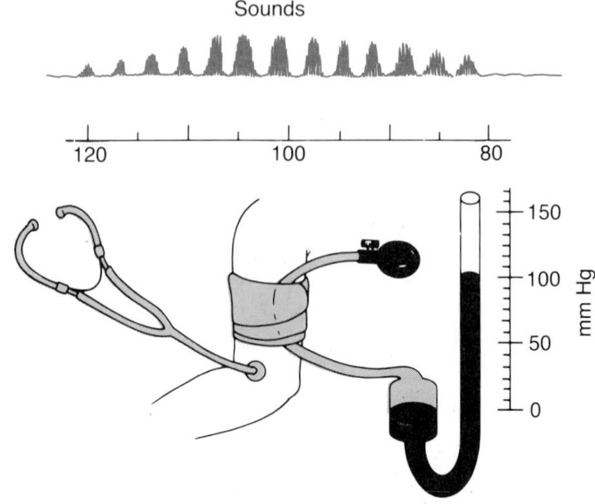

Figure 12-4. The auscultatory method of measuring systolic and diastolic pressures.

pressure cycle, a sound is then heard with each pulsation. These sounds are called *Korotkoff sounds.*

The Korotkoff sounds are believed to be caused by blood jetting through the partly occluded vessel. The jet causes turbulence in the open vessel beyond the cuff, and this sets up the vibrations heard through the stethoscope.

In determining blood pressure by the auscultatory method, the pressure in the cuff is first elevated well above arterial systolic pressure. As long as this pressure is higher than systolic pressure, the brachial artery remains collapsed and no blood whatsoever flows into the lower artery during any part of the pressure cycle. Therefore, no Korotkoff sounds are heard in the lower artery. But then the cuff pressure is gradually reduced. Just as soon as the pressure in the cuff falls below systolic pressure, blood slips through the artery beneath the cuff during the peak of systolic pressure, and one begins to hear *tapping* sounds in the antecubital artery in synchrony with the heartbeat. As soon as these sounds are heard, the pressure level indicated by the manometer connected to the cuff is approximately equal to the systolic pressure.

As the pressure in the cuff is lowered still more, the Korotkoff sounds change in quality, having less of the tapping quality but more of a rhythmic, harsher quality. Then, finally, when the pressure in the cuff falls to equal diastolic pressure, the artery no longer closes during diastole, which means that the basic factor causing the sounds (the jetting of blood through a squeezed artery) is no longer present. Therefore, the sounds suddenly change to a muffled quality and then usually disappear entirely after another 5 to 10 mm drop in cuff pressure. One notes the manometer pressure when the Korotkoff sounds change to the muffled quality, and this pressure is approximately equal to the diastolic pressure.

The auscultatory method for determining systolic and diastolic pressures is not entirely accurate, but it usually gives values within 10 per cent of those determined by direct measurement from the arteries.

Normal Arterial Pressures As Measured by the Auscultatory Method. Figure 12–5 illustrates the normal ranges of systolic and diastolic pressures at different ages. The progressive increase in pressure with age results from the effects of aging on the long-term blood pressure control mechanisms. We see in Chapter 16 that the kidneys primarily are responsible for this long-term regulation of arterial pressure; it is well known that the kidneys do indeed exhibit definitive changes with age, especially after the age of 50 years.

The exceptional rise in *systolic* pressure beyond the age of 60 years results from hardening of the arteries, which itself is an end-stage result of *atherosclerosis.* This causes a bounding systolic pressure and also considerable increase in the pulse pressure.

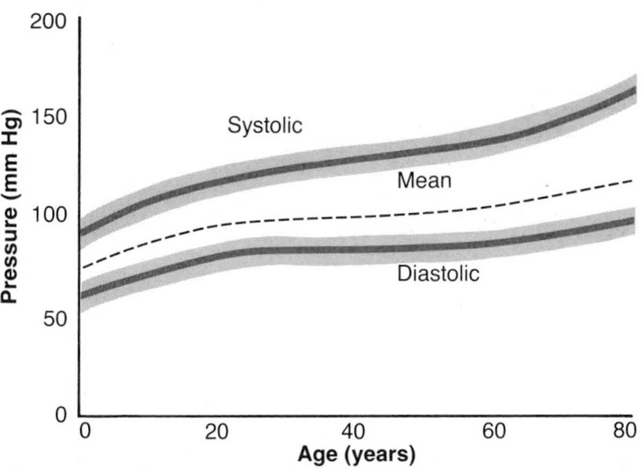

Figure 12–5. Changes in systolic, diastolic, and mean arterial pressures with age. The shaded areas show the normal range.

The Mean Arterial Pressure. The mean arterial pressure is the average of all the pressures measured millisecond by millisecond over a period of time. It is not equal to the average of systolic and diastolic pressure, however, because the pressure remains nearer to diastolic pressure than to systolic pressure during the greater part of the cardiac cycle. Therefore, the mean arterial pressure is determined about 60 per cent by the diastolic pressure and 40 per cent by the systolic pressure. Note in Figure 12–5 that the mean pressure, the dashed line, at all ages is nearer to the diastolic pressure than to the systolic pressure, especially so at older ages.

THE VEINS AND THEIR FUNCTIONS

For years the veins have been considered to be nothing more than passageways for flow of blood into the heart, but it is rapidly becoming apparent that they perform many functions that are necessary to the operation of the circulation. Especially important, they are capable of constricting and enlarging, of storing large quantities of blood and making this blood available when it is required by the remainder of the circulation, of actually propelling blood forward by means of a so-called venous pump, and even of helping regulate cardiac output, an exceedingly important function that is described in Chapter 17.

Venous Pressures—Right Atrial Pressure (Central Venous Pressure) and Peripheral Pressures

Blood from all the systemic veins flows into the right atrium; therefore, the pressure in the right atrium is frequently called the *central venous pressure.* Obviously, anything that affects right atrial pressure usually affects venous pressure everywhere in the body.

Right atrial pressure is regulated by a balance between the ability of the heart to pump blood out of the right atrium and, second, *the tendency for blood to flow from the peripheral vessels back into the right atrium.*

The *normal right atrial pressure* is approximately 0 mm Hg, which is about equal to the atmospheric pressure around the body. However, it can rise to as high as 20 to 30 mm Hg under very abnormal conditions, such as (1) serious heart failure or (2) following massive transfusion of blood, which will cause excessive quantities of blood to attempt to flow into the heart from the peripheral vessels.

The lower limit to the right atrial pressure is usually about −3 to −5 mm Hg, which is the pressure in the chest cavity that surrounds the heart. The right atrial pressure approaches these very low values when the heart pumps with exceptional vigor or when the flow of blood into the heart from the peripheral vessels is greatly depressed, such as following severe hemorrhage.

Venous Resistance and Peripheral Venous Pressure

Large veins have almost no resistance *when they are distended.* However, as illustrated in Figure 12–6, most of the large veins entering the thorax are compressed at many points by the surrounding tissues, so that blood flow is impeded. For instance, the veins from the arms are compressed by their sharp angulation over the first rib. Second, the pressure in the neck veins often falls so low that the atmospheric pressure on the outside of the neck causes them to collapse. Finally, veins coursing through the abdomen are often compressed by different organs and by the intra-abdominal pressure, so that usually they are at least partially collapsed to an ovoid or slitlike state. For these reasons, the *large veins do usually offer considerable resistance to blood flow,* and because of this the pressure in the peripheral veins is usually 4 to 7 mm Hg greater than the right atrial pressure.

Effect of High Right Atrial Pressure on Peripheral Venous Pressure. When the right atrial pressure rises above its normal value of 0 mm Hg, blood begins to back up in the large veins and to open them up. The pressures in the peripheral veins do not rise until all the collapsed points between the peripheral veins and the large veins have opened up. This usually occurs when the right atrial pressure rises to about + 4 to 6 mm Hg. Then, as the right atrial pressure rises still further, the additional increase in pressure is reflected by a corresponding rise in peripheral venous pressure. Because the heart must be greatly weakened to cause a rise in right atrial pressure to as high as 4 to 6 mm Hg, one often finds that the peripheral venous pressure is not elevated in the early stages of heart failure.

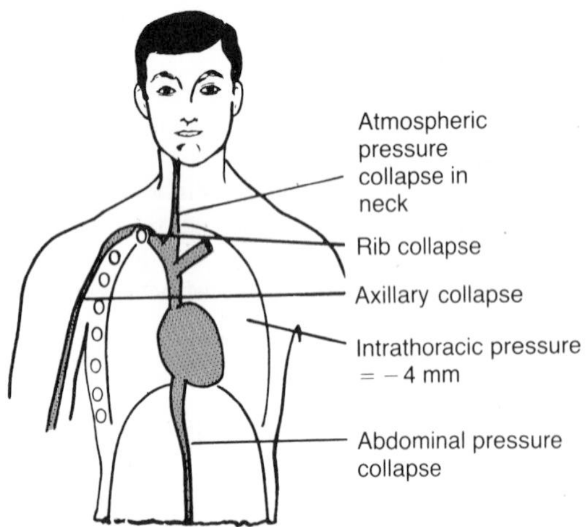

Figure 12–6. Factors tending to collapse the veins entering the thorax.

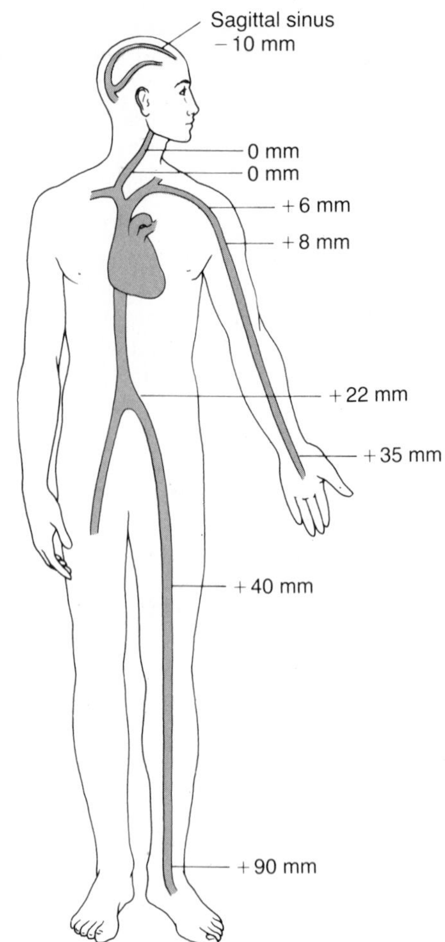

Figure 12–7. Effect of hydrostatic pressure on the venous pressures throughout the body.

Effect of "Hydrostatic" Pressure on Venous Pressure

In any body of water, the pressure at the surface of the water is equal to atmospheric pressure, but the pressure rises 1 mm Hg for each 13.6 mm distance below the surface. This pressure results from the weight of the water and therefore is called *hydrostatic pressure.*

Hydrostatic pressure also occurs in the vascular system of the human being because of the weight of the blood in the vessels, as illustrated in Figure 12–7. When a person is standing, the pressure in the right atrium remains approximately 0 mm Hg because the heart pumps into the arteries any excess blood that attempts to accumulate at this point. However, in an adult *who is standing absolutely still* the pressure in the veins of the feet is approximately +90 mm Hg simply because of the weight of the blood in the veins between the heart and the feet. The venous pressures at other levels of the body below the heart lie proportionately between 0 and 90 mm Hg.

Effect of the Hydrostatic Factor on Arterial and Other Pressures

The hydrostatic factor also affects the peripheral pressures in the arteries and capillaries as well as in the veins. For instance, a standing person who has an arterial pressure of 100 mm Hg at the level of the heart has an arterial pressure in the feet of about 190 mm Hg. Therefore, when one states that the arterial pressure is 100 mm Hg, it generally means that this is the pressure at the hydrostatic level of the heart.

Venous Valves, the "Venous Pump," and the Venous Pressure

Were it not for valves in the veins, the hydrostatic pressure effect would cause the venous pressure in the feet always to be about +90 mm Hg in a standing adult. However, every time one moves the legs one tightens the muscles and compresses the veins either in the muscles or adjacent to them, and this squeezes the blood out of the veins. The valves in the veins, illustrated in Figure 12-8, are arranged so that the direction of blood flow can be only toward the heart. Consequently, every time a person moves the legs or even tenses the muscles, a certain amount of blood is propelled toward the heart, and the pressure in the veins is lowered. This pumping system is known as the "venous pump" or "muscle pump," and it is efficient enough that under ordinary circumstances the venous pressure in the feet of a walking adult remains less than 25 mm Hg.

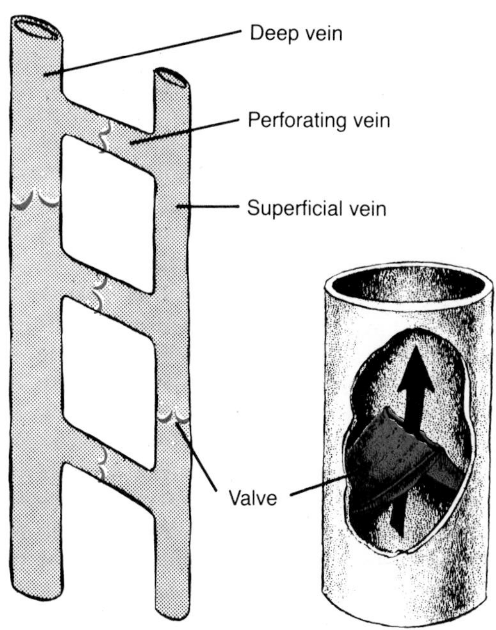

Figure 12-8. The venous valves of the leg.

If the human being stands perfectly still, the venous pump does not work, and the venous pressures in the lower part of the leg will rise to the full hydrostatic value of 90 mm Hg in about 30 seconds. The pressures in the capillaries also increase greatly, causing fluid to leak from the circulatory system into the tissue spaces. As a result, the legs swell, and the blood volume diminishes. Indeed, as much as 15 to 20 per cent of the blood volume is frequently lost from the circulatory system within the first 15 minutes of standing absolutely still, as often occurs when a soldier is made to stand at absolute attention.

Venous Valve Incompetence and Varicose Veins. The valves of the venous system frequently become "incompetent" or sometimes are even destroyed. This is especially true when the veins have been overstretched by excess venous pressure lasting weeks or months, as occurs in pregnancy or when one stands most of the time. When valve incompetence develops, the pressure in the veins of the legs increases still more owing to failure of the venous pump; this further increases the size of the veins and finally destroys the function of the valves entirely. Thus, the person develops "varicose veins," which are characterized by large, bulbous protrusions of the veins beneath the skin of the entire leg and particularly of the lower leg. The venous and capillary pressures become very high, and leakage of fluid from the capillaries causes constant edema in the legs whenever these persons stand for more than a few minutes. The edema in turn prevents adequate diffusion of nutritional materials from the capillaries to the muscle and skin cells, so that the muscles become painful and weak, and the skin frequently becomes gangrenous and ulcerates. Obviously, the best treatment for such a condition is continual elevation of the legs to a level at least as high as the heart, but tight binders on the legs are also of considerable aid in preventing the edema and its sequelae.

Clinical Estimation of Venous Pressure

The venous pressure can often be estimated by simply observing the degree of distention of the peripheral veins—especially the neck veins. For instance, in the sitting position, the neck veins are never distended in the normal person. However, when the right atrial pressure becomes increased to as much as 10 mm Hg, the lower veins of the neck begin to protrude, and at 15 mm Hg essentially all the veins in the neck become distended.

Direct Measurement of Venous Pressure and Right Atrial Pressure. Venous pressure can be measured with ease by inserting a syringe needle directly into a vein and connecting it to a pressure recorder.

The only means by which *right atrial pressure* can be measured accurately is by inserting a catheter through the veins into the right atrium. Pressures measured through such "central venous catheters" are used almost routinely in hospitalized cardiac patients to provide constant assessment of heart pumping ability.

Blood Reservoir Function of the Veins

It was pointed out in the previous chapter that over 60 per cent of all the blood in the circulatory system is in the veins. For this reason, and also because the veins are so compliant, it is frequently said that the venous system serves as a *blood reservoir* for the circulation.

When blood is lost from the body and the arterial pressure begins to fall, pressure reflexes are elicited from the carotid sinuses and other pressure-sensitive areas of the circulation, as is discussed in Chapter 15; these in turn send sympathetic nerve signals to the veins, causing them to constrict, and this takes up much of the slack in the circulatory system caused by the lost blood. Indeed, even after as much as 20 per cent of the total blood volume has been lost, the circulatory system often functions almost normally because of this variable reservoir system of the veins.

Specific Blood Reservoirs. Certain portions of the circulatory system are so extensive and so compliant that they are called specific "blood reservoirs." These include (1) the *spleen,* which can sometimes decrease in size sufficiently to release as much as 100 milliliters of blood into other areas of the circulation; (2) the *liver,* the sinuses of which can release several hundred milliliters of blood into the remainder of the circulation; (3) the *large abdominal veins,* which can contribute as much as 300 milliliters; and (4) the *venous plexus beneath the skin,* which can also contribute several hundred milliliters. The *heart* and the *lungs,* though not parts of the systemic venous reservoir system, must also be considered to be blood reservoirs. The heart, for instance, becomes reduced in size during sympathetic stimulation and in this way can contribute some 50 to 100 milliliters of blood, and the lungs can contribute another 100 to 200 milliliters when the pulmonary pressures fall to low values.

THE MICROCIRCULATION

In the microcirculation, illustrated in Figure 12–9, the most purposeful function of the circulation occurs, transport of nutrients to the tissues and removal of cellular excreta. The small arterioles control the blood flow to each tissue area, and local conditions in the tissues themselves control the diameters of the arterioles in turn. Thus, each tissue in most instances controls its own blood flow in relation to its needs, a subject that is discussed in detail in Chapter 14.

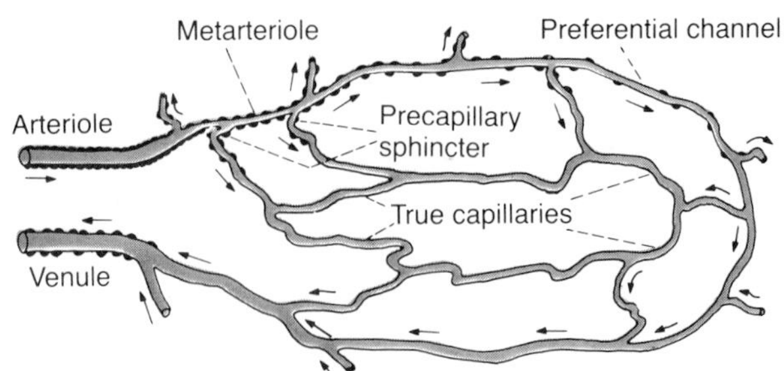

Figure 12–9. Structure of the mesenteric capillary bed. (From Zweifach: Factors Regulating Blood Pressure. New York, Josiah Macy, Jr., Foundation, 1950.)

Structure of the Microcirculation and Capillary System

The microcirculation of each organ is specifically organized to serve that organ's own special needs. In general, each nutrient artery entering an organ branches six to eight times before the arteries become small enough to be called "arterioles," which have internal diameters generally less than 20 micrometers. Then the arterioles themselves branch two to five times, reaching diameters of 5 to 9 micrometers at their ends, where they supply blood to the capillaries.

Figure 12–9 illustrates the structure of a representative capillary bed as seen in the mesentery, showing that blood enters the capillaries through an *arteriole* and leaves by way of a *venule.* Blood from the arteriole passes into a series of *metarterioles,* which are called by some physiologists *terminal arterioles* and which have a structure midway between that of arterioles and capillaries. After leaving the metarteriole, the blood enters the *capillaries,* some of which are large and are called *preferential channels* and others of which are small and are *true capillaries.* After passing through the capillaries, the blood enters the venule and returns to the general circulation.

The arterioles are highly muscular, and their diameters can change manyfold. The metarterioles (the terminal arterioles) do not have a continuous muscular coat, but smooth muscle fibers encircle the vessel at intermediate points, as illustrated in Figure 12–9 by the large black dots to the sides of the metarteriole.

At the point where the true capillaries originate from the metarterioles a smooth muscle fiber usually encircles the capillary. This is called the *precapillary sphincter.* This sphincter can open and close the entrance to the capillary.

The venules are considerably larger than the arterioles and have a much weaker muscular coat. Yet, it must be remembered that the pressure in the venules is much less than that in the arterioles, so that the venules can still contract considerably.

This typical arrangement of the capillary bed is not found in all parts of the body; however, some similar arrangement serves the same purposes. Most important of all, the metarterioles (and the precapillary sphincters when they also exist) are in extremely close contact with the tissues that they serve. Therefore, the local conditions of the tissues—the concentrations of nutrients, end products of metabolism, hydrogen ions, and so forth—can cause direct effects on these in controlling the local blood flow in each minute tissue area.

Blood Flow in the Capillaries—Vasomotion

Blood usually does not flow continuously through the capillaries. Instead, it flows intermittently, turning on and off every few seconds or minutes. The cause of this intermittency is the phenomenon called *vasomotion,* which means intermittent contraction of the metarterioles and precapillary sphincters.

Regulation of Vasomotion. The most important factor found thus far to affect the degree of opening and closing of the metarterioles and precapillary sphincters is the concentration of *oxygen* in the tissues. When the rate of oxygen usage is great, the intermittent periods of blood flow occur more often, and the duration of each period of flow lasts for a longer time, thereby allowing the blood to carry increased quantities of oxygen (as well as other nutrients) to the tissues. This effect as well as multiple other factors that control local tissue blood flow is discussed in Chapter 14.

Average Function of the Capillary System

Despite the fact that blood flow through each capillary is intermittent, so many capillaries are present in the tissues that their overall function becomes averaged. That is, there is an *average rate of blood flow* through each tissue capillary bed, an *average capillary pressure* within the capillaries, and an *average rate of transfer of substances* between the blood of the capillaries and the surrounding interstitial fluid. In the following chapter, we are concerned with these averages, though one must remember that the average functions are in reality the functions of literally billions of individual capillaries, each operating intermittently in response to the local conditions in the tissues.

REFERENCES

Chien, S.: Red cell deformability and its relevance to blood flow. Annu. Rev. Physiol., 49:177, 1987.

Chien, S., et al.: Blood flow in small tubes. In Renkin, E. M., and Michel, C. C. (eds).: Handbook of Physiology. Sec. 2, Vol. IV. Bethesda, Md., American Physiological Society, 1984, p. 217.

Fronek, A. (ed.): Noninvasive Diagnostics in Vascular Disease. New York, McGraw-Hill Book Co., 1989.

Goerke, J., and Mines, A. H.: Cardiovascular Physiology. New York, Raven Press, 1988.

Green, H. D.: Circulation: Physical principles. In Glasser, O. (ed.): Medical Physics. Chicago, Year Book Medical Publishers, 1944.

Guyton, A. C.: Arterial Pressure and Hypertension. Philadelphia, W. B. Saunders Co., 1980.

Guyton, A. C., and Jones, C. E.: Central venous pressure: Physiological significance and clinical implications. Am. Heart J., 86:431, 1973.

Guyton, A. C., et al.: Cardiac Output and Its Regulation. Philadelphia, W. B. Saunders Co., 1973.

Guyton, A. C., et al.: Pressure-volume curves of the entire arterial and venous systems in the living animal. Am. J. Physiol., 184:253, 1956.

Guyton, J. R.: Mechanical control of smooth muscle growth. In Seidel, C. L., and Weisbrodt, N. W.: Hypertrophic Response in Smooth Muscle. Boca Raton, Fla., CRC Press, 1987, p. 121.

Hochmuth, R. M., and Waugh, R. E.: Erythrocyte membrane elasticity and viscosity. Annu. Rev. Physiol., 49:209, 1987.

Milnor, W. R.: Hemodynamics. 2nd ed. Baltimore, Williams & Wilkins, 1989.

Rothe, C. F.: Reflex control of veins and vascular capacitance. Physiol. Rev., 63:1281, 1983.

Vanhoutte, P. M.: Vasodilation: Vascular Smooth Muscle, Peptides, Autonomic Nerves, and Endothelium. New York, Raven Press, 1988.

QUESTIONS

1. Draw a normal pressure pulse contour for the ascending aorta and point out systolic pressure, diastolic pressure, and the incisura, the point where the aortic valve closes. What are the major factors that affect the pulse pressure?
2. Explain the changes in the pressure pulse contour as the pressure pulse is transmitted into the peripheral arteries.
3. Describe the auscultatory method for measuring systolic and diastolic pressures.
4. Describe the changes in systolic and diastolic pressures with age and the causes of these changes.
5. Discuss the various factors that alter venous resistance.
6. List the different factors that affect peripheral venous pressure. How do "hydrostatic" factors affect the peripheral venous pressures?
7. Discuss and explain the important factors that determine the right atrial pressure.
8. Explain the importance of the venous valves and how they function as part of the "venous pump."
9. Why do the veins more than any other portion of the circulation serve as blood reservoirs?
10. Describe a typical capillary bed.
11. What is meant by vasomotion, and how is capillary blood flow controlled by the arterioles, metarterioles, and precapillary sphincters?

13

Capillary Fluid Exchange, Interstitial Fluid Dynamics, and Lymph Flow

It is in the capillaries that the most purposeful function of the circulation occurs, namely, interchange of nutrients and cellular excreta between the tissues and the circulating blood. About 10 billion capillaries, which have a total surface area of probably 500 to 700 square meters, provide this function. Indeed, it is rare that any single functional cell of the body is more than 20 to 30 microns away from a capillary.

The purpose of this chapter is to discuss the transfer of substances between the blood and interstitial fluid. The factors that affect the transfer of fluid volume between the circulating blood and the interstitial fluid are discussed especially, as well as return of fluid from the interstitium to the circulation through the lymphatic system.

Structure of the Capillary

The capillaries are extremely thin structures with walls of a single layer of highly permeable endothelial cells. Here interchange of nutrients and cellular excreta occurs between the tissues and the circulating blood. About 10 billion capillaries with a total surface area estimated to be 500 to 700 square meters (approximately the surface area of a football field) provide this function for the whole body. Indeed, it is rare that any single functional cell of the body is more than 20 to 30 micrometers away from a capillary.

Figure 13–1 illustrates the ultramicroscopic structure of a typical capillary wall as found in most organs of the body, especially in the muscles and connective tissue. Note that the wall is composed of a unicellular layer of endothelial cells and is surrounded by a basement membrane on the outside. The total thickness of the wall is about 0.5 micrometer.

The diameter of the capillary is 4 to 9 micrometers, barely large enough for red blood cells and other blood cells to squeeze through.

"Pores" in the Capillary Membrane. Studying Figure 13–1, one sees two minute passageways connecting the interior of the capillary with the exterior. One of these is the *intercellular cleft,* which is the thin slit that lies between adjacent endothelial cells. Each of these clefts is interrupted periodically by short ridges of protein attachments that hold the endothelial cells together, but each ridge in turn is broken after a short distance, so that in between them fluid can percolate freely through the cleft. The cleft normally has a very uniform spacing with a width of approximately 6 to 7 nanometers (60 to 70 angstroms), slightly smaller than the diameter of an albumin protein molecule.

Because the intercellular clefts are located only at the edges of the endothelial cells, they usually represent no more than 1/1000 of the total surface area of the capillary. Nevertheless, the rate of thermal motion of water molecules, as well as of most other water-soluble ions and small solutes, is so rapid that all these diffuse with ease between the interior and exterior of the capillaries through these "slit-pores," the intercellular clefts.

Also present in the endothelial cells are many minute *plasmalemmal vesicles.* These form at one surface of the cell by imbibing small packets of plasma or extracellular fluid. They can then move slowly through the endothelial cell, and it has been postulated that they transport significant amounts of substances through the capillary wall.

The "pores" in the capillaries of some organs have special characteristics to meet the peculiar needs of the organs. To give an example, in the *brain,* the junc-

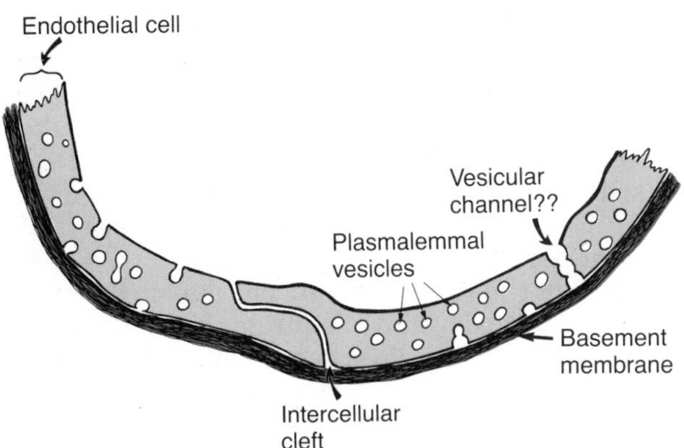

Figure 13-1. Structure of the capillary wall. Note especially the *intercellular cleft* at the junction between adjacent endothelial cells; it is believed that most water-soluble substances diffuse through the capillary membrane along this cleft.

tions between the capillary endothelial cells are mainly "tight" junctions that will allow only very small molecules to pass into the brain tissues. This is called the *blood-brain barrier* and is discussed further in Chapter 41.

EXCHANGE OF NUTRIENTS AND OTHER SUBSTANCES BETWEEN THE BLOOD AND INTERSTITIAL FLUID

Diffusion Through the Capillary Membrane

By far the most important means by which substances are transferred between the plasma and interstitial fluid is by *diffusion.* Figure 13-2 illustrates this process, showing that, as the blood traverses the capillary, tremendous numbers of water molecules and dissolved particles diffuse back and forth through the capillary wall, providing continual mixing between the interstitial fluid and the plasma. Diffusion results from thermal motion of the water molecules and the dissolved substances in the fluid, the different particles moving first in one direction, then another, moving randomly in every direction.

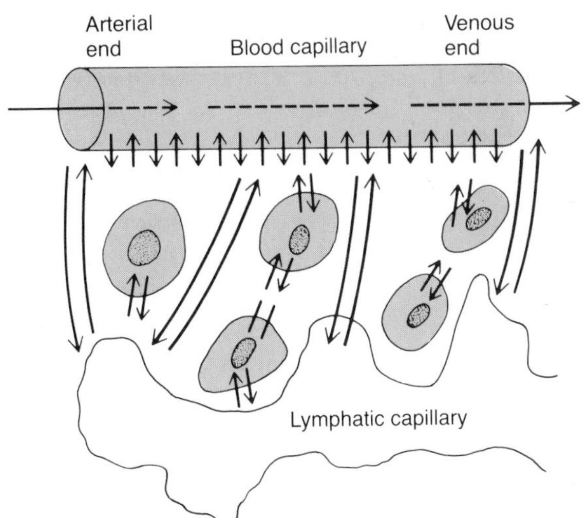

Figure 13-2. Diffusion of fluid and dissolved substances between the capillary and interstitial fluid spaces.

Diffusion of Lipid-Soluble Substances Through the Capillary Membrane. If a substance is lipid-soluble, it can diffuse directly through the cell membranes of the capillary without having to go through the pores. Such substances include especially oxygen and carbon dioxide. Because these can permeate all areas of the capillary membrane, their rates of transport through the capillary membrane are many times the rates for lipid-insoluble substances, such as sodium ions, glucose, and so forth.

Diffusion of Water-Soluble Substances Through the Capillary Membrane. Many substances needed by the tissues are soluble in water but cannot pass through the lipid membranes of the endothelial cells; such substances include water molecules themselves, sodium ions, chloride ions, and glucose. Despite the fact that not over 1/1000 of the surface area of the capillaries is represented by the intercellular junctions, the velocity of thermal molecular motion is so great that even this small area is sufficient to allow tremendous diffusion of water and water-soluble substances through these pores. To give one an idea of the extreme rapidity with which these substances diffuse, *the rate at which water molecules diffuse through the capillary membrane is approximately 80 times as great as the rate at which plasma itself flows linearly along the capillary.* That is, the water of the plasma is exchanged with the water of the interstitial fluid 80 times before the plasma can go the entire distance through the capillary.

Effect of Molecular Size on Passage Through the Pores. The width of the capillary intercellular slit-pores, 6 to 7 nanometers, is about 20 times the diameter of the water molecule, which is the smallest molecule that normally passes through the capillary pores. On the other hand, the diameters of plasma protein molecules are slightly greater than the width of the pores. Other substances, such as sodium ions, chloride ions, glucose, and urea, have intermediate diameters. Therefore, it is obvious that the permeabil-

Table 13-1 RELATIVE PERMEABILITY OF MUSCLE CAPILLARY PORES TO DIFFERENT-SIZED MOLECULES

Substance	Molecular Weight	Permeability
Water	18	1.00
NaCl	58.5	0.96
Urea	60	0.8
Glucose	180	0.6
Sucrose	342	0.4
Inulin	5000	0.2
Myoglobin	17,600	0.03
Hemoglobin	68,000	0.01
Albumin	69,000	.0001

Based mainly on data from Pappenheimer: *Physiol. Rev. 33*:389, 1953.

ity of the capillary pores for different substances varies according to their molecular diameters.

Table 13-1 gives the relative permeabilities of the capillary pores in muscle for substances commonly encountered by the capillary membrane, illustrating, for instance, that the permeability for glucose molecules is 0.6 times that for water molecules, whereas the permeability for albumin molecules is very, very slight.

Effect of Concentration Difference on Net Rate of Diffusion Through the Capillary Membrane. The "net" rate of diffusion of a substance through any membrane is proportional to the *concentration difference* between the two sides of the membrane. That is, the greater the difference between the concentrations of any given substance on the two sides of the capillary membrane, the greater will be the net movement of the substance through the membrane. Thus, the concentration of oxygen in the blood is normally greater than that in the interstitial fluid. Therefore, large quantities of oxygen normally move from the blood toward the tissues. Conversely, the concentration of carbon dioxide is greater in the tissues than in the blood, which obviously causes carbon dioxide to move into the blood and to be carried away from the tissues.

THE INTERSTITIUM AND THE INTERSTITIAL FLUID

Approximately one sixth of the body consists of spaces between cells, which collectively are called the *interstitium.* The fluid in these spaces is the *interstitial fluid.*

The structure of the interstitium is illustrated in Figure 13-3. It has two major types of solid structures: (1) collagen fiber bundles and (2) proteoglycan filaments. The collagen fiber bundles extend long distances in the interstitium. They are extremely strong and therefore provide most of the tensional strength of the tissues. The proteoglycan filaments, on the other hand, are extremely thin, coiled molecules composed of about 98 per cent hyaluronic acid and 2 per cent protein. These molecules are so thin that they can never be seen with a light microscope and are very difficult to demonstrate even with the electron microscope. Nevertheless, they form a filler of very fine reticular filaments aptly described as a "brush pile."

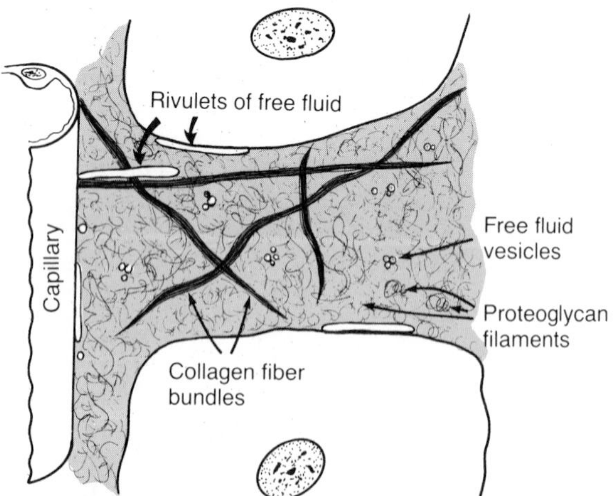

Figure 13-3. Structure of the interstitium. Proteoglycan filaments fill the spaces between the collagen fiber bundles. Free fluid vesicles are seen and small amounts of free fluid in the form of rivulets.

"Gel" in the Interstitium. The fluid in the interstitium is derived by filtration from the capillaries. It contains almost the same constituents as plasma except for lower concentrations of proteins because these do not filter out of the capillaries with ease. This fluid is mainly entrapped in the minute spaces among the proteoglycan filaments. This combination of the proteoglycan filaments and the fluid entrapped within them has the characteristics of a *gel* and therefore is often called the *tissue gel.*

Because of the large number of proteoglycan filaments, fluid *flows* through the tissue gel only very poorly. Instead, it mainly *diffuses* through the gel; that is, it moves molecule by molecule from one place to another by the process of kinetic motion rather than by large numbers of molecules moving together.

Fortunately, diffusion through the gel occurs about 95 to 99 per cent as rapidly as it does through free fluid. For the short distances between the capillaries and the tissue cells, this diffusion allows rapid transport through the interstitium not only of the water molecules but also of electrolytes, nutrients, cellular excreta, oxygen, carbon dioxide, and so forth.

"Free" Fluid in the Interstitium. Although almost all the fluid in the interstitium is normally entrapped within the tissue gel, occasionally small *rivulets of "free" fluid* and small *free fluid vesicles* are also present, which means fluid that is free of the proteoglycan molecules and therefore can flow freely. When a dye is injected into the circulating blood, it can often be seen to flow through the interstitium in the small rivulets, usually coursing along the surfaces of collagen fibers or surfaces of cells. However, the amount of "free" fluid present in *normal* tissues is very slight, usually much less than 1 per cent. On the other hand, when the tissues develop *edema, these small pockets and rivulets of free fluid often expand to equal more than half of the interstitial fluid,* as we shall discuss later in the chapter.

DISTRIBUTION OF FLUID VOLUME BETWEEN THE PLASMA AND THE INTERSTITIAL FLUID

The pressure in the capillaries tends to force fluid and its dissolved substances through the capillary pores into the interstitial spaces. In contrast, osmotic pressure caused by the plasma proteins (called *colloid* osmotic pressure) tends to cause fluid movement by osmosis from the interstitial spaces into the blood; it is this osmotic pressure that prevents significant loss of fluid volume from the blood into the interstitial spaces. Yet, also important is the lymphatic system to return back to the circulation the small amounts of protein and fluid that do leak into the interstitial spaces. In the following few paragraphs we discuss the factors that determine the movement, or lack of movement, of fluid volume through the capillary membrane, and later in the chapter, we discuss the role of the lymphatic system in this overall mechanism.

The Four Primary Forces That Determine Fluid Movement Through the Capillary Membrane. Figure 13–4 illustrates the four primary forces that determine whether fluid will move out of the blood into the interstitial fluid or in the opposite direction; these, called "Starling forces" in honor of the physiologist who first demonstrated their importance, are:

1. The *capillary pressure* (Pc), which tends to force fluid outward through the capillary membrane.
2. The *interstitial fluid pressure* (Pif), which tends to force fluid inward through the capillary membrane when Pif is positive but outward when Pif is negative.
3. The *plasma colloid osmotic pressure* (Πp), which tends to cause osmosis of fluid inward through the membrane.
4. The *interstitial fluid colloid osmotic pressure* (Πif), which tends to cause osmosis of fluid outward through the membrane.

Capillary Pressure

Two different methods have been used to estimate the capillary pressure: (1) *direct cannulation of the capillaries,* which has given an average mean capillary pressure of about 25 mm Hg, and (2) *indirect functional measurement of the capillary pressure,* which has given a capillary pressure averaging about 17 mm Hg. These methods are the following:

Micropipet Method for Measuring Capillary Pressure. To measure pressure in a capillary by cannulation, a microscopic glass pipet is thrust directly into the capillary, and the pressure is measured by an appropriate micromanometer system. Using this method, capillary pressures have been measured in capillaries of exposed tissues of lower animals and in large capillary loops of the eponychium at the base of

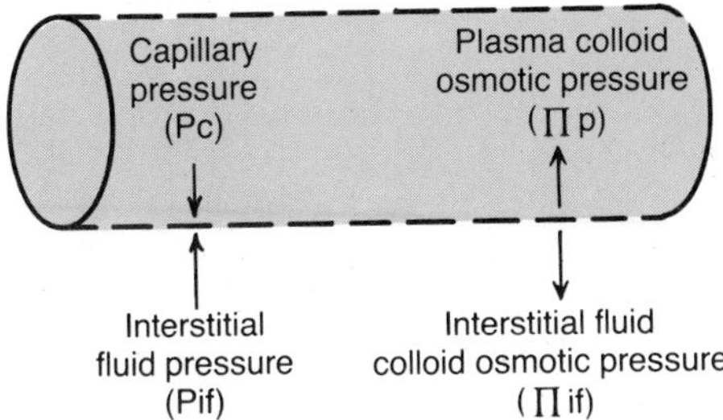

Figure 13–4. Forces operative at the capillary membrane tending to move fluid either outward or inward through the membrane.

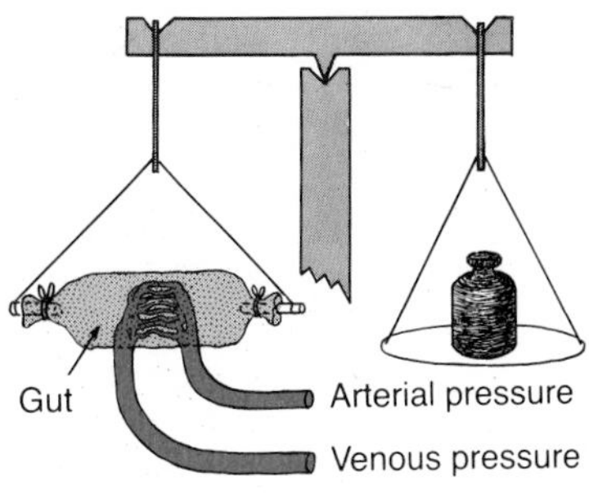

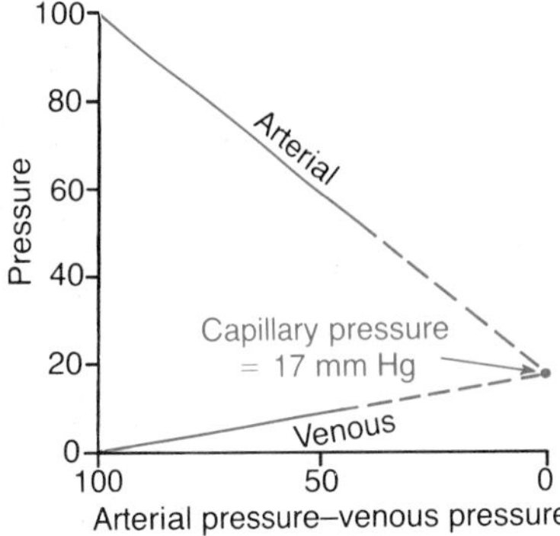

Figure 13–5. Isogravimetric method for measuring capillary pressure (explained in the text).

the fingernail in humans. These measurements have given pressures of 30 to 40 mm Hg in the arterial ends of the capillaries, 10 to 15 mm Hg in the venous ends, and about 25 mm Hg in the middle.

Isogravimetric Method for Indirectly Measuring "Functional" Capillary Pressure. Figure 13–5 illustrates an *isogravimetric* method for estimating capillary pressure. This figure shows a section of gut held by one arm of a gravimetric balance. Blood is perfused through the gut. When the arterial pressure is decreased, the resulting decrease in capillary pressure allows the osmotic pressure of the plasma proteins to cause absorption of fluid out of the gut wall and makes the weight of the gut decrease. This immediately causes displacement of the balance arm. However, to prevent this weight decrease, the venous pressure is raised an amount sufficient to overcome the effect of decreasing the arterial pressure. In other words, the capillary pressure is kept constant while decreasing the arterial pressure but raising the venous pressure.

In the lower part of the figure, the changes in arterial and venous pressures that exactly nullify all weight changes are illustrated. The arterial and venous lines meet each other at a value of 17 mm Hg. Therefore, the capillary pressure must have remained at this same level of 17 mm Hg throughout these maneuvers, or otherwise filtration or absorption of fluid through the capillary walls would have occurred. Thus, in a roundabout way, the "functional" capillary pressure is measured to be about 17 mm Hg.

The Functional Capillary Pressure. It is clear that the aforementioned two methods do not give the same capillary pressure. However, the isogravimetric method determines the capillary pressure that exactly balances all the other forces tending to move fluid into or out of the capillaries. Since such a balance of forces is the normal state, the average functional capillary pressure must be very close to the pressure measured by the isogravimetric method. Therefore, one is justified in believing that the true functional capillary pressure averages about 17 mm Hg.

It is very easy to explain why the cannulation methods give higher pressure values. The most important reason is that these measurements are usually made in capillaries whose arterial ends are open, with blood actively flowing into the capillary. However, it should be recalled from the earlier discussion of capillary vasomotion that the metarterioles and precapillary sphincters are normally closed during a very large part of the vasomotion cycle. When closed, the pressure in the capillaries beyond the closures should be almost equal to the pressure at the venous ends of the capillaries, about 10 mm Hg. Therefore, when averaged over a period of time, one would expect the *functional* mean capillary pressure to be much nearer to the pressure in the venous ends of the capillaries than to the pressure in the arterial ends.

Also, there are two other reasons why the functional capillary pressure is less than the values measured by cannulation. One of these is that there are far more venous capillaries than arterial capillaries. Second, the venous capillaries are several times as permeable as the arterial capillaries. Both of these effects further weight the functional capillary pressure to a lower value.

Interstitial Fluid Pressure

As is true for the measurement of capillary pressure, there have also been several different methods for measuring interstitial fluid pressure, and each of these gives slightly different values but usually slightly *negative,* less than atmospheric pressure. The two methods most widely used have been (1) direct cannulation of the tissues with a micropipet, and (2) measurement of the pressure from implanted perforated capsules.

Measurement of Interstitial Fluid Pressure Using the Micropipet. The same type of micropipet used for measuring capillary pressure can also be used in some tissues for measuring interstitial fluid pressure. The tip of the micropipet is about 1 micron in diameter, but even this is 20 or more times larger than the sizes of the spaces between the proteoglycan filaments of the interstitium. Therefore, the pressure that is measured is probably the pressure in a free fluid pocket.

The most recent pressures measured using the micropipet method have averaged about −1 mm Hg but have ranged between −4 and +1, giving average pressure values in *loose* tissues that are slightly less than atmospheric pressure.

Measurement of Interstitial Free Fluid Pressure in Implanted Perforated Hollow Capsules. Figure 13–6 illustrates an indirect method for measuring interstitial fluid pressure that may be explained as follows: A small hollow plastic capsule perforated by several hundred small holes is implanted in the tissues, and the surgical wound is allowed to heal for approximately 1 month. At the end of that time, tissue will have grown inward through the holes to line the inner surface of the sphere. Furthermore, the cavity is filled with fluid that flows freely through the perforations back and forth between the fluid in the interstitial spaces and the fluid in the cavity. Therefore, the pressure in the cavity should equal the free fluid pressure in the interstitial fluid spaces. A needle is inserted through the skin and through one of the perforations to the interior of the cavity, and the pressure is measured by use of an appropriate manometer.

Interstitial free fluid pressure measured by this method in normal *loose* subcutaneous tissue averages about −6 mm Hg. That is, the pressure is *less than atmospheric pressure*—in other words, is a semivacuum or a suction.

Is the True Interstitial Fluid Pressure in Subcutaneous Tissue Subatmospheric?

The concept that the interstitial fluid pressure is subatmospheric in many tissues of the body began with clinical observations that could not be explained by the previously held concept that interstitial fluid

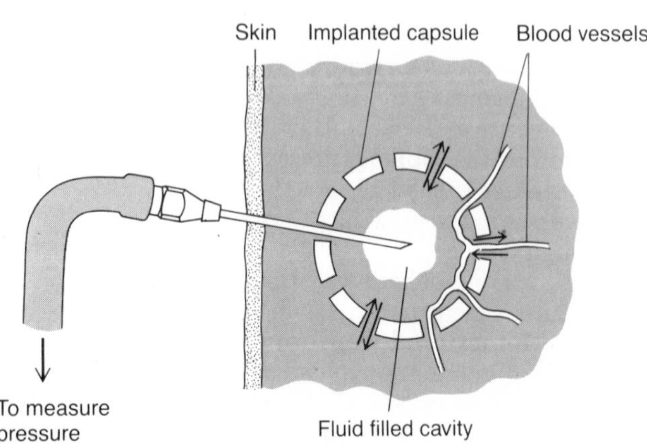

Figure 13–6. The perforated capsule method for measuring interstitial fluid pressure.

pressure was always positive. Two pertinent observations are the following:

1. When a skin graft is placed on a concave surface of the body, such as in an eye socket after removal of the eye, before the skin becomes attached to the sublying socket, fluid tends to collect underneath the graft. Nevertheless, some negative force underneath the skin causes absorption of the fluid and usually will literally pull the skin back into the concavity.
2. In most natural cavities of the body where there is free fluid in dynamic equilibrium with the surrounding interstitial fluids, the pressures that have been measured have been negative. Some of these are the following:

   Intrapleural space: −8 mm Hg.
   Joint synovial spaces: −4 to −6 mm Hg.
   Epidural space: −4 to −6 mm Hg.

Summary—An Average Value for Interstitial Fluid Pressure in Loose Subcutaneous Tissue. Although the aforementioned different methods give slightly different values for interstitial fluid pressure, there is now a general belief among most physiologists that the true interstitial fluid pressure in *loose* subcutaneous tissue is slightly less than atmospheric pressure. A pressure value that many are beginning to accept is an average value of about −3 mm Hg. However, in all tissues with tight fibrous or fascial coverings that hold the tissues together, the pressures underneath these constrictive coverings are usually more positive.

Pumping by the Lymphatic System Is the Basic Cause of the Negative Pressure

The lymphatic system is discussed later in the chapter, but we need to understand here the basic role that this system plays in determining interstitial fluid pressure. The lymphatic system is a "scavenger" system that removes excess fluid, debris, and other matter from the tissue spaces. When the amount of fluid leaking from the blood capillaries is very slight, as is true for most tissues, research evidence suggests that the lymphatic capillaries can actually pump a slight intermittent negative pressure that gives the average negativity observed in the loose tissues. The details of this lymphatic pumping system are discussed later in the chapter.

Plasma Colloid Osmotic Pressure

Colloid Osmotic Pressure Caused by Proteins. The proteins are the only dissolved substances in the plasma and interstitial fluid that do not diffuse readily through the capillary membrane. Furthermore, when small quantities of protein do diffuse into the interstitial fluid, these are soon removed from the interstitial spaces by way of the lymph vessels. Therefore, the concentration of protein in the plasma averages two to three times that in the interstitial fluid, 7.3 gm/dl in the plasma versus 2 to 3 gm/dl in the interstitial fluid.

In the basic discussion of osmotic pressure in Chapter 4, it was pointed out that only those substances that fail to pass through the pores of a semipermeable membrane exert osmotic pressure. Since the proteins are the only dissolved constituents that do not readily penetrate the pores of the capillary membrane, it is the dissolved proteins of the plasma and interstitial fluids that are responsible for the osmotic pressure at the capillary membrane. To distinguish this osmotic pressure from that which occurs at the cell membrane, it is called either *colloid osmotic pressure* or *oncotic pressure.* The term "colloid" osmotic pressure is derived from the fact that a protein solution resembles a colloidal solution despite the fact that it is actually a true solution. (The osmotic pressure that results at the cell membrane is often called *total osmotic pressure* to distinguish it from the colloid osmotic pressure because essentially all dissolved substances of the body fluids exert osmotic pressure at the cell membrane.)

Normal Values for Plasma Colloid Osmotic Pressure. The colloid osmotic pressure of normal human plasma averages approximately 28 mm Hg. Note particularly that this value is only 1/200 the total osmotic pressure that would develop at a *cell* membrane if normal interstitial fluid were on one side of the cell membrane and pure water on the other side. Thus, the colloid osmotic pressure of the plasma is actually a weak osmotic force; but, even so, it plays an exceedingly important role in the maintenance of normal blood and interstitial fluid volumes.

Effect of the Different Plasma Proteins on Colloid Osmotic Pressure. The plasma proteins are a mixture of proteins that contain albumin, with an average molecular weight of 69,000; globulins, 140,000; and fibrinogen, 400,000. Thus, 1 gram of globulin contains only half as many molecules as 1 gram of albumin, and 1 gram of fibrinogen contains only one sixth as many molecules as 1 gram of albumin. (It should be recalled from the discussion of osmotic pressure in Chapter 4 that the osmotic pressure is determined by the *number of molecules* dissolved in a fluid rather than by the weight of these molecules.) The average relative concentrations of the different types of proteins in the plasma and their respective colloid osmotic pressures are:

	gm/dl	*Πp (mm Hg)*
Albumin	4.5	21.8
Globulins	2.5	6.0
Fibrinogen	0.3	0.2
Total	7.3	28.0

Thus, about 75 per cent of the total colloid osmotic pressure of the plasma results from the albumin fraction, 25 per cent from the globulins, and almost none from the fibrinogen. Therefore, from the point of view of capillary dynamics, it is mainly albumin that is important.

Interstitial Fluid Colloid Osmotic Pressure

Although the size of the usual capillary pore is smaller than the molecular sizes of the plasma proteins, this is not true of all the pores. Therefore, small amounts of plasma proteins do leak through the pores into the interstitial spaces.

The total quantity of protein in the entire 12 liters of interstitial fluid of the body is actually greater than the total quantity of protein in the plasma itself, but since this volume is four times the volume of plasma, the average protein *concentration* of the interstitial fluid is usually about 40 per cent of that in plasma, or approximately 3 gm/dl. The average colloid osmotic pressure for this concentration of proteins in the interstitial fluids is approximately 8 mm Hg.

Exchange of Fluid Volume Through the Capillary Membrane

Now that the different factors affecting capillary membrane dynamics have been discussed, it is possible to put all these together to see how normal capillaries function.

The average capillary pressure at the arterial ends of the capillaries is 15 to 25 mm Hg greater than at the venous ends. Because of this difference, fluid "filters" out of the capillaries at their arterial ends and then is reabsorbed into the capillaries at their venous ends. This causes a small amount of fluid actually to "flow" through the tissues from the arterial ends of the capillaries to the venous ends. The dynamics of this flow are the following:

Analysis of the Forces Causing Filtration at the Arterial End of the Capillary. The approximate average forces operative at the arterial end of the capillary that cause movement through the capillary membrane are:

	mm Hg
Forces tending to move fluid outward:	
Capillary pressure	30
Negative interstitial free fluid pressure	3
Interstitial fluid colloid osmotic pressure	8
TOTAL OUTWARD FORCE	41
Forces tending to move fluid inward:	
Plasma colloid osmotic pressure	28
TOTAL INWARD FORCE	28
Summation of forces:	
Outward	41
Inward	28
NET OUTWARD FORCE	13

Thus, the summation of forces at the arterial end of the capillary shows a net *filtration pressure* of 13 mm Hg, tending to move fluid in the outward direction.

This 13 mm Hg filtration pressure causes, on the average, about 0.5 per cent of the plasma to filter out of the arterial end of the capillaries into the interstitial spaces.

Analysis of Reabsorption at the Venous End of the Capillary. The low pressure at the venous end of the capillary changes the balance of forces in favor of absorption as follows:

	mm Hg
Forces tending to move fluid inward:	
Plasma colloid osmotic pressure	28
TOTAL INWARD FORCE	28
Forces tending to move fluid outward:	
Capillary pressure	10
Negative interstitial free fluid pressure	3
Interstitial fluid colloid osmotic pressure	8
TOTAL OUTWARD FORCE	21
Summation of forces:	
Inward	28
Outward	21
NET INWARD FORCE	7

Thus, the force that causes fluid to move into the capillary, 28 mm Hg, is greater than that opposing reabsorption, 21 mm Hg. The difference, 7 mm Hg, is the *reabsorption pressure*. This reabsorption pressure is considerably less than the filtration pressure, but remember that the venous capillaries are more numerous and more permeable than the arterial capillaries, so that less pressure is required to cause the inward movement of fluid.

The reabsorption pressure causes about nine tenths of the fluid that has filtered out of the arterial ends of the capillaries to be reabsorbed at the venous ends. The other one tenth flows into the lymph vessels.

The Starling Equilibrium for Capillary Exchange

E. H. Starling pointed out almost a century ago that under normal conditions a state of near equilibrium exists at the capillary membrane, whereby the amount of fluid filtering outward from some capillaries equals almost exactly that quantity of fluid that is returned to the circulation by absorption through other capillaries. The very slight disequilibrium that does occur accounts for the small amount of fluid that is eventually returned by way of the lymphatics. The following chart shows the normal mean dynamics of the capillary system; however, note this time that we assume the mean *functional* capillary pressure to be 17.3 mm Hg, a slightly higher value than assumed in the earlier analyses, this time to emphasize the very slight disequilibrium:

	mm Hg
Mean forces tending to move fluid outward:	
Mean capillary pressure	17.3
Negative interstitial free fluid pressure	3.0
Interstitial fluid colloid osmotic pressure	8.0
TOTAL OUTWARD FORCE	28.3
Mean force tending to move fluid inward:	
Plasma colloid osmotic pressure	28.0
TOTAL INWARD FORCE	28.0
Summation of mean forces:	
Outward	28.3
Inward	28.0
NET OUTWARD FORCE	0.3

Thus, we find a near-equilibrium but nevertheless a slight imbalance of forces, 0.3 mm Hg, that causes slightly more filtration of fluid into the interstitial spaces than reabsorption. This slight excess of filtration is called the *net filtration,* and it is balanced by fluid return to the circulation through the lymphatics. The normal rate of net filtration in the entire body is only about 2 ml/min.

Effect of Excessive Imbalance of Forces at the Capillary Membrane

If the mean capillary pressure rises above 17 mm Hg, the net force tending to cause filtration of fluid into the tissue spaces obviously rises. Thus, a 20 mm Hg rise in mean capillary pressure causes an increase in the net filtration pressure from 0.3 mm Hg to 20.3 mm Hg, which results in 68 times as much net filtration of fluid into the interstitial spaces as normally occurs, and this would require also 68 times the normal flow of fluid into the lymphatic system, an amount that is usually too much for the lymphatics to carry away. As a result, fluid begins to accumulate in the interstitial spaces, and edema results.

Conversely, if the capillary pressure falls very low, net reabsorption of fluid into the capillaries occurs instead of net filtration, and the blood volume increases at the expense of the interstitial fluid volume. The effects of these imbalances at the capillary membrane are discussed in Chapter 20 in relation to the formation of edema.

THE LYMPHATIC SYSTEM

The lymphatic system represents an accessory route by which fluids can flow from the interstitial spaces into the blood. And, most important of all, the lymphatics can carry proteins and large particulate matter away from the tissue spaces, neither of which can be removed by absorption directly into the blood capillary. This removal of proteins from the interstitial spaces is an absolutely essential function, without which we would die within about 24 hours.

The Lymph Channels of the Body

With the exception of a very few, almost all tissues of the body have lymphatic channels that drain excess fluid directly from the interstitial spaces. Essentially all the lymph from the lower part of the body — even most of that from the legs — flows up the *thoracic duct* and empties into the venous system at the juncture of the *left* internal jugular vein and subclavian vein, as illustrated in Figure 13–7. Lymph from the left side of the head, the left arm, and parts of the chest region also enters the thoracic duct before it empties into the veins. Lymph from the right side of the neck and head, from the right arm, and from parts of the thorax enters the *right lymph duct,* which then empties into the venous system at the juncture of the *right* subclavian vein and internal jugular vein.

The Lymphatic Capillaries and Their Permeability. Most of the fluid filtering from the arterial capillaries flows among the cells and is finally reabsorbed back into the *venous ends* of the *blood capillaries;* but about *one tenth* of the fluid enters the *lymphatic capillaries* instead and returns to the blood through the lymphatic system rather than through the venous capillaries.

The minute quantity of fluid that returns to the circulation by way of the lymphatics is extremely important because substances of high molecular weight, such as proteins, cannot be reabsorbed into the venous capillaries, but they can enter the lymphatic capillaries almost completely unimpeded. The reason for this is a special structure of the lymphatic capillaries, illustrated in Figure 13–8. This figure shows the endothelial cells of the capillary attached by *anchoring filaments* to the surrounding connective tissue. At the junctions of adjacent endothelial cells, the edge of one endothelial cell usually overlaps the edge of the adjacent one in such a way that the overlapping edge is free to flap inward, thus forming a minute valve that opens to the interior of the capillary. Interstitial fluid, along with its suspended particles, can push the valve open and flow directly into the lymphatic capillary. But this fluid has difficulty leaving the capillary once it has entered because any backflow will close the flap valve. Thus, the lymphatics have valves at the very tips of the terminal lymphatic capillaries as well as valves along their larger vessels up to the point where they empty into the blood circulation.

Formation of Lymph

Lymph is derived from interstitial fluid that flows into the lymphatics. Therefore, lymph as it first flows

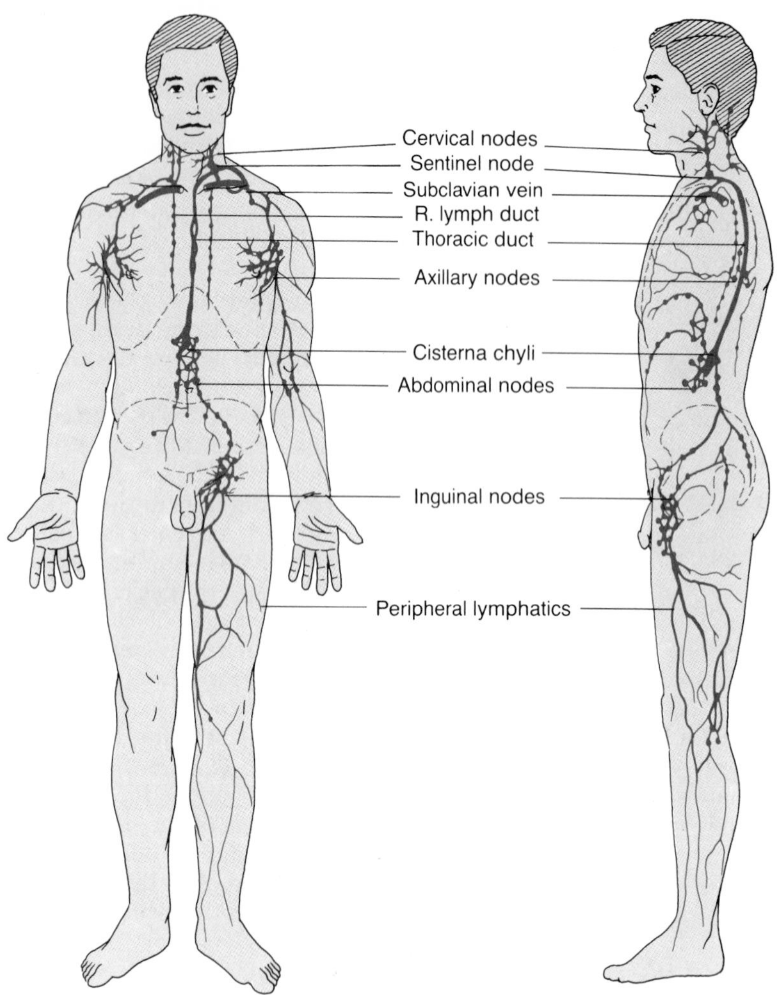

Figure 13-7. The lymphatic system.

from each tissue has almost the same composition as the interstitial fluid.

The protein concentration in the interstitial fluid of most tissues averages about 2 gm/dl, and the protein concentration of lymph flowing from these tissues is near this value. On the other hand, lymph formed in the liver has a protein concentration as high as 6 gm/dl, and lymph formed in the intestines has a protein concentration as high as 3 to 4 gm/dl. Because about two thirds of all lymph is derived from the liver and intestines, the thoracic lymph, which is a mixture of lymph from all areas of the body, usually has a protein concentration of 3 to 5 gm/dl.

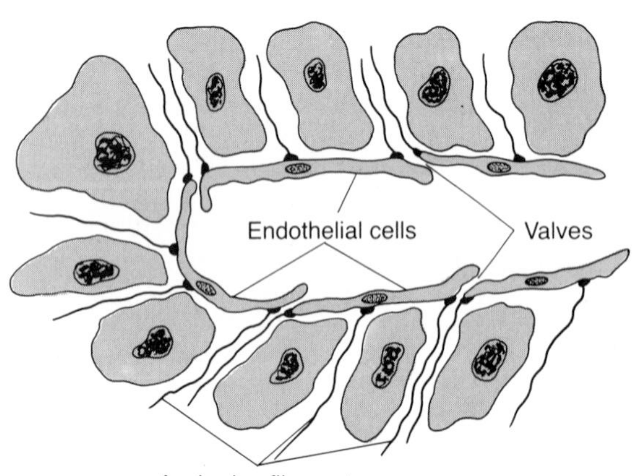

Figure 13-8. Special structure of the lymphatic capillaries that permits passage of substances of high molecular weight back into the circulation.

The lymphatic system is also one of the major routes for absorption of nutrients from the gastrointestinal tract, being responsible principally for the absorption of fats, as is discussed in Chapter 44. Indeed, after a fatty meal, thoracic duct lymph sometimes contains as much as 1 to 2 per cent fat.

Finally, even large particles, such as bacteria, can push their way between the endothelial cells of the lymphatic capillaries and in this way enter the lymph. As the lymph passes through the lymph nodes, these particles are removed and destroyed, as discussed in Chapter 24.

Rate of Lymph Flow

Approximately 100 milliliters of lymph flow through the *thoracic duct* of a resting human per hour, and perhaps another 20 milliliters flow into the circulation each hour through other channels, making a

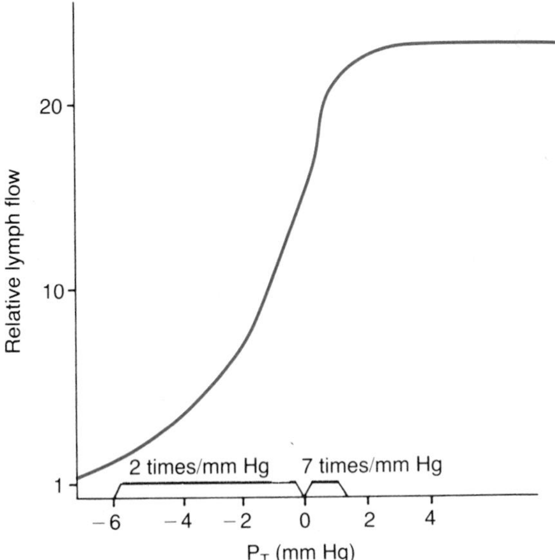

Figure 13-9. Relationship between interstitial fluid pressure and lymph flow. Note that lymph flow reaches a maximum as the interstitial pressure rises slightly above atmospheric pressure (0 mm Hg). (Courtesy of Drs. Harry Gibson and Aubrey Taylor.)

total estimated lymph flow of perhaps 120 ml/hr. This is only one tenth the rate of fluid *filtration* from the arterial ends of the capillaries into the tissue spaces in the entire body.

The rate of lymph flow is determined mainly by two factors: (1) the interstitial fluid pressure and (2) the degree of activity of the lymphatic pump.

Effect of Interstitial Fluid Pressure on Lymph Flow. Figure 13-9 illustrates the effect of different levels of interstitial fluid pressure on lymph flow as measured in dog legs. Note that the lymph flow is very slight at interstitial fluid pressures more negative than −6 mm Hg. Then, as the pressure rises to values slightly greater than 0 mm Hg (atmospheric pressure), the flow increases more than 20-fold. Therefore, any factor that increases interstitial fluid pressure will normally also increase the lymph flow.

However, note that when the interstitial fluid pressure reaches a millimeter or two greater than atmospheric pressure (0 mm Hg), lymph flow fails to rise further at still higher pressures. This probably results from the fact that the increasing tissue pressure not only increases entry of fluid into the lymphatic capillaries, but also compresses the outside surfaces of the larger lymphatics, thus impeding lymph flow. These two factors appear to balance each other almost exactly.

Effect of the Lymphatic Pump. Valves exist in all lymph channels; typical valves are illustrated in Figure 13-10 in *collecting lymphatics* into which the lymphatic capillaries empty. In the large lymphatics, valves exist every few millimeters and in the smaller lymphatics much closer than this.

Motion pictures of exposed lymph vessels, both in animals and humans, show that when a lymph vessel becomes stretched with fluid, the smooth muscle in the wall of the vessel automatically contracts. Furthermore, each segment of the lymph vessel between successive valves functions as a separate automatic pump. That is, filling of a segment causes it to contract, and the fluid is pumped through the valve into the following lymphatic segment. This fills the subsequent segment, and a few seconds later it too contracts, the process continuing all along the lymph vessel until the fluid is finally emptied. In a large lymph vessel, this lymphatic pump can generate pressures as high as 25 to 50 mm Hg if the outflow from the vessel becomes blocked.

Pumping Caused by External Compression of the Lymphatics. In addition to the pumping caused by intrinsic contraction of the lymph vessel walls, any external factor that compresses the lymph vessel can also cause pumping. In order of their importance, such factors are

Contraction of muscles.
Movement of the parts of the body.
Arterial pulsations.
Compression of the tissues by objects outside the body.

Obviously, the lymphatic pump becomes very active during exercise, often increasing lymph flow as much as 10-fold to 30-fold. On the other hand, during periods of rest, lymph flow is very sluggish.

The Lymphatic Capillary Pump. The lymphatic capillary endothelial cells contain contractile

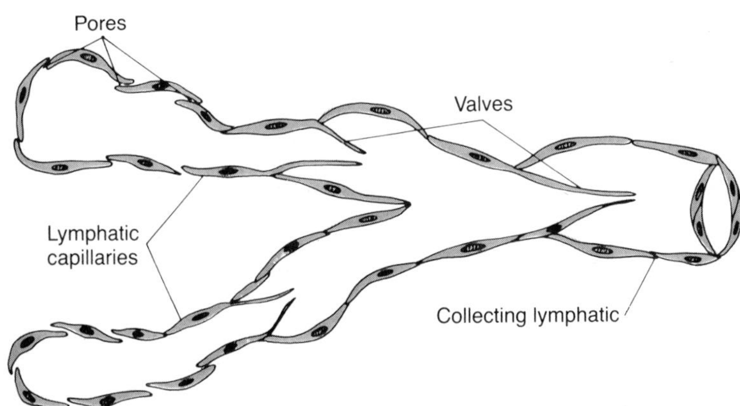

Figure 13-10. Structure of lymphatic capillaries and a collecting lymphatic, showing also the lymphatic values.

actomyosin filaments. In some animals these have been observed to cause rhythmical contraction of the lymphatic capillaries in the same way that many of the small blood vessels contract rhythmically. Therefore, it is possible that at least part of the lymph pumping results from lymph capillary contraction as well as contraction of the larger lymphatics.

Summary of Factors That Determine Lymph Flow. From the previous discussion one can see that the two primary factors that determine lymph flow are the interstitial fluid pressure and the activity of the lymphatic pump. Therefore, one can state that, roughly, *the rate of lymph flow is determined by the product of interstitial fluid pressure and the activity of the lymphatic pump.*

Role of the Lymphatic System in Controlling Interstitial Fluid Protein Concentration, Interstitial Fluid Volume, and Interstitial Fluid Pressure

It is already clear that the lymphatic system functions as an "overflow mechanism" to return to the circulation excess proteins and excess fluid volume from the tissue spaces. Therefore, the lymphatic system also plays a central role in controlling (1) the concentration of proteins in the interstitial fluids, (2) the volume of interstitial fluid, and (3) the interstitial fluid pressure. Let us explain how these different factors interact.

First, remember that small amounts of proteins leak continuously out of the blood capillaries into the interstitium. Only very minute amounts of the leaked proteins return to the circulation by way of the venous ends of the blood capillaries. Therefore, these proteins tend to accumulate in the interstitial fluid, and this in turn increases the colloid osmotic pressure of the interstitial fluids.

Second, the increasing colloid osmotic pressure in the interstitial fluid shifts the balance of forces at the blood capillary membranes in favor of fluid filtration into the interstitium. Therefore, fluid is pulled osmotically by these proteins into the interstitium, thus increasing both the interstitial fluid volume and the interstitial fluid pressure.

Third, the increasing interstitial fluid pressure greatly increases the rate of lymph flow. This in turn carries away the excess volume and excess protein that has accumulated in the spaces.

Thus, once the interstitial fluid protein concentration reaches a certain level and causes a comparable increase in interstitial fluid volume and interstitial fluid pressure, the return of protein and fluid by way of the lymphatic system becomes great enough to balance exactly the rate of leakage of these from the blood capillaries.

REFERENCES

Bassingthwaighte, J. B., and Sparks, H. V., Jr.: Indicator dilution estimation of capillary endothelial transport. Annu. Rev. Physiol., 48:321, 1986.

Brace, R. A., and Guyton, A. C.: Interaction of transcapillary Starling forces in the isolated dog forelimb. Am. J. Physiol., 233:H136, 1977.

Chien, S. (ed.): Vascular Endothelium in Health and Disease. New York, Plenum Publishing Corp., 1988.

Crone, C.: Modulation of solute permeability in microvascular endothelium. Fed. Proc., 45:77, 1986.

Folkman, J., and Klagsbrun, M.: Angiogenic factors. Science, 235:442, 1987.

Guyton, A. C.: Interstitial fluid pressure: II. Pressure-volume curves of interstitial space. Circ. Res., 16:452, 1965.

Guyton, A. C.: Concept of negative interstitial pressure based on pressures in implanted perforated capsules. Circ. Res., 12:399, 1963.

Guyton, A. C., et al.: Circulatory Physiology II. Dynamics and Control of the Body Fluids. Philadelphia, W. B. Saunders Co., 1975.

Guyton, A. C., et al.: Interstitial fluid pressure. Physiol. Rev., 51:527, 1971.

Haraldsson, B.: Physiological studies of macromolecular transport across capillary walls. Acta Physiol. Scand., 128:1, 1986.

Hoppeler, H., and Kayar, S. R.: Capillarity and oxidative capacity of muscles. News Physiol. Sci., 3:113, 1988.

Landis, E. M., and Pappenheimer, J. R.: Exchange of substances through the capillary walls. In Hamilton, W. F. (ed.): Handbook of Physiology. Sec. 2, Vol. 2. Baltimore, Williams & Wilkins, 1963, p. 961.

Marx, J. L.: Angiogenesis research comes of age. Res. News, 237:23, 1987.

Pappenheimer, J. R.: Passage of molecules through capillary walls. Physiol. Rev., 33:387, 1953.

Rippe, B., and Haraldsson, B.: How are macromolecules transported across the capillary wall? News Physiol. Sci., 2:135, 1987.

Taylor, A. E., and Townsley, M. I.: Evaluation of the Starling fluid flux equation. News Physiol. Sci., 2:48, 1987.

QUESTIONS

1. Describe the structure of a representative capillary bed, such as that in the mesentery.
2. Describe the pores in the capillary membrane.
3. Explain how nutrients and other substances pass from the capillaries to the tissues by diffusion.
4. What is the relative permeability of the capillary membrane to plasma proteins in comparison with water and the electrolytes of plasma?
5. Characterize the *interstitium* and the *interstitial fluid.*
6. Name the four *primary forces* that determine fluid movement through the capillary membrane, and explain why each of these causes fluid movement.
7. What is the normal *capillary pressure?* How is it measured?
8. What is the normal *interstitial fluid pressure?* How is it measured?
9. What are some of the reasons for believing that the true interstitial fluid pressure in the soft tissues of the body is subatmospheric?
10. What is the normal plasma colloid osmotic pressure?
11. What is the normal interstitial fluid colloid osmotic pressure?
12. State the quantitative values for the four forces that cause fluid absorption at the arterial ends of the capillaries.
13. State the quantitative values for the four primary forces that cause fluid absorption at the venous ends of the capillaries.

14. State quantitative values for the balance of the mean forces in the entire capillary bed.
15. Describe the anatomy of the lymphatic system. How are the *lymphatic capillaries* different from *blood capillaries*?
16. What is the relationship between *interstitial fluid pressure* and lymph flow?
17. Describe the lymphatic pump. What are the different external effects that can compress the lymph vessels and cause lymphatic pumping?
18. Why is the concentration of proteins higher in the lymph than in the fluid that filters out of the arterial ends of the capillaries?
19. Why does leakage of protein out of the capillaries into the interstitial spaces increase lymph flow?
20. Explain the mechanism and the importance of lymph flow in regulating tissue fluid protein concentration.
21. What causes *negative* interstitial fluid pressure?
22. Why is it important for the interstitial spaces to be normally compacted in a so-called "dry" state?

14

Local Control of Blood Flow by the Tissues and Humoral Regulation

The circulatory system is provided with a complex system for control of blood flow to the different parts of the body. In general, the controls are of three major types:

1. Local control of blood flow in each individual tissue, the flow being controlled mainly in proportion to that tissue's need for blood perfusion.
2. Nervous control of blood flow, which often affects blood flow in large segments of the systemic circulation, such as shifting blood flow from the nonmuscular vascular beds to the muscles during exercise or changing the blood flow in the skin to control body temperature.
3. Humoral control, in which various substances dissolved in the blood such as hormones, ions, or other chemicals can cause either local increase or decrease in tissue flow or widespread generalized changes in flow.

LOCAL CONTROL OF BLOOD FLOW IN RESPONSE TO TISSUE NEED

One of the most fundamental and important characteristics of the circulation is the ability of each tissue to control its own local blood flow in proportion to its need. Furthermore, as the need changes, the flow follows the change.

What are some of the specific needs of the tissues for blood flow? The answer to this is manifold, including especially the following:

1. Delivery of oxygen to the tissues.
2. Delivery of other nutrients, like glucose, amino acids, fatty acids, and so forth.
3. Removal of carbon dioxide from the tissues.
4. Removal of hydrogen ions from the tissues.

Variations in Blood Flow in Different Tissues and Organs. In general, the greater the degree of metabolism in an organ, the greater its blood flow. Note, for instance, in Table 14–1 the very large blood flows in the various glandular organs—for example, several hundred ml/min per 100 grams of thyroid or adrenal gland tissue and a blood flow of 95 ml/min per 100 grams of liver.

Also note the extremely large blood flow through the kidneys, 360 ml/min per 100 grams. This extreme amount of flow is required for the kidneys to perform their function of cleansing the blood of waste products.

On the other hand, most surprising is the low blood flow to the resting muscles of the body, even though they constitute between 30 and 40 per cent of the total body mass. However, in the resting state the metabolic activity of the muscles is very low, and so also is the blood flow, only 4 ml/min per 100 grams. Yet, during very heavy exercise, the metabolic activity can increase as much as 50-fold and the blood flow as much as 20-fold, rising to as high as 80 ml/min per 100 grams.

Mechanisms of Local Blood Flow Control

Local blood flow control can be divided into two different phases: (1) acute control, and (2) long-term control. Acute control means rapid changes in local blood flow control, occurring within seconds to minutes to provide a rapid means for maintaining appropriate local tissue conditions. Long-term control, on

Table 14–1 BLOOD FLOW TO DIFFERENT ORGANS AND TISSUES UNDER BASAL CONDITIONS

	Per cent	Ml/min	Ml/min/ 100 gm
Brain	14	700	50
Heart	4	200	70
Bronchi	2	100	25
Kidneys	22	1100	360
Liver	27	1350	95
Portal	(21)	(1050)	
Arterial	(6)	(300)	
Muscle (inactive state)	15	750	4
Bone	5	250	3
Skin (cool weather)	6	300	3
Thyroid gland	1	50	160
Adrenal glands	0.5	25	300
Other tissues	3.5	175	1.3
TOTAL	100.0	5000	—

Based mainly on data compiled by Dr. L. A. Sapirstein.

the other hand, means slow changes in flow over a period of days, weeks, or even months. In general, the long-term changes come about as a result of an increase or decrease in the sizes and numbers of actual blood vessels supplying the tissues.

Acute Control of Local Blood Flow

Local Blood Flow Regulation When Oxygen Availability Changes. One of the most necessary of the nutrients is oxygen. Whenever the availability of oxygen to the tissues decreases, such as at high altitude, in pneumonia, in carbon monoxide poisoning (which poisons the ability of hemoglobin to transport oxygen), or in cyanide poisoning (which poisons the ability of the tissues to use oxygen), the blood flow through the tissues increases markedly. Figure 14–1 shows that as the arterial oxygen saturation falls to about 25 per cent of normal, the blood flow through an isolated leg increases about threefold; that is, the blood flow increases almost enough, but not quite, to make up for the decreased amount of oxygen in the blood, thus automatically maintaining an almost constant supply of oxygen to the tissues. Cyanide poisoning of local tissue areas can cause a local blood flow increase as much as sevenfold, thus illustrating the extreme effect of oxygen deficiency in increasing blood flow.

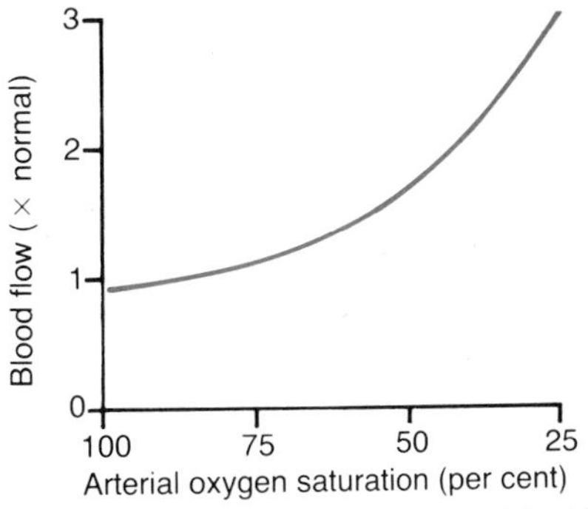

Figure 14–1. Effect of arterial oxygen saturation on blood flow through an isolated dog leg.

There are two basic theories for the regulation of local blood flow when either the rate of tissue metabolism changes or the availability of oxygen changes. These are (1) the *vasodilator theory* and (2) the *oxygen demand theory.*

The Vasodilator Theory for Local Blood Flow Regulation. According to this theory, the greater the rate of metabolism, the less the blood flow, or the less the availability of oxygen and other nutrients to a tissue, the greater becomes the rate of formation of a *vasodilator substance.* The vasodilator substance then is believed to diffuse back to the precapillary sphincters, metarterioles, and arterioles to cause dilatation. Some of the different vasodilator substances that have been suggested are *adenosine, carbon dioxide, lactic acid, adenosine phosphate compounds, histamine, potassium ions,* and *hydrogen ions.*

Most of the vasodilator theories assume that the vasodilator substance is released from the tissue mainly in response to oxygen deficiency. Many physiologists have suggested that the substance *adenosine* is perhaps the most important of the local vasodilators for controlling local blood flow. For instance, minute quantities of adenosine are released from heart muscle cells whenever coronary blood flow becomes too little, and it is believed that this causes local vasodilation in the heart and thereby returns the blood flow back toward normal. Also, whenever the heart becomes overly active and the heart's metabolism increases, this too causes excessive utilization of oxygen, followed by decreased oxygen concentration in the heart muscle with consequent degradation of adenosine triphosphate (ATP) and increased formation of adenosine. Here again it is believed that some of this adenosine leaks out of the cells to cause coronary vasodilation, with increased coronary blood flow to supply the nutrient demands of the active heart.

Unfortunately, it has been difficult to prove that sufficient quantities of any single vasodilator substance are indeed formed in the tissues to cause all of the measured increase in blood flow either in states of increased tissue metabolic demand or in decreased tissue oxygen. On the other hand, perhaps a combination of all the different vasodilators could increase the blood flow sufficiently.

The Oxygen Demand Theory for Local Blood Flow Control. Although the vasodilator theory is accepted by most physiologists, several critical facts have made a few physiologists favor still another theory, which can be called either the oxygen demand theory or, more accurately, the *nutrient demand theory* (because probably other nutrients besides oxygen are involved). Oxygen (and other nutrients as well) is required to maintain vascular muscle contraction. Therefore, in the absence of an adequate supply of oxygen and other nutrients, it is reasonable to believe that the blood vessels would naturally dilate. Also, increased utilization of oxygen in the tissues as a result of increased metabolism would theoretically decrease the local tissue oxygen availability, and this too would cause local vasodilation.

A mechanism by which the oxygen demand theory could operate is illustrated in Figure 14-2. This figure shows what might be called a "tissue unit," consisting of a metarteriole, a single capillary, and its surrounding tissue. At the origin of the capillary is a *precapillary sphincter,* and around the metarteriole are several smooth muscle fibers. Observing under a microscope a thin tissue, such as a bat's wing, one sees that the precapillary sphincters are normally either completely open or completely closed, and the degree of constriction of the metarteriole also varies with time. The number of precapillary sphincters that are open at any given time is approximately proportional to the requirements of the tissue for nutrition.

Now, let us explain how oxygen concentration in the local tissue could regulate blood flow through the area. Since smooth muscle requires oxygen (or other nutrients or both) to remain contracted, one might assume that the strength of contraction of the sphincters would increase with an increase in oxygen concentration. Consequently, when the oxygen concentration in the tissue rises above a certain level, the precapillary and metarteriole sphincters presumably close and remain closed until the tissue cells consume the excess oxygen. When the oxygen concentration falls low enough, the sphincters open once more to begin the cycle again.

Thus, on the basis of presently available data, either a vasodilator theory or an oxygen demand theory could explain local blood flow regulation in response to the metabolic needs of the tissues. Perhaps the truth lies in a combination of the two mechanisms.

"Autoregulation" of Blood Flow When the Arterial Pressure Changes From Normal—"Metabolic" Versus "Myogenic" Mechanisms

In most tissues of the body, an acute increase or decrease in arterial pressure will cause an immediate

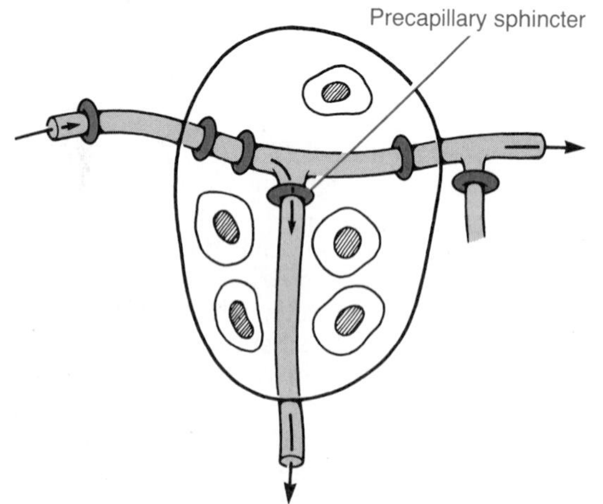

Figure 14-2. Diagram of a tissue unit area for explanation of local feedback control of blood flow.

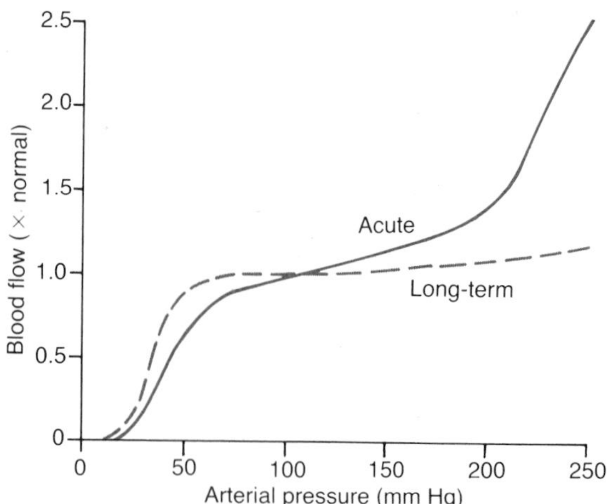

Figure 14-3. Effect of increasing arterial pressure on blood flow through a muscle. The solid curve shows the effect if the arterial pressure is raised over a period of a few minutes. The dashed curve shows the effect if the arterial pressure is raised extremely slowly over a period of many weeks.

increase or decrease in blood flow. However, within less than a minute, the blood flow usually returns most of the way back toward the normal level. Therefore, if a few minutes are allowed for the local blood flow control mechanisms to function properly, the blood flow will be related to arterial pressure approximately in accord with the solid curve labeled "acute" in Figure 14-3. Note that between an arterial pressure of approximately 70 mm Hg and 175 mm Hg the blood flow increases only about 30 per cent. This maintenance of the flow at relatively normal levels despite marked changes in arterial pressure is called *autoregulation of blood flow.* For almost a century, two different views have been proposed to explain the acute autoregulation mechanism. These have been called (1) the metabolic theory and (2) the myogenic theory.

The *metabolic theory* can be understood very easily by simply applying the basic principles of local blood flow regulation already discussed in earlier sections. That is, when the arterial pressure becomes too great, the excess flow provides too many nutrients to the tissues and also flushes vasodilator substances out of the tissues; both these effects will then cause the blood vessels to constrict and the flow to return nearly to normal despite the increased pressure.

The *myogenic theory,* on the other hand, suggests that still another mechanism not at all related to tissue metabolism explains the phenomenon of autoregulation. This theory is based on the observation that sudden stretch of small blood vessels will cause the smooth muscle of the vessel wall to contract. Therefore, it is believed that when high arterial pressure stretches the vessel, this in turn causes vascular constriction and reduces the blood flow nearly back to normal. Conversely, at low pressures, the degree of stretch of the vessel is less, so that the smooth muscle relaxes and allows increased flow.

Certainly, some experiments are difficult to explain without invoking the myogenic theory of autoregulation. Yet it is doubtful that myogenic autoregulation is a very powerful functional mechanism in most of the body, for a very clear reason. A strong myogenic mechanism everywhere in the body could rapidly lead to death in the following way: An increase in pressure would stretch the blood vessels, which would then cause vasoconstriction. The increased constriction would increase the peripheral resistance and raise the blood pressure still more. This secondary increase in pressure would cause another cycle of stretch followed by still more vasoconstriction and then still more increase in pressure. Thus, a vicious circle would ensue, and if this should occur strongly in all the body at once, the arterial pressure would rise suddenly to such a high level that the heart would fail.

It has been suggested especially that the myogenic mechanism protects the capillaries from excessively high blood pressures. That is, if the pressure in the small arteries and arterioles rises too high, these vessels would simply constrict and prevent this high pressure from being transmitted into the capillaries, which are so weak that excessive pressure could rupture them.

A Mechanism for Secondary Dilatation of the Larger Arteries When Microvascular Blood Flow Increases — The Endothelium-Derived Relaxing Factor

The local mechanisms for controlling tissue blood flow can dilate only the very small microvessels located in the immediate tissue itself because local feedback caused by vasodilator substances or oxygen deficiency can affect only these vessels, not the larger arteries back upstream. Yet, when blood flow through the microvascular portion of the circulation increases, this is believed to entrain secondarily another mechanism that dilates the larger vessels as well. This mechanism is the following:

The endothelial cells lining the arterioles and small arteries synthesize several different substances that, when released, can affect the degree of contraction of the arterial wall. The most important of these is a vasodilator substance called *endothelium-derived relaxing factor (EDRF).* Rapid flow of blood through the arteries causes "sheer-stress" on the endothelial cells because of viscous drag of the blood against the vascular walls. This stress contorts the endothelial cells in the direction of flow and causes greatly increased release of EDRF. The EDRF then relaxes the arterial wall, causing it to dilate.

This is a fortunate mechanism because it causes a secondary increase in the dimensions of the larger blood vessels whenever the microvascular blood flow increases. Without such a response, the effectiveness of local blood flow control would be greatly compromised because much of the resistance to blood flow is in the upstream arterioles and small arteries.

Long-Term Vascular Dilatation of Upstream Vessels. When the blood flow through an arteriole, small artery, or even larger artery continues at excessive velocity for days, weeks, or months, the structural dimensions of the vessel enlarge — not merely relaxation of the smooth muscle in the vessel wall. This is caused either by some effect of the EDRF mechanism or perhaps by the prolonged physical overdilation itself of the vessel wall. The sizes of all the different arteries throughout the body appear to be continually adjusted and readjusted throughout the lifetime of the person, so that the velocity of blood flow is never great enough to cause an inordinate amount of blood flow resistance.

Long-Term Blood Flow Regulation

Thus far, most of the mechanisms for local blood flow regulation that we have discussed act within a few seconds to a few minutes after the local tissue conditions have changed. Yet, even after full function of these acute mechanisms, the blood flow usually is adjusted only about three quarters of the way to the exact requirement of the tissues.

However, over a period of hours, days, and weeks a long-term type of local blood flow regulation develops in addition to the acute regulation. This long-term regulation gives far more complete regulation than the acute mechanism. Figure 14–3 illustrates by the dashed curve the extreme effectiveness of this long-term local blood flow regulation. Note that once the long-term regulation has had time to occur, changes in arterial pressure between 50 and 250 mm Hg have very little effect on the rate of local blood flow.

Mechanism of Long-Term Regulation — Change in Tissue Vascularity

The mechanism of long-term local blood flow regulation is a change in the degree of vascularity of the tissues. That is, if the arterial pressure falls to 60 mm Hg and remains at this level for many weeks, the physical structural sizes of the vessels in the tissue increase, and under some conditions even the numbers of vessels increase as well; if the pressure then rises to a very high level, the number and sizes of vessels decrease. Likewise, if the metabolism in a given tissue is increased for a prolonged period of time, vascularity increases; if the metabolism is decreased, vascularity decreases.

Role of Oxygen in Long-Term Regulation. A probable stimulus for increased or decreased vascularity in many instances is need of the tissue for oxygen. One reason for believing this is that increased vascularity occurs in the tissues of many animals that live at high altitudes, where the atmospheric oxygen is low. A second reason is that fetal chicks hatched in low oxygen have up to two times as much vascular conductivity as is normally seen.

Growth of New Vessels—Angiogenesis and Angiogenic Factors

The term "angiogenesis" means growth of new blood vessels. Angiogenesis occurs mainly in response to the presence of angiogenic factors released from (1) ischemic tissues, (2) tissues that are growing rapidly, or (3) tissues that have excessively high metabolic rates.

A dozen or more such angiogenic factors have been found, almost all of which are small peptides. Three of those that have been best characterized are *endothelial cell growth factor (ECGF), fibroblast growth factor (FGF),* and *angiogenin,* each of which has been isolated either from tumors or from other tissues that are growing rapidly or that generally have inadequate blood supply. Presumably it is the deficiency of tissue oxygen, other nutrients, or both that leads to the formation of the angiogenic factors.

Essentially all the angiogenic factors promote new vessel growth in the same manner. They cause new vessels to sprout from either small venules or occasionally capillaries. The first step is dissolution of the basement membrane of the endothelial cells. This is followed by rapid reproduction of new endothelial cells that then stream out of the vessel wall in extended cords directed toward the source of the angiogenic factor. The cells in each cord continue to divide and eventually fold over into a tube. Next, the tube connects up with another tube budding from another donor vessel and forms a capillary loop through which blood begins to flow. If the flow is great enough, smooth muscle cells eventually invade the wall, so that some of the new vessels eventually grow to be small arterioles or perhaps even larger arteries. Thus, this process of angiogenesis explains the manner in which metabolic factors in local tissues can cause the growth of new vessels.

HUMORAL REGULATION OF THE CIRCULATION

Humoral regulation of the circulation means regulation by substances secreted into or absorbed into the body fluids, such as by hormones, ions, or so forth. Some of these substances are formed by special glands and then transported in the blood throughout the entire body. Others are formed in local tissue areas in response to local tissue conditions or are released by excited nerves. They then cause local circulatory effects. Among the most important of the humoral factors that affect circulatory function are the following:

Vasoconstrictor Agents

Norepinephrine and Epinephrine. Norepinephrine is an especially powerful vasoconstrictor hormone; epinephrine is less so and in some instances even causes mild vasodilation. When the sympathetic nervous system is generally stimulated during stress or exercise, the sympathetic nerves directly release norepinephrine, which excites the heart, the veins, and the arterioles. They also cause the adrenal medullae to secrete both norepinephrine and epinephrine. These then circulate in the blood and cause almost the same excitatory effects on the circulation as the direct stimulation, thus providing a dual system of control.

Angiotensin. Angiotensin is one of the most powerful vasoconstrictor substances known. As little as *one millionth* of a gram can increase the arterial pressure of a human as much as 50 or more mm Hg.

The effect of angiotensin is to constrict very powerfully the small arterioles. The real importance of angiotensin is that it normally acts simultaneously on all the arterioles of the body to increase the *total* peripheral resistance, thereby increasing the arterial pressure. Because of this plus several renal and adrenocortical stimulatory effects of angiotensin, this hormone plays an integral role in the regulation of the arterial pressure, as is discussed in detail in the following two chapters.

Vasopressin. Vasopressin, also called *antidiuretic hormone,* is formed in the hypothalamus (see Chapter 49) but is transported down the center of nerve axons to the posterior pituitary gland, where it is eventually secreted into the blood. Vasopressin is even more powerful than angiotensin as a vasoconstrictor, thus making it perhaps the body's most potent constrictor substance. Normally, only very minute amounts of vasopressin are secreted. However, following severe hemorrhage the concentration of vasopressin can rise enough to increase the arterial pressure as much as 60 mm Hg; in many instances this can by itself bring the arterial pressure almost back up to normal.

Also, vasopressin has an *all-important* function in controlling water reabsorption in the renal tubules, which is discussed in Chapter 22, and therefore to help control body fluid volume. That is why this hormone is also called antidiuretic hormone.

Vasodilator Agents

Bradykinin. Several substances called *kinins* that can cause powerful vasodilation are frequently formed in the blood and tissue fluids. One of these substances is *bradykinin.*

The kinins are small polypeptides that are split away by proteolytic enzymes from alpha$_2$-globulins in the plasma or tissue fluids. An enzyme of particular importance is *kallikrein,* which is present in the blood and tissue fluids in an inactive form. Kallikrein is activated by maceration of the blood, tissue inflammation, and other similar chemical and physical effects on the blood. As kallikrein becomes activated, it acts immediately on the alpha$_2$-globulin to release a kinin called *kallidin* that is then converted by tissue enzymes into *bradykinin.* Once formed, the bradykinin persists for only a few minutes because it is digested by the enzyme *carboxypeptidase* or by *converting enzyme,* an enzyme that also plays an essential role in activating angiotensin, as discussed in Chapter 16.

Bradykinin causes very powerful *arteriolar dilatation* and also *increased capillary permeability.* For instance, injection of 1 *microgram* of bradykinin into the brachial artery of a person increases the blood flow through the arm as much as sixfold, and even smaller amounts injected locally into tissues can cause marked edema because of the increase in capillary pore size.

There is reason to believe that kinins play special roles in regulating blood flow and capillary leakage of fluids in inflamed tissues. It is also believed that bradykinin plays a role in regulating blood flow in the skin and also in the salivary and gastrointestinal glands.

Histamine. Histamine is released in essentially every tissue of the body when it becomes damaged, inflamed, or is the subject of an allergic reaction. Most of the histamine is derived from mast cells in the damaged tissues and from basophils in the blood.

Histamine has a powerful vasodilator effect on the arterioles and, like bradykinin, also has the ability to greatly increase capillary porosity, allowing leakage of both fluid and plasma protein into the tissues. In many pathological conditions, the intense arteriolar dilatation and increased capillary porosity caused by histamine cause tremendous quantities of fluid to leak out of the circulation into the tissues, inducing edema. The local vasodilatory and edema-producing effects of histamine are especially prominent in allergic reactions and are discussed in Chapter 25.

Prostaglandins. Almost every tissue of the body contains small to moderate amounts of several chemically related substances called prostaglandins. These substances probably have especially important intracellular effects, but some of them are also released into the local tissue fluids and into the circulating blood under both physiological and pathological conditions. Although some of the prostaglandins cause vasoconstriction, most of the more important ones seem to be mainly vasodilator agents. Thus far, no specific pattern of function of the prostaglandins in circulatory control has been found. However, their widespread prevalence and their myriad effects on the circulation make them ideal candidates for special roles in circulatory control, especially for control in local vascular areas. For this reason, these substances are presently under intensive research investigation.

Effects of Different Ions and Other Chemical Factors on Vascular Control

Many different ions and other chemical factors can either dilate or constrict local blood vessels. Most of them have little function in the overall *regulation* of the circulation, but their specific effects can be listed as follows:

An increase in *calcium ion* concentration causes vasoconstriction. This results from the general effect of calcium to stimulate smooth muscle contraction, as discussed in Chapter 7.

An increase in *potassium ion* concentration causes vasodilation. This results from the ability of potassium ions to inhibit smooth muscle contraction.

An increase in *magnesium ion* concentration causes powerful vasodilation, for magnesium ions inhibit smooth muscle generally.

Increased *sodium ion* concentration causes mild arteriolar dilatation. This results mainly from an increase in osmolality of the fluids rather than from a specific effect of sodium ion itself. *Increased osmolality* of the blood caused by increased quantities of *glucose* or other nonvasoactive substances also causes arteriolar dilatation. Decreased osmolality causes arteriolar constriction.

The only anions to have significant effects on blood vessels are *acetate* and *citrate,* both of which cause mild degrees of vasodilation.

An *increase in hydrogen ion* concentration (decrease in pH) causes dilatation of the arterioles. A slight *decrease in hydrogen ion* concentration causes arteriolar constriction, but an intense decrease causes dilatation, which is the same effect as that which occurs with increased hydrogen ion concentration.

An increase in carbon dioxide concentration causes moderate vasodilation in most tissues and marked vasodilation in the brain. However, carbon dioxide, acting on the vasomotor center, has an extremely powerful indirect vasoconstrictor effect that is transmitted through the sympathetic vasoconstrictor system.

REFERENCES

Banchero, N.: Cardiovascular responses to chronic hypoxia. Annu. Rev. Physiol., 49:465, 1987.

Chien, S. (ed.): Vascular Endothelium in Health and Disease. New York, Plenum Publishing Corp., 1988.

Cowley, A. W., Jr., et al: Vasopressin: Cellular and Integrative Functions. New York, Raven Press, 1988.

Davies, P. F.: How do vascular endothelial cells respond to flow? News Physiol. Sci., 4:22, 1989.

Folkman, J.: Angiogenesis: What makes blood vessels grow? News Physiol. Sci., 1:199, 1986.

Fridovich, I., et al.: Endothelium-derived relaxing factor: In search of the endogenous nitroglycerin. News Physiol. Sci., 2:61, 1987.

Furchgott, R. F., and Vanhoutte, P. M.: Endothelium-derived relaxing and contracting factors. FASEB J., 3:1007, 1989.

Guyton, A. C., et al.: Cardiac Output and Its Regulation. Philadelphia, W. B. Saunders Co., 1973.

Guyton, A. C., et al.: Circulation: Overall regulation. Annu. Rev. Physiol., 34:13, 1972.

Harris, P. D.: Movement of oxygen in skeletal muscle. News Physiol. Sci., 1:147, 1986.

Schmid-Schonbein, G. W.: Granulocyte: Friend and foe. News Physiol. Sci., 3:144, 1988.

Seidel, C. L., and Schildmeyer, L. A.: Vascular smooth muscle adaptation to increased load. Annu. Rev. Physiol., 49:489, 1987.

Steranka, L. R., et al.: Antagonists of B_2 bradykinin receptors. FASEB J., 3:2019, 1989.

Vallee, B. L., et al.: Tumor derived angiogenesis factors from rat Walker 256 carcinoma: An experimental investigation and review. Experientia, 41:1, 1985.

Vanhoutte, P. M.: Vasodilation: Vascular Smooth Muscle, Peptides, Autonomic Nerves, and Endothelium. New York, Raven Press, 1988.

Vanhoutte, P. M.: Endothelium and the control of vascular tissue. News Physiol. Sci., 2:18, 1987.

QUESTIONS

1. What are some of the special "needs" of the tissues that play a significant role in controlling local tissue blood flow?
2. Describe the typical structure of a microcirculatory bed.
3. What is the specific anatomy of the small arteries and arterioles, and what are their nervous connections that allow these to be especially important in controlling blood flow?
4. What are the specific characteristics of the *metarterioles* and *precapillary sphincters* that allow them to control local blood flow in response to local humoral factors?
5. What is the special importance of oxygen in the control of local blood flow? Explain both the *vasodilator theory* and the *oxygen demand theory* for control of local blood flow.
6. Explain the mechanisms of *reactive hyperemia* and *active hyperemia.*
7. Explain what is meant by *autoregulation.*
8. Explain the difference between long-term blood flow regulation and short-term regulation. What is the function of angiogenesis factor in long-term blood flow regulation?
9. What are the roles of *epinephrine, norepinephrine, angiotensin, vasopressin, bradykinin, serotonin, histamine,* and the *prostaglandins* in the control of blood flow?
10. How do each of the following ions and other chemical factors affect vascular control: *calcium ion, potassium ion, magnesium ion, sodium ion, osmolality of the blood, hydrogen ion, carbon dioxide concentration?*

15

Nervous Regulation of the Circulation, and Rapid Control of Arterial Pressure

NERVOUS REGULATION OF THE CIRCULATION

In addition to the all-important regulation of blood flow by each local tissue, as discussed in the previous chapter, the nervous system provides additional powerful control of the circulation but usually quite a different kind of control. Nervous control normally has little to do with adjustment of blood flow tissue by tissue — this is the function of the local tissue blood flow control. Instead, nervous control mainly affects more global functions, such as redistributing the blood flow to different areas of the body, increasing the pumping activity of the heart, and especially providing very rapid control of arterial pressure.

The means by which the nervous system controls the circulation is almost entirely through the autonomic nervous system. The total function of this system is presented in Chapter 41. Yet, its specific anatomical and functional characteristics relating to circulatory control require special attention here as well.

The Autonomic Nervous System

By far the most important part of the autonomic nervous system for regulation of the circulation is the *sympathetic nervous system.* However, the *parasympathetic nervous system* is also important for its regulation of heart function, as we see later in the chapter.

The Sympathetic Nervous System. Figure 15-1 illustrates the anatomy of sympathetic nervous control of the circulation. Sympathetic vasomotor nerve fibers leave the spinal cord through all the thoracic and the first one to two lumbar spinal nerves. These pass into the sympathetic chain and thence by two routes to the circulation: (1) through specific *sympathetic nerves* that innervate mainly the vasculature of the internal viscera and the heart and (2) through the *spinal nerves* that innervate mainly the vasculature of the peripheral areas. The precise pathways of these fibers in the spinal cord and in the sympathetic chains are discussed in Chapter 41.

Sympathetic Innervation of the Blood Vessels. All the vessels except the capillaries, precapillary sphincters, and most of the metarterioles are innervated by the sympathetic nerves.

The innervation of the *small arteries* and *arterioles* allows sympathetic stimulation to increase the *resistance* and thereby to change the rate of blood flow through the tissues.

The innervation of large vessels, particularly of the *veins,* makes it possible for sympathetic stimulation to change the volume of these vessels and thereby to alter the volume of the peripheral circulatory system. This can translocate blood into the heart and thereby play a major role in the regulation of cardiovascular function, as we see later in this and subsequent chapters.

Sympathetic Nerve Fibers to the Heart. In addition to sympathetic nerve fibers supplying the blood vessels, other sympathetic fibers go to the heart, as was discussed in Chapter 8. It should be recalled that sympathetic stimulation markedly increases the activity of the heart, increasing the heart rate and enhancing its strength of pumping.

Parasympathetic Control of Heart Function, Especially Heart Rate. Although the parasympathetic nervous system is exceedingly important for many other autonomic functions of the body, it plays

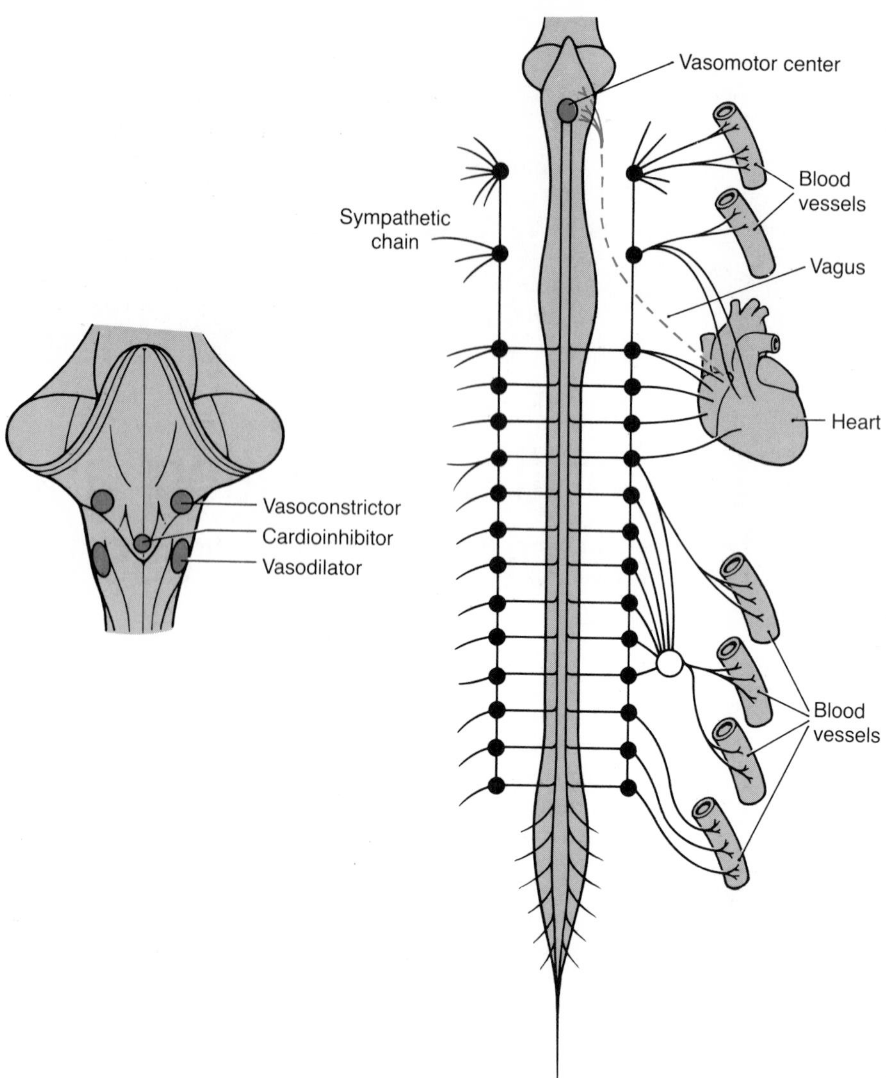

Figure 15-1. Anatomy of sympathetic nervous control of the circulation.

only a minor role in regulation of the circulation. Its only really important circulatory effect is its control of heart rate by way of parasympathetic fibers carried to the heart in the *vagus nerves,* shown in Figure 15-1 by the dashed nerve from the medulla directly to the heart.

The effects of parasympathetic stimulation on heart function are discussed in detail in Chapter 8. Principally, parasympathetic stimulation causes a marked *decrease* in heart rate and a slight decrease in contractility.

The Sympathetic Vasoconstrictor System and Its Control by the Central Nervous System

The sympathetic nerves carry tremendous numbers of *vasoconstrictor fibers* and only a very few vasodilator fibers. The vasoconstrictor fibers are distributed to essentially all segments of the circulation. However, this distribution is greater in some tissues than in others. It is especially powerful in the kidneys, the gut, the spleen, and the skin but less potent in skeletal muscle and in the brain.

The Vasomotor Center and Its Control of the Vasoconstrictor System. Located bilaterally in the reticular substance of the medulla and lower third of the pons, illustrated in Figure 15-2, is an area called the *vasomotor center.* The center transmits impulses downward through the cord and thence through the sympathetic vasoconstrictor fibers to all or almost all the blood vessels of the body.

Although the total organization of the vasomotor center is still unclear, experiments have made it possible to identify certain important areas in the center, as follows:

1. A *vasoconstrictor area,* called area "C-1," located bilaterally in the anterolateral portions of the upper medulla. The neurons in this area secrete *norepinephrine;* their fibers are distributed throughout the cord, where they excite the vasoconstrictor neurons of the sympathetic nervous system.
2. A *vasodilator area,* called area "A-1," located bilaterally in the anterolateral portions of the lower half of the medulla. The fibers from these

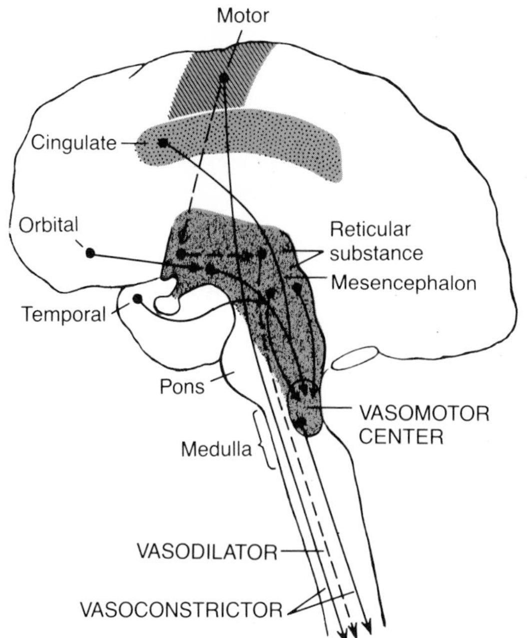

Figure 15-2. Areas of the brain that play important roles in the nervous regulation of the circulation. The dashed lines represent inhibitory pathways.

neurons project upward to the vasoconstrictor area (C-1) and inhibit the vasoconstrictor activity of that area, thus causing vasodilation.

3. A *sensory area,* area "A-2," located bilaterally in the *tractus solitarius* in the posterolateral portions of the medulla and lower pons. The neurons of this area receive sensory nerve signals mainly from the vagus and glossopharyngeal nerves, and the output signals from this sensory area then help to control the activities of both the vasoconstrictor and vasodilator areas, thus providing "reflex" control of many circulatory functions. An example is the baroreceptor reflex for controlling arterial pressure, which we describe later in the chapter.

Continuous Partial Constriction of the Blood Vessels Caused by Sympathetic Vasoconstrictor Tone. Under normal conditions, the vasoconstrictor area of the vasomotor center transmits signals continuously to the sympathetic vasoconstrictor nerve fibers, causing continuous slow firing of these fibers at a rate of about one half to two impulses per second. This continual firing is called *sympathetic vasoconstrictor tone.* These impulses maintain a partial state of contraction in the blood vessels, a state called *vasomotor tone.*

Figure 15-3 demonstrates the significance of vasoconstrictor tone. In the experiment of this figure, total spinal anesthesia was administered to an animal, which completely blocked all transmission of nerve impulses from the central nervous system to the periphery. As a result, the arterial pressure fell from 100 to 50 mm Hg, illustrating the effect of loss of vasoconstrictor tone throughout the body. A few minutes later a small amount of the hormone norepinephrine was injected intravenously—norepinephrine is the substance secreted at the endings of sympathetic vasoconstrictor nerve fibers throughout the body. As this hormone was transported in the blood to all the blood vessels, the vessels once again became constricted, and the arterial pressure rose to a level even greater than normal for a minute or two until the norepinephrine was destroyed.

Control of Heart Activity by the Vasomotor Center. At the same time that the vasomotor center is controlling the degree of vascular constriction, it also controls heart activity. The lateral portions of the vasomotor center transmit excitatory impulses through the sympathetic nerve fibers to the heart to increase heart rate and contractility, whereas the medial portion of the vasomotor center, which lies in immediate apposition to the *dorsal motor nucleus of*

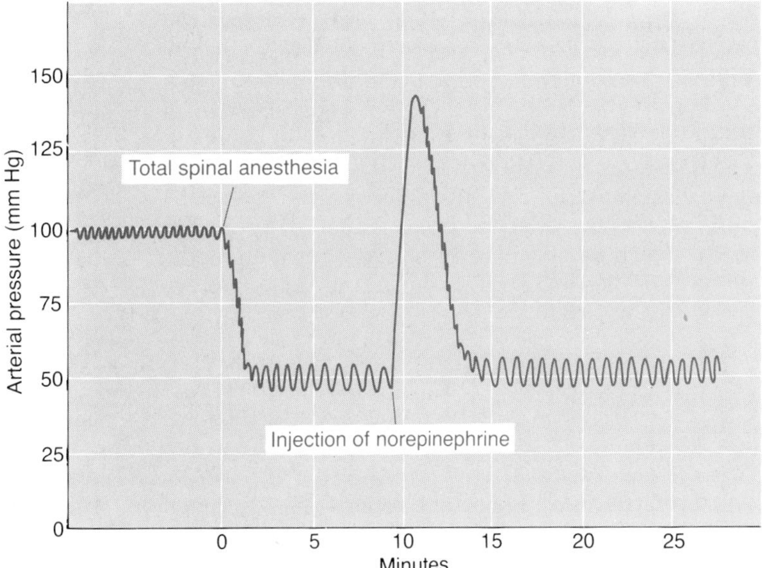

Figure 15-3. Effect of total spinal anesthesia on the arterial pressure, showing a marked fall in pressure resulting from loss of vasomotor tone.

the vagus nerve, transmits impulses through the vagus nerve to the heart to decrease heart rate. Therefore, the vasomotor center can either increase or decrease heart activity, this ordinarily increasing at the same time that vasoconstriction occurs throughout the body and ordinarily decreasing at the same time that vasoconstriction is inhibited.

Control of the Vasomotor Center by Higher Nervous Centers. Large numbers of areas throughout the *reticular substance* of the *pons, mesencephalon,* and *diencephalon* can either excite or inhibit the vasomotor center. This reticular substance is illustrated in Figure 15–2 by the diffuse shaded area. In general, the more lateral and superior portions of the reticular substance cause excitation, whereas the more medial and inferior portions cause inhibition.

The *hypothalamus* plays a special role in the control of the vasoconstrictor system, for it can exert powerful excitatory or inhibitory effects on the vasomotor center. The *posterolateral portions* of the hypothalamus cause mainly excitation, whereas the *anterior part* can cause mild excitation or inhibition, depending on the precise part of the anterior hypothalamus stimulated.

Many different parts of the *cerebral cortex* can also excite or inhibit the vasomotor center. Stimulation of the *motor cortex,* for instance, excites the vasomotor center because of impulses transmitted downward into the hypothalamus and thence to the vasomotor center.

Thus, widespread areas of the brain can have profound effects on cardiovascular function.

Norepinephrine—The Sympathetic Vasoconstrictor Transmitter Substance. The substance secreted at the endings of the vasoconstrictor nerves is norepinephrine. Norepinephrine acts directly on the so-called alpha receptors of the vascular smooth muscle to cause vasoconstriction, as is discussed in Chapter 41.

The Adrenal Medullae and Their Relationship to the Sympathetic Vasoconstrictor System. Sympathetic impulses are usually transmitted to the adrenal medullae at the same time that they are transmitted to the blood vessels. These cause the medullae to secrete both epinephrine and norepinephrine into the circulating blood. These two hormones are carried in the blood stream to all parts of the body, where they act directly on the blood vessels usually to cause vasoconstriction, but sometimes the epinephrine causes vasodilation because it has a potent "beta"-receptor stimulatory effect, which often dilates vessels, as is discussed in Chapter 41.

ROLE OF THE NERVOUS SYSTEM FOR RAPID CONTROL OF ARTERIAL PRESSURE

One of the most important functions of nervous control of the circulation is its capability to cause very rapid increases in arterial pressure. For this purpose, the entire vasoconstrictor and cardioaccelerator functions of the sympathetic nervous system are stimulated as a unit. At the same time there is reciprocal inhibition of the normal parasympathetic vagal inhibitory signals to the heart. In consequence, three major changes occur simultaneously, each of which helps increase the arterial pressure. These are as follows:

1. *Almost all arterioles of the body are constricted.* This greatly increases the total peripheral resistance, impeding the run-off of blood from the arteries and thereby increasing the arterial pressure.
2. *The veins especially but the other large vessels of the circulation as well are strongly constricted.* This displaces blood out of the circulation toward the heart, thus increasing the volume of blood in the heart chambers. This then causes the heart to beat with far greater force and therefore to pump increased quantities of blood. This, too, increases the arterial pressure.
3. Finally, *the heart itself is directly stimulated by the autonomic nervous system, further enhancing cardiac pumping.* Much of this is caused by an increase in the heart rate sometimes to as great as three times normal. In addition, sympathetic nervous signals have a direct effect to increase the contractile force of the heart muscle, this too increasing the capability of the heart to pump larger volumes of blood.

Rapidity of Nervous Control of Arterial Pressure. An especially important characteristic of nervous control of arterial pressure is its rapidity of response, beginning within seconds and often increasing the pressure to two times normal within 5 to 15 seconds. Conversely, sudden inhibition of nervous stimulation can decrease the arterial pressure to as little as one half normal within 10 to 40 seconds.

Increase in Arterial Pressure During Muscle Exercise and Other Types of Stress

An important example of the ability of the nervous system to increase the arterial pressure is the increased pressure during muscle exercise. During heavy exercise, the muscles require greatly increased blood flow. Part of this increase results from local vasodilation of the muscle vasculature caused by increased metabolism of the muscle cells, as explained in the previous chapter. However, still additional increase results from simultaneous elevation of arterial pressure during the exercise. In most heavy exercise, the arterial pressure rises about 30 to 40 per cent, which will increase blood flow by approximately an additional twofold.

The increase in arterial pressure during exercise results mainly from the following effect: At the same time that the motor areas of the nervous system become activated to cause exercise, most of the reticular activating system of the brain stem is also activated, which includes greatly increased stimulation of the vasoconstrictor and cardioacceleratory areas of the vasomotor center. These raise the arterial pressure instantaneously to keep pace with the increase in muscle activity.

In many other types of stress besides muscle exercise, a similar rise in pressure can also take place. For instance, during extreme fright, the arterial pressure often rises to as high as double normal within a few seconds. This is called the *alarm reaction,* and it obviously provides a head of pressure that can immediately supply blood to any or all muscles of the body that might wish to respond instantly to cause flight from danger.

The Reflex Mechanisms for Maintaining Normal Arterial Pressure

Aside from the exercise and stress functions of the autonomic nervous system to raise the arterial pressure, there are also multiple subconscious nervous mechanisms for maintaining the arterial pressure at or near its normal operating level. Almost all of these are *negative feedback reflex mechanisms,* which we explain in the following sections.

The Arterial Baroreceptor Control System — Baroreceptor Reflexes

By far the best known of the mechanisms for arterial pressure control is the *baroreceptor reflex.* Basically, this reflex is initiated by stretch receptors, called either *baroreceptors* or *pressoreceptors,* which are located in the walls of the large systemic arteries. A rise in pressure stretches the baroreceptors and causes them to transmit signals into the central nervous system, and "feedback" signals are then sent back through the autonomic nervous system to the circulation to reduce arterial pressure downward toward the normal level.

Physiologic Anatomy of the Baroreceptors, and Their Innervation. Baroreceptors are spray-type nerve endings lying in the walls of certain arteries; they are stimulated when stretched. As illustrated in Figure 15-4, baroreceptors are extremely abundant in (1) the wall of each internal carotid artery slightly above the carotid bifurcation, an area known as the *carotid sinus,* and (2) the wall of the aortic arch.

Figure 15-4 also shows that signals are transmitted from each carotid sinus through the very small *Hering's nerve* to the glossopharyngeal nerve and thence to the *tractus solitarius* in the medullary area of the brain stem. Signals from the arch of the aorta are transmitted through the vagus nerves also into this area of the medulla.

Response of the Baroreceptors to Pressure. Normally, the carotid sinus baroreceptors are not stimulated at all by pressures between 0 and 60 mm Hg, but above 60 mm Hg they respond progressively more and more rapidly and reach a maximum at about 180 mm Hg. The responses of the aortic baroreceptors are similar to those of the carotid receptors except that they operate, in general, at pressure levels about 30 mm Hg higher.

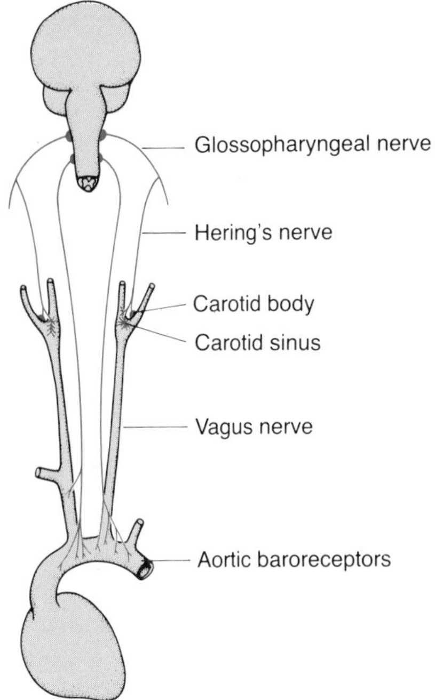

Figure 15-4. The baroreceptor system.

The baroreceptors respond extremely rapidly to changes in arterial pressure; in fact, the rate of impulse firing even increases during systole and decreases again during diastole.

The Reflex Initiated by the Baroreceptors. After the baroreceptor signals have entered the tractus solitarius of the medulla, secondary signals *inhibit the vasoconstrictor center* of the medulla and *excite the vagal center.* The net effects are (1) *vasodilation* of the veins and the arterioles throughout the peripheral circulatory system and (2) *decreased heart rate* and *strength of heart contraction.* Therefore, excitation of the baroreceptors by increased pressure in the arteries reflexly *causes the arterial pressure to decrease* because of both a decrease in peripheral resistance and a decrease in cardiac output. Conversely, low pressure has opposite effects, reflexly causing the pressure to rise back toward normal.

Figure 15-5 illustrates a typical reflex change in arterial pressure caused by occluding the common carotid arteries. This reduces the carotid sinus pressure; as a result, the baroreceptors become inactive and lose their inhibitory effect on the vasomotor center. The vasomotor center then becomes much more active than usual, causing the arterial pressure to rise and to remain elevated during the 10 minutes that the carotids are occluded. Removal of the occlusion allows the pressure to fall immediately to slightly below normal as a momentary overcompensation and then to return to normal in another minute or so.

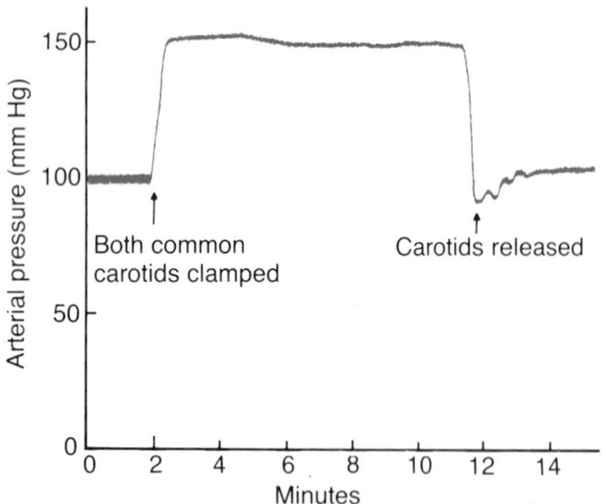

Figure 15-5. Typical carotid sinus reflex effect on arterial pressure, caused by clamping both common carotids (after the two vagus nerves have been cut).

Function of the Baroreceptors During Changes in Body Posture. The ability of the baroreceptors to maintain relatively constant arterial pressure is extremely important when a person sits or stands after having been lying down. Immediately upon standing, the arterial pressure in the head and upper part of the body obviously tends to fall, and marked reduction of this pressure can cause loss of consciousness. Fortunately, however, the falling pressure at the baroreceptors elicits an immediate reflex, resulting in strong sympathetic discharge throughout the body, and this minimizes the decrease in pressure in the head and upper body.

The "Buffer" Function of the Baroreceptor Control System. Because the baroreceptor system opposes either increases or decreases in arterial pressure, it is often called a *pressure buffer system,* and the nerves from the baroreceptors are called *buffer nerves.*

Figure 15-6 illustrates the importance of this buffer function of the baroreceptors. The upper record in this figure shows an arterial pressure recording for 2 hours from a normal dog and the lower record from a dog whose baroreceptor nerves from both the carotid sinuses and the aorta had previously been removed. Note the extreme variability of pressure in the denervated dog caused by simple events of the day, such as lying down, standing, excitement, eating, defecation, noises, and so forth.

In summary, a primary purpose of the arterial baroreceptor system is to reduce the daily variation in arterial pressure to about one half to one third that which would occur were the baroreceptor system not present.

Unimportance of the Baroreceptor System for Long-Term Regulation of Arterial Pressure—"Resetting" of the Baroreceptors. The baroreceptor control system is probably of little or no importance in long-term regulation of arterial pressure for a very simple reason: The baroreceptors themselves reset in 1 to 2 days to whatever pressure level they are exposed. That is, if the pressure rises from the normal value of 100 mm Hg to 200 mm Hg, extreme numbers of baroreceptor impulses are at first transmitted. During the next few seconds, the rate of firing diminishes considerably; then it diminishes much more slowly during the next 1 to 2 days, at the end of which time the rate will have returned essentially to the normal level despite the fact that the arterial pressure now remains 200 mm Hg. Conversely, when the arterial pressure falls to a very low level, the baroreceptors at first transmit no impulses at all, but gradually over a day or two the rate of baroreceptor firing returns again to the original control level.

This "resetting" of the baroreceptors obviously prevents the baroreceptor reflex from functioning as a control system for arterial pressure changes that last longer than a few days at a time. In fact, animal experiments have shown that the average arterial pressure over any prolonged period of time is almost exactly the same whether the baroreceptors are present or not. This illustrates the *unimportance of the baroreceptor system for long-term regulation of the arterial pressure* even though it is a potent and almost necessary mechanism for preventing the rapid changes of arterial pressure that occur moment by moment or hour by hour. Prolonged regulation of arterial pressure requires other control systems, principally the renal-body fluid-pressure control system (along with its associated hormonal mechanisms), discussed in the following chapter.

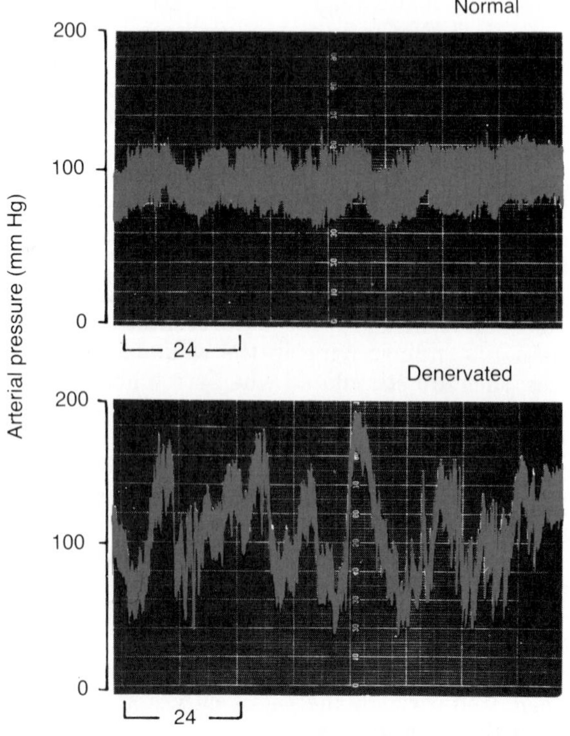

Figure 15-6. Two-hour records of arterial pressure in a normal dog (above) and in the same dog (below) several weeks after the baroreceptors had been denervated. (From Cowley, Liard, and Guyton: *Circ. Res.,* *32*:564, 1973. By permission of the American Heart Association, Inc.)

Control of Arterial Pressure by the Carotid and Aortic Chemoreceptors—Effect of Oxygen Lack on Arterial Pressure

Closely associated with the baroreceptor pressure control system is a chemoreceptor reflex that operates in much the same way as the baroreceptor reflex except that instead of stretch receptors initiating the response, *chemoreceptors* do this.

The chemoreceptors are chemosensitive cells sensitive to oxygen lack, carbon dioxide excess, or hydrogen ion excess. They are located in several small organs 1 to 2 millimeters in size: two *carotid bodies,* one of which lies in the bifurcation of each common carotid artery, and several *aortic bodies* adjacent to the aorta. The chemoreceptors excite nerve fibers that pass along with the baroreceptor fibers through Hering's nerves and the vagus nerves into the vasomotor center.

Each carotid or aortic body is supplied with an abundant blood flow through a small nutrient artery, so that the chemoreceptors are always in close contact with the arterial blood. Whenever the arterial pressure falls below a critical level, the chemoreceptors become stimulated because of diminished blood flow to the bodies and therefore diminished availability of oxygen and excess buildup of carbon dioxide and hydrogen ions that are not removed by the slow flow of blood.

The signals transmitted from the chemoreceptors into the vasomotor center *excite* the vasomotor center, and this elevates the arterial pressure. Obviously, this reflex helps to return the arterial pressure back toward the normal level whenever it falls too low.

However, the chemoreceptor reflex is not a powerful arterial pressure controller in the normal arterial pressure range because the chemoreceptors themselves are not stimulated strongly until the arterial pressure falls below 80 mm Hg. Therefore, it is at the lower pressures that this reflex becomes important to help prevent still further fall in pressure.

The chemoreceptors are discussed in much more detail in Chapter 29 in relation to respiratory control, in which they play a much more important role than in pressure control.

Atrial and Pulmonary Artery Reflexes That Help Regulate Arterial Pressure and Other Circulatory Factors

Both the atria and the pulmonary arteries have stretch receptors, called *low pressure receptors,* in their walls similar to the baroreceptor stretch receptors of the large systemic ateries. These low pressure receptors play an important role in minimizing arterial pressure changes in response to changes in blood volume. To give an example, if 300 milliliters of blood are infused into a dog with all the receptors intact, the arterial pressure wll rise only 15 mm Hg. With the arterial baroreceptors denervated, the pressure will rise 50 mm Hg. If the low pressure receptors are also denervated, the pressure may rise 120 mm Hg.

Thus, one can see that even though the low pressure receptors in the pulmonary artery and in the atria cannot detect the systemic arterial pressure, these receptors nevertheless do detect simultaneous increases in pressure in the low pressure areas of the circulation caused by an increase in volume, and they elicit reflexes parallel to the baroreceptor reflexes to make the total reflex system much more potent for control of arterial pressure.

The Central Nervous System Ischemic Response—Control of Arterial Pressure by the Vasomotor Center in Response to Diminished Brain Blood Flow

Normally, most nervous control of blood pressure is achieved by reflexes originating in the baroreceptors, the chemoreceptors, and the low pressure receptors, all of which are located in the peripheral circulation outside the brain. However, when blood flow to the vasomotor center in the lower brain stem becomes decreased enough to cause nutritional deficiency, that is, to cause *cerebral ischemia,* the neurons in the vasomotor center itself respond directly to the ischemia and become strongly excited. When this occurs, the systemic arterial pressure often rises to a level as high as the heart can possibly pump. This effect is believed by some physiologists to be caused by failure of the slowly flowing blood to carry carbon dioxide away from the vasomotor center; the local concentration of carbon dioxide then increases greatly and has an extremely potent effect in stimulating the sympathetic nervous system. It is possible that other factors, such as the buildup of lactic acid and other acidic substances, also contribute to the marked stimulation of the vasomotor center and to the elevation in pressure. This arterial pressure elevation in response to cerebral ischemia is known as the *central nervous system ischemic response* or simply *CNS ischemic response.*

The magnitude of the ischemic effect on vasomotor activity is tremendous; it can elevate the mean arterial pressure for as long as 10 minutes sometimes to as high as 250 mm Hg.

Importance of the CNS Ischemic Response as a Regulator of Arterial Pressure. Despite the extremely powerful nature of the CNS ischemic response, it does not become very active until the arterial pressure falls far below normal, down to 60 mm Hg and below, reaching its greatest degree of stimulation at a pressure of 15 to 20 mm Hg. Therefore, it is not one of the usual mechanisms for regulating normal arterial pressure. Instead, it operates principally as an *emergency arterial pressure control system that acts rapidly and extremely powerfully to prevent further decrease in arterial pressure whenever blood flow to the brain decreases dangerously close to the lethal level.* It is sometimes called the "last ditch stand" pressure control mechanism.

The Cushing Reaction. The so-called Cushing reaction is a special type of CNS ischemic response that results from increased pressure in the cranial vault. For instance, when the cerebrospinal fluid pressure rises to equal the arterial pressure, it compresses the arteries in the brain and cuts off the blood supply to the brain. Obviously, this initiates a CNS ischemic response, which causes the arterial pressure to rise. When the arterial pressure has risen to a level higher than the cerebrospinal fluid pressure, blood flows once again into the vessels of the brain to relieve the ischemia. Ordinarily, the blood pressure comes to a new equilibrium level slightly higher than the cerebrospinal fluid pressure, thus allowing blood to continue flowing to the brain.

Depressant Effect of Extreme, Prolonged Ischemia on the Vasomotor Center. If cerebral ischemia becomes so severe that maximum rise in mean arterial pressure still cannot relieve the ischemia, the neuronal cells begin to suffer metabolically, and within 3 to 10 minutes they become totally inactive. The arterial pressure then falls to about 40 to 50 mm Hg, which is the level to which the pressure falls when the vasomotor center loses all its control of the circulation, so that all tonic vasoconstrictor activity is lost. Therefore, it is fortunate that the ischemic response is extremely powerful, so that arterial pressure can usually rise high enough to correct brain ischemia before it causes nutritional depression and death of the neuronal cells.

REFERENCES

Buckley, J. P., et al. (eds.): Brain Peptides and Catecholamines in Cardiovascular Regulation. New York, Raven Press, 1987.

Calaresu, F. R., and Yardley, C. P.: Medullary basal sympathetic tone. Annu. Rev. Physiol., 50:511, 1988.

Cushing, H.: Concerning a definite regulatory mechanism of the vasomotor center which controls blood pressure during cerebral compression. Bull. Johns Hopkins Hosp., 12:290, 1901.

Dampney, R. A., et al.: Identification of cardiovascular cell groups in the brain stem. Clin. Exp. Hypertens., 6:205, 1984.

Guyton, A. C.: Arterial Pressure and Hypertension. Philadelphia, W. B. Saunders Co., 1980.

Guyton, A. C.: Acute hypertension in dogs with cerebral ischemia. Am. J. Physiol., 154:45, 1948.

Mathias, C. J., and Frankel, H. L.: Cardiovascular control in spinal man. Annu. Rev. Physiol., 50:577, 1988.

Persson, P. B., et al.: Cardiopulmonary-arterial baroreceptor interaction in control of blood pressure. News Physiol. Sci., 4:56, 1989.

Regoli, D.: Neurohumoral regulation of precapillary vessels: The kallikrein-kinin system. J. Cardiovasc. Pharmacol., 6:(Suppl. 2) S401, 1984.

Reid, J. L., and Rubin, P. C.: Peptides and central neural regulation of the circulation. Physiol. Rev., 67:725, 1987.

Share, L.: Role of vasopressin in cardiovascular regulation. Physiol. Rev., 68:1246, 1988.

Vanhoutte, P. M.: Vasodilation: Vascular Smooth Muscle, Peptides, Autonomic Nerves, and Endothelium. New York, Raven Press, 1988.

QUESTIONS

1. Describe the organization of the autonomic nervous system, especially the sympathetic portion, for circulatory control.
2. What is meant by *vasomotor tone,* and why is this important?
3. What is the role of the higher nervous centers in the control of the circulation?
4. Describe the anatomy of the baroreceptor reflex mechanism for controlling arterial pressure.
5. When the arterial pressure rises too high, what are the reflex effects on the circulatory system caused by excitation of the baroreceptors?
6. Explain the role of the baroreceptor pressure control system in relation to body posture, and also explain the buffer function of the baroreceptor system.
7. Why is the baroreceptor system not of importance for long-term regulation of arterial pressure?
8. Explain the CNS ischemic response, and tell why it is frequently called the "last ditch stand" pressure control mechanism.
9. What is the role of the epinephrine and norepinephrine hormonal system in the reflex control of arterial pressure?
10. How does the vasopressin-vasoconstrictor mechanism contribute to arterial pressure regulation?

16

Role of the Kidneys in Long-Term Regulation of Arterial Pressure and in Hypertension

Although we saw in the previous chapter that the nervous system has powerful capabilities for rapid, short-term control of arterial pressure, when the arterial pressure changes slowly over many hours or days the nervous mechanisms gradually lose their ability to oppose the changes. Therefore, what is it, week after week or month after month, that sets long-term arterial pressure level? We see in this chapter that the kidneys play the dominant role in this control.

THE RENAL-BODY FLUID SYSTEM FOR ARTERIAL PRESSURE CONTROL

The renal-body fluid system for arterial pressure control is a very simple one: When the body contains too much extracellular fluid, the arterial pressure rises. The rising pressure in turn has a direct effect to cause the kidneys to excrete the excess extracellular fluid, thus returning the pressure back to normal. Indeed, an increase in arterial pressure in the human of only a few millimeters of mercury can double the output of water, which is called *pressure diuresis,* and also double the output of salt, which is called *pressure natriuresis.* However, multiple refinements have been added to make this system much more exact in its control. An especially important refinement, as we see, has been the addition of the renin-angiotensin mechanism.

Quantification of Pressure Diuresis as a Basis for Arterial Pressure Control

Figure 16-1 illustrates the approximate average effect of different arterial pressures on urinary volume output, illustrating markedly increased output of volume as the pressure rises, which is the phenomenon of *pressure diuresis.* The curve in this figure is called either a *renal output curve* or a *renal function curve.* At an arterial pressure of 50 mm Hg, the urinary output is essentially zero. At 100 mm Hg, it is normal and at 200 mm Hg, about six to eight times normal. Furthermore, not only does increasing the pressure increase the urinary volume output, but also there is an approximately equal effect on sodium output, which is the phenomenon of *pressure natriuresis.*

An Experiment Demonstrating the Renal-Body Fluid System for Arterial Pressure Control. Figure 16-2 illustrates an experiment in dogs in which all the nervous reflex mechanisms for blood pressure control were blocked, and the arterial pressure was then suddenly elevated by infusing about 400 milliliters of blood. Note the instantaneous increase in cardiac output to approximately double its normal level and the increase in mean arterial pressure to 205 mm Hg, 115 mm Hg above its resting level. Shown by the middle curve is the effect of this increased arterial pressure on urinary output, which increased 12-fold. Along with this tremendous loss of fluid, both the cardiac output and the arterial pressure returned to normal during the subsequent hour. Thus, one sees the extreme capability of the kidneys to eliminate fluid volume from the body and in so doing to return the arterial pressure back to normal.

Graphical Analysis of Pressure Control by the Renal-Body Fluid Mechanism, Demonstrating Its "Infinite Gain" Feature. Figure 16-3 illustrates a graphical method that can be used for analyzing arterial pressure control by the renal-body fluid system. This analysis is based on two separate curves that intersect each other: (1) the renal output

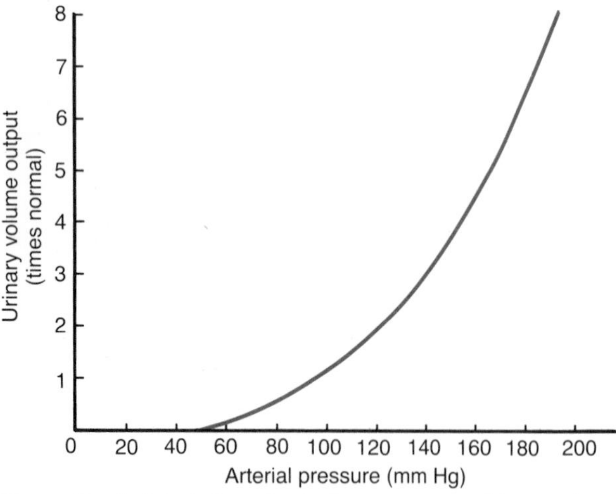

Figure 16-1. A typical renal output curve measured in a perfused isolated kidney, showing pressure diuresis when the arterial pressure rises above normal.

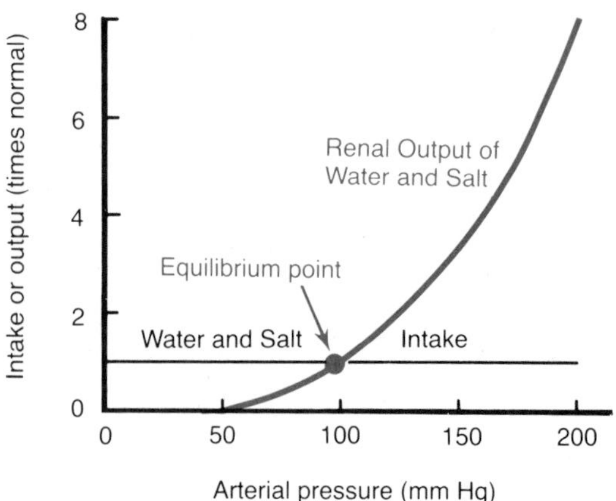

Figure 16-3. Analysis of arterial pressure regulation by equating the renal output curve with the salt and water intake curve. The "equilibrium point" describes the level to which the arterial pressure will be regulated. (That portion of the salt and water intake that is lost from the body through nonrenal routes is ignored in this and other similar figures of this chapter.)

curve for water and salt, which is the same renal output curve as that illustrated in Figure 16-1, and (2) the curve (or line) that represents the water and salt intake minus the amount of water and salt lost from the body in ways other than through the kidneys.

Obviously, over a long period of time the water and salt output must equal the intake. Furthermore, the only place on the graph in Figure 16-3 at which the output equals the intake is where the two curves intersect, which is called the *equilibrium point.* Now, let us see what will happen if the arterial pressure becomes some value that is different from that at the equilibrium point.

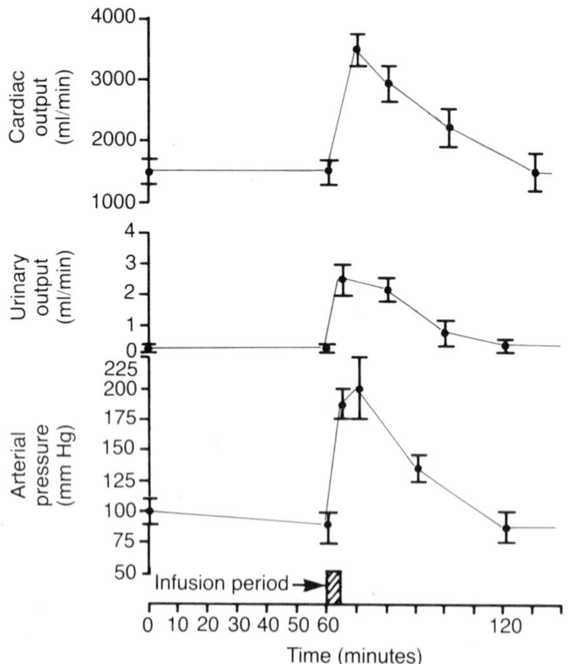

Figure 16-2. Increase in cardiac output, arterial pressure, and urinary output caused by increased blood volume in animals whose nervous pressure control mechanisms had been blocked. This figure shows the return of arterial pressure to normal after about an hour of fluid loss into the urine. (Courtesy of Dr. William Dobbs.)

First, assume that the arterial pressure rises to 150 mm Hg. At this level, the graph shows that renal output of water and salt is about three times as great as the intake. Therefore, the body loses fluid, the blood volume decreases, and the arterial pressure decreases. Furthermore, this "negative balance" of fluid will not cease until the pressure falls *all the way* back exactly to the equilibrium point. Indeed, even when the arterial pressure is only 1 mm Hg greater than the equilibrium point, there will still be more loss of water and salt than intake, so that the pressure will still continue to fall that last 1 mm Hg *until the pressure returns exactly to the equilibrium point.*

Now, let us see what will happen if the arterial pressure falls below the equilibrium point. This time, the intake of water and salt is greater than the output. Therefore, the body fluid volume increases, the blood volume increases, and the arterial pressure rises until once again it returns *exactly* to the equilibrium point.

This return of the arterial pressure always exactly back to the equilibrium point is the *infinite gain principle* for control of arterial pressure by the renal-body fluid mechanism.

The Two Determinants of the Long-Term Arterial Pressure Level. In Figure 16-3 one can also see that two basic long-term factors determine the long-term arterial pressure level. These are:

1. The *degree of shift of the renal output curve* for water and salt along the arterial pressure axis.
2. The *level of the water and salt intake line.*

The operation of these two determinants in the control of arterial pressure is illustrated in Figure 16-4. In Figure 16-4A, some abnormality of the kidney has caused the renal output curve to shift 50 mm Hg in the high pressure direction (to the right). Note that the equilibrium point has also shifted to 50 mm Hg higher than normal. Therefore, one can state that if the intake of salt and water remains constant but the renal output curve shifts to a new pressure level, so also will the arterial pressure

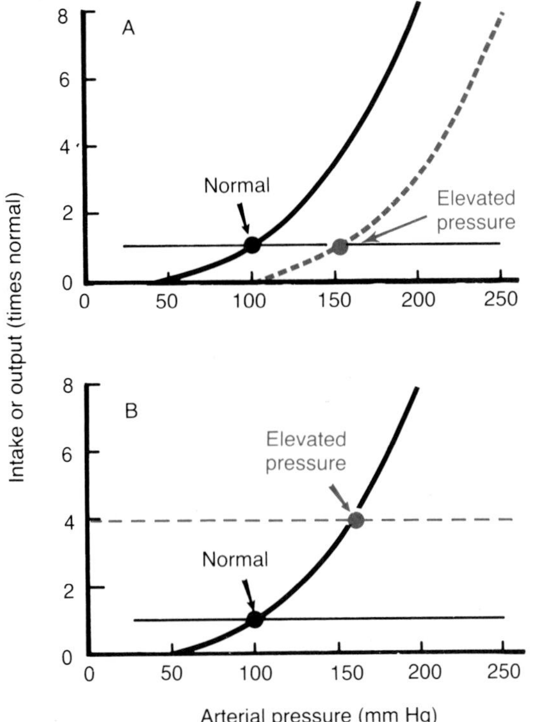

Figure 16-4. Demonstration of the two ways in which the arterial pressure can be increased: *A*, by shifting the renal output curve in the right-hand direction toward a higher pressure level and *B*, by increasing the intake level of salt and water.

follow to this new pressure level within a few days' time.

Figure 16-4B illustrates how a change in the level of salt and water intake can change the arterial pressure when the renal output curve remains undisturbed. In this case, the intake has increased fourfold, and the equilibrium point has shifted to a pressure level of 160 mm Hg, 60 mm Hg above the normal level.

Therefore, it is *impossible* to change the long-term mean arterial pressure level to a new value without changing one or both of the two basic determinants of the long-term arterial pressure level, either the level of salt and water intake or the degree of shift of the renal function curve along the pressure axis. However, if either of these is changed, one would expect the arterial pressure thereafter to be regulated at a new pressure level, at the pressure level at which these two new curves intersect.

Failure of Increased Total Peripheral Resistance to Elevate the Long-Term Level of Arterial Pressure If Fluid Intake and Renal Function Do Not Change

Now is the chance for the reader to see whether or not he or she really understands the renal-body fluid mechanism for arterial pressure control. Recalling the basic equation for arterial pressure, *arterial pressure* equals *cardiac output* times *total peripheral resistance,* it is clear that an increase in total peripheral resistance should elevate the arterial pressure. Indeed, when the total peripheral resistance is acutely increased, the arterial pressure does rise immediately. Yet, if the kidneys continue to function normally, the acute rise in arterial pressure is not maintained. Instead the arterial pressure returns to normal within a day or so. Why?

The answer to this is as follows: Increasing the resistance in the blood vessels everywhere else in the body besides in the kidneys does not change the equilibrium point for blood pressure control (see again Figs. 16-3 and 16-4). Therefore, the kidneys immediately begin to respond to the high arterial pressure with pressure diuresis and pressure natriuresis. Within hours or days, large amounts of salt and water are lost from the body, and this continues until the arterial pressure returns to the pressure level of the equilibrium point.

As proof of this principle that changes in total peripheral resistance will not affect the long-term level of arterial pressure, carefully study Figure 16-5. This figure shows the approximate cardiac outputs and the arterial pressures in different clinical conditions in which the *long-term* total peripheral resistance is either much less than or much greater than normal, but kidney excretion of salt and water is normal or nearly normal. Note in all the different conditions that the arterial pressure is also normal.

However, note also in Figure 16-5 that a *long-term decrease* in total peripheral resistance causes an exact reciprocal *increase* in cardiac output, whereas a long-term *increase* in total peripheral resistance causes an exact reciprocal *decrease* in cardiac output. We leave it to the reader to figure out how it is that the renal-body fluid mechanism automatically adjusts the cardiac output to the reciprocal level that will balance exactly the changes in total peripheral resistance. Just apply the principle of infinite gain of the renal-

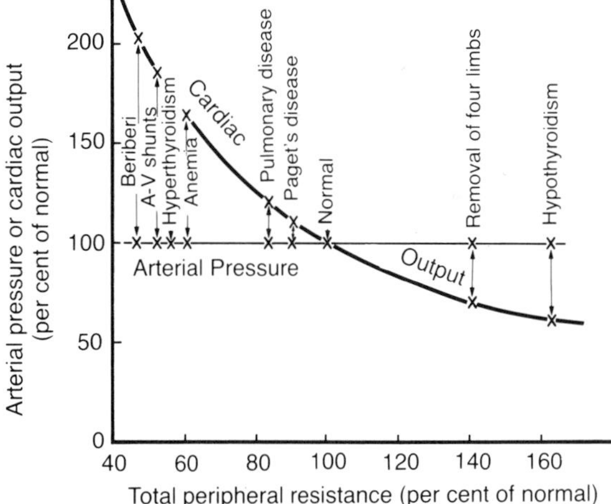

Figure 16-5. Relationships of total peripheral resistance to the long-term levels of arterial pressure and cardiac output in different clinical abnormalities. In these conditions, the kidneys were functioning normally. Note that the changes in total peripheral resistance caused equal and opposite changes in cardiac output but had no effect on the arterial pressure. (Reprinted from Guyton: Arterial Pressure and Hypertension. Philadelphia, W. B. Saunders Company, 1980.)

body fluid mechanism for pressure control, and the result is inevitable. Until this is clear, one can be certain that he or she still does not understand the renal–body fluid mechanism for arterial pressure control.

(Yet, a word of caution! Many times when the total peripheral resistance increases, this increases the intrarenal vascular resistance at the same time, which alters the function of the kidney and can cause hypertension by shifting the renal function curve to a higher pressure level, in the manner illustrated in Figure 16–4A. We see an example of this later in this chapter when we discuss hypertension caused by vasoconstrictor mechanisms. But it is the increase in renal resistance that is the culprit, not the increased total peripheral resistance — a very important distinction!)

How Increased Fluid Volume Elevates the Arterial Pressure — The Role of Autoregulation

The overall mechanism by which increased extracellular volume elevates arterial pressure is given in the schema of Figure 16–6. The sequential events are (1) increased extracellular fluid volume, which (2) increases the blood volume, which (3) increases the mean circulatory filling pressure, which (4) increases the venous return of blood to the heart, which (5) increases the cardiac output, which (6) increases the arterial pressure.

Note especially in this schema the two different ways in which an increase in cardiac output can increase the arterial pressure. One of these is (1) the direct effect of increased cardiac output in increasing the pressure, and the other is (2) an indirect effect resulting from local tissue autoregulation of blood flow. This second effect can be explained as follows:

Referring back to Chapter 14, let us recall that whenever an excess amount of blood flows through a tissue, the local vasculature constricts and decreases the blood flow back toward normal. This phenomenon is called "autoregulation," which simply means regulation of blood flow by the tissue itself. When increased blood volume increases the cardiac output, the blood flow increases in all the tissues of the body, so that this autoregulation mechanism will constrict the blood vessels all over the body. This, in turn, will also increase the total peripheral resistance.

Finally, since arterial pressure is equal to cardiac output times total peripheral resistance, the secondary increase in total peripheral resistance that results from the autoregulation mechanism helps greatly in increasing the arterial pressure, often accounting for as much as 80 to 90 per cent of the pressure rise.

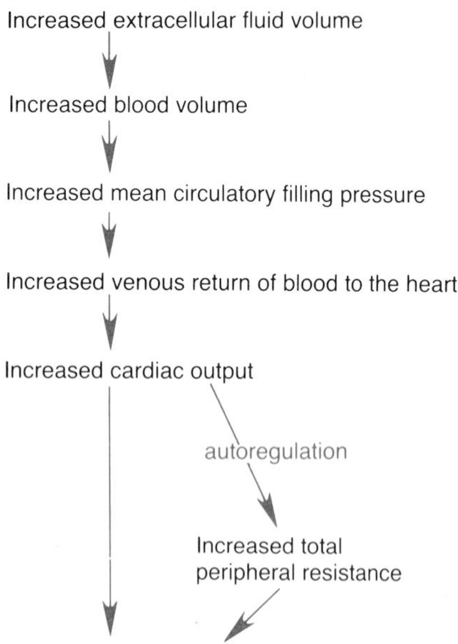

Figure 16–6. The sequential steps by which increased extracellular fluid volume increases the arterial pressure. Note especially that increased cardiac output has both a direct effect of increasing arterial pressure and an indirect effect of increasing the total peripheral resistance.

Importance of Salt in the Renal–Body Fluid Schema for Arterial Pressure Regulation

Although the discussions thus far have emphasized the importance of volume in the regulation of arterial pressure, experimental studies have shown that an increase in salt intake is far more likely to elevate the arterial pressure than is an increase in water intake. The reason for this is that water is normally excreted by the kidneys almost as rapidly as it is ingested, but salt often is not excreted so easily. As it accumulates in the body, salt indirectly increases the extracellular fluid volume for two basic reasons:

1. When there is excess salt in the body, the osmolality of the body fluids increases, and this in turn *stimulates the thirst center,* making the person drink extra amounts of water to dilute the extracellular salt to a normal concentration. This obviously increases the extracellular fluid volume.
2. The increase in osmolality in the extracellular fluid also stimulates the hypothalamic–posterior pituitary gland secretory mechanism to secrete increased quantities of *antidiuretic hormone.* This is discussed fully in Chapter 22. The antidiuretic hormone in turn causes the kidneys to reabsorb greatly increased quantities of water from the renal tubular fluid before it is excreted as urine, thereby diminishing the volume of urine while increasing the extracellular fluid volume.

Thus, for these two important reasons, the amount of salt that accumulates in the body is the main determinant of the extracellular fluid volume. Because only small increases in extracellular fluid can often increase the arterial pressure greatly, the accumulation of even a small amount of extra salt in the body can lead to considerable elevation of the arterial pressure.

Hypertension (High Blood Pressure) Caused by Excessive Extracellular Fluid Volume

When a person is said to have hypertension (or "high blood pressure"), it is meant that his or her mean arterial pressure is greater than the upper range of accepted normality. Usually, a mean arterial pressure greater than 110 mm Hg under resting conditions is considered to be hypertensive; this level normally occurs when the diastolic blood pressure is greater than 90 mm Hg and the systolic pressure is greater than about 135 to 140 mm Hg. In very severe hypertension, the mean arterial pressure can rise to as high as 150 to 170 mm Hg, with diastolic pressures as high as 130 mm Hg and systolic arterial pressures occasionally as great as 250 mm Hg.

Even moderate elevation of the arterial pressure leads to shortened life expectancy; at very high pressures—mean arterial pressures 50 per cent or more above normal—a person can expect to live no more than a few more years at most. The lethal effects of hypertension are caused mainly in three ways: (1) Excess workload on the heart leads to early development of congestive heart disease, coronary heart disease, or both, often causing death as a result of a heart attack. (2) The high pressure frequently ruptures a major blood vessel in the brain, followed by clotting of the blood and death of major portions of the brain; this is a *cerebral infarct.* Clinically it is called a "stroke." Depending on what part of the brain is involved, a stroke can cause paralysis, dementia, blindness, or multiple other serious brain disorders. (3) Very high pressure almost always causes multiple hemorrhages in the kidneys, producing many areas of renal destruction and eventually kidney failure, uremia, and death.

The lessons learned from one type of hypertension called "volume-loading hypertension" have been crucial in understanding the role of the renal–body fluid volume mechanism for arterial pressure regulation. Volume-loading hypertension means hypertension caused by excess accumulation of extracellular fluid in the body, some examples of which follow.

The Sequential Changes in Circulatory Function During the Development of Volume-Loading Hypertension. It is especially instructive to study the sequential changes in circulatory function during the progressive development of volume-loading hypertension. Figure 16–7 illustrates these sequential changes. A week or so prior to the point labeled "0" days, the kidney mass in dogs had been decreased to only 30 per cent of normal. Then at this point, the intake of salt and water was increased to about six times normal. The acute effect was increases in extracellular fluid volume, blood volume, and cardiac output to 20 to 40 per cent above normal. Simultaneously, the arterial pressure began to rise as well but not nearly so much at first as did the fluid volumes and cardiac output. The reason for this can be discerned by studying the total peripheral resistance curve, which shows an initial *decrease* in total peripheral resistance. This decrease was caused by the baroreceptor mechanism, discussed in the previous chapter, which tried to prevent the rise in pressure. However, after a few days, the baroreceptors adapted (reset) and no longer opposed the rise in pressure. By this time, the arterial pressure had risen almost to its full height because of the increase in cardiac output, even though the total peripheral resistance was still almost at the normal level.

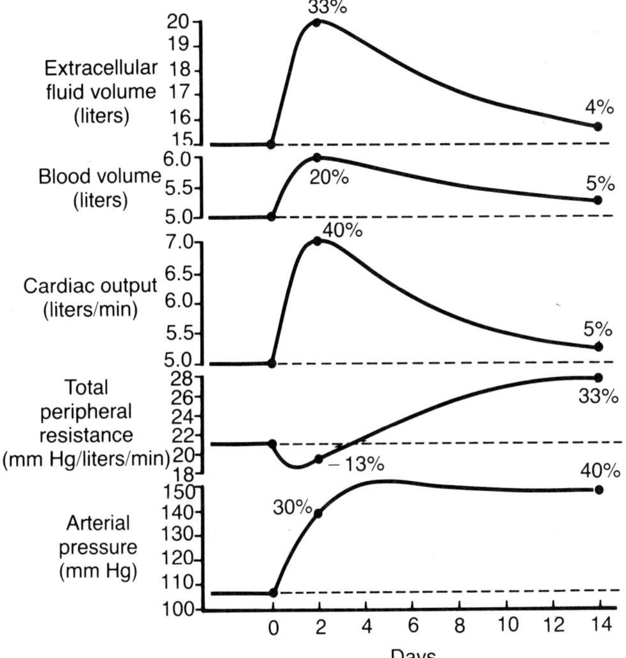

Figure 16–7. Progressive changes in important circulatory system variables during the first few weeks of *volume-loading hypertension.* Note especially the initial rise in cardiac output as the basic cause of the hypertension. Subsequently, the autoregulation mechanism returns the cardiac output almost to normal while at the same time causing a *secondary increase in total peripheral resistance.* (Modified from Guyton: Arterial Pressure and Hypertension. Philadelphia, W. B. Saunders Company, 1980.)

After these early acute changes in the circulatory variables had occurred, more prolonged secondary changes occurred during the next few days and weeks. Especially important was a *progressive increase in total peripheral resistance,* while at the same time *the cardiac output decreased almost all the way back to normal.* Multiple experiments have now shown that these changes were almost certainly caused mainly by *the long-term autoregulation* mechanism that is discussed in Chapter 14 as well as earlier in this chapter. That is, after the cardiac output had risen to a high level and had initiated the hypertension, the excess blood flow through the tissues then caused progressive constriction of the local arterioles, thus returning the cardiac output almost all the way back to normal but simultaneously causing a *secondary increase in total peripheral resistance.*

Note also that the extracellular fluid volume and blood volume returned almost all the way back to normal along with the decrease in cardiac output. This resulted from two factors: First, the increase in arteriolar resistance decreased the capillary pressure, which allowed the fluid in the tissue spaces to be absorbed back into the blood. Second, the elevated arterial pressure now caused the kidneys to excrete the excess volume of fluid that had initially accumulated in the body.

Finally, let us take stock of the final state of the circulation several weeks after the initial onset of volume loading. We find the following effects:

1. *Hypertension.*
2. *Marked increase in total peripheral resistance.*
3. *Almost complete return of the extracellular fluid volume, blood volume, and cardiac output back to normal.*

Therefore, we can divide volume-loading hypertension into two separate sequential stages:

The first stage results from increased fluid volumes and increased cardiac output. It is this increase in cardiac output that causes the hypertension.

The second stage in volume-loading hypertension is characterized by high blood pressure and high total peripheral resistance but return of the cardiac output so near to normal that the usual measuring techniques most frequently cannot detect an abnormally elevated output.

It should be especially noted that *the increased total peripheral resistance in volume-loading hypertension occurs* ***after*** *the hypertension has developed and therefore is* ***secondary*** *to the hypertension rather than being the cause of the hypertension.*

THE RENIN-ANGIOTENSIN SYSTEM: ITS ROLE IN PRESSURE CONTROL AND IN HYPERTENSION

Aside from the capability to control arterial pressure through changes in extracellular fluid volume, the kidneys also have another powerful mechanism for controlling pressure. This is the renin-angiotensin system.

Renin is a small protein enzyme released by the kidneys when the arterial pressure falls too low. In turn, it raises the arterial pressure in several different ways, thus helping to correct the initial fall in pressure.

The Components of the Renin-Angiotensin System

Figure 16–8 illustrates the functional steps by which the renin-angiotensin system helps to regulate arterial pressure.

Renin is synthesized and stored in an inactive form called *prorenin* in the *juxtaglomerular cells* of the kidneys, which are modified smooth muscle cells located in the walls of the afferent arterioles immediately proximal to the glomeruli. When the arterial pressure falls, intrinsic reactions in the kidneys themselves cause many of these prorenin molecules to split and release *renin.* Most of the renin enters the blood and circulates throughout the entire blood stream, although a small amount remains in the local fluids of the kidney and initiates several intrarenal functions.

Renin is an enzyme, not a vasoactive substance itself. Instead, as illustrated in the schema of Figure 16–8, it acts enzymatically on another plasma protein, a globulin called *renin substrate* (or *angiotensinogen*), to release a 10–amino acid peptide, *angiotensin* I. Angiotensin I has mild vasoconstrictor properties but not enough to cause significant functional changes in circulatory function.

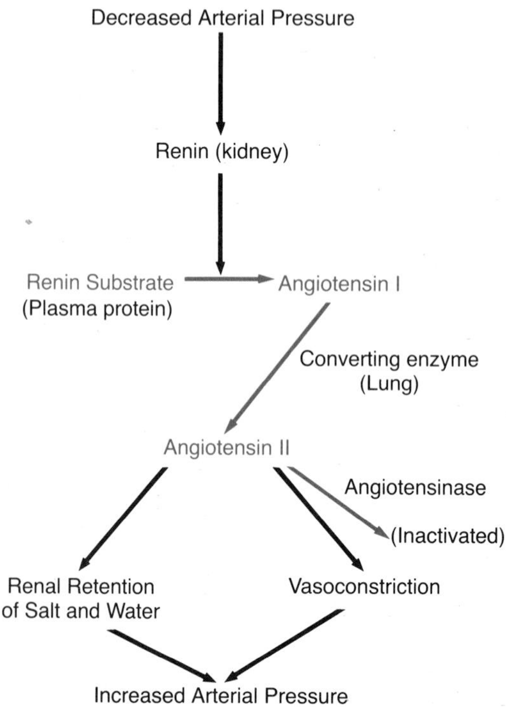

Figure 16–8. The renin-angiotensin-vasoconstrictor mechanism for arterial pressure control.

Within a few seconds after formation of the angiotensin I, two additional amino acids are split from it to form the 8-amino acid peptide *angiotensin II.* This conversion occurs almost entirely in the small vessels of the lungs, catalyzed by the enzyme *converting enzyme* that is present in the endothelium of the lung vessels. Angiotensin II is an extremely powerful vasoconstrictor agent and has other effects as well that affect the circulation. However, it persists in the blood only for a minute or two because it is rapidly inactivated by multiple blood and tissue enzymes collectively called *angiotensinase.*

During its persistence in the blood, angiotensin II has two principal effects that can elevate arterial pressure. The first of these, *vasoconstriction,* occurs very rapidly, within seconds. Vasoconstriction occurs very intensely in the arterioles and to considerably less extent in the veins. Constriction of the arterioles increases the peripheral resistance, thereby raising the arterial pressure back toward normal, as illustrated at the bottom of the schema in Figure 16-8. Also, the mild constriction of the veins promotes increased venous return of blood to the heart, thereby helping the heart pump against the increasing pressure.

The second principal means by which angiotensin increases the arterial pressure is to act on the kidneys to *decrease the excretion of both salt and water.* This increases the extracellular fluid volume, which then increases the arterial pressure slowly over a period of hours and days. This long-term effect, acting through the extracellular fluid volume mechanism, is even more powerful than the acute vasoconstrictor mechanism in eventually returning the arterial pressure back to normal.

Effect of Angiotensin to Cause Renal Retention of Salt and Water—An Especially Important Means for Long-Term Control of Arterial Pressure

Angiotensin causes the kidneys to retain both salt and water in two different ways:

1. Angiotensin *acts directly on the kidneys to cause salt and water retention.*
2. Angiotensin *causes the adrenal glands to secrete aldosterone, and the aldosterone in turn increases salt and water reabsorption by the kidney tubules.*

Obviously, to achieve balance between fluid intake and output, the arterial pressure must rise to a considerably increased level to overcome these two fluid-retaining effects of angiotensin. For this reason, whenever excess amounts of angiotensin circulate in the blood, the entire long-term renal-body fluid mechanism for arterial pressure control automatically becomes set to a higher than normal arterial pressure level.

Mechanisms of the Direct Renal Effects of Angiotensin to Cause Renal Retention of Salt and Water. Angiotensin has several intrarenal effects that make the kidneys retain salt and water. Probably the most important is to constrict the renal blood vessels, thereby diminishing blood flow through the kidneys. As a result, less fluid filters through the glomeruli into the tubules. Also, the slow flow of blood in the peritubular capillaries reduces their pressure, which allows rapid osmotic reabsorption of fluid from the tubules. Thus, for both of these reasons, less urine is excreted. In addition, angiotensin has a weak effect on the tubular cells themselves to increase tubular reabsorption of sodium and water. The total result of all these effects is very significant, sometimes decreasing urinary output as much as fourfold to sixfold.

Stimulation of Aldosterone Secretion by Angiotensin, and the Effect of Aldosterone in Increasing Salt and Water Retention by the Kidneys. Angiotensin is also one of the most powerful controllers of aldosterone secretion, as we discuss in relation to body fluid regulation in Chapter 22. Therefore, when the renin-angiotensin system becomes activated, the rate of aldosterone secretion usually increases at the same time. One of the most important functions of aldosterone is to cause marked increase in sodium reabsorption by the kidney tubules, thus increasing the extracellular fluid sodium. This then causes water retention, as already explained, thus increasing the extracellular fluid volume and leading secondarily to still more long-term elevation of the arterial pressure.

Quantitative Analysis of Arterial Pressure Changes Caused by Angiotensin. Figure 16-9 illustrates a quantitative analysis of the effect of angiotensin arterial pressure control. This figure shows two separate renal output curves and also illustrates the normal level of sodium intake. The left-hand renal output curve is approximately that measured in dogs whose renin-angiotensin system has been blocked by

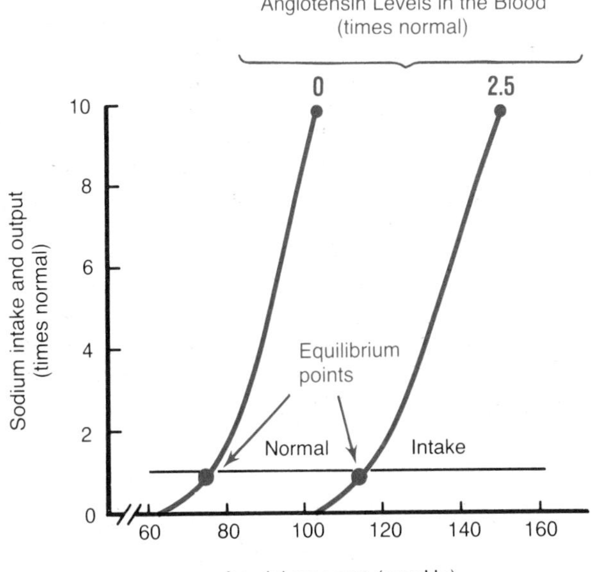

Figure 16-9. Effect of two different angiotensin levels on the renal output curve, showing regulation of the arterial pressure at an "equilibrium point" of 75 mm Hg when the angiotensin level is low and at 115 mm Hg when the angiotensin level is high.

the drug captopril (which blocks the conversion of angiotensin I to angiotensin II). The right-hand curve is that measured in dogs infused continuously with angiotensin II at a level about 2.5 times the normal rate of angiotensin formation in the blood. Note the obvious shift of the renal output curve toward higher pressure levels under the influence of angiotensin. This shift is caused by both the direct effect of angiotensin on the kidney and the indirect effect acting through aldosterone secretion, as explained previously.

Finally, note the two separate equilibrium points, one for zero angiotensin at an arterial pressure level of 75 mm Hg and one for elevated angiotensin at a pressure level of 115 mm Hg.

Therefore, even though the vasoconstrictor effect of angiotensin on all the *nonrenal* blood vessels of the body cannot cause a long-term increase in arterial pressure, the effects of angiotensin on renal retention of water and salt can have a very powerful effect in causing chronic elevation of the arterial pressure.

Role of the Renin-Angiotensin System in Maintaining a Normal Arterial Pressure Despite Wide Variations in Salt Intake

Probably the most important function of the renin-angiotensin system is to allow a person to eat either a very small or a very large amount of salt without causing great changes in either extracellular fluid volume or arterial pressure. This function is explained by the analysis illustrated in Figure 16–10. This figure presents a graphical analysis of the automatic renin-angiotensin feedback mechanism for preventing excessive rise in arterial pressure when sodium intake increases. It shows four separate levels of salt intake, as illustrated by the four separate horizontal lines. To the right of each line is shown the approximate level of

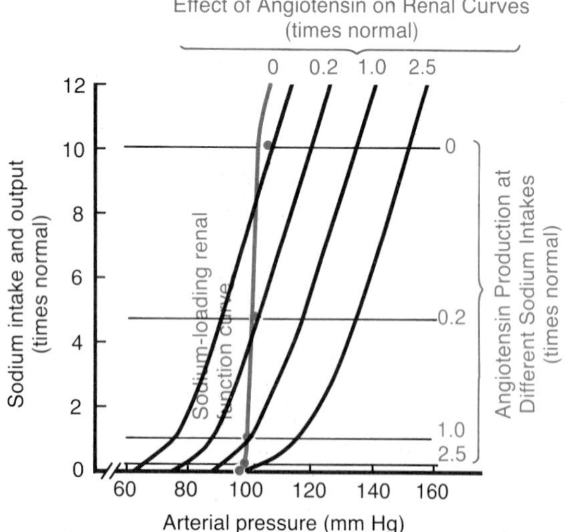

Figure 16–10. The effect of different levels of salt intake on the arterial pressure. The lighter curves are renal output curves. The very dark red curve is the "sodium-loading renal function curve" for a person with normal kidneys. See text for explanation.

circulating angiotensin that one finds in the blood at each of these salt intake levels. Note that at very low salt intake, the concentration of angiotensin in the blood increases to about 2.5 times normal. On the other hand, when the sodium intake is 50 times greater, the level of circulating angiotensin becomes essentially zero.

Now, observe the four separate renal output curves (the black curves). These are the renal output curves caused by the four different levels of angiotensin that occur respectively at the different levels of salt intake. Thus, when the level of angiotensin in the blood is high, it is the renal output curve to the far right that depicts the relationship between arterial pressure and sodium output. Conversely, when the circulating level of angiotensin is zero, the far left renal output curve depicts this relationship.

Now, finally, match the appropriate levels of sodium intake with the appropriate renal output curves at the different levels of angiotensin and you will be able to determine the equilibrium point for these four separate pairs of intake and output curves. These equilibrium points are illustrated by the very heavy red points on the graph.

As a final maneuver, draw a heavy line connecting the four separate equilibrium points, as is illustrated in red in the figure. This line represents the relationship between long-term sodium intake and long-term level of arterial pressure, called the *salt-loading renal function curve*. In other words, this salt-loading renal function curve shows the relationship between arterial pressures and the renal sodium outputs that are recorded when the initial factor that is changed is the salt intake. Note that despite an approximate 50-fold change in sodium intake, as depicted in the figure, the arterial pressure change is only 4 mm Hg. These are the results that have been observed in animals when the sodium intake has been changed as much as 50-fold. Furthermore, the same experiment performed in humans has shown that changing the sodium intake from 1/15 normal to 10 times normal—a total range of 150-fold—changes the arterial pressure only by about 17 mm Hg.

Goldblatt Hypertension—A Hypertension Involving Both Renin-Angiotensin and Fluid Retention

When one kidney is removed and a constrictor is placed on the renal artery of the remaining kidney, as illustrated in Figure 16–11, the immediate effect is greatly reduced pressure in the renal artery beyond the constrictor, as shown by the dashed curve in the figure. Then, within a few minutes the systemic arterial pressure, shown by the upper solid curve, begins to rise and continues to rise for several days. The pressure usually rises rapidly for the first hour or so, and this is followed by a slower rise over a period of several days to a much higher pressure level. When the systemic arterial pressure reaches its new stable

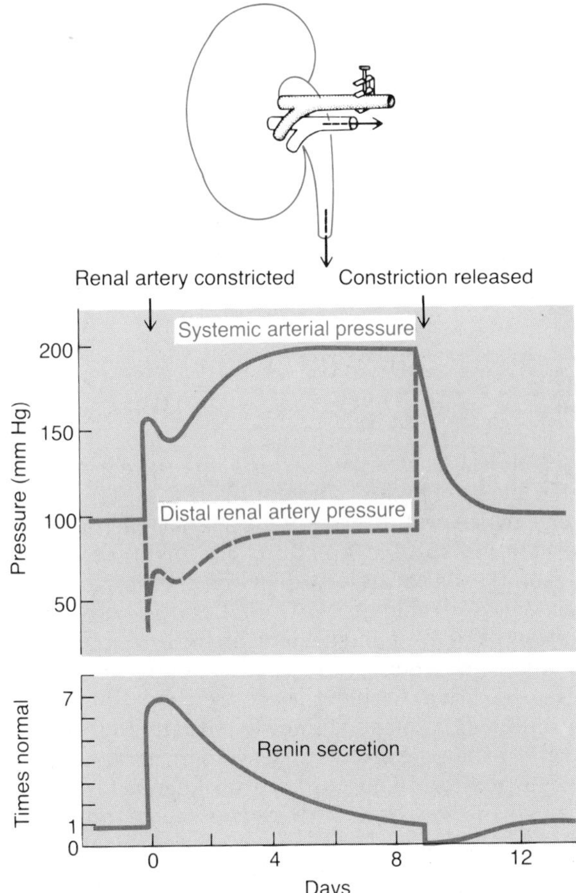

Figure 16-11. Effect of placing a constricting clamp on the renal artery of one kidney after the other kidney has been removed. Note the changes in systemic arterial pressure, renal artery pressure distal to the clamp, and rate of renin secretion. The resulting hypertension is called "one-kidney Goldblatt hypertension."

pressure level, the renal arterial pressure will have returned either all the way or almost all the way back to normal. The hypertension produced in this way is called *"one-kidney" Goldblatt hypertension* in honor of Goldblatt, who first studied the important quantitative features of hypertension caused by renal artery constriction.

The early rise in arterial pressure in Goldblatt hypertension is caused by the renin-angiotensin vasoconstrictor mechanism. Because of the poor blood flow through the kidney after acute reduction of renal arterial pressure, large quantities of renin are secreted by the kidneys, as illustrated by the lowermost curve in Figure 16–11, and this causes angiotensin to be formed in the blood, as described earlier in the chapter; the angiotensin in turn raises the arterial pressure acutely. The secretion of renin rises to a peak in a few hours but returns all the way back to normal within 5 to 7 days because the renal arterial pressure by that time has also risen back to normal, so that the kidney is no longer ischemic.

The second rise in arterial pressure is caused by fluid retention resulting from the initially low renal arterial pressure; within 5 to 7 days the fluid volume has increased enough to raise the arterial pressure to its new sustained level. The quantitative value of this sustained pressure level is determined by the degree of constriction of the renal artery. That is, the aortic pressure must rise to a much higher than normal level in order to make the renal arterial pressure distal to the constrictor rise high enough to cause normal urinary output.

Note especially that one-kidney Goldblatt hypertension has two phases. The first phase is a vasoconstrictor type of hypertension caused by angiotensin, but this is only transient. The second stage is a volume-loading type of hypertension. However, it is often very difficult to tell that this second stage is true volume-loading hypertension because neither the blood volume nor the cardiac output is significantly elevated. Instead, the total peripheral resistance is increased. To understand this, recall that in pure volume-loading hypertension blood volume and cardiac output are elevated only the first few days during the onset; after the first few days, volume-loading hypertension is a high resistance hypertension exactly as seen in the second stage of one-kidney Goldblatt hypertension. The transient increases in blood volume and cardiac output that are normally seen in pure volume-loading hypertension are obscured by the angiotensin vasoconstriction that occurs in Goldblatt hypertension during these early days.

Essential Hypertension

Approximately 90 per cent of all persons who have hypertension are said to have "essential hypertension." This term means simply that *the hypertension is of unknown origin.*

Some of the characteristics of severe essential hypertension are the following:

1. The mean arterial pressure is increased 40 to 60 per cent.
2. The renal blood flow in the later stages is decreased to about one half normal.
3. The resistance to blood flow through the kidneys is increased twofold to fourfold.
4. Despite the great decrease in renal blood flow, the glomerular filtration rate is often very near normal. The reason for this is that the high arterial pressure still causes adequate filtration of fluid through the glomeruli into the renal tubules.
5. The cardiac output is approximately normal.
6. The total peripheral resistance is increased about 40 to 60 per cent, about the same amount that the arterial pressure is increased.

Finally, the most important finding of all in persons with essential hypertension is the following:

7. The kidneys will not excrete adequate amounts of salt and water unless the arterial pressure is high. In other words, if the mean arterial pressure in the essential hypertensive person is

150 mm Hg, reduction of the arterial pressure artificially to the normal value of 100 mm Hg (but without otherwise altering renal function except for the decreased pressure) will cause almost total anuria, and the person will retain salt and water until the pressure rises back to the elevated value of 150 mm Hg.

The exact reason for this failure of the kidneys of essential hypertensive persons to excrete salt and water at normal pressure levels is unknown. However, the very significant vascular changes in the kidneys listed earlier in this section suggest that decreased renal blood flow is the cause of this.

Graphical Analysis of Arterial Pressure Control in Essential Hypertension. Figure 16–12 is a graphical analysis of essential hypertension. The curves of this figure are not the same renal output curves that have been used in the early figures of this chapter. Instead, these curves are *sodium-loading renal function curves* of the type shown for the normal kidney by the heavy red curve in Figure 16–10. The reason for using this curve rather than the renal output curve is the following: It is very easy to determine the sodium-loading type of curve by simply increasing the level of sodium intake to a new level every few days, then waiting for the renal output of sodium to come into balance with the intake, and finally recording the changes in arterial pressure. When this procedure is employed in essential hypertensive patients, the two curves to the right in Figure 16–12 are recorded in two different groups of essential hypertensive patients, one called (1) *non–salt-sensitive* patients, and the other (2) *salt-sensitive.* Note in both instances that the curves are shifted to a much higher pressure level than for normal persons. Now, let us plot on this same graph (1) a normal level of salt intake, and (2) a high level of salt intake representing 3.5 times the normal intake. In the case of the person with non–salt-sensitive essential hypertension, the arterial pressure does not increase significantly when

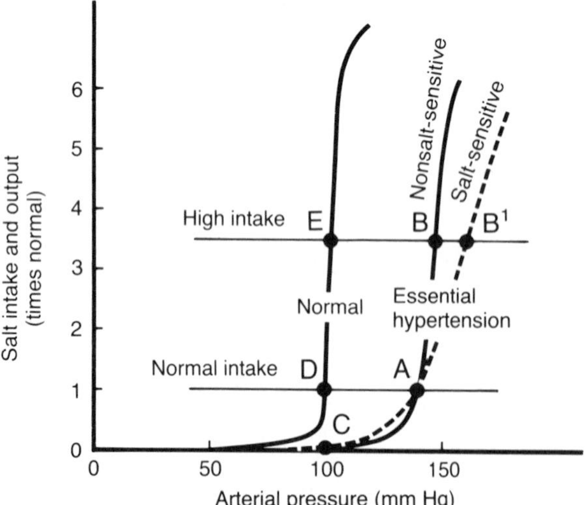

Figure 16–12. Analysis of arterial pressure regulation in "non–salt-sensitive" essential hypertension and "salt-sensitive" essential hypertension. Explained in the text. (From Guyton et al.: *Annu. Rev. Med. 31*:15, 1980.)

changing from normal salt intake to high salt intake. On the other hand, in those patients who have salt-sensitive essential hypertension, the high salt intake further exacerbates the hypertension.

The reason for the difference between non–salt-sensitive essential hypertension and salt-sensitive hypertension is presumably structural or functional differences in the kidneys of these two types of hypertensive patients.

SUMMARY OF THE INTEGRATED, MULTIFACETED SYSTEM FOR ARTERIAL PRESSURE REGULATION

By now, it is clear that arterial pressure is not regulated by a single pressure controlling system but instead by several interrelated systems, each of which performs a specific function. For instance, when a person bleeds severely so that the pressure falls suddenly, two problems confront the pressure control system. The first is survival, to return the arterial pressure immediately to a high enough level that the person can live through the acute episode. The second is to return the blood volume eventually to its normal level, so that the circulatory system can re-establish full normality, including return of the arterial pressure all the way back to its normal value, not merely back to a pressure level required for survival.

In the previous chapter we saw that the first line of defense against acute changes in arterial pressure is the nervous control system. In the present chapter we have emphasized the role of the kidneys in long-term control of arterial pressure.

Figure 16–13 illustrates the approximate control responses, expressed as feedback gain, of eight different arterial pressure control mechanisms. These mechanisms can be divided into three separate groups: (1) those that react very rapidly, within seconds or minutes; (2) those that respond over an intermediate time period, minutes or hours; and (3) those that provide long-term arterial pressure regulation, days, months, and years. Let us see how these all fit together as a total, concerted system for pressure control.

The Rapidly Acting Pressure Control Mechanisms, Acting Within Seconds or Minutes. The rapidly acting pressure control mechanisms are almost entirely acute nervous reflexes or other nervous responses. Note in Figure 16–13 the three mechanisms that show responses within seconds. These are (1) the baroreceptor feedback mechanism, (2) the central nervous system ischemic mechanism, and (3) the chemoreceptor mechanism. These not only begin to react within seconds, but they are also very powerful. After any acute fall in pressure, as might be caused by severe hemorrhage, the nervous mechanisms combine to cause constriction of the veins to provide increased transfer of blood into the heart, increased heart rate and contractility of the heart to provide greater pumping capacity by the heart, and constriction of the arterioles to impede the flow of the blood

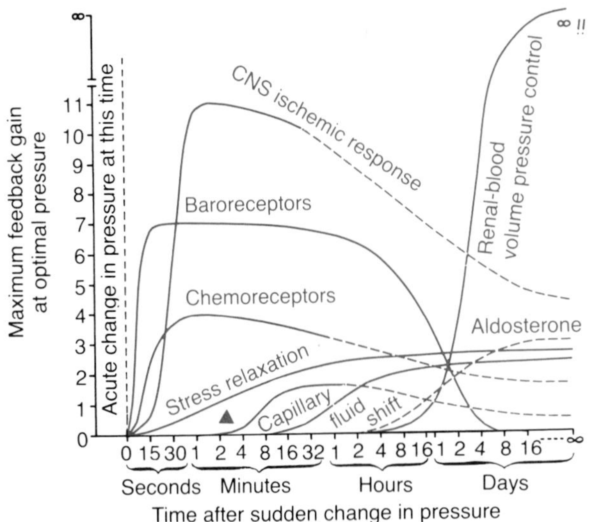

Figure 16-13. Approximate patency of various arterial pressure control mechanisms at different time intervals after the onset of a disturbance to the arterial pressure. Note especially the infinite gain of the renal-body fluid pressure control mechanism that occurs after a few days' time. (Reprinted from Guyton: Arterial Pressure and Hypertension. Philadelphia, W. B. Saunders Company, 1980.)

out of the arteries; all these effects occur almost instantly to raise the arterial pressure back into a survival range.

The Intermediate Time-Period Pressure Control Mechanisms. Several pressure control mechanisms exhibit significant responses only after a few minutes following an acute arterial pressure change. Three of these, illustrated in Figure 16-13, are (1) the renin-angiotensin vasoconstrictor mechanism, (2) stress-relaxation of the vasculature, and (3) shift of fluid through the capillary walls in and out of the circulation to readjust the blood volume as needed.

These three intermediate mechanisms become mostly activated within 30 minutes to several hours. Their effect can last for long periods of time, days if necessary. During this time, the nervous mechanisms usually fatigue and become less and less effective, which explains the importance of these intermediate pressure control measures.

The Long-Term Mechanisms for Arterial Pressure Regulation. The goal of the present chapter has been to explain the role of the kidneys in long-term control of arterial pressure. To the far right in Figure 16-13 is shown the renal-blood volume pressure control mechanism (which is the same as the renal-body fluid pressure control mechanism), illustrating that it takes a few hours to show any significant response. Yet, it eventually develops a feedback gain for control of arterial pressure equal to infinity. This means that this mechanism can eventually return the arterial pressure *all the way* back to that pressure level that will provide normal output of salt and water by the kidneys. By now, the reader should be fully familiar with this concept, which has been the major point of the present chapter.

However, it must also be remembered that many different factors can affect the pressure regulating level of the renal-body fluid mechanism. One of these, illustrated in Figure 16-13, is aldosterone. And another is the interaction of the renin-angiotensin system with the aldosterone and renal fluid mechanism.

Thus, arterial pressure control begins with the lifesaving measures of the nervous pressure controls, then continues with the sustaining characteristics of the intermediate pressure controls, and, finally is stabilized at the long-term pressure level by the renal-body fluid mechanism. This long-term mechanism, in turn, has multiple interactions with the renin-angiotensin-aldosterone system, the nervous system, and several other factors that provide special control capabilities for special purposes.

REFERENCES

Bohr, D. F.: Cell membrane in hypertension. News Physiol. Sci., 4:85, 1989.

Coleman, T. G., and Guyton, A. C.: Hypertension caused by salt loading in the dog. III. Onset transients of cardiac output and other circulatory variables. Circ. Res., 25:153, 1969.

Cowley, A. W., Jr., et al.: Vasopressin: Cellular and Integrative Functions. New York, Raven Press, 1988.

Folkman, J.: Angiogenesis: What makes blood vessels grow? News Physiol. Sci., 1:199, 1986.

Glorioso, N., et al.: Renovascular Hypertension. New York, Raven Press, 1987.

Guyton, A. C.: Arterial Pressure and Hypertension. Philadelphia, W. B. Saunders Co., 1980.

Guyton, A. C., and Coleman, T. G.: Quantitative analysis of the pathophysiology of hypertension. Circ. Res., 24:1, 1969.

Guyton, A. C., et al.: A systems analysis approach to understanding long-range arterial blood pressure control and hypertension. Circ. Res., 35:159, 1974.

Kaplan, N. M., et al.: The Kidney in Hypertension. New York, Raven Press, 1987.

Laragh, J. H., et al.: Endocrine Mechanisms in Hypertension (Perspectives in Hypertension, Vol. 2). New York, Raven Press, 1989.

Meyer, P., and Marche, P.: Blood Cells and Arteries in Hypertension and Atherosclerosis (Atherosclerosis Reviews, Vol. 19). New York, Raven Press, 1989.

Reid, J. L., and Rubin, P. C.: Peptides and central neural regulation of the circulation. Physiol. Rev., 67:725, 1987.

Vanhoutte, P. M.: Calcium-entry blockers, vascular smooth muscle and systemic hypertension. Am. J. Cardiol., 55:17B, 1985.

QUESTIONS

1. Describe the overall renal-body fluid system for arterial pressure control.
2. Describe the renal function curve.
3. Describe graphical analysis of arterial pressure control by the renal-body fluid mechanism, using the renal function curve and the curve (or line) that represents the level of water and salt intake.

4. What is meant by the *infinite gain principle* for control of arterial pressure by the renal–body fluid mchanism?
5. What are the two determinants of the long-term arterial pressure level?
6. Explain the role of autoregulation in increasing the total peripheral resistance in volume-loading hypertension.
7. Why does the autoregulation mechanism reduce to a very small amount the volume accumulation that is required to cause hypertension?
8. Explain how angiotensin alters the renal function curve and why this causes a long-term increase in arterial pressure.
9. Explain how aldosterone alters the renal function curve and why this causes a long-term increase in arterial pressure.
10. What are the basic differences between volume-loading hypertension and vasoconstrictor hypertension?
11. Explain why the renal–body fluid pressure control mechanism plays an essential role in determining the long-term arterial pressure level even in the vasoconstrictor types of hypertension.
12. Describe Goldblatt hypertension.
13. What are the characteristics of essential hypertension?
14. How is renal function altered in essential hypertension?

17

Cardiac Output and Circulatory Shock

Cardiac output is the quantity of blood pumped by the left ventricle into the aorta each minute. It is perhaps the single most important factor that we have to consider in relation to the circulation, for it is cardiac output that is responsible for transport of substances to and from the tissues.

Normal Values for Cardiac Output

The normal cardiac output for the young healthy male adult averages approximately 5.6 liters per minute. However, if we consider all adults, including older people and women, the average cardiac output is very close to 5 liters per minute. In general, the cardiac output of women is about 10 per cent less than that of men of the same body size.

The cardiac output increases approximately in proportion to the surface area of the body. Therefore, the cardiac output is frequently stated in terms of the *cardiac index,* which is the *cardiac output per square meter of body surface area.* The normal human being weighing 70 kilograms has a body surface area of approximately 1.7 square meters, which means that the normal average cardiac index for adults of all ages is approximately 3.0 liters per minute per square meter.

CONTROL OF CARDIAC OUTPUT BY VENOUS RETURN—ROLE OF THE FRANK-STARLING MECHANISM OF THE HEART

When one states that cardiac output is controlled by venous return, one means that it is not the heart itself that is the primary controller of cardiac output, but instead it is the various factors of the peripheral circulation that affect the flow of blood into the heart from the veins, called *venous return,* that are the primary controllers.

The main reason why peripheral factors are normally more important in controlling cardiac output is that the heart has a built-in mechanism that allows it to pump automatically whatever amount of blood flows into the right atrium from the veins. This mechanism, called the *Frank-Starling law of the heart,* was discussed in Chapter 8. Basically, when increased quantities of blood flow into the heart, this stretches the walls of the heart chambers. As a result of the stretch, the cardiac muscle contracts with increased force and empties the chambers almost as much as ever. Therefore, all the extra blood flowing into the heart is automatically pumped without delay on into the aorta and flows again through the systemic circulation.

Therefore, under most normal unstressful conditions, the cardiac output is controlled mainly by peripheral factors that determine the venous return. We see later in the chapter that when the returning blood is more than the heart can pump, the heart does then become a major factor in cardiac output regulation.

Cardiac Output Regulation Is the Sum of All Local Blood Flow Regulations—Effect of Body Metabolism

The venous return to the heart is the sum of all the local blood flows from the individual segments of the peripheral circulation. Therefore, it follows that cardiac output regulation is the sum of all the local blood flow regulations. Chapter 14 discussed the mechanisms of local blood flow regulation. In most tissues, the blood flow increases mainly in proportion to the tissue's metabolism. For instance, the blood flow almost always increases when tissue oxygen consumption increases, which is illustrated in Figure 17–1, during different levels of exercise. Note that, at each increasing level of exercise, both the oxygen consumption and the cardiac output increase in a parallel manner.

Therefore, normally the cardiac output is determined principally by the sum of the various factors throughout the body that control local blood flow. All the different local blood flows summate to form the venous return, and the heart automatically pumps this returning blood back into the arteries to flow around the system again.

The Heart Has a Pumping Limit—The Plateau Level of the Cardiac Output Curve

What we have said thus far about cardiac output control has assumed that the heart has the strength to cope with whatever amount of blood returns to it from the periphery and can pump all of this blood from the veins into the arteries as it returns. However, there are definite limits to the amount of blood that the heart can pump, which are best expressed in the form of cardiac output curves.

Figure 17–2 illustrates by the central heavy black curve the normal cardiac output curve, showing the cardiac output per minute at each level of right atrial pressure. This is one type of *cardiac function curve,* which was discussed in Chapter 8. Note that the plateau level of this normal cardiac output curve is about 13 liters/min, two and one half times the normal cardiac output of about 5 liters/min. This means that the normal heart, functioning without any excess nervous stimulation, can pump an amount of venous return up to about two and one half times the normal venous return before the heart becomes a limiting factor in the control of cardiac output.

Shown in red in Figure 17–2 are several other cardiac output curves for hearts not pumping normally. The uppermost curves are for *hypereffective* hearts

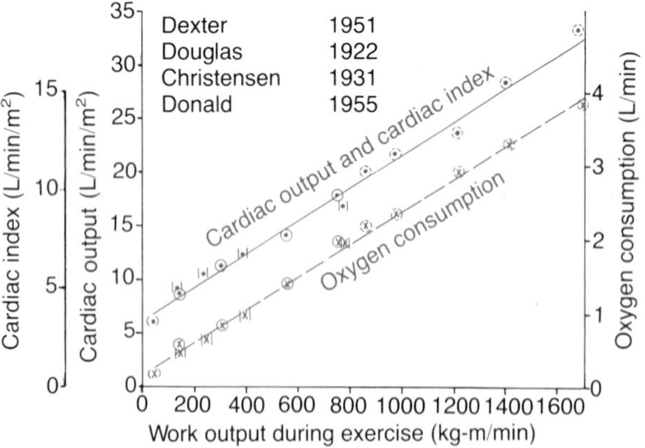

Figure 17–1. Relationships between cardiac output and work output (solid curve) and between oxygen consumption and work output (dashed curve) during different levels of exercise. (From Guyton, Jones, and Coleman: Circulatory Physiology: Cardiac Output and Its Regulation. Philadelphia, W. B. Saunders Company, 1973.)

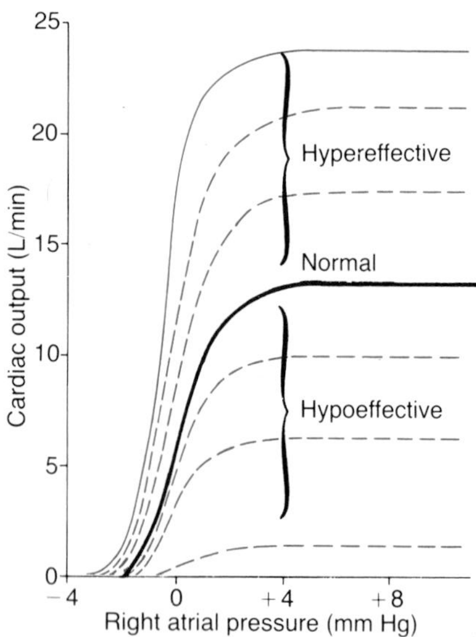

Figure 17–2. Cardiac output curves for the normal heart and for hypoeffective and hypereffective hearts. (From Guyton, Jones, and Coleman: Circulatory Physiology: Cardiac Output and Its Regulation. Philadelphia, W. B. Saunders, 1973.)

that are pumping better than normal. The lowermost curves are for *hypoeffective hearts,* pumping at levels below normal.

The Hypereffective Heart and Factors That Can Cause Hypereffectivity

Only two types of factors can make the heart a better pump than normal. These are (1) nervous stimulation and (2) hypertrophy of the heart muscle.

Effect of Nervous Excitation to Increase Heart Pumping. In Chapter 8, we saw that a combination of sympathetic *stimulation* and parasympathetic *inhibition* will do two things to increase the pumping effectiveness of the heart: (1) greatly increase the heart rate—sometimes to as much as 180 to 200 beats per minute—and (2) increase the strength of heart contraction, which is called increased "contractility," to as much as two times the normal strength. Combining these two effects, maximal nervous excitation of the heart can raise the plateau level of the cardiac output curve to almost two times the plateau of the normal curve, as illustrated by the 25-liter level of the uppermost curve.

Increased Pumping Effectiveness Caused by Heart Hypertrophy. A heart that is subjected to increased workload, but not so much excess load that it damages the heart, will cause the heart muscle to increase in mass and contractile strength in the same way that heavy exercise causes skeletal muscles to hypertrophy. For instance, it is common for the hearts of marathon runners to be increased in mass as much as 50 to 75 per cent. This increases the plateau level of the cardiac output curve, sometimes by as much as 50 to 100 per cent, and therefore allows the heart to pump much greater than usual amounts of cardiac output.

When one combines both nervous excitation of the

heart plus hypertrophy, as occurs in marathon runners, the combined effect can allow the heart to pump as much as 30 to 35 liters/min; this increased level of pumping is one of the most important factors in determining the running time of the runner.

Factors That Cause a Hypoeffective Heart

Obviously, any factor that decreases the ability of the heart to pump blood will cause hypoeffectivity. Some of the numerous factors are

- Inhibition of nervous excitation of the heart.
- Pathological factors that cause abnormal rhythm or rate of heart beat.
- Valvular heart disease.
- Increased arterial pressure against which the heart must pump, such as in hypertension.
- Congenital heart disease.
- Myocarditis.
- Cardiac anoxia.
- Diphtheritic or other types of myocardial damage or toxicity.

What is the Role of the Nervous System in Controlling Cardiac Output?

Importance of the Nervous System to Maintain the Arterial Pressure When Tissue Blood Flow Increases

Figure 17–3 illustrates an important difference in cardiac output control with and without a functioning autonomic nervous system. The solid curves show the effect in the normal animal of intense dilatation of the peripheral blood vessels caused by administering the drug dinitrophenol, which increased the metabolism of virtually all tissues of the body about fourfold. Note that with normal nervous control, dilating all of the peripheral blood vessels caused almost no change in arterial pressure but increased the cardiac output almost fourfold. However, after autonomic control of the nervous system had been totally blocked, none of the normal circulatory reflexes for maintaining the arterial pressure could function, and vasodilation of the vessels with dinitrophenol (dashed curves) then caused a profound fall in arterial pressure to about one half normal, while the cardiac output rose only 1.6-fold instead of 4-fold.

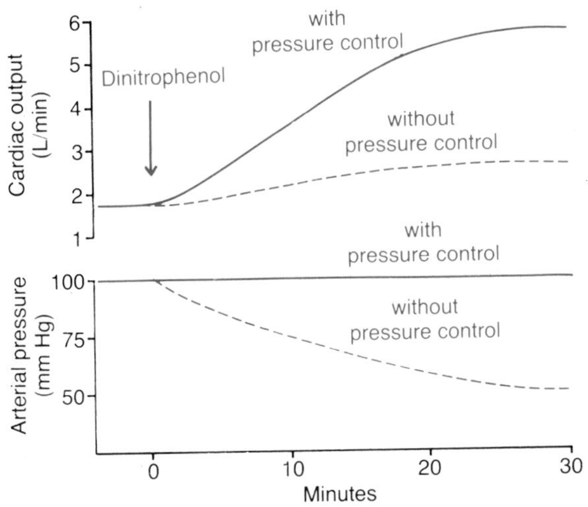

Figure 17–3. An experiment in a dog to demonstrate the importance of nervous control of arterial pressure as a prerequisite for cardiac output control. Note that with pressure control, the metabolic stimulant dinitrophenol increases cardiac output; without pressure control, the arterial pressure falls and the cardiac output rises very little. (Drawn from experiments by Dr. M. Banet.)

Therefore, maintenance of a normal arterial pressure by the nervous reflexes, by mechanisms explained in Chapter 15, is essential to achieve high cardiac outputs when the peripheral tissues dilate their vessels to increase their local blood flow.

Effect of the Nervous System to *Increase* the Arterial Pressure and Cardiac Output During Exercise. During exercise, the nervous system not only prevents the arterial pressure from falling, but it also actually *increases* the pressure. The cause of this is mainly the following: The same brain activity that sends signals to the peripheral muscles to cause exercise also sends simultaneous signals into the autonomic centers to excite circulatory activity, causing venous constriction, increased heart rate, and increased contractility of the heart; all these changes acting together increase the arterial pressure even above normal, which in turn forces more blood flow through the tissues. This increased pressure often allows the cardiac output to increase during exercise at least an extra 50 per cent or more.

In summary, when the local tissue vessels dilate and attempt to increase the cardiac output above normal, the nervous system plays an exceedingly important role in preventing the arterial pressure from falling to disastrously low levels. In fact, in exercise, the nervous system goes even further, providing additional signals to raise the arterial pressure above normal, which serves to increase the cardiac output an extra 50 per cent or more.

PATHOLOGICALLY HIGH AND PATHOLOGICALLY LOW CARDIAC OUTPUTS

In normal human beings, the cardiac outputs are surprisingly constant from one person to another. However, multiple clinical abnormalities can cause either high or low cardiac outputs. Some of the more important of these are illustrated in Figure 17–4.

High Cardiac Output—Virtually Always Caused by Reduced Total Peripheral Resistance

The left side of Figure 17–4 identifies pathological conditions that commonly cause cardiac outputs higher than normal. One of the distinguishing features of these is that *they all result from chronically reduced total peripheral resistance.* None of them result from excessive excitation of the heart itself, which we explain subsequently. For the present, let us

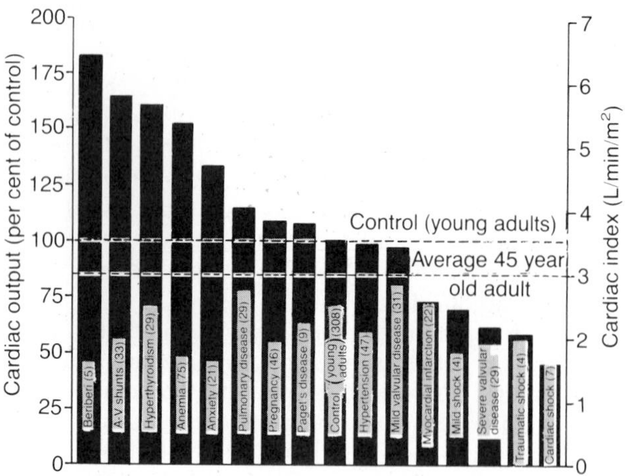

Figure 17-4. Cardiac output in different pathological conditions. The numbers in parentheses indicate number of patients studied in each condition. (From Guyton, Jones, and Coleman: Circulatory Physiology: Cardiac Output and Its Regulation. Philadelphia, W. B. Saunders Company, 1973.)

look at some of the peripheral factors that can increase the cardiac output to above normal:

1. *Beriberi.* This is a disease caused by insufficient quantity of the vitamin *thiamine* in the diet. Lack of this vitamin causes diminished ability of the tissues to use cellular nutrients, and the local tissue blood flow mechanisms in turn cause marked peripheral vasodilation. The total peripheral resistance decreases sometimes to as little as one half normal. Consequently, the long-term level of cardiac output also often increases to as much as two times normal.
2. *Arteriovenous fistula (shunt).* Whenever a fistula (also called a shunt) occurs between a major artery and a major vein, tremendous amounts of blood will flow directly from the artery into the vein. This, too, greatly decreases the total peripheral resistance and likewise increases the venous return and cardiac output.
3. *Hyperthyroidism.* In hyperthyroidism, the metabolism of all the tissues of the body becomes greatly increased. Oxygen usage increases, and vasodilator products are released from the tissues. Therefore, the total peripheral resistance decreases markedly, again because of the local tissue blood flow control reactions throughout the body. The cardiac output often increases to as much as 40 to 80 per cent above normal.
4. *Anemia.* In anemia, two peripheral effects greatly decrease the total peripheral resistance. One of these is reduced viscosity of the blood, resulting from the decreased concentration of red blood cells. The other is diminished delivery of oxygen to the tissues because of the decreased hemoglobin, which causes local vasodilation. As a consequence, the cardiac output increases greatly.

Any other factor that decreases the total peripheral resistance chronically will also increase the cardiac output.

Failure of Increased Cardiac Pumping to Cause Prolonged Increase of the Cardiac Output. If the heart is suddenly stimulated excessively, the cardiac output often increases by as much as 20 to 30 per cent. However, even this small increase is maintained no longer than a few minutes, even though the heart continues to be strongly stimulated. There are two reasons for this: (1) Excess blood flow through the tissues causes automatic vasoconstriction of the blood vessels because of the autoregulation mechanism discussed in previous chapters, and this reduces the venous return and cardiac output back toward normal. (2) The slightly increased arterial pressure that results following acute cardiac stimulation raises the capillary pressure, and fluid filters out of the capillaries into the tissues, thereby decreasing the blood volume and also decreasing the venous return back toward normal. Over a period of hours and days, the increased pressure also causes the kidneys to lose fluid volume until the arterial pressure and cardiac output return to normal.

Thus, all the known conditions that cause *chronic* elevation of the cardiac output result from decreased total peripheral resistance and not increased cardiac activity.

Low Output

Figure 17-4 illustrates to the far right the conditions that cause abnormally low cardiac output. These fall into two categories: (1) abnormalities that cause the pumping effectiveness of the heart to fall too low and (2) those that cause venous return to fall too low.

Decreased Cardiac Output Caused by Cardiac Factors. Whenever the heart becomes severely damaged, from whatever cause, its limiting level of pumping may fall below that needed for adequate blood flow to the tissues. Some examples of this include *severe myocardial infarction, severe valvular heart disease, myocarditis, cardiac tamponade,* and certain *cardiac metabolic derangements.* The effect of several of these is illustrated on the right in Figure 17-4, showing the low cardiac outputs that result.

Decrease in Cardiac Output Caused by Peripheral Factors—Decreased Venous Return. Any factor that interferes with venous return also can lead to decreased cardiac output. Two of the most important of these are: (1) *decreased blood volume,* and (2) *acute venous dilation.* These will be discussed fully later in the chapter in relation to circulatory shock, which results when the cardiac output falls so low that the tissues begin to suffer and even die for lack of adequate nutrition.

METHODS FOR MEASURING CARDIAC OUTPUT

In animal experiments, one can cannulate the aorta, the pulmonary artery, or the great veins entering the heart and measure the cardiac output using any type of flowmeter. For instance, an electromagnetic or ultrasonic flowmeter can be placed on the aorta or pulmonary artery to measure cardiac output. However, except in rare instances, in the human, cardiac output is measured by indirect methods that do not require surgery. Two of the methods commonly used are the *oxygen Fick method* and the *indicator dilution method.*

Measurement of Cardiac Output by the Oxygen Fick Method

The Fick procedure is explained by Figure 17–5. This figure shows that 200 milliliters of oxygen are being absorbed from the lungs into the pulmonary blood each minute. It also illustrates that the blood entering the right side of the heart has an oxygen concentration of 160 milliliters per liter of blood, whereas that leaving the left side has an oxygen concentration of 200 milliliters per liter of blood. From these data one can calculate that each liter of blood passing through the lungs picks up 40 milliliters of oxygen. Since the total quantity of oxygen absorbed into the blood from the lungs each minute is 200 milliliters, a total of five 1-liter portions of blood must pass through the pulmonary circulation each minute to absorb this amount of oxygen. Therefore, the quantity of blood flowing through the lungs each minute is 5 liters, which is also a measure of the cardiac output. Thus, the cardiac output can be calculated by the following formula:

$$\text{Cardiac output (liters/min)} = \frac{O_2 \text{ absorbed per minute by the lungs (ml/min)}}{\text{Arteriovenous } O_2 \text{ difference (ml/liter of blood)}}$$

In applying the Fick procedure, mixed venous blood is usually obtained through a catheter inserted up the brachial vein of the forearm, through the subclavian vein, down to the right atrium, and finally into the right ventricle or pulmonary artery. Arterial blood can be obtained from any artery in the body, and the rate of oxygen absorption by the lungs is measured by the disappearance of oxygen from the respired air, using any of many types of oxygen meters.

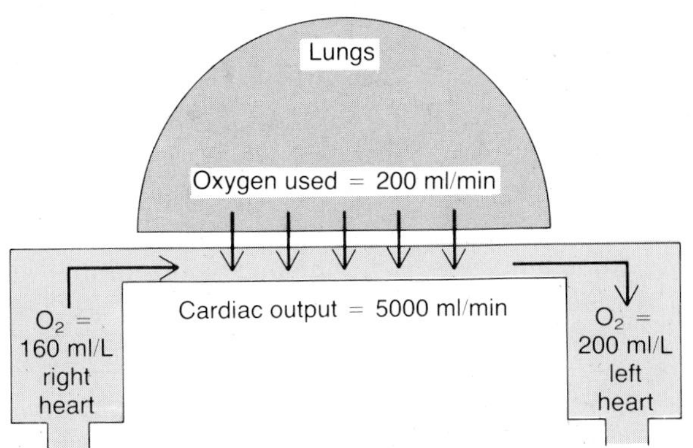

Figure 17–5. The Fick principle for determining cardiac output.

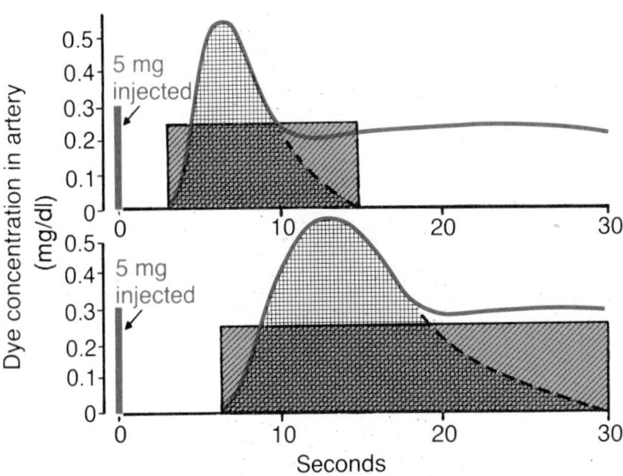

Figure 17–6. Dye concentration curves used to calculate the cardiac output by the dilution method. (The rectangular areas are the calculated average concentrations of dye in the arterial blood for the durations of the respective curves.)

The Indicator Dilution Method

In measuring the cardiac output by the indicator dilution method, a small amount of *indicator,* such as a dye, is injected into a large vein or preferably into the right side of the heart itself. This passes rapidly through the right heart, the lungs, the left heart, and finally into the arterial system. Then one records the concentration of the dye as it passes through one of the peripheral arteries, giving a curve such as one of the two red curves illustrated in Figure 17–6. In each of these instances, 5 milligrams of Cardio-Green dye was injected at zero time. In the top recording, none of the dye passed into the arterial tree until approximately 3 seconds after the injection, but then the arterial concentration of the dye rose rapidly to a maximum in approximately 6 to 7 seconds. After that, the concentration fell rapidly. However, before the concentration reached the zero point, some of the dye had already circulated all the way through some of the peripheral vessels and returned through the heart for a second time. Consequently, the dye concentration in the artery began to rise again. For the purpose of calculation, however, it is necessary to extrapolate the early downslope of the curve to the zero point, as shown by the dashed portion of the curve. In this way, the *time-concentration curve* of the dye in an artery can be measured in its first portion and estimated reasonably accurately in its latter portion.

Once the time-concentration curve has been determined, one can then calculate the mean concentration of dye in the arterial blood for the duration of the curve. In Figure 17–6, this was done by measuring the area under the entire curve and then averaging the concentration of dye for the duration of the curve; one can see from the shaded rectangle straddling the upper curve of the figure that the average concentration of dye was approximately 0.25 mg/dl of blood and that the duration of this average value was 12 seconds. A total of 5 mg of dye was injected at the beginning of the experiment. In order for blood carrying only 0.25 mg of dye in each deciliter to carry the entire 5 mg of dye through the heart and lungs in 12 seconds, it would be necessary for a total of 20 1-deciliter portions of blood to pass through the heart during this time, which would be the same as a cardiac output of 2 liters per 12 seconds, or 10 liters/min.

We leave it to the reader to calculate the cardiac output from the bottom curve of Figure 17–6.

To summarize, the cardiac output can be determined using the following formula:

$$\text{Cardiac output (ml/min)} = \frac{\text{Milligrams of dye injected} \times 60}{\left(\begin{array}{c}\text{Average concentration of}\\ \text{dye in each milliliter of blood}\\ \text{for the duration of the curve}\end{array}\right) \times \left(\begin{array}{c}\text{Duration of}\\ \text{the curve}\\ \text{in seconds}\end{array}\right)}$$

CIRCULATORY SHOCK

Circulatory shock means generalized inadequacy of blood flow throughout the body to the extent that the tissues are damaged because of too little flow, especially too little delivery of oxygen and other nutrients to the tissue cells. Even the cardiovascular system itself—the heart musculature, the walls of the blood vessels, the vasomotor system, and other circulatory parts—begins to deteriorate, so that the shock becomes progressively worse.

Circulatory Shock Caused by Decreased Cardiac Output

Shock usually results from inadequate cardiac output. Therefore, any factor that reduces the cardiac output will likely lead to circulatory shock. Basically, two types of factors can severely reduce the cardiac output; these are

1. *Cardiac abnormalities that decrease the ability of the heart to pump blood.* These include especially *myocardial infarction* but also *toxic states of the heart, severe heart valve dysfunction,* heart *arrhythmias,* and other conditions. The circulatory shock that results from diminished cardiac pumping ability is called *cardiogenic shock.* This is discussed also in Chapter 19, where it is pointed out that about 85 per cent of persons who develop cardiogenic shock do not survive.
2. *Factors that decrease the venous return.* The most common cause of this is *diminished blood volume,* but venous return also can be reduced as a result of decreased *vasomotor tone* or *obstruction to blood flow* at some point in the circulation, especially in the venous return pathway to the heart.

What Happens to the Arterial Pressure in Circulatory Shock?

In the minds of many physicians, the arterial pressure is the principal measure of the adequacy of circulatory function. However, the arterial pressure often can be seriously misleading because many times a person may be in severe shock and still have almost a normal pressure because powerful nervous reflexes often keep the pressure from falling. Yet at other times the arterial pressure can fall to as low as one-half normal, but the person still has normal tissue perfusion and is not in shock.

Nevertheless, it is true that in most types of shock, especially that caused by severe blood loss, the arterial blood pressure usually does decrease at the same time that the cardiac output decreases, though usually not as much as the decrease in output.

The End-Stages of Circulatory Shock, Whatever the Cause

Once circulatory shock reaches a critical state of severity, regardless of its initiating cause, *the shock itself breeds more shock.* That is, the inadequate blood flow causes the circulatory system itself to begin to deteriorate. This in turn causes even more decrease in cardiac output, and a vicious circle ensues, with progressively increasing circulatory shock, still less adequate tissue perfusion, still more shock, and so forth until death. It is with this late stage of the circulatory shock that we are especially concerned because appropriate physiological treatment can often reverse the rapid slide to oblivion.

The Stages of Shock. Because the characteristics of circulatory shock change at different degrees of severity, shock is generally divided into three major stages:

1. A *nonprogressive stage* (sometimes called the *compensated stage*), from which the normal circulatory compensatory mechanisms will eventually cause full recovery without any help from outside therapy.
2. A *progressive stage,* in which the shock becomes steadily worse until death.
3. An *irreversible stage,* in which the shock has progressed to such an extent that all forms of known therapy will be inadequate to save the life of the person even though for the moment the person is still alive.

Now, let us discuss the different stages of circulatory shock caused by decreased blood volume, which will illustrate the basic principles. Then we can consider the special characteristics of other initiating causes of shock.

SHOCK CAUSED BY HYPOVOLEMIA—HEMORRHAGIC SHOCK

Hypovolemia means diminished blood volume, and hemorrhage is the most common cause of hypovolemic shock.

Hemorrhage *decreases* the degree of filling of all the blood vessels in the body and as a consequence decreases venous return. As a result, the cardiac output falls below normal, and shock ensues. Obviously, all degrees of shock can result from hemorrhage, from the mildest diminishment of cardiac output to almost complete cessation of output.

Relationship of Bleeding Volume to Cardiac Output and Arterial Pressure

Figure 17-7 illustrates the approximate effect on both cardiac output and arterial pressure of removing blood from the circulatory system over a period of about half an hour. Approximately 10 per cent of the total blood volume can be removed with no significant effect on either arterial pressure or cardiac output, but greater blood loss usually diminishes the cardiac output first and later the pressure, both of these falling to zero when about 35 to 45 per cent of the total blood volume has been removed.

Sympathetic Reflex Compensation in Shock. Fortunately, the decrease in arterial pressure as well as decrease in pressures in the low pressure areas of the thorax following hemorrhage initiates powerful sympathetic reflexes (initiated mainly by the baroreceptors and the low pressure stretch receptors). These reflexes stimulate the sympathetic vasoconstrictor system throughout the body, resulting in three important effects: (1) The arterioles constrict in most parts of the body, thereby greatly increasing the total peripheral resistance. (2) The veins and venous reservoirs constrict, thereby helping to maintain adequate venous return despite diminished blood volume. (3) Heart activity increases markedly, sometimes increasing the heart rate from the normal value of 72 beats per minute to as much as 170 to 200 beats per minute.

Value of the Reflexes. In the absence of the sympathetic reflexes, only 15 to 20 per cent of the blood volume can be removed over a period of half an hour before a person will die; this is in contrast to a 30 to 40 per cent loss of blood volume that a person can sustain when the reflexes are intact. Therefore, the reflexes extend the amount of blood loss that can occur without causing death to about two times that which is possible in their absence.

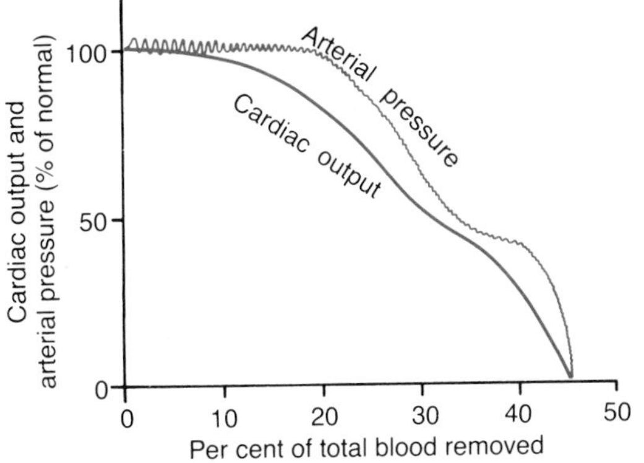

Figure 17-7. Effect of hemorrhage on cardiac output and arterial pressure.

Protection of Coronary and Cerebral Blood Flow by the Reflexes. A special value of the maintenance of normal arterial pressure even in the face of decreasing cardiac output is protection of blood flow through the coronary and cerebral circulatory systems. Sympathetic stimulation does not cause significant constriction of either the cerebral or the cardiac vessels. In addition, in both these vascular beds local autoregulation is excellent, which prevents moderate decreases in arterial pressure from significantly affecting their blood flows. Therefore, blood flow through the heart and brain is maintained essentially at normal levels as long as the arterial pressure does not fall below about 70 mm Hg, despite the fact that blood flow in many other areas of the body might be decreased to as little as one-quarter normal by this time because of vasospasm.

Nonprogressive Shock—Compensated Shock

If shock is not too severe, the person eventually recovers. Therefore, shock of this lesser degree can be called *nonprogressive shock.* It is also frequently called *compensated shock,* meaning that the sympathetic reflexes and other factors have compensated enough to prevent further deterioration of the circulation.

The factors that cause a person to recover from moderate degrees of shock are all the negative feedback control mechanisms of the circulation that attempt to return cardiac output and arterial pressure to normal levels. These include

1. The *baroreceptor reflexes,* which elicit powerful sympathetic stimulation of the circulation.
2. The *central nervous system ischemic response,* which elicits even more powerful sympathetic stimulation throughout the body but is not activated significantly until the arterial pressure falls below 50 mm Hg.
3. *Formation of angiotensin,* which constricts the peripheral arteries and causes increased conservation of water and salt by the kidneys, both of which help prevent progression of the shock.
4. *Formation of vasopressin (antidiuretic hormone),* which constricts the peripheral arteries and veins and also greatly increases water retention by the kidneys.
5. *Compensation mechanisms that return the blood volume back toward normal,* including absorption of large quantities of fluid from the intestinal tract, absorption of fluid from the interstitial spaces of the body, conservation of water and salt by the kidneys, and increased thirst and increased appetite for salt, which make the person drink water and eat salty foods if able.

Progressive Shock—The Vicious Circle of Cardiovascular Deterioration

Once shock has become severe enough, the structures of the circulatory system themselves begin to deteriorate, and various types of positive feedback develop that can cause a vicious circle of progressively decreasing cardiac output. Figure 17–8 illustrates some of these positive feedbacks that further depress the cardiac output in shock. Among the more important of these are the following:

Cardiac Depression. When the arterial pressure falls low enough, *coronary blood flow decreases below that required for adequate nutrition of the myocardium* itself. This obviously weakens the heart and thereby decreases the cardiac output still more. Thus, a positive feedback cycle has developed whereby the shock becomes more and more severe.

Vasomotor Failure. In the early stages of shock, various circulatory reflexes cause intense activity of the sympathetic nervous system. This, as discussed previously, helps delay depression of the cardiac output and especially helps prevent decreased arterial pressure. However, there comes a point at which diminished blood flow to the vasomotor center itself so depresses the center that it becomes progressively less active and finally totally inactive. For instance, complete circulatory arrest to the brain causes, during the first 4 to 8 minutes, the most intense of all sympathetic discharges, but by the end of 10 to 15 minutes, the vasomotor center becomes so depressed that no evidence of sympathetic discharge at all can be demonstrated. Fortunately, though, the vasomotor center does not usually fail in the early stages of shock—only in the late stages.

Release of Toxins by Ischemic Tissues. Throughout the history of research in the field of shock, it has been suggested time and again that shock causes tissues to release toxic substances, such as histamine, serotonin, tissue enzymes, and so forth, that then cause further deterioration of the circulatory system. Quantitative studies have especially proved the significance of at least one toxin, *endotoxin,* in many types of shock.

Endotoxin. Endotoxin is a toxin released from the bodies of dead gram-negative bacteria in the intestines. Diminished blood flow to the intestines causes enhanced formation and absorption of this toxic substance, and it then causes extensive vascular dilatation, greatly increased cellular metabolism despite the inadequate nutrition of the cells, and cardiac depression. This toxin can play a major role in some types of shock, especially septic shock, discussed later in the chapter.

Generalized Cellular Deterioration. As shock becomes very severe, many signs of generalized cellular deterioration occur throughout the body. One organ especially affected is the *liver,* primarily because of the lack of enough nutrients to support the normally high rate of metabolism in liver cells, but also partly because of the extreme vascular exposure of the liver cells to any toxic or other abnormal metabolic factor in shock.

Among the different damaging cellular effects that are known to occur are the following:

1. Active transport of sodium and potassium through the cell membrane is greatly diminished. As a result, sodium and chloride accumulate in the cells and potassium is lost from the cells. In addition, the cells begin to swell.
2. Mitochondrial activity in the liver cells as well as in many other tissues of the body becomes severely depressed.
3. Lysosomes begin to split in widespread tissue areas, with intracellular release of hydrolases that cause further intracellular deterioration.

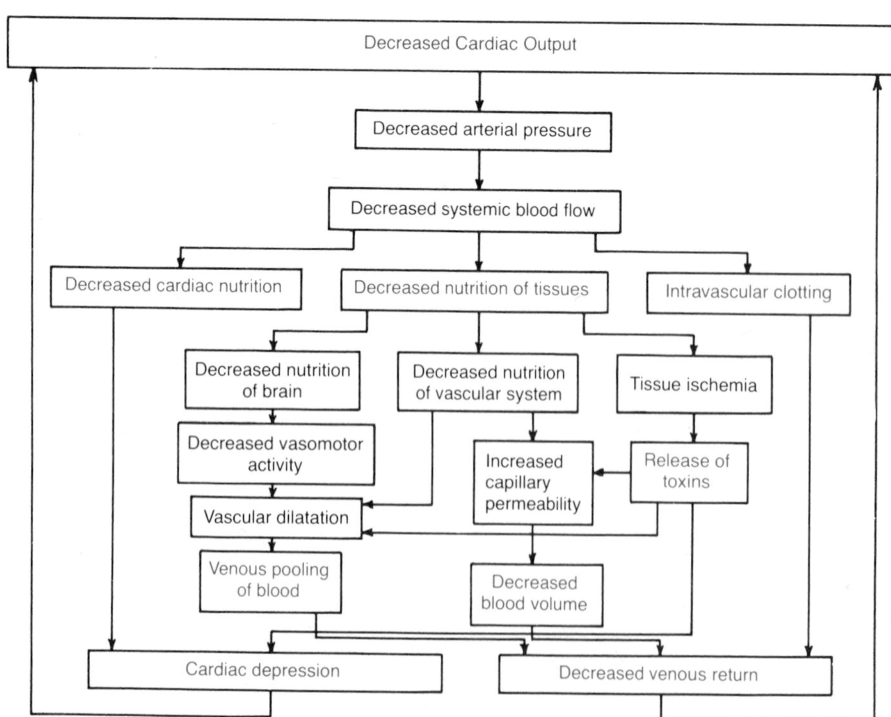

Figure 17–8. Different types of feedback that can lead to progression of shock.

4. Cellular metabolism of nutrients, such as glucose, eventually becomes greatly depressed in the last stages of shock.

Obviously, all these effects contribute to further deterioration of many different organs of the body, including especially (1) the *liver*, with depression of its many metabolic and detoxification functions; (2) the lungs, with eventual development of pulmonary edema and poor ability to oxygenate the blood; and (3) the heart, thereby further depressing the contractility of the heart.

Irreversible Shock

After shock has progressed to a certain stage, transfusion or any other type of therapy becomes incapable of saving the life of the person. Therefore, the person is then said to be in the *irreversible stage of shock.* Ironically, even in this irreversible stage, therapy can on occasion still return the arterial pressure and even the cardiac output to normal for short periods of time, but the circulatory system nevertheless continues to deteriorate, and death ensues in another few minutes to a few hours. The reason for this is that, beyond a certain point, so much tissue damage has occurred, so many destructive enzymes have been released into the body fluids, and so many other destructive factors are now in progress that even a normal cardiac output cannot reverse the continuing deterioration. Therefore, in severe shock a stage is eventually reached beyond which the person is destined to die even though vigorous therapy can still return the cardiac output to normal for short periods of time.

Hypovolemic Shock Caused by Plasma Loss

Loss of plasma from the circulatory system, even without the loss of whole blood, can sometimes be severe enough to reduce the total blood volume markedly, in this way causing typical hypovolemic shock similar in almost all details to that caused by hemorrhage. Severe plasma loss occurs especially in the following conditions:

1. *Intestinal obstruction*, in which distention of the intestine causes fluid to leak from the intestinal capillaries into the intestinal walls and intestinal lumen.
2. In patients who have *severe burns* or other denuding conditions of the skin, so much plasma almost always is lost through the exposed areas that the plasma volume becomes markedly reduced.

SEPTIC SHOCK

The condition that was formerly known by the popular name of "blood poisoning" is now called *septic shock* by most clinicians. This simply means widely disseminated infection to many areas of the body, with the infection being borne through the blood from one tissue to another and causing extensive damage. Actually, there are many different varieties of septic shock because of the many different types of bacterial infection that can cause it and also because infection in one part of the body will produce different effects from those caused by infection elsewhere in the body.

Septic shock causes patient death in the modern hospital more frequently than any other kind of shock besides cardiogenic shock. Some of the typical causes of septic shock include

1. Peritonitis caused by spread of infection from the uterus and fallopian tubes, frequently resulting from instrumental abortion.
2. Peritonitis resulting from rupture of the gut, sometimes caused by intestinal disease and sometimes by wounds.
3. Generalized infection resulting from spread of a simple skin infection, such as streptococcal or staphylococcal infection.
4. Generalized gangrenous infection resulting specifically from gas gangrene bacilli, spreading first through the tissues themselves and finally by way of the blood to the internal organs, especially to the liver.
5. Infection spreading into the blood from the kidney or urinary tract, often caused by colon bacilli.

Special Features of Septic Shock. Because of the multiple types of septic shock, it is difficult to categorize this condition. However, some features are

1. High fever.
2. Marked vasodilation throughout the body, especially in the infected tissues.
3. High cardiac output in perhaps half of the patients, caused by vasodilation in the infected tissues and also by high metabolic rate and vasodilation elsewhere in the body, resulting from bacterial toxin stimulation of cellular metabolism and from the high body temperature.
4. Development of microclots in widespread areas of the body, a condition called *disseminated intravascular coagulation.* Also, this causes the clotting factors to be used up so that hemorrhages occur into many tissues, especially into the gut wall and into the intestinal tract.

In the early stages of septic shock, the patient usually does not have signs of circulatory collapse but, instead, only signs of the bacterial infection itself. However, as the infection becomes more severe, the circulatory system usually becomes involved either directly or as a secondary result of toxins from the bacteria, and *there finally comes a point at which deterioration of the circulation becomes progressive in the same way that progression occurs in all other types of shock. Therefore, the end-stages of septic shock are not greatly different from the end-stages of hemorrhagic shock,* even though the initiating factors are markedly different in the two conditions.

Endotoxin Shock. A special type of septic shock is known as endotoxin shock. It frequently occurs when a large segment of the gut becomes strangulated and loses most of its blood supply. The gut rapidly becomes gangrenous, and the bacteria in the gut multiply rapidly. Most of these bacteria are so-called "gram-negative" bacteria, mainly colon bacilli, that contain a toxin called *endotoxin.*

On entering the circulation, endotoxin causes severe dilation of many or most of the blood vessels of the body, often resulting in severe shock. Also, further compounding the circulatory depression is a direct effect of endotoxin on the heart to decrease myocardial contractility.

EFFECTS OF SHOCK ON THE BODY

In virtually all types of shock, the delivery of both oxygen and other nutrients to the tissues becomes inadequate. This in turn reduces the metabolism of virtually all cells of the body, leading to multiple types of cellular damage, including (1) decreased ability of the mitochondria to synthesize ATP, (2) decreased ability of the cell's membrane pump to keep the sodium concentration low and the potassium concentration high inside the cell, (3) depressed processing of nutrients by the cell's metabolic machinery, and (4) eventual rupture of many lysosomes, releasing digestive enzymes within the cells that cause intracellular destruction and even death of cells. Obviously, all these effects lead to still greater cellular deterioration and further decrease in total bodily metabolism. Usually a person can continue to live for only a few hours if the cardiac output falls to as low as 40 per cent of normal.

Some of the more generalized effects on the body are (1) extreme muscular weakness, (2) sometimes reduced body temperature except in septic shock, (3) depressed brain function with stupor and sometimes coma, and (4) decreased excretion of body waste products by the kidneys, as well as eventual deterioration and self-destruction of the kidney tissue cells.

CIRCULATORY ARREST

A condition closely allied to circulatory shock is circulatory arrest, in which all blood flow completely stops. This occurs frequently on the surgical operating table as a result of *cardiac arrest* or of *ventricular fibrillation.*

Ventricular fibrillation can usually be stopped by strong electroshock of the heart, the basic principles of which were described in Chapter 9.

Cardiac arrest usually results from too little oxygen in the anesthetic gaseous mixture or from a depressant effect of the anesthesia itself. A normal cardiac rhythm can usually be restored by removing the anesthetic and then applying cardiopulmonary resuscitation procedures for a few minutes while supplying the patient's lungs with adequate quantities of ventilatory oxygen.

Effect of Circulatory Arrest on the Brain

A special problem in circulatory arrest is to prevent detrimental effects in the brain as a result of the arrest. In general, 4 to 5 minutes of circulatory arrest causes permanent brain damage in over half the patients. Circulatory arrest for as long as 10 minutes almost universally destroys most, if not all, of the mental powers.

For many years it was taught that this detrimental effect on the brain was caused by the cerebral hypoxia that occurs during circulatory arrest. However, experiments have shown that, if a drug is used to prevent blood clots from occurring in the blood vessels of the brain, this will delay the very rapid deterioration of the brain during circulatory arrest. Therefore, it is likely that the severe brain damage that occurs following circulatory arrest results mainly from permanent blockage of many small or even large blood vessels by blood clots, thus causing prolonged ischemia and eventual death of the neurons.

REFERENCES

Cardiac Output

Coleman, T. G., et al.: Control of cardiac output of regional blood flow distribution. Ann. Biomed. Eng., 2:149, 1974.

Donald, D. E., and Shepherd, J. T.: Response to exercise in dogs with cardiac denervation. Am. J. Physiol., 205:393, 1963.

Grodins, F. S.: Integrative cardiovascular physiology: A mathematical synthesis of cardiac and blood vessel hemodynamics. Q. Rev. Biol., 34:93, 1959.

Guyton, A. C.: Essential cardiovascular regulation—the control linkages between bodily needs and circulatory function. In Dickinson, C. J., and Marks, J. (eds.): Developments in Cardiovascular Medicine. Lancaster, England, MTP Press, 1978, p. 265.

Guyton, A. C.: Venous return. In Hamilton, W. F. (ed.): Handbook of Physiology. Sec. 2, Vol. 2. Baltimore, Williams & Wilkins, 1963, p. 1099.

Guyton, A. C.: Determination of cardiac output by equating venous return curves with cardiac response curves. Physiol. Rev., 35:123, 1955.

Guyton, A. C., et al: Cardiac Output and Its Regulation. Philadelphia, W. B. Saunders Co., 1973.

Lyons, K. P.: Cardiovascular Nuclear Medicine. East Norwalk, Conn., Appleton & Lange, 1988.

Rothe, C. F.: Reflex control of veins and vascular capacitance. Physiol. Rev., 63:1281, 1983.

Sarnoff, S., and Mitchell, J. H.: The regulation of the performance of the heart. Am. J. Med., 30:747, 1961.

Circulatory Shock

Achauer, B. M.: Management of the Burned Patient. East Norwalk, Conn., Appleton & Lange, 1987.

Braunwald, E. (ed.): Heart Disease. A Textbook of Cardiovascular Medicine. Philadelphia, W. B. Saunders Co., 1988.

Heffernan, J. J., et al.: Clinical Problems in Acute Care Medicine. Philadelphia, W. B. Saunders Co., 1989.

Jones, C. E., et al.: A cause-effect relationship between oxygen deficit and irreversible hemorrhagic shock. Surgery, 127:93, 1968.

Luce, J. M., and Pierson, D. J.: Critical Care Medicine. Philadelphia, W. B. Saunders Co., 1988.
Shoemaker, W. C., et al. (eds.): Society of Critical Care Medicine, The Textbook of Critical Care. Philadelphia, W. B. Saunders Co., 1988.
Sibbald, W. J. (ed.): Synopsis of Critical Care. Baltimore, Williams & Wilkins, 1988.
Tintinalli, J. E.: Emergency Medicine: A Comprehensive Study Guide. 2nd ed. New York, McGraw-Hill Book Co., 1988.

QUESTIONS

1. What are the approximate normal values for cardiac output both at rest and during very heavy exercise?
2. Explain why increased metabolism in any given tissue of the body increases both the local blood flow and the cardiac output by approximately the same amount?
3. List and explain the different factors that cause the extreme increases in cardiac output during strenuous exercise.
4. Discuss the different conditions that can cause greatly decreased cardiac output.
5. Discuss the different conditions that can cause high cardiac outputs.
6. Why does increased pumping activity by the heart fail to cause a prolonged increase in cardiac output?
7. If the amount of oxygen absorbed by the lungs per minute is 150 ml and the arteriovenous oxygen difference (arterial oxygen minus venous oxygen) is 60 ml per liter of blood, what is the cardiac output?
8. Explain the indicator dilution method for measuring cardiac output.
9. Give a definition of "circulatory shock."
10. What are the relationships of arterial pressure and cardiac output to circulatory shock?
11. List and explain the different *negative* feedback mechanisms that help to compensate for circulatory shock.
12. List and explain the important *positive* feedback mechanisms that occur in circulatory shock and can lead to progressive shock.
13. What are some of the cellular effects in circulatory shock that lead to generalized cellular deterioration?
14. What causes shock in its extremely severe stages to become irreversible?
15. Explain the causes and special features of *septic shock*.
16. What are the important effects of circulatory shock on bodily function?

18

Muscle Blood Flow and Cardiac Output During Exercise; the Coronary Circulation; Ischemic Heart Disease

In the present chapter we consider blood flow to the skeletal muscles and coronary blood flow to the heart. Regulation of both of these is achieved mainly by local control of vascular resistance by tissue metabolic needs. In addition, related subjects such as cardiac output control during exercise, the characteristics of heart attacks, and the pain of angina pectoris are discussed.

BLOOD FLOW IN SKELETAL MUSCLES AND ITS REGULATION IN EXERCISE

Very strenuous exercise is the most stressful condition that the normal circulatory system faces. This is true because the blood flow in muscles can increase more than 20-fold (a greater increase than in any other tissue of the body) and also because there is such a very large mass of skeletal muscle in the body. The product of these two factors can increase the cardiac output to as much as five times normal, and in the well-trained athlete to as much as six to seven times normal.

Rate of Blood Flow Through the Muscles

During rest, blood flow through skeletal muscle averages 3 to 4 ml/min per 100 grams of muscle. However, during extreme exercise, this rate can increase as much as 15-fold to 25-fold, rising to 50 to 80 milliliters per 100 grams of muscle. Even moderate exercise can increase the flow 8-fold to 10-fold, as illustrated in Figure 18–1.

Opening of Muscle Capillaries During Exercise. During rest, only 20 to 25 per cent of the muscle capillaries have flowing blood. But during strenuous exercise, all the capillaries open. This opening of dormant capillaries also diminishes the distance that oxygen and other nutrients must diffuse from the capillaries to the muscle fibers and contributes a much increased surface area through which nutrients can diffuse from the blood.

Control of Blood Flow Through the Skeletal Muscles

Local Regulation. The tremendous increase in muscle blood flow that occurs during skeletal muscle activity is caused primarily by local effects in the muscles acting directly on the arterioles to cause vasodilation.

This local increase in blood flow during muscle contraction is probably caused by several different factors all operating at the same time. One of the most important of these is reduction of oxygen in the muscle tissues. That is, during muscle activity the muscle uses oxygen very rapidly, thereby decreasing the oxygen concentration in the tissue fluids. This in turn causes vasodilation either because the vessel walls cannot maintain contraction in the absence of oxygen or because oxygen deficiency causes release of vasodilator substances. The vasodilator substance that has been suggested most widely in recent years has been

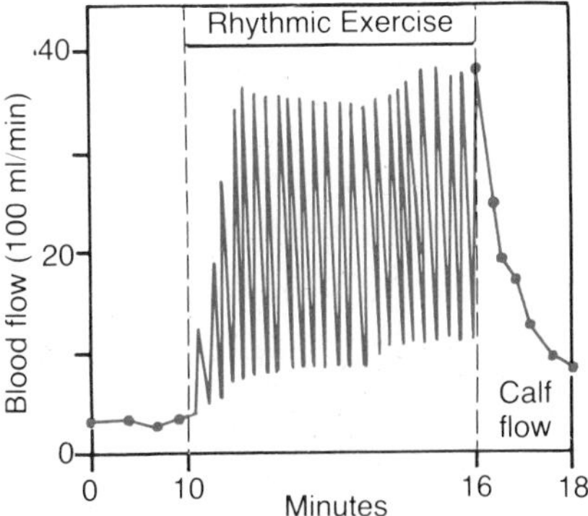

Figure 18-1. Effects of muscle exercise on blood flow in the calf of a leg during strong rhythmic contraction. The blood flow was much less during contraction than between contractions. (From Barcroft and Dornhorst: *J. Physiol.*, *109*:402, 1949.)

adenosine, but experiments have shown that even large amounts of adenosine infused directly into a muscle artery cannot cause long-sustained vasodilation in skeletal muscle. Furthermore, even after the muscle blood vessels have become insensitive to the vasodilator effects of adenosine, these same vessels will still dilate fully in response to muscle activity.

Other vasodilator substances released during muscle contraction include potassium ions, acetylcholine, adenosine triphosphate, lactic acid, and carbon dioxide. Unfortunately, we still do not know quantitatively how great a role each of these plays in increasing muscle blood flow during muscle activity; this subject is discussed in more detail in Chapter 14.

Nervous Control of Muscle Blood Flow. In addition to the local tissue regulatory mechanism, the skeletal muscles are also provided with sympathetic vasoconstrictor nerves and, in some species of animals, sympathetic vasodilator nerves as well.

Sympathetic Vasoconstrictor Nerves. The sympathetic vasoconstrictor nerve fibers secrete norepinephrine and when maximally stimulated can decrease blood flow through the muscles to perhaps one half to one fourth normal. This represents rather poor vasoconstriction in comparison with that caused by sympathetic nerves in some other areas of the body in which blood flow can be almost completely blocked. Yet even this degree of vasoconstriction is of physiological importance in circulatory shock and during other periods of stress when it is desirable to reduce blood flow through the many muscles of the body.

In addition to the norepinephrine secreted at the sympathetic vasoconstrictor nerve endings, the adrenal medullae secrete large amounts of additional norepinephrine plus epinephrine into the circulating blood during strenuous exercise. The circulating norepinephrine acts on the muscle vessels to cause a vasoconstrictor effect similar to that caused by direct sympathetic nerve stimulation. The epinephrine, on the other hand, often has a slight vasodilator effect because epinephrine excites the *beta* receptors of the vessels, which are vasodilator receptors, in contrast to the *alpha* vasoconstrictor receptors excited by the norepinephrine. These receptors are discussed in Chapter 41.

Circulatory Readjustments During Exercise

Three major effects occur during exercise that are essential for the circulatory system to supply the tremendous blood flow required by the muscles. These effects are (1) mass discharge of the sympathetic nervous system throughout the body with consequent stimulatory effects on the circulation, (2) increase in arterial pressure, and (3) increase in cardiac output.

Mass Sympathetic Discharge

At the onset of exercise, signals are transmitted from the higher levels of the brain into the vasomotor center to initiate mass sympathetic discharge. Simultaneously, the parasympathetic signals to the heart are greatly attenuated. Therefore, three major circulatory effects result.

First, the *heart is stimulated* to greatly increased heart rate and pumping strength as a result of the sympathetic drive to the heart as well as release of the heart from the normal parasympathetic inhibition.

Second, most of the arterioles of the peripheral circulation are strongly contracted except the arterioles in the active muscles, which are strongly vasodilated by the local vasodilator effects in the muscles themselves. Thus, the heart is stimulated to supply the increased blood flow required by the muscles, and blood flow through most nonmuscular areas of the body is temporarily reduced, thereby temporarily "lending" their blood supply to the muscles.

Third, the muscular walls of the *veins and other capacitative areas of the circulation are contracted powerfully,* which translocates large amounts of blood from the blood vessels into the heart. As we learned in the previous chapter, this is one of the most important factors in promoting extra contractile strength of the heart and therefore in increasing the cardiac output as well.

Increase in Arterial Pressure—An Important Result of Increased Sympathetic Activity

One of the most important effects of increased sympathetic activity in exercise is to increase the arterial pressure. This results from multiple stimulatory effects, including (1) vasoconstriction of the arterioles and small arteries in most of the tissues of the body besides the active muscles, (2) increased pumping activity by the heart, and (3) a great increase in venous contraction. These effects working together virtually always increase the arterial pressure during exercise. This increase can be as little as 20 or as great as 80 mm Hg, depending on the conditions under which the exercise is performed. When a person performs exercise under very tense conditions but uses only a few muscles, the sympathetic response still occurs everywhere in the body, but vasodilation occurs in only a few muscles. Therefore, the net effect is mainly one of vasoconstriction, often increasing the mean arterial pressure to as high as 170 mm Hg. Such a condition occurs in a person standing on a ladder and nailing with a hammer on the ceiling above. The tenseness of the situation is obvious, and yet the amount of muscle vasodilation is relatively slight.

On the other hand, when a person performs whole-body exercise, such as running or swimming, the increase in arterial pressure is often only 20 to 40 mm Hg. The lack of a tremendous rise in pressure results from the extreme vasodilation occurring in large masses of muscle.

In rare instances, persons are found in whom the sympathetic nervous system is absent, either congenitally or because of surgical removal. When such a person exercises, instead of the arterial pressure rising, the pressure actually falls — sometimes to as low as one-half normal, and the cardiac output rises only about one third as much as it does normally. Therefore, one can readily understand the major importance of increased sympathetic activity during exercise.

Why Is the Arterial Pressure Rise Important During Exercise? When muscles are stimulated maximally in a laboratory experiment, but without allowing the arterial pressure to rise, the blood flow will rarely rise more than about eightfold. Yet, we know from studies of marathon runners that the blood flow through the muscles can increase from as little as 1 liter/min for the whole body during rest to at least 20 liters/min during maximal activity. Therefore, it is clear that the muscle blood flow can increase much more than occurs in simple laboratory experiments. What is the difference? The difference is mainly that in physiologic exercise the arterial pressure rises at the same time. Let us assume, for instance, that the arterial pressure rises 30 per cent, a common rise during exercise. This 30 per cent increase causes 30 per cent more force to push the blood through the tissue vessels. However, this is not the only effect of the increasing pressure, for the pressure also dilates the blood vessels and allows about another 100 per cent increase in flow. Thus, a 30 per cent increase over the original 8-fold increase in blood flow would increase the flow to 10.4-fold, and doubling this again would increase the flow to more than 20-fold.

The Increase in Cardiac Output in Exercise

Many different physiological effects occurring together during exercise cause the cardiac output to increase almost in proportion to the degree of exercise. This increase in output, in turn, is essential to supply the large amounts of oxygen and other nutrients needed by the working muscles. In fact, the ability of the circulatory system to provide increased cardiac output in heavy exercise is as important as the strength of the muscles themselves in setting the limit for the performance of muscle work. For instance, those marathon runners who can increase their cardiac outputs the most are generally the same ones who have the record-breaking times.

THE CORONARY CIRCULATION

Approximately one third of all deaths in the affluent society of the Western world result from coronary artery disease, and almost all elderly persons have at least some impairment of the coronary artery circulation. For this reason, the normal and pathological physiology of the coronary circulation is one of the most important subjects in the entire field of medicine and physiology.

Physiological Anatomy of the Coronary Blood Supply

Figure 18-2 illustrates the heart with its coronary blood supply. Note that the main coronary arteries lie on the surface of the heart, and small arteries penetrate into the cardiac muscle mass. It is almost entirely through these arteries that the heart receives its nutritive blood supply. Only the inner 75 to 100 micrometers of the endocardial surface can obtain significant amounts of nutrition directly from the blood in the cardiac chambers.

The *left coronary artery* supplies mainly the anterior and lateral portions of the left ventricle, whereas the *right coronary artery* supplies most of the right ventricle as well as the posterior part of the left ventricle in 80 to 90 per cent of all persons.

Most of the venous blood flow from the left ventricle leaves by way of the *coronary sinus* — which is about 75 per cent of the total coronary blood flow — and most of the venous blood from the right ventricle flows through the small *anterior cardiac veins* directly into the right atrium, which are not connected with the coronary sinus.

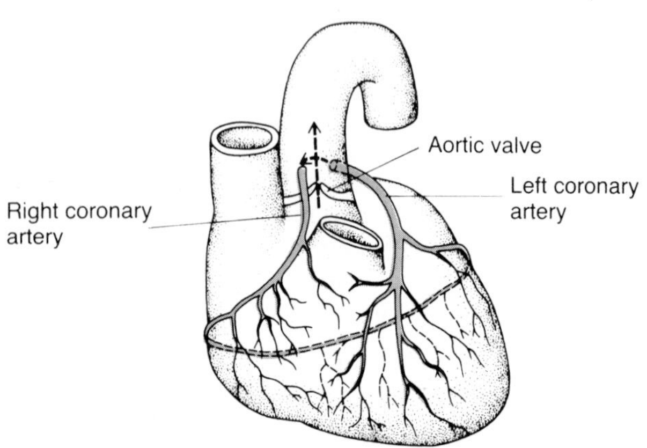

Figure 18-2. The coronary vessels.

Normal Coronary Blood Flow

The resting coronary blood flow in the human averages approximately 225 ml/min, which is about 0.7 to 0.8 milliliter per gram of heart muscle, or 4 to 5 per cent of the total cardiac output.

In strenuous exercise, the heart increases its cardiac output as much as fourfold to sevenfold, and it pumps this blood against a higher than normal arterial pressure. Consequently, the work output of the heart muscle under severe conditions may increase as much as sixfold to eightfold. The coronary blood flow increases threefold to fourfold to supply the extra nutrients needed by the heart. Obviously, this increase is not as much as the increase in work load, which means that the ratio of coronary blood flow to energy expenditure by the heart decreases. However, the "efficiency" of cardiac utilization of energy increases to make up for this relative deficiency of blood supply.

Phasic Changes in Coronary Blood Flow—Effect of Cardiac Muscle Compression. Figure 18–3 illustrates the average blood flow *through the nutrient capillaries* of the left ventricular coronary system in milliliters per minute in the human heart during systole and diastole, as *calculated* from experiments in lower animals. Note from this diagram that the blood flow in the left ventricle falls to a low value during *systole,* which is opposite to the flow in other vascular beds of the body. The reason for this is the strong compression of the left ventricular muscle around the intramuscular vessels during systole.

During *diastole,* the cardiac muscle relaxes completely and no longer obstructs the blood flow through the left ventricular capillaries, so that blood now flows rapidly during all of diastole.

Blood flow through the coronary capillaries of the right ventricle also undergoes phasic changes during the cardiac cycle, but, because the force of contraction of the right ventricle is far less than that of the left ventricle, the inverse phasic changes are only rarely observed.

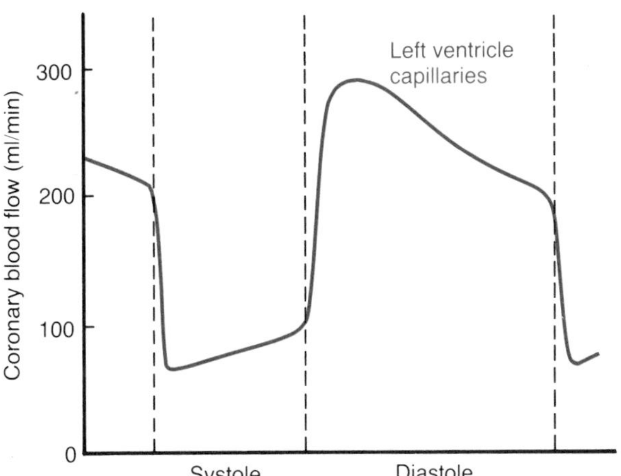

Figure 18–3. Phasic flow of blood through the coronary capillaries of the human left ventricle (as extrapolated from studies in dogs).

Control of Coronary Blood Flow

Local Metabolism as the Primary Controller of Coronary Flow

Blood flow through the coronary system is regulated almost entirely by vascular response to the local needs of the cardiac musculature for nutrition. This mechanism works equally well when the nerves to the heart are intact or are removed. That is, whenever the vigor of contraction is increased, regardless of cause, the rate of coronary blood flow simultaneously increases, and, conversely, decreased activity is accompanied by decreased coronary flow. It is immediately obvious that this local regulation of blood flow is almost identical with that occurring in many other tissues, especially in the skeletal muscles of all the body.

Oxygen Demand as a Major Factor in Local Blood Flow Regulation. Blood flow in the coronaries is regulated almost exactly in proportion to the need of the cardiac musculature for oxygen. Even in the normal resting state, about 70 per cent of the oxygen in the arterial blood is removed as the blood passes through the heart; and, because not much oxygen is left, not much additional oxygen can be supplied to the heart musculature unless the blood flow increases. Fortunately, the blood flow does increase almost directly in proportion to the metabolic consumption of oxygen by the heart.

Yet, the exact means by which increased oxygen consumption causes coronary dilatation has not been determined. It is speculated that a decrease in the oxygen concentration in the heart causes vasodilator substances to be released from the muscle cells, and that these dilate the arterioles. The substance with the greatest vasodilator propensity is *adenosine.* In the presence of very low concentrations of oxygen in the muscle cells, a large proportion of the cell's adenosine triphosphate (ATP) degrades to adenosine monophosphate; then small portions of this are further degraded to release adenosine into the tissue fluids of the heart muscle. After the adenosine causes vasodilation, much of it is reabsorbed back into the cardiac cells to be reused.

Adenosine is not the only vasodilator product that has been identified. Others include adenosine phosphate compounds, potassium ions, hydrogen ions, carbon dioxide, bradykinin, and possibly prostaglandins.

Yet, difficulties still exist with the vasodilator hypothesis. For one, agents that block or partially block the vasodilator effect of adenosine do not prevent the coronary vasodilation caused by increased muscle activity. Second, studies in skeletal muscle have shown that adenosine will maintain vascular dilatation for only 1 to 3 hours, and yet muscle activity will still dilate the local blood vessels even when the adenosine can no longer dilate them.

Therefore, yet another theory to explain the coronary artery dilatation should be remembered until proved false: In the absence of adequate amounts of oxygen in the cardiac muscle, not only does the muscle itself suffer oxygen deficiency, but so do the arteriolar muscle walls as well. This could easily cause local vasodilation because of lack of the required energy to keep the coronary vessels contracted against the high arterial pressure. But this, too, has its problems because the coronary arteries require only minute amounts of oxygen to maintain full contraction.

Nervous Control of Coronary Blood Flow

Stimulation of the autonomic nerves to the heart can affect coronary blood flow in two ways — directly and indirectly. The direct effects result from direct action of the nervous transmitter substances, acetylcholine from the vagus nerves and norepinephrine from the sympathetic nerves, on the coronary vessels themselves. The indirect effects result from secondary changes in coronary blood flow caused by increased or decreased activity of the heart.

The indirect effects, which are mostly opposite to the direct effects, play by far the more important role in normal control of coronary blood flow. Thus, sympathetic stimulation, which releases norepinephrine, increases both heart rate and heart contractility as well as its rate of metabolism. In turn, the increased activity of the heart sets off local blood flow regulatory mechanisms for dilating the coronary vessels, and the blood flow increases approximately in proportion to the metabolic needs of the heart muscle. In contrast, vagal stimulation, with its release of acetylcholine, slows the heart and also has a slight depressive effect on cardiac contractility. Both these effects decrease cardiac oxygen consumption and therefore indirectly constrict the coronaries.

Direct Effects of Nervous Stimuli on the Coronary Vasculature. The distribution of parasympathetic (vagal) nerve fibers to the ventricular coronary system is so slight that parasympathetic stimulation has only a *very slight* direct effect to *dilate* the coronaries.

On the other hand, there is much more extensive sympathetic innervation of the coronary vessels. In Chapter 41 we see that the sympathetic transmitter substances norepinephrine and epinephrine can have either constrictor or dilator effects, depending on the presence or absence of specific receptors in the blood vessel walls. The constrictor receptors are called *alpha receptors,* and the dilator receptors are called *beta receptors.* Both alpha- and beta-receptors are known to exist in the coronary vessels. In general, the epicardial coronary vessels have a preponderance of alpha-receptors and therefore constrict, whereas the intramuscular arteries may have a preponderance of beta-receptors and therefore dilate.

It must be pointed out again, however, that metabolic factors — especially myocardial oxygen consumption — are the major controllers of myocardial blood flow. Therefore, whenever the direct effects of nervous stimulation alter the coronary blood flow, the metabolic factors usually override these direct coronary nervous effects and return the flow most of the way back toward normal within seconds.

Ischemic Heart Disease

The single most common cause of death in Western culture is ischemic heart disease, which results from insufficient coronary blood flow. Approximately 35 per cent of all humans in the United States die of this cause. Some deaths occur suddenly as a result of an acute coronary occlusion or of fibrillation of the heart, whereas others occur slowly over a period of weeks to years as a result of progressive weakening of the heart pumping process. In the present chapter, we discuss the coronary ischemia problem itself as well as acute coronary occlusion and myocardial infarction. In the following chapter, we discuss cardiac failure, the most frequent cause of which is progressive coronary ischemia.

Atherosclerosis as the Cause of Ischemic Heart Disease. The most frequent cause of diminished coronary blood flow is atherosclerosis. The atherosclerotic process is discussed in connection with lipid metabolism in Chapter 46; briefly, this process is the following: In certain persons who have a genetic predisposition to atherosclerosis or in persons who eat excessive quantities of cholesterol and other fats, large quantities of cholesterol gradually become deposited beneath the intima at many points in the arteries. Later, these areas of deposit become invaded by fibrous tissue, and they also frequently become calcified. The net result is the development of atherosclerotic plaques that protrude into the vessel lumens and either block or partially block blood flow.

A very common site for development of atherosclerotic plaques is the first few centimeters of the coronary arteries.

Acute Coronary Occlusion

Acute occlusion of a coronary artery frequently occurs in a person who already has serious underlying atherosclerotic coronary heart disease but almost never in a person with a normal coronary circulation. Most important, the atherosclerotic plaque can cause a local blood clot called a *thrombus,* which in turn occludes the artery. The thrombus usually begins where the plaque has broken through the intima, thus coming in contact with the flowing blood. Because the plaque presents an unsmooth surface, platelets begin to adhere to it, fibrin begins to be deposited, and blood cells become entrapped to form a clot that grows until it occludes the vessel. Or, occasionally the clot breaks away from its attachment on the atherosclerotic plaque and flows to a more peripheral branch of the coronary arterial tree, where it blocks the artery at that point. A thrombus that flows along the artery in this way and occludes the vessel more distally is called an *embolus.*

The Lifesaving Value of Collateral Circulation in the Heart. The degree of damage to the heart caused either by slowly developing atherosclerotic constriction of the coronary arteries or by sudden occlusion is determined to a great extent by the degree of collateral circulation that is already developed or that can develop within a short period of time after the occlusion.

Unfortunately, in a normal heart, almost no communications exist among the larger coronary arteries. But many anastomoses do exist among the smaller arteries sized 20 to 250 micrometers in diameter, as shown in Figure 18-4.

When a sudden occlusion occurs in one of the larger coronary arteries, these small anastomoses dilate within a few seconds. The blood flow through these minute collaterals is usually less than one half that needed to keep alive the cardiac muscle that they supply; unfortunately, the diameters of the collateral vessels do not enlarge farther for the next 8 to 24 hours. But then collateral flow does begin to increase, doubling by the second or third day and often reaching normal or almost normal coronary flow in the previously ischemic muscle within about 1 month. It is because of these developing collateral channels that a patient often recovers almost completely from various types of coronary occlusion when the area of muscle involved is not too great.

When atherosclerosis constricts the coronary arteries slowly over a period of many years rather than suddenly, collateral vessels can develop at the same time that the atherosclerosis does. Therefore, the person may never experience an acute episode of cardiac dysfunction. Eventually, however, the sclerotic process develops beyond the limits of even the collateral blood supply to provide the needed blood flow, and even the collaterals sometimes develop atherosclerosis. When this occurs, the heart muscle becomes severely limited in its work output, often so much so that the heart cannot pump even the normally required amounts of blood flow. This is the most common cause of cardiac failure and occurs in vast numbers of older persons.

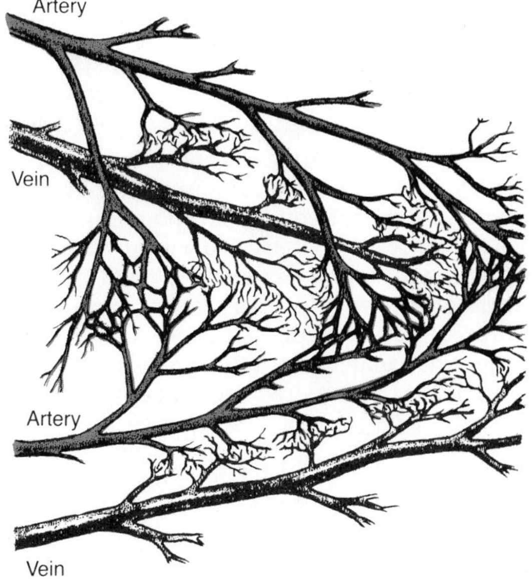

Figure 18-4. Minute anastomoses of the coronary arterial system.

Myocardial Infarction

Immediately after an acute coronary occlusion, blood flow ceases in the coronary vessels beyond the occlusion except for small amounts of collateral flow from surrounding vessels. The area of muscle that has either zero flow or so little flow that it cannot sustain cardiac muscle function is said to be *infarcted.* The overall process is called a *myocardial infarction.*

Cardiac muscle requires approximately 1.3 milliliters of oxygen per 100 grams of muscle tissue per minute simply to remain alive. This is in comparison with approximately 8 milliliters of oxygen per 100 grams delivered to the normal resting left ventricle each minute. Therefore, if there is even as much as 15 to 30 per cent of normal resting coronary blood flow, the muscle will not die. In the central portion of a large infarct, however, the blood flow is usually less than this, so that this muscle does die.

Causes of Death Following Acute Coronary Occlusion

The four major causes of death following acute myocardial infarction are decreased cardiac output; damming of blood in the pulmonary or systemic veins with death resulting from edema, especially pulmonary edema; fibrillation of the heart; and, occasionally, rupture of the heart.

Decreased Cardiac Output—Cardiac Shock. When some of the cardiac muscle fibers are not functioning at all and others are too weak to contract with great force, the overall pumping ability of the affected ventricle is proportionately depressed.

When the heart becomes incapable of contracting with sufficient force to pump enough blood into the arterial tree, cardiac failure and death of the peripheral tissues ensue as a result of peripheral ischemia. This condition is called *coronary shock, cardiogenic shock, cardiac shock,* or *low cardiac output failure.* Cardiac shock almost always occurs when more than 40 per cent of the left ventricle is infarcted. Death occurs in about 85 per cent of those patients who develop cardiac shock.

Damming of Blood in the Venous System. When the heart is not pumping blood forward, it must be damming blood in the blood vessels of the lungs or in the systemic circulation. Obviously, this increases both the left and right atrial pressures and also leads to increased capillary pressures, particularly in the lungs. Many patients who seemingly are getting along well develop acute pulmonary edema several days after a myocardial infarction and often die within a few hours after appearance of the initial edema symptoms.

Rupture of the Infarcted Area. During the first day of an acute infarct there is little danger of rupture of the ischemic portion of the heart, but a few days after a large infarct occurs, the dead muscle fibers begin to degenerate, and the dead tissue is likely to become very thin. If this happens, the dead muscle bulges outward severely with each heart contraction, and the systolic stretch becomes greater and greater until finally the heart ruptures. In fact, one of the means used in assessing the progress of a severe myocardial infarction is to record by radiograph whether the degree of systolic stretch is getting worse.

When a ventricle does rupture, the loss of blood into the pericardial space causes rapid development of *cardiac tamponade*—that is, compression of the heart from the outside by blood collecting in the pericardial cavity. Because the heart is compressed, blood cannot flow into the right atrium, and the patient dies of suddenly decreased cardiac output.

Fibrillation of the Ventricles Following Myocardial Infarction. Many persons who die of coronary occlusion die because of ventricular fibrillation. There are two especially dangerous periods during which fibrillation is most likely to occur. The first is during the first 10 minutes after the infarction occurs. Then there is a short period of relative safety, followed by a secondary period of cardiac irritability beginning an hour or so later and lasting for another few hours. However, fibrillation can occur many days after the infarct.

Ischemia causes an "injury current," in the affected heart muscle. That is, the ischemic musculature cannot repolarize its membranes, so that the external surface of this muscle remains negative with respect to the normal cardiac muscle membrane elsewhere in the heart. Therefore, electrical current flows from this ischemic area of the heart to the normal area and can elicit abnormal impulses that can cause fibrillation.

The Stages of Recovery from Acute Myocardial Infarction

The upper part of Figure 18-5 illustrates the effects of acute coronary occlusion, on the left, in a patient with a small area of muscle ischemia and, on the right, in a patient with a large area of ischemia. When the area of ischemia is small, little or no death of the muscle cells may occur, but part of the muscle often does become temporarily nonfunctional because of inadequate nutrition to support muscle contraction.

When the area of ischemia is large, some of the muscle fibers in the very center of the area die rapidly, within 1 to 3 hours in an area of total cessation of coronary blood supply. Immediately around the dead area is a nonfunctional area because of failure of contraction and usually also failure of impulse conduction. Then, extending circumferentially around the nonfunctional area is an area that is still contracting but weakly so because of mild ischemia.

Replacement of Dead Muscle by Scar Tissue. In the lower part of Figure 18-5, the various stages of

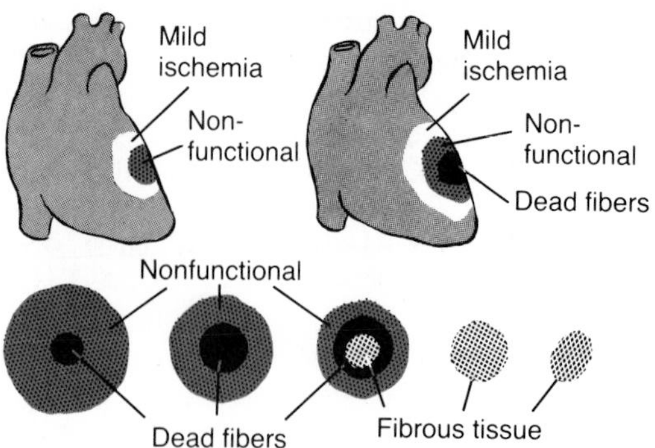

Figure 18-5. *Top,* Small and large areas of coronary ischemia. *Bottom,* Stages of recovery from myocardial infarction.

recovery following a myocardial infarction are illustrated. Shortly after the occlusion, the muscle fibers die in the very center of the ischemic area. Then during the ensuing days, this area of dead fibers grows because many of the marginal fibers finally succumb to the prolonged ischemia. At the same time, owing to the enlargement of the collateral arterial channels growing into the outer rim of the infarcted area, the nonfunctional area of muscle becomes smaller and smaller. After a few days to 3 weeks, most of the nonfunctional area of muscle becomes functional again or dead—one or the other. In the meantime, fibrous tissue begins developing among the dead fibers, for ischemia stimulates growth of fibroblasts and promotes development of greater than normal quantities of fibrous tissue. Therefore, the dead muscular tissue is gradually replaced by fibrous tissue. Then, because it is a general property of fibrous tissue to undergo progressive elastomeric contraction and dissolution, the size of the fibrous scar may become smaller over a period of several months to a year.

Finally, the normal areas of the heart gradually hypertrophy to compensate at least partially for the lost cardiac musculature. By these means the heart recovers.

Function of the Heart Following Recovery from Myocardial Infarction

Occasionally, a heart that has recovered from a large myocardial infarction returns to full functional capability, but more frequently its pumping capability is permanently decreased below that of a normal heart. This does not mean that the person is necessarily a cardiac invalid or that the resting cardiac output is depressed below normal, because the normal person's heart is capable of pumping about four times as much blood as the body requires under resting conditions.

Pain in Coronary Disease

Normally, a person cannot "feel" his or her heart, but ischemic cardiac muscle does produce pain sensation. It is believed that ischemia causes the muscle to release acidic substances, such as lactic acid, or other pain-promoting products, such as histamine, kinins, or cellular proteolytic enzymes, that are not removed rapidly enough by the slowly moving blood. The high concentrations of these abnormal products then stimulate the pain endings in the cardiac muscle, and pain impulses are conducted through the sympathetic afferent nerve fibers into the central nervous system.

Angina Pectoris

In most persons who develop progressive constriction of their coronary arteries, cardiac pain, called *angina pectoris,* begins to appear whenever the load on the heart becomes too great in relation to the coronary blood flow. This pain is usually felt beneath the upper sternum and is often also referred to surface areas of the body, most often to the left arm and left shoulder but also frequently to the neck and even to the side of the face or to the opposite arm and shoulder. The reason for this distribution of pain is that the heart originates during embryonic life in the neck, as do the arms. Therefore, both of these structures receive pain nerve fibers from the same spinal cord segments.

In general, most persons who have chronic angina pectoris feel the pain when they exercise and also when they experience emotions that increase metabolism of the heart or temporarily constrict the coronary vessels because of sympathetic vasoconstrictor nerve signals. Usually the pain lasts for only a few minutes. However, some patients have such severe and lasting ischemia that the pain is present all the time. The pain is frequently described as hot, pressing, and constricting; it is of such quality that it usually makes the patient stop all activity and come to a complete state of rest.

When a person has frequent attacks of angina, the likelihood of developing an acute coronary occlusion is generally very great.

Treatment with Drugs. Several vasodilator drugs, when administered during an acute anginal attack, will usually give immediate relief from the pain. Commonly used vasodilators are *nitroglycerin* and *other nitrate drugs.*

A second class of drugs that are used for prolonged treatment of angina pectoris is the *beta-blockers,* such as propranolol. These block the sympathetic beta-receptors, which prevents sympathetic stimulation of heart rate and cardiac metabolism during exercise or emotional episodes. Therefore, therapy with a beta blocker decreases the need of the heart for metabolic oxygen during stressful conditions. For obvious reasons, this can greatly reduce the number of anginal attacks as well as their severity.

Surgical Treatment of Coronary Disease

Aortic-Coronary Bypass Surgery. In many patients with coronary ischemia, the constricted areas of the coronary vessels are located at only a few discrete points, and the coronary vessels beyond these points are normal or almost normal. A surgical procedure has been developed in the past 25 years, called *aortic-coronary bypass,* for anastomosing small vein grafts to the aorta and to the sides of the more peripheral coronary vessels. Usually, one to five such grafts are performed during the operation, each of which supplies a peripheral coronary artery beyond a block.

The acute results from this type of surgery have been especially good, causing this to be the most common cardiac operation performed. Anginal pain is relieved in most patients. Also, in patients whose hearts have not become too severely damaged prior to the operation, the coronary bypass procedure often can provide the patient with a normal survival expectation.

REFERENCES

Braunwald, E.: Heart Disease. Philadelphia, W. B. Saunders Co., 1988.
Chapman, C. B.: The physiology of exercise. Sci. Am., 212:88, 1986.
Chilian, W. M., and Marcus, M. L.: Coronary vascular adaptations to myocardial hypertrophy. Annu. Rev. Physiol., 49:477, 1987.
Feigl, E. O.: Coronary physiology. Physiol. Rev., 63:1, 1983.
Gregg, D. E.: Coronary Circulation in Health and Disease. Philadelphia, Lea & Febiger, 1950.
Guyton, A. C., et al.: Cardiac Output and Its Regulation. Philadelphia, W. B. Saunders Co., 1973.
Guyton, R. A., and Daggett, W. M.: The evolution of myocardial infarction: Physiological basis for clinical intervention. Int. Rev. Physiol., 9:305, 1976.
Lawrie: Coronary Artery Bypass Surgery. Chicago, Year Book Medical Publishers, 1985.
Miller, A. J.: Diagnosis of Chest Pain. New York, Raven Press, 1988.
Roberts, L.: Study bolsters case against cholesterol. Science, 237:28, 1987.
Virmani, R., and Forman, M. B.: Nonatherosclerotic Ischemic Heart Disease. New York, Raven Press, 1989.
Vogel, J. H. K., and King, S. B., III: Interventional Cardiology: Future Directions. St. Louis, C. V. Mosby Co., 1989.

QUESTIONS

1. Approximately how much can the blood flow through an exercising muscle increase above the normal resting level?
2. What proportion of the muscle capillaries is open during rest? What happens to the capillary blood flow during exercise?
3. What causes the blood vessels of the muscles to dilate during exercise?
4. What other circulatory adjustments besides the local vasodilation of the muscles must occur if the circulatory system is to be able to cope with the increased flow required by the muscles?

5. Discuss the role of the sympathetic nervous system during exercise.
6. What is the normal blood flow through the coronary system, and how much can this increase during exercise?
7. Why is blood flow through the left ventricular coronary vessels greater during diastole than during systole?
8. What factors control the coronary blood flow?
9. What causes *atherosclerosis*?
10. Describe what happens when an *acute coronary occlusion* occurs? Describe recovery for this occlusion by the development of collateral vessels.
11. What are the various effects of coronary occlusion that frequently lead to death?
12. What are the causes of *angina pectoris*?
13. Describe the surgical treatment for coronary disease using the *aortic-coronary bypass* operation.

19

Heart Sounds; Valvular and Congenital Heart Defects; Cardiac Failure

THE HEART SOUNDS

The function of the heart valves was discussed in Chapter 8. It was pointed out that closure of the valves is associated with audible sounds. On the other hand, no sounds occur when the valves open. The purpose of the first section of this chapter is to discuss the factors that cause the sounds in the heart, under both normal and abnormal conditions.

Normal Heart Sounds

Listening with a stethoscope to a normal heart, one hears a sound usually described as "lub, dub, lub, dub . . ." The "lub" is associated with closure of the A-V valves at the beginning of systole and the "dub" with closure of the semilunar valves at the end of systole. The "lub" sound is called the *first heart sound* and the "dub" the *second heart sound* because the normal cycle of the heart is considered to start with the beginning of systole.

Causes of the First and Second Heart Sounds. The earliest suggestion for the cause of the heart sounds was that the slapping together of the valve leaflets sets up vibrations, but this has been shown to cause little if any of the sound because of the cushioning effect of the blood. Instead, the cause is *vibration of the taut valves immediately after closure* along with *vibration of the adjacent blood, walls of the heart, and major vessels around the heart.* That is, in generating the first heart sound, contraction of the ventricles causes sudden backflow of blood against the A-V valves (the tricuspid and mitral valves), causing them to bulge toward the atria until the chordae tendineae abruptly stop the backbulging. The elastic tautness of the valves then causes the backsurging blood to bounce forward again into each respective ventricle. This sets the blood and the ventricular walls as well as the valves into vibration and also causes vibrating turbulence in the blood. The vibrations then travel through the adjacent tissues to the chest wall, where they can be heard as sound by the stethoscope for about a tenth of a second.

The second heart sound results from sudden closure of the semilunar valves (the aortic and pulmonary valves). When the semilunar valves close, they bulge backward toward the ventricles, and their elastic stretch recoils the blood back into the arteries, which causes a short period of reverberation of blood back and forth between the walls of the arteries and the valves and also between the valves and the ventricular walls.

The Third Heart Sound. Occasionally a very weak rumbling third heart sound is heard at the beginning of the *middle third of diastole.* A logical, but yet unproved, explanation of this sound is oscillation of blood back and forth between the walls of the ventricles initiated by inrushing blood from the atria. The reason the third heart sound does not occur until the middle third of diastole is presumably that in the early part of diastole the heart is not filled sufficiently to create even the small amount of elastic tension in the ventricles necessary for reverberation. The frequency of this sound is usually so low that the ear cannot hear the sound; yet it can often be recorded in the phonocardiogram.

The Atrial Heart Sound (Fourth Heart Sound). An atrial heart sound can be recorded in many persons in the phonocardiogram, but it can almost never be heard with a stethoscope because of its low frequency — usually 20 cycles per second or less.

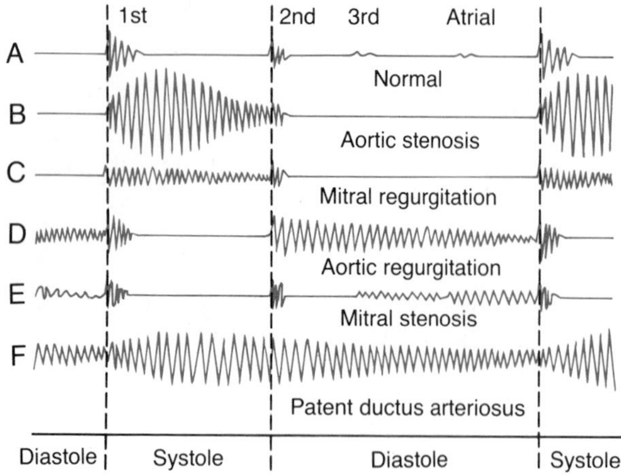

Figure 19–1. Phonocardiograms from normal and abnormal hearts.

This sound occurs when the atria contract, and presumably it is caused by inrush of blood into the ventricles, which initiates vibrations similar to those of the third heart sound.

The Phonocardiogram

If a microphone specially designed to detect low frequency sound is placed on the chest, the heart sounds can be amplified and recorded by a high-speed recording apparatus. The recording is called a *phonocardiogram,* and the heart sounds appear as waves, as illustrated schematically in Figure 19–1. Record A is a recording of normal heart sounds, showing the vibrations of the first, second, and third heart sounds and even the atrial sound. Note specifically that the third and atrial heart sounds are each a very low rumble. The third heart sound can be recorded in only one third to one half of all persons, and the atrial heart sound can be recorded in perhaps one fourth of all persons.

VALVULAR LESIONS

Rheumatic Valvular Lesions

By far the greatest number of valvular lesions results from rheumatic fever. Rheumatic fever is an autoimmune disease in which the heart valves are likely to be damaged or destroyed. It is initiated by streptococcal toxin in the following manner:

The sequence of events almost always begins with a preliminary streptococcal infection caused specifically by group A hemolytic streptococci, such as a sore throat, scarlet fever, or middle ear infection. The streptococci release several different proteins against which antibodies are formed, the most important of which seems to be a protein called the "M" antigen. The antibodies then react not only with this M antigen, but unfortunately also with different tissues of the body, including the heart valves, often causing severe damage. These reactions continue to take place as long as the antibodies persist in the blood—6 months or more. The degree of heart valve damage is directly correlated with the titer and the persistence of these antibodies.

In rheumatic fever, large hemorrhagic, fibrinous, bulbous lesions grow along the inflamed edges of the heart valves. Because the mitral valve receives more trauma during valvular action than any of the other valves, this valve is the one most often seriously damaged, and the aortic valve is the second most frequently damaged.

Scarring of the Valves. The lesions of acute rheumatic fever frequently occur on adjacent valve leaflets simultaneously, so that the edges of the leaflets become stuck together. Then, weeks, months, or years later, the lesions become scar tissue, permanently fusing portions of the leaflets. Also, the free edges of the leaflets, which are normally filmy and free-flapping, become solid, scarred masses.

A valve in which the leaflets adhere to each other so extensively that blood cannot flow through satisfactorily is said to be *stenosed.* On the other hand, when the valve edges are so destroyed by scar tissue that they cannot close when the ventricles contract, *regurgitation,* or backflow, of blood occurs when the valve should be closed.

Other Causes of Valvular Lesions. Stenosis or lack of one or more leaflets of a valve frequently occurs as a congenital defect. Complete lack of leaflets is rare, though stenosis is common.

Heart Murmurs Caused by Valvular Lesions

As illustrated by the phonocardiograms in Figure 19–1, many abnormal heart sounds, known as "heart murmurs," occur when there are abnormalities of the valves, as follows:

The Murmur of Aortic Stenosis. In aortic stenosis, blood is ejected from the left ventricle through only a small opening of the aortic valve. Because of the resistance to ejection, the pressure in the left ventricle rises sometimes as high as 300 mm Hg, while the pressure in the aorta is still normal. Thus, a nozzle effect is created *during systole,* with blood jetting at tremendous velocity through the small opening of the valve. This causes *severe turbulence* of the blood in the root of the aorta, and a loud, harsh murmur is transmitted throughout the upper aorta and even into the larger arteries of the neck.

The Murmur of Aortic Regurgitation. In aortic regurgitation, no sound is heard during systole, but *during diastole* blood flows backward from the aorta into the left ventricle, causing a "blowing" murmur of relatively high pitch and with a swishing quality heard maximally over the left ventricle. This murmur results from *turbulence* of blood jetting backward into the blood already in the left ventricle.

The Murmur of Mitral Regurgitation. In mitral regurgitation, blood flows backward through the mitral valve *during systole.* This also causes a high frequency "blowing," swishing sound similar to that of aortic regurgitation, transmitted most strongly into the left atrium. However, the left atrium is so deep within the chest that it is difficult to hear this sound directly over the atrium. As a result, the sound of mitral regurgitation is transmitted to the chest wall mainly through the left ventricle instead, and it is usually heard best at the apex of the heart.

The Murmur of Mitral Stenosis. In mitral stenosis, blood passes with difficulty from the left atrium into the left ventricle. Yet, because the pressure in the left atrium rarely rises above 35 mm Hg except for short periods of time, a great pressure differential forcing blood from the left atrium into the left ventricle never develops. Consequently, the abnormal sounds heard in mitral stenosis are usually weak and of very low frequency, so that most of the sound spectrum is below the low frequency end of human hearing.

Phonocardiograms of Valvular Murmurs. Phonocardiograms B, C, D, and E of Figure 19–1 illustrate, respectively, idealized records obtained from patients with aortic stenosis, mitral regurgitation, aortic regurgitation, and mitral stenosis. It is obvious from these phonocardiograms that the aortic stenotic lesion causes the loudest of all the murmurs, and the mitral stenotic lesion the weakest. The phonocardiograms show how the intensity of the murmurs varies during different portions of systole and diastole, and the relative timing of each murmur is also evident. Note especially that the murmurs of aortic stenosis and mitral regurgitation occur only during systole, whereas the murmurs of aortic regurgitation and mitral stenosis occur only during diastole — if the reader does not understand this timing, a moment's pause should be taken until it is understood.

ABNORMAL CIRCULATORY DYNAMICS IN VALVULAR HEART DISEASE

In general, it is easy to understand the derangements of the circulation caused by heart valve lesions. If a valve becomes stenosed, blood will not flow through the valve easily, so that blood dams up behind the valve. In the case of regurgitation, the blood passes through the velve satisfactorily but then also flows backward when the valve should close. Thus, the effect on the circulation is almost the same in each instance, poor pumping by the heart.

Obviously, in aortic valve lesions, blood tends to dam up in the left ventricle. This enlarges the ventricle, stretches its muscle, and causes muscle hypertrophy. Sometimes the hypertrophy is great enough to overcome partially the detrimental effects of the valve lesion. At other times the lesion is so severe that even with maximal amounts of hypertrophy, the ventricle cannot pump adequate amounts of blood, thus causing heart failure.

In the case of mitral valvular lesions, blood does not flow easily from the left atrium into the left ventricle. Therefore, tremendous amounts of blood accumulate in the left atrium and lungs. Often the atrium is enlarged severalfold. Two major consequences usually result: First, the enlarged atrial wall provides an extremely long pathway for passage of action potentials within the atrial muscle. Referring back to Chapter 10 on the discussion of cardiac fibrillation, a long pathway can cause fibrillation to develop. Therefore, most patients with very severe mitral valvular disease eventually develop persistent atrial fibrillation, and thereafter the atria no longer function as primer pumps for the ventricles. This weakens the overall pumping activity of the heart. Yet, because of the large reserve pumping capability of the ventricles, many of these patients still live for months or even years even without atrial pumping. The second serious effect of mitral valvular lesions is very high pressures in the pulmonary veins and pulmonary capillaries. When the pulmonary capillary pressure rises above about 20 to 30 mm Hg, pulmonary edema usually develops. Sometimes this can be lethal within a few hours. In other instances, the pulmonary edema persists for many months, especially in the lower areas of the lung that lie beneath the level of the heart.

ABNORMAL CIRCULATORY DYNAMICS IN CONGENITAL HEART DEFECTS

Occasionally, the heart or its associated blood vessels are malformed during fetal life; the defect is called a *congenital anomaly*. Let us consider two common types of congenital heart defects: first, *patent ductus arteriosus* and second, *tetralogy of Fallot*.

Patent Ductus Arteriosus — A Left-to-Right Shunt

During fetal life the lungs are collapsed, and the elastic factors that keep the alveoli collapsed also keep the blood vessels collapsed. Therefore, the resistance to blood flow through the lungs is so great that the pulmonary arterial pressure is high in the fetus. On the other hand, because of very low resistance to blood flow from the aorta through the large vessels of the placenta, the pressure in the aorta is lower than in the pulmonary artery, causing almost all the pulmonary arterial blood to flow through a special artery that is present in the fetus connecting the pulmonary artery with the aorta (Fig. 19–2), called the *ductus arteriosus,* thus bypassing the lungs. This allows immediate recirculation of the blood through the systemic arteries of the fetus. Obviously, this lack of blood flow through the lungs is not detrimental to the fetus because the blood is oxygenated by the placenta of the mother.

Closure of the Ductus After Birth. As soon as a baby is born, the lungs inflate; not only do the alveoli fill with air but also the resistance to blood flow through the pulmonary vascular tree decreases tremendously, allowing pulmonary arterial pressure to

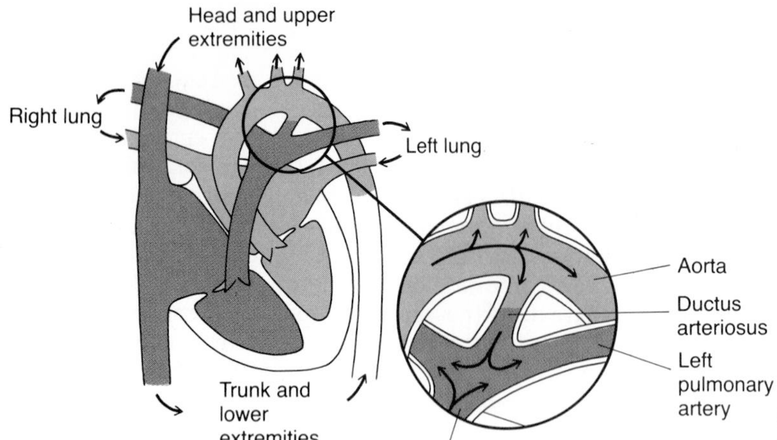

Figure 19–2. Patent ductus arteriosus, illustrating the degree of blood oxygenation in the different parts of the circulation.

fall. Simultaneously, the aortic pressure rises because of sudden cessation of blood flow through the placenta. Thus, the pressure in the pulmonary artery falls, while that in the aorta rises. As a result, forward blood flow through the ductus ceases suddenly at birth, and blood begins to flow backward from the aorta into the pulmonary artery. This new state of blood flow causes the ductus arteriosus to become occluded within a few hours to a few days in most babies, so that blood flow through the ductus does not persist. The ductus is believed to close because the aortic blood now flowing through the ductus has about two times as high an oxygen concentration as the pulmonary artery blood (which was actually venous blood) that had been flowing in the ductus during fetal life. The oxygen in turn constricts the ductus muscle.

Unfortunately, in about 1 of every 5500 babies the ductus never closes, causing the condition known as *patent ductus arteriosus,* which is illustrated in Figure 19–2.

Dynamics of Persistent Patent Ductus. In the child with a patent ductus, as much as half to two thirds of the aortic blood flows through the ductus into the pulmonary artery, then through the lungs, into the left atrium, and finally back into the left ventricle, passing through the lungs and left heart two or more times for every one time that it passes through the systemic circulation.

These persons do not show cyanosis until the heart fails or until the lungs become congested. Yet, because of the tremendous accessory flow of blood around and around through the lungs and left side of the heart, the output of the left ventricle in patent ductus arteriosus is often two to three times normal. Eventually, though, as a result of the increased load on the heart and especially because pulmonary congestion develops and becomes progressively more severe with age, most patients with uncorrected patent ductus die between the ages of 20 and 40 years.

Surgical Treatment. Surgical treatment of patent ductus arteriosus is extremely simple, for all one needs to do is to ligate the patent ductus or to divide it and sew the two ends.

Tetralogy of Fallot—A Right-to-Left Shunt

Tetralogy of Fallot is illustrated in Figure 19–3. This is the most common cause of the "blue baby" in which most of the blood by-passes the lungs, and therefore the aortic blood is mainly still unoxygenated venous blood. In this condition, four different abnormalities of the heart occur simultaneously.

1. The aorta originates from the right ventricle rather than the left, or it overrides the septum as shown in the figure, receiving blood from both ventricles.
2. The pulmonary artery is stenosed, so that much less than normal amounts of blood pass from the right ventricle into the lungs; instead the blood passes into the aorta.

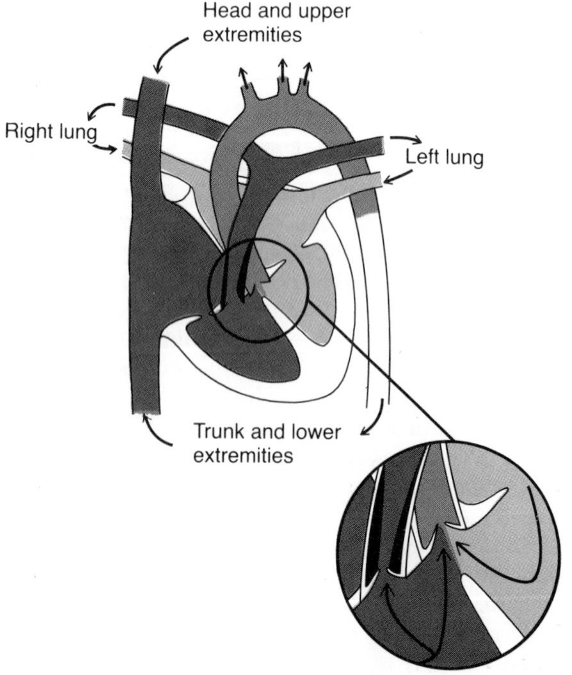

Figure 19–3. Tetralogy of Fallot, illustrating the degree of blood oxygenation in the different parts of the circulation.

3. Blood from the left ventricle flows either through a ventricular septal defect into the right ventricle and then into the aorta or directly into the overriding aorta.
4. Because the right side of the heart must pump large quantities of blood against the high pressure in the aorta, its musculature is highly developed, causing an enlarged right ventricle.

Abnormal Dynamics. It is readily apparent that the major physiological difficulty caused by tetralogy of Fallot is the shunting of blood past the lungs without its becoming oxygenated. As much as 75 per cent of the venous blood returning to the heart may pass directly from the right ventricle into the aorta without becoming oxygenated.

A diagnosis of tetralogy of Fallot is usually based on (1) the fact that the baby is *cyanotic* (blue), (2) records of high systolic pressure in the right ventricle recorded through a catheter, (3) characteristic changes in the radiological silhouette of the heart showing an enlarged right ventricle, and (4) angiograms showing abnormal blood flow through the interventricular septal defect into the overriding aorta and less flow through the stenosed pulmonary artery.

Surgical Treatment. Tetralogy of Fallot has been treated very successfully by surgery. The usual operation is to open the pulmonary stenosis, close the septal defect, and reconstruct the flow pathway into the aorta. When surgery is successful, the average life expectancy increases from only 3 to 4 years to 50 or more years.

Causes of Congenital Anomalies

One of the most common causes of congenital heart defects is a virus infection in the mother during the first trimester of pregnancy when the fetal heart is being formed. Defects are particularly prone to develop when the mother contracts German measles at this time — so often indeed that obstetricians advise termination of pregnancy if German measles occurs in the first trimester. However, some congenital defects of the heart are hereditary, for the same defect has been known to occur in identical twins and also in succeeding generations.

USE OF EXTRACORPOREAL CIRCULATION DURING CARDIAC SURGERY

It is almost impossible to repair intracardiac defects while the heart is still pumping. Therefore, many different types of artificial *heart-lung machines* have been developed to take the place of the heart and lungs during the course of operation. Such a system is called an *extracorporeal circulation.* The system consists principally of (1) a pump and (2) an oxygenating device. Almost any type of pump that does not cause hemolysis of the blood seems to be suitable.

The different principles that have been used for oxygenating blood are (1) bubbling oxygen through the blood and then removing the bubbles from the blood before passing it back into the patient, (2) dripping the blood downward over the surfaces of large areas of plastic sheet in the presence of oxygen, (3) passing the blood over the surfaces of rotating discs, and (4) passing the blood between thin membranes or through thin tubes that are porous to oxygen and carbon dioxide.

In the hands of experts, patients can be kept on artificial heart-lung machines for many hours while operations are performed on the inside of the heart.

CARDIAC FAILURE

Perhaps the most important ailment that must be treated by the physician is cardiac failure, which can result from any heart condition that reduces the ability of the heart to pump blood. Usually the cause is decreased contractility of the myocardium, resulting from diminished coronary blood flow, but failure to pump can also be caused by damage to the heart valves, external pressure around the heart, vitamin deficiency, primary cardiac muscle disease, or any other abnormality that makes the heart a hypoeffective pump.

Definition of Cardiac Failure. The term "cardiac failure" means simply *failure of the heart, usually because of some malfunction of the heart itself, to pump enough blood to satisfy the needs of the body.* Cardiac failure may be manifested in either of two ways: (1) by a decrease in cardiac output or (2) by a damming of the blood in the veins behind the left or right heart — even though the cardiac output may be normal or at times even above normal.

DYNAMICS OF THE CIRCULATION IN CARDIAC FAILURE

Acute Effects of Moderate Cardiac Failure

If a heart suddenly becomes severely damaged, such as by myocardial infarction, the pumping ability of the heart is immediately depressed. As a result, two essential effects occur: (1) reduced cardiac output and (2) damming of blood in the veins, resulting in increased systemic venous pressure. These two effects are shown graphically in Figure 19–4. This figure illustrates, first, a normal cardiac output curve, and point A on this curve is the normal operating point, with a normal cardiac output under resting conditions of 5 liters/minute and a right atrial pressure of 0 mm Hg.

Immediately after the heart becomes damaged, the cardiac output curve becomes greatly reduced, falling to the lower, short-dashed curve at the very bottom of the graph. Within a few seconds, a new circulatory state is established at point B rather than point A,

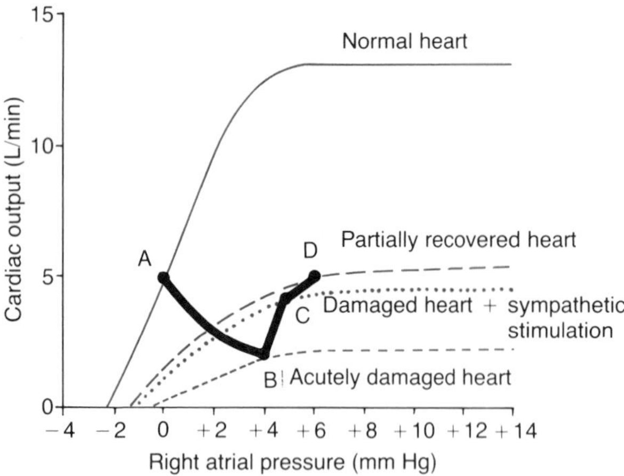

Figure 19-4. Progressive changes in the cardiac output curve following acute myocardial infarction. The cardiac output and right atrial pressure change progressively from point A to point D, as explained in the text.

showing that the cardiac output has fallen to 2 liters/min, about two-fifths normal, while the right atrial pressure has risen to 4 mm Hg because blood returning to the heart is dammed up in the right atrium. This low cardiac output is still sufficient to sustain life, but it is likely to be associated with fainting. Fortunately, this acute stage lasts for only a few seconds because sympathetic reflexes occur immediately that can compensate to a great extent for the damaged heart, as follows:

Compensation for Acute Cardiac Failure by Sympathetic Reflexes. When the cardiac output falls precariously low, many of the different circulatory reflexes discussed in Chapter 15 are immediately activated. The best known of these is the baroreceptor reflex, which is activated by diminished arterial pressure. It is probable that the chemoreceptor reflex, the central nervous system ischemic response, and even reflexes originating in the damaged heart itself also contribute to the nervous response. But whatever all the reflexes might be, the sympathetics become strongly stimulated within a few seconds, and the parasympathetics become reciprocally inhibited at the same time.

Strong sympathetic stimulation has two major effects on the circulation: first, on the heart itself and, second, on the peripheral vasculature. If all the heart musculature is diffusely damaged but is still functional, sympathetic stimulation strengthens this damaged musculature. If part of the muscle is totally nonfunctional, while part of it is still normal, the normal muscle is strongly stimulated by sympathetic stimulation, in this way compensating for the nonfunctional muscle. Thus, *the heart one way or another becomes a stronger pump, often as much as 100 per cent stronger, under the influence of the sympathetic impulses.* This effect is also illustrated in Figure 19-4, which shows elevation of the cardiac output curve after sympathetic compensation (the dotted curve).

Sympathetic stimulation also increases the tendency for venous return, for it increases the tone of most of the blood vessels of the circulation, especially of the veins, *raising the peripheral venous pressures* to about 100 per cent above normal. As should be recalled from the discussion in Chapter 17, this greatly increases the tendency for blood to flow back to the heart. Therefore, the damaged heart becomes primed with more inflowing blood than usual, and the right atrial pressure rises still further, which helps the heart pump larger quantities of blood. Thus, in Figure 19-4 the new circulatory state is depicted by point C, showing a cardiac output of 4.2 liters/min and a right atrial pressure of 5 mm Hg.

The sympathetic reflexes become maximally developed in about 30 seconds. Therefore, a person who has a sudden moderate heart attack might experience nothing more than cardiac pain and a few seconds of fainting. Shortly thereafter, with the aid of the sympathetic reflex compensations, the cardiac output may return to a level entirely adequate to sustain the person who remains quiet, though the pain might persist.

The Chronic Stage of Failure

After the first few minutes of an acute heart attack, a prolonged secondary state begins. This is characterized mainly by two events: (1) retention of fluid by the kidneys and (2) usually progressive recovery of the heart itself over a period of several weeks to months, as discussed in the previous chapter.

Renal Retention of Fluid and Increase in Blood Volume

A low cardiac output has a profound effect on renal function, sometimes causing anuria when the cardiac output falls to as low as one-half to two-thirds normal. In general, the urinary output remains reduced as long as the cardiac output is significantly less than normal, and it usually does not return to normal after an acute heart attack until the cardiac output rises either all the way back to normal or almost to normal.

The Beneficial Effects of Moderate Fluid Retention in Cardiac Failure. Although many cardiologists formerly considered fluid retention always to have a detrimental effect in cardiac failure, it is now known that a moderate increase in body fluid and blood volume is actually a very important factor helping to compensate for the diminished pumping ability of the heart. It does this by increasing the tendency for venous return. That is, the increased blood volume increases the venous return in two ways: First, it increases the pressure in virtually all the peripheral blood vessels, especially the veins, which *increases the pressure gradient for causing flow of blood toward the heart.* Second, it distends the veins, which *reduces the venous resistance* and thereby allows increased ease of flow of blood to the heart.

If the heart is not too greatly damaged, this increased tendency for venous return can often fully compensate for the heart's diminished pumping ability — so much so, in fact, that if the heart's pumping ability is reduced to as little as 40 to 50 per cent of normal, still the increased venous return can often cause an entirely normal cardiac output.

On the other hand, when the heart's maximum pumping ability is reduced to less than 25 to 45 per cent of normal, the blood flow to the kidneys becomes too low for the urinary output of salt and water ever to equal the intake. Therefore, fluid retention begins and will continue indefinitely unless major therapeutic procedures are employed to prevent this. Furthermore, because the heart is already pumping at its maximum pumping capacity, this excess fluid no longer has a beneficial effect on the circulation. Instead, very severe edema develops throughout the body, which can be very detrimental in itself and can lead to death.

Detrimental Effects of Excess Fluid Retention in the Severe Stages of Cardiac Failure. In contrast to the beneficial effects of moderate fluid retention in cardiac failure, in severe failure with extreme excesses of fluid retention, the fluid then begins to have very serious physiological consequences, including overstretching of the heart, thus weakening the heart still more; filtration of fluid into the lungs to cause pulmonary edema and consequent deoxygenation of the blood; and, often, development of extensive edema in all of the peripheral tissues of the body as well. These detrimental effects of excessive fluid are discussed in subsequent sections of the chapter.

Recovery of the Myocardium Following Myocardial Infarction

After a heart becomes suddenly damaged as a result of myocardial infarction, the natural reparative processes of the body begin immediately to help restore normal cardiac function. Thus, a new collateral blood supply begins to penetrate the peripheral portions of the infarcted area, often causing much of the muscle in the fringe areas to become functional again. Also, the undamaged musculature hypertrophies, in this way offsetting much of the cardiac damage.

Obviously, the degree of recovery depends on the type of cardiac damage, and it varies from no recovery at all to almost complete recovery. Ordinarily, after myocardial infarction the heart recovers rapidly during the first few days and weeks and will have achieved most of its final state of recovery within 5 to 7 weeks, though some recovery continues for months.

Cardiac Output Curve After Partial Recovery. The long-dashed curve of Figure 19-4 illustrates function of the partially recovered heart a week or so after the acute myocardial infarction. By this time, considerable fluid also has been retained in the body, and the tendency for venous return has increased markedly; therefore, the right atrial pressure has risen even more. As a result, the state of the circulation is now changed from point C to point D, which represents a *normal* cardiac output of 5 liters/minute but a right atrial pressure elevated to 6 mm Hg.

Because the cardiac output has returned to normal, renal output also will have returned to normal, and no further fluid retention will occur. Therefore, except for the high right atrial pressure represented by point D in this figure, the person now has essentially normal cardiovascular dynamics *as long as he remains at rest.*

If the heart itself recovers to a significant extent and if adequate fluid retention occurs, the sympathetic stimulation gradually abates toward normal for the following reasons: The partial recovery of the heart can do the same thing for the cardiac output curve as sympathetic stimulation, and the increased blood volume can do the same thing for venous return as sympathetic contraction of the veins. Thus, as these two factors develop, the fast pulse rate, cold skin, and pallor resulting from sympathetic stimulation in the acute stage of cardiac failure gradually disappear.

Summary of the Changes That Occur Following Acute Cardiac Failure — "Compensated Heart Failure"

To summarize the events discussed in the past few sections describing the dynamics of circulatory changes following an acute, moderate heart attack, we may divide the stages into (1) the instantaneous effect of the cardiac damage; (2) compensation by the sympathetic nervous system, which occurs mainly within the first 30 seconds to 1 minute; and (3) chronic compensations resulting from partial cardiac recovery and renal retention of fluid. These progressive changes are shown graphically by the very heavy line in Figure 19-4. The progression of this line shows the normal state of the circulation (point A), the state a few seconds after the heart attack but before sympathetic reflexes have occurred (point B), the rise in cardiac output toward normal caused by sympathetic stimulation (point C), and final return of the cardiac output to normal following several days to several weeks of heart muscle recovery and fluid retention (point D). This final state is called *compensated heart failure.*

Compensated Heart Failure. Note especially in Figure 19-4 that the pumping ability of the heart, as depicted by the cardiac output curve, is still depressed to less than one half normal. This illustrates that factors that increase the right atrial pressure (principally the increased blood volume caused by retention of fluid) can maintain the cardiac output at a normal level despite continued weakness of the heart itself. However, one of the results of chronic cardiac weakness is this chronic increase in right atrial pressure itself; in Figure 19-4 it is shown to be 6 mm Hg. Many persons, especially in old age, have completely normal resting cardiac outputs but mildly to moderately elevated right atrial pressures because of compensated heart failure. These persons may not know that they have cardiac damage because the damage more often than not has occurred a little at a time, and the compensation has occurred concurrently with the progressive stages of damage.

When a person is in compensated heart failure, any attempt to perform heavy exercise will usually cause immediate return of the symptoms of acute failure because the heart simply is not able to increase its pumping capacity to the levels required to sustain the exercise. Therefore, it is said that the *cardiac reserve* is reduced in compensated heart failure.

Dynamics of Severe Cardiac Failure—Decompensated Heart Failure

If the heart becomes severely damaged, no amount of compensation, either by sympathetic nervous reflexes or by fluid retention, can make this weakened heart pump a normal cardiac output. As a consequence, the cardiac output cannot rise to a high enough value to bring about return of normal renal function. Fluid continues to be retained, the person develops progressively more and more edema, and this state of events eventually leads to death. This is called *decompensated heart failure.*

Thus, the main basis of decompensated heart failure is *failure of the heart to pump sufficient blood to make the kidneys function adequately.*

Analysis of Decompensated Heart Failure. Figure 19–5 illustrates a greatly depressed cardiac output curve, depicting the function of a heart that has become extremely weakened and cannot be strengthened. Point A on this curve represents the approximate state of the circulation before any compensation has occurred, and point B the state after the first few minutes of acute compensation by sympathetic stimulation, as described previously. At point B, the cardiac output has risen to 4 liters/min and the right atrial pressure to 5 mm Hg. The person appears to be in reasonably good condition, but this state will not remain static for the following reason: The cardiac output has not risen quite high enough to cause adequate kidney excretion of fluid; therefore, fluid retention continues unabated and can eventually be the cause of death. These events can be explained quantitatively in the following way:

Note the dashed line at a cardiac output level of 5 liters in Figure 19–5. This is the critical cardiac output level that is required to allow the kidneys to reestablish normal fluid balance—that is, for the output of salt and water to become as great as the intake of these. At any cardiac output below this level, all the fluid-retaining mechanisms discussed in the earlier section remain in play, and the body fluid volumes increase progressively. Because of this progressive increase in fluid volume, the state of the circulation changes in Figure 19–5 from point B to point C—the right atrial pressure rising to 7 mm Hg and the cardiac output to 4.2 liters/min. However, note again that the cardiac output is still not high enough to cause normal renal output of fluid; therefore, fluid continues to be retained, and after another day or so the right atrial pressure rises to 9 mm Hg, and the circulatory state becomes that depicted by point D. Still, the cardiac output is not enough to establish normal fluid balance.

After another few days of fluid retention, the right atrial pressure has risen still further, but by now the cardiac function curve is beginning to decline toward a lower level. This decline is caused by overstretch of the heart, edema of the heart muscle, and other factors that diminish the pumping performance of the heart. It is now clear that further retention of fluid will be more detrimental than beneficial to the circulation. Yet, the cardiac output still is not high enough to bring about normal renal function, and fluid retention not only continues but actually accelerates because of the falling cardiac output. Consequently, within a few days the state of the circulation has reached point F on the curve, with the cardiac output less than 2.5 liters/min and the right atrial pressure 16 mm Hg. This is a state that now has reached incompatibility with life, and the patient dies. This state of heart failure in which the failure continues to worsen is called *decompensated heart failure.*

Thus, one can see from this analysis that failure of the cardiac output ever to rise to the critical level required for normal renal function results in (1) progressive retention of fluid, which causes (2) progressive elevation of the right atrial pressure until finally the heart is so overstretched or so edematous that it becomes unable to pump even moderate quantities of blood and, therefore, fails completely. Clinically, one detects this serious condition of decompensation principally by the progressive edema, especially edema of the lungs, which leads to bubbling rales in the lungs and dyspnea (air hunger). All clinicians

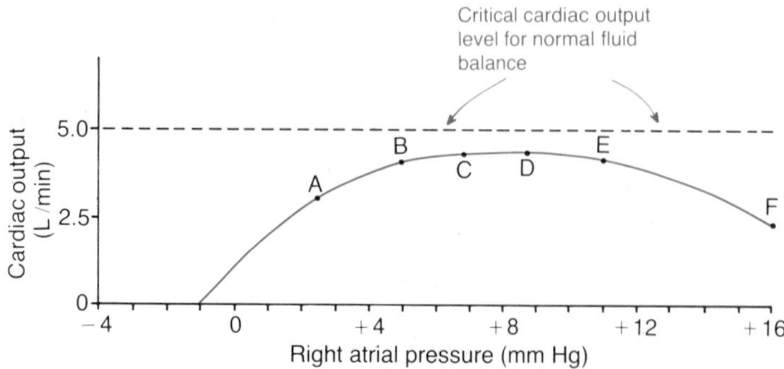

Figure 19–5. Greatly depressed cardiac output curve that indicates decompensated heart disease. Progressive fluid retention raises the right atrial pressure, and the cardiac output progresses from point A to point F, as explained in the text.

know that lack of appropriate therapy when this state of events occurs leads to rapid death.

Treatment of Decompensation. The two ways in which the decompensation process can often be stopped are (1) by strengthening the heart in any one of several ways, especially by administration of a cardiotonic drug, such as digitalis, so that it can pump adequate quantities of blood to make the kidneys function normally again, or (2) by administering diuretics and reducing water and salt intake, which brings about a balance between fluid intake and output despite the low cardiac output.

Both methods stop the decompensation process by re-establishing normal fluid balance, so that at least as much fluid leaves the body as enters it.

UNILATERAL LEFT HEART FAILURE

In the discussions thus far in this chapter, we have considered failure of the heart as a whole. Yet in a large number of patients, especially those with early acute failure, left-sided failure predominates over right-sided failure, and only in rare instances will the right side fail without significant failure of the left side. Therefore, we need especially to discuss the special features of unilateral left heart failure.

When the left side of the heart fails without concomitant failure of the right side, blood continues to be pumped into the lungs with usual right heart vigor, whereas it is not pumped adequately out of the lungs into the systemic circulation. As a result, the pressures in all the blood vessels in the lungs rise because of shift of large volumes of blood from the systemic circulation into the pulmonary circulation.

As the volume of blood in the lungs increases, the pulmonary capillary pressure also increases, and if this rises above a value approximately equal to the colloid osmotic pressure of the plasma, about 28 mm Hg, fluid begins to filter out of the capillaries into the interstitial spaces and alveoli, resulting in pulmonary edema.

Thus, among the most important problems of left heart failure are *pulmonary vascular congestion* and *pulmonary edema*. In severe acute left heart failure, pulmonary edema occasionally occurs so rapidly that it causes death by suffocation in as little as 20 to 30 minutes.

LOW OUTPUT CARDIAC FAILURE—"CARDIOGENIC SHOCK"

In many instances after acute heart attacks, and even sometimes after prolonged periods of slow progressive cardiac deterioration, the heart becomes incapable of pumping even the minimal amount of blood flow required to keep the body alive. Consequently, all the body tissues begin to suffer and even to deteriorate, often leading to death within a few hours to a few days. The picture then is one of circulatory shock, as explained in Chapter 17. Even the cardiovascular system itself suffers from lack of nutrition, and it, too, deteriorates, along with the remainder of the body, thus hastening the death. This circulatory shock syndrome caused by inadequate cardiac pumping is called *cardiogenic shock* or simply *cardiac shock*. Once a person develops cardiogenic shock, the survival rate even with the best of therapy is usually less than 15 per cent.

Vicious Circle of Cardiac Deterioration in Cardiogenic Shock. The discussion of circulatory shock in Chapter 17 emphasizes the tendency of the heart itself to become progressively more damaged during the course of shock. That is, the low arterial pressure that occurs during shock reduces the coronary supply, which makes the heart still weaker, which makes the shock still worse, the process eventually becoming a vicious circle of cardiac deterioration. In cardiogenic shock caused by myocardial infarction, this problem is greatly compounded by the already existing coronary thrombosis. For instance, in a normal heart, the arterial pressure usually must be reduced below about 45 mm Hg before cardiac deterioration sets in. However, in a heart that already has a blocked major coronary vessel, deterioration will set in when the arterial pressure falls to as low as 80 to 90 mm Hg. In other words, even the minutest amount of fall in arterial pressure can set off a vicious circle of cardiac deterioration following myocardial infarction. For this reason, in treating myocardial infarction it is extremely important to prevent even short periods of hypotension.

Physiology of Treatment. Often a patient dies of cardiogenic shock before the various compensatory processes can return the cardiac output to a life-sustaining level. Therefore, treatment of this condition is one of the most important problems in the management of acute heart attacks. Immediate digitalization of the heart is often employed for strengthening the heart if the remaining functioning ventricular muscle shows signs of deterioration. Also, infusion of whole blood, plasma, or a blood pressure-raising drug is used to sustain the arterial pressure. If the arterial pressure can be raised high enough, the coronary blood flow may be elevated to a high enough value to prevent the vicious circle of deterioration until appropriate compensatory mechanisms in the body can correct the shock. Even with the best therapy, however, once the shock syndrome has begun, with the arterial pressure remaining as much as 20 mm Hg below normal for as long as an hour, 85 per cent of the patients die.

EDEMA IN PATIENTS WITH CARDIAC FAILURE—ROLE OF THE KIDNEYS

When the heart fails acutely, the formation of urine by the kidneys almost always falls drastically, and this causes the water and salt that we drink and eat to begin accumulating in the body. There are three known causes of the reduced renal output, all of which are perhaps equally important though in different ways.

1. Decreased Glomerular Filtration. A decrease in cardiac output has a tendency to reduce the glomerular pressure in the kidneys because of (1) *reduced arterial pressure* and (2) *intense sympathetic constriction of the afferent arterioles of the kidney.* As a consequence, except in the mildest degrees of heart failure, the glomerular filtration rate becomes less than normal. It should become evident from the discussion of kidney function in Chapters 21 and 22 that *even a very slight decrease in glomerular filtration often decreases urine output markedly.* When the cardiac output falls to about one half normal, this factor alone can result in almost complete anuria.

2. Activation of the Renin-Angiotensin System and Increased Reabsorption of Water and Salt by the Renal Tubules. The reduced blood flow to the kidneys causes marked increase in renin output, and this in turn causes the formation of angiotensin by the mechanism described in Chapter 16. The angiotensin has a direct effect on the arterioles of the kidneys to decrease further the blood flow through the kidneys. Therefore, the net loss of water and salt into the urine is greatly decreased, and the quantities of salt and water in the body fluids increase.

3. Increased Aldosterone Secretion. In the chronic stage of heart failure, large quantities of aldosterone are secreted by the adrenal cortex. This results mainly from the effect of angiotensin in stimulating aldosterone secretion. The elevated aldosterone, in turn, further increases the reabsorption of sodium and water from the renal tubules.

Acute Pulmonary Edema in Chronic Heart Failure — A Lethal Vicious Circle

A frequent cause of death is acute pulmonary edema occurring in patients who have had chronic heart failure for a long time. When this occurs in a person without new cardiac damage, it usually is set off by some temporary overload of the heart, such as might result from a bout of heavy exercise, some emotional experience, or even a severe cold. This acute pulmonary edema is believed to result from the following vicious circle:

1. A temporarily increased load on the already weak left ventricle results from increased venous return from the peripheral circulation. Because of the limited pumping capacity of the left heart, blood begins to dam up in the lungs.
2. The increased blood in the lungs elevates the pulmonary capillary pressure, and a small amount of fluid begins to transude into the lung tissues and alveoli.
3. The increased fluid in the lungs diminishes the degree of oxygenation of the blood.
4. The decreased oxygen in the blood further weakens the heart and also causes peripheral vasodilatation.
5. The peripheral vasodilatation increases venous return from the peripheral circulation still more.
6. The increased venous return further increases the damming of the blood in the lungs, leading to still more transudation of fluid, more arterial oxygen desaturation, more venous return, and so forth. Thus, a vicious circle has been established.

Once this vicious circle has proceeded beyond a certain critical point, it will continue until death of the patient unless heroic therapeutic measures are employed. The types of heroic therapeutic measures that can reverse the process and save the life of the patient include

1. Putting tourniquets on all four limbs to sequester much of the blood in the veins and therefore to decrease the workload on the left heart.
2. Bleeding the patient.
3. Giving a rapidly acting diuretic, such as furosemide, to cause rapid loss of fluid from the body.
4. Giving the patient pure oxygen to breathe to reverse the blood desaturation, the heart deterioration, and the peripheral vasodilatation.
5. Giving the patient a rapidly acting cardiotonic drug, such as ouabain, to strengthen the heart.

Unfortunately, this vicious circle of acute pulmonary edema can proceed so rapidly that death can occur within 20 minutes to an hour. Therefore, any procedure that is to be successful must be instituted immediately.

CARDIAC RESERVE

The maximum percentage that the cardiac output can increase above normal is called the *cardiac reserve.* Thus, in the normal young adult the cardiac reserve is 300 to 400 per cent. In the athletically trained person, it is occasionally as high as 500 to 600 per cent, whereas in the asthenic or elderly person, it may be as low as 200 per cent. In heart failure, there is no reserve at all.

Any factor that prevents the heart from pumping

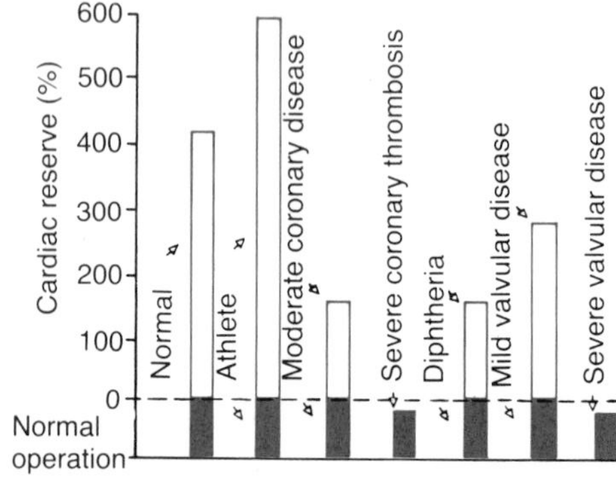

Figure 19-6. Cardiac reserve in different conditions.

blood satisfactorily decreases the cardiac reserve. This can result from ischemic heart disease, primary myocardial disease, vitamin deficiency, damage to the myocardium, valvular heart disease, and many other factors, some of which are illustrated in Figure 19–6.

Diagnosis of Low Cardiac Reserve—The Exercise Test. So long as people with low cardiac reserve remain in a state of rest, they usually will not know that they have heart disease. However, a diagnosis of low cardiac reserve can usually be made easily by requiring a person to exercise either on a treadmill or by walking up and down steps. The increased load on the heart rapidly uses up the small amount of reserve that is available, and the cardiac output fails to rise high enough to sustain the body's new level of activity. The acute effects are

1. Immediate and sometimes extreme shortness of breath (dyspnea) resulting from the heart's not pumping sufficient blood to the tissues, thereby causing tissue ischemia and creating a sensation of air hunger.
2. Extreme muscle fatigue resulting from muscle ischemia, thus limiting the person's ability to continue with the exercise.
3. Excessive increase in heart rate because the nervous reflexes overreact in an attempt to overcome the inadequate cardiac output.

Therefore, exercise tests are part of the armamentarium of the cardiologist. These tests take the place of cardiac output measurements that unfortunately cannot be made with ease in most clinical settings.

REFERENCES

Heart Sounds and Valvular and Congenital Heart Defects

Dunn, J. M.: Cardiac Valve Disease in Children. New York, Elsevier Science Publishing Co., 1988.
Hallman, G. L., et al.: Surgical Treatment of Congenital Heart Disease. 3rd ed. Philadelphia, Lea & Febiger, 1987.
Montgomery, W. H., and Atkins, J. A.: Decision Making in Emergency Cardiology. St. Louis, C. V. Mosby Co., 1989.
Rutherford, R. B.: Vascular Surgery. 3rd ed. Philadelphia, W. B. Saunders Co., 1989.
Shields, T. W. (ed.): General Thoracic Surgery. 3rd ed. Philadelphia, Lea & Febiger, 1989.
Simpson, P. C.: Proto-oncogenes and cardiac hypertrophy. Annu. Rev. Physiol., 51:189, 1989.
Weyman, A. E.: Principles and Practice of Echocardiography, 2nd ed. Philadelphia, Lea & Febiger, 1989.

Cardiac Failure

Braunwald, E.: Heart Disease. Philadelphia, W. B. Saunders Co., 1988.
Francis, G. S.: Neurohumoral mechanisms involved in congestive heart failure. Am. J. Cardiol., 55:15A, 1985.
Goldberger, E.: Treatment of Cardiac Emergencies. St. Louis, C. V. Mosby Co., 1989.
Guyton, A. C., et al.: Cardiac Output and Its Regulation. Philadelphia, W. B. Saunders Co., 1973.
Miller, A. J.: Diagnosis of Chest Pain. New York, Raven Press, 1988.
Shoemaker, W. C., et al.: Society of Critical Care Medicine, The Textbook of Critical Care. 2nd ed. Philadelphia, W. B. Saunders Co., 1988.
Tintinalli, J. E., et al.: Emergency Medicine: A Comprehensive Study Guide. 2nd ed. New York, McGraw-Hill Book Co., 1988.
Wasserman, K., et al.: Principles of Exercise Testing and Interpretation. Philadelphia, Lea & Febiger, 1987.
Weisfeldt, M. L.: The aging heart. Hosp. Pract., 20:115, 1985.

QUESTIONS

1. What causes the normal first and second heart sounds?
2. What is the cause of rheumatic valvular heart disease? What is the difference between a *stenosed valve* and a *regurgitating valve*?
3. Describe the *heart murmurs* caused by different valvular lesions.
4. Describe the dynamics of the circulation in *aortic stenosis, aortic regurgitation, mitral stenosis,* and *mitral regurgitation.*
5. Why do fatigue and pulmonary edema freqently occur in valvular heart disease patients during exercise?
6. Describe the cause and circulatory effects of *patent ductus arteriosus.*
7. Describe the congenital abnormality of the heart called *tetralogy of Fallot.* Explain why this is called a *right-to-left shunt* and why it is so detrimental to the circulatory system.
8. Describe the sequential changes that occur in circulation function after an *acute myocardial infarction* and the development of acute cardiac failure and subsequent recovery of circulatory function.
9. Explain why moderate fluid retention can be of value in helping the circulatory system to compensate for moderate degrees of heart failure, whereas extreme retention of fluid in severe degrees of heart failure can be lethal.
10. What are the specific characteristics of *unilateral left heart failure*? Explain why pulmonary edema is usually worse in unilateral left heart failure than in generalized heart failure.
11. What is meant by *cardiogenic shock*? Why does this condition frequently lead to a vicious circle of cardiac deterioration?
12. What is meant by *cardiac reserve*? What are some of the causes of very low cardiac reserve?

V

The Body Fluids and the Kidneys

20

The Body Fluid Compartments: Extracellular and Intracellular Fluids and Edema

The body fluids are so important to the basic physiology of bodily function that we discuss them at several points in this text but each time in different contexts. In the present chapter and in the following chapters on the kidneys, we are concerned with the body fluids from the total point of view, including regulation of body fluid volume, regulation of the constituents in the extracellular fluid, regulation of acid-base balance, and factors that govern gross interchange of fluid between the extracellular and intracellular compartments.

Total Body Water

The total amount of water in a man of average weight (70 kilograms) is approximately 40 liters (Fig. 20–1), averaging 57 per cent of his total body weight.

Daily Intake of Water. Most of our daily intake of water enters the body by the oral route. Approximately two thirds is in the form of pure water or some other beverage, and the remainder is in the food that is eaten. A small amount is also synthesized in the body as the result of oxidation of hydrogen in the food; this quantity ranges between 150 and 250 ml/day, depending on the rate of metabolism. The normal intake of fluid, including that synthesized, averages about 2300 ml/day.

Daily Loss of Body Water. Table 20–1 shows the routes by which water is lost from the body under different conditions. Normally, at an atmospheric temperature of about 68°F (20°C), approximately 1400 of the 2300 milliliters of water intake is lost in the *urine,* 100 milliliters is lost in the *sweat,* and 100 milliliters in the *feces.* The remaining 700 milliliters is lost by *evaporation from the respiratory tract* or by *diffusion through the skin.*

Loss of Water in Hot Weather and During Exercise. In very hot weather, water loss in sweat occasionally rises to as much as 1.5 to 2.0 liters an hour, which obviously can rapidly deplete the body fluids. Sweating is discussed in Chapter 47 in relation to body temperature regulation.

Exercise increases the loss of water in two ways. First, exercise increases the rate of respiration, which promotes increased water evaporation from the respiratory tract in proportion to the increased ventilatory rate. Second, and much more important, exercise increases the body heat and consequently is likely to result in excessive sweating to lower the body temperature.

BODY FLUID COMPARTMENTS

The Intracellular Fluid Compartment

About 25 of the 40 liters of fluid in the body are inside the approximately 100 trillion cells of the body and are collectively called the *intracellular fluid.* The fluid of each cell contains its own individual mixture of different constituents, but the concentrations of these constituents are reasonably similar from one cell to another. For this reason the intracellular fluid of all the different cells together is considered to be one large fluid compartment.

The Extracellular Fluid Compartment

All the fluids outside the cells are called *extracellular fluid,* and these fluids are constantly mixing, as explained in Chapter 1. The total amount of fluid in the extracellular compartment averages about 15 liters in a 70-kilogram adult.

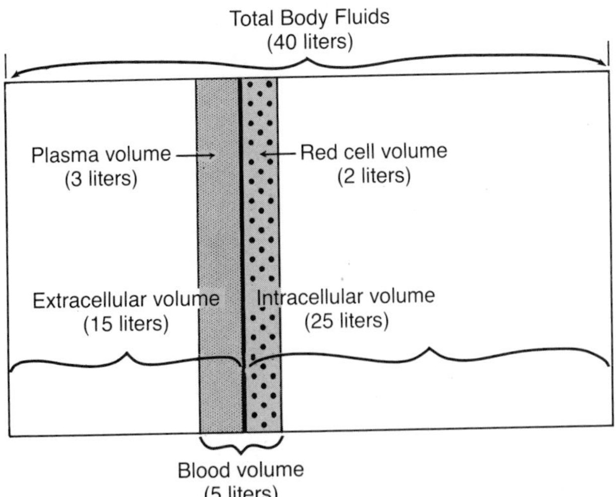

Figure 20-1. The body fluids diagrammed, showing the extracellular fluid volume, intracellular fluid volume, blood volume, and total body fluids.

The extracellular fluid can be divided into *interstitial fluid, plasma, cerebrospinal fluid, intraocular fluid, fluids of the gastrointestinal tract,* and *fluids of the potential spaces.*

Plasma. The plasma is the noncellular portion of blood. It is part of the extracellular fluid and communicates continually with the interstitial fluid through pores in the capillaries. The plasma volume averages 3 liters in the normal adult.

Blood Volume

Blood contains both extracellular fluid (the fluid of the plasma) and intracellular fluid (the fluid in the red blood cells). However, since blood is contained in a closed chamber all its own—the circulatory system—its volume and its special dynamics are exceedingly important.

The average blood volume of normal adult is almost exactly 5000 milliliters. On the average, approximately *3000 milliliters of this is plasma,* and the remainder, *2000 milliliters, is red blood cells.* However, these values vary greatly in different individuals; also, sex, weight, and many other factors affect the blood volume.

Table 20-1 DAILY LOSS OF WATER (IN MILLILITERS)

	Normal Temperature	Hot Weather	Prolonged Heavy Exercise
Insensible loss:			
Skin	350	350	350
Respiratory tract	350	250	650
Urine	1400	1200	500
Sweat	100	1400	5000
Feces	100	100	100
TOTAL	2300	3300	6600

The Hematocrit. The hematocrit is the percentage of red blood cells in the blood as determined by centrifuging blood in a "hematocrit tube" until the cells become packed tightly in the bottom of the tube. The hematocrit (H) is approximately 42 for a normal man and 38 for a normal woman.

In severe anemia, the hematocrit may fall to as low as 10, but this small quantity of red blood cells is barely sufficient to sustain life. On the other hand, a few conditions cause excessive production of red blood cells, resulting in polycythemia. In these instances, the hematocrit occasionally rises to 65. Obviously, there is an upper limit to the level of the hematocrit in polycythemic blood, because excessive hematocrit causes the blood to become so viscous that death ensues as a result of multiple plugging of the peripheral vascular tree.

Measurement of Body Fluid Volumes

The Dilution Principle for Measuring Fluid Volumes

The volume of any fluid compartment of the body can be measured by placing a substance in the compartment, allowing it to disperse evenly throughout the fluid, and then measuring the extent to which the substance has become diluted. Figure 20-2 illustrates this "dilution" principle for measuring the volume of any fluid compartment of the body. In this example, a small quantity of dye or other foreign substance is placed in fluid chamber A, and the substance is allowed to disperse throughout the chamber until it becomes mixed in equal concentrations in all areas, as shown in chamber B. Then a sample of the dispersed fluid is removed and the concentration of the substance is analyzed chemically, photoelectrically, or by any other means. The volume of the chamber can then be determined from the following formula:

$$\text{Volume in milliliters} = \frac{\text{Quantity of test substance instilled}}{\text{Concentration per ml of dispersed fluid}}$$

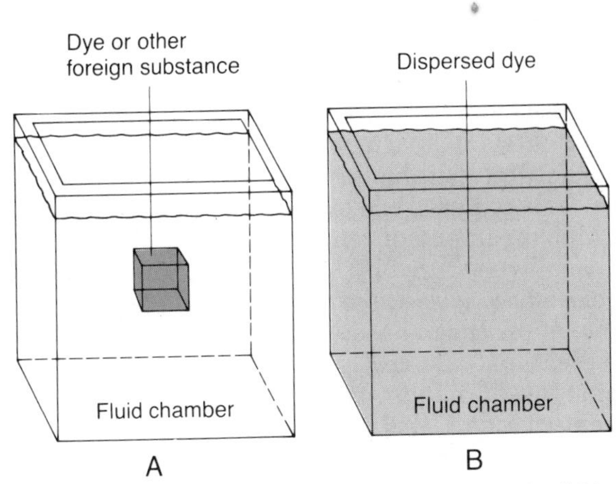

Figure 20-2. Principles of the dilution method for measuring fluid volumes (explained in the text).

Note that all one needs to know is (1) the *total quantity of the test substance* put into the chamber and (2) the *concentration in the fluid after dispersement.* As an example, if 10 milligrams of dye is dispersed in a chamber and the final concentration is 0.01 milligram for each milliliter of fluid, then the volume calculates to be 10 divided by 0.01, or 1000 milliliters.

Determination of Volumes of Different Body Fluid Compartments

Fortunately, certain substances remain in specific fluid compartments without diffusing into the other compartments. Therefore, by choosing the appropriate "marker substance," the fluid volume of almost any compartment of the body can be measured using the dilution principle. Some of the substances used for measuring fluid volumes are as follows:

Total Body Water. Radioactive water or heavy water contains respectively radioactive *tritium* (H^3) or *deuterium* (H^2). These mix with the total body water within a few hours after being injected into the blood, and the dilution principle can be used to calculate the total body water.

Extracellular Fluid Volume. Multiple substances diffuse into most of the extracellular fluids, with only small amounts diffusing into the cells; these include *radioactive sodium, radioactive chloride, radioactive bromide, radioiothalamate, thiosulfate ion, thiocyanite ion, inulin,* and *sucrose.* When any one of these is injected into the blood, it will usually mix almost completely with the extracellular fluids within 30 minutes to an hour, and the dilution principle can then be used to calculate the extracellular fluid volume.

Calculation of Intracellular Volume. Obviously, by subtracting the extracellular fluid volume from the total body water, one can calculate the intracellular fluid volume.

Measurement of Plasma Volume. Any substance that attaches strongly to the plasma proteins will diffuse throughout the plasma with only small amounts leaking into the interstitium. Therefore, radioactive plasma protein, such as ^{131}I-protein, or plasma protein to which a so-called vital dye has been attached can be used to measure plasma volume. A vital dye often used is *T-1824,* also called *Evans blue.*

Calculation of Interstitial Fluid Volume. To calculate interstitial fluid volume, the plasma volume is subtracted from the extracellular fluid volume.

Measurement of Blood Volume. Blood volume is usually measured by injecting into the circulation *radioactively labeled red cells.* After these mix in the circulation, the radioactivity of a sample of blood can be measured and the total blood volume calculated using the dilution principle. The substance most frequently used to label the red blood cells is *radioactive chromium* (^{51}Cr), which binds tightly with the red blood cells.

CONSTITUENTS OF EXTRACELLULAR AND INTRACELLULAR FLUIDS

The constituents of extracellular and intracellular fluids are illustrated diagrammatically and quantitatively in Figures 20–3 and 20–4 and in Table 20–2. Figure 20–3 gives the compositions of plasma, interstitial fluid, and intracellular fluid in milliequivalents per liter. Figure 20–4 shows the concentrations of the nonelectrolytes in plasma, expressed as milligrams per deciliter of plasma. Finally, Table 20–2 gives the constituents of plasma, interstitial fluid, and intracellular fluid in terms of their milliosmolar concentrations.

Important Constituents of the Extracellular Fluid. Referring again to Figure 20–3, one sees that extracellular fluid, both that of the blood plasma and that of the interstitial fluid, contains large quantities of *sodium* and *chloride ions,* reasonably large quantities of *bicarbonate ion,* but only small quantities of potassium, calcium, magnesium, phosphate, sulfate, and organic acid ions. In addition, plasma contains a large amount of protein, whereas interstitial fluid contains much less.

In Chapter 1, it is pointed out that the extracellular fluid is called the *internal environment* of the body and that its constituents are accurately regulated, mainly by the kidneys, so that the cells remain bathed continually in a fluid containing the proper electrolytes and nutrients for continued cellular function.

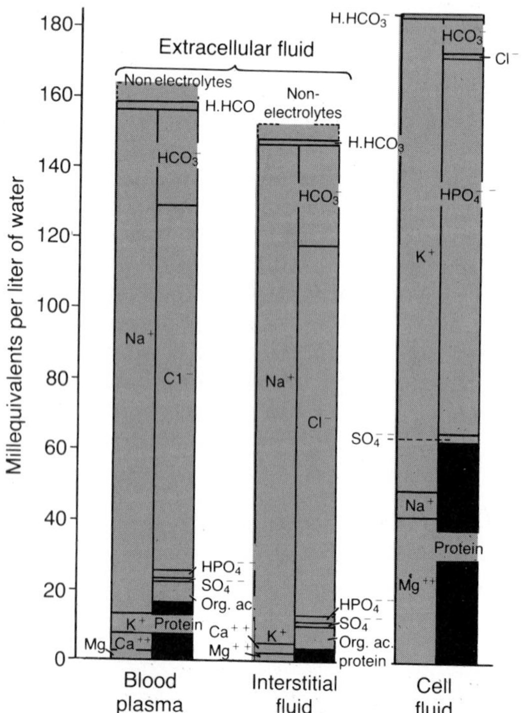

Figure 20–3. The compositions of plasma, interstitial fluid, and intracellular fluid. (Modified from Gamble: Chemical Anatomy, Physiology, and Pathology of Extracellular Fluid: A Lecture Syllabus. Cambridge, Mass., Harvard University Press, 1954. Reprinted with permission.)

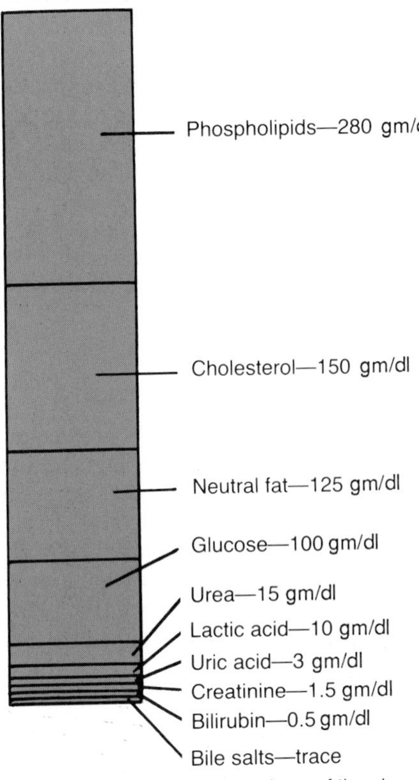

Figure 20-4. The nonelectrolytes of the plasma.

The regulation of most of these constituents is presented in Chapter 22.

Important Constituents of the Intracellular Fluid. From Figure 20-3 it is also clear that the intracellular fluid contains only small quantities of sodium and chloride ions and almost no calcium ions; but it does contain large quantities of *potassium* and *phosphate* and moderate quantities of *magnesium* and *sulfate ions,* all of which are present in only small concentrations in the extracellular fluid. In addition, cells contain very large amounts of protein, approximately four times as much as in plasma.

OSMOTIC EQUILIBRIA AND FLUID SHIFTS BETWEEN THE EXTRACELLULAR AND INTRACELLULAR FLUIDS

One of the most troublesome of all problems in clinical medicine is maintenance of adequate body fluids and proper balance between the extracellular and intracellular fluid volumes in seriously ill patients. The purpose of the following discussion, therefore, is to explain the interrelationships between extracellular and intracellular fluid volumes and the osmotic factors that cause shifts of fluid between the extracellular and intracellular compartments.

Basic Principles of Osmosis and Osmotic Pressure

The basic principles of osmosis and osmotic pressure are presented in Chapter 4. The essence of these is reviewed here briefly.

Whenever a membrane between two fluid compartments is permeable to water but not to some of the

Table 20-2 OSMOLAR SUBSTANCES IN EXTRACELLULAR AND INTRACELLULAR FLUIDS

	Plasma (mOsm/liter of H_2O)	Interstitial (mOsm/liter of H_2O)	Intracellular (mOsm/liter of H_2O)
Na^+	143	140	14
K^+	4.2	4.0	140
Ca^{++}	1.3	1.2	0
Mg^{++}	0.8	0.7	20
Cl^-	108	108	4
HCO_3^-	24	28.3	10
HPO_4^{--}, $H_2PO_4^{--}$	2	2	11
SO_4	0.5	0.5	1
Phosphocreatine			45
Carnosine			14
Amino acids	2	2	8
Creatine	0.2	0.2	9
Lactate	1.2	1.2	1.5
Adenosine triphosphate			5
Hexose monophosphate			3.7
Glucose	5.6	5.6	
Protein	1.2	0.2	4
Urea	4	4	4
Others	4.8	3.9	11
TOTAL mOsm/liter	302.8	301.8	302.2
Corrected osmolar activity (mOsm/liter)	282.5	281.3	281.3
Total osmotic pressure at 37°C (mm Hg)	5450	5430	5430

dissolved solutes—that is, the membrane is selectively *permeable*—and the concentration of the solutes is greater on one side of the membrane than on the other, water passes through the membrane toward the side with the greater concentration of solutes. This phenomenon is called *osmosis.*

Osmosis results from the kinetic motion of the individual particles—both the molecules and the ions—in the solutions on the two sides of the membrane. This can be explained in the following way: When the temperature is the same in both solutions, the particles on both sides of the membrane, on the average, all have the same amount of kinetic energy of motion. However, the nonpermeant particles in the two solutions displace some of the water molecules. As a result, the so-called *chemical potential* of the water is reduced on each side of the membrane in direct proportion to the concentration of nonpermeant particles. Therefore, on the side of the membrane where there is the lower concentration of nonpermeant particles, the concentration of water molecules is the greater; that is, the chemical potential of the water is greater. This means that more water molecules will strike each pore of the membrane each second on the side of the membrane that has the lower concentration of nonpermeant solutes. As a result, net diffusion of water molecules will occur from this side toward the solution on the opposite side of the membrane, where the concentration of nonpermeant particles is greater. This net rate of diffusion is called the *rate of osmosis.*

Osmotic Pressure. Osmosis of water molecules can be opposed by applying a pressure across the selectively permeable membrane in the direction opposite that of the osmosis. The amount of pressure required to oppose the osmosis exactly is called the *osmotic pressure.*

Osmotic Effect of Ions. Nonpermeant ions cause osmosis and osmotic pressure in exactly the same manner as do nonpermeant molecules. Furthermore, when a molecule dissociates into two or more ions, each of the ions then exerts osmotic pressure individually. Therefore, to determine the osmotic effect, all the nonpermeant ions must be added to all the nonpermeant molecules; but note that a bivalent ion, such as calcium, exerts no more osmotic pressure than does a univalent ion, such as sodium.

Osmoles. The ability of solutes to cause osmosis and osmotic pressure is measured in terms of "osmoles"; the osmole is a measure of the total number of particles. *One gram mole of nonpermeant and nonionizable substance is equal to 1 osmole.* On the other hand, if a substance ionizes into two ions (sodium chloride into sodium and chloride ions, for instance), 0.5 gram mole of the substance equals 1 osmole. The obvious reason for using the osmole is that osmotic pressure is determined by the number of particles instead of the mass of the solute.

In general, the osmole is too large a unit for satisfactory use in expressing osmotic activity of solutes in the body. Therefore, the term *milliosmole,* which equals 1/1000 osmole, is commonly used.

Osmolality and Relation to Osmotic Pressure. The osmolal concentration of a solution is called its *osmolality* when the concentration is expressed in osmoles per kilogram of water. The osmotic pressure of a solution *at body temperature of 98.6° F (37° C)* can be determined approximately from the following formula:

$$\text{Osmotic pressure (mm Hg)} = 19.3 \times \text{Osmolality (milliosmole/kg water)}$$

Osmolality of the Body Fluids

Table 20–2 lists the osmotically active substances in plasma, interstitial fluid, and intracellular fluid. The approximate milliosmoles of each of these per liter of water is given. Note especially that approximately *four fifths* of the total osmolality of the interstitial fluid and plasma is caused by sodium and chloride ions, whereas almost *half* of the intracellular osmolality is caused by potassium ions; the remainder is divided among the many other intracellular substances.

As noted at the bottom of Table 20–2, the total osmolality of each of the three compartments is approximately 300 mOsm/liter, with that of the plasma being 1.3 milliosmoles greater than that of the interstitial and intracellular fluids. This slight difference between plasma and interstitial fluid is caused by the osmotic effect of the plasma proteins, which maintains about 20 mm Hg greater pressure in the capillaries than in the surrounding interstitial fluid spaces, as explained in Chapter 13.

Maintenance of Osmotic Equilibrium Between Extracellular and Intracellular Fluids

The tremendous osmotic pressure that can develop across the cell membrane when one side of the membrane is exposed to pure water—more than 5400 mm Hg—illustrates how much force can become available to move water molecules through the membrane when the solutions on the two sides of the membrane are not in osmotic equilibrium. For instance, in Figure 20–5A, a cell is placed in a solution that has an osmolality far less than that of the intracellular fluid. As a result, osmosis of water into the cell begins immediately, causing the cell to swell and *within seconds* diluting the intracellular fluid while concentrating the extracellular fluid. When the fluid inside the cell becomes diluted sufficiently to equal the osmolal concentration of the fluid on the outside, as shown in Figure 20–5B, further osmosis then ceases.

In Figure 20–5C, a cell is placed in a solution having a much higher concentration outside the cell than inside. This time, water passes by osmosis to the exterior, concentrating the intracellular fluid and diluting

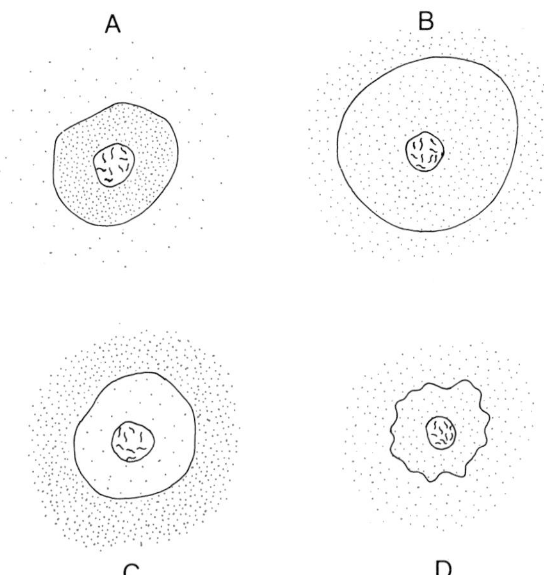

Figure 20-5. Establishment of osmotic equilibrium when cells are placed in a hypotonic or hypertonic solution.

the extracellular fluid. This time the cell shrinks until the two concentrations become equal, as shown in Figure 20-5D.

Isotonicity, Hypotonicity, and Hypertonicity. A fluid into which normal body cells can be placed without causing either swelling or shrinkage of the cells is said to be *isotonic* with the cells. A 0.9 per cent solution of sodium chloride or a 5 per cent glucose solution is approximately isotonic. Isotonic solutions are especially important in clinical medicine because they can be infused into the blood without danger of upsetting the osmotic equilibria between the fluids outside and inside the cells.

A solution that will cause the cells to swell is said to be *hypotonic;* any solution of sodium chloride with less than 0.9 per cent concentration is hypotonic.

A solution that will cause the cells to shrink is said to be *hypertonic;* sodium chloride solutions of greater than 0.9 per cent concentration are hypertonic.

Glucose and Other Solutions Administered for Nutritive Purposes

Many different types of solutions are often administered intravenously to provide nutrition to patients who cannot otherwise take adequate amounts of food. Especially used are *glucose solutions* and to a lesser extent *amino acid* solutions. Rarely used are *homogenized fat solutions.* When these are administered, their concentrations of osmotically active substances are adjusted nearly to isotonicity, or they are given slowly enough that they do not upset the osmotic equilibria of the body fluids. However, after the glucose or other nutrient is metabolized, an excess of water often remains. Ordinarily, the kidneys excrete this in the form of very dilute urine. Thus, the net result is only addition of the nutrient to the body.

EDEMA

Edema means the presence of excess fluid in the tissues of the body. In many instances edema occurs mainly in the extracellular fluid compartment, but it can involve the intracellular fluids as well. Two conditions are prone to cause intracellular swelling.

First, *depression of the metabolic systems of the tissues or lack of adequate nutrition to the cells* can cause serious intracellular edema. This especially occurs in any area of the body where the local blood flow is depressed and the delivery of oxygen and other nutrients is too low to maintain normal tissue metabolism. This depresses the cell membrane ionic pumps, especially the pump that removes sodium from the cells. Then, when sodium ions leak into the interior of the cells, the pump fails to remove these; instead, they cause osmosis of water into the cells as well. This can sometimes increase the intracellular volume of a tissue area, even an entire ischemic leg, for instance, to as much as two or more times normal. It is usually a prelude to death of the tissues.

Second, *intracellular edema also occurs in inflamed tissue areas.* The inflammation usually has a direct effect on the cell membranes to increase their permeability, allowing sodium and other ions to diffuse to the interior, with subsequent osmosis of water also into the cells.

Extracellular Fluid Edema

Aside from the instances that cause intracellular edema, a great host of conditions can cause extracellular edema. These can usually be classified into two different types: (1) edema caused by abnormal leakage of fluid from the blood capillaries or failure of the lymphatic system to return fluid from the interstitium, and (2) edema caused by renal retention of salt and water.

Edema Caused by Abnormal Leakage of Fluid from the Capillaries or by Lymphatic Obstruction

Obviously, excess interstitial fluid will accumulate and cause extracellular edema if either too much fluid filters from the capillaries into the interstitium or lymphatic blockage prevents the return of interstitial fluid and protein to the circulation. The following is a partial list of the different conditions that can cause extracellular edema by one of these two methods.

I. Increased Capillary Pressure
   A. Excessive kidney retention of salt and water
   B. High venous pressure
      1. Heart failure
      2. Local venous block
      3. Failure of venous pumps
         (a) Paralysis of muscles
         (b) Immobilized parts of body
         (c) Failure of venous valves

II. Decreased Plasma Proteins
   A. Loss of proteins in urine (nephrosis)
   B. Loss of protein from denuded skin areas
      1. Burns
      2. Wounds
   C. Failure to produce proteins
      1. Liver disease
      2. Serious protein or caloric malnutrition
III. Increased Capillary Permeability
   A. Immune reactions that cause release of histamine and other immune products
   B. Toxins
   C. Bacterial infections
IV. Blockage of Lymph Return
   A. Blockage of lymph nodes by cancer
   B. Blockage of lymph nodes by infection—especially with filaria nematodes

One of the most prevalent causes of edema in the whole body is *heart failure*, which causes edema for several reasons. First, the heart fails to pump blood normally from the veins into the arteries; this causes the venous pressure and capillary pressure both to increase. Second, the arterial pressure tends to fall; this decreases the urinary output of water and salt by the kidneys.

In those heart failure patients in whom the left heart fails without significant failure of the right heart, blood is pumped into the lungs normally by the right heart but cannot escape easily from the pulmonary veins through the left heart. Consequently, all the pulmonary pressures, including the pulmonary capillary pressure, rise far above normal and cause serious pulmonary edema. This is discussed in Chapter 27.

Edema Caused by Renal Retention of Salt and Water

In the discussions earlier in this chapter, it has already become clear that sodium chloride normally remains almost entirely in the extracellular fluid compartment, with only small amounts entering the cells. Also, we learn in the following chapters that most diseases that compromise renal function have an extreme tendency to reduce the excretion of salt and water into the urine. Therefore, the quantity of sodium chloride and water in the extracellular fluid often increases drastically. The effects of this are twofold: (1) widespread extracellular edema and (2) hypertension because of the increased blood volume (if all other aspects of the circulation are functioning normally), as explained in Chapter 16. To give an example, children who develop acute glomerulonephritis, in which the renal glomeruli are blocked by inflammation and therefore fail to filter adequate quantities of fluid, develop serious extracellular fluid edema in the entire body, and along with this they also develop hypertension.

Relationship Between Interstitial Fluid Pressure and Interstitial Fluid Volume

In Chapter 13, we noted that the interstitial fluid pressure in most loose subcutaneous tissues of the body is slightly less than atmospheric pressure—that is, a slight *suction* in the tissues averaging about −3 mm Hg that helps hold the tissues together. Figure 20–6 illustrates the approximate effects of different levels of interstitial fluid pressure on the interstitial fluid volume, as extrapolated to the human from animal studies. Note that at −3 mm Hg the interstitial fluid volume is approximately 12 liters. Furthermore, virtually all of this fluid is in a *gel* form. That is, the fluid is *bound in a proteoglycan filament meshwork,* so that there are virtually no "free" fluid spaces larger than a few hundredths of a micron in diameter. The importance of the gel is that it prevents the fluid from flowing easily through the tissues because of the impediment of the "brushpile" of trillions of proteoglycan filaments. Also, when the interstitial fluid pressure falls to very negative values, the gel fluid does not contract greatly because the meshwork of proteoglycan filaments offers an elastic resistance to compression. Therefore, in the negative interstitial fluid pressure range, the interstitial fluid volume does not change greatly regardless of whether the degree of suction is only a millimeter or so of negative pressure or as much as 10 to 20 mm Hg negative pressure.

Effect of Positive Pressure on Interstitial Volume—"Free Fluid" and Pitting Edema. Note to the right in Figure 20–6 the sudden increase in total interstitial fluid volume when the interstitial

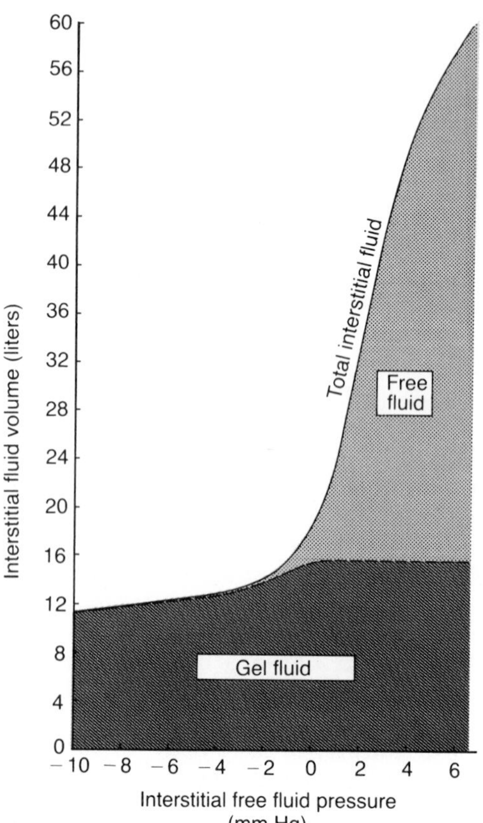

Figure 20–6. Effect of increasing interstitial fluid pressure on the volumes of total interstitial fluid, gel fluid, and free fluid. Note that significant amounts of free fluid occur only when the interstitial free fluid pressure becomes positive. (Modified from Guyton, Granger, and Taylor: *Physiol. Rev., 51:* 527, 1971.)

fluid pressure rises above atmospheric pressure (above zero pressure level). Because the loose subcutaneous tissues of the body are highly distensible, even 2, 3, or 4 mm Hg of positive pressure often can increase the interstitial fluid volume from its normal level of 12 liters up to two to three times normal. Furthermore, most of the extra fluid is "free fluid" that forms large free fluid spaces in the tissues that are no longer enmeshed tightly within a meshwork of the tissue gel. This fluid can now flow freely through the tissue spaces. When this occurs, the edema is said to be "pitting" edema because one can press the thumb against a tissue area and push the fluid out of that area into other areas. Then, when the thumb is removed, a pit is left in the skin for a few seconds, or sometimes as long as a minute, until the pit fills again with fluid that flows back from the surrounding tissues.

The Concept of an "Edema Safety Factor"

Even though any one of many abnormalities can cause edema, usually the abnormality must become quite severe before edema actually occurs. The reason for this is that there is a so-called edema safety factor. This safety factor is made up of three different components:

1. Figure 20–6 illustrates that edema does not begin to appear until the interstitial fluid pressure rises above the atmospheric pressure level. Therefore, *all of the negative interstitial fluid pressure must be dissipated,* and the pressure must rise into the positive range before edema will occur. Obviously, this allows at least some degree of capillary filtration abnormality or even some degree of lymphatic obstruction before edema would occur.
2. *Lymph flow can increase as much as 10-fold to 50-fold.* This constitutes another safety factor because the lymph vessels can carry away large amounts of fluid as they are formed and help to prevent the interstitial fluid pressure from rising into the positive pressure range.
3. As the lymph flow increases, it also carries protein away from the interstitium, thus reducing the interstitial fluid colloid osmotic pressure. This is called *"washdown" of the interstitial fluid protein.* As washdown occurs, the differential between plasma colloid osmotic pressure and the colloid osmotic pressure in the interstitium increases, thus increasing the osmotic absorption of fluid from the interstitium into the capillaries. This, too, increases the safety factor against edema.

Putting all these factors together, we find that the capillary pressure in a peripheral tissue of an otherwise normal person could theoretically rise to as high as 34 mm Hg, to approximately double its normal value of 17 mm Hg, before edema would occur.

Thus, the concept of a safety factor against edema explains why we are not continuously edematous.

REFERENCES

Gilmore, J. P.: Neural control of extracellular volume in the human and nonhuman primate. In Shepherd, J. T., and Abboud, F. M. (eds.): Handbook of Physiology. Sec. 2, Vol. III. Bethesda, Md., American Physiological Society, 1983, p. 885.

Guyton, A. C., et al.: Circulatory Physiology II: Dynamics and Control of Body Fluids. Philadelphia, W. B. Saunders Co., 1975.

Guyton, A. C., et al.: Interstitial fluid pressure. Physiol. Rev., 51:527, 1971.

Haas, M.: Properties and diversity of (Na-K-Cl) cotransporters. Annu. Rev. Physiol., 51:443, 1989.

Kokko, J. P., and Tannen, R. L.: Fluids and Electrolytes. Philadelphia, W. B. Saunders Co., 1986.

Lebenthal, E.: Total Parenteral Nutrition: Indications, Utilization, Complications, and Pathophysiological Considerations. New York, Raven Press, 1986.

Maxwell, M. H., et al. (eds.): Clinical Disorders of Fluid and Electrolyte Metabolism, 4th ed. New York, McGraw-Hill Book Co., 1987.

Post, R. L.: Seeds of sodium, potassium ATPase. Annu. Rev. Physiol., 51:1, 1989.

Rose, B. D. (ed.): Clinical Physiology of Acid-Base and Electrolyte Disorders, 3rd ed. New York, McGraw-Hill Book Co., 1989.

QUESTIONS

1. What percentage of the body is composed of water, and how is this distributed between the intracellular and extracellular fluids?
2. List the different components of the extracellular fluid.
3. How much is the blood volume, how much of this is plasma and red blood cells, and explain what is meant by the "hematocrit."
4. Explain the dilution principle for measuring a body fluid volume. Give an example as well as the mathematical formula for calculating the volume.
5. What are the most important constituents of the extracellular fluid?
6. What are the most important constituents of the intracellular fluid?
7. What is the approximate osmotic pressure of the body fluids? In the extracellular fluids, about how much of the total osmotic pressure is contributed by sodium and chloride ions?
8. Explain what is meant by isotonicity, hypotonicity, and hypertonicity.
9. Why does inflammation or depression of the metabolic system of the tissues cause intracellular edema?
10. List the capillary and lymphatic abnormalities that can cause edema and explain how each does so.
11. What is the relationship between *positive* tissue pressure and edema?
12. Explain the importance of the proteoglycan filament meshwork of the interstitial spaces.
13. Explain what is meant by "edema safety factor," and what are the different mechanisms that provide this safety factor?

21

Formation of Urine by the Kidneys

The kidneys perform two major functions. First, they excrete most of the end-products of bodily metabolism, and second, they control the concentrations of most of the constituents of the body fluids. The purpose of this chapter is to discuss the basic principles of urine formation. Then, in the following chapters, we present detailed mechanisms for processing and control of excretion of the individual constituents in the urine.

Physiological Anatomy of the Kidney

The two kidneys together contain about 2,000,000 nephrons, and each nephron is capable of forming urine by itself. Therefore, in most instances, it is not necessary to discuss the entire kidney but merely the function of a single nephron to explain the function of the kidney. The nephron is composed basically of (1) a *glomerulus* through which fluid is filtered from the blood, and (2) a long *tubule* in which the filtered fluid is converted into urine on its way to the *pelvis* of the kidney.

Figure 21–1 shows the general organizational plan of the kidney and urinary tract, illustrating especially the distinction between the *cortex* of the kidney and the *medulla.* Figure 21–2A illustrates the basic anatomy of the nephron, which may be described as follows: Blood enters the glomerulus through the *afferent arteriole* and then leaves through the *efferent arteriole.* The glomerulus is a network of up to 50 parallel branching and anastomosing capillaries covered by epithelial cells and encased in *Bowman's capsule.* Pressure of the blood in the glomerulus causes fluid to filter into Bowman's capsule, and from here the fluid flows into the *proximal tubule* that lies in the *cortex* of the kidney along with the glomerulus.

From the proximal tubule the fluid passes into the *loop of Henle* that dips deeply into the kidney mass, some of the loops passing all the way to the bottom of the renal medulla. Each loop is divided into the *descending limb* and the *ascending limb.* The wall of the descending limb and the lower end of the ascending limb is very thin and therefore is called the *thin segment* of the loop of Henle. However, after the ascending limb of the loop has returned part way back in the cortical direction, its wall once again becomes thick like that of the other portions of the tubular system; this portion of the loop of Henle is called the *thick segment of the ascending limb.*

After passing through the loop of Henle, the fluid then enters the *distal tubule,* which, like the proximal tubule, lies in the renal cortex. Then, still in the cortex, as many as eight of the distal tubules coalesce to form the *cortical collecting duct,* the end of which turns once again away from the cortex and passes downward into the medulla, where it becomes the *medullary collecting duct* but is usually called simply the *collecting duct.* Successive generations of collecting ducts coalesce to form progressively larger collecting ducts that penetrate all the way through the medulla, parallel to the loops of Henle. The largest collecting ducts empty into the *renal pelvis* through the tips of the *renal papillae;* these are conical projections of the medulla that protrude into the *renal calyces,* which are themselves recesses of the *renal pelvis.* In each kidney there are about 250 of these very large collecting ducts, each of which transmits the urine from about 4000 nephrons.

As the glomerular filtrate flows through the tubules, over 99 per cent of its water and varying amounts of its solutes are normally reabsorbed into the vascular system, and small amounts of a few substances are also *secreted* through the tubular epithelial cells into the tubules. The remaining tubular water and dissolved substances become the urine.

The Peritubular Capillary Network and the Vasa Recta. Surrounding the entire tubular system

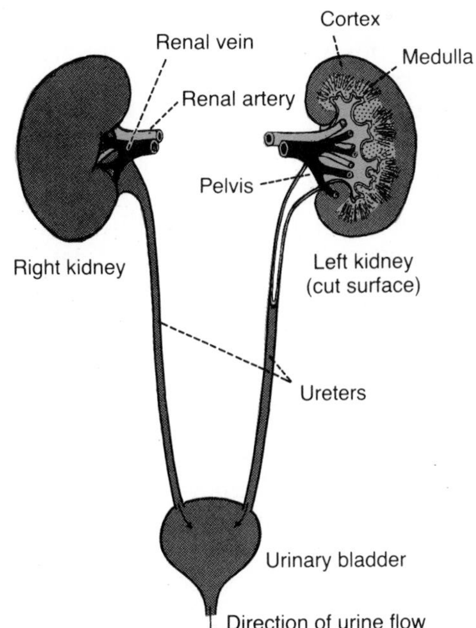

Figure 21-1. The general organizational plan of the urinary system.

of the kidney is an extensive network of capillaries called the *peritubular capillary network.* This network is supplied with blood from the *efferent arterioles,* blood that has already passed through the glomerulus. Most of the peritubular capillary network lies in the renal cortex alongside the proximal tubules, distal tubules, and cortical collecting ducts. However, from the deeper portions of this peritubular network, long branching capillary loops called *vasa recta* extend downward into the medulla to lie side by side with the juxtaglomerular loops of Henle all the way to the renal papillae. Then, like the loops of Henle, they also loop back toward the cortex and empty into the cortical veins.

Functional Diagram of the Nephron. Figure 21-3 illustrates a simplified diagram of the "physiological nephron." This diagram contains most of the nephron's functional structures, and it is used in the present discussion to explain many aspects of renal function.

Basic Theory of Nephron Function

The basic function of the nephron is to clean, or "clear," the blood plasma of unwanted substances as it passes through the kidney. The substances that must be cleared include particularly the end-products of metabolism, such as urea, creatinine, uric acid, and urates. In addition, many other substances, such as sodium ions, potassium ions, chloride ions, and hydrogen ions, tend to accumulate in the body in excess quantities; it is the function of the nephron also to clear the plasma of these excesses.

The principal mechanism by which the nephron clears the plasma of unwanted substances is as follows: (1) It filters a large proportion of the plasma in the flowing glomerular blood, usually about one fifth of it, through the glomerular capillary membrane into the tubular system of the nephron. (2) Then, as this filtered fluid flows through the tubules, the *unwanted substances fail to be reabsorbed* while the *wanted substances, especially almost all of the water and many of the electrolytes, are reabsorbed* back into the plasma of the peritubular capillaries. In other words, the wanted

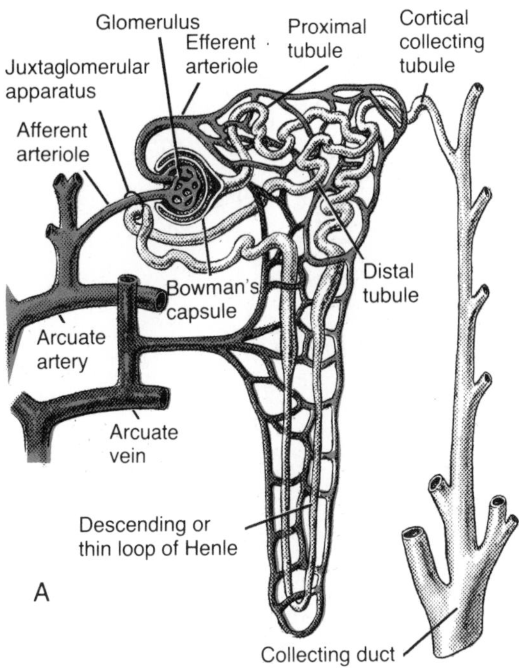

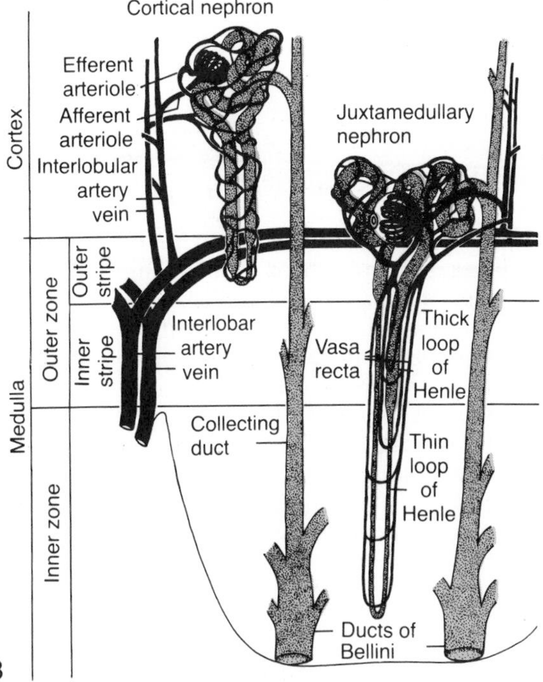

Figure 21-2. *A,* The nephron. (From Smith: The Kidney: Structure and Functions in Health and Disease. New York, Oxford University Press, 1951.) *B,* Differences between a cortical and a juxtamedullary nephron. (From Pitts: Physiology of the Kidney and Body Fluids. Chicago, Year Book Medical Publishers, 1974.)

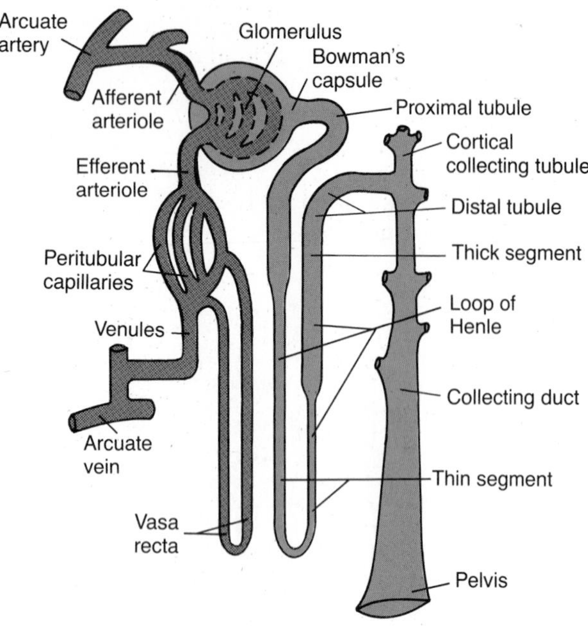

Figure 21-3. The functional nephron.

portions of the tubular fluid are returned to the blood and the unwanted portions pass into the urine.

A second mechanism by which the nephron clears the plasma of other unwanted substances is by *secretion.* That is, substances are secreted from the plasma directly through the epithelial cells lining the tubules into the tubular fluid. Thus, the urine that is eventually formed is composed mainly of *filtered* substances but also of small amounts of *secreted* substances.

RENAL BLOOD FLOW AND PRESSURES

Blood Flow Through the Kidneys

The rate of blood flow through both kidneys of a 70-kilogram man is about 1200 ml/min.

The proportion of the total cardiac output that passes through the kidneys is about 21 per cent. This can vary from as little as 12 per cent to as high as 30 per cent in the normal resting person.

Special Aspects of Blood Flow Through the Renal Vasculature. Note in Figure 21-3 that there are two capillary beds associated with the nephron: (1) the *glomerulus* and (2) the *peritubular capillaries.* The glomerular capillary bed receives its blood from the *afferent arteriole,* and from this bed the blood flows into the peritubular capillary bed through the *efferent arteriole,* which offers considerable resistance to blood flow. As a result, the glomerular capillary bed is a *high pressure bed,* whereas the peritubular capillary bed is a *low pressure bed.* Because of the high pressure in the glomerulus, it functions in much the same way as the usual arterial ends of the tissue capillaries, with fluid filtering continually out of the glomerulus into Bowman's capsule. On the other hand, the low pressure in the peritubular capillary system causes it to function in much the same way as the venous ends of the tissue capillaries, with fluid being absorbed continually into the capillaries.

Blood Flow in the Vasa Recta. A special portion of the peritubular capillary system is the vasa recta, which are a network of capillaries that descend into the medulla around the loops of Henle. These capillaries form loops in the medulla of the kidney and then return to the cortex before emptying into the veins. The vasa recta play a special role in the formation of concentrated urine, which is discussed in Chapter 22.

Only a small proportion of the total renal blood flow, about 1 to 2 per cent, flows through the vasa recta. In other words, blood flow through the medulla of the kidney is sluggish in contrast to the rapid blood flow in the cortex.

Pressures in the Renal Circulation

Figure 21-4 gives the approximate pressures in different parts of the renal circulation and tubules, showing an initial pressure of approximately 100 mm Hg in the large arcuate arteries and about 8 mm Hg in the veins into which the blood finally drains. The two major areas of resistance to blood flow through the nephron are (1) the *small renal arteries and afferent arteriole* and (2) the *efferent arteriole.* In the small arteries and afferent arteriole, the pressure falls from 100 mm Hg at its arterial end to an estimated mean pressure of about 60 mm Hg in the glomerulus. As the blood flows through the efferent arterioles from the glomerulus to the peritubular capillary system, the pressure falls another 47 mm Hg to a mean peritubular capillary pressure of 13 mm Hg. Thus, the high pressure capillary bed in the glomerulus operates at a mean pressure of about 60 mm Hg and therefore causes rapid filtration of fluid, whereas the low pressure capillary bed in the peritubular capillary system operates at a mean capillary pressure of about 13 mm Hg, therefore allowing rapid absorption of fluid because of the high osmotic pressure of the plasma.

Function of the Peritubular Capillaries

Tremendous quantities of fluid, about 180 liters each day, are filtered through all the glomeruli; all but the 1 to 1.5 liters of this that becomes urine is reabsorbed from the tubules into the renal interstitial spaces and thence into the peritubular capillaries. This represents about four times as much fluid as that reabsorbed at the venous ends of all the other capillaries of the entire body.

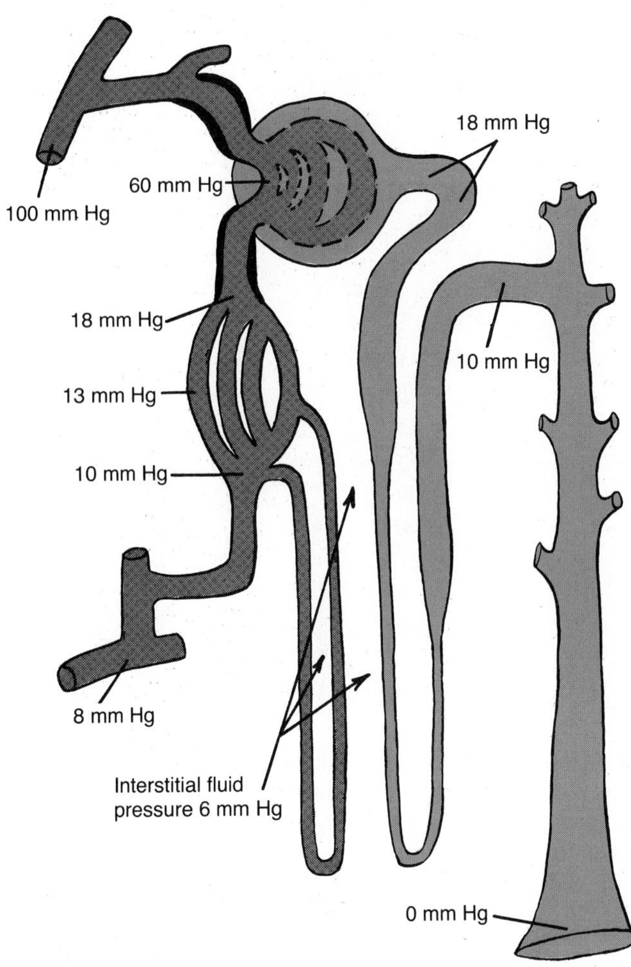

Figure 21-4. Approximate pressures at different points in the vessels and tubules of the functional nephron and in the interstitial fluid.

GLOMERULAR FILTRATION AND THE GLOMERULAR FILTRATE

The Glomerular Membrane and Glomerular Permeability. The fluid that filters through the glomerulus into Bowman's capsule is called *glomerular filtrate,* and the membrane of the glomerular capillaries is called the *glomerular membrane.* Although, in general, this membrane is similar to that of other capillaries throughout the body, it has several differences, as illustrated in Figure 21-5. First, it has three major layers: (1) the endothelial layer of the capillary itself, (2) a basement membrane, and (3) a layer of epithelial cells that is illustrated on the outer surfaces of the glomerular capillaries in the figure. Yet, despite the number of layers, the permeability of the glomerular membrane is from 100 to 500 times as great as that of the usual capillary.

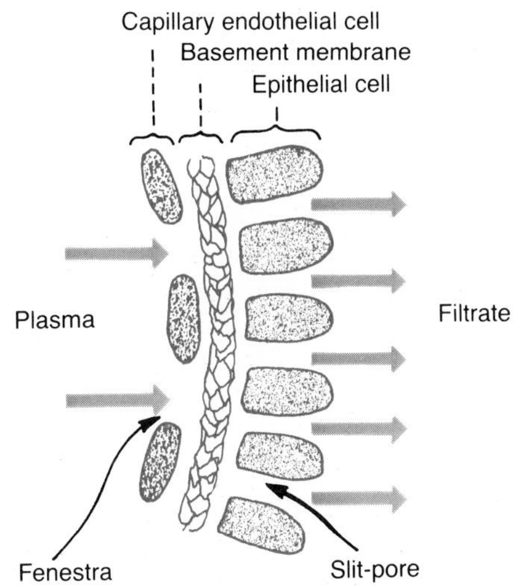

Figure 21-5. Functional structure of the glomerular membrane.

The tremendous permeability of the glomerular membrane is caused by its special structure. The capillary *endothelial cells* lining the glomerulus are perforated by literally thousands of small holes called *fenestrae.* Then, outside the endothelial cells is a *basement membrane,* composed mainly of a meshwork of collagen and proteoglycan fibrillae that also has large spaces through which fluid can filter. A final layer of the glomerular membrane is a layer of *epithelial cells* that line the outer surfaces of the glomerulus. However, these cells are not continuous but instead consist mainly of finger-like projections that cover the basement membrane. Figure 21-6 is a scanning electron micrograph of the outer surfaces of the glomerular

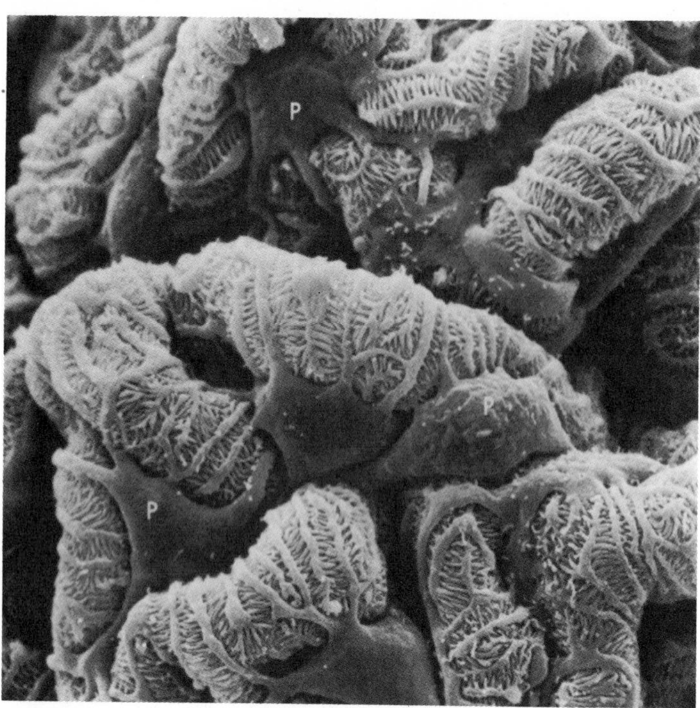

Figure 21–6. Scanning electron micrograph of a glomerulus from a normal rat kidney. The visceral epithelial cells, or podocytes (P), extend multiple processes outward from the main cell body, which wrap around the individual capillary loops. Note that immediately adjacent pedicles, or foot processes, arise from different podocytes. (Magnification, × 3300.) (From Brenner and Rector: The Kidney. Philadelphia, W. B. Saunders Company, 1986.)

capillaries, illustrating thousands to millions of minute parallel "fingers" of the epithelial cells. These fingers form slits called *slit-pores* through which the glomerular filtrate filters.

Thus, the glomerular filtrate passes through three different layers before entering Bowman's capsule, but each of these layers is several hundred times as porous as the usual capillary membrane, which accounts for the tremendous volume of glomerular filtrate that can be formed each minute. Yet, despite the tremendous permeability of the glomerular membrane, it has an extremely high degree of selectivity for the sizes of molecules that it allows to pass.

Overall, the permeability of the glomerular membrane to substances of different molecular weights (expressed as the ratio of concentration of the dissolved substance on the filtrate side of the membrane to its concentration on the plasma side) is approximately as follows:

Molecular Weight	*Permeability*	*Example Substance*
5200	1.00	Inulin
30,000	0.5	Very small protein
69,000	0.005	Albumin

This means that at a molecular weight of 5200, the dissolved substance filters 100 per cent as easily as water, but at the protein molecular weight of 69,000 only 0.5 per cent of the protein molecules filter. Note that the molecular weight of the smallest plasma protein, albumin, is 69,000. Therefore, for practical purposes the glomerular membrane is almost completely impermeable to all plasma proteins but is highly permeable to essentially all other dissolved substances in normal plasma.

There are two basic reasons for the high degree of molecular selectivity by the glomerular membrane. First is the sizes of the pores in the membrane itself. That is, the pores of the membrane are large enough to allow molecules with diameters up to about 8 nanometers (80 angstroms) to pass through. Yet, the molecular diameter of the plasma protein albumin molecule is only about 6 nanometers, which is somewhat smaller than the sizes of these large pores. Therefore, why do the protein molecules not pass through in great quantity? The answer to this is the second factor that determines the permeability of the membrane: The *basement membrane portions of the glomerular pores are lined with a complex of proteoglycans that have very strong negative electrical charges.* The plasma proteins also have strong negative electrical charges. Therefore, electrostatic repulsion of the molecules by the pore walls keeps virtually all protein molecules larger than 69,000 molecular weight from passing through.

Composition of the Glomerular Filtrate. The glomerular filtrate has almost exactly the same composition as the fluid that filters from the arterial ends of the capillaries into the interstitial fluids. It contains no red blood cells and about 0.03 per cent protein, or about 1⁄240 the protein in the plasma.

For all practical purposes, *glomerular filtrate is the same as plasma, except that it has no significant amount of proteins.*

The Glomerular Filtration Rate

The quantity of glomerular filtrate formed each minute in all nephrons of both kidneys is called the *glomerular filtration rate.* In the normal person, this averages approximately 125 ml/min. To express this differently, the total quantity of glomerular filtrate formed each day averages about 180 liters, or more than two times the total weight of the body. Over 99 per cent of the filtrate is normally reabsorbed in the tubules, with the remaining small portion passing into the urine.

The Filtration Fraction. The filtration fraction is the fraction of the renal plasma flow that becomes glomerular filtrate. Since the normal plasma flow through both kidneys is 650 ml/min and the normal glomerular filtration rate in both kidneys is 125 milliliters, *the average filtration fraction is approximately 1/5 or 19 per cent.*

Dynamics of Filtration Through the Glomerular Membrane

The same forces that cause fluid to filter from any high pressure capillary also apply to filtration from the glomerulus into Bowman's capsule. Thus, the forces are as follows:

1. The *pressure inside the glomerular capillaries* promotes filtration through the glomerular membrane.
2. The *pressure in Bowman's capsule* outside the capillaries opposes filtration.
3. The *colloid osmotic pressure of the plasma proteins inside the capillary membrane* also opposes filtration.
4. The *colloid osmotic pressure of the proteins in Bowman's capsule* outside the capillaries promotes filtration; however, so little protein normally filters into the glomerular filtrate that this factor usually has no significant effect and is actually considered to be zero.

Glomerular Pressure. The glomerular pressure is the average pressure in the glomerular capillaries. This unfortunately has been measured directly only in one mammal, the rat, in which the average value is about 45 mm Hg. However, from various indirect measurements it has been calculated to be about 60 mm Hg in the dog. Because humans are also large mammals, *a reasonable average value can be considered to be 60 mm Hg,* though, as noted later, this can increase or decrease considerably under varying conditions.

Pressure in Bowman's Capsule. In lower animals, pressure measurements actually have been made in Bowman's capsule and at different points along the renal tubules by inserting micropipets into the lumen. On the basis of these studies, *capsular pressure in the human being is estimated to be about 18 mm Hg.*

Colloid Osmotic Pressure in the Glomerular Capillaries. Because approximately one fifth of the plasma in the capillaries filters into the capsule, the protein concentration increases about 20 per cent as the blood passes from the arterial to the venous ends of the glomerular capillaries. If the normal colloid osmotic pressure of blood entering the capillaries is 28 mm Hg, it rises to approximately 36 mm Hg by the time the blood reaches the venous ends of the capillaries, and the average colloid osmotic pressure is about 32 mm Hg.

Factors That Affect the Glomerular Filtration Rate

Effect of Renal Blood Flow on Glomerular Filtration Rate. An increase in the rate of blood flow through the nephrons greatly elevates the glomerular filtration rate. One of the reasons for this is that the increasing flow elevates the glomerular pressure, which obviously enhances filtration. However, a second reason that is not quite so easily understood is the following: At normal renal blood flow, about 20 per cent of the plasma is filtered through the glomerular membrane; therefore, the concentration of the plasma proteins becomes considerably increased before the blood leaves the glomerulus and, consequently, the colloid osmotic pressure increases. This rising colloid osmotic pressure exerts a strong influence on reducing further filtration. Now let us see what effect increased blood flow will have on this. As the flow increases, greater quantities of plasma enter the glomeruli, so that filtration of fluid from the plasma causes a smaller percentage increase in protein concentration and colloid osmotic pressure. Therefore, the colloid osmotic pressure rises much less and now exerts far less inhibitory influence on glomerular filtration. Consequently, even when the

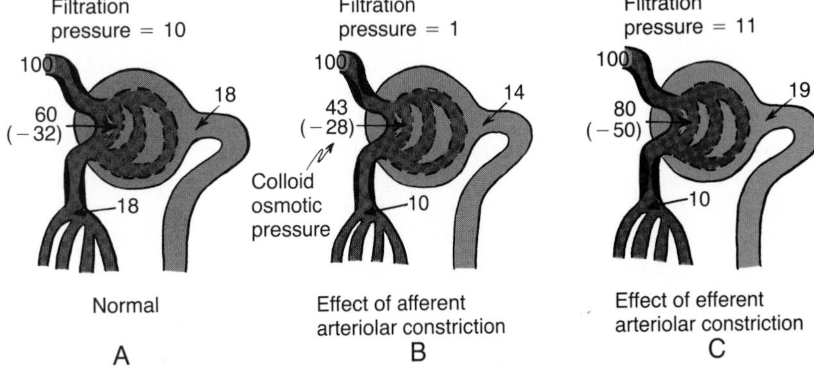

Figure 21-7. *A,* Normal pressures at different points in the nephron and the normal filtration pressure. *B,* Effect of afferent arteriolar constriction on pressures in the nephron and on filtration pressure. *C,* Effect of efferent arteriolar constriction on pressures in the nephron and on filtration pressure.

glomerular pressure remains constant, the greater the rate of blood flow into the glomerulus, the greater the glomerular filtration rate.

Effect of Afferent Arteriolar Constriction on Glomerular Filtration Rate. Afferent arteriolar constriction decreases the rate of blood flow into the glomerulus and also decreases the glomerular pressure; both of these effects decrease the filtration rate. This effect is illustrated in Figure 21–7B. Conversely, dilatation of the afferent arteriole increases the glomerular filtration rate.

Effect of Efferent Arteriolar Constriction on Glomerular Filtration Rate. Constriction of the efferent arteriole increases the resistance to outflow from the glomeruli. This obviously increases the glomerular pressure and at small increases in efferent resistance causes a slight increase in glomerular filtration rate, as illustrated in Figure 21–7C. *However,* the blood flow decreases at the same time, and if the increase in efferent arteriolar constriction is moderate or severe, the plasma will remain for a longer period of time in the glomerulus, and extra large portions of plasma will filter out. This will increase the plasma colloid osmotic pressure to excessive levels, which will cause a paradoxical decrease in the glomerular filtration rate despite the elevated glomerular pressure.

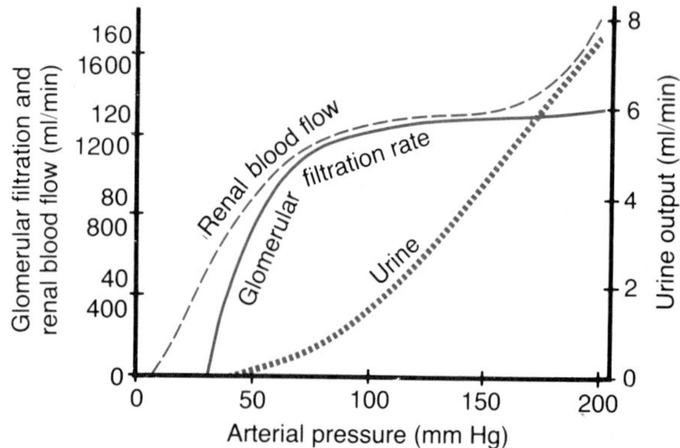

Figure 21–8. Autoregulation of glomerular filtration rate (GFR) and renal blood flow (RBF) when the arterial pressure is increased, but there is lack of autoregulation of urine flow.

CONTROL OF GLOMERULAR FILTRATION RATE AND RENAL BLOOD FLOW

For the most part, renal blood flow and glomerular filtration rate are controlled together by local feedback control mechanisms within the kidney that keep both flow and filtration rate at very constant levels. Therefore, it is said that glomerular filtration and blood flow are both "autoregulated." The mechanisms of these autoregulation processes are the following:

Autoregulation of Glomerular Filtration Rate

The glomerular filtration rate normally remains very nearly constant hour after hour, usually varying very little either above or below the normal value of about 125 ml/min for the two kidneys. Even a change in arterial pressure from as little as 75 mm Hg to as high as 160 mm Hg hardly changes the glomerular filtration rate. This effect is illustrated in Figure 21–8, and it is called *autoregulation of glomerular filtration rate.*

Why Is It Important for the Glomerular Filtration Rate to Be Autoregulated? To understand the importance of maintaining a constant glomerular filtration rate, let us consider what would happen if the glomerular filtration rate should become, first, very slight or, second, very great.

At a very slight glomerular filtration rate, the tubular fluid would pass through the tubules so slowly that essentially all of it would be reabsorbed. Therefore, the kidney would fail to eliminate the necessary waste products.

At the other extreme, with a much too high glomerular filtration rate, the fluid would pass so rapidly through the tubules that they would be unable to reabsorb those substances that need to be conserved in the body.

Thus, one can readily see that the glomerular filtrate must flow into the tubular system at an appropriate rate (1) to allow the unwanted substances to pass on into the urine while (2) reabsorbing the wanted substances. However, it is often not appreciated how narrow the range of glomerular filtration rate must be if optimal function of the tubular system is to occur. To emphasize this narrow range, analyses of tubular function have shown that even a 5 per cent too great or too little rate of glomerular filtration can have considerable effects in causing either excess loss of solutes and water into the urine or, at the other extreme, too little of the necessary excretion of waste products.

Mechanism of Autoregulation of Glomerular Filtration Rate — Tubuloglomerular Feedback

The precision with which glomerular filtration rate must be autoregulated demands that there be a highly efficient control system for controlling this filtration rate. Fortunately, each nephron is provided with not one but *two* special feedback mechanisms from the distal tubule to the periglomerular arterioles; these add together to provide the degree of glomerular filtration autoregulation that is required. These two mechanisms are (1) an *afferent arteriolar vasodilator feedback mechanism* and (2) an *efferent arteriolar vasoconstrictor feedback mechanism.* The combination of these is called *tubuloglomerular feedback.* The feedback process occurs either entirely or almost entirely at the *juxtaglomerular complex,* which has the following characteristics:

The Juxtaglomerular Complex. Figure 21-9 illustrates the juxtaglomerular complex, showing that the initial portion of the distal tubule, immediately after the upper end of the thick segment of the ascending limb of the loop of Henle, passes in the angle between the afferent and efferent arterioles, actually abutting each of these two arterioles. Furthermore, those epithelial cells of the distal tubule that come in contact with the arterioles are more dense than the other tubular cells and are collectively called the *macula densa.* The macula densa cells appear to secrete some substance toward the arterioles because the Golgi apparatus, an intracellular secretory organelle, is directed toward the arterioles and not toward the lumen of the tubule, in contrast to all the other tubular epithelial cells. Note also in Figure 21-9 that the smooth muscle cells of both the afferent and efferent arterioles are swollen and contain dark granules where they come in contact with the macula densa. These cells are called *juxtaglomerular cells,* and the granules are composed mainly of inactive *renin.* The whole complex of macula densa and juxtaglomerular cells is called the *juxtaglomerular complex.*

Thus, the anatomical structure of the juxtaglomerular apparatus suggests strongly that the fluid in the distal tubule in some way plays an important role in helping to control nephron function by providing feedback signals to both the afferent and the efferent arterioles.

The Afferent Arteriolar Vasodilator Feedback Mechanism

A low rate of tubular fluid flow causes overreabsorption of sodium and chloride ions in the ascending limb of the loop of Henle and therefore decreases the ionic concentration at the macula densa. This decrease in ions in turn initiates a signal from the macula densa to dilate the afferent arteriole. This in turn allows increased blood flow into the glomerulus, which increases the glomerular filtration rate back toward the required level.

Thus, this is a typical negative feedback mechanism for controlling the glomerular filtration rate at a steady rate. This mechanism *also helps autoregulate the renal blood flow at the same time.*

The Efferent Arteriolar Vasoconstrictor Feedback Mechanism

Too few sodium and chloride ions at the macula densa also cause the juxtaglomerular cells to release active renin, and this in turn causes formation of angiotensin. The angiotensin then constricts mainly the efferent arteriole because it is highly sensitive to angiotensin II, much more so than is the afferent arteriole.

With these facts in mind, we can now describe the efferent arteriolar vasoconstrictor mechanism that helps maintain a constant glomerular filtration rate:

1. A too low glomerular filtration rate causes excess reabsorption of sodium and chloride ions in the ascending limb of the loop of Henle, reducing the ionic concentration at the macula densa.
2. The low concentration of ions then causes the juxtaglomerular cells to release renin from their granules.
3. The renin causes formation of angiotensin II.
4. The angiotensin II constricts the efferent arteri-

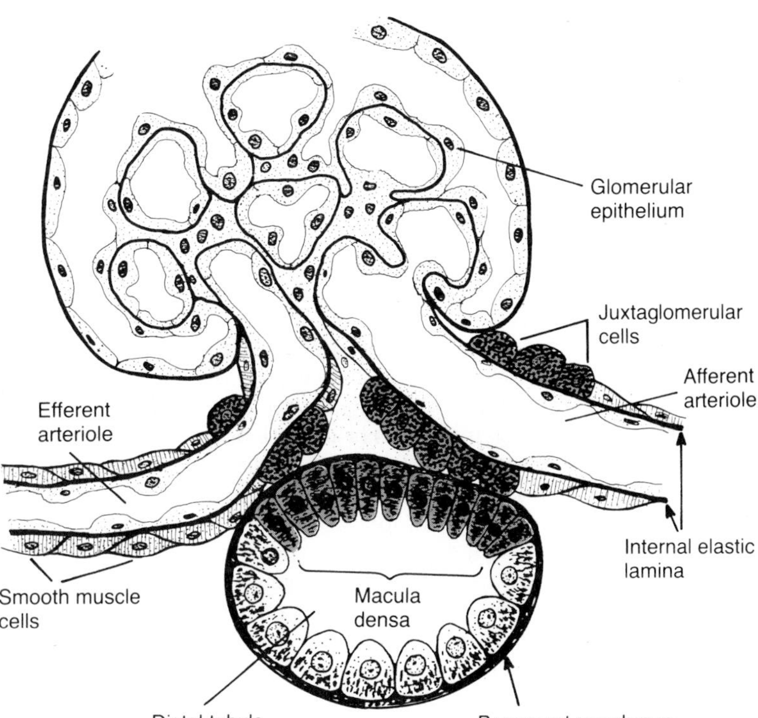

Figure 21-9. Structure of the juxtaglomerular apparatus, illustrating its possible feedback role in the control of nephron function. (Modified from Ham: Histology. Philadelphia, J. B. Lippincott Company, 1971.)

oles, which causes the pressure in the glomerulus to rise and the glomerular filtration rate to return back toward normal.

Thus, this is still another negative feedback mechanism that helps to maintain a very constant glomerular filtration rate. When both these mechanisms function together, the glomerular filtration rate increases only a few per cent, as shown in Figure 21–8, even though the arterial pressure changes between the limits of 75 and 160 mm Hg.

Effect of Arterial Pressure on Urinary Output—The Phenomenon of "Pressure Diuresis"

Because of the autoregulation phenomenon, increasing the arterial pressure between the limits of 75 mm Hg and 160 mm Hg usually has only a slight effect on renal blood flow and glomerular filtration rate. However, the very slight increase in glomerular filtration rate that does occur is nevertheless enough to cause marked increase in urinary output, an effect that is illustrated by the dotted curve in Figure 21–8. This curve shows that a decrease in the mean arterial pressure from its normal value of about 100 mm Hg down to about 50 mm Hg causes complete cessation of urine output, whereas an increase in arterial pressure to double normal (to 200 mm Hg) increases the urine output as much as sevenfold to eightfold. As we study tubular reabsorptive mechanisms it becomes clear that tubular reabsorption does not necessarily increase when the arterial pressure rises. Therefore, all or most of the increase in glomerular filtration becomes also an increase in urinary output. This large effect that arterial pressure has on urinary output is called *pressure diuresis.*

Effect of Sympathetic Stimulation on Renal Blood Flow and Glomerular Filtration Rate

The sympathetic nerves innervate both the afferent arterioles and the efferent arterioles and to a lesser extent some of the renal tubules as well. Even so, slight to moderate degrees of sympathetic stimulation usually have only mild effects on either renal blood flow or glomerular filtration. The reason for this is probably that the renal autoregulation mechanisms override the nervous stimuli.

On the other hand, strong acute sympathetic stimulation can constrict the renal arterioles so greatly that urine output may decrease all the way to zero for a few minutes. Then, over prolonged periods, urine flow can remain seriously reduced for several hours until the arterial pressure rises high enough to overcome the effects of continued sympathetic vasoconstriction.

REABSORPTION OF FLUID BY THE PERITUBULAR CAPILLARIES

As the glomerular filtrate passes through the renal tubular system, the tubular epithelium reabsorbs more than 99 per cent of the water in the filtrate as well as large quantities of electrolytes and other substances. This absorbed fluid passes first into the interstitium and is absorbed from there into the peritubular capillaries, thus returning to the blood, as illustrated in Figure 21–10.

Note in the figure that the normal peritubular capillary pressure averages about 13 mm Hg, whereas the renal interstitial fluid pressure averages about 6 mm Hg. Thus, there is a positive pressure gradient from the peritubular capillary to the interstitial fluid of 7 mm Hg that opposes fluid reabsorption. However, this is more than overbalanced by the colloid osmotic pressures, with −32 mm Hg in the plasma and −15 mm Hg in the interstitium, giving a net −17 mm Hg osmotic force to reabsorb the interstitial fluid into the capillary blood. Combining the 7 mm Hg pressure gradient and the −17 mm Hg colloid osmotic pressure gradient, the result is −10 mm Hg net absorption pressure. It is this large absorption pressure that causes continual reabsorption by the peritubular capillaries of the large amounts of fluid entering the interstitium from the renal tubules.

Reabsorption and Secretion in the Tubules

The glomerular filtrate entering the tubules of the nephron flows (1) through the *proximal tubule,* (2)

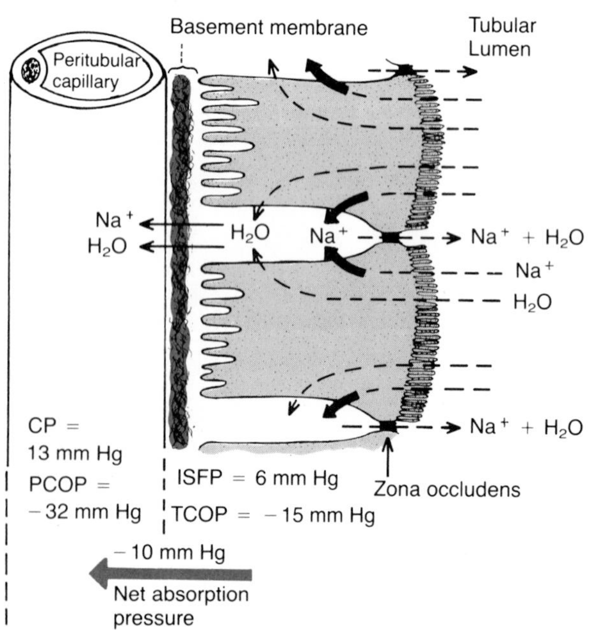

Figure 21–10. Absorption of fluid at the peritubular capillary membrane and the effect of this on the absorption of water and sodium through the tubular epithelium.

through the *loop of Henle,* (3) through the *distal tubule,* (4) through the *cortical collecting duct,* and (5) through the *collecting duct* into the pelvis of the kidney. Along this course, substances are selectively reabsorbed or secreted by the tubular epithelium, and the resultant fluid after this processing enters the renal pelvis as *urine.* Reabsorption plays a much greater role than does secretion in this formation of urine, but secretion is especially important in determining the amounts of potassium ions, hydrogen ions, and a few other substances in the urine, as discussed later.

Ordinarily, more than 99 per cent of the water in the glomerular filtrate is reabsorbed as it is processed in the tubules. Therefore, if some dissolved constituent of the glomerular filtrate is not reabsorbed at all along the entire course of the tubules, this reabsorption of water obviously concentrates the substance more than 99-fold.

Active Transport Through the Tubular Membrane

As explained in Chapter 4, there are two basic mechanisms of active transport, *primary active transport* and *secondary active transport.* These two types can best be explained by considering actual examples.

Primary Active Transport of Sodium Ions Through the Tubular Membrane — Function of Na^+,K^+-ATPase

The basic mechanism for transporting sodium ions through the tubular membrane, which always occurs in the direction from the tubular lumen to the interstitium, is illustrated in Figure 21–11A. On the basal and lateral surfaces of the tubular epithelial cell, the cell membrane contains an extensive Na^+,K^+-ATPase system that is capable of cleaving adenosine trisphosphate (ATP) and using the released energy to transport sodium ions out of the cell into the interstitium, while at the same time transporting potassium ions from the interstitium to the interior of the cell. However, the basolateral sides of the tubular epithelial cell are so permeable to potassium that virtually all the potassium immediately diffuses back out of the cell into the interstitium. Therefore, the net effect, illustrated in Figure 21–11A, is to pump so much sodium out that this reduces the sodium inside the cell to a very low concentration. Also, because three positive electrical charges are pumped out of the cell along with the sodium ions, the interior of the cell is left with a very negative potential of about −70 millivolts. Therefore, two factors now cause sodium ions to *diffuse* through the cell's *luminal* membrane *from the tubular lumen to the interior* of the cell: (1) the very large sodium concentration gradient across the membrane, with high sodium concentration in the tubular lumen and low sodium concentration inside the cell, and (2) the attraction of the positive sodium ions in the tubular lumen to the interior of the cell by the −70 millivolts intracellular potential.

Secondary Active Absorption from the Tubular Lumen

In secondary active transport, no energy is used directly from ATP or any other high-energy phosphate source. Instead, the movement of sodium ions from the tubular lumen to the interior of the cell energizes most of the secondary transport of other substances. This is achieved by multiple different types of sodium carrier proteins in the epithelial cell brush

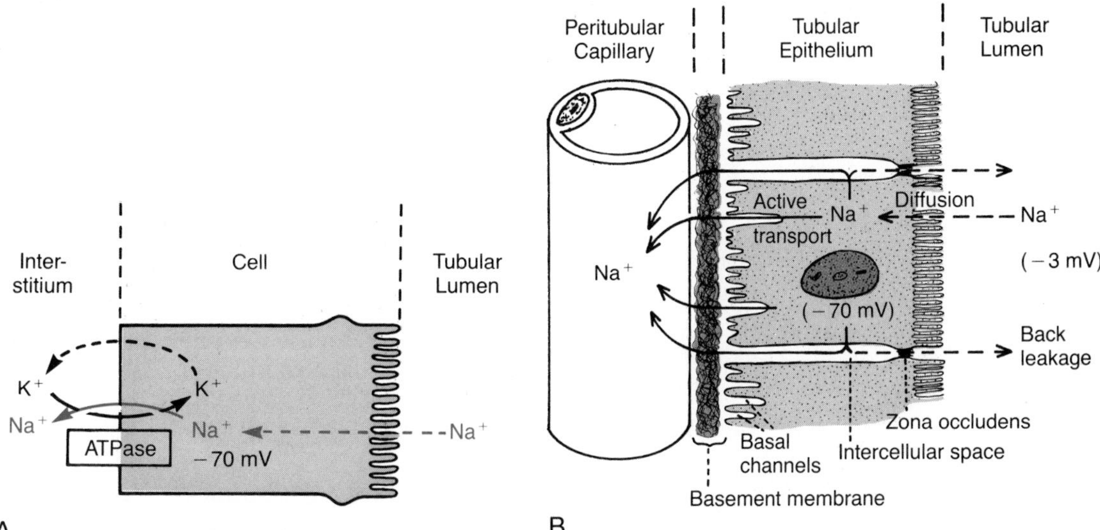

Figure 21–11. *A,* Basic mechanism for active transport of sodium through the tubular epithelial cell. This figure shows active transport by the sodium-potassium pump, which pumps sodium out of the basolateral membrane of the cell and simultaneously creates a very low intracellular sodium concentration as well as a negative intracellular potential. The low intracellular sodium concentration and the negative potential then cause sodium ions to diffuse from the tubular lumen into the cell through the brush border. *B,* The net mechanism for active transport of sodium from the tubular lumen all the way into the peritubular capillary.

border. For instance, in Figure 21–12, the uppermost cell illustrates secondary active transport of glucose, and the second cell illustrates secondary active transport of amino acid ions. In each case, the carrier protein in the brush border membrane combines with both the substance to be transported and a sodium ion at the same time. As the sodium moves down its electrochemical gradient to the interior of the cell, it pulls the glucose or the amino acid ion along with it. Usually, each type of carrier protein is specific for transport of each different substance or for a class of substances. This type of secondary active transport, in which the sodium ion pulls a substance along with it through the membrane, is called *co-transport.*

Glucose, amino acids, and several other organic compounds are especially strongly co-transported in the proximal tubules. Chloride ions are co-transported mainly in the thick segment of the ascending limb of the loop of Henle. Other substances also co-transported at some point in the tubular system include phosphate, calcium, magnesium, and hydrogen ions.

Once the glucose, amino acid, or other substance has been co-transported from the tubular lumen into the epithelial cell, it then usually moves through the basolateral border of the cell by facilitated diffusion in conjunction with another carrier protein.

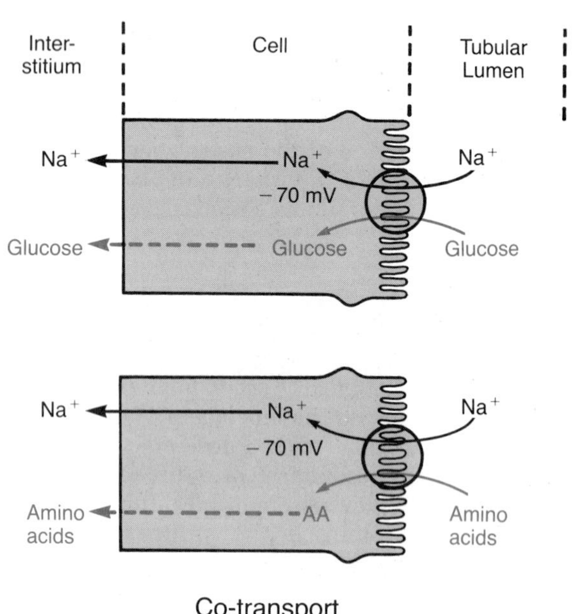

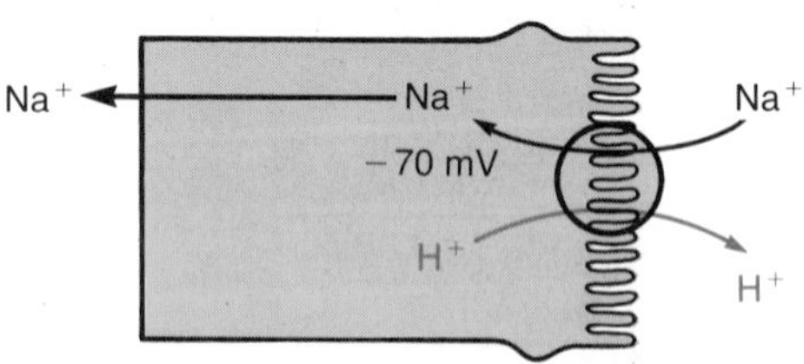

Figure 21–12. Mechanisms of secondary active transport. The upper two cells show *co-transport* of glucose and amino acids through the brush border of the epithelial cells along with sodium ions, followed by facilitated diffusion through the basolateral membranes. The third cell shows *counter-transport* of hydrogen ions through the brush border into the tubular lumen; inward movement of sodium ions provides the energy for outward movement of the hydrogen ions.

Secondary Active Secretion into the Tubules

A few substances are secondarily actively *secreted* into the tubules. In general, the process is the reverse of that discussed in the previous paragraphs for secondary absorption. Some of the important substances that are secreted this way in specific portions of the tubules are hydrogen ions, potassium ions, and urate ions. As an example, the lowermost cell in Figure 21–12 illustrates secondary active secretion of hydrogen ions into the proximal tubules.

Passive Absorption of Water: Osmosis Through the Tubular Epithelium

When the different solutes are transported out of the tubule by either primary or secondary active transport, their total concentration decreases inside the tubular lumen but increases in the interstitium. This obviously creates a concentration difference that causes osmosis of water in the same direction that the solutes have been transported.

A large share of this osmosis occurs through the so-called tight junctions between the epithelial cells rather than through the cells themselves. The reason for this is that these junctions are not nearly so tight as their name would imply but instead allow rapid diffusion of water as well as some of the small ions. This is especially true of the proximal tubules, where the "tight" junctions are very, very loose. As solutes are absorbed through the proximal tubular epithelial cells, this increases the osmolality in the interstitium, which then causes almost instantaneous osmosis of a commensurate volume of water to go along with the solutes.

In the more distal parts of the tubular system, beginning in the loop of Henle and extending through the remaining tubules, the "tight" junctions are much tighter, and the epithelial cells also have much less extensive membrane surfaces. Therefore, in general, the latter portions of the tubular system are far less permeable to water than are the proximal tubules.

Passive Absorption of Chloride Ions, Urea, and Other Solutes by the Process of Diffusion

When sodium ions are transported through the tubular epithelial cell, a negative ion, such as the *chlo-*

ride ion, is usually transported along with each sodium ion to maintain electrical neutrality. This occurs especially through the "tight" junctions of the proximal tubules but also to a lesser extent through the "tight" junctions of the later portions of the tubular system.

Urea is another substance that is passively reabsorbed but to a much lesser degree than are chloride ions. Actually, one of the principal functional purposes of the kidneys is *not* to reabsorb urea but instead to allow as much as possible of this waste product of metabolism to pass on into the urine. Unfortunately, though, the urea molecule is very small, and the tubules are partially permeable to it. Therefore, usually, as water is reabsorbed from the tubules, about half the urea in the glomerular filtrate is passively reabsorbed by diffusing along with the water, while the other half passes on into the urine.

Another waste product of metabolism is *creatinine.* However, its molecule is somewhat larger than that of urea, so that virtually none of it is reabsorbed; instead, virtually all creatinine that is filtered in the glomerular filtrate passes on through the tubular system and is excreted in the urine.

Absorptive Capabilities of Different Tubule Segments

In subsequent chapters, the absorption and secretion of specific substances in different segments of the tubular system are discussed. However, it is important first to point out basic differences between the absorptive and secretory capabilities of the different tubular segments.

Proximal Tubular Epithelium. Figure 21–13 illustrates the cellular characteristics of the tubular membrane in (1) the proximal tubule, (2) the thin segment of the loop of Henle, (3) the distal tubule, and (4) the collecting duct. The proximal tubular cells have the appearance of being highly metabolic cells, having large numbers of mitochondria to support extremely rapid active transport processes; true enough, one finds that *about 65 per cent of the glomerular filtrate normally is reabsorbed before reaching the loops of Henle.*

The extensive membrane surface of the proximal tubular epithelial cell brush border is literally loaded with protein carrier molecules that promote either *co-transport* for absorbing substances from the tubular lumen into the interstitium or *counter-transport* for secreting other substances into the tubules. The most important substances that are specifically absorbed by secondary active transport in the proximal tubules are *glucose* and the *amino acids.* The most important substance that is secreted by secondary active transport is *hydrogen ions.*

Thin Segment of the Loop of Henle. The epithelium of the thin segment of the loop of Henle, as the name implies, is very thin. The cells have no brush border and very few mitochondria, indicating a minimal level of metabolic activity. The *descending portion* of this thin segment is highly permeable to water and moderately permeable to urea, sodium, and most other ions. Therefore, it appears to be adapted primarily for simple diffusion of substances through its walls.

The ascending portion of the thin segment, on the other hand, is believed to be different in one very important characteristic; it is believed to be far less permeable to water than is the descending portion. This difference is important for explaining the mechanism for concentrating urine, as we discuss later.

Thick Segment of the Loop of Henle. The thick segment of the loop of Henle begins about halfway up the ascending limb of the loop, where the epithelial cells become grossly thickened, as illustrated in Figure 21–2. This segment then ascends all the way back to the same glomerulus from which the tubule originated and passes snugly through the angle between the afferent and efferent arterioles, forming a complex with these arterioles called the *juxtaglomerular complex,* discussed earlier in this chapter. Beyond this point, the tubule becomes the distal tubule.

The epithelial cells of the thick segment of the loop of Henle are similar to those of the proximal tubules. They are especially adapted for strong active transport of sodium and chloride ions, transporting these from the tubular lumen into the interstitial fluid.

On the other hand, this thick segment is almost entirely impermeable to both water and urea. Therefore, even though over three quarters of all the ions in the tubular fluid are transported out of the thick segment into the interstitium, almost all the water and urea remain in the tubule. Thus, the ascending limb tubular fluid becomes very dilute except that its concentration of urea is high. This thick segment plays an exceedingly important role under different conditions in the renal mechanisms for diluting or concentrating the urine that is eventually formed by the kidney.

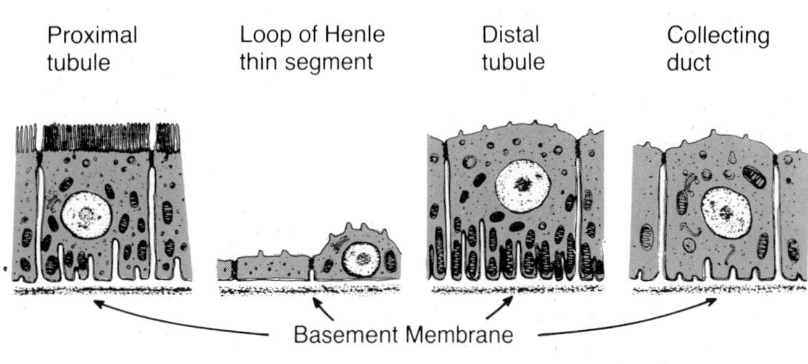

Figure 21–13. Characteristics of the epithelial cells in different tubular segments.

The Distal Tubule. The distal tubule is divided into two important functional segments, the *diluting segment* and the *late distal tubule.*

The Diluting Segment. The first half of the distal tubule has almost the same characteristics as the thick segment of the ascending limb of the loop of Henle. It absorbs most of the ions avidly but is almost entirely impermeable to both water and urea. Therefore, this diluting segment, too, contributes to the dilution of the tubular fluid in the same way as the thick segment of the ascending limb of the loop of Henle.

The Late Distal Tubule and Cortical Collecting Duct. The functional characteristics of the late distal tubule and the cortical collecting duct are similar to each other; even their lining epithelial cells are similar. Several important characteristics of these tubular segments are the following:

1. The epithelium of both is almost entirely impermeable to urea, the same as in the diluting segment of the distal tubule, so that essentially all the urea passes on into the collecting duct, eventually to be excreted in the urine.
2. These two segments reabsorb *sodium ions* avidly, but the rate of this reabsorption is controlled to a very great extent by aldosterone, as we discuss in more detail in the following chapter. Simultaneously with the pumping of sodium out of the tubular lumen into the peritubular interstitium, *potassium ions* are transported in the opposite direction into the tubular lumen; this too is controlled by aldosterone and by several other factors, including the concentration of potassium ions in the body fluids. Thus, potassium ions are actively secreted into these tubular segments, and *it is mainly by this means that the potassium ion concentration is controlled in the extracellular fluids of the body.*
3. The late distal tubule and the cortical collecting duct also contain a special type of epithelial cell called *intercalated cells,* or "brown cells," that secrete hydrogen ions by primary active secretion. These cells can secrete hydrogen ions against a concentration gradient of as much as a thousand to one. Therefore, the intercalated cells play an absolutely essential role in the final high degrees of acidification that can occur in the urine.
4. The late distal tubule and the cortical collecting duct differ from the diluting segment in still another very important aspect: They are *permeable to water in the presence of antidiuretic hormone* but *impermeable when this hormone is absent,* providing a method for controlling the degree of dilution of the urine, a subject that we discuss in detail later. The collecting duct also shares this responsiveness to antidiuretic hormone.

The Collecting Duct. The epithelial cells of the collecting duct have two especially important characteristics for renal function:

1. The permeability of the collecting duct to water is controlled mainly by the level of antidiuretic hormone in the circulating blood, as just mentioned. When excessive amounts of antidiuretic hormone are available, water is reabsorbed into the medullary interstitium with great avidity, thus reducing the volume of urine and concentrating the dissolved substances in the urine.
2. The second important characteristic of the collecting duct epithelium is that it too is capable of secreting hydrogen ions against a very high hydrogen ion gradient. Therefore, the late distal tubule and the collecting duct system play an exceedingly important role in controlling the acid-base balance of the body fluids.

Reabsorption of Water in Different Segments of the Tubules

Water transport occurs entirely by osmotic diffusion. That is, whenever some solute in the glomerular filtrate is absorbed, the resulting decreased concentration of solute in the tubular fluid and increased concentration in the interstitial fluid causes osmosis of water out of the tubules. Therefore, the volume of tubular fluid progressively diminishes along the tubular system.

The following table shows the volumes of fluid that flow per minute at different points in the tubular system.

	ml/min
Glomerular filtrate	125
Flowing into the loops of Henle	45
Flowing into the distal tubules	25
Flowing into the collecting tubules	12
Flowing into the urine	1

From this chart one can also deduce the approximate percentage of the glomerular filtrate water that is reabsorbed in each segment of the tubules, as follows:

	Per cent
Proximal tubules	65
Loops of Henle	15
Distal tubules	10
Collecting ducts	9.3
Passing into the urine	0.7

We see later in this and the following chapters that some of these values vary greatly under different operational conditions of the kidney, particularly when the kidney is forming very dilute or very concentrated urine.

Reabsorption of Specific Substances at Different Points Along the Tubular System

Reabsorption of Substances of Nutritional Value to the Body — Glucose, Proteins, Amino Acids, Acetoacetate Ions, and Vitamins. Five different substances in the glomerular filtrate of particular importance to bodily nutrition are *glucose, proteins, amino acids, acetoacetate ions,* and *the vitamins.* Normally, all these are completely or almost completely *reabsorbed by active processes in the proximal tubules* of the kidney. Thus, Figure 21-14 shows that the concentrations of glucose, protein, and amino acids all decrease to the vanishing point before the tubular fluid has passed through the proximal tubules. Therefore, almost none of these substances remain in the fluid entering the loop of Henle.

Poor Reabsorption of the Metabolic End-Products: Urea and Creatinine. Figure 21-14 also illustrates the concentrations of two major metabolic end-products in the different segments of the tubular system—urea and creatinine. Only small quantities of *urea* are reabsorbed during the entire course through the tubular system. Yet, about 99.3 per cent of the water is reabsorbed. The removal of all this water therefore concentrates the urea about 65-fold.

Creatinine is not reabsorbed in the tubules at all; indeed, small quantities of creatinine are actually secreted into the tubules by the proximal tubules, so that the concentration of creatinine increases about 140-fold.

Reabsorption of Inulin and Para-Aminohippuric Acid by the Tubules. Note also in Figure 21-14 that when the substance *inulin,* a large polysaccharide, is infused into the blood and is then filtered in the glomerular filtrate, its concentration increases 125-fold by the time it reaches the urine. The cause of this is simply that inulin is neither reabsorbed nor secreted in any segment of the tubules, whereas all but 1 milliliter of the 125 milliliters of water in the glomerular filtrate is reabsorbed.

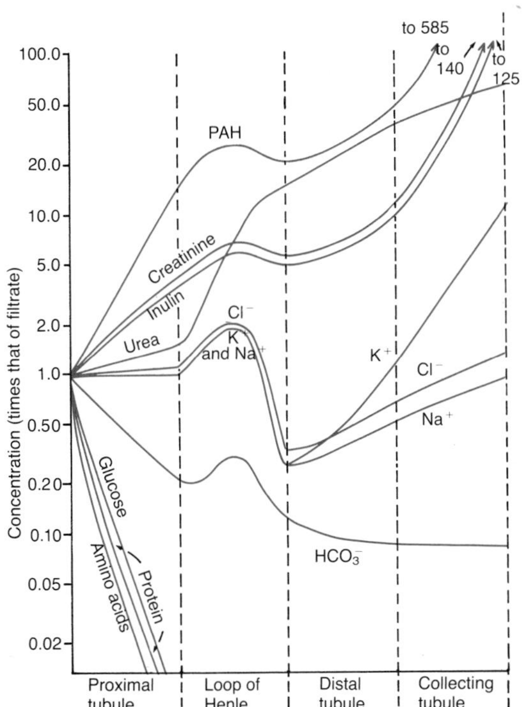

Figure 21-14. Composite figure showing average concentrations of different substances at different points in the tubular system.

Also, Figure 21-14 shows that when *para-aminohippuric acid* (PAH) is infused into the blood and then excreted by the kidneys, its concentration increases 585-fold as the tubular fluid passes through the tubular system. This is because large quantities of PAH are *secreted* into the tubular fluid by the proximal tubular epithelial cells, and it is not reabsorbed in any segment of the tubular system.

These two substances play an important role in experimental studies of tubular function, as is discussed later in the chapter.

Reabsorption of Different Ions by the Tubules—Sodium, Potassium, Chloride, Bicarbonate, Potassium, and Others. Finally, note in Figure 21-14 the concentration changes of several important ions—sodium, potassium, chloride, and bicarbonate. Some of the concentrations rise above 1.0, which means greater concentration than in the glomerular filtrate, whereas others fall below 1.0. The degree of concentration or dilution depends on various mechanisms that increase or decrease reabsorption of the different ions for the purpose of controlling their extracellular fluid concentrations. In the following chapters we are particularly concerned with several of these control systems.

To excrete enough potassium and hydrogen ions, it is necessary for both of these to be actively secreted into the tubular system; the amounts of secretion are precisely determined by the potassium and hydrogen ion concentrations in the extracellular fluids.

Bicarbonate ion is transported in a very peculiar way, by converting the bicarbonate ion into carbon dioxide and then allowing the carbon dioxide simply to diffuse through the tubular wall into the interstitial fluid. The method for converting the bicarbonate ion into carbon dioxide is first to secrete a hydrogen ion into the tubule; this then binds with the bicarbonate ion to form H_2CO_3. In turn, the H_2CO_3 dissociates into water and carbon dioxide. After the carbon dioxide diffuses through the tubular membrane, on the other side it recombines with water to form new bicarbonate ion.

Finally, both calcium and magnesium ions are actively reabsorbed in some of the tubules, and many negative ions, especially chloride ions, are reabsorbed mainly by passive diffusion as a result of the electrical gradient that develops across the tubular wall when positive ions are reabsorbed. In addition, some negative ions—urate, phosphates, sulfate, and nitrate—can be reabsorbed by active transport, occurring to the greatest extent in the proximal tubules.

THE CONCEPT OF "PLASMA CLEARANCE"—ITS USE IN ASSESSING RENAL FUNCTION

The term "plasma clearance" is used to express the ability of the kidneys to clean, or "clear," the plasma of various substances. Thus, if the plasma passing through the kidneys contains 0.1 gram of a substance in each deciliter, and 0.1 gram of this substance also passes into the urine each minute, 1 deciliter of the plasma is cleaned or "cleared" of the substance per minute.

To give an example, the normal concentration of urea in each milliliter of plasma and glomerular filtrate is 0.26 milligram, and the quantity of urea that passes into the urine each minute is approximately 18.2 milligrams. Therefore, the equivalent quantity of plasma that completely loses its entire content of urea each minute can be calculated by dividing the quantity of urea entering the urine each minute by the quantity of urea in each milliliter of plasma. Thus $18.2 \div 0.26 = 70$; that is, 70 milliliters of plasma is *cleaned* or *cleared* of urea each minute. This amount that is cleared each minute is known as the *plasma clearance of urea.* Obviously, therefore, the plasma clearance of each substance is a measure of the effectiveness of the kidney in removing that substance from the extracellular fluid.

Plasma clearance for any substance can be calculated by the following formula:

$$\text{Plasma clearance (ml/min)} = \frac{\text{Urine flow (ml/min)} \times \text{Concentration in urine}}{\text{Concentration in plasma}}$$

Inulin Clearance as a Measure of Glomerular Filtration Rate

Inulin is a polysaccharide that has the specific attributes of not being reabsorbed to a significant extent by the tubules of the nephron and yet being of small enough molecular weight (about 5200) that it passes through the glomerular membrane as freely as the crystalloids and water of the plasma. Also, inulin is not actively secreted even in the minutest amount by the tubules. Consequently, glomerular filtrate contains virtually the same concentration of inulin as does plasma, and as the filtrate flows down the tubules, all the filtered inulin continues on into the urine. Thus, *all the glomerular filtrate formed is cleared of inulin.* Therefore, the *plasma clearance per minute of inulin is equal to the glomerular filtration rate.*

As an example, let us assume that chemical analysis shows the inulin concentration in the plasma to be 0.001 gram in each milliliter and that 0.125 gram of inulin passes into the urine per minute. By dividing 0.001 into 0.125, one finds that 125 ml of glomerular filtrate must be formed each minute in order to deliver to the urine the analyzed quantity of inulin. In other words, by measuring the plasma clearance of inulin, we have determined that the glomerular filtration rate is 125 ml/min.

Para-Aminohippuric Acid (PAH) Clearance as a Measure of Plasma Flow Through the Kidneys

PAH, like inulin, passes through the glomerular membrane with perfect ease. However, it is different from inulin in that most of the PAH remaining in the plasma after the glomerular filtrate is formed is secreted from the peritubular capillaries into the tubules by the proximal tubular epithelium (if the plasma concentration of PAH is very low). Indeed, only about one tenth of the original PAH remains in the plasma by the time the blood leaves the kidneys.

One can use the clearance of PAH for estimating the *flow of plasma* through the kidneys. As an example, let us assume that 585 ml of plasma is cleared of PAH each minute. Obviously, if this much plasma is cleared of PAH, *at least this much plasma must have passed through the kidneys* in this same period of time. And, to be still more accurate, one can correct for the average amount of PAH that is still in the blood when it leaves the kidney. In different experiments the PAH clearance has been found to be about 91 per cent of the plasma load of PAH entering the kidneys; thus, dividing 585 by 0.91 gives a total plasma flow per minute of approximately 650 milliliters.

One can then calculate the *total blood flow* through the kidneys each minute from the plasma flow and the hematocrit (the percentage of red blood cells in the blood). If the hematocrit is 45 per cent and the plasma flow 650 ml/min, the total blood flow through both kidneys is $650 \times 100 \div 55$, or 1182 ml/min.

REFERENCES

Aronson, P. S.: The renal proximal tubule: A model for diversity of anion exchangers and stilbene-sensitive anion transporters. Annu. Rev. Physiol., 51:419, 1989.

Brenner, B. M., and Rector, F. C., Jr.: The Kidney. 3rd ed. Philadelphia, W. B. Saunders Co., 1986.

Edwards, R. M.: Direct assessment of glomerular arteriole reactivity. News Physiol. Sci., 3:216, 1988.

Greger, R.: Chloride transport in thick ascending limb, distal convolution, and collecting duct. Annu. Rev. Physiol., 50:111, 1988.

Guyton, A. C., et al.: Dynamics and Control of the Body Fluids. Philadelphia, W. B. Saunders Co., 1975.

Mandel, L. J.: Metabolic substrates, cellular energy production, and the regulation of proximal tubular transport. Annu. Rev. Physiol., 47:85, 1985.

Massry, S. G., and Gassock, R. J. (eds.): Textbook of Nephrology. Baltimore, Williams & Wilkins, 1988.

Pinter, G. G.: Renal lymph: Vital for the kidney and valuable for the physiologist. News Physiol. Sci., 3:189, 1988.

Post, R. L.: Seeds of sodium, potassium ATPase. Annu. Rev. Physiol., 51:1, 1989.

Schild, L., et al.: Chloride transport in the proximal renal tubule. Annu. Rev. Physiol., 50:97, 1988.

QUESTIONS

1. Describe the functional anatomy of the kidney, paying special attention to the arrangements of the separate segments of the nephron.
2. Describe the relationship of the *vasa recta* to the loops of Henle.
3. State approximate values in the human being for *rate of*

blood flow through the kidneys, *glomerular filtration rate,* and *rate of urine excretion.*

4. Approximately what proportion of the glomerular filtrate is normally reabsorbed during the formation of urine?
5. Explain the effects on glomerular filtration of afferent arteriolar constriction and of efferent arteriolar constriction.
6. Describe the characteristics of the glomerular membrane and its permeability to various substances.
7. Compare the composition of glomerular filtrate with that of plasma.
8. State approximate values for the forces at the glomerular membrane that determine glomerular filtration.
9. Describe the chemical and physical events causing active transport of sodium ions through the tubular epithelium.
10. Why does absorption of osmotic substances through the tubular epithelium cause osmosis of water through the epithelium as well?
11. Explain why urea and other waste products become concentrated as they pass through the tubular system.
12. What are the specific characteristics of absorption of each of the following substances through the tubular epithelium: glucose; proteins; amino acids; and sodium, chloride, bicarbonate, and potassium ions?
13. What important ions are secreted into the tubular fluid through the tubular epithelium?
14. Explain the effect of arterial pressure on the volume of urine excretion. Why is this relationship very important to the overall control of circulatory function?
15. Describe the *juxtaglomerular complex* and its relationship to the autoregulation of glomerular filtration rate.
16. Explain the differences between the afferent and the efferent arteriolar feedback mechanisms for control of glomerular filtration rate.
17. Why is the *renin-angiotensin system* of importance in allowing a person to conserve water and electrolytes in low blood pressure states while at the same time continuing to excrete waste products?
18. Explain the concept of *plasma clearance.*
19. If the concentration of inulin in the blood is 0.05 g in each 100 ml of plasma and a total of 0.02 g of inulin passes into the urine per minute, what is the glomerular filtration rate?

22

Renal and Associated Mechanisms for Controlling the Body Fluids and Their Constituents

The principal function of the kidneys is to control almost all the characteristics of the body fluids, such characteristics as volume, composition, and osmolality. This chapter will discuss these fluids and the roles of the kidneys and the thirst mechanism in their control.

THE MECHANISM FOR EXCRETING EXCESS WATER: EXCRETION OF A DILUTE URINE

One of the most important functions of the kidney is to control the osmolality of the body fluids. When the osmolality falls too low—that is, when the fluids become too dilute—nervous and hormonal feedback mechanisms cause the kidneys to excrete a great excess of water in the urine. This obviously causes a dilute urine, but it also removes water from the body, in this way increasing the body fluid osmolality back toward normal. Conversely, when the osmolality of the body fluids is too great, the kidneys excrete an excess of solutes, thereby reducing the body fluid osmolality again back toward normal but at the same time excreting a concentrated urine.

Role of Antidiuretic Hormone in Controlling Urine Concentration. The signal that tells the kidney whether to excrete a dilute or a concentrated urine is the hormone called *antidiuretic hormone* (ADH) (also called "vasopressin") that is secreted by the posterior pituitary gland. When the body fluids are too concentrated, the posterior pituitary gland secretes large amounts of ADH, which allows the kidneys to continue excreting large amounts of solutes but to conserve water. Conversely, in the absence of ADH, the kidneys excrete a dilute urine, thus losing excess water from the body. The feedback mechanisms for controlling this system are described later in the chapter; for now, let us discuss the renal mechanisms for excreting a dilute or a concentrated urine.

The Renal Mechanism for Excreting a Dilute Urine. Figure 22–1 illustrates the mechanism for excreting a dilute urine. When the glomerular filtrate is initially formed by the glomerulus, its osmolality is almost exactly the same as that of the plasma, approximately 300 mOsm/liter. To excrete excess water, it is necessary to dilute the filtrate as it passes through the tubules. This is achieved by reabsorbing a higher proportion of solutes than water.

The distal segments of the tubular system are depicted in Figure 22–1 with thickened, darkened walls to indicate that their epithelia are almost completely impermeable to water when the kidneys are excreting a dilute urine. The ascending limb of the loop of Henle and the diluting segment of the distal tubule even normally are very impermeable to water, whereas the late distal tubule, the cortical collecting duct, and the collecting duct also become almost completely impermeable to water *when ADH is not present* in the circulating body fluids.

The reabsorption of solutes in these distal segments of the tubular system is strong and active. In the thick segment of the ascending limb of the loop of Henle, active reabsorption of sodium, potassium, and chloride ions is especially powerful, and one can see from

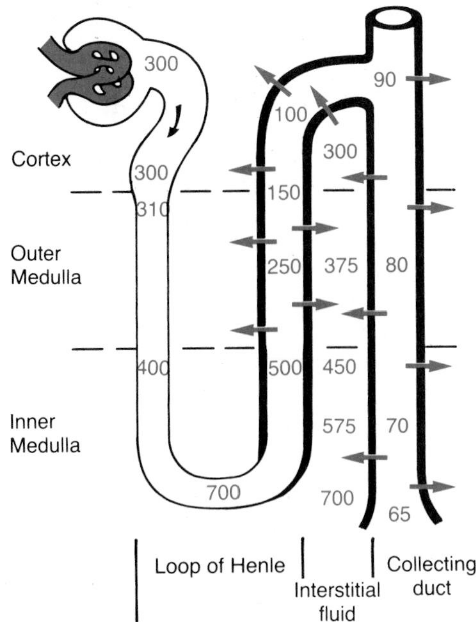

Figure 22-1. The renal mechanism for forming a dilute urine. The darkened walls of the distal portions of the tubular system indicate that these portions of the tubules are relatively impermeable to the reabsorption of water in the absence of antidiuretic hormone. The solid arrows indicate active processes for absorption of most of the solutes besides the urinary waste products. (Numerical values are in milliosmoles per liter.)

the numerical values in the figure that the osmolality of the fluid in the ascending limb of the loop of Henle decreases progressively to about 100 mOsm/liter by the time the fluid leaves this tubular segment. That is, most of the solutes besides the waste products are reabsorbed, but the water remains behind. Then, as this remaining dilute fluid passes through the distal tubule, cortical collecting duct, and collecting duct, some additional reabsorption of solutes, especially of sodium ions, causes still more dilution of the tubular fluid, often decreasing its osmolality to as little as 65 mOsm/liter and rarely to levels below 50 mOsm/liter by the time it leaves the collecting duct to enter the urine.

To summarize, the process for excreting a dilute urine is very simple; it is one of absorbing solutes from the distal segments of the tubular system while leaving the water in the tubules. However, this failure of water to be reabsorbed occurs only in the absence of ADH.

THE MECHANISM FOR EXCRETING EXCESS SOLUTES: THE COUNTERCURRENT MECHANISM FOR EXCRETING A CONCENTRATED URINE

The process for concentrating the urine is not nearly so simple as for diluting it. Yet, at times it is exceedingly important to concentrate the urine as much as possible, so that excess solutes can be eliminated with as little loss of water from the body as possible — for instance, when one is exposed to desert conditions with an inadequate supply of water. Fortunately, the kidneys have developed a special, though very complex, mechanism for concentrating the urine, called the *countercurrent mechanism.*

The countercurrent mechanism depends on a peculiar anatomical arrangement of the loops of Henle and the vasa recta in the renal medulla, as illustrated in Figure 22-2. In the human, the loops of Henle of one third to one fifth of the nephrons dip deep into the

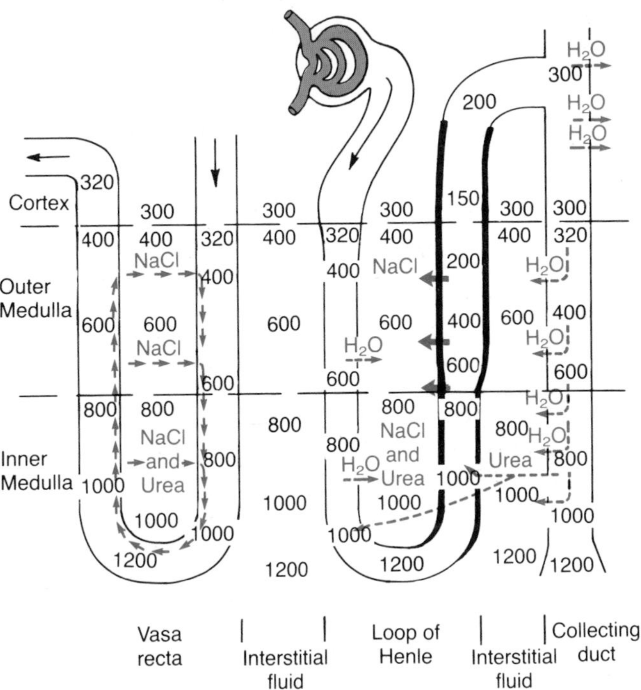

Figure 22-2. The countercurrent mechanism for concentrating the urine. (Numerical values are in milliosmoles per liter.)

medulla and then return to the cortex. Paralleling the long loops of Henle are loops of peritubular capillaries called the *vasa recta;* these also loop down into the medulla from the cortex and then back out to the cortex.

Hyperosmolality of the Medullary Interstitial Fluid, and Mechanisms for Achieving It

The first step in the excretion of excess solutes in the urine—that is, for excreting a concentrated urine—is to create a very high osmotic pressure (hyperosmolality) of the medullary interstitial fluid. Let us explain the mechanism for creating this hyperosmolality.

The normal osmolality of the fluids in almost all parts of the body is about 300 mOsm/liter. However, as shown by the numbers in Figure 22-2, the osmolality of the interstitial fluid in the medulla of the kidney is much higher than this, and it becomes progressively greater the deeper one goes into the medulla, increasing from 300 mOsm/liter in the cortex to 1200 mOsm/liter (occasionally as high as 1400 mOsm/liter) in the pelvic tip of the medulla.

The principal cause of the greatly increased medullary osmolality is active transport of sodium ions (plus co-transport of potassium, chloride, and other ions) out of the thick portion of the ascending limb of the loop of Henle and also out of the collecting duct into the interstitium. The large colored arrows shown in Figure 22-2 illustrate this transport into the outer medullary interstitial fluid. The sodium and its associated ions become concentrated in this fluid. Also, they are carried downward into the inner medulla by the downward flowing blood in the descending limbs of the vasa recta and also by diffusing into the descending thin limb of the loop of Henle, as we see shortly.

Mechanism by Which Antidiuretic Hormone Increases Water Reabsorption. ADH acts on the basolateral membrane of the epithelial cells in the late distal tubules, cortical collecting ducts, and medullary collecting ducts. It activates the enzyme *adenyl cyclase* in this membrane, which then causes formation of *cyclic adenosine monophosphate* (cyclic AMP) in the cell cytoplasm. This then diffuses to the luminal side of the cell and within minutes causes elongated vesicular structures in the cytoplasm to develop and fuse with the cell's luminal membrane. In this way the membranes of these vesicles become part of the luminal cell membrane, providing patches of membrane containing aggregates of protein particles that have very large water-conducting channels. Therefore, the luminal membrane becomes highly water-permeable in contrast to its normal state of almost total impermeability.

When ADH is no longer present, the vesicular structures detach from the luminal membrane within 10 to 15 minutes and return to their internal position in the cytoplasm; the tubules again become water impermeable.

Countercurrent Exchange Mechanism in the Vasa Recta—A Mechanism for Holding Solutes in the Medulla

We have now discussed the mechanisms by which high concentrations of solutes are achieved in the medullary interstitium. However, without a special medullary vascular system as well, the flow of blood through the interstitium would rapidly remove the excess solutes and keep the concentration from rising very high. Fortunately, the medullary blood flow has two characteristics, both exceedingly important, for maintaining the high solute concentration in the medullary interstitial fluids. These are as follows:

First, the inner medullary blood flow is very slight in quantity, amounting to only 1 to 2 per cent of the total blood flow of the kidney. Because of this very sluggish blood flow, removal of solutes is minimized.

Second, the vasa recta capillaries function as a *countercurrent exchanger* that also minimizes the washout of solutes from the medulla. This can be explained as follows: A countercurrent fluid exchange mechanism is one in which fluid flows through a long, highly permeable U-tube, with the two arms of the U lying in close proximity to each other, so that fluid and solutes can exchange readily between the two arms. Because the fluids and solutes in the two parallel streams of flow can exchange rapidly, tremendous concentrations of solute can be maintained at the tip of the loop with negligible washout of solute.

Thus, in Figure 22-2, as blood flows down the descending limbs of the vasa recta, sodium chloride and urea diffuse into the blood from the interstitial fluid, while water diffuses outward into the interstitium. These two effects cause the osmolal concentration in the capillary blood to rise progressively higher, to a maximum concentration of 1200 mOsm/liter at the tips of the vasa recta. Then, as the blood flows back up the ascending limbs, the extreme diffusibility of all molecules through the capillary membrane allows almost all the extra sodium chloride and urea to diffuse back out of the blood into the interstitial fluid, while water diffuses back into the blood. Therefore, by the time the blood finally leaves the medulla, its osmolal concentration is only slightly greater than that of the blood that had initially entered the vasa recta. As a result, the blood flowing through the vasa recta carries only a minute amount of the medullary interstitial solutes away from the medulla.

Mechanism for Excreting a Concentrated Urine—Role of Antidiuretic Hormone

Now that we have explained how the kidney creates hyperosmolality in the medullary interstitium, it becomes a simple matter to explain the mechanism for excreting a concentrated urine.

When the concentration of ADH in the blood is high, the epithelium of the cortical collecting duct, the collecting duct, and in some species of animals the late distal tubule as well become highly permeable to water. This is illustrated in Figure 22-2 by the thin walls of these segments of the tubular system. Most important, as the tubular fluid flows through the collecting duct, water is pulled by osmosis into the highly concentrated fluid of the medullary interstitium. The loss of this water from the duct causes the collecting duct fluid to become highly concentrated, and it issues from the papilla into the pelvis of the kidney at a concentration of about 1200 mOsm/liter, almost exactly equal to the osmolal concentration of the solutes in the medullary interstitium near the papilla.

CONTROL OF EXTRACELLULAR FLUID OSMOLALITY AND SODIUM CONCENTRATION

Now that the mechanisms by which the kidney can excrete either a dilute or a concentrated urine have been discussed, in the next few pages we explain how these mechanisms are manipulated to control extracellular fluid osmolality and sodium concentration.

The osmolality of the extracellular fluid averages almost exactly 300 mOsm/liter, and the sodium ion concentration 142 mEq/liter. These rarely change more than ±3 per cent day in and day out, which gives one an idea how tightly both of these are controlled.

Relationship Between Extracellular Fluid Osmolality and Sodium Concentration. The osmolality of the extracellular fluids is determined almost entirely by the extracellular fluid sodium concentration. The reason for this is that sodium is by far the most abundant positive ion of the extracellular fluid, representing over 90 per cent of these ions. Furthermore, every time a positive ion is reabsorbed by the renal tubules, a negative ion also is reabsorbed. Therefore, in effect, the control of the positive ions controls the total ion concentration. Also, the glucose and urea, which are the most abundant of the nonionic osmolar solutes in the extracellular fluids, normally represent only 3 per cent of the total osmolality, and even then the urea exerts very little *effective* osmotic pressure because it penetrates cells too easily to cause significant osmotic results. Therefore, *the sodium ions of the extracellular fluid determine either directly or indirectly over 90 per cent of the osmotic pressure of the extracellular* fluid. Consequently, we can generally talk in terms of control of osmolality and control of sodium ion concentration at the same time.

Three separate control systems operate in close association to regulate extracellular osmolality and sodium concentration. These are (1) the osmoreceptor-antidiuretic hormone system, (2) the thirst mechanism, and (3) the salt appetite mechanism.

The Osmoreceptor-Antidiuretic Hormone Feedback Control System

Figure 22-3 illustrates the osmoreceptor-antidiuretic hormone system for control of extracellular fluid sodium concentration and osmolality. It is a typical feedback control system that operates by the following steps:

1. An increase in osmolality (mainly excess sodium and the negative ions that go with it) excites *osmoreceptors* located in the anterior hypothalamus near to the supraoptic nuclei.
2. Excitation of the osmoreceptors in turn stimulates the supraoptic nuclei, which then cause the posterior pituitary gland to release ADH.
3. The ADH increases the permeability of the late distal tubules, the cortical collecting ducts, and the collecting ducts to water, as explained earlier, and therefore *causes increased conservation of water by the kidneys.*
4. The conservation of water but *loss of sodium and other osmolar substances in the urine* causes dilution of the sodium and other substances in the extracellular fluid, thus correcting the initial, excessively concentrated extracellular fluid.

Conversely, when the extracellular fluid becomes too dilute (hypo-osmotic), less ADH is formed, and

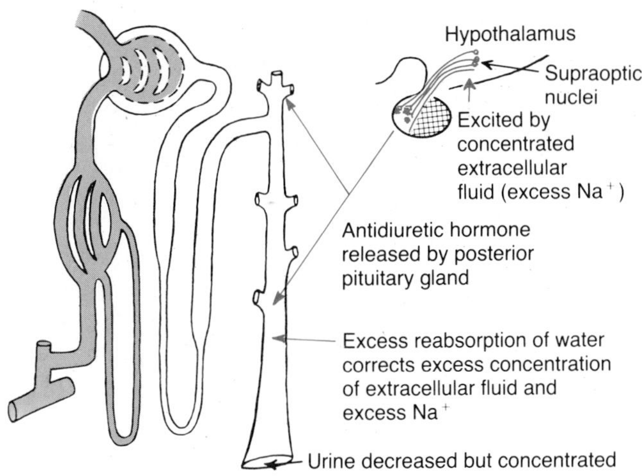

Figure 22-3. Control of extracellular fluid osmolality and sodium ion concentration by the osmosodium receptor-antidiuretic hormone feedback control system.

excess water is lost in comparison with the extracellular fluid solutes, thus concentrating the body fluids back toward normal.

The Osmoreceptors (or Osmosodium Receptors)—The "AV3V Region" of the Brain. Figure 22–4 illustrates the hypothalamus and the pituitary gland. The hypothalamus contains two areas that are important in controlling ADH secretion and also in controlling thirst. One of these is the *supraoptic nuclei.* Here about five sixths of the ADH is formed in the cell bodies of large neuronal cells; the remaining one sixth is formed in the nearby *paraventricular nuclei.* This hormone is transported down the axons of the neurons to their tips, terminating in the posterior pituitary gland. When the supraoptic and paraventricular nuclei are stimulated, nerve impulses pass to these nerve endings and cause ADH to be released into the capillary blood of the posterior pituitary gland.

A second neuronal area important in controlling osmolality is a broad area located along the anteroventral border of the third ventricle, called the *AV3V region,* also illustrated in Figure 22–4. Either in the AV3V region or in its vicinity are neuronal cells that are excited by very minute increases in extracellular fluid osmolality and, conversely, inhibited by decreases in osmolality. These neurons are called *osmoreceptors.* They in turn send nerve signals to the supraoptic nuclei to control the secretion of ADH. It is likely that they also induce thirst as well.

Summary of the Antidiuretic Hormone Mechanism for Controlling Extracellular Fluid Osmolality and Extracellular Fluid Sodium Concentration. From these discussions, we can reiterate once again the importance of the ADH mechanism for controlling at the same time both extracellular fluid osmolality and extracellular fluid sodium concentration. That is, an increase in sodium concentration causes almost an exactly parallel increase in osmolality, which in turn excites the osmoreceptors of the hypothalamus. These receptors then cause the secretion of ADH, which markedly increases the reabsorption of water in the renal tubules. Consequently, very little water is lost into the urine, but the urinary solutes continue to be lost. Therefore, the relative proportion of water in the extracellular fluid increases, whereas the proportion of solutes decreases. In this way, the sodium ion concentration of the extracellular fluid, and the osmolality as well, decrease toward the normal level. This is a very powerful mechanism for controlling both the extracellular fluid osmolality and the extracellular fluid sodium concentration.

Thirst and Its Role in Controlling Extracellular Fluid Osmolality and Sodium Concentration

The phenomenon of thirst is equally as important for regulating body water, osmolality, and sodium concentration as is the osmoreceptor-renal mechanism previously discussed, because the amount of water in the body at any one time is determined by the balance between both *intake* and *output* of water.

Neural Integration of Thirst—The "Thirst" Center

Referring again to Figure 22–4, note that the same area along the anteroventral wall of the third ventricle that promotes antidiuresis can also cause thirst. Also located anterolaterally in the preoptic hypothalamus are other small areas that, when stimulated electrically, will cause immediate onset of drinking that continues as long as the stimulation lasts. All these areas together are called the *thirst center.*

Injection of hypertonic salt solution into portions of the center causes osmosis of water out of the neuronal cells, and this causes the desire for drinking. Therefore, these cells function as *osmoreceptors* to activate the thirst mechanism. Probably these are the same osmoreceptors that activate the antidiuretic system as well.

Basic Stimulus for Exciting Thirst—Intracellular Dehydration. Any factor that will cause *intracellular dehydration* will in general cause the sensation of thirst. The most common cause of this is increased osmolar concentration of the extracellular fluid, especially increased sodium concentration, which causes osmosis of fluid out of the neuronal cells of the thirst center. However, another important cause is excessive loss of potassium from the body, which reduces the intracellular potassium of the thirst cells and therefore also decreases their volume.

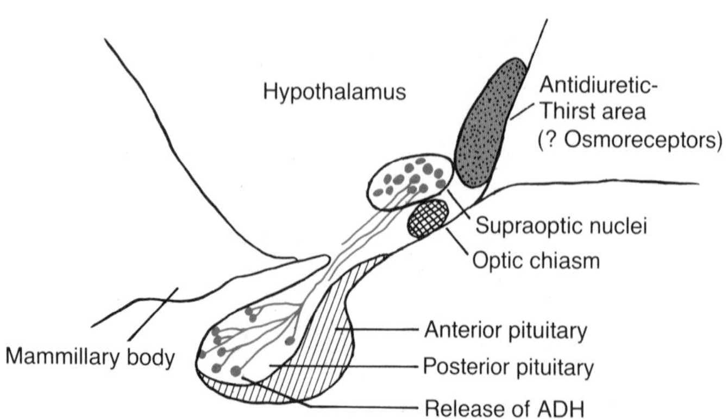

Figure 22–4. The supraopticopituitary antidiuretic system and its relationship to the thirst center in the hypothalamus.

Role of Thirst in Controlling Extracellular Fluid Osmolality and Sodium Concentration

Threshold for Drinking — The Tripping Mechanism. The kidneys are continually excreting fluid; also water is lost by evaporation from the skin and lungs. Therefore, a person is continually being dehydrated, causing the volume of extracellular fluid to decrease and its concentration of sodium and other osmolar elements to rise. When the sodium concentration rises approximately 2 mEq/liter above normal (or the osmolality rises approximately 4 mOsm/liter above normal), the drinking mechanism becomes "tripped"; that is, the person then reaches a level of thirst that is strong enough to activate the necessary motor effort to cause drinking. This is called the *threshold for drinking.* The person ordinarily drinks precisely the required amount of fluid to bring the extracellular fluids back to normal — that is, to a state of *satiety.* Then the process of dehydration and sodium concentration begins again, and after a period of time the drinking act is tripped again, the process continuing on and on indefinitely.

In this way, both the osmolality and the sodium concentration of the extracellular fluid are very precisely controlled.

Effect of Cardiovascular Reflexes on the ADH-Thirst Control System

Two cardiovascular reflexes also have powerful effects on the ADH-thirst mechanism: (1) the *arterial baroreceptor reflex* and (2) the *volume receptor reflex,* activated by changes in the volume-stretch of the atria of the heart; these reflexes are discussed in Chapter 15. A decrease in blood volume causes the arterial pressure to fall and activates the arterial baroreceptor reflex. And the volume receptor reflex is activated when the pressures in the two atria, in the pulmonary artery, and in other low pressure areas of the lesser circulation fall below normal, all a common result of too little volume in the circulation. The net result is to activate the ADH-thirst system and thereby to increase the body fluid volume.

SODIUM EXCRETION AND ITS CONTROL BY ALDOSTERONE

The glomerular filtrate normally contains about 26,000 mEq of sodium each day, and yet the average intake of sodium per day is only 150 mEq. Therefore, the kidneys can be allowed to excrete only about 150 of the total 26,000 mEq; otherwise the body would become depleted of sodium. Consequently, the principal role of the tubular system in sodium excretion is to reabsorb sodium, not to excrete it.

Reabsorption of Most of the Tubular Sodium in the Proximal Tubules and Loops of Henle. By the time the tubular fluid reaches the distal tubules, all but about 8 per cent of the sodium has already been reabsorbed. About 65 per cent of this is reabsorbed in the proximal tubules because of the active transport of sodium by the proximal tubular epithelial cells.

In the thick portion of the ascending limb of the loop of Henle approximately another 27 per cent of the sodium is reabsorbed, leaving only 8 per cent to enter the distal tubules.

Variable Reabsorption of Sodium in the Late Distal Tubules and Cortical Collecting Ducts — Role of Aldosterone

Sodium reabsorption in the late distal tubules and in the cortical collecting ducts is highly variable. The rate of reabsorption is controlled mainly by the concentration in the blood of *aldosterone,* a hormone secreted by the adrenal cortex. In the presence of large amounts of aldosterone, almost the last vestiges of tubular sodium are reabsorbed from these portions of the tubular system so that essentially none of the sodium enters the urine. On the other hand, in the absence of aldosterone, almost all of the sodium that enters the late distal tubules, about 800 mEq/day, is not reabsorbed and does then pass into the urine. Thus, the sodium excretion may be as little as 0.1 gram per day or as great as 20 grams per day, depending inversely on the amount of aldosterone that is secreted.

Mechanism by Which Aldosterone Enhances Sodium Transport. Upon entering a tubular epithelial cell, aldosterone combines with a *receptor protein;* this combination diffuses within minutes into the nucleus, where it activates the DNA molecules to form one or more types of messenger RNA. The RNA is then believed to cause formation of carrier proteins or protein enzymes that are necessary for the sodium transport process.

Ordinarily, aldosterone has no effect on sodium transport for the first 45 minutes after it is administered; after this time the specific proteins important for transport begin to appear in the epithelial cells, followed by progressive increase in transport during the ensuing few hours.

Control of Aldosterone Secretion. Aldosterone is secreted by the zona glomerulosa cells in the outer cortex of the adrenal glands, as is discussed in much greater detail in Chapter 51. Three different factors are known to stimulate this secretion of aldosterone. These are (1) increased angiotensin II in the blood, (2) increased extracellular fluid potassium ion concentration, and (3) decreased extracellular fluid sodium ion concentration. The second of these is important for the control of potassium ion concentration, as discussed later. The first and the third factors are especially important for the control of both sodium excretion by the kidneys and extracellular fluid volume.

When the extracellular fluid volume falls too low, the resulting effects on the circulatory system are to decrease the arterial pressure and to increase the reflex stimulation of the sympathetic nervous system.

Both of these reduce blood flow through the kidneys and excite the secretion of renin, as is explained in Chapter 16. The renin in turn causes the formation of angiotensin I, which is later converted to angiotensin II. Finally, the angiotensin II has a direct effect on the zona glomerulosa cells to increase the secretion of aldosterone.

In addition, a decrease in extracellular fluid sodium ion concentration also seems to have a direct weak stimulatory effect on aldosterone secretion, though this effect is much, much less potent than the effect of angiotensin II.

Thus, whenever either the extracellular fluid volume or the extracellular fluid sodium ion concentration falls below normal, aldosterone is secreted and the renal tubules reabsorb extra quantities of sodium and water, leading to return of both extracellular fluid sodium and extracellular fluid volume back toward normal.

Relative Unimportance of the Aldosterone Feedback Mechanism for Determining Sodium Ion *Concentration* Under Normal Conditions. Although aldosterone increases the *quantity* of sodium in the extracellular fluid, the increased reabsorption of water along with the sodium usually prevents a rise in sodium *concentration* but instead mainly increases the total quantity of extracellular fluid.

This lack of importance of aldosterone feedback control of sodium concentration seems to be a paradox, but it results from the following simple effect: When the aldosterone causes increased sodium reabsorption from the tubules, as discussed earlier, this causes a simultaneous reabsorption of water and an increase in extracellular fluid volume. An increase of only a few per cent in the extracellular fluid volume eventually leads to an increase in arterial pressure, and the increase in arterial pressure leads to increased excretion of both sodium and water together, so that the concentration changes very little.

Indeed, even in patients who have *primary aldosteronism* (these patients secrete tremendous quantities of aldosterone), the sodium concentration still rises only 2 to 3 mEq/liter above normal.

CONTROL OF SODIUM INTAKE BY THE SALT APPETITE MECHANISM

Maintenance of normal extracellular sodium requires not only control of sodium excretion but also control of sodium intake. Fortunately, the body uses the salt appetite mechanism to control sodium intake, which is analogous to the thirst mechanism for control of water intake.

In the same way that two major stimuli elicit thirst, two major stimuli also excite salt appetite: (1) decreased sodium concentration in the extracellular fluid and (2) circulatory insufficiency, often caused by decreased blood volume. However, a major difference between thirst and salt appetite is that thirst is elicited almost immediately, whereas the craving for salt usually begins only after several hours, then builds progressively more and more.

The neuronal mechanism for salt appetite also is analogous to that of the thirst mechanism. Some of the same neuronal centers in the AV3V region of the brain seem to be involved, for lesions in this region frequently affect both thirst and salt appetite together.

The importance of salt craving is especially illustrated in persons who have Addison's disease. In persons with this disease, the adrenal glands secrete virtually no aldosterone, which causes excessive loss of salt in the urine and leads to both low sodium ion concentration in the extracellular fluid and decreased blood volume; both of these strongly excite the desire for salt. Likewise, it is well known that animals living in the wild where often little salt is in the food will actively search out mineral deposits called "salt licks" that contain concentrated salt.

CONTROL OF BLOOD VOLUME

One mechanism above all others dominates the control of blood volume and extracellular fluid volume. This is the effect of blood volume on arterial pressure, on the one hand, and the effect, on the other hand, of arterial pressure on urinary excretion of sodium and water. This interplay between the kidneys and the circulatory system is so powerful in controlling blood volume — and secondarily extracellular fluid volume as well — that it dominates over the other mechanisms that help control salt and water intake or salt and water excretion.

Pressure Natriuresis and Pressure Diuresis as the Major Basis for Blood Volume Control

The overall mechanism for blood volume control is essentially the same as the basic mechanism for arterial pressure control that was presented in Chapter 16. It was pointed out in that chapter that extracellular fluid volume, blood volume, cardiac output, arterial pressure, and urine output are all controlled at the same time as separate parts of a common basic feedback mechanism. To summarize the principles, we can trace what happens when the blood volume becomes abnormal.

When the blood volume becomes too great, the cardiac output also becomes too great and therefore increases the arterial pressure.

The increased pressure, in turn, has a profound effect on the kidneys, causing loss of fluid from the body and returning the blood volume to normal. This very large effect of increasing pressure on volume output in the urine is illustrated in Figure 22-5.

Conversely, if the blood volume falls below normal, the cardiac output and arterial pressure decrease, the kidneys retain fluid, and progressive accumulation of the ingested fluid builds the blood volume eventually back to normal.

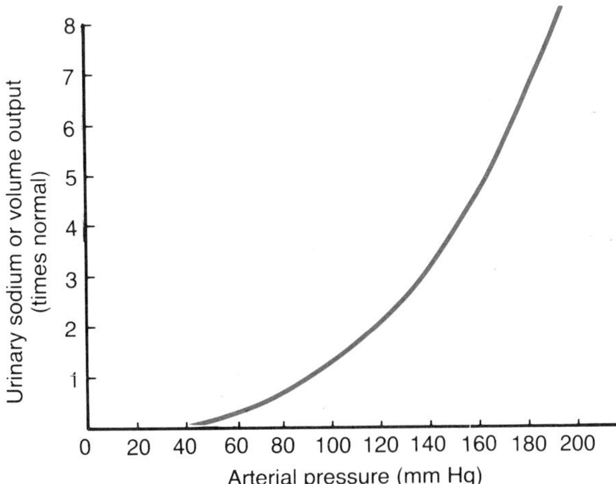

Figure 22-5. Effect of arterial pressure change on urinary output.

Usually, parallel processes will also occur to reconstitute red cell mass, plasma proteins, and so forth if these have become abnormal at the same time. However, if the red cell volume remains abnormal, the plasma volume will simply make up the difference, the volume becoming essentially normal despite the low red cell mass.

Effect of Nervous and Hormonal Factors on the Control of Blood Volume

The discussions of the previous chapter made it clear that both nervous and hormonal factors can cause acute changes in salt and water excretion by the kidneys. These acute effects are often dramatic in short-term experiments; therefore, most physiology texts emphasize greatly these mechanisms of blood volume control. However, after full adjustment of the basic renal mechanism for blood volume control discussed above, the chronic changes in blood volume caused by any one of the nervous or hormonal factors are usually no more than 5 to 10 percent. Let us speak of each of these separately.

Arterial Baroreceptor and Low Pressure Stretch Receptor Reflexes—The "Volume Reflex." When the blood volume becomes too great, the arterial pressure rises; also, the pressures in the pulmonary artery and other low pressure regions of the thorax increase. The stretch of the arterial baroreceptors and of the low pressure stretch receptors in turn cause reflex inhibition of the sympathetic nervous system, which acutely dilates the renal arterioles and often allows an immediate severalfold increase in urinary output. For this reason, this set of reflexes is sometimes called the *volume reflex*. However, this reflex rarely changes the blood volume more than a few percentage points.

Effect of Atrial Natriuretic Factor. Overstretching the two atria as a result of excess blood volume causes the release of ANF into the blood. This acts on the kidneys acutely to increase sodium and volume excretion as much as threefold to tenfold. However, this extreme effect on urine output does not last, so that in the chronic state, there is only a suggestion of slightly reduced blood volume associated with a slight reduction in arterial pressure as well.

Effect of Aldosterone. Aldosterone causes very strong reabsorption of sodium in the distal segments of the renal tubular system. As a result, the blood volume increases by as much as 10 to 20 per cent during the first day or two after aldosterone increases. Then, as the arterial pressure rises in response to the increasing blood volume, the phenomenon of "aldosterone escape" occurs, which means that the kidneys, in response to the rising pressure, begin to excrete thereafter an amount of sodium equal to the daily intake despite the continued presence of aldosterone.

After aldosterone escape, the blood volume returns within a few days to only 5 to 10 per cent above normal, which is associated with continued moderate elevation of the arterial pressure.

Effect of Antidiuretic Hormone. Infusion of large amounts of ADH (also called *vasopressin*) into animals can cause so much renal retention of water that the blood volume increases 15 to 25 per cent during the first few days. However, the arterial pressure also rises and then causes excretion of the excess volume. After several weeks of continued infusion, the blood volume measures no more than 5 to 10 per cent above normal, and the arterial pressure also returns to within 10 mm Hg of normal. Thus, there is not a serious volume change.

In patients who have lost their ability to secrete ADH because of destruction of the supraoptic nuclei, the urine output may be as great as 5 to 10 times normal day in and day out, but this is virtually always compensated for by ingestion of enough water to make up the difference. Therefore, the blood volume is rarely decreased more than 5 per cent as long as sufficient water is available.

Summary

In summary, within the normal ranges of operation of the nervous reflexes and the various hormonal factors that affect urinary sodium and fluid volume output, these rarely affect the blood volume more than plus or minus 5 to 10 per cent. However, even these slight changes in volume can sometimes have considerable effect on the long-term arterial pressure level, which was discussed in Chapter 16.

Increased Blood Volume Caused by Heart Disease

The blood volume is often increased as much as 15 to 20 per cent as a result of heart disease, and occasionally as much as 30 to 40 per cent. The reason is that a weak heart often cannot attain a high enough arterial pressure to cause necessary urinary output of fluid. Therefore, in myocardial failure, in heart valvular disease, and in congenital abnormalities of the heart—in all of these—one of the most important circulatory compensations is increased blood volume.

This often allows even the weakened heart to pump a life-sustaining level of cardiac output.

CONTROL OF EXTRACELLULAR FLUID VOLUME

It is clear from the foregoing discussion of the basic mechanisms for blood volume control that extracellular fluid volume is controlled at the same time. That is, fluid first goes into the blood, but it rapidly becomes distributed between the interstitial spaces and the plasma. Therefore, it is generally impossible to control blood volume to any given level without controlling the extracellular fluid volume at the same time. Yet the relative volumes of distribution between the interstitial spaces and the blood can vary greatly, depending on the physical characteristics of the circulatory system and of the interstitial spaces.

Under normal conditions, virtually all the fluid in the interstitial spaces is bound in a gel-like matrix of proteoglycan molecules, and there is essentially no free fluid. At other times, however, abnormal conditions can cause edema to occur. These abnormal conditions were discussed in detail in Chapter 20. The principal factors that can cause edema are (1) increased capillary pressure, (2) decreased plasma colloid osmotic pressure, (3) increased tissue colloid osmotic pressure, and (4) increased permeability of the capillaries. Whenever any one of these conditions occurs, a very high proportion of the extracellular fluid becomes distributed to the interstitial spaces.

Normal Distribution of Fluid Volume Between the Interstitial Spaces and Vascular System. Figure 22-6 illustrates the approximate normal relationship between extracellular fluid volume and blood volume. When an extra amount of fluid accumulates in the extracellular fluid space, either as a result of intake of too much fluid or because of decreased kidney output of fluid, about one sixth to one third of the extra fluid normally stays in the blood and increases the blood volume. The remainder of the fluid is distributed to the interstitial spaces. However, when the extracellular fluid volume rises more than 30 to 50 per cent above normal, as shown in the figure, very little of the additional fluid then remains in the blood—almost all of it instead goes into the interstitial spaces. This occurs because the interstitial fluid pressure rises from its normal negative (subatmospheric) value to a positive value, which causes the loose tissues to swell rapidly and allows fluid literally to pour out of the capillaries. That is, the interstitial spaces literally become an "overflow" reservoir for excess fluid, sometimes increasing in volume as much as 10 to 30 liters. This obviously causes edema, as was explained in Chapter 20, but it also acts as an important overflow release valve for the circulatory system, a well-known phenomenon that is utilized daily by the clinician to allow administration of almost unlimited quantities of intravenous fluid and yet not force the heart into cardiac failure.

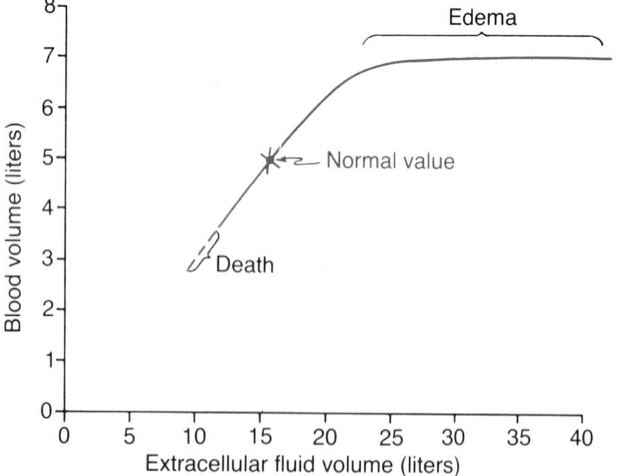

Figure 22-6. Approximate relationship between extracellular fluid volume and blood volume, showing a nearly linear relationship in the normal range but indicating failure of the blood volume to continue rising when the extracellular fluid volume becomes excessive.

To summarize, extracellular fluid volume is controlled simultaneously with the control of blood volume, but the relative ratio of the extracellular fluid volume to blood volume depends on the physical properties of the circulation and of the interstitial spaces.

UREA EXCRETION

The body forms an average of 25 to 30 grams of urea each day—more than this in persons who eat a very high protein diet and less in persons who are on a low protein diet. All this urea must be excreted in the urine; otherwise, it will accumulate in the body fluids. Its normal concentration in plasma is approximately 26 mg/dl, but patients with renal insufficiency frequently have levels as high as 200 mg/dl, and it has been recorded as high as 800 mg/dl.

The two major factors that determine the rate of urea excretion are (1) the concentration of urea in the plasma, and (2) the glomerular filtration rate. These factors increase urea excretion mainly because the "load" of urea entering the proximal tubules is equal to the *product of the plasma urea concentration and the glomerular filtration rate.* In general, the quantity of urea that passes on through the tubules into the urine averages between 40 and 60 per cent of the total urea that enters the proximal tubules. Only when the function of kidneys is abnormal does this fraction change much from this normal range.

Effect of Decreased Glomerular Filtration Rate on Urea Excretion and on Plasma Urea Concentration. In many renal diseases, the glomerular filtration rate of the two kidneys falls considerably below normal. Because urea excretion is directly related to the glomerular filtration of urea, there is decreased excretion of urea when the glomerular filtration decreases. However, the body continues to form large quantities of urea, which means that urea will progressively collect in the body fluids until its plasma concentration rises very high. Then the urea filtered in the glomerular filtrate, which is equal to the plasma urea concentration times the glomerular filtration rate, eventually will become great enough to allow excretion of the urea as rapidly as it is formed. Yet one will recognize that this occurs only because the plasma concentration of urea has risen very high, and this in itself is a very abnormal state that can be severely damaging to the body.

Therefore, probably the most important reason for forming large amounts of glomerular filtrate each day by the two kidneys is to excrete the necessary amounts of urea.

Many of the other waste products that must be excreted by the kidneys obey the same principles of excretion as urea, for their rates of excretion also depend highly upon the amount of glomerular filtrate formed each day. Such substances include creatinine, uric acid, and various other toxic waste products.

The Mechanism for Excreting Large Quantities of Urea but Minimal Quantities of Water. Were it not for the ability of the tubular system to concentrate urea, the kidneys could excrete the necessary urea only by passing large amounts of water into the urine at the same time. Instead, urea is normally concentrated at least 50-fold and when water is being conserved by the body and a concentrated urine is excreted, sometimes as much as several hundredfold.

POTASSIUM EXCRETION

The amount of potassium entering the glomerular filtrate each day is about 800 mEq, while the daily intake of potassium is only about 100 mEq. Therefore, to maintain normal body potassium balance, one eighth of the total daily tubular load of potassium must be excreted. Furthermore, as is true for sodium excretion, the rate of potassium excretion must be carefully controlled so that it will exactly match the daily potassium intake.

Reabsorption of Large Amounts of Potassium in the Proximal Tubules and Loops of Henle. Large amounts of potassium are reabsorbed as a result of potassium co-transport with sodium in both the proximal tubules and the thick ascending limbs of the loops of Henle. Active transport by the proximal tubular epithelial cells reabsorbs about 65 per cent of all the filtered potassium. Then, approximately another 27 per cent is reabsorbed in the thick portion of the ascending limb of the loop of Henle, leaving about 8 per cent of the original filtered potassium to enter the distal tubules. This represents only 65 mEq of potassium per day, which is actually less than the average daily intake of 100 mEq of potassium for most people.

Therefore, when the extracellular fluid potassium concentration is normal or high, large amounts of potassium need to be excreted into the urine simply to rid the body of the normal amounts of potassium ingested each day. For this purpose, the distal tubular segments have evolved a specific mechanism for secreting potassium, as follows.

Secretion of Potassium in the Late Distal Tubules and Cortical Collecting Ducts

In the *late distal tubules,* and even more so in the *cortical collecting ducts,* so-called *principal cells,* which make up about 90 per cent of the epithelial cells in these regions, have the special capability of secreting large quantities of potassium into the tubular lumen. However, this secretion occurs only when the extracellular fluid potassium concentration is higher than a critical level. The mechanism of this secretion is illustrated in Figure 22–7. It begins with the usual Na^+-K^+-adenosine triphosphatase (ATPase) pump in the basolateral membrane of the cell, which pumps sodium out of the cell into the interstitium and at the same time pumps potassium to the interior of the cell. In contrast to the epithelial cells elsewhere in the renal tubules, the luminal border of the principal cells is very permeable to potassium. Therefore, the great increase in potassium inside the cell promotes rapid diffusion of potassium also into the tubular lumen.

Thus, the basic driving force for the potassium secretory mechanism is the Na^+-K^+ pump in the basolateral membrane. For this pump to work, sodium ions must continually diffuse from the tubular lumen into the cell and then be exchanged at the basolateral membrane for potassium ions. Therefore, the greater the quantity of sodium that is available in the tubular lumen to diffuse into the cell, the greater also is the rate of potassium secretion. This is sometimes important clinically because persons on a low sodium diet often fail to excrete adequate amounts of potassium and therefore develop hyperkalemia.

Control of Potassium Excretion and Potassium Concentration in the Extracellular Fluid

It is especially important to control the extracellular fluid potassium ion concentration because very slight changes in concentration can alter nervous and cardiac functions seriously, as discussed in Chapter 5 for nerves and Chapter 9 for the heart. The normal

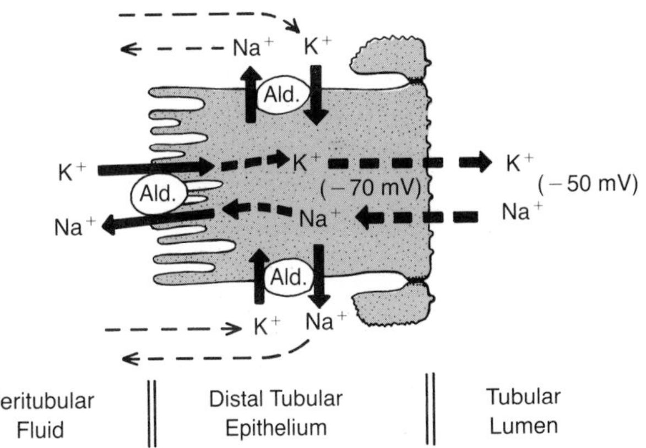

Figure 22–7. Mechanisms of Na^+ and K^+ transport through the distal tubular epithelium.

concentration is about 4.5 mEq/liter, and this rarely rises or falls more than ±0.3 mEq.

Two major factors play important roles in controlling the potassium ion concentration: (1) the direct effect of increased extracellular fluid potassium concentration in causing increased secretion of potassium into the tubules, and (2) the effect of aldosterone in increasing potassium secretion.

Direct Effect of Extracellular Potassium Concentration on Potassium Secretion

The rate of secretion of potassium ions into the late distal tubules and cortical collecting ducts is directly stimulated by increased extracellular fluid potassium ion concentration (as illustrated by the *black curve* in Figure 22–8)—in fact, drastically so after the extracellular potassium concentration rises above about 4.1 mEq/liter. Unfortunately, the mechanism of this effect on secretion is still unknown. Nevertheless, the effect serves as one of the two very important feedback mechanisms for controlling the extracellular fluid potassium ion concentration.

Effect of Aldosterone in Controlling Potassium Ion Secretion

Earlier in the chapter we learned that active reabsorption of sodium ions by the principal cells in the late distal tubules and cortical collecting ducts is strongly controlled by the hormone aldosterone. Aldosterone also has a very powerful effect of controlling *potassium ion secretion* by these same cells, for it activates the Na^+,K^+-ATPase pump that pumps sodium from the tubular fluid into the interstitial fluid

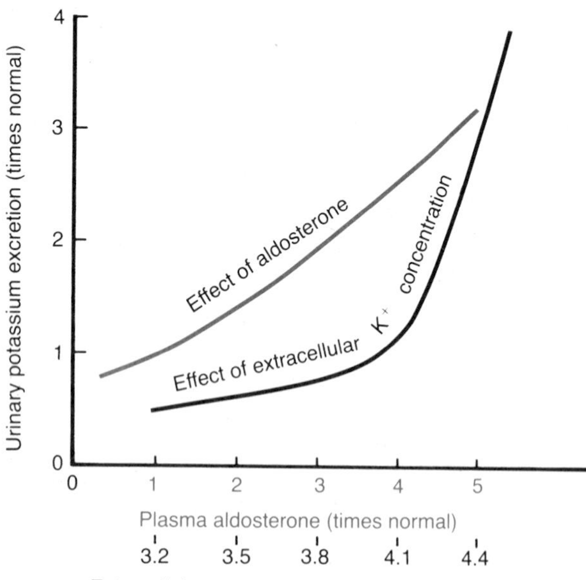

Figure 22–8. Effect of (1) plasma aldosterone concentration and (2) extracellular potassium ion concentration on the rate of urinary potassium excretion. These are the two most important factors regulating the rate of potassium excretion in the urine. (Drawn from data in Young: *Am. J. Physiol. 244:*F28, 1983.)

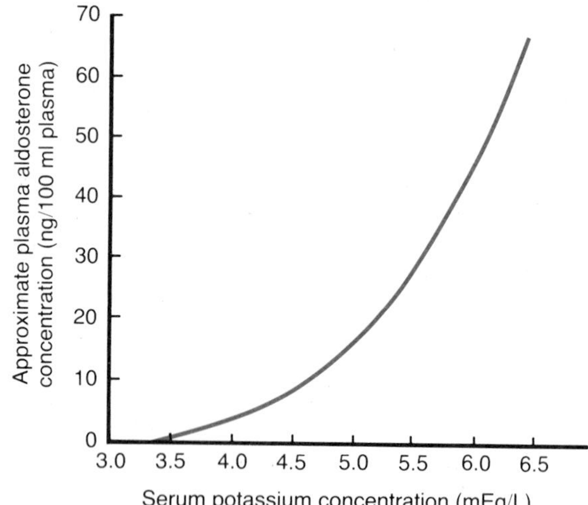

Figure 22–9. Effect on extracellular fluid aldosterone concentration of potassium ion concentration changes. Note the extreme change in aldosterone concentration for very minute changes in potassium concentration.

and potassium in the opposite direction both at the same time. The *red curve* in Figure 22–8 illustrates this, showing a threefold increase in urinary excretion of potassium when aldosterone is increased.

Therefore, aldosterone is the second important factor that controls potassium excretion; thus, it also helps greatly in controlling extracellular fluid potassium ion concentration, as we discuss more fully in the following sections.

Effect of Potassium Ion Concentration on the Rate of Aldosterone Secretion. In any properly functioning feedback control system, the factor that is controlled almost invariably has a feedback effect for control of the controller. In the case of the aldosterone-potassium control system, the rate of aldosterone secretion by the zona glomerulosa cells of the adrenal cortex is controlled very strongly by the extracellular fluid potassium concentration. Figure 22–9 illustrates this, showing that an increase in the potassium concentration of about 3 mEq/liter can increase the plasma aldosterone concentration from almost 0 to as high as 60 ng/dl of plasma, a concentration almost ten times normal.

Thus, to summarize, an increase in potassium concentration causes an increase in aldosterone concentration in the circulating blood. The increase in aldosterone then causes a marked increase in potassium excretion by the kidneys. And, finally, the increased potassium excretion decreases the extracellular fluid potassium concentration back toward normal.

Effect of Primary Aldosteronism and Addison's Disease on Extracellular Fluid Potassium Concentration. *Primary aldosteronism* is caused by a tumor of the zona glomerulosa of one of the adrenal glands, the tumor secreting tremendous quantities of aldosterone. One of the most important effects of this disease is a marked increase in aldosterone-stimulated potassium excretion; this causes a severe decrease in extracellular fluid potassium concentration, so that many of these patients experience paralysis caused by failure of nerve transmission, as was explained in Chapter 5.

Conversely, in *Addison's disease* the adrenal glands have been destroyed, aldosterone secretion approaches zero, renal potassium secretion becomes very poor, and the extracellular fluid potassium concentration frequently rises to as high as double normal. This is often the cause of death in these patients, resulting in cardiac arrest.

CONTROL OF THE EXTRACELLULAR CONCENTRATIONS OF OTHER IONS

Regulation of Calcium Ion Concentration

The role of calcium in the body and control of its concentration in the extracellular fluid are discussed in detail in Chapter 53 in relation to the endocrinology of parathyroid hormone, calcitonin, and bone. The most important mechanism of control is the following:

The *day-to-day* calcium ion concentration remains within a few per cent of 2.4 mEq/liter and is *controlled principally by the effect of parathyroid hormone on bone reabsorption.* When the extracellular fluid concentration of calcium falls too low, the parathyroid glands are directly stimulated to promote increased secretion of parathyroid hormone. This hormone in turn acts directly on the bones to increase the reabsorption of bone salts, thus releasing large amounts of calcium into the extracellular fluid and elevating the calcium level back to normal. On the other hand, when the calcium concentration becomes too great, parathyroid hormone secretion becomes depressed so that almost no bone reabsorption then occurs. Yet the osteoblastic system for forming new bone does continue to deposit calcium, thus removing calcium from the extracellular fluid, in this way reducing the calcium ion concentration to its normal level.

However, the bones do not have an inexhaustible supply of calcium, and eventually they will run out of calcium. Therefore, *long-term control* of calcium ion concentration results from the effect of parathyroid hormone on reabsorption of calcium from the kidney tubules and absorption of calcium from the gut through the gastrointestinal mucosa, both of which effects are markedly increased by parathyroid hormone.

The effect of parathyroid hormone on calcium handling by the kidneys closely parallels the effect of aldosterone on sodium handling. That is, even in the absence of parathyroid hormone, much of the calcium is reabsorbed from the tubular fluid in the proximal tubules, the loop of Henle, and the diluting segment of the distal tubules, but about 10 per cent of the filtered load of calcium still remains to enter the late distal tubules. Then, if large amounts of parathyroid hormone are present in the body fluids, essentially all of the remaining calcium will be reabsorbed from the late distal tubules and cortical collecting ducts, thus conserving the calcium in the body. These and other control factors will be discussed in more detail in Chapter 53.

Regulation of Magnesium Ion Concentration

Much less is known about the regulation of magnesium ion concentration than of calcium ion concentration. Magnesium ions are reabsorbed by all portions of the renal tubules. However, increased magnesium ion concentration directly affects the tubular epithelial cells by decreasing this reabsorption. Therefore, when the extracellular fluid magnesium concentration is high, excessive amounts of magnesium are excreted; conversely, when the magnesium concentration is low, magnesium is conserved.

REFERENCES

Briggs, J. P., and Schnermann, J.: The tubuloglomerular feedback mechanism: Functional and biochemical aspects. Annu. Rev. Physiol., 49:251, 1987.

Cowley, A. W., Jr., et al.: Vasopressin: Cellular and Integrative Functions. New York, Raven Press, 1988.

Gash, D. M., and Boer, G. J. (eds.): Vasopressin. New York, Plenum Publishing Corp., 1987.

Greenwald L., and Stetson, D.: Urine concentration and the length of the renal papilla. News Physiol. Sci., 3:46, 1988.

Greger, R., and Valazquez, H.: The cortical thick ascending limb and early distal convoluted tubule in the urinary concentration mechanism. Kidney Int., 31:590, 1987.

Guyton, A. C., et al.: Dynamics and Control of the Body Fluids. Philadelphia, W. B. Saunders Co., 1975.

Guyton, A. C., et al.: Theory for renal autoregulation by feedback at the juxtaglomerular apparatus. Circ. Res., 14:187, 1964.

Hall, J. E., et al.: Control of glomerular filtration rate by the renin-angiotensin system. Am. J. Physiol., 233:F366, 1977.

Hays, R. M., et al.: Effects of antidiuretic hormone on the collecting duct. Kidney Int., 31:530, 1987.

Imai, M., et al.: Function of thin loops of Henle. Kidney Int., 31:565, 1987.

Kokko, J. P.: The role of the collecting duct in urinary concentration. Kidney Int., 31:606, 1987.

Marsh, D. J.: Functional transitions in the renal countercurrent system. Kidney Int., 31:668, 1987.

Seldin, D. W., and Giebisch, G.: The Regulation of Potassium Balance. New York, Raven Press, 1989.

Stricker, E. M., and Verbalis, J. G.: Hormones and behavior: The biology of thirst and sodium appetite. Am. Scientist, 76:261, 1988.

Young, D. B., et al.: Effectiveness of the aldosterone-sodium-potassium feedback control system. Am. J. Physiol., 231:945, 1976.

QUESTIONS

1. Explain how the kidney excretes a dilute urine.
2. Explain how the kidney excretes a concentrated urine.
3. Explain the concept of the *countercurrent phenomenon* that occurs in the renal medulla.

4. What is the role of antidiuretic hormone in shifting renal function from excreting a dilute urine to excreting a concentrated urine?
5. Describe the manner in which the kidneys excrete urea.
6. Explain overall control of the blood volume.
7. What is the relationship of the extracellular fluid volume to the blood volume?
8. Explain the antidiuretic hormone and thirst mechanisms for controlling the sodium concentration in the extracellular fluid.
9. Why does the sodium concentration in the extracellular fluid determine most of the osmolar concentration of the body fluids?
10. What is meant by the tripping mechanism of thirst control?
11. Explain the feedback mechanisms by which the body controls the extracellular potassium concentration. Why is aldosterone especially involved with potassium concentration control but not to a great extent with sodium concentration control?

23

Regulation of Acid-Base Balance; Renal Disease; Micturition

When one speaks of the regulation of acid-base balance, regulation of hydrogen ion concentration in the body fluids is actually meant. Just slight changes from the normal value in hydrogen ion concentration can cause marked alterations in the rates of chemical reactions in the cells, some being depressed and others accelerated. For this reason, the regulation of hydrogen ion concentration is one of the most important aspects of homeostasis.

Normal Hydrogen Ion Concentration and Normal pH of the Body Fluids—Acidosis and Alkalosis. The hydrogen ion concentration in the extracellular fluid is normally regulated at a constant value of approximately 4×10^{-8} Eq/liter; this value can vary from as low as 1×10^{-8} to as high as 1.6×10^{-7} without causing death.

From these values, it is already apparent that expressing hydrogen ion concentration in terms of actual concentrations is a cumbersome procedure. Therefore, the symbol *pH* has come into use for expressing the concentration; pH is related to actual hydrogen ion concentration by the following formula (when H^+ concentration is expressed in equivalents per liter):

$$pH = \log \frac{1}{H^+ \text{ conc.}} = -\log H^+ \text{ conc.} \qquad (1)$$

Note from this formula that a low pH corresponds to a high hydrogen ion concentration, which is called *acidosis;* and, conversely, a high pH corresponds to a low hydrogen ion concentration, which is called *alkalosis.*

The normal pH of arterial blood is 7.4, while the pH of venous blood and of interstitial fluids is about 7.35 because of extra quantities of carbon dioxide that form carbonic acid in these fluids.

Since the normal pH of the arterial blood is 7.4, a person is considered to have acidosis whenever the pH is below this value and to have alkalosis when it rises above 7.4. The lower limit at which a person can live more than a few hours is about 6.8, and the highest limit approximately 8.0.

Defense Against Changes in Hydrogen Ion Concentration

To prevent acidosis or alkalosis, three principal control systems are available: (1) All the body fluids are supplied with acid-base *buffer systems* that immediately combine with any acid or alkali to prevent excessive changes in hydrogen ion concentration. (2) If the hydrogen ion concentration does change measurably, the *respiratory center is immediately stimulated* to alter the rate of breathing. This changes the rate of carbon dioxide removal from the body fluids, which, for reasons that will be presented later, causes the hydrogen ion concentration to return toward normal. (3) When the hydrogen concentration changes from normal, *the kidneys excrete either an acid or an alkaline urine,* thereby also helping to readjust the hydrogen ion concentration of the body fluids back toward normal.

The buffer systems can act within a fraction of a second to prevent excessive changes in hydrogen ion concentration. On the other hand, it takes 1 to 12 minutes for the respiratory system to function fully to readjust the hydrogen ion concentration after a sudden change has occurred. Finally, the kidneys, though providing the most powerful of all the acid-base regulatory systems, require several hours to several days to readjust fully the hydrogen ion concentration.

FUNCTION OF ACID-BASE BUFFERS

An acid-base buffer is a solution containing a combination of two or more chemical compounds that prevent marked changes in hydrogen ion concentration when either an acid or a base is added to the solution. An *acid* is defined as a substance that can contribute hydrogen ions to a solution. A *base* is defined as a substance that will combine with hydrogen ions in a solution and will thereby remove them. The alkaline chemicals are types of bases, which gives rise to the term *alkalosis,* a state in which there are too few hydrogen ions in the body fluids.

If only a few drops of concentrated hydrochloric acid are added to a beaker of pure water, the pH of the water might immediately fall to as low as 1.0. However, if a satisfactory buffer system is present, the hydrochloric acid combines instantaneously with the buffer, and the pH falls only slightly. Perhaps the best way to explain the action of an acid-base buffer is to consider an actual simple buffer system, such as the bicarbonate buffer, which is extremely important in regulation of acid-base balance in the body.

The Bicarbonate Buffer System

A typical bicarbonate buffer system consists of a *mixture* of carbonic acid (H_2CO_3) and sodium bicarbonate ($NaHCO_3$) in the same solution. It must first be noted that carbonic acid is a very weak acid, for its degree of dissociation into hydrogen ions and bicarbonate ions is poor in comparison with that of many other acids.

When a strong acid, such as hydrochloric acid, is added to the bicarbonate buffer solution, the following reaction takes place:

$$HCl + NaHCO_3 \rightarrow H_2CO_3 + NaCl \qquad (2)$$

From this equation it can be seen that the strong hydrochloric acid is converted into the very weak carbonic acid. Therefore, addition of the HCl lowers the pH of the solution only slightly.

Now let us see what happens when a strong base, such as sodium hydroxide, is added to a buffer solution containing carbonic acid. The following reaction takes place:

$$NaOH + H_2CO_3 \rightarrow NaHCO_3 + H_2O \qquad (3)$$

This equation shows that the hydroxyl ion of the sodium hydroxide combines with a hydrogen ion from the carbonic acid to form water and that the other product formed is sodium bicarbonate. The net result is exchange of the strong base NaOH for the weak base $NaHCO_3$.

Thus, the mixture of carbonic acid and sodium bicarbonate acts as a buffer to prevent either a marked rise or fall in pH. Fortunately, this buffer is present in all the fluids of the body, both extracellular and intracellular, and it plays an important role in maintaining normal acid-base balance.

Relationship of Bicarbonate and Carbon Dioxide Concentrations to pH—the Henderson-Hasselbalch Equation. There is always a definite mathematical relationship between the ratio of the concentrations of the acidic and basic elements of each buffer system on the one hand and the pH of the solution on the other hand. The following equation, called the *Henderson-Hasselbalch equation,* gives this relationship for the bicarbonate buffer system:

$$pH = 6.1 + \log \frac{HCO_3^-}{CO_2} \qquad (4)$$

In this equation, the carbon dioxide concentration represents the acidic element—because carbon dioxide (CO_2) combines with water to form carbonic acid, H_2CO_3—and the bicarbonate ion (HCO_3^-) represents the basic element. Note that pH changes in direct proportion to the change in the *logarithm of the ratio* between the basic and acid elements of the buffer system. Thus, when the ratio is in favor of the basic element (HCO_3^-), the pH increases, denoting alkalosis. When the ratio is in favor of the acidic element (CO_2), the pH decreases, denoting acidosis.

The Phosphate Buffer System

Another buffer system, the phosphate buffer system, acts in an almost identical manner, but it is composed of the following two elements: $H_2PO_4^-$ and HPO_4^{--}. When a strong acid, such as hydrochloric acid, is added to a mixture of these two substances, the following reaction occurs:

$$HCl + Na_2HPO_4 \rightarrow NaH_2PO_4 + NaCl \qquad (5)$$

The net result of this reaction is that the hydrochloric acid is removed, and in its place an additional quantity of NaH_2PO_4 is formed. NaH_2PO_4 is only weakly acidic, so that the added strong acid is immediately traded for a very weak acid, and the pH changes relatively slightly.

The Protein Buffer System

The most plentiful buffer of the body is the proteins of the cells and plasma, mainly because of their very high concentrations. There is a slight amount of diffusion of hydrogen ions through the cell membrane; even more important, carbon dioxide can diffuse within seconds through cell membranes, and even bicarbonate ions can diffuse to some extent. This diffusion of hydrogen ions and of the two elements of the bicarbonate buffer system causes the pH in the intracellular fluids to change approximately in proportion to the changes in pH in the extracellular fluids. Thus, all the buffer systems inside the cells help buffer the extracellular fluids as well but may take several hours to do so. Indeed, experimental studies have shown that about three quarters of all the *chemical* buffering power of the body fluids is inside the cells, and most of this results from the intracellular proteins. However, except for the red blood cells, the slowness of movement of hydrogen and bicarbonate ions through the cell membranes often delays the ability of the intracellular buffers to buffer extracellular acid-base abnormalities for several hours.

The method by which the protein buffer system operates is precisely the same as that of the bicarbonate buffer system. It will be recalled that a protein is composed of amino acids bound together by peptide linkages, but some of the different amino acids, especially histidine, have free acidic radicals that can dissociate to form a weak base plus H^+, which can serve in a manner similar to carbonic acid as the basis of a buffer system.

RESPIRATORY REGULATION OF ACID-BASE BALANCE

In the discussion of the Henderson-Hasselbalch equation, it was noted that an *increase in carbon dioxide concentration in the body fluids decreases the pH toward the acidic side,* whereas a *decrease in carbon dioxide raises the pH toward the alkaline side.* On the basis of this effect, the respiratory system is capable of altering the pH either up or down.

Balance Between Metabolic Formation of Carbon Dioxide and Pulmonary Expiration of Carbon Dioxide. Carbon dioxide is continually being formed in the body by the different intracellular metabolic processes, the carbon in the foods being oxidized by oxygen to form carbon dioxide. This in turn diffuses into the interstitial fluids and blood and is transported to the lungs, where it diffuses into the alveoli and then is transferred to the atmosphere by pulmonary ventilation. However, several minutes are required for this passage of carbon dioxide from the cells to the atmosphere, so that an average of 1.2 mmol/liter of dissolved carbon dioxide is normally in the extracellular fluids at all times.

If the rate of metabolic formation of carbon dioxide becomes increased, its concentration in the extracellular fluids is likewise increased. Conversely, decreased metabolism decreases the carbon dioxide concentration.

On the other hand, if the rate of pulmonary ventilation is increased, carbon dioxide is blown off from the lungs, and the amount of carbon dioxide in the extracellular fluids decreases.

Effect of Hydrogen Ion Concentration on Alveolar Ventilation

Not only does the rate of alveolar ventilation affect the hydrogen ion concentration of the body fluids but, in turn, the hydrogen ion concentration affects the rate of alveolar ventilation. This results from a *direct action of hydrogen ions on the respiratory center in the medulla oblongata* that controls breathing, which will be discussed in detail in Chapter 29.

Figure 23-1 illustrates the changes in alveolar ventilation caused by changing the pH of arterial blood from 7.0 to 7.6. From this graph it is evident that a decrease in pH from the normal value of 7.4 to the strongly acidic level of 7.0 can increase the rate of alveolar ventilation to as much as four to five times normal, whereas an increase in pH into the alkaline range can decrease the rate of alveolar ventilation to only a fraction of the normal level.

Feedback Control of Hydrogen Ion Concentration by the Respiratory System. Because of the ability of the respiratory center to respond to hydrogen ion concentration, and because changes in alveolar ventilation in turn alter the hydrogen ion concentration in the body fluids, the respiratory system acts as a typical feedback controller of hydrogen ion concentration. That is, any time the hydrogen ion

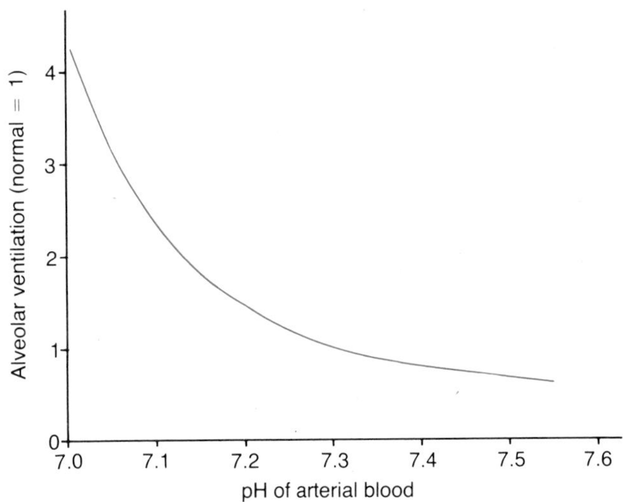

Figure 23-1. Effect of blood pH on the rate of alveolar ventilation. (Constructed from data obtained by Gray: Pulmonary Ventilation and Its Regulation. Springfield, Ill., Charles C Thomas.)

concentration becomes high, the respiratory system becomes more active, and alveolar ventilation increases. As a result, the carbon dioxide concentration and the carbonic acid concentration in the extracellular fluids decrease, thus reducing the hydrogen concentration back toward normal. Conversely, if the hydrogen ion concentration falls too low, the respiratory center becomes depressed, alveolar ventilation also decreases, and the hydrogen ion concentration rises back toward normal.

Effectiveness of Respiratory Control of Hydrogen Ion Concentration. Unfortunately, respiratory control cannot return the hydrogen ion concentration all the way to the normal value of 7.4 when some abnormality outside the respiratory system has altered the pH from normal. The reason for this is that as the pH returns toward normal, the stimulus that has been causing either increased or decreased respiration will itself begin to be lost. Ordinarily, the respiratory mechanism for controlling hydrogen ion concentration has a control effectiveness of between 50 and 75 per cent. That is, if the hydrogen ion concentration should suddenly be decreased from 7.4 to 7.0 by some extraneous factor, the respiratory system, in 1 to 12 minutes, returns the pH to a value of about 7.2 to 7.3.

RENAL CONTROL OF HYDROGEN ION CONCENTRATION

The kidneys control extracellular fluid hydrogen ion concentration by excreting either an acidic urine or a basic urine. Excreting an acidic urine reduces the amount of acid in the extracellular fluids, whereas excreting a basic urine removes base from the extracellular fluids.

The body's means for determining whether the urine will be acidic or basic is as follows: Large numbers of bicarbonate ions are filtered continually into the glomerular filtrate, which removes base from the blood. On the other hand, large numbers of hydrogen ions are secreted at the same time into the tubular lumens by the tubular epithelium, thus removing acid. If more hydrogen ions are secreted than bicarbonate ions are filtered, there will be a net loss of acid from the extracellular fluids. Conversely, if more bicarbonate is filtered than hydrogen is secreted, there will be a net loss of base. The following sections describe the different renal mechanisms that accomplish these events.

Tubular Secretion of Hydrogen Ions

The epithelial cells everywhere in the tubular system, except in the thin limb of the loop of Henle, secrete hydrogen ions into the tubular fluid. However, in different tubular segments there are two quite different methods for doing this, each of which has separate characteristics and even separate purposes.

Secondary Active Transport of Hydrogen Ions in the Early Tubular Segments. The epithelial cells of the proximal tubule, the thick segment of the ascending limb of the loop of Henle, and the distal tubule all secrete hydrogen ions into the tubular fluid by secondary active transport; the mechanism of this is illustrated in Figure 23–2. Tremendous numbers of hydrogen ions are secreted in this manner, several thousand milliequivalents per day, but never against a very high hydrogen ion gradient, because the tubular fluid becomes very acidic only in the latter segments of the tubular system.

Figure 23–2 shows that hydrogen ions are secreted into the tubule by a mechanism of *Na^+-H^+ countertransport.* That is, when sodium moves from the lumen of the tubule to the interior of the cell, it first combines with a *carrier protein* in the luminal border of the cell membrane, and at the same time a hydrogen ion inside the cell combines with the opposite side of the same carrier protein. Then, because the concentration of sodium is much lower inside the cell than in the tubular lumen, this causes movement of the sodium down the concentration gradient to the interior, providing at the same time the energy for moving the hydrogen ion in the opposite direction (the "counter" direction) into the tubular lumen.

Primary Active Transport of Hydrogen Ions in the Late Tubular Segments. Beginning in the late distal tubules and then continuing all the way through the collecting duct system to the renal pelvis, the tubules secrete hydrogen ions by *primary active transport.* The characteristics of this transport are quite different from the secondary active transport system in the earlier tubular segments. First, it normally accounts for less than 5 per cent of the total hydrogen ions excreted. On the other hand, it can concentrate hydrogen ions as much as 900-fold, in contrast to only 3- to 4-fold concentrations that can be achieved in the proximal tubules and 10- to 15-fold concentrations in the early distal tubules by the secondary transport mechanism. The 900-fold concentration of the hydrogen ions can decrease the pH of the tubular fluid to about 4.5, which therefore is the lower limit of pH that can be achieved in the excreted urine.

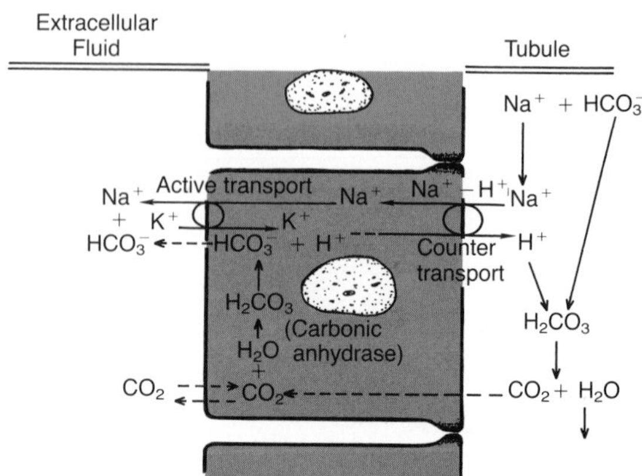

Figure 23–2. Chemical reactions for (1) secondary active secretion of hydrogen ions into the tubule, (2) sodium ion reabsorption in exchange for the hydrogen ions secreted, and (3) combination of hydrogen ions with bicarbonate ions in the tubules to form carbon dioxide and water.

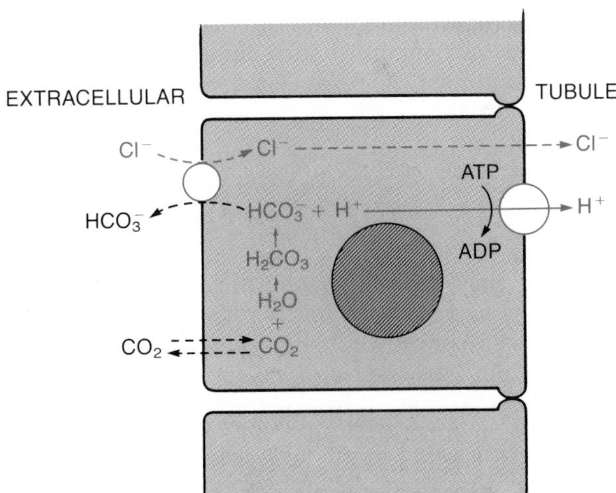

Figure 23-3. Primary active transport of hydrogen ions through the luminal membrane of the tubular epithelial cell. Note that one bicarbonate ion is absorbed for each hydrogen ion secreted, and a chloride ion is secreted passively along with the hydrogen ion.

The mechanism of primary active hydrogen ion transport is illustrated in Figure 23-3. It occurs at the luminal membrane of the tubular cell, where hydrogen ions are transported directly by a specific transport protein, *a hydrogen-transporting adenosine triphosphatase (ATPase).*

Regulation of Hydrogen Ion Secretion by the Hydrogen Ion Concentration in the Extracellular Fluids

The rate of hydrogen ion secretion into the tubules increases markedly in response to only slight increases in extracellular fluid hydrogen ion concentration. The control of this is achieved in the following way:

In acidosis, the *ratio* of carbon dioxide to bicarbonate ions in the extracellular fluid is above normal, as one can determine by referring again to the Henderson-Hasselbalch equation. Also, a similar ratio occurs inside the epithelial secretory cell, giving a high level of hydrogen ions and a correspondingly high rate of hydrogen ion secretion into the tubular lumen. In alkalosis, exactly the opposite occurs, with a resulting decrease in hydrogen ion secretion.

At normal extracellular fluid pH, the rate of hydrogen ion secretion is about 3.5 mM/min, but this rises or falls almost directly in proportion to the change in extracellular hydrogen ion concentration.

Titration of Bicarbonate Ions Against Hydrogen Ions in the Tubules

Under normal conditions the *rate of hydrogen ion secretion is about 3.5 mmol/min* and the *rate of filtration of bicarbonate ions in the glomerular filtrate is about 3.46 mmol/min.* Thus, the quantities of the two ions entering the tubules are almost equal, and they combine with each other and actually annihilate each other, the end products being carbon dioxide and water. Therefore, it is said that the bicarbonate ions and hydrogen ions normally "titrate" each other in the tubules.

However, note also that this titration process is not quite exact, for usually a slight excess of hydrogen ions (3.5 minus 3.46 equals 0.04 mmol/min) remains in the tubules to be excreted in the urine. The reason for this is that under normal conditions a person's metabolic processes continually form a small amount of excess acid (about 60 mEq/day) that gives rise to the slight excess of hydrogen ions over bicarbonate ions in the tubules.

On rare occasions the bicarbonate ions are in excess, as we shall see in subsequent discussions. When this occurs, the titration process again is not quite complete; this time, excess bicarbonate ions (the basic component) are left in the tubules to pass into the urine.

Thus, the basic mechanism by which the kidney corrects either acidosis or alkalosis is by incomplete titration of hydrogen ions against bicarbonate ions, leaving one or the other of these to pass into the urine and therefore to be removed from the extracellular fluid.

Renal Correction of Acidosis

Now that we have described the mechanisms by which the renal tubules titrate hydrogen ions against bicarbonate ions, we can explain the manner in which the kidneys readjust the pH of the extracellular fluids when it becomes abnormal.

First, let us consider *acidosis.* Referring again to Equation 5, the Henderson-Hasselbalch equation, we see that in *acidosis* the ratio of *carbon dioxide to bicarbonate ions* in the extracellular fluid increases. Therefore, the *rate of hydrogen ion secretion* rises to a level greater than the *rate of bicarbonate ion filtration* into the tubules. As a result, an excess of hydrogen ions is secreted into the tubules, while diminished quantities of bicarbonate ions enter the glomerular filtrate, so that now there are far too few bicarbonate ions to react with the hydrogen ions. The excess hydrogen ions combine with buffers in the tubular fluid and are excreted into the urine.

Renal Correction of Alkalosis

In *alkalosis,* the *ratio* of bicarbonate ions to dissolved carbon dioxide molecules in the extracellular fluid increases. The effect of this on the titration process in the tubules is to increase the bicarbonate ions filtered into the tubules and to decrease the hydrogen ions secreted. Therefore, far greater quantities of bicarbonate ions than hydrogen ions now enter the tubules. After titration of the hydrogen and bicarbonate ions, all the excess bicarbonate ions pass into the urine and carry with them sodium ions or other positive ions. Thus, in effect, sodium bicarbonate is removed from the extracellular fluid. Loss of sodium bicarbonate from the extracellular fluid decreases the bicarbonate ion portion of the bicarbonate buffer system, and, in accordance with the Henderson-Hasselbalch equation, this shifts the pH of the body fluids back in the acid direction.

Combination of Excess Hydrogen Ions with Tubular Buffers and Transport into the Urine

When excess hydrogen ions are secreted into the tubules, only a small portion of these can be carried in the free form by the tubular fluid into the urine. The reason for this is that the maximum hydrogen ion concentration that the tubular system can achieve corresponds to a pH of 4.5. At normal daily urine flows, only 1 per cent of the daily excretion of excess hydrogen ions can be transported into the urine at this concentration.

Therefore, to carry the excess hydrogen ions into the urine the hydrogen ions must be carried in some form other than free hydrogen ions. This is achieved by the hydrogen ions' first combining with intratubular buffers and then being transported in this form.

The tubular fluids have two very important buffer systems that transport the excess hydrogen ions into the urine: (1) the phosphate buffer and (2) the ammonia buffer.

The phosphate buffer is composed of a mixture of HPO_4^{--} and $H_2PO_4^-$. Both become considerably concentrated in the tubular fluid because of their relatively poor reabsorption and because of removal of water from the tubular fluid. Therefore, even though the phosphate buffer is very weak in the blood, it is a much more powerful buffer in the tubular fluid.

The ammonia buffer is composed of ammonia (NH_3) and the ammonium ion (NH_4^+). The epithelial cells of all the tubules besides those of the thin segment of the loop of Henle continually synthesize ammonia, and this diffuses into the tubules. The ammonia then reacts with hydrogen ions to form ammonium ions. These are then excreted into the urine in combination with chloride ions and other tubular anions. This ammonium ion mechanism for transport of excess hydrogen ions in the tubules is especially important, for two reasons: (1) Each time an ammonia molecule (NH_3) combines with a hydrogen ion to form an ammonium ion (NH_4^+), the concentration of ammonia in the tubular fluid becomes decreased, which causes still more ammonia to diffuse from the epithelial cells into the tubular fluid. Thus, the rate of ammonia secretion into the tubular fluid is actually controlled by the amount of excess hydrogen ions to be transported. (2) Most of the negative ions of the tubular fluid are chloride ions. Only a few hydrogen ions could be transported into the urine in direct combination with chloride, because hydrochloric acid is a very strong acid and the tubular pH would fall rapidly below the *critical value of 4.5, below which further hydrogen ion secretion ceases.* However, when hydrogen ions combine with ammonia and the resulting ammonium ions then combine with chloride, the pH does not fall significantly, because ammonium chloride is only very weakly acidic.

Rapidity of Acid-Base Regulation by the Kidneys

The kidney mechanism for regulating acid-base balance cannot readjust the pH within seconds, as can the extracellular fluid buffer systems, nor within minutes, as can the respiratory compensatory mechanism; but it is different from these other two in that it can keep on functioning for hours or days until it brings the pH almost exactly back to normal. In other words, its ultimate capability to regulate the body fluid pH, though it is slow to act, is infinitely more powerful than that of the other two regulatory mechanisms.

CLINICAL ABNORMALITIES OF ACID-BASE BALANCE

Respiratory Acidosis and Alkalosis

From the discussions earlier in the chapter it is obvious that any factor that decreases the rate of pulmonary ventilation increases the concentration of dissolved carbon dioxide in the extracellular fluid. And this in turn leads to increased carbonic acid and hydrogen ions, thus resulting in acidosis. Because this type of acidosis is caused by an abnormality of respiration, it is called *respiratory acidosis.*

On the other hand, excessive pulmonary ventilation reverses the process and decreases the hydrogen ion concentration, thus resulting in alkalosis; this condition is called *respiratory alkalosis.*

A person can cause respiratory acidosis in himself by simply holding his breath, which he can do until the pH of the body fluids falls to as low as perhaps 7.0. On the other hand, he can voluntarily overbreathe and cause alkalosis to a pH of about 7.9.

Respiratory acidosis frequently results from pathological conditions. For instance, damage to the respiratory center in the medulla oblongata that causes reduced breathing, obstruction of the passageways in the respiratory tract, pneumonia, decreased pulmonary membrane surface area, or any other factor that interferes with the exchange of gases between the blood and alveolar air can result in respiratory acidosis.

On the other hand, only rarely do pathological conditions cause *respiratory alkalosis.* However, occasionally a psychoneurosis causes overbreathing to the extent that a person becomes alkalotic. Also, a physiologic type of respiratory alkalosis occurs when a person ascends to a *high altitude.* The low oxygen content of the air stimulates respiration, which causes excess loss of carbon dioxide and development of mild respiratory alkalosis.

Metabolic Acidosis and Alkalosis

The terms *metabolic acidosis* and *metabolic alkalosis* refer to all other abnormalities of acid-base balance besides those caused by excess or insufficient carbon dioxide in the body fluids. Use of the word "metabolic" in this instance is unfortunate, because carbon dioxide is also a metabolic product. Yet, by convention, carbonic acid resulting from dissolved carbon dioxide is called a *respiratory acid* while any other acid in the body, whether it be formed by metabolism or simply ingested by the person, is called a *metabolic acid.*

Causes of Metabolic Acidosis

Diarrhea. Severe diarrhea is one of the most frequent causes of metabolic acidosis for the following reasons: The gastrointestinal secretions normally contain large amounts of sodium bicarbonate. Therefore, excessive loss of these secretions during a bout of diarrhea is exactly the same as excretion of large amounts of sodium bicarbonate into the urine. In accordance with the Henderson-Hasselbalch equation, this results in a shift of the bicarbonate buffer system toward the acid side and results in metabolic acidosis. In fact, acidosis resulting from severe diarrhea can be so serious that it is one of the most common causes of death in young children.

Uremia. A third common type of acidosis is uremic acidosis, which occurs in severe renal disease. The cause of this is failure of the kidneys to rid the body of even the normal amounts of acids formed each day by the metabolic processes of the body.

Diabetes Mellitus. A fourth and extremely important cause of metabolic acidosis is diabetes mellitus. In this condition, lack of insulin secretion by the pancreas prevents normal use of glucose for metabolism. Instead, some of the fats are split into acetoacetic acid, and this in turn is metabolized by the tissues for energy in place of glucose. Simultaneously, the concentration of acetoacetic acid in the extracellular fluids often rises very high and causes very severe acidosis. Also, large quantities of the acetoacetic acid are excreted in the urine, sometimes as much as 500 to 1000 mmol/day.

Causes of Metabolic Alkalosis

Metabolic alkalosis does not occur nearly as often as metabolic acidosis. However, there are several common causes of metabolic alkalosis.

Excessive Ingestion of Alkaline Drugs. One of the most common causes of alkalosis is excessive ingestion of alkaline drugs, such as sodium bicarbonate, for the treatment of gastritis or peptic ulcer.

Alkalosis Caused by Loss of Chloride Ions. Excessive vomiting of gastric contents *without* vomiting of lower gastrointestinal contents causes excessive loss of hydrochloric acid secreted by the stomach mucosa. The net result is loss of acid from the extracellular fluid and development of metabolic alkalosis. This type of alkalosis occurs in newborn children who have pyloric obstruction caused by a greatly hypertrophied pyloric sphincter muscle.

Alkalosis Caused by Excess Aldosterone. When excess quantities of aldosterone are secreted by the adrenal glands, the extracellular fluid becomes slightly alkalotic. This is caused in the following way: The aldosterone promotes extensive reabsorption of sodium ions from the distal segments of the tubular system, but coupled with this is increased secretion of hydrogen ions as well, which promotes alkalosis.

Effects of Acidosis and Alkalosis on the Body

Acidosis. The major clinical effect of acidosis is depression of the *central nervous system.* When the pH of the blood falls below 7.0, the nervous system becomes so depressed that the person first becomes disoriented and later comatose. Therefore, patients dying of diabetic acidosis, uremic acidosis, and other types of acidosis usually die in a state of coma.

In metabolic acidosis, the high hydrogen ion concentration causes increased rate and depth of respiration. Therefore, one of the diagnostic signs of *metabolic* acidosis is increased pulmonary ventilation. On the other hand, *in respiratory acidosis,* the cause of the acidosis is *depressed respiration,* which is opposite to the effect in metabolic acidosis.

Alkalosis. The major clinical effect of alkalosis is *overexcitability of the nervous system.* This occurs both in the central nervous system and in the peripheral nerves, but usually the peripheral nerves are affected before the central nervous system. The nerves sometimes become so excitable that they automatically and repetitively fire even when they are not stimulated by normal stimuli. As a result, the muscles go into a state of *tetany,* which means a state of tonic spasm. This tetany usually appears first in the muscles of the forearm, then spreads to the muscles of the face and finally all over the body. Extremely alkalotic patients may die of tetany of the respiratory muscles.

Occasionally an alkalotic person develops severe symptoms of central nervous system overexcitability. The symptoms may manifest themselves as extreme nervousness or, in susceptible persons, as convulsions. For instance, in persons who are predisposed to epileptic seizures, simply overbreathing often results in an attack. Indeed, this is one of the clinical methods for assessing one's degree of epileptic predisposition.

Physiology of Treatment in Acidosis or Alkalosis

Obviously, the best treatment for acidosis or alkalosis is to remove the condition causing the abnormality, but if this cannot be effected, different drugs can be used to neutralize the excess acid or alkali.

To neutralize excess acid, large amounts of *sodium bicarbonate* can be ingested by mouth. This is absorbed into the blood stream and increases the bicarbonate ion portion of the bicarbonate buffer, thereby shifting the pH toward the alkaline side. Sodium bicarbonate is occasionally used also for intravenous therapy, but this has such strong and often dangerous physiological effects that other substances are often used instead, such as *sodium lactate* or *sodium gluconate.* The lactate and gluconate portions of the molecules are metabolized in the body, leaving the sodium in the extracellular fluids in the form of sodium bicarbonate, and thereby shifting the pH of the fluids in the alkaline direction.

For treatment of alkalosis, ammonium chloride is often administered by mouth. When this is absorbed into the blood, the ammonia portion of the ammonium chloride is converted by the liver into urea; this reaction liberates hydrochloric acid, which immediately reacts with the buffers of the body fluids to shift the hydrogen ion concentration in the acid direction.

RENAL DISEASE

It will not be possible to discuss here the great numbers of kidney diseases. However, of special physiological importance are (1) renal failure and (2) the nephrotic syndrome.

Renal Failure

Renal Failure Caused by Acute Glomerulonephritis. Acute glomerulonephritis is a disease caused by an abnormal immune reaction. In about 95 per cent of the patients, this occurs 1 to 3 weeks following an infection elsewhere in the body caused by certain types of group A beta streptococci. The infection may have been a streptococcal sore throat, streptococcal tonsillitis, or even streptococcal infection of the skin. It is not the infection itself that causes damage to the kidneys. Instead, as antibodies develop during the succeeding few weeks against the streptococcal antigen, it is believed that the antibodies and antigen react with each other to form an insoluble immune complex that becomes entrapped in the glomerulus, especially in the basement membrane portion of the glomerulus.

Once the immune complex has deposited in the glomeruli, all the cells of the glomerulus begin to proliferate, but mainly the epithelial cells and the mesangial cells that lie between the endothelium and epithelium. In addition, large numbers of white blood cells become entrapped in the glomeruli. Many of the glomeruli become blocked entirely by this inflammatory reaction, and those that are not blocked usually become excessively permeable, allowing both protein and red blood cells to leak into the glomerular filtrate. In a few of the severest cases, either total or almost total renal shutdown occurs.

The acute inflammation of the glomeruli usually subsides in 10 days to 2 weeks, and in most patients the kidneys return to normal function within the next few weeks to few months. Sometimes, however, many of the glomeruli are destroyed beyond repair, and in a small percentage of patients progressive renal deterioration continues indefinitely, similar to that described for chronic glomerulonephritis in a subsequent section.

Chronic Glomerulonephritis. Chronic glomerulonephritis is caused by any one of many diseases that damage principally the glomeruli but often the tubules as well. The basic glomerular lesion is usually very similar to that which occurs in acute glomerulonephritis. The glomerular membrane becomes progressively thickened and is eventually invaded by fibrous tissue. In the later stages of the disease, glomerular filtration becomes greatly reduced because of decreased numbers of filtering capillaries in the glomerular tufts and because of thickened glomerular membranes. In the final stages of the disease many of the glomeruli are completely replaced by fibrous tissue.

Pyelonephritis. Pyelonephritis is an infectious and inflammatory process that usually begins with bacterial infection in the renal pelvis and then extends progressively into the renal parenchyma. The infection can result from many different types of bacteria, but especially from the colon bacillus that originates from fecal contamination of the urinary tract. Invasion of the kidneys by these bacteria results in progressive destruction of renal tubules, glomeruli, and any other structures in the path of the invading organisms. Consequently, large portions of the functional renal tissue are lost.

A particularly interesting feature of pyelonephritis is that the invading infection usually affects the medulla of the kidney more than it affects the cortex. Because one of the primary functions of the medulla is to provide the counter-current mechanism for concentrating the urine, patients with pyelonephritis sometimes have reasonably normal renal function except for reduced ability to concentrate the urine.

Effect of Renal Failure on the Body Fluids — Uremia

The effect of renal failure on the body fluids depends to a great extent on water and food intake. Assuming that the person continues to ingest moderate amounts of water and food after complete renal shutdown, the concentration changes of different substances in the extracellular fluid are approximately those shown in Figure 23–4. The most important effects are (1) *generalized edema* resulting from water and salt retention; (2) *acidosis* resulting from failure of the kidneys to rid the body of normal acidic products; (3) *high concentrations of the nonprotein nitrogens,* especially *urea, creatinine,* and *uric acid,* resulting from failure of the body to excrete the metabolic end-products of proteins; and (4) *high concen-*

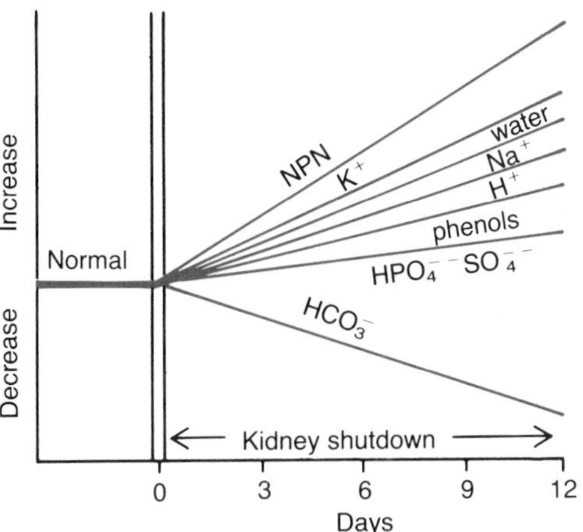

Figure 23-4. Effect of kidney shutdown on extracellular fluid constituents.

trations of other urinary retention products, including *phenols, guanidine bases, sulfates, phosphates,* and *potassium.* This condition is called *uremia* because of the high concentration of urea in the body fluids.

Acidosis in Renal Failure. Each day the metabolic processes of the body normally produce 50 to 80 millimoles more metabolic acid than metabolic alkali. Therefore, any time the kidneys fail to function, acid begins to accumulate in the body fluids. Normally, the buffers of the fluids can buffer up to a total of 500 to 1000 millimoles of acid without lethal depression of the extracellular fluid pH, and the phosphate compounds in the bones can buffer an additional few thousand millimoles, but gradually this buffering power is used up so that the pH falls drastically. The patient becomes *comatose* at about this same time, mainly because of acidosis, as is discussed subsequently.

Increase in Urea and Other Nonprotein Nitrogens (Azotemia) in Uremia. The nonprotein nitrogens include urea, uric acid, creatinine, and a few less important compounds. These, in general, are the end-products of protein metabolism and must be removed from the body continually to ensure continued protein metabolism in the cells. The concentrations of these, particularly of urea, can rise to as high as ten times normal during 1 to 2 weeks of renal failure. However, even these high levels do not seem to affect physiological function nearly so much as do the high concentrations of hydrogen ions and some of the other less obvious substances, such as very toxic guanidine bases, ammonium ions, and others. Yet one of the most important means of assessing the degree of renal failure is to measure the concentrations of urea and creatinine.

Uremic Coma. After a week or more of renal failure the sensorium becomes clouded, and the patient soon progresses into a state of coma. The acidosis is believed to be the principal factor responsible for the coma, because acidosis caused by other conditions, such as severe diabetes mellitus, also causes coma.

The respiration usually is deep and rapid in coma, which is a respiratory attempt to compensate for the metabolic acidosis. In addition to this, during the last day or so before death, the arterial pressure falls progressively, then rapidly in the last few hours. Death occurs usually when the pH of the blood falls to about 6.8.

Dialysis of Patients with the Artificial Kidney

Artificial kidneys have now been used for almost 40 years to treat patients with severe renal failure. In certain types of acute renal failure, such as that following mercury poisoning of the kidneys or following circulatory shock, the artificial kidney is used simply to tide the patient over for a few weeks until the renal damage heals so that the kidneys can resume function. However, the artificial kidney has now been developed to the point that thousands of persons with permanent renal failure or even total kidney removal are being maintained in health for years at a time, their lives depending entirely on the artificial kidney.

The basic principle of the artificial kidney is to pump blood for a few hours several times a week through very minute blood channels bounded by a thin membrane. On the other side of the membrane is a *dialyzing fluid* into which unwanted substances in the blood pass by diffusion.

Figure 23-5 illustrates the components of one type of artificial kidney in which blood flows continually between two thin membranes of cellophane; on the outside of the membranes is the dialyzing fluid. The cellophane is porous enough to allow all constituents of the plasma except the plasma proteins to diffuse in both directions—from plasma into the dialyzing fluid and from the dialyzing fluid back into the plasma. If the concentration of a substance is greater in the plasma than in the dialyzing fluid, there will be net transfer of the substance from the plasma into the dialyzing fluid. The amount of the substance that is transferred depends on (1) the permeability characteristics of the membrane as well as its surface area; (2) the difference between the concentrations on the two sides of the membrane; (3) molecular size, the smaller molecules diffusing more rapidly than larger ones; and (4) the length of time that the blood and the fluid remain in contact with the membrane.

In the normal operation of the artificial kidney, blood flows continually or intermittently back into a vein. The total amount of blood in the artificial kidney at any one time is usually less than 500 milliliters. To prevent coagulation of blood in the artificial kidney, a small amount of heparin is infused into the blood as it enters the "kidney."

The Dialyzing Fluid. Table 23-1 compares the constituents in a typical dialyzing fluid with those in normal plasma and uremic plasma. Note that the concentrations of the ions and other substances in the dialyzing fluid are not the same as the concentrations in normal plasma or in uremic plasma. Instead, they are adjusted to levels that are needed to cause appropriate movement of water and each solute through the membrane during the dialysis period.

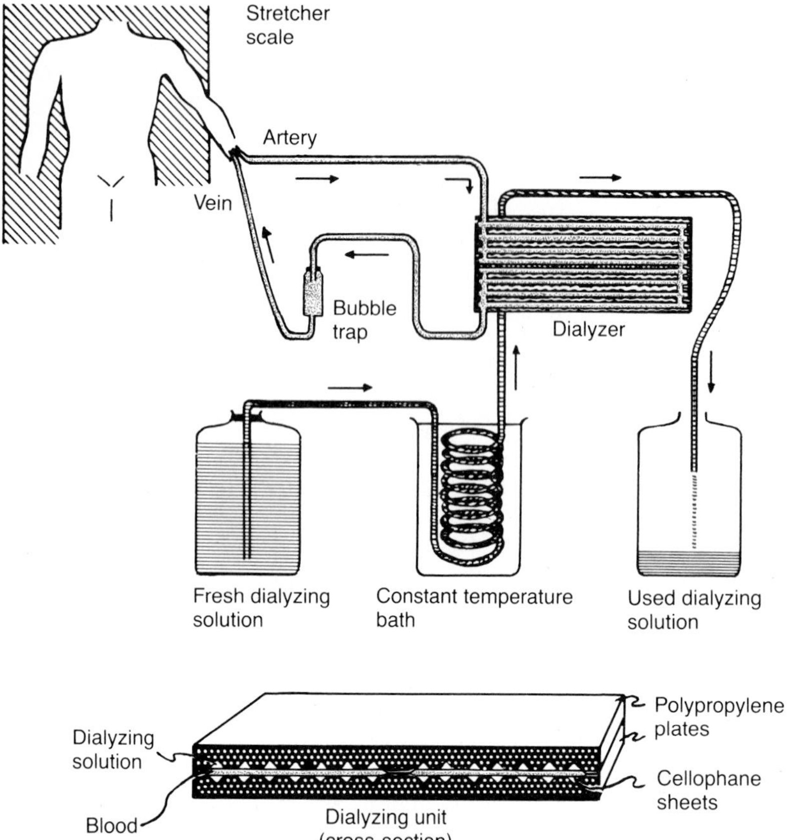

Figure 23-5. Principles of the artificial kidney.

Note also that there is no phosphate, urea, urate, sulfate, or creatinine in the dialyzing fluid, but they are present in high concentrations in the uremic blood. Therefore, when the uremic patient is dialyzed, these substances are lost in large quantities into the dialyzing fluid; thereby major proportions of them are removed from the plasma. Even so, the overall plasma clearance is still considerably limited when the artificial kidney replaces the normal kidneys.

Table 23-1 COMPARISON OF DIALYZING FLUID WITH NORMAL AND UREMIC PLASMA

Constituent	Normal Plasma	Dialyzing Fluid	Uremic Plasma
Electrolytes (mEq/liter)			
Na^+	142	133	142
K^+	5	1.0	7
Ca^{++}	3	3.0	2
Mg^{++}	1.5	1.5	1.5
Cl^-	107	105	107
HCO_3^-	27	35.7	14
Lactate$^-$	1.2	1.2	1.2
HPO_4^{--}	3	0	9
Urate$^-$	0.3	0	2
Sulfate^{--}	0.5	0	3
Nonelectrolytes (mg/dl)			
Glucose	100	125	100
Urea	26	0	200
Creatinine	1	0	6

The Nephrotic Syndrome — Increased Glomerular Permeability

Large numbers of patients with renal disease develop a so-called *nephrotic syndrome,* which is characterized especially by *loss of large quantities of plasma proteins into the urine.* In some instances this occurs without evidence of any other abnormality of renal function, but more often it is associated with some degree of renal failure.

The cause of the protein loss in the urine is increased permeability of the glomerular membrane. Therefore, any disease condition that can increase the permeability of this membrane can cause the nephrotic syndrome. Such diseases include *chronic glomerulonephritis* (in the previous discussion, it was noted that this disease primarily affects the glomeruli and often causes a greatly increased permeability of the glomerular membrane); *amyloidosis,* which results from deposition of an abnormal proteinoid substance in the walls of the blood vessels and seriously damages the basement membrane of the glomerulus; and *minimal change nephrotic syndrome,* a disease found mainly in young children.

"Minimal Change" Nephrotic Syndrome. In so-called minimal change nephrotic syndrome, one can rarely discern with the light microscope any abnormality of the glomerular membrane. However, with special study techniques, it has been found that the negative electrical charge normally exhibited by the glomerular membrane is reduced or lacking. Also, immunologic studies show abnormal immune reactions in some cases, suggesting that the loss of the negative charge might have resulted from antibody attack on the membrane.

Loss of the negative charge allows proteins, especially albumin, to pass through the glomerular membrane with ease, for it will be recalled that this negative charge normally repulses the negatively charged plasma protein molecules, which is a principal means of preventing leakage of proteins into the urine.

Minimal change nephrotic syndrome occurs mainly in children between the ages of 2 and 6 years, but it occurs occasionally in adults as well.

The greatly increased permeability of the glomerular membrane occasionally allows as much as 40 grams of plasma protein loss into the urine each day, which is an extreme amount for a young child. Therefore, the plasma proteins often fall below 2 gm/dl, and the colloid osmotic pressure falls from a normal of 28 to as low as 6 to 8 mm Hg. A consequence of this is that the blood capillaries all over the body leak tremendous quantities of fluid into all tissues, causing very severe *low protein edema.* Even in the very young child, as much as 10 liters of extra tissue fluid are sometimes present, as well as an additional 10 liters of *ascites* in the abdomen. Also, the joints swell, and the pleural cavity and the pericardium can become partially filled with fluid.

Approximately 90 per cent of these children respond exceedingly well to the administration of glucocorticoid steroids, which are known to alter certain types of immunologic abnormalities. However, the cellular mechanism of the glucocorticoid effect is not understood.

In all types of nephrosis in which plasma albumin concentration falls very low, large quantities of lipids appear in the blood plasma, with especially greatly increased blood cholesterol. This is believed to be caused by a direct effect of low plasma albumin on the liver to increase the production of the plasma lipoproteins.

MICTURITION

Micturition is the process by which the urinary bladder empties when it becomes filled. Basically the bladder (1) progressively fills until the tension in its walls rises above a threshold value, at which time (2) a nervous reflex called the "micturition reflex" occurs that either causes micturition or, if it fails in this, at least causes a conscious desire to urinate.

Physiological Anatomy and Nervous Connections of the Bladder

The urinary bladder, illustrated in Figure 23–6, is a smooth muscle chamber composed of two principal parts: (1) the *body,* which is the major part of the bladder, in which the urine collects, and (2) the *neck,* which is a funnel-shaped extension of the body, passing inferiorly to the urethra.

The smooth muscle of the bladder is known as the *detrusor muscle.* Its muscle fibers extend in all directions and, when contracted, can increase the pressure in the bladder sometimes to as high as 40 to 60 mm Hg. An action potential can spread throughout the detrusor muscle to cause contraction of the entire bladder at once.

On the posterior wall of the bladder, immediately above the bladder neck, the two ureters enter the bladder. Where each ureter enters the bladder, it courses obliquely through the detrusor muscle and then passes still another 1 to 2 cm underneath the bladder mucosa before emptying into the bladder.

The bladder neck muscle is frequently called the

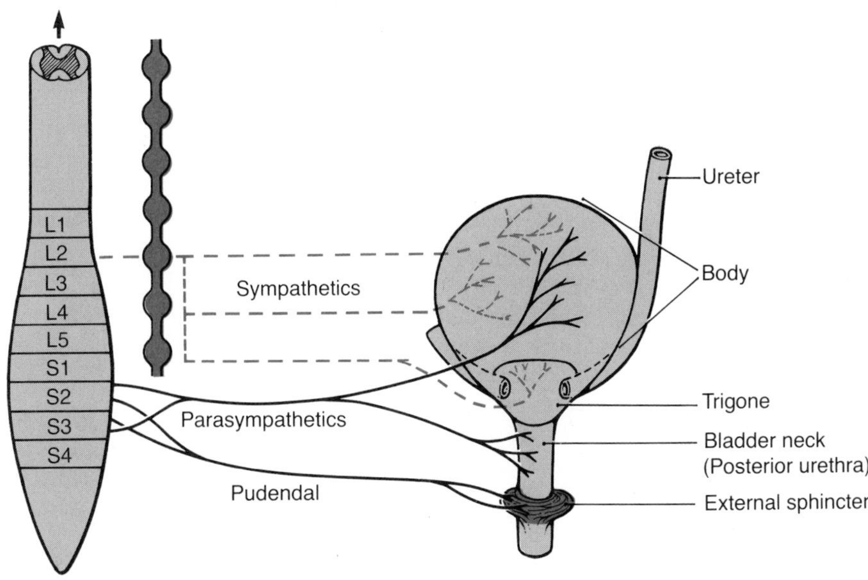

Figure 23–6. The urinary bladder and its innervation.

internal sphincter. Its natural tone normally keeps the bladder neck and posterior urethra empty of urine and therefore prevents emptying of the bladder until the pressure in the body of the bladder rises above a critical threshold.

Beyond the posterior urethra, the urethra passes through the *urogenital diaphragm,* which contains a layer of muscle called the *external sphincter* of the bladder. This muscle is a voluntary skeletal muscle in contrast to the muscle of the bladder body and bladder neck, which is entirely smooth muscle. This external muscle is under voluntary control of the nervous system and can be used to prevent urination even when the involuntary controls are attempting to empty the bladder.

Innervation of the Bladder. The principal nerve supply to the bladder is by way of the *pelvic nerves,* which connect with the spinal cord through the sacral plexus, mainly connecting with cord segments S-2 and S-3. Coursing through the pelvic nerves are both *sensory nerve fibers* and *motor fibers.* The sensory fibers mainly detect the degree of stretch of the bladder wall. Stretch signals from the posterior urethra are especially strong and are mainly responsible for initiating the reflexes that cause bladder emptying.

The motor nerve fibers transmitted in the pelvic nerves are *parasympathetic fibers.* These terminate on ganglion cells located in the wall of the bladder. Short postganglionic nerves then innervate the *detrusor muscle.*

Apart from the pelvic nerves are skeletal motor fibers transmitted through the *pudendal nerve* to the *external bladder sphincter.* These are *somatic* nerve fibers that innervate and control the voluntary skeletal muscle of this sphincter.

Transport of Urine Through the Ureters

The ureters are small smooth muscle tubes that originate in the pelves of the two kidneys and pass downward to enter the bladder. As urine collects in the pelvis, the pressure in the pelvis increases and initiates a peristaltic contraction beginning in the pelvis and spreading downward along the ureter to force urine toward the bladder. The peristaltic wave can move urine against an obstruction with a pressure as high as 50 to 100 mm Hg. Transmission of the peristaltic wave is probably caused by action potentials passing along the smooth muscle syncytium of the ureteral wall. However, parasympathetic stimulation can increase and sympathetic stimulation can decrease the frequency of the waves and probably also can affect the intensity of contraction.

At the lower end, the ureter penetrates the bladder obliquely, as illustrated in Figure 23-6. The ureter courses for several centimeters under the bladder epithelium so that pressure in the bladder compresses the ureter, thereby preventing backflow of urine when pressure builds up in the bladder during micturition.

Tone of the Bladder Wall, and the Cystometrogram During Bladder Filling

The solid curve of Figure 23-7 is called the *cystometrogram* of the bladder. It shows the approximate changes in intravesical pressure as the bladder fills with urine. By the time 30 to 50 milliliters of urine has collected, the pressure will have risen to 5 to 10 centimeters of water. Additional urine up to 200 to 300 milliliters can collect with only a small amount of additional rise in pressure; this constant level of pressure is caused by *intrinsic tone* of the bladder wall itself. Beyond 300 to 400 milliliters, collection of more urine causes the pressure to rise very rapidly.

Superimposed on the tonic pressure changes during filling of the bladder are *micturition waves* in the cystometrogram caused by the micturition reflex, which is discussed next.

The Micturition Reflex

Referring again to Figure 23-7, one sees that as the bladder fills, many superimposed *micturition contractions* begin to appear, as denoted by the dashed spikes. These are the result of a stretch reflex initiated by sensory stretch receptors in the bladder wall, especially by the receptors in the posterior urethra when this begins to fill with urine at the higher bladder pressures. *Sensory signals* are conducted to the sacral segments of the cord through the *pelvic nerves* and then back again to the bladder through the *parasympathetic fibers* in these same nerves.

Once a micturition reflex begins, it is "self-regenerative." That is, initial contraction of the bladder further activates the receptors to cause still further increase in sensory impulses from the bladder and posterior urethra, which causes further increase in reflex contraction of the bladder, the cycle thus repeating itself again and again until the bladder has

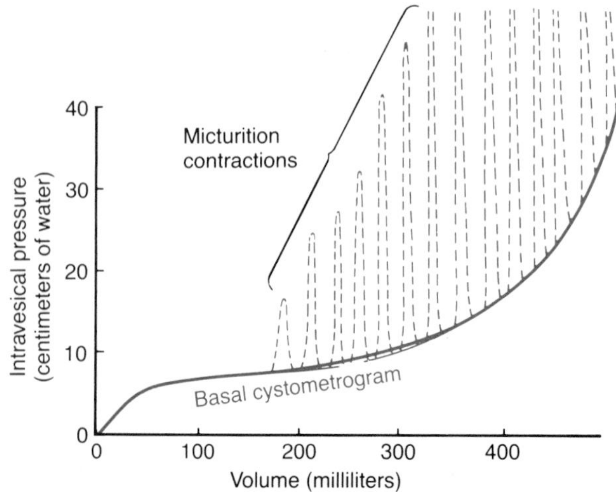

Figure 23-7. A normal cystometrogram showing also acute pressure waves (the dashed spikes) caused by micturition reflexes.

reached a strong degree of contraction. Then, after a few seconds to more than a minute, the reflex begins to fatigue, and the regenerative cycle of the micturition reflex ceases, allowing rapid reduction in bladder contraction. Once a micturition reflex has occurred but has not succeeded in emptying the bladder, the nervous elements of this reflex usually remain in an inhibited state for at least a few minutes to sometimes as long as an hour or more before another micturition reflex occurs. However, as the bladder becomes more and more filled, micturition reflexes occur more and more often and more powerfully, until still another reflex occurs, which passes through the *pudendal nerves* to the *external sphincter* to inhibit it. If this inhibition is more potent than the voluntary constrictor signals to the external sphincter from the brain, urination will occur. If not, urination will not occur until the bladder fills still more and the micturition reflex becomes more powerful.

Control of Micturition by the Brain. The micturition reflex is a completely automatic cord reflex, but it can be inhibited or facilitated by centers in the brain. These include (1) strong *facilitatory and inhibitory centers in the brain stem,* probably located in the pons, and (2) several *centers located in the cerebral cortex* that are mainly inhibitory but can at times become excitatory.

The micturition reflex is the basic cause of micturition, but the higher centers normally exert final control of micturition by the following means:

1. The higher centers keep the micturition reflex partially inhibited all the time except when micturition is desired.
2. The higher centers prevent micturition, even if a micturition reflex occurs, by continual tonic contraction of the external bladder sphincter until a convenient time presents itself.
3. When the time to urinate arrives, the cortical centers can (a) facilitate the sacral micturition centers to help initiate a micturition reflex and (b) inhibit the external urinary sphincter so that urination can occur.

Abnormalities of Micturition

The Atonic Bladder. Destruction of the sensory nerve fibers from the bladder to the spinal cord prevents transmission of stretch signals from the bladder and, therefore, also prevents micturition reflex contractions. Therefore, the person loses all bladder control despite intact efferent fibers from the cord to the bladder and despite intact neurogenic connections with the brain. Instead of emptying periodically, the bladder fills to capacity and overflows a few drops at a time through the urethra. This is called *outflow incontinence,* or simply *overflow dribbling.*

The Automatic Bladder. If the spinal cord is damaged above the sacral region but the sacral segments are still intact, typical micturition reflexes still occur. However, they are no longer controllable by the brain. During the first few days to several weeks after the damage to the cord has occurred, the micturition reflexes are completely suppressed because of the state of "spinal shock" caused by the sudden loss of facilitatory impulses from the brain stem and cerebrum. However, if the bladder is emptied periodically by catheterization to prevent physical bladder injury, the excitability of the micturition reflex gradually increases until typical micturition reflexes return.

It is especially interesting that stimulating the skin in the genital region can sometimes elicit a micturition reflex in this condition, thus providing a means by which some patients can still control urination.

REFERENCES

de Roufignac, C., and Ealouf, J-M.: Hormonal regulation of chloride transport in the proximal and distal nephron. Annu. Rev. Physiol., 50:123, 1988.

Dirks, J. H., and Sutton, R. A.: Diuretics: Physiology, Pharmacology and Clinical Use. Philadelphia, W. B. Saunders Co., 1986.

DuBose, T. D., Jr., and Bidani, A.: Kinetics of CO_2 exchange in the kidney. Annu. Rev. Physiol., 50:653, 1988.

Galla, J. H., and Luke, R. G.: Chloride transport and disorders of acid-base balance. Annu. Rev. Physiol., 50:141, 1988.

Halperin, M. L., and Goldstein, M. B.: Fluid, Electrolyte, and Acid-Base Emergencies. Philadelphia, W. B. Saunders Co., 1988.

Knepper, M. A., et al.: Ammonium transport in the kidney. Physiol. Rev., 69:179, 1989.

Massry, S. G., and Glassock, R. J. Textbook of Nephrology. 2nd ed. Baltimore, Williams & Wilkins, 1988.

Maren, T. H.: The kinetics of HCO_3^- synthesis related to fluid secretion, pH control, and CO_2 elimination. Annu. Rev. Physiol., 50:695, 1988.

Murer, H., and Malmstrom, K.: How renal phosphate transport is regulated. News Physiol. Sci., 2:45, 1987.

Rose, B. D. (ed.): Clinical Physiology of Acid-Base and Electrolyte Disorders. 3rd ed. New York, McGraw-Hill Book Co., 1989.

Seldin, D. W., and Giebisch, G.: The Regulation of Acid-Base Balance. New York, Raven Press, 1989.

Shah, S. V.: Oxidant mechanisms in glomerular injury. News Physiol. Sci., 3:254, 1988.

QUESTIONS

1. What is the relationship between the hydrogen ion concentration and the pH of a fluid?
2. Explain how the bicarbonate buffer system buffers the hydrogen ion concentration.
3. Give the Henderson-Hasselbalch equation for the relationship between pH and the two elements of the bicarbonate buffer system.
4. Explain how the phosphate and protein systems buffer the hydrogen ion concentration.
5. What is the feedback mechanism controlling respiration that also helps control the hydrogen ion concentration of the extracellular fluids?
6. Explain the mechanism for hydrogen ion secretion by the renal tubular epithelium.

7. Explain the "titration" of hydrogen ions against bicarbonate ions in the renal tubules as a means for controlling extracellular fluid hydrogen ion concentration.
8. Why is the phosphate buffer system of special importance for transport of hydrogen ions from the tubules into the urine?
9. How does the ammonia buffer system increase the transport of hydrogen ions from the tubules into the urine as much as tenfold?
10. What is the difference between metabolic acidosis and respiratory acidosis?
11. Explain the various causes of respiratory acidosis and alkalosis and of metabolic acidosis and alkalosis.
12. Why can either acidosis or alkalosis be fatal?
13. Give the sequence of events in the development of acute renal failure caused by acute glomerulonephitis.
14. How does pyelonephritis differ in its effects on renal function from glomerular nephritis?
15. What are the effects on the body of uremia?
16. Explain the manner in which the artificial kidney removes unwanted substances from the body fluids.
17. What is "minimal change" nephrotic syndrome, and how does it affect renal function?
18. Explain the mechanism by which the ureters transport urine from the kidneys to the urinary bladder.
19. Describe the anatomy and the function of the *micturition reflex.*
20. How is micturition controlled?

VI

Blood Cells, Immunity, and Blood Clotting

24

Red Blood Cells, White Blood Cells, and Resistance of the Body to Infection

With this chapter we begin a discussion of the blood cells and of other cells closely related to those of the blood: the cells of the macrophage system and of the lymphatic system.

THE RED BLOOD CELLS

The major function of red blood cells is to transport hemoglobin, which in turn carries oxygen from the lungs to the tissues. Normal red blood cells are biconcave discs having a mean diameter of approximately 8 microns and a thickness at the thickest point of 2 microns and in the center of 1 micron or less. The shapes of red blood cells can change remarkably as the cells pass through capillaries. Actually, the red blood cell is a "bag" that can be deformed into almost any shape. Furthermore, because the normal cell has a great excess of cell membrane for the quantity of material inside, deformation does not stretch the membrane and consequently does not rupture the cell, as would be the case with many other cells.

In normal men, the average number of red blood cells per cubic millimeter is 5,200,000 and in normal women, 4,700,000. Also, the altitude at which the person lives affects the number of red blood cells; this is discussed later.

Quantity of Hemoglobin in the Cells and Transport of Oxygen. When the hematocrit (defined as the percentage of the blood that is red cells—normally 40 to 45 per cent) and the quantity of hemoglobin in each respective cell are normal, the blood contains an average of 15 grams of hemoglobin in every 100 milliliters. As will be discussed in connection with the transport of oxygen in Chapter 28, each gram of pure hemoglobin is capable of combining with approximately 1.39 milliliters of oxygen. Therefore, in a normal person, over 20 ml of oxygen can be carried in combination with hemoglobin in each 100 milliliters of blood.

Genesis of Blood Cells

Pluripotential Hemopoietic Stem Cells, Growth Inducers, and Differentiation Inducers. In the bone marrow are cells called *pluripotential hemopoietic stem cells* (PHSCs), from which all the cells in the circulating blood are derived. Figure 24–1 illustrates the successive divisions of the pluripotential cells to form the different peripheral blood cells. As these cells reproduce, continuing throughout the life of the person, a portion of them are exactly like the original pluripotential cells and are retained in the bone marrow to maintain a supply of these, though their numbers do diminish with age. The larger portion of the reproduced stem cells, however, differentiate to form the other cells illustrated to the right in Figure 24–1. The early offspring still cannot be recognized as the different types of blood cells, even though they have already become committed to a particular line of cells and are called *committed stem cells.*

A committed stem cell that produces erythrocytes is called a *colony-forming unit–erythrocyte,* and the abbreviation CFU-E is used to designate this type of stem cell. Likewise, colony-forming units that form granulocytes and monocytes have the designation CFU-GM, and so forth.

Growth and reproduction of the different stem cells are controlled by multiple proteins called *growth inducers.* Four major growth inducers have been described, each having different characteristics. One of these, *interleukin-3,* promotes growth and reproduc-

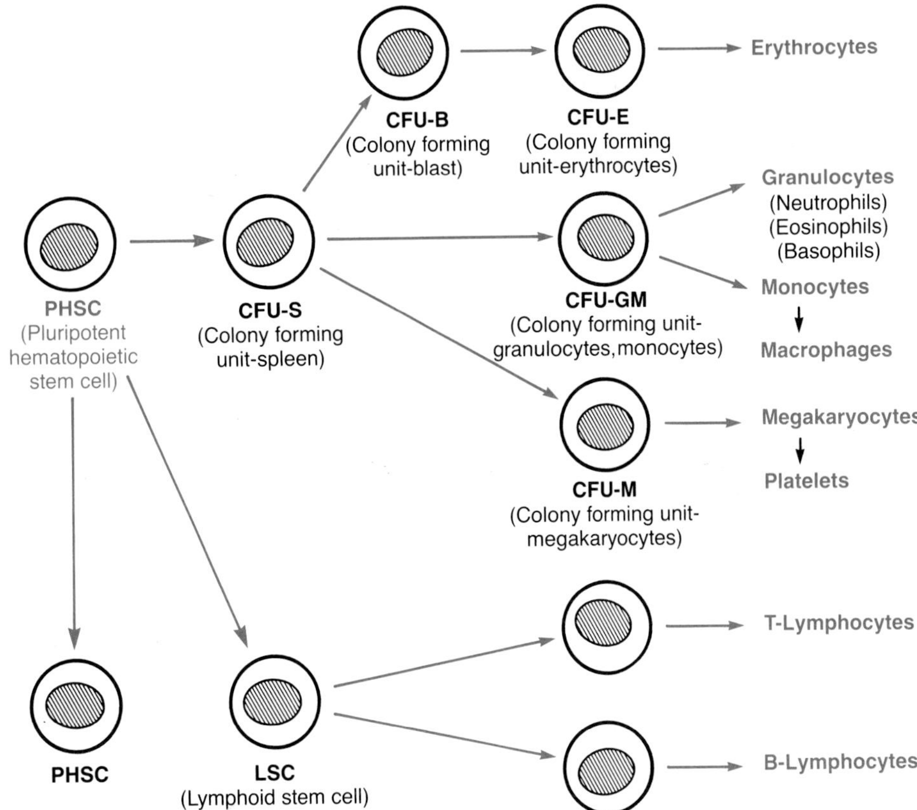

Figure 24-1. Formation of the multiple different peripheral blood cells from the original pluripotential hematopoietic stem cell (PHSC) in the bone marrow.

tion of virtually all the different types of stem cells, whereas the others induce growth of only specific types of committed stem cells.

The growth inducers promote growth but not differentiation of the cells. Instead, this is the function of still another set of proteins, called *differentiation inducers.* Each of these causes one type of stem cell to differentiate one or more steps toward a final type of adult blood cell.

Formation of the growth inducers and differentiation inducers is itself controlled by factors outside the bone marrow. For instance, in the case of red blood cells, exposure to low oxygen for a long period of time results in growth induction, differentiation, and production of greatly increased numbers of erythrocytes, as we shall discuss later in the chapter. In the case of some of the white blood cells, infectious diseases cause growth, differentiation, and eventual formation of the specific types of white blood cells that are needed to combat the infection.

Stages of Differentiation of Red Blood Cells

The first cell that can be identified as belonging to the red blood cell series is the *proerythroblast,* illustrated in Figure 24-2. Under appropriate stimulation, large numbers of these cells are formed from the CFU-E stem cells.

Once the proerythroblast has been formed, it divides several more times, eventually forming many mature red blood cells. The first-generation cells are called *basophil erythroblasts* because they stain with basic dyes; the cell at this time has accumulated very little hemoglobin. However, in the succeeding generations, as illustrated in the figure, the cells become filled with hemoglobin to a concentration of approximately 34 per cent, the nucleus condenses to a small size, and its final remnant is extruded from the cell. At this stage the cells pass into the blood capillaries by diapedesis (squeezing through the pores of the membrane).

Regulation of Red Blood Cell Production— The Role of Erythropoietin

The total mass of red blood cells in the circulatory system is regulated within very narrow limits, so that an adequate number of red cells is always available to provide sufficient tissue oxygenation and yet so that the cells do not become so concentrated that they impede blood flow. What we know about this control mechanism is diagrammed in Figure 24-3 and is as follows.

Tissue Oxygenation as the Basic Regulator of Red Blood Cell Production. Any condition that causes the quantity of oxygen transported to the tissues to decrease ordinarily increases the rate of red blood cell production. Thus, when a person becomes extremely *anemic* as a result of hemorrhage or any other condition, the bone marrow immediately begins

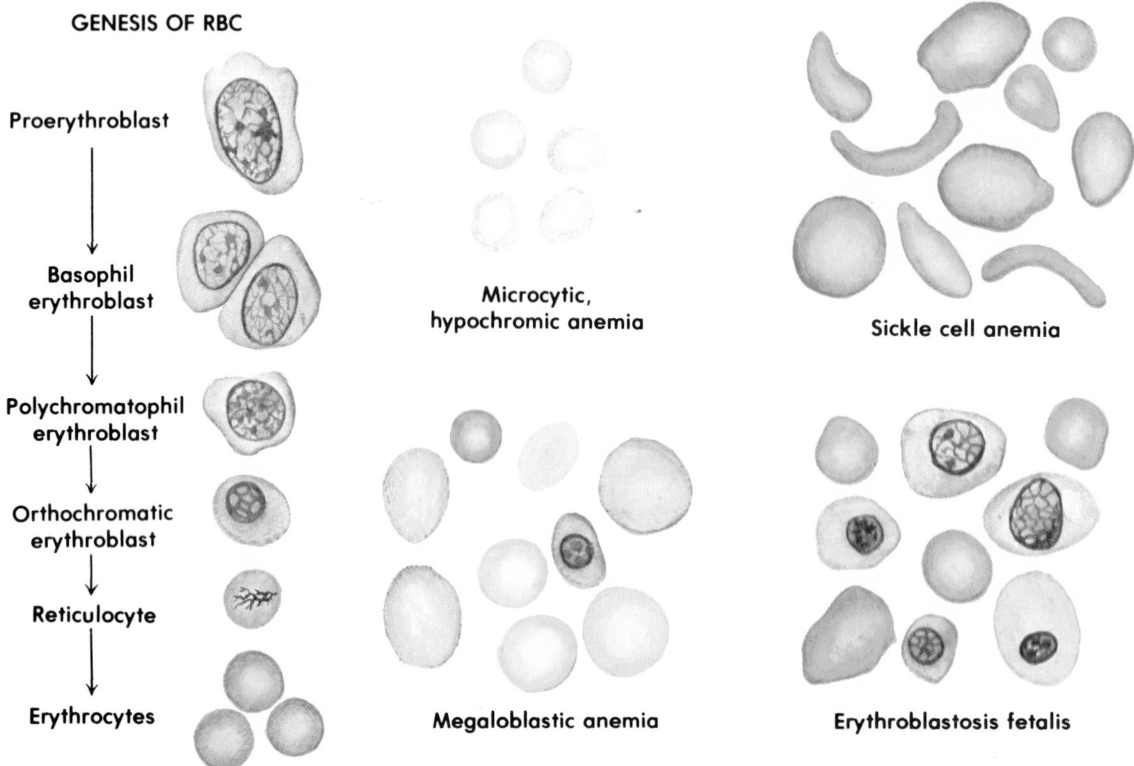

Figure 24-2. Genesis of red blood cells, and red blood cells in different types of anemias.

to produce large quantities of red blood cells. Also, at *high altitudes,* where the quantity of oxygen in the air is greatly decreased, insufficient oxygen is transported to the tissues, and red cells are produced so rapidly that their number in the blood is considerably increased.

Therefore, it is obvious that it is not the concentration of red blood cells in the blood that controls the rate of red cell production, but instead it is the functional ability of the cells to transport oxygen to the tissues in relation to the tissue demand for oxygen.

Erythropoietin, Its Formation in Response to Hypoxia, and Its Function in Regulating Red Blood Cell Production. The principal factor that stimulates red blood cell production is a circulating hormone called *erythropoietin,* a glycoprotein with a molecular weight of about 34,000. In the absence of erythropoietin, hypoxia has either no effect or very little effect in stimulating red blood cell production. On the other hand, when the erythropoietin system is functional, hypoxia causes marked increase in erythropoietin production, and the erythropoietin in turn enhances red blood cell production until the hypoxia is relieved.

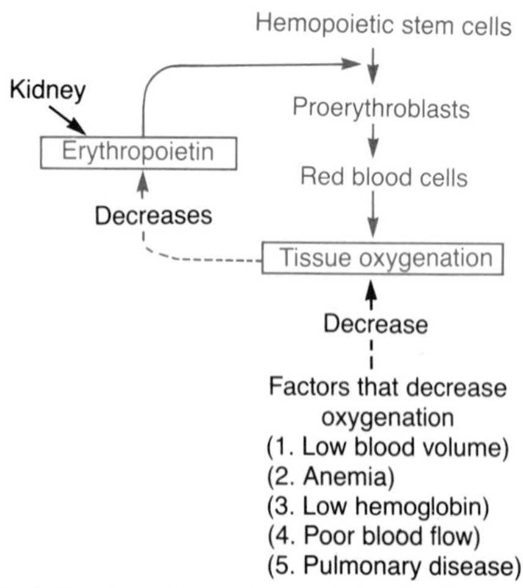

Figure 24-3. Function of the erythropoietin mechanism to increase the production of red blood cells when various factors decrease tissue oxygenation.

Role of the Kidneys in the Formation of Erythropoietin. In the normal person, 80 to 90 per cent of all erythropoietin is formed in the kidneys; the remainder is formed mainly in the liver. However, it is not known exactly where in the kidney the erythropoietin is formed. One possibility is the mesangial cells located at the pole of the glomerulus and extending also into the tuft of glomerular capillaries.

When both kidneys are removed from a person or when the kidneys are destroyed by renal disease, the person invariably becomes very anemic because the 10 to 20 per cent of the normal erythropoietin formed in other tissues (mainly in the liver) is sufficient to cause only one third to one half as much red blood cell formation as needed by the body.

Maturation of Red Blood Cells — Requirement for Vitamin B_{12} (Cyanocobalamin) and Folic Acid

Especially important for final maturation of the red blood cells are the two vitamins *vitamin B_{12}* and *folic* *acid.* Both of these are essential for the synthesis of DNA, for each in a different way is required for the formation of thymidine triphosphate, one of the essential building blocks of DNA. Therefore, lack of either vitamin B_{12} or folic acid causes diminished DNA and consequently failure of nuclear maturation and division. Furthermore, the erythroblastic cells of the bone marrow, in addition to failing to proliferate rapidly, become larger than normal, developing into so-called *megaloblasts,* and the adult erythrocyte has a flimsy membrane and is often irregular, large, and oval instead of the usual biconcave disc. These poorly formed cells, after entering the circulating blood, are capable of carrying oxygen normally but their fragility causes them to have a short life, one half to one third of normal. Therefore, it is said that vitamin B_{12} or folic acid deficiency causes *maturation failure* in the process of erythropoiesis.

Maturation Failure Caused by Poor Absorption of Vitamin B_{12}—Pernicious Anemia. A common cause of maturation failure is failure to absorb vitamin B_{12} from the gastrointestinal tract. This often occurs in the disease called *pernicious anemia,* in which the basic abnormality is an *atrophic gastric mucosa* that fails to secrete normal gastric secretions. The parietal cells of the gastric glands secrete a glycoprotein called *intrinsic factor,* which combines with vitamin B_{12} of the food and makes the B_{12} available for absorption by the gut. It does this in the following way: (1) The intrinsic factor binds tightly with the vitamin B_{12}. In this bound state the B_{12} is protected from digestion by the gastrointestinal enzymes. (2) Still in the bound state, the intrinsic factor binds to specific receptor sites on the brush border membranes of the mucosal cells in the ileum. (3) Vitamin B_{12} is then transported into the blood during the next few hours by the process of pinocytosis, carrying the intrinsic factor and the vitamin together through the membrane.

Lack of intrinsic factor, therefore, causes loss of much of the vitamin because of both enzyme action in the gut and failure of its absorption.

Formation of Hemoglobin

Synthesis of hemoglobin begins in the proerythroblasts and continues until a few days after the cells leave the bone marrow and pass into the blood stream.

Figure 24–4 shows the basic chemical steps in the formation of hemoglobin. An important stage is the formation of *heme,* which contains one atom of iron. Next, each heme molecule combines with a very long polypeptide chain, called a *globin,* forming a subunit of hemoglobin called a *hemoglobin chain* (Fig. 24–5). Each of these chains has a molecular weight of about 16,000; four of them in turn bind together loosely to form the whole hemoglobin molecule.

Because each chain has a heme prosthetic group, there are four separate iron atoms in each hemoglobin molecule; each of these can bind with 1 molecule of oxygen, making a total of 4 molecules of oxygen (or 8 atoms) that can be transported by each hemoglobin molecule. Hemoglobin has a molecular weight of 64,458.

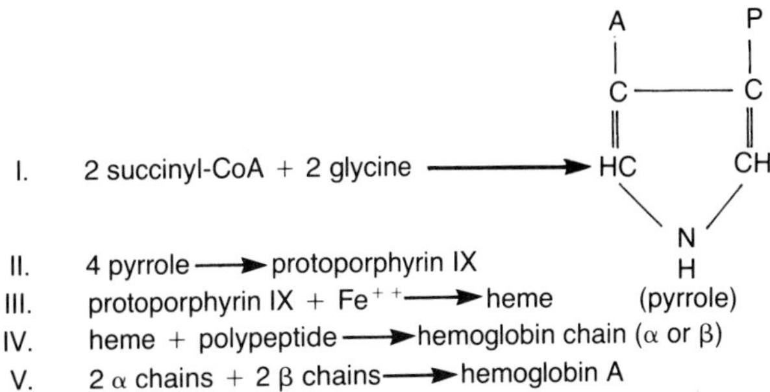

Figure 24–4. Formation of hemoglobin.

Combination of Hemoglobin with Oxygen. The most important feature of the hemoglobin molecule is its ability to combine loosely and reversibly with oxygen. This ability is discussed in detail in Chapter 28 in relation to respiration, for the primary function of hemoglobin in the body depends upon its ability to combine with oxygen in the lungs and then to release this oxygen readily in the tissue capillaries where the gaseous tension of oxygen is lower than in the lungs.

Oxygen *does not* combine with the two positive bonds of the iron in the hemoglobin molecule. Instead, it binds loosely with one of the six "coordination" bonds of the iron atom. This is an extremely loose bond so that the combination is easily reversible, releasing oxygen into the tissue fluids in the form of dissolved molecular oxygen, rather than ionic oxygen.

Iron Metabolism

Because iron is important for formation of hemoglobin, myoglobin, and other substances such as the

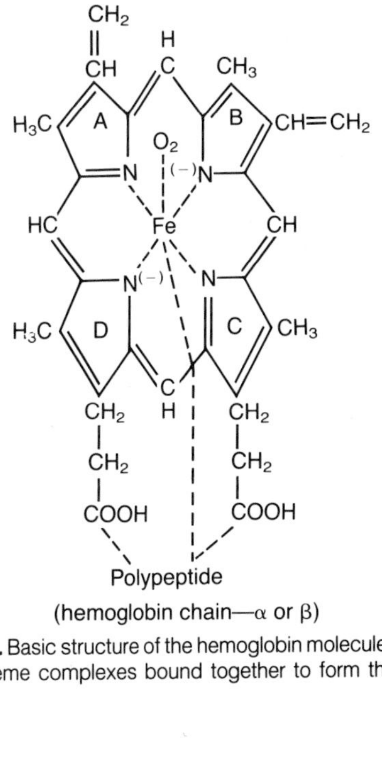

Figure 24–5. Basic structure of the hemoglobin molecule, showing one of the four heme complexes bound together to form the hemoglobin molecule.

cytochromes, cytochrome oxidase, peroxidase, and catalase, it is essential to understand the means by which iron is utilized in the body.

The total quantity of iron in the body averages about 4 grams, approximately 65 per cent of which is present in the form of hemoglobin. About 4 per cent is present in the form of myoglobin, 1 per cent in the form of the various heme compounds that promote intracellular oxidation, 0.1 per cent combined with the protein transferrin in the blood plasma, and 15 to 30 per cent stored mainly in the liver in the form of ferritin.

Transport and Storage of Iron. Transport, storage, and metabolism of iron in the body are illustrated in Figure 24-6, and may be explained as follows: When iron is absorbed from the small intestine, it immediately combines in the blood plasma with a beta-globulin, *apotransferrin,* to form *transferrin,* which is then transported in the plasma. The iron is only loosely bound and, consequently, can be released to any of the tissue cells *but especially* the reticuloendothelial cells and liver hepatocytes. In the cell cytoplasm, it combines mainly with a protein, *apoferritin,* to form *ferritin.* Apoferritin has a molecular weight of approximately 460,000, and varying quantities of iron can combine in clusters of iron radicals with this large molecule; therefore, ferritin may contain only a small amount of iron or a large amount. This iron stored in ferritin is called *storage iron.*

When the quantity of iron in the plasma falls very low, iron is removed from ferritin quite easily and can again be transported by transferrin in the plasma to the portions of the body where it is needed.

A unique characteristic of the transferrin molecule is that it binds especially strongly with receptors in the cell membranes of erythroblasts in the bone marrow. Then, along with its bound iron, it is ingested into the erythroblasts by endocytosis. There the transferrin delivers the iron directly to the mitochondria, where heme is synthesized. In persons who do not have adequate quantities of transferrin in their blood, failure to transport iron to the erythroblasts in this manner can cause severe hypochromic anemia—that is, decreased numbers of red cells containing very little hemoglobin.

When red blood cells have lived their life span and are destroyed, the hemoglobin released from the cells is ingested by the cells of the monocyte-macrophage system. There free iron is liberated, and it can then be either stored in the ferritin pool or reused for formation of hemoglobin.

Daily Loss of Iron. About 1 milligram of iron is excreted each day by men, mainly into the feces. Additional quantities of iron are lost whenever bleeding occurs. In women, the menstrual loss of blood brings the average iron loss to a value of approximately 2 mg/day.

Regulation of Total Body Iron by Alteration of Rate of Absorption. When the body has become saturated with iron so that essentially all the apoferritin in the iron storage areas is already combined with iron, the rate of absorption of iron from the intestinal tract becomes greatly decreased. The principal reason for this is the following: When essentially all the apoferritin in the body has become saturated with iron, it becomes difficult for plasma transferrin to release iron to the tissues. As a consequence, the transferrin, which is normally only one third saturated with iron, now becomes almost fully bound with iron, so that the transferrin accepts almost no new iron from the intestinal mucosal cells.

DESTRUCTION OF RED BLOOD CELLS

When red blood cells are delivered from the bone marrow into the circulatory system, they normally circulate an average of 120 days before being destroyed. Even though mature red cells do not have a nucleus, mitochondria, or endoplasmic reticulum, they nevertheless have cytoplasmic enzymes that are capable of metabolizing glucose and forming small amounts of adenosine triphosphate (ATP). The ATP in turn helps preserve the red cell. Even so, the metabolic systems of the red cell become progressively less active with time, and the cells become more and more fragile.

Once the red cell membrane becomes very fragile, the cell ruptures during passage through some tight spot of the circulation. Many of the red cells fragment

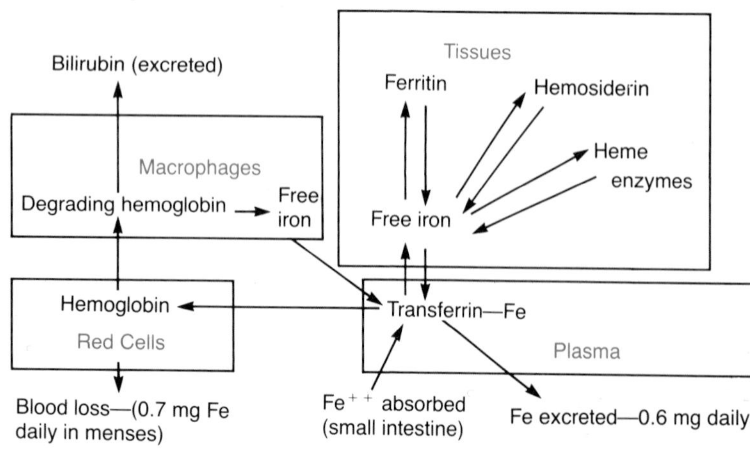

Figure 24-6. Iron transport and metabolism.

in the spleen, where they squeeze through the red pulp of the spleen. Here the spaces between the structural trabeculae of the pulp are only 3 micrometers wide, in comparison with the 8-micrometer diameter of the red cell. When the spleen is removed, the number of abnormal cells and old cells circulating in the blood increases considerably.

Destruction of Hemoglobin. The hemoglobin released from the cells when they burst is phagocytized almost immediately by macrophages in many parts of the body, but especially in the liver (the Kupffer cells), spleen, and bone marrow. During the next few hours to days, the macrophages release the iron from the hemoglobin back into the blood to be carried by transferrin either to the bone marrow for production of new red blood cells or to the liver and other tissues for storage in the form of ferritin. The porphyrin portion of the hemoglobin molecule is converted by the macrophages, through a series of stages, into the bile pigment *bilirubin,* which is released into the blood and later secreted by the liver into the bile; this will be discussed in relation to liver function in Chapter 43.

THE ANEMIAS

Anemia means a deficiency of red blood cells, which can be caused either by too rapid loss or too slow production of red blood cells. Some types of anemia and their physiological causes are the following:

Blood Loss Anemia. After rapid hemorrhage the body replaces the plasma within 1 to 3 days, but this leaves a low concentration of red blood cells. If a second hemorrhage does not occur, the red blood cell concentration returns to normal within 3 to 4 weeks.

Aplastic Anemia. *Bone marrow aplasia* means lack of a functioning bone marrow. For instance, the person exposed to gamma ray radiation from a nuclear bomb blast is likely to sustain complete destruction of bone marrow, followed in a few weeks by lethal anemia. Likewise, excessive x-ray treatment, certain industrial chemicals, and even drugs to which the person might be sensitive can cause the same effect.

Megaloblastic Anemia. From the earlier discussion in this chapter of vitamin B_{12}, folic acid, and intrinsic factor from the stomach mucosa, one can readily understand that loss of any one of these factors can lead to very slow reproduction of the erythroblasts in the bone marrow. As a result, these grow too large, with odd shapes, and are called *megaloblasts.* Thus, atrophy of the stomach mucosa, as occurs in *pernicious anemia,* or loss of the entire stomach as the result of total gastrectomy can lead to megaloblastic anemia.

Hemolytic Anemia. Many different abnormalities of the red blood cells, many of which are hereditarily acquired, make the cells very fragile, so that they rupture easily as they go through the capillaries, especially through the spleen. Therefore, even though the number of red blood cells formed is completely normal, or even vastly excessive in some hemolytic diseases, the red cell life span is so short that serious anemia results. One of these types of anemia is sickle cell anemia.

In *sickle cell anemia,* which is present in 0.3 to 1.0 per cent of West African and American blacks, the cells contain an abnormal type of hemoglobin called *hemoglobin S,* caused by abnormal composition of the globin chains of the hemoglobin. When this hemoglobin is exposed to low concentrations of oxygen, it precipitates into long crystals inside the red blood cell. These crystals elongate the cell and give it the appearance of being a sickle, rather than a biconcave disc. The precipitated hemoglobin also damages the cell membrane so that the cells become highly fragile, leading to serious anemia. Such patients frequently go into a vicious circle called a sickle cell disease "crisis," in which low oxygen tension in the tissues causes sickling, which causes impediment of blood flow though the tissues, in turn causing still further decrease in oxygen tension. Thus, once the process starts, it progresses rapidly, leading to a serious decrease in red blood cell mass within a few hours and, often, to death.

EFFECTS OF ANEMIA ON THE CIRCULATORY SYSTEM

The viscosity of the blood, which was discussed in Chapter 11, depends almost entirely on the concentration of red blood cells. In severe anemia the blood viscosity may fall to as low as 1.5 times that of water rather than the normal value of approximately 3. This decreases the resistance to blood flow in the peripheral vessels so that far greater than normal quantities of blood return to the heart. Moreover, hypoxia due to diminished transport of oxygen by the blood causes the tissue vessels to dilate, allowing still further increase in return of blood to the heart, increasing the cardiac output to a still higher level. Thus, one of the major effects of anemia is greatly *increased work load on the heart.* This can be especially serious when the anemic person begins to exercise, for the heart is not capable of pumping much greater quantities of blood than it is already pumping. Consequently, during exercise, which greatly increases the tissue demand for oxygen, extreme tissue hypoxia results, and acute cardiac failure often ensues.

WHITE BLOOD CELLS AND RESISTANCE OF THE BODY TO INFECTION

Our bodies normally are exposed to bacteria, viruses, fungi, and parasites, which occur especially in the skin, the mouth, the respiratory passageways, the intestinal tract, the lining membranes of the eyes, and even the urinary tract. Many of these agents are capable of causing serious disease if they invade the deeper tissues. In addition, we are exposed intermittently to other highly infectious bacteria and viruses besides those that are normally present in our bodies, and these cause lethal diseases such as pneumonia, streptococcal infection, and typhoid fever.

Fortunately, our bodies have a special system for combating the different infectious and toxic agents. This is composed of the blood leukocytes (the white blood cells) and tissue cells derived from the leukocytes. These cells all work together in two different ways to prevent disease: (1) by actually destroying invading agents by the process of phagocytosis and (2) by forming antibodies and sensitized lymphocytes, one or both of which may destroy the invader.

THE LEUKOCYTES (WHITE BLOOD CELLS)

The leukocytes are the *mobile units* of the body's protective system. They are formed partially in the bone marrow (the *granulocytes* and *monocytes,* and a few *lymphocytes*) and partially in the lymph tissue (*lymphocytes* and *plasma cells*). The real value of the white blood cells is that most of them are specifically transported in the blood to areas of serious inflammation, thereby providing a rapid and potent defense against any infectious agent that might be present. As we see later, the granulocytes and monocytes have a special capability to "seek out and destroy" any foreign invader.

General Characteristics of Leukocytes

The Types of White Blood Cells. Six different types of white blood cells are normally found in the blood. These are *polymorphonuclear neutrophils, polymorphonuclear eosinophils, polymorphonuclear basophils, monocytes, lymphocytes,* and occasional *plasma cells.* In addition, there are large numbers of *platelets,* which are fragments of a seventh type of white cell found in the bone marrow, the *megakaryocyte.* The three types of polymorphonuclear cells have a granular appearance, as illustrated in Figure 24–7, for which reason they are called *granulocytes,* or, in clinical terminology, simply "polys."

The granulocytes and the monocytes protect the body against invading organisms by ingesting them—that is, by the process of *phagocytosis.* The lymphocytes and plasma cells function mainly in connection with the immune system; this is discussed in the following chapter. However, a function of certain lymphocytes is to attach themselves to specific invading organisms and destroy them, an action similar to those of the granulocytes and monocytes. Finally, the function of platelets is mainly to activate the blood-clotting mechanism, which is discussed in Chapter 26.

Concentrations of the Different White Blood Cells in the Blood. The adult human being has approximately 7000 white blood cells per microliter of blood. The normal percentages of the different types of white blood cells are approximately the following:

Polymorphonuclear neutrophils	62.0%
Polymorphonuclear eosinophils	2.3%
Polymorphonuclear basophils	0.4%
Monocytes	5.3%
Lymphocytes	30.0%

The number of platelets, which are only cell fragments, in each microliter of blood is normally about 300,000.

Genesis of the Leukocytes

The early differentiation of the pluripotential hemopoietic stem cell into the different types of committed stem cells was illustrated in Figure 24–1 earlier in the chapter. Aside from those cells committed to the formation of red blood cells, two major lineages of *white blood cells* are also formed, the myelocytic and the lymphocytic lineages. To the left in Figure 24–7 is illustrated the *myelocytic lineage* beginning with the *myeloblast;* to the right is illustrated the *lymphocytic lineage* beginning with the *lymphoblast.*

The granulocytes and monocytes are formed only in the bone marrow. Lymphocytes and plasma cells are produced mainly in the various lymphogenous organs, including the lymph glands, the spleen, the thymus, the tonsils, and various lymphoid rests in the bone marrow, gut, and elsewhere.

The white blood cells formed in the bone marrow, especially the granulocytes, are stored within the marrow until they are needed in the circulatory system. Then when the need arises, various factors that are discussed later cause them to be released. Normally, about three times as many granulocytes are stored in the marrow as circulate in the entire blood. This represents about a 6-day supply of granulocytes.

Life Span of the White Blood Cells

The main reason white blood cells are present in the blood is simply to be transported from the bone marrow or lymphoid tissue to the areas of the body where they are needed. The life of the granulocytes once released from the bone marrow is normally 4 to 8 hours circulating in the blood and another 4 to 5 days in the tissues. In times of serious tissue infection, this total life span is often shortened to only a few hours because the granulocytes then proceed rapidly to the infected area, perform their functions, and in the process are themselves destroyed.

The monocytes also have a short transit time, 10 to 20 hours, in the blood before wandering through the capillary membranes into the tissues. However, once in the tissues they swell to much larger sizes to become *tissue macrophages* and in this form can live for months or even years unless destroyed by performing phagocytic function.

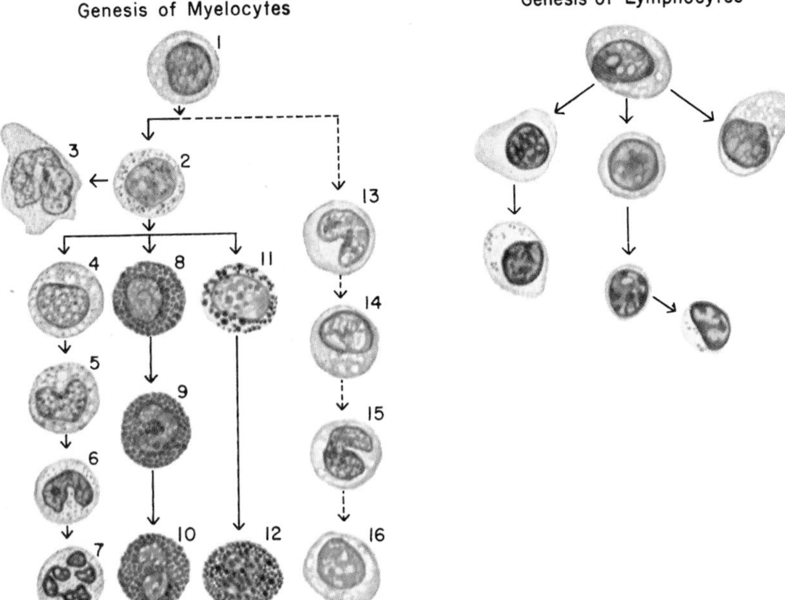

Figure 24-7. Genesis of the white blood cells. The different cells of the myelogenous series are 1, myeloblast; 2, promyelocyte; 3, megakaryocyte; 4, neutrophil myelocyte; 5, young neutrophil metamyelocyte; 6, "band" neutrophil metamyelocyte; 7, polymorphonuclear neutrophil; 8, eosinophil myelocyte; 9, eosinophil metamyelocyte; 10, polymorphonuclear eosinophil; 11, basophil myelocyte; 12, polymorphonuclear basophil; 13-16, stages of monocyte formation.

Lymphocytes enter the circulatory system continually along with the drainage of lymph from the lymph nodes. Then, after a few hours, they pass back into the tissues by diapedesis, then re-enter the lymph and return to the blood again and again; thus, there is continual circulation of the lymphocytes through the tissues. The lymphocytes have life spans of months or even years, but this depends on the body's need for these cells.

DEFENSIVE PROPERTIES OF NEUTROPHILS AND MONOCYTE-MACROPHAGES

It is mainly the neutrophils and the monocytes that attack and destroy invading bacteria, viruses, and other injurious agents. The neutrophils are mature cells that can attack and destroy bacteria and viruses even in the circulating blood. On the other hand, the blood monocytes are immature cells that have very little ability to fight infectious agents. However, once they enter the tissues, they begin to swell, sometimes increasing their diameters as much as fivefold, to as great as 80 micrometers, a size that can be seen with the naked eye. Also, extremely large numbers of lysosomes develop in the cytoplasm, giving the cytoplasm the appearance of a bag filled with granules. These cells are now called *macrophages,* and they are extremely capable of combating disease agents.

Ameboid Motion. Both neutrophils and macrophages move through the tissues by ameboid motion, which was described in Chapter 2. Some of the cells can move at velocities as great as 40 μm/min, several times their own length each minute.

Chemotaxis. Many different chemical substances in the tissues cause both neutrophils and macrophages to move toward the source of the chemical. This phenomenon, illustrated in Figure 24-8, is known as *chemotaxis.* When a tissue becomes inflamed, at least a dozen different products are formed that can cause chemotaxis toward the inflamed area. These include especially (1) some of the bacterial toxins, (2) degenerative products of the inflamed tissues themselves, and (3) several reaction products of the "complement complex" (discussed in the following chapter).

Phagocytosis

The most important function of the neutrophils and macrophages is phagocytosis.

Obviously, phagocytes must be selective of the material that is phagocytized, or otherwise some of the normal cells and structures of the body would be in-

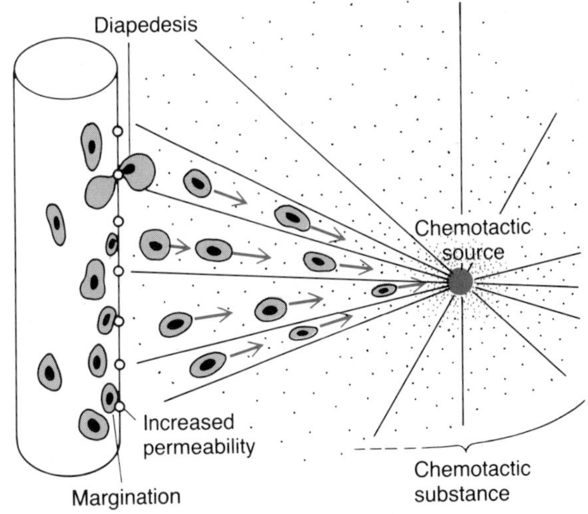

Figure 24-8. Movement of neutrophils by the process of *chemotaxis* toward an area of tissue damage.

gested. Whether or not phagocytosis will occur depends especially upon three selective procedures. First, if the surface of a particle is rough, the likelihood of phagocytosis is increased. Second, most natural substances of the body have protective protein coats that repel the phagocytes. On the other hand, dead tissues and foreign particles frequently have no protective coats, and many are also strongly electrically charged, which also makes them subject to phagocytosis. Third, the body has a specific means of recognizing certain foreign materials. This is a function of the immune system that is described in the following chapter. The immune system develops antibodies against infectious agents like bacteria. A portion of the antibody then adheres to the bacterial membrane and thereby makes the bacterium especially susceptible to phagocytosis.

Phagocytosis by Neutrophils. The neutrophils entering the tissues are already mature cells that can immediately begin phagocytosis. On approaching a particle to be phagocytized, the neutrophil first attaches itself to the particle, then projects pseudopodia in all directions around the particle, and the pseudopodia meet each other on the opposite side and fuse. This creates an enclosed chamber containing the phagocytized particle. Then the chamber invaginates to the inside of the cytoplasmic cavity and breaks away from the outer cell membrane to form a free-floating *phagocytic vesicle* (also called a *phagosome*) inside the cytoplasm.

A neutrophil can usually phagocytize 5 to 20 bacteria before the neutrophil itself becomes inactivated and dies.

Phagocytosis by Macrophages. Macrophages, when activated by the immune system as described in the following chapter, are much more powerful phagocytes than the neutrophils, often capable of phagocytizing as many as 100 bacteria. They also have the ability to engulf much larger particles, even whole red blood cells, or malarial parasites; whereas neutrophils are not capable of phagocytizing particles much larger than bacteria. Also, macrophages, after digesting particles, can extrude the residual products and often survive many more months.

Enzymatic Digestion of the Phagocytized Particles. Once a foreign particle has been phagocytized, lysosomes and other cytoplasmic granules immediately come in contact with the phagocytic vesicle, and their membranes fuse with those of the vesicle, thereby dumping many digestive enzymes and bactericidal agents into the vesicle. Thus, the phagocytic vesicle now becomes a *digestive vesicle,* and digestion of the phagocytized particle occurs almost immediately.

THE MONOCYTE-MACROPHAGE SYSTEM—THE "RETICULOENDOTHELIAL SYSTEM"

In the above paragraphs we have described the macrophages mainly as mobile cells that are capable of wandering through the tissues. However, a large portion of the monocytes, on entering the tissues and after becoming macrophages, become attached to the tissues and remain attached for months or perhaps even years unless they are called upon to perform specific protective functions. They have the same capabilities as the mobile macrophages to phagocytize large quantities of bacteria, viruses, necrotic tissue, or other foreign particles in the tissue. When appropriately stimulated, they can break away from their attachments and become mobile macrophages.

The combination of monocytes, mobile macrophages, fixed tissue macrophages, and a few specialized endothelial cells in the bone marrow, spleen, and lymph nodes constitutes the *monocyte-macrophage system,* but it is also frequently called the *reticuloendothelial system* because it was formerly believed that the macrophages originated from endothelial cells.

Macrophages of the Lymph Nodes. Essentially no particulate matter that enters the tissues can be absorbed directly through the capillary membranes into the blood. Instead, if the particles are not destroyed locally in the tissues, they enter the lymph and flow through the lymphatic vessels to the lymph nodes located intermittently along the course of the lymph vessel. The foreign particles are trapped there in a meshwork of sinuses lined by *tissue macrophages.*

Figure 24–9 illustrates the general organization of the lymph node, showing lymph entering by way of the *afferent lymphatics,* flowing through the *medullary sinuses,* and finally passing out of the *hilus* into the *efferent lymphatics.* Large numbers of macrophages line the sinuses, and, if any particles enter the sinuses, the macrophages phagocytize them and prevent general dissemination throughout the body.

Alveolar Macrophages. Another route by which invading organisms frequently enter the body is through the respiratory system. Fortunately, large numbers of tissue macrophages are also present as integral components of the alveolar walls. These can phagocytize particles that become entrapped in the alveoli, especially bacteria from the inspired air.

Tissue Macrophages (Kupffer's Cells) in the Liver Sinuses. Still another favorite route by which bacteria invade the body is through the gastrointesti-

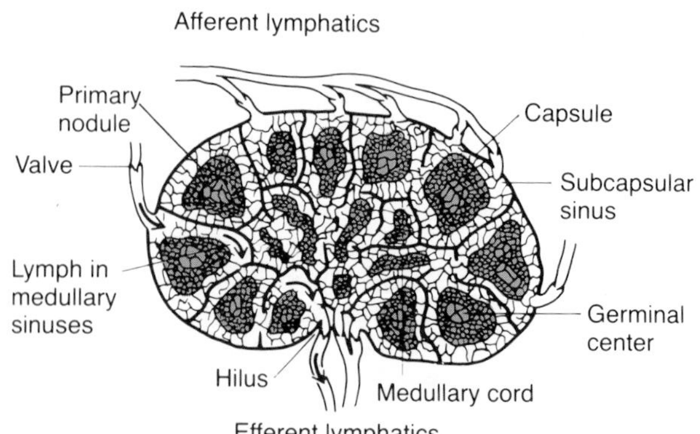

Figure 24–9. Functional diagram of a lymph node. (Redrawn from Ham: Histology. Philadelphia, J. B. Lippincott Company, 1971.)

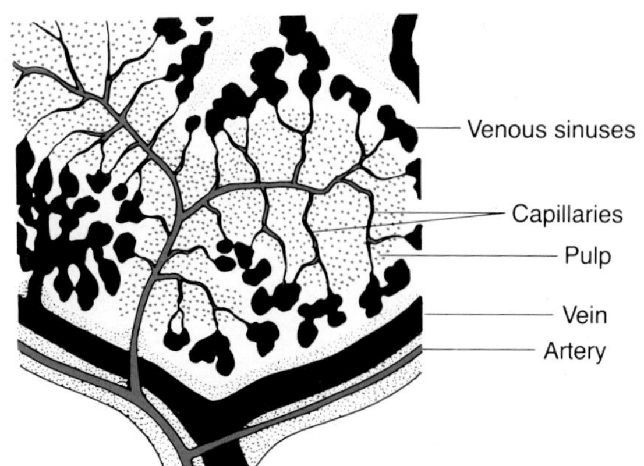

Figure 24-10. Functional structures of the spleen. (Modified from Bloom and Fawcett: Textbook of Histology. Philadelphia, W. B. Saunders Company, 1975.)

nal tract. Large numbers of bacteria constantly pass through the gastrointestinal mucosa into the portal blood. However, before this blood enters the general circulation, it must pass through the sinuses of the liver; these sinuses are lined with tissue macrophages called *Kupffer's cells.* These cells form such an effective particulate filtration system that almost none of the bacteria from the gastrointestinal tract succeeds in passing from the portal blood into the general systemic circulation.

Macrophages of the Spleen and Bone Marrow. If an invading organism does succeed in entering the general circulation, there still remain other lines of defense by the tissue macrophage system, especially by macrophages of the spleen and bone marrow.

The spleen is similar to the lymph nodes, except that blood, instead of lymph, flows through the substance of the spleen. Figure 24-10 illustrates the spleen's general structure, showing a small peripheral segment. Note that a small artery penetrates from the splenic capsule into the *splenic pulp* and terminates in small capillaries. The capillaries are highly porous, allowing large numbers of whole blood cells to pass out of the capillaries into the *cords of the red pulp.* These cells then gradually *squeeze* through the trabecular meshwork of the cords and eventually return to the circulation through the endothelial walls of the *venous sinuses.* The trabeculae of the red pulp are lined with vast numbers of macrophages, and the venous sinuses are also lined with macrophages. This peculiar passage of blood through the cords of the red pulp provides an exceptional means of phagocytosis of unwanted debris in the blood, especially old and abnormal red blood cells.

INFLAMMATION AND FUNCTION OF NEUTROPHILS AND MACROPHAGES

The Process of Inflammation

When tissue injury occurs, whether caused by bacteria, trauma, chemicals, heat, or any other phenomenon, multiple substances that cause dramatic secondary changes in the tissues are released by the injured tissues. The entire complex of tissue changes is called *inflammation.*

The "Walling-Off" Effect of Inflammation. One of the first results of inflammation is to "wall off" the area of injury from the remaining tissues. The tissue spaces and the lymphatics in the inflamed area are blocked by fibrinogen clots so that fluid barely flows through the spaces. Therefore, this walling-off process delays the spread of bacteria or toxic products.

The intensity of the inflammatory process is usually proportional to the degree of tissue injury. For instance, staphylococci invading the tissues liberate extremely lethal cellular toxins. As a result, the process of inflammation develops rapidly—indeed, much more rapidly than the staphylococci themselves can multiply and spread. Therefore, staphylococcal infection is characteristically walled off rapidly. On the other hand, streptococci do not cause such intense local tissue destruction. Therefore, the walling-off process develops slowly. As a result, streptococci have a far greater tendency to spread through the body and cause death than do staphylococci, even though staphylococci are far more destructive to the tissues.

The Macrophage and Neutrophil Response to Inflammation

The Tissue Macrophage as the First Line of Defense. Within minutes after inflammation begins, those macrophages already present in the tissues immediately begin their phagocytic actions. Next, many of the previously sessile macrophages break loose from their attachments and become mobile, forming the first line of defense against infection during the first hour or so.

Neutrophil Invasion of the Inflamed Area—The Second Line of Defense. Also within the first hour or so after inflammation begins, large numbers of neutrophils begin to invade the inflamed area from the blood. This is caused by products from the inflamed tissues that attract these cells and cause chemotaxis toward the point of inflammation.

Acute Increase in Neutrophils in the Blood—"Neutrophilia." Also within a few hours after the onset of acute, severe inflammation, the number of neutrophils in the blood sometimes increases as much as four- to fivefold—to as high as 15,000 to 25,000 per microliter. This is called *neutrophilia,* which means an increase in the number of neutrophils in the blood. Neutrophilia is caused by products of the inflammation that enter the blood stream, then are transported to the bone marrow, and there act on the marrow capillaries and on stored neutrophils to mobilize these immediately into the circulating blood. This obviously makes more neutrophils available to the inflamed tissue area.

Monocyte-Macrophage Invasion of the Inflamed Tissue—The Third Line of Defense. Along with the invasion of neutrophils, monocytes from the blood also enter the inflamed tissue. However, the number of monocytes in the circulating blood is low; also, the storage pool of monocytes in the bone marrow is much less than that of neutrophils. Therefore, the buildup of monocytes in the inflamed tissue area is much slower than that of neutrophils. Yet after several days to several weeks, the macrophages finally come to dominate the phagocytic cells of the inflamed area because of greatly increased bone marrow production of monocytes, as explained below.

Increased Production of Granulocytes and Monocytes by the Bone Marrow—The Fourth Line of Defense. The fourth line of defense is greatly increased production of granulocytes and monocytes by the bone marrow. This results from stimulation of the committed granulocytic and monocytic stem cells. However, it takes 3 to 4 days before newly formed granulocytes and monocytes reach the stage of leaving the bone marrow. If the stimulus from the inflamed tissue continues, the bone marrow can continue to produce these cells, especially monocytes, in tremendous quantities for months and even for years, sometimes at rates of production as great as 50 times normal.

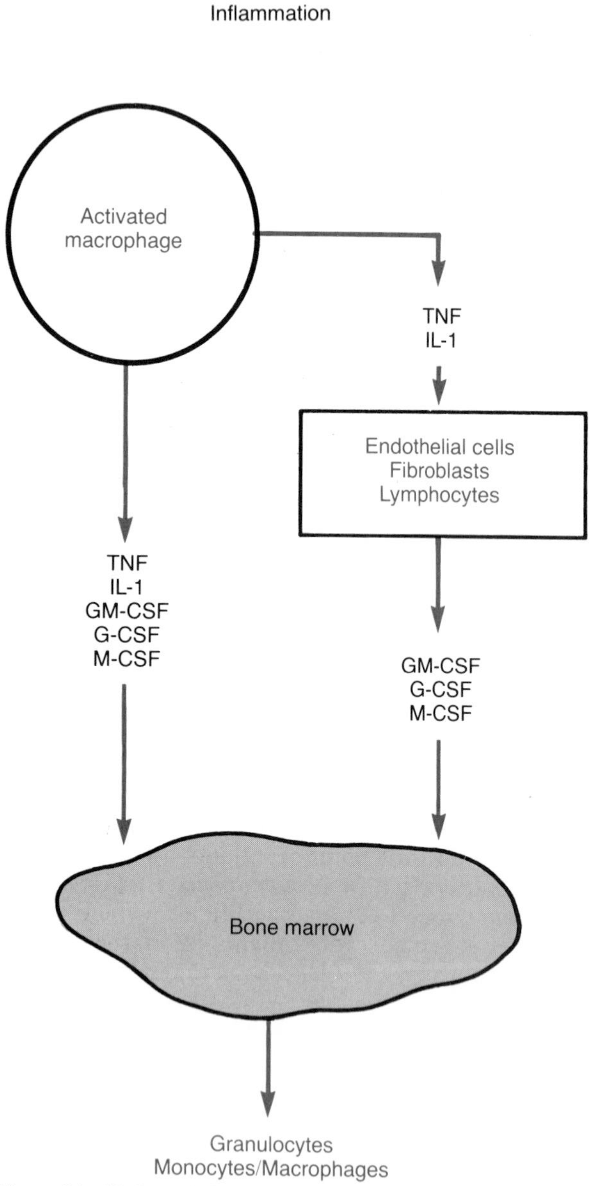

Figure 24-11. Control of bone marrow production of granulocytes and monocyte-macrophages in response to multiple growth factors released from activated macrophages in an inflamed tissue. (TNF, tissue necrosis factor; IL-1, interleukin-1; GM-CSF, granulocyte-monocyte colony-stimulating factor; G-CSF, granulocyte colony-stimulating factor; M-CSF, monocyte-macrophage colony-stimulating factor.)

Feedback Control of the Macrophage and Neutrophil Responses

Though more than two dozen different factors have been implicated in the control of the macrophage-neutrophil response to inflammation, five of these are believed to play dominant roles. These are illustrated in Figure 24-11: (1) *tumor necrosis factor* (TNF), (2) *interleukin-1* (IL-1), (3) *granulocyte-monocyte colony-stimulating factor* (GM-CSF), (4) *granulocyte colony-stimulating factor* (G-CSF), and (5) *monocyte colony-stimulating factor* (M-CSF).

Thus, a powerful feedback mechanism begins with tissue inflammation, then formation of defensive white blood cells, and finally removal of the cause of the inflammation by the activated monocyte-macrophage system.

THE EOSINOPHILS

The eosinophils normally comprise 2 to 3 per cent of all the blood leukocytes. Eosinophils are weak phagocytes, and they exhibit chemotaxis, but in comparison with the neutrophils it is doubtful that the eosinophils are of significant importance in protection against the usual types of infection.

On the other hand, eosinophils are often produced in very large numbers in persons with parasitic infections, and they migrate into tissues diseased by parasites. Though most of the parasites are too large to be phagocytized by the eosinophils or by any other phagocytic cells, nevertheless the eosinophils attach themselves to the parasites and release substances that kill many of them.

Eosinophils also have a special propensity to collect in tissues in which allergic reactions have occurred, such as in the peribronchial tissues of the lungs in asthmatic persons, in the skin after allergic skin reactions, and so forth. The eosinophils are believed to detoxify some inflammation-inducing substances, thus preventing spread of the local inflammatory process.

THE BASOPHILS

The basophils in the circulating blood are very similar to, though not identical with, the large *mast* cells located immediately outside many of the capillaries in the body. Both these cells liberate *heparin* into the blood, a substance that can prevent blood coagulation and that can also speed the removal of fat particles from the blood after a fatty meal.

The mast cells and basophils play an exceedingly potent role in some types of allergic reactions because the type of antibody that causes allergic reactions, the IgE type (see Chapter 25), has a special propensity to become attached to mast cells and basophils. Then, when the specific antigen subsequently reacts with the antibody, the mast cell or basophil ruptures and releases exceedingly large quantities of histamine, bradykinin, serotonin, heparin, slow-reacting substance of anaphylaxis, and a number of lysosomal enzymes. These in turn cause local vascular and tissue reactions that cause the allergic manifestations. These are discussed in greater detail in the following chapter.

LEUKOPENIA

A clinical condition known as leukopenia (or *agranulocytosis*) occasionally occurs, in which the bone marrow stops producing white blood cells, leaving the body unprotected against bacteria and other agents that might invade the tissues.

Normally, the human body lives in symbiosis with many bacteria, for all the mucous membranes of the body are constantly exposed to large numbers of bacteria. The mouth almost always contains various spirochetal, pneumococcal, and streptococcal bacteria, and these same bacteria are present to a lesser extent in the entire respiratory tract. The gastrointestinal tract is especially loaded with colon bacilli. Furthermore, one can always find bacteria in the eyes, the urethra, and the vagina. Therefore, any decrease in the number of white blood cells immediately allows invasion of the tissues by the bacteria that are already present in the body. Within 2 days after the bone marrow stops producing white blood cells, ulcers may appear in the mouth and colon, or the person develops some form of severe respiratory infection. Bacteria from the ulcers then rapidly invade the surrounding tissues and the blood. Without treatment, death often ensues 3 to 6 days after acute total leukopenia begins.

Irradiation of the body by gamma rays caused by a nuclear explosion, or exposure to drugs and chemicals containing benzene or anthracene nuclei, is especially likely to cause aplasia of the bone marrow.

THE LEUKEMIAS

Types of Leukemia. Leukemias are divided into two general types: the *lymphogenous leukemias* and the *myelogenous leukemias.* The lymphogenous leukemias are caused by uncontrolled cancerous production of lymphoid cells, usually beginning in a lymph node or other lymphogenous tissue and then spreading to other areas of the body. The second type of leukemia, myelogenous leukemia, begins by cancerous production of young myelogenous cells in the bone marrow and then spreads throughout the body so that white blood cells are produced in many extramedullary organs.

Leukemic cells are usually nonfunctional, so they cannot provide the usual protection against infection associated with white blood cells.

The first effect of leukemia usually is metastatic growth of leukemic cells in abnormal areas of the body. The leukemic cells of the bone marrow may reproduce so greatly that they invade the surrounding bone, causing pain and eventually a tendency to easy fracture. Almost all leukemias spread to the spleen, the lymph nodes, the liver, and other especially vascular regions, regardless of whether the origin of the leukemia is in the bone marrow or in the lymph nodes. In each of these areas the rapidly growing cells invade the surrounding tissues, utilizing the metabolic elements of these tissues and consequently causing tissue destruction.

Very common effects in leukemia are the development of infections, severe anemia, and bleeding tendency caused by thrombocytopenia (lack of platelets). These effects result mainly from displacement of the normal bone marrow by the nonfunctional leukemic cells.

Finally, perhaps the most important effect of leukemia on the body is the excessive use of metabolic substrates by the growing cancerous cells. The leukemic tissues reproduce new cells so rapidly that tremendous demands are made on the body fluids for foodstuffs, especially the amino acids and vitamins. Consequently, the energy of the patient is greatly depleted, and the excessive utilization of amino acids causes rapid deterioration of the normal protein tissues of the body.

REFERENCES

Red Blood Cells

Barnes, D. M.: Blood-forming stem cells purified. Science, 241:24, 1988.

Bauer, C., and Kurtz, A.: Oxygen sensing in the kidney and its relation to erythropoietin production. Annu. Rev. Physiol., 51:845, 1989.

Clark, M. R.: Senescence of red blood cells: Progress and problems. Physiol. Rev., 68:503, 1988.

Golde, D. W., and Gasson, J. C.: Hormones that stimulate the growth of blood cells. Sci. Am., July 1988, p. 62.

Huebers, H. A., and Finch, C. A.: The physiology of transferrin and transferrin receptors. Physiol. Rev., 67:520, 1987.

Lee, G. R., et al.: Wintrobe's Clinical Hematology. 9th ed. Philadelphia, Lea & Febiger, 1989.

Miller, D. R., et al. (eds.): Blood Diseases of Infancy and Childhood. St. Louis, C. V. Mosby Co., 1989.

White Blood Cells

Dinarello, C. A.: Biology of interleukin-1. FASEB J., 2:108, 1988.
Gallin, J. I., et al.: Inflammation: Basic Principles and Clinical Correlates. New York, Raven Press, 1988.
Henderson, E. S., and Lister, T. A.: Leukemia. 5th ed. Philadelphia, W. B. Saunders Co., 1989.
Hogg, J. C.: Neutrophil kinetics and lung injury. Physiol. Rev., 67:1249, 1987.
Pardoll, D. M., et al.: The unfolding story of T cell receptor c. FASEB J., 1:103, 1987.
Schmid-Schonbein, G. W.: Granulocyte: Friend and foe. News Physiol. Sci., 3:144, 1988.
Williams, W. J., et al. (eds.): Hematology. 4th ed. New York, McGraw-Hill Book Co., 1990.
Young, J. D.: Killing of target cells by lymphocytes: A mechanistic view. Physiol. Rev., 69:250, 1989.

QUESTIONS

1. Describe the functions of the red blood cells.
2. Where are the red blood cells formed, and what are the stages of their formation?
3. Explain the roles of tissue oxygenation and *erythropoietin* in the regulation of red blood cell production.
4. What important vitamins are required for proper formation of red blood cells and why?
5. List the important features of the hemoglobin molecule, and describe its chemical method for transporting oxygen to the tissues.
6. Describe the mechanisms of absorption of iron from the gut, its transport in the blood, and its storage in the liver.
7. How is the total body iron controlled?
8. What is the average life span of the red blood cell, and how are the old cells destroyed? What happens to the hemoglobin and the iron of the destroyed cells?
9. Describe the characteristics of several types of anemia.
10. Describe the different types of white blood cells, and state their relative percentages in the blood.
11. Describe the formation and life span of the different white blood cells.
12. List the specific properties of *neutrophils* and *macrophages* for the phagocytosis of bacteria and tissue debris.
13. Describe the anatomy and the function of the *monocyte-macrophage system* of the body.
14. Discuss the roles of the neutrophils and macrophages in *inflammation.*
15. What controls the numbers of neutrophils and macrophages?
16. Discuss the role of the *eosinophils* for protection against parasites and the role of these white blood cells in allergy.
17. Discuss the roles of the *basophils* in blood coagulation and in allergy.
18. What types of *leukemic cells* are frequently formed, and what are the effects of leukemia on the body?

25

Immunity, Allergy, Blood Groups, and Transfusion

INNATE IMMUNITY

The human body has the ability to resist almost all types of organisms or toxins that tend to damage the tissues and organs. This capacity is called *immunity.* Much of immunity is caused by a special immune system that forms antibodies and activated lymphocytes that attack and destroy the specific organisms or toxins. This type of immunity is called *acquired immunity.* However, an additional portion of immunity results from general processes, rather than from processes directed at specific disease organisms. This is called *innate immunity.* It includes the following:

1. Phagocytosis of bacteria and other invaders by white blood cells and cells of the tissue macrophage system, as described in the previous chapter.
2. Destruction by the acid secretions of the stomach and by the digestive enzymes of organisms swallowed into the stomach.
3. Resistance of the skin to invasion by organisms.
4. Presence in the blood of certain chemical compounds that attach to foreign organisms or toxins and destroy them.

This innate immunity makes the human body resistant to such diseases as some paralytic viral infections of animals, hog cholera, cattle plague, and distemper — a viral disease that kills a large percentage of dogs that become afflicted with it. On the other hand, lower animals are resistant or even completely immune to many human diseases, such as poliomyelitis, mumps, human cholera, measles, and syphilis, which are very destructive or even lethal to the human being.

ACQUIRED IMMUNITY

In addition to its innate immunity, the human body also has the ability to develop extremely powerful specific immunity, called *acquired immunity*, against individual invading agents such as lethal bacteria, viruses, toxins, and even foreign tissues from other animals.

Acquired immunity can often bestow extreme protection. For instance, certain toxins such as the paralytic toxin of botulinum or the tetanizing toxin of tetanus can be protected against in doses as high as 100,000 times the amount that would be lethal without immunity. This is the reason the process known as "vaccination" is so extremely important in protecting human beings against disease and against toxins, as is explained in the course of this chapter.

Two Basic Types of Acquired Immunity

Two basic, but closely allied, types of acquired immunity occur in the body. In one of these the body develops circulating *antibodies,* which are globulin molecules that are capable of attacking the invading agent. This type of immunity is called *humoral immunity* or *B cell immunity.* The second type of acquired immunity is achieved through the formation of large numbers of *activated lymphocytes* that are specifically designed to destroy the foreign agent. This type of immunity is called *cell-mediated immunity* or *T cell immunity.*

We shall see shortly that both the antibodies and the activated lymphocytes are formed in the lymphoid tissue of the body. First, let us discuss the initiation of the immune process by *antigens.*

Antigens

Because acquired immunity does not occur until after invasion by a foreign organism or toxin, it is clear that the body must have some mechanism for recognizing the invasion. Each toxin or each type of organism almost always contains one or more specific chemical compounds in its makeup that are different from all other compounds. In general, these are proteins or large polysaccharides, and these are what initiate the acquired immunity. These substances are called *antigens.*

For a substance to be antigenic it usually must have a high molecular weight, usually 8000 or greater. Furthermore, the process of antigenicity depends upon regularly recurring molecular groups, called *epitopes,* on the surface of the large molecule, which explains why proteins and large polysaccharides are almost always antigenic, for they both have this type of stereochemical characteristic.

Role of Lymphocytes in Acquired Immunity

Acquired immunity is the product of the body's lymphocyte system. The lymphocytes are located most extensively in the *lymph nodes,* but they are also found in special lymphoid tissues such as the *spleen, submucosal areas of the gastrointestinal tract,* and the *bone marrow.* The lymphoid tissue is distributed very advantageously in the body to intercept the invading organisms or toxins before they can spread too widely. For instance, the lymphoid tissue of the gastrointestinal tract is exposed immediately to antigens invading through the gut. The lymphoid tissue of the throat and pharynx (the tonsils and adenoids) is extremely well located to intercept antigens that enter by way of the upper respiratory tract. The lymphoid tissue in the lymph nodes is exposed to antigens that invade the peripheral tissues of the body. And, finally, the lymphoid tissue of the spleen and bone marrow plays the specific role of intercepting antigenic agents that have succeeded in reaching the circulating blood.

Two Types of Lymphocytes That Promote, Respectively, Cell-Mediated Immunity and Humoral Immunity—The T and the B Lymphocytes. Though most of the lymphocytes in normal lymphoid tissue look alike when studied under the microscope, these cells are distinctly divided into two major populations. One of the populations is responsible for forming the activated lymphocytes that provide *cell-mediated immunity* and the other for forming the antibodies that provide *humoral immunity.*

Both of these types of lymphocytes are derived originally in the embryo from *pluripotent hemopoietic stem cells* that differentiate and become committed to form lymphocytes. The lymphocytes that are formed eventually end up in the lymphoid tissue, but before doing so they are further differentiated or "preprocessed," as illustrated in Figure 25–1, in the following ways:

Those lymphocytes that are eventually destined to form activated lymphocytes first migrate to and are preprocessed in the *thymus* gland, for which reason they are called *T lymphocytes.* These are responsible for cell-mediated immunity.

The other population of lymphocytes—those that are destined to form antibodies—are preprocessed in the liver during midfetal life and in the bone marrow in late fetal life and after birth. However, this population of cells was first discovered in birds in which the preprocessing occurs in the *bursa of Fabricius,* a structure not found in mammals. For this reason these lymphocytes are called B lymphocytes, and they are responsible for humoral immunity.

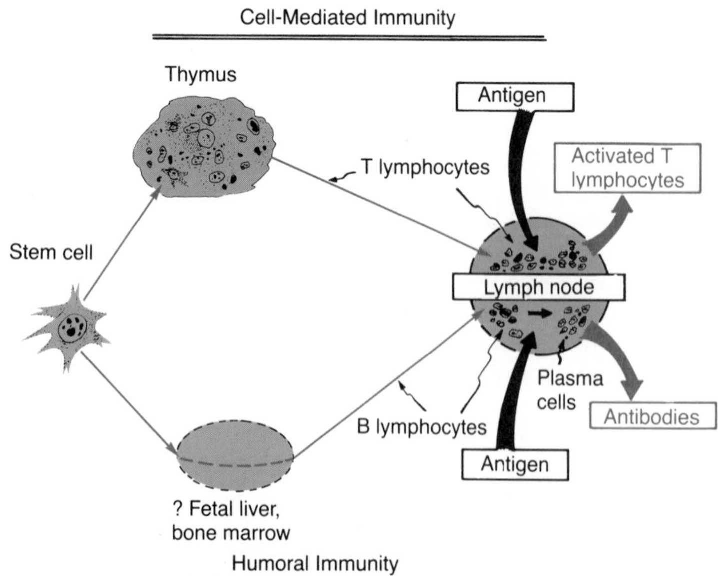

Figure 25–1. Formation of antibodies and sensitized lymphocytes by a lymph node in response to antigens. This figure also shows the origin of *thymic* (T) and *bursal* (B) lymphocytes that are responsible for the cell-mediated and humoral immune processes of the lymph nodes.

Preprocessing of the T and B Lymphocytes

Though all the lymphocytes of the body originate from the lymphocytic committed stem cells of the embryo, these stem cells are themselves incapable of forming either activated lymphocytes or antibodies. Before they can do so, they must be further differentiated in appropriate processing areas in the thymus or in the B cell processing area.

Role of the Thymus Gland in Preprocessing the T Lymphocytes. Most of the preprocessing of the T lymphocytes of the thymus gland occurs shortly before the birth of the baby and for a few months after birth. Therefore, beyond this period of time, removal of the thymus gland usually will not seriously impair the T lymphocytic immune system, the system necessary for cell-mediated immunity. However, removal of the thymus several months before birth can completely prevent development of all cell-mediated immunity.

Thymic Hormone. In addition to preprocessing the T lymphocytes, the thymus is believed by some research workers to secrete one or more stimulatory factors, collectively called *thymic hormone.* This hormone supposedly spreads through the body fluids and increases the activity of the T lymphocytes that have already left the thymus gland and have migrated to the lymphoid tissue. This hormone is believed to cause further proliferation and increased activity of these lymphocytes. Otherwise, little is known about either the nature or the function of this hormone.

Role of the Bursa of Fabricius for Preprocessing B Lymphocytes in Birds. During the latter part of fetal life the bursa of Fabricius preprocesses the B lymphocytes and prepares them to manufacture antibodies. Here again, this preprocessing continues for a while after birth. In mammals, it is believed that the B cells are preprocessed during midfetal life in the liver but thereafter in the bone marrow.

Spread of Processed Lymphocytes to the Lymphoid Tissue. After formation of processed lymphocytes in both the thymus and the bursa, these first circulate freely in the blood for a few hours but then become entrapped in the lymphoid tissue. Thus, lymphocytes do not originate primordially in the lymphoid tissue but, instead, are transported to this tissue by way of the preprocessing areas of the thymus and probably fetal liver and bone marrow.

Specificity of T Lymphocytes and Antibodies — Role of Lymphocyte Clones

When a specific antigen comes in contact with the T and B lymphocytes in the lymphoid tissue, certain of the T lymphocytes become activated to form "T cells," and certain of the B lymphocytes form antibodies. The T cells and antibodies in turn then react highly specifically against the particular type of antigen that initiated their development. The mechanism of this specificity is the following:

Millions of Preformed Specific Lymphocytes in the Lymphoid Tissue. There are at least a million different types of preformed B lymphocytes and equally as many preformed T lymphocytes that are capable of forming highly specific antibodies or T cells when stimulated by the appropriate antigens. Each one of these preformed lymphocytes is capable of forming only one type of antibody or one type of T cell with a single type of specificity. And only the specific type of antigen with which it can react can activate it. However, once the specific lymphocyte is activated by its antigen, it reproduces wildly, forming tremendous numbers of duplicate lymphocytes. If it is a B lymphocyte, its progeny will eventually secrete antibodies that then circulate throughout the body. If it is a T lymphocyte, its progeny are sensitized T cells that are released into the lymph and carried to the blood, then circulated through all the tissue fluids and back into the lymph, circulating around and around in this circuit sometimes for months or years.

All the different lymphocytes that are capable of forming one specificity of antibody or T cell are called a *clone of lymphocytes.* That is, the lymphocytes in each clone are alike and are derived originally from one or a few early lymphocytes of its specific type.

Origin of the Many Clones of Lymphocytes

Only about a thousand genes code for the different types of antibodies and T lymphocytes. At first, it was a mystery how it was possible for so few genes to code for the million or more different specificities of antibody molecules or T cells that can be produced by the lymphoid tissue, especially when one considers that a single gene is usually necessary for the formation of each different type of protein. However, the answer to this has now been discovered. During the preprocessing stage, the genes cause the formulation of large RNA molecules containing many small functional segments, each of which codes for an individual portion of an antibody or of a T cell "marker" (the protein on the T cell surface that gives it specificity), but not for the entire antibody or T cell marker. Then, while still in the nucleus, the RNA molecules are cut by enzymes into segments and respliced to form the final messenger RNA molecules. However, during this cutting and splicing the individual segments of the original RNA molecules are spliced in different combinations in different ones of the processed lymphocytes. And when one realizes that there are a thousand or more different genes, each coding for multiple segments of antibodies or cell markers, one can understand what a vast number of different combinations can be formed, giving rise to literally millions of possible antibody and T cell specificities.

Mechanism for Activating a Clone of Lymphocytes

Each clone of lymphocytes is responsive to only a single type of antigen (or to similar antigens that have almost exactly the same stereochemical characteristics). The reason for this is the following: In the case of the B lymphocytes, each one has on the surface of its cell membrane about 100,000 antibody molecules that will react highly specifically with only the one specific type of antigen. Therefore, when the appropriate antigen comes along, it immediately attaches to the cell membrane; this leads to the activation process, which we will describe in more detail subsequently. In the case of the T lymphocytes, molecules very similar to antibodies, called *surface receptor proteins* (or T cell markers), are on the surface of the cell membrane, and these too are highly specific for the one specified activating antigen.

Specific Attributes of the B Lymphocyte System — Humoral Immunity and the Antibodies

Formation of Antibodies by Plasma Cells. Prior to exposure to a specific antigen, the clones of B lymphocytes remain dormant in the lymphoid tissue. However, upon entry of a foreign antigen, the lymphoid tissue macrophages phagocytize the antigen and then present it to the adjacent B lymphocytes. In addition, the antigen is also presented to T cells at the same time, and activated "helper" T cells then also contribute to the activation of the B lymphocytes, as we discuss more fully later. Those B lymphocytes specific for the antigen immediately enlarge and take on the appearance of *lymphoblasts.* Some of these then further differentiate to form *plasma cells.* In these cells the cytoplasm expands and the rough endoplasmic reticulum vastly proliferates. The cells then divide at a rate of approximately once every 10 hours for about nine divisions, giving in 4 days a total population of about 500 plasma cells. The mature plasma cell then produces gamma globulin antibodies at an extremely rapid rate — about 2000 molecules per second for each plasma cell. The antibodies are secreted into the lymph and are carried to the circulating blood. This process continues for several days or weeks until death of the plasma cells.

Formation of "Memory" Cells — Difference Between the Primary Response and the Secondary Response. Some of the lymphoblasts formed by activation of a clone of B lymphocytes do not go on to form plasma cells, but, instead, form new B lymphocytes similar to those of the original clone. In other words, the population of the specifically activated clone becomes greatly enhanced. And the new B lymphocytes are added to the original lymphocytes of the clone. They also circulate throughout the body to inhabit all the lymphoid tissue, but immunologically they remain dormant until activated once again by a new quantity of the same antigen. They are called *memory cells.* Obviously, subsequent exposure to the same antigen will then cause a much more rapid and much more potent antibody response, because there are many more memory cells than there were original lymphocytes of the specific clone.

The increased potency and duration of the secondary response explains why *vaccination* is usually accomplished by injecting antigen in multiple doses with periods of several weeks or several months between injections.

The Nature of the Antibodies

The antibodies are gamma globulins called *immunoglobulins,* and they have molecular weights between approximately 150,000 and 900,000. Usually they constitute about 20 per cent of all the plasma proteins.

All the immunoglobulins are composed of combinations of *light* and *heavy polypeptide chains;* most are a combination of two light and two heavy chains, as illustrated in Figure 25 – 2. Some of the immunoglobulins, though, have combinations of as many as ten heavy and ten light chains, which gives rise to the much larger molecular weight immunoglobulins. Yet in all immunoglobulins, each heavy chain is paralleled by a light chain at one of its ends, thus forming a heavy-light pair, and there are always at least two such pairs in each immunoglobulin molecule.

Figure 25 – 2 shows a designated end of each of the light and each of the heavy chains, called the *variable portion;* the remainder of each chain is called the *constant portion.* The variable portion is different for each specificity of antibody, and it is this portion that attaches specifically to a particular type of antigen. The constant portion of the antibody determines other properties of the antibody, establishing such factors as diffusivity of the antibody in the tissues, adherence of the antibody to specific structures within the tissues, the ease with which the antibodies pass through membranes, and other biological properties of the antibody.

Specificity of Antibodies. Each antibody is specific for a particular antigen; this is caused by its unique structural organization of amino acids in the variable portions of both the light and heavy chains.

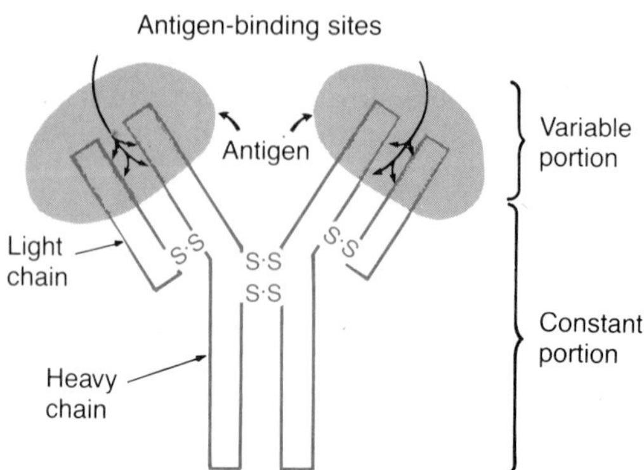

Figure 25 – 2. Structure of the typical IgG antibody, showing it to be composed of two heavy polypeptide chains and two light polypeptide chains. The antigen binds at two different sites on the variable portions of the chains.

These have a different steric shape for each antigen specificity, so that when an antigen comes in contact with it, the prosthetic groups of the antigen fit as a mirror image with those of the antibody, thus allowing rapid bonding between the antibody and the antigen. When the antibody is highly specific, there are so many bonding sites that the antibody-antigen coupling is exceedingly strong.

Note, especially, in Figure 25–2 that there are two variable sites on the illustrated antibody for attachment of antigens, making this type of antibody *bivalent.* However, a small proportion of the antibodies, which consist of combinations of up to 10 light and 10 heavy chains, have as many as ten *binding* sites.

Mechanisms of Action of Antibodies

Antibodies act mainly in two different ways to protect the body against invading agents: (1) by direct attack on the invader and (2) by activation of the complement system that then destroys the invader.

Direct Action of Antibodies on Invading Agents. Because of the bivalent nature of the antibodies and the multiple antigen sites on most invading agents, the antibodies can inactivate the invading agent in one of several ways, as follows:

1. *Agglutination,* in which multiple large particles with antigens on their surfaces, such as bacteria or red cells, are bound together into a clump.
2. *Precipitation,* in which the molecular complex of soluble antigen (such as tetanus toxin) and antibody becomes so large that it is rendered insoluble and precipitates.
3. *Neutralization,* in which the antibodies cover the toxic sites of the antigenic agent.
4. *Lysis,* in which some very potent antibodies are occasionally capable of directly attacking membranes of cellular agents and thereby causing rupture of the cell.

However, the direct actions of antibodies attacking the antigenic invaders, under normal conditions, are not strong enough to play a major role in protecting the body against the invader. Most of the protection comes through the *amplifying* effects of the complement system described next.

The Complement System for Antibody Action

"Complement" is a collective term to describe a system of about 20 different proteins, many of which are enzyme precursors. The principal actors in this system are 11 proteins designated C1 through C9, B, and D, illustrated in Figure 25–3. All these are present normally among the plasma proteins and also among the plasma proteins that leak out of the capillaries into the tissue spaces. The enzyme precursors are normally inactive, but they can be activated by the antigen-antibody reaction. That is, when an antibody binds with an antigen, a specific reactive site on the "constant" portion of the antibody becomes uncovered, or activated, and this in turn binds directly with the C1 molecule of the complement system, setting into motion a "cascade" of sequential reactions, illustrated in Figure 25–3, beginning with activation of the proenzyme C1 itself. A single antigen-antibody combination can activate many molecules of proenzyme. The C1 enzymes thus formed *then activate successively increasing quantities of enzymes* in each successive stage of the system, so that from a very small beginning an extremely large "amplified" reaction occurs. Multiple end-products are formed, as illustrated in the figure, and several of these cause important effects that help prevent damage by the invading organism or toxin. Among the more important effects are the following:

1. *Opsonization* and *phagocytosis.* One of the products of the complement cascade, C3b, strongly activates phagocytosis by both neutrophils and

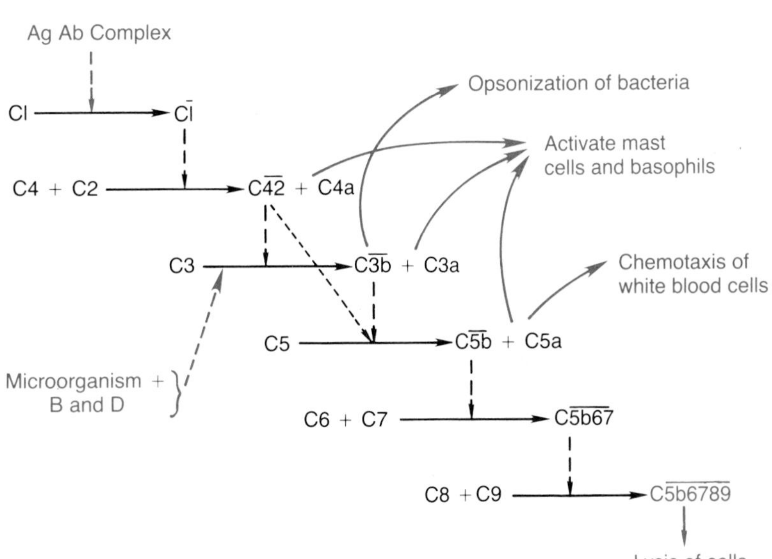

Figure 25–3. Cascade of reactions during activation of the classical pathway of complement. (Modified from Alexander and Good: Fundamentals of Clinical Immunology. Philadelphia, W. B. Saunders Company, 1977.)

macrophages, causing them to engulf the bacteria to which the antigen-antibody complexes are attached. This process is called *opsonization.* It often enhances the number of bacteria that can be destroyed by many hundredfold.

2. *Lysis.* One of the most important of all the products of the complement cascade is the *lytic complex,* which is a combination of multiple complement factors and is designated C5b6789. This has a direct effect of rupturing the cell membranes of bacteria or other invading organisms.
3. *Agglutination.* The complement products also change the surfaces of the invading organisms, causing them to adhere to each other, thus promoting agglutination.
4. *Neutralization of viruses.* The complement enzymes and other complement products can attack the structures of some viruses and thereby render them nonvirulent.
5. *Activation of mast cells and basophils.* Fragments C3a, C4a, and C5a all activate mast cells and basophils, causing them to release histamine and several other substances into the local fluids. These substances in turn cause increased local blood flow, increased leakage of fluid and plasma protein into the tissue, and other local tissue reactions that help inactivate or immobilize the antigenic agent.

Special Attributes of the T Lymphocyte System—Activated T Cells and "Cell-Mediated Immunity"

Release of Activated T Cells from Lymphoid Tissue, and Formation of Memory Cells. Upon exposure to the proper antigens, as presented by adjacent macrophages, the T lymphocytes of the lymphoid tissue proliferate and release large numbers of activated T cells in ways that parallel antibody release. The principal difference is that instead of releasing antibodies, whole activated T cells are formed and released into the lymph. These then pass into the circulation and are distributed throughout the body, passing through the capillary walls into the tissue spaces, back into the lymph and blood once again, and circulating again and again throughout the body, sometimes lasting for months or even years.

Also, *T lymphocyte memory cells* are formed in the same way that memory cells are formed in the humoral antibody system. Therefore, on subsequent exposure to the same antigen, the release of activated T cells occurs far more rapidly and much more powerfully than in the first response.

Antigen Receptors on the T Lymphocytes. Antigens bind with *receptor molecules* on the surfaces of T cells in the same way that they bind with antibodies. These receptor molecules are composed of a variable unit similar to the variable portion of the humoral antibody, but its stem section is firmly bound to the cell membrane. Therefore, it is never secreted from the cell into the body fluids. There are as many as 100,000 receptor sites on a single T cell.

The Many Types of T Cells and Their Functions

In the last few years it has become clear that there are many different types of T cells. These are classified into three major groups: *(1) helper T cells, (2) cytotoxic T cells,* and *(3) suppressor T cells.* The functions of each of these are quite distinct.

The Helper T Cells—Their Role in Overall Regulation of Immunity

The helper T cells are by far the most numerous of the T cells, usually constituting more than three quarters of all of them. As their name implies, they help in the functions of the immune system in many ways. In fact, they serve as the major regulator of virtually all immune functions, as illustrated in Figure 25–4. They do this by forming a series of protein mediators, called *lymphokines,* that act on other cells of the immune system.

Among the functions of the helper cells are (1) stim-

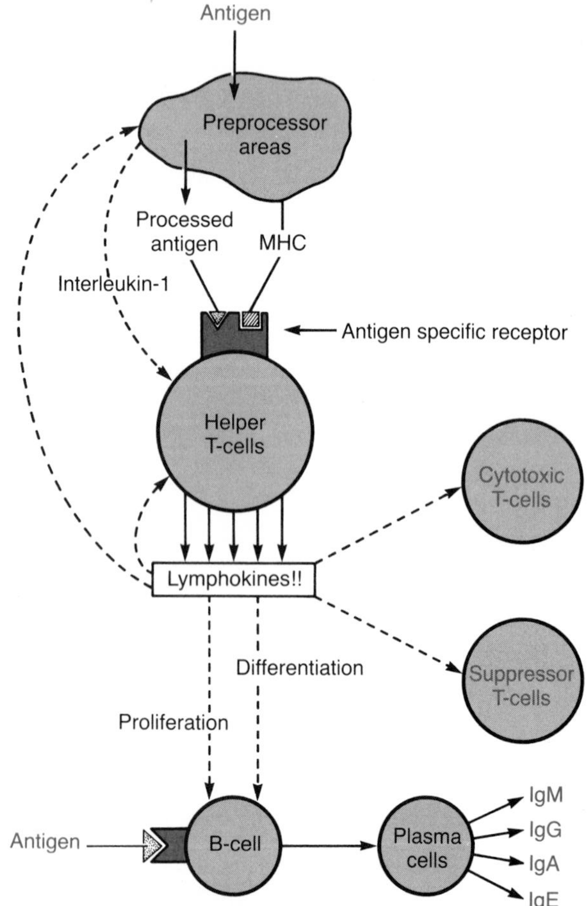

Figure 25–4. Regulation of the immune system, emphasizing the pivotal role of the helper T cells.

ulation of growth and proliferation of *cytotoxic T cells,* (2) stimulation of growth and proliferation of *suppressor T cells,* and (3) activation of macrophages throughout the body.

Cytotoxic T Cells

The cytotoxic T cell is a direct attack cell, capable of killing microorganisms and at times even some of the body's own cells. For this reason, these cells are frequently called *killer cells.* The receptor proteins on the surfaces of the cytotoxic cells cause them to bind tightly to those organisms or cells that contain their binding-specific antigen. After binding, the cytotoxic T cell secretes *hole-forming proteins,* called *perforins,* that literally punch large round holes in the membrane of the attacked cell. Then the cytotoxic cell releases cytotoxic substances directly into the attacked cell. Almost immediately, the attacked cell becomes greatly swollen and usually dissolves entirely shortly thereafter.

The cytotoxic cells also play an important role in destroying cancer cells, heart transplant cells, or other types of cells that are "foreign" to the person's own body.

Suppressor T Cells

Much less is known about the suppressor T cells than about the others, but they are capable of suppressing the functions of both cytotoxic and helper T cells. It is believed that these suppressor functions serve the purpose of regulating the activities of the other cells, keeping them from causing excessive immune reactions that might be severely damaging to the body.

Tolerance of the Acquired Immunity System to One's Own Tissues—Role of Preprocessing in the Thymus and Bone Marrow

Obviously, if a person should become immune to his or her own tissues, the process of acquired immunity would destroy the individual's own body. Fortunately, the immune mechanism normally "recognizes" a person's own tissues as being completely distinctive from those of invaders, and the immunity system forms very few antibodies or activated T cells against its own antigens. This phenomenon is known as *self-tolerance* to the body's own tissues.

The Clone Selection Mechanism of Self-Tolerance. It is believed that most of the phenomenon of tolerance develops during the processing of the T lymphocytes in the thymus and the B lymphocytes in the B lymphocyte processing area.The reason for this belief is that injecting a strong antigen into a fetus at the time that the lymphocytes are being processed in these two areas will prevent the development of clones of lymphocytes in the lymphoid tissue that are specific for the injected antigen. Also, experiments have shown that specific immature lymphocytes in the thymus, when exposed to a strong antigen, become lymphoblastic, proliferate considerably, and then combine with the stimulating antigen — an effect that is believed to cause the cells themselves to be destroyed by the thymic epithelial cells before they can migrate to and colonize the lymphoid tissue.

Therefore, it is believed that during the processing of lymphocytes in the thymus and in the B lymphocyte processing area, all or most of those clones of lymphocytes that are specific for the body's own tissues are self-destroyed because of their continual exposure to the body's antigens.

Failure of the Tolerance Mechanism—Autoimmune Diseases. Unfortunately, people frequently lose some of their immune tolerance to their own tissues — that is, they do form immunity against certain of their own tissues. This is called *autoimmunity.* This occurs to a greater extent the older a person becomes. It usually occurs after destruction of some of the body's tissues, which releases considerable quantities of antigens that circulate in the body and presumably cause acquired immunity in the form of either activated T cells or antibodies.

Diseases that result from autoimmunity include *rheumatic fever,* in which the body becomes immunized against tissues in the joints and heart, especially the heart valves, following exposure to a specific type of streptococcal toxin; one type of *glomerulonephritis,* in which the person becomes immunized against the basement membranes of the glomeruli; *myasthenia gravis,* in which immunity develops against the acetylcholine receptor proteins of the neuromuscular junction, causing paralysis; and *lupus erythematosus,* in which the person becomes immunized against many different body tissues at the same time, a disease that causes extensive damage and often rapid death.

Vaccination

The process of vaccination has been used for many years to cause acquired immunity against specific diseases. A person can be vaccinated by injecting dead organisms that are no longer capable of causing disease but which still have their chemical antigens. This type of vaccination is used to protect against typhoid fever, whooping cough, diphtheria, and many other types of bacterial diseases. Also, immunity can be achieved against toxins that have been treated with chemicals so that their toxic nature has been destroyed even though their antigens for causing immunity are still intact. This procedure is used in vaccinating against tetanus, botulism, and other similar toxic diseases. And, finally, a person can be vaccinated by infection with live organisms that have been "attenuated." That is, these organisms either have been grown in special culture media or have been passed through a series of animals until they have mutated enough that they will not cause disease but do still carry the specific antigens. This procedure is used to protect against poliomyelitis, yellow fever, measles, smallpox, and many other viral diseases.

ALLERGY

Some persons have an "allergic" tendency that is genetically passed on from parent to child, and it is characterized by the presence of large quantities of IgE *antibodies.* These antibodies are called *reagins,* or *sensitizing antibodies,* to distinguish them from the more common IgG antibodies. When an *allergen* (defined as an antigen that reacts specifically with a specific type of IgE reagin antibody) enters the body, an allergen-reagin reaction takes place, and a subsequent allergic reaction occurs.

A special characteristic of the IgE antibodies (the reagins) is a strong propensity to attach to mast cells and basophils. Indeed, a single mast cell or basophil can bind as many as half a million molecules of IgE antibodies. Then, when an antigen (an allergen) that has multiple binding sites binds with several of the IgE antibodies attached to a mast cell or basophil, this causes an immediate change in the membrane of the cell, perhaps resulting from a simple physical effect of the antibody molecules being pulled together by the antigen. At any rate, many of the mast cells and basophils rupture; others release their granules without rupturing and also secrete additional substances not already preformed in the granules. Some of the many different substances that are either released immediately or secreted shortly thereafter include *histamine, slow-reacting substance of anaphylaxis* (which is a mixture of toxic substances called leukotrienes), *eosinophil chemotactic substance,* a *protease,* a *neutrophil chemotactic substance, heparin,* and *platelet-activating factors.* These substances cause such phenomena as dilatation of the local blood vessels, attraction of eosinophils and neutrophils to the reactive site, damage to the local tissues by the protease, increased permeability of the capillaries and loss of fluid into the tissues, and contraction of local smooth muscle cells. Therefore, any number of different types of abnormal tissue responses can occur, depending upon the type of tissue in which the allergen-reagin reaction occurs. Among the different types of allergic reactions caused in this manner are the following:

Anaphylaxis. When a specific allergen is injected directly into the circulation, it can react in widespread areas of the body with the basophils of the blood and the mast cells located immediately outside the small blood vessels. Therefore, a widespread allergic reaction occurs throughout the vascular system and in closely associated tissues. This is called *anaphylaxis.* The *histamine* released into the circulation causes widespread peripheral vasodilation as well as increased permeability of the capillaries and marked loss of plasma from the circulation. Often, persons experiencing this reaction die of circulatory shock within a few minutes unless treated with norepinephrine to oppose the effects of the histamine.

Urticaria. Urticaria results from antigen entering specific skin areas and causing localized anaphylactoid reactions. *Histamine* released locally causes (1) vasodilatation that induces an immediate *red flare* and (2) increased local permeability of the capillaries that leads to local circumscribed areas of swelling of the skin in another few minutes. The swellings are commonly called *hives.* Administration of antihistamine drugs to a person prior to exposure will prevent the hives.

Hay Fever. In hay fever, the allergen-reagin reaction occurs in the nose. *Histamine* released in response to this causes rapid fluid leakage into the tissues of the nose, and the nasal linings become swollen and secretory. Here again, use of antihistamine drugs can prevent this swelling reaction.

Asthma. In asthma, the allergen-reagin reaction occurs in the bronchioles of the lungs. Here, the most important product released from the mast cells seems to be the *slow-reacting substance of anaphylaxis,* which causes spasm of the bronchiolar smooth muscle. Consequently, the person has difficulty breathing until the reactive products of the allergic reaction have been removed.

BLOOD GROUPS AND BLOOD TRANSFUSION

Antigenicity and Immune Reactions of Blood

When blood transfusions from one person to another were first attempted the transfusions were successful in some instances, but in many more immediate or delayed agglutination and hemolysis of the red blood cells occurred. Soon it was discovered that the bloods of different persons usually have different antigenic and immune properties, so that antibodies in the plasma of one blood react with antigens on the surfaces of the red cells of another. Furthermore, the antigens and antibodies are almost never precisely the same in one person as in another. For this reason, it is easy for blood from a donor to be mismatched with that of a recipient. Fortunately, if proper precautions are taken, one can determine ahead of time whether or not specific antibodies and antigens are present in the blood of the donor and the recipient to cause a reaction, but, on the other hand, lack of proper precautions often results in varying degrees of red cell agglutination and hemolysis, resulting in a typical *transfusion reaction* that can lead to death.

Multiplicity of Antigens in the Blood Cells. At least 30 commonly occurring antigens, each of which can at times cause antigen-antibody reactions, have been found in human blood cells, especially on the surfaces of the cell membranes.

Two particular groups of antigens are more likely

than the others to cause blood transfusion reactions. These are the so-called *O-A-B* system of antigens and the *Rh* system. Bloods are divided into different *groups* and *types* in accordance with the types of antigens present in the cells.

O-A-B Blood Groups

The A and B Antigens, Called Agglutinogens

Two related antigens—type A and type B—occur on the surfaces of the red blood cells in a large proportion of the population. Because of the way these antigens are inherited, people may have neither of them on their cells, they may have one, or they may have both simultaneously.

Strong antibodies that react specifically with either the type A or type B antigen almost always *occur in the plasmas of persons who do not have the antigens on their red cells.* These antibodies bind with the red cell antigens to cause agglutination of the red cells. Therefore, the type A and type B antigens are called *agglutinogens,* and the plasma antibodies that cause the agglutination are called *agglutinins.* It is on the basis of the presence or absence of the agglutinogens in the red blood cells that blood is grouped for the purpose of transfusion.

The Four Major O-A-B Blood Groups. In transfusing blood from one person to another, the bloods of donors and recipients are normally classified into four major O-A-B groups, as illustrated in Table 25-1, depending on the presence or absence of the two agglutinogens. When neither A nor B agglutinogen is present, the blood group is *group O.* When only type A agglutinogen is present, the blood is *group A.* When only type B agglutinogen is present, the blood is *group B.* And when both A and B agglutinogens are present, the blood is *group AB.*

The Agglutinins

When type A agglutinogen *is not present* in a person's red blood cells, antibodies known as anti-A agglutinins develop in the plasma. Also, when type B agglutinogen *is not present* in the red blood cells, antibodies known as anti-B agglutinins develop in the plasma.

Thus, referring once again to Table 25-1, it will be observed that group O blood, though containing no agglutinogens, does contain both *anti-A* and *anti-B agglutinins;* group A blood contains type A agglutinogens and *anti-B agglutinins;* and group B blood contains type B agglutinogens and *anti-A agglutinins.* Finally, group AB blood contains both A and B agglutinogens but no agglutinins at all.

Origin of Agglutinins in the Plasma. The agglutinins are gamma globulins, as are other antibodies, and are produced by the same cells that produce antibodies to any other antigens. Most of them are IgM and IgG immunoglobulin molecules.

But why are these agglutinins produced in individuals who do not have the antigenic substances in their red blood cells? The answer to this seems to be that small numbers of group A and B antigens enter the body in the food, in bacteria, and in other ways, and these substances initiate the development of the anti-A or anti-B agglutinins. One of the reasons for believing this is that injection of group A or group B antigen into a recipient having another blood type causes a typical immune response with formation of greater quantities of agglutinins than ever. Also, the newborn baby has few if any agglutinins, showing that agglutinin formation occurs almost entirely after birth.

Table 25-1 THE BLOOD GROUPS WITH THEIR GENOTYPES AND THEIR CONSTITUENT AGGLUTINOGENS AND AGGLUTININS

Genotypes	Blood Types	Agglutinogens	Agglutinins
OO	O	—	Anti-A and Anti-B
OA or AA	A	A	Anti-B
OB or BB	B	B	Anti-A
AB	AB	A and B	—

The Agglutination Process in Transfusion Reactions

When bloods are mismatched so that anti-A or anti-B plasma agglutinins are mixed with red blood cells containing A or B agglutinogens, respectively, the red cells agglutinate by the following process: The agglutinins attach themselves to the red blood cells. Because the agglutinins have two binding sites (IgG type) or ten sites (IgM type), a single agglutinin can attach to two or more different red blood cells at the same time, thereby causing the cells to adhere to each other. This causes the cells to clump. Then these clumps plug small blood vessels throughout the circulatory system. During the ensuing few hours to a few days, the phagocytic white blood cells and the reticuloendothelial system destroy the agglutinated cells, releasing hemoglobin into the plasma.

Hemolysis in Transfusion Reactions. Sometimes, when recipient and donor bloods are mismatched, immediate hemolysis of red cells occurs in the circulating blood. In this case the antibodies cause lysis of the red blood cells by activating the complement system. This in turn releases proteolytic enzymes (the *lytic complex*) that rupture the cell membranes, as was described earlier in the chapter.

However, *immediate* intravascular hemolysis is far less common than agglutination followed by *delayed* hemolysis, because not only does there have to be a very high titer of antibodies for this to occur but also a different type of antibody seems to be required, mainly the IgM antibodies; these antibodies are called *hemolysins.*

Acute Kidney Shutdown Following Transfusion Reactions. One of the most lethal effects of transfusion reactions is kidney shutdown, which can begin within a few minutes to a few hours and continue until the person dies of renal failure.

The kidney shutdown results from multiple effects, but one of these is the following: If the total amount of free hemoglobin in the blood rises above a critical level, much of the excess leaks through the glomerular membranes into the kidney tubules. If this amount is still slight, it can be reabsorbed through the tubular epithelium into the blood and will cause no harm; but if it is great, then only a small percentage is reabsorbed. Yet water continues to be reabsorbed, causing the tubular hemoglobin concentration to rise so high that it precipitates and blocks many of the tubules. If renal shutdown is complete and fails to open up, the patient dies within a week to 12 days.

THE Rh BLOOD TYPES

Along with the O-A-B blood group system, the most important other system in the transfusion of blood is the Rh system. The one major difference between the O-A-B system and the Rh system is the following: In the O-A-B system, the agglutinins responsible for causing transfusion reactions develop spontaneously, whereas in the Rh system spontaneous agglutinins almost never occur. Instead, the person must first be massively exposed to an Rh antigen, usually by transfusion of blood or by having a baby with the antigen, before enough agglutinins to cause a significant transfusion reaction will develop.

The Rh Antigens—"Rh Positive" and "Rh Negative" Persons. There are six common types of Rh antigens, but one type, called *type D,* is widely prevalent in the population, and it is also considerably more antigenic than the other Rh antigens. Therefore, anyone who has this type of antigen is said to be *Rh positive,* whereas those persons who do not have type D antigen are said to be *Rh negative.* However, it must be noted that even in Rh negative persons some of the other Rh antigens can still cause transfusion reactions, though usually much milder.

Approximately 85 per cent of all whites are Rh positive and 15 per cent, Rh negative. In American blacks, the percentage of Rh positives is about 95, whereas in African blacks it is virtually 100 per cent.

The Rh Immune Response

Formation of Anti-Rh Agglutinins. When red blood cells containing Rh factor are injected into a person without the factor—that is, into the Rh negative person—anti-Rh agglutinins develop very slowly, the maximum concentration of agglutinins occurring approximately 2 to 4 months later. This immune response occurs to a much greater extent in some people than in others. On multiple exposure to the Rh factor, the Rh negative person eventually becomes strongly "sensitized" to Rh factor.

Characteristics of Rh Transfusion Reactions. If an Rh negative person has never before been exposed to Rh positive blood, transfusion of Rh positive blood into him or her causes no immediate reaction at all. However, in some of these persons anti-Rh antibodies develop in sufficient quantities during the next 2 to 4 weeks to cause agglutination of the transfused cells that are still in the blood. These cells are then hemolyzed by the tissue macrophage system. Thus, a delayed transfusion reaction occurs, though it is usually mild. Yet on subsequent transfusion of Rh positive blood into the same person, who is now immunized against the Rh factor, the transfusion reaction is greatly enhanced and can be as severe as the reactions that occur with blood of types A and B.

Erythroblastosis Fetalis

Erythroblastosis fetalis is a disease of the fetus and newborn infant characterized by progressive agglutination and subsequent phagocytosis of the red blood cells. In most instances of erythroblastosis fetalis the mother is Rh negative and the father is Rh positive. The baby has inherited the Rh positive antigen from the father, and the mother has developed anti-Rh agglutinins that diffuse through the placenta into the fetus to cause red blood cell agglutination.

Effect of the Mother's Antibodies on the Fetus. After anti-Rh antibodies have formed in the mother, they diffuse slowly through the placental membrane into the fetus' blood. There they cause agglutination of the fetus' blood. The agglutinated red blood cells subsequently hemolyze, releasing hemoglobin into the blood. The macrophages then convert the hemoglobin into bilirubin, which causes yellowness (jaundice) of the skin. The antibodies probably also attack and damage some other cells of the body.

Clinical Picture of Erythroblastosis. The newborn, jaundiced, erythroblastotic baby is usually anemic at birth, and the anti-Rh agglutinins from the mother usually circulate in the baby's blood for 1 to 2 months after birth, destroying more and more red blood cells.

The hematopoietic tissues of the baby attempt to replace the hemolyzing red blood cells. The liver and the spleen become greatly enlarged and produce red blood cells in the same manner that they normally do during the middle of gestation. Because of the very rapid production of cells, many early forms, including many nucleated blastic forms, are emptied into the circulatory system, and it is because of the presence of these that the disease is called erythroblastosis fetalis.

Although the severe anemia of erythroblastosis fetalis is usually the cause of death, many children who barely survive the anemia exhibit permanent mental impairment or damage to motor areas of the brain because of precipitation of bilirubin in the neuronal cells, causing their destruction.

Treatment of the Erythroblastotic Baby. The usual treatment for erythroblastosis fetalis is to replace the newborn infant's blood with Rh negative blood. Approximately 400 ml of Rh negative blood is infused over a period of 1.5 or more hours while the baby's own Rh positive blood is being removed. This procedure may be repeated several times during the first few weeks of life, mainly to keep the bilirubin level low and thereby to prevent brain damage. By the time these transfused Rh negative cells are replaced with the baby's own Rh positive cells, a process that requires 6 or more weeks, the anti-Rh agglutinins that had come from the mother will have been destroyed.

REFERENCES

Bierman, C. W., and Pearlman, D. S.: Allergic Diseases from Infancy to Adulthood. 2nd ed. Philadelphia, W. B. Saunders Co., 1988.

Blalock, J. E.: A molecular basis for bidirectional communication between the immune and neuroendocrine systems. Physiol. Rev., 69:1, 1989.

Evans, A. S. (ed.): Viral Infections of Humans. 3rd ed. New York, Plenum Publishing Corp., 1989.

Graziano, F. M., and Lemanske, R. F., Jr., (eds.): Clinical Immunology. Baltimore, Williams & Wilkins, 1988.

Lessof, M. H., et al.: Allergy: Immunological and Clinical Aspects. 2nd ed. Baltimore, Williams & Wilkins, 1988.

Lockey, R. F., and Bukantz, S. C.: Principles of Immunology and Allergy. Philadelphia, W. B. Saunders Co., 1987.

Marx, J. L.: What T cells see and how they see it. Science, 242:863, 1988.

Metzger, H., and Kinet, J.-P.: How antibodies work: Focus on Fc receptors. FASEB J., 2:3, 1988.

Miller, D. R., et al. (eds.): Blood Diseases of Infancy and Childhood. St. Louis, C. V. Mosby Co., 1989.

Miyajima, A., et al.: Coordinate regulation of immune and inflammatory responses by T cell–derived lymphokines. FASEB J., 2:2462, 1988.

Nossal, G. J. V.: Immunologic tolerance: Collaboration between antigen and lymphokines. Science, 245:147, 1989.

Paige, C. J., and Wu, G. E.: The B cell repertoire. FASEB J., 3:1818, 1989.

Smith, K. A.: Interleukin-2: Inception, impact, and implications. Science, 240:1169, 1988.

Williams, W. J., et al. (eds.): Hematology. 4th ed. New York, McGraw-Hill Book Co., 1990.

QUESTIONS

1. What is the difference between *innate immunity* and *acquired immunity*?
2. Characterize the two different types of acquired immunity.
3. What is an *antigen,* and what are its characteristics?
4. What are the roles of lymphoid tissue in acquired immunity?
5. What are the differences between *T lymphocytes* and *B lymphocytes*?
6. Explain the preprocessing of T lymphocytes in the thymus gland.
7. Explain the preprocessing of B lymphocytes in other tissues of the body, probably the liver and bone marrow.
8. What is meant by a *lymphocyte clone*?
9. Explain how a clone of lymphocytes is activated. What is the role of macrophages in this activation?
10. Describe the antibodies. What are the *light* and *heavy polypeptide chains?* Also, what is meant by the *variable portion* and the *constant portion* of the light and heavy polypeptide chains?
11. What are the different actions of antibodies?
12. How does the complement system enter into antibody actions?
13. What are the three different types of T cells?
14. Explain how *cytotoxic T cells* kill microorganisms.
15. Explain how *helper T cells* help other portions of the immune system to become activated.
16. What are possible regulatory functions of the *suppressor T cells?*
17. What is the mechanism of *tolerance?*
18. Explain how *autoimmune diseases* develop.
19. What type of antibodies frequently causes allergy, and what is the relationship of these antibodies to mast cells and basophils?
20. What are some of the allergic conditions experienced by different persons?
21. Characterize the *O-A-B blood group system.*
22. What are the *agglutinogens* and the *agglutinins?*
23. Explain how transfusion reactions occur.
24. Explain the differences between transfusion reactions caused by the Rh blood types and those caused by the O-A-B blood types.
25. Explain the development of *erythroblastosis fetalis.*
26. Why do transfusion reactions occasionally cause acute kidney shutdown?

26

Hemostasis and Blood Coagulation

EVENTS IN HEMOSTASIS

The term *hemostasis* means prevention of blood loss. Whenever a vessel is severed or ruptured, hemostasis is achieved by several different mechanisms, including (1) vascular spasm, (2) formation of a platelet plug, (3) blood coagulation, and (4) eventual growth of fibrous tissue into the blood clot to close the hole in the vessel permanently.

Vascular Constriction

Immediately after a blood vessel is cut or ruptured, the stimulus of the traumatized vessel causes the wall of the vessel to contract; this instantaneously reduces the flow of blood from the vessel rupture. The contraction results from nervous reflexes, local myogenic spasm, and local humoral factors from the traumatized tissues and blood platelets.

Formation of the Platelet Plug

If the rent in the blood vessel is very small — and many very small vascular holes do develop each day — it is often sealed by a *platelet plug,* rather than by a blood clot. To understand this it is important that we first discuss the nature of platelets themselves.

Physical and Chemical Characteristics of Platelets

Platelets are minute round or oval discs 2 to 4 micrometers in diameter. They are formed in the bone marrow from *megakaryocytes,* which are extremely large cells of the hematopoietic series in the bone marrow that fragment into platelets either in the bone marrow or soon after entering the blood. The normal concentration of platelets in the blood is between 150,000 and 300,000 per microliter.

In the platelet's cytoplasm are such active factors as (1) *actin* and *myosin molecules,* similar to those found in muscle cells, that can cause the platelets to contract; (2) residuals of both the *endoplasmic reticulum* and the *Golgi apparatus* that synthesize various enzymes and store large quantities of calcium ions; (3) mitochondria and enzyme systems that are capable of forming *adenosine triphosphate (ATP)* and *adenosine diphosphate (ADP);* (4) enzyme systems that synthesize *prostaglandins,* which are local hormones that cause many different types of vascular and other local tissue reactions; and (5) an important protein called *fibrin-stabilizing factor,* which we discuss later in relation to blood coagulation.

Thus, the platelet is a very active structure. It has a half-life in the blood of 8 to 12 days, at the end of which time its life processes run out. More than half the platelets are removed by the macrophages in the spleen, where the blood passes through a latticework of tight trabeculae.

Mechanism of the Platelet Plug

When platelets come in contact with a damaged vascular surface, such as the collagen fibers in the vascular wall or even damaged endothelial cells, they immediately change their characteristics drastically. They begin to swell; they assume irregular forms with numerous irradiating processes protruding from their surfaces; their contractile proteins contract forcefully and cause the release of granules containing multiple active factors; they become sticky so that they stick to the collagen fibers; they secrete large quantities of *ADP;* and their enzymes form *thromboxane A_2,* which is also secreted into the blood. The ADP and thromboxane, in turn, act on nearby platelets to activate

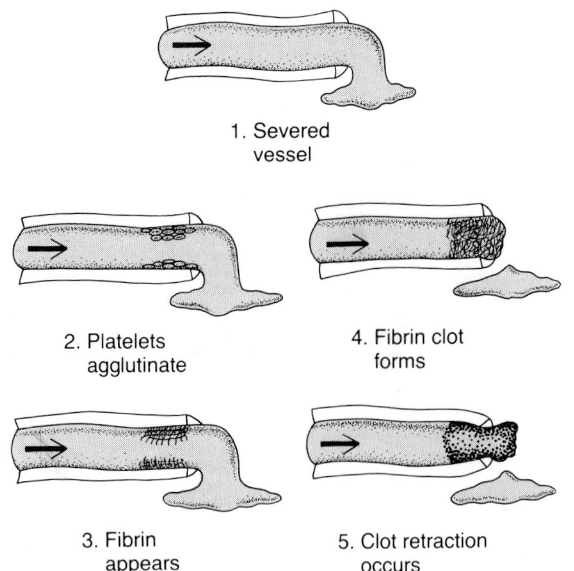

Figure 26-1. The clotting process in the traumatized blood vessel. (Modified from Seegers: Hemostatic Agents. Springfield, Ill., Charles C Thomas.)

them as well, and the stickiness of these additional platelets causes them to adhere to the originally activated platelets. Therefore, at the site of any rent in a vessel, the damaged vascular wall or extravascular tissues elicit a vicious cycle of activation of successively increasing numbers of platelets that themselves attract more and more additional platelets, thus forming a *platelet plug.*

Importance of the Platelet Method for Closing Vascular Holes. If the rent in a vessel is small, the platelet plug by itself can stop blood loss completely, but if there is a large hole, a blood clot in addition to the platelet plug is required to stop the bleeding. A person who has very few platelets develops literally hundreds of small hemorrhagic areas under the skin and throughout the internal tissues, but this does not occur in the normal person.

Blood Coagulation in the Ruptured Vessel

The third mechanism for hemostasis is formation of the blood clot. The clot begins to develop in 15 to 20 seconds if the trauma of the vascular wall has been severe and in 1 to 2 minutes if the trauma has been minor. Activator substances both from the traumatized vascular wall and from platelets and blood proteins adhering to the traumatized vascular wall initiate the clotting process. The physical events of this process are illustrated in Figure 26-1, and the chemical events will be discussed in detail later in the chapter.

Within 3 to 6 minutes after rupture of a vessel, if the vessel opening is not too large, the entire opening or broken end of the vessel is filled with clot. After 20 minutes to an hour, the clot retracts; this closes the vessel still further. Platelets play an important role in this clot retraction, as is also discussed later.

MECHANISM OF BLOOD COAGULATION

Basic Theory. Over 50 important substances that affect blood coagulation have been found in the blood and tissues, some promoting coagulation, called *procoagulants,* and others inhibiting coagulation, called *anticoagulants.* Whether or not the blood will coagulate depends on the degree of balance between these two groups of substances.

General Mechanism. All research workers in the field of blood coagulation agree that clotting takes place in three essential steps: (1) A complex of substances called *prothrombin activator* is formed in response to rupture of the vessel or damage to the blood itself. (2) The prothrombin activator catalyzes the conversion of *prothrombin* into *thrombin.* (3) The thrombin acts as an enzyme to convert *fibrinogen* into *fibrin threads* that enmesh platelets, blood cells, and plasma to form the clot itself.

Let us discuss first the mechanism by which the blood clot itself is formed, beginning with the conversion of prothrombin to thrombin; then we will come back to the initiating stages in the clotting process by which prothrombin activator is formed.

Conversion of Prothrombin to Thrombin

After prothrombin activator has been formed as a result of rupture of the blood vessel or as a result of damage to special activator substances in the blood, the prothrombin activator then causes conversion of prothrombin to thrombin (Fig. 26-2), which in turn causes polymerization of fibrinogen molecules into fibrin threads within another 10 to 15 seconds to cause the actual clot.

Prothrombin and Thrombin. Prothrombin is a plasma protein, an alpha$_2$-globulin, having a molecular weight of 68,700. It is an unstable protein that can split easily into smaller compounds, one of which is *thrombin,* which has a molecular weight of 33,700, almost exactly half that of prothrombin.

Prothrombin is formed continually by the liver, and it is continually being used throughout the body for blood clotting. If the liver fails to produce prothrombin, its concentration in the plasma falls too low to provide normal blood coagulation within 24 hours. Vitamin K is required by the liver for normal forma-

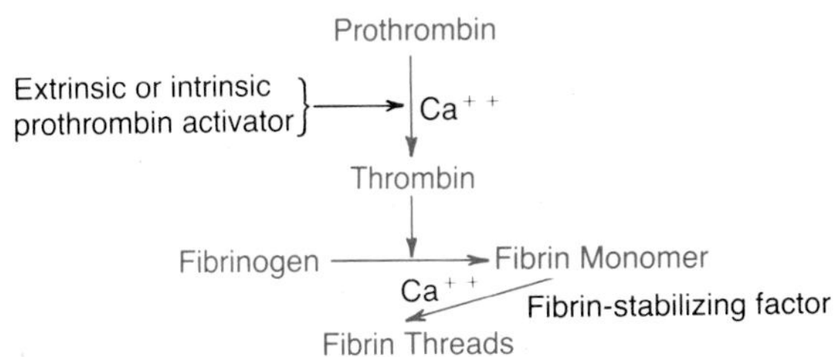

Figure 26-2. Schema for conversion of prothrombin to thrombin and polymerization of fibrinogen to form fibrin threads.

tion of prothrombin as well as three other clotting factors that we discuss later; therefore, either lack of vitamin K or the presence of liver disease that prevents normal prothrombin formation can often decrease the prothrombin level to such a low level that a bleeding tendency results.

Conversion of Fibrinogen to Fibrin— Formation of the Clot

Fibrinogen. Fibrinogen is a high molecular weight protein (340,000) occurring in the plasma in quantities of 100 to 700 mg/dl. Fibrinogen is formed in the liver, and liver disease occasionally decreases the concentration of circulating fibrinogen, as it does the concentration of prothrombin, as was pointed out previously.

Because of its large molecular size, very little fibrinogen normally leaks through the capillary pores into the interstitial fluids; and since it is one of the essential factors in the coagulation process, interstitial fluids ordinarily coagulate poorly if at all. Yet when the permeability of the capillaries becomes pathologically increased, fibrinogen does then leak into the tissue fluids in sufficient quantities to allow clotting in much the same way that plasma and whole blood clot.

Action of Thrombin on Fibrinogen to Form Fibrin. Thrombin is a protein *enzyme* with proteolytic capabilities. It acts on the fibrinogen molecule to remove four low molecular weight peptides, forming a molecule of *fibrin monomer* that has the automatic capability of polymerizing with other fibrin monomer molecules. Therefore, many fibrin monomer molecules polymerize within seconds into *long fibrin threads* that form the *reticulum* of the clot.

Then, still another process occurs during the following few minutes that greatly strengthens the fibrin reticulum. This involves a substance called *fibrin-stabilizing factor* that is normally present in small amounts in the plasma globulins but that is also released from platelets entrapped in the clot. This substance operates as an enzyme to cause *covalent bonds* between the fibrin monomer molecules as well as multiple cross-linkages between the adjacent fibrin threads, thus adding tremendously to the three-dimensional strength of the fibrin meshwork.

The Blood Clot. The clot is composed of a meshwork of fibrin threads running in all directions and entrapping blood cells, platelets, and plasma. The fibrin threads adhere to damaged surfaces of blood vessels; therefore, the blood clot becomes adherent to any vascular opening and thereby prevents blood loss.

Clot Retraction. Within a few minutes after a clot is formed, it begins to contract and usually expresses most of the fluid from the clot within 20 to 60 minutes.

Platelets are necessary for clot retraction to occur. Therefore, failure of clot retraction is an indication that the number of platelets in the circulating blood is low. Electron micrographs of platelets in blood clots show that they become attached to the fibrin threads in such a way that they actually bond different threads together. Furthermore, platelets entrapped in the clot continue to release procoagulant substances, one of which is fibrin-stabilizing factor, which causes more and more cross-linking bonds between the adjacent fibrin threads.

As the clot retracts, the edges of the broken blood vessel are pulled together, thus contributing still more to the ultimate state of hemostasis.

Initiation of Coagulation: Formation of Prothrombin Activator Complex

Now that we have discussed the clotting process initiated by the formation of thrombin from prothrombin, we must turn to the more complex mechanisms that activate the prothrombin and cause it to form thrombin. These mechanisms can be set into play by trauma to the vascular wall and adjacent tissues, trauma to the blood, or contact of the blood with damaged tissue cells. In each instance, they lead to the formation of *prothrombin activator complex,* which then causes prothrombin conversion to thrombin.

Prothrombin activator is generally considered to be formed in two basic ways, although in reality these interact constantly with each other: (1) by the *extrinsic pathway* that begins with trauma to the vascular wall and surrounding tissues, and (2) by the *intrinsic pathway* that begins in the blood itself.

In both the extrinsic and intrinsic pathways a series

Table 26-1 CLOTTING FACTORS IN THE BLOOD AND THEIR SYNONYMS

Clotting Factor	Synonyms
Factor I	Fibrinogen
Factor II	Prothrombin
Factor III; tissue factor	Tissue thromboplastin
Factor IV	Calcium
Factor V	Proaccelerin; labile factor; Ac-globulin (Ac-G)
Factor VII	Serum prothrombin conversion accelerator (SPCA); proconvertin; stable factor
Factor VIII	Antihemophilic factor (AHF); antihemophilic globulin (AHG); antihemophilic factor A
Factor IX	Plasma thromboplastin component (PTC); Christmas factor; antihemophilic factor B
Factor X	Stuart factor; Stuart-Prower factor
Factor XI	Plasma thromboplastin antecedent (PTA); antihemophilic factor C
Factor XII	Hageman factor
Factor XIII	Fibrin-stabilizing factor
Prekallikrein	Fletcher factor
High molecular weight kininogen	Fitzgerald factor; HMWK
Platelets	

of different plasma proteins, especially beta-globulins, play major roles. These, along with the other factors already discussed that enter into the clotting process, are called *blood-clotting factors*. For the most part they are *inactive* forms of proteolytic enzymes. When converted to the active forms, their enzymatic actions cause the successive, cascading reactions of the clotting process.

The important clotting factors are listed in Table 26-1. Most of them are designated by Roman numerals.

The Extrinsic Mechanism for Initiating Clotting

The extrinsic mechanism for initiating the formation of prothrombin activator begins with a traumatized vascular wall or extravascular tissues and occurs according to the following three basic steps, as illustrated in Figure 26-3.

1. *Release of tissue thromboplastin.* Traumatized tissue releases a complex of several factors called *tissue thromboplastin.* This includes especially *phospholipids* from the membranes of the tissues and a *lipoprotein complex* containing an important glycoprotein that functions as a *proteolytic enzyme.*
2. *Activation of factor X to form activated factor X — role of factor VII and tissue thromboplastin.* The lipoprotein complex of tissue thromboplastin further complexes with blood coagulation factor VII, and, in the presence of tissue phospholipids and calcium ions acts enzymatically on factor X to form *activated factor X.*
3. *Effect of activated factor X to form prothrombin activator—role of factor V.* The activated factor X complexes immediately with the tissue phospholipids released as part of the tissue thromboplastin and also with factor V to form a complex called *prothrombin activator.* Within a few seconds this splits prothrombin to form thrombin, and the clotting process proceeds as has already been explained. Thus, activated factor X is the actual protease that causes splitting of prothrombin to thrombin.

The Intrinsic Mechanism for Initiating Clotting

The second mechanism for initiating the formation of prothrombin activator, and therefore for initiating clotting, begins with trauma to the blood itself or exposure of the blood to collagen in a traumatized vascular wall. Then, it continues through the following series of cascading reactions illustrated in Figure 26-4:

1. *Activation of factor XII and release of platelet phospholipids.* Trauma to the blood or exposure of the blood to vascular wall collagen alters two

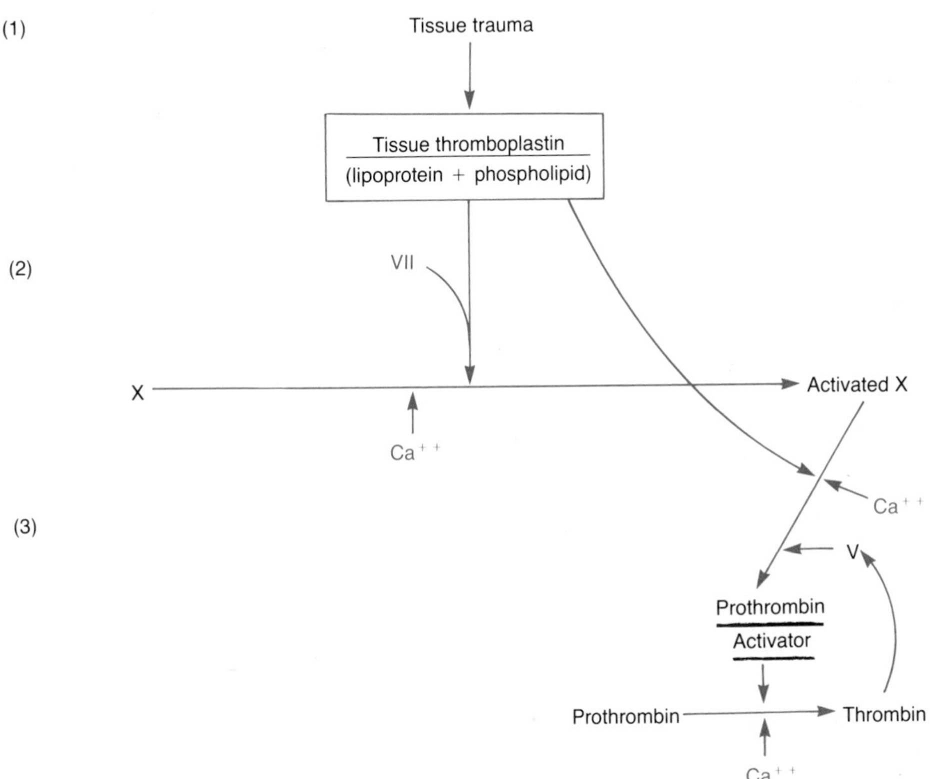

Figure 26-3. The extrinsic pathway for initiating blood clotting.

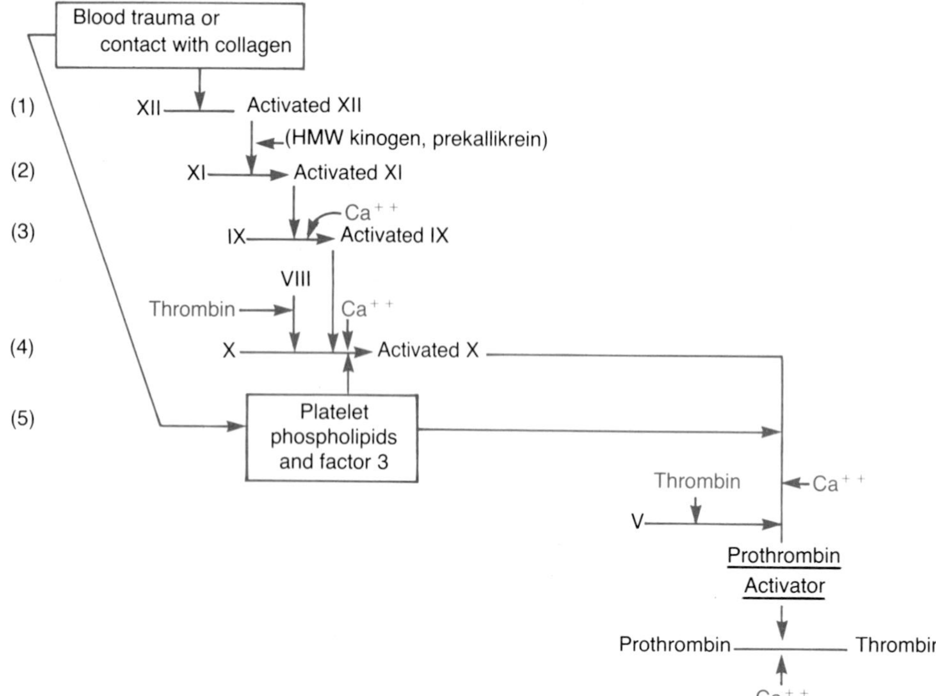

Figure 26-4. The intrinsic pathway for initiating blood clotting.

important clotting factors in the blood—factor XII and the platelets. When factor XII is disturbed, it takes on a new configuration that converts it into a proteolytic enzyme called "activated factor XII." Simultaneously, the blood trauma also damages the platelets, because of adherence either to collagen or to a wettable surface (or by damage in other ways), and this releases platelet phospholipid containing the lipoprotein called platelet factor 3, which also plays a role in subsequent clotting reactions.

2. *Activation of factor XI.* The activated factor XII acts enzymatically on factor XI to activate this as well, which is the second step in the intrinsic pathway.
3. *Activation of factor IX by activated factor XI.* The activated factor XI then acts enzymatically on factor IX to activate this factor, also.
4. *Activation of factor X—role of factor VIII.* The activated factor IX, acting in concert with factor VIII and with platelet phospholipids and factor 3 from the traumatized platelets, activates factor X. It is clear that when either factor VIII or platelets are in short supply, this step is deficient. Factor VIII is the factor that is missing in the person who has classic *hemophilia,* for which reason it is called *antihemophilic factor.* Platelets are the clotting factor that is lacking in the bleeding disease called *thrombocytopenia.*
5. *Action of activated factor X to form prothrombin activator—role of factor V.* This step in the intrinsic pathway is the same as the last step in the extrinsic pathway. That is, activated factor X combines with factor V and platelet or tissue phospholipids to form the complex called *prothrombin activator.* The prothrombin activator in turn initiates within seconds the cleavage of prothrombin to form thrombin, thereby setting into motion the final clotting process, as described earlier.

Role of Calcium Ions in the Intrinsic and Extrinsic Pathways

Except for the first two steps in the intrinsic pathway, calcium ions are required for promotion of all the reactions. Therefore, in the absence of calcium ions, blood clotting will not occur.

Fortunately, in the living body the calcium ion concentration rarely falls low enough to affect significantly the kinetics of blood clotting. On the other hand, when blood is removed from a person, it can be prevented from clotting by reducing the calcium ion concentration below the threshold level for clotting, either by deionizing the calcium by reacting it with substances such as *citrate ion* or by precipitating the calcium with substances such as *oxalate ion.*

Interaction Between the Extrinsic and Intrinsic Pathways—Summary of Blood-Clotting Initiation

It is clear from the above schemas of the intrinsic and extrinsic systems that after blood vessels rupture, clotting is initiated by both pathways simultaneously. The tissue thromboplastin initiates the extrinsic pathway, whereas contact of factor XII and the platelets with collagen in the vascular wall initiates the intrinsic pathway.

When blood is removed from the body and held in a test tube, the intrinsic pathway alone must elicit the clotting. This usually results from contact of factor XII and platelets with the wall of the vessel, which activates both of these and initiates the intrinsic mechanism. If the surface of the container is very "nonwettable," such as a siliconized surface, blood clotting is delayed for up to an hour or more.

An especially important difference between the extrinsic and intrinsic pathways is that *the extrinsic pathway* can be explosive in nature; once initiated, its speed of occurrence is limited only by the amount of tissue thromboplastin released from the traumatized tissues and by the quantities of factors X, VII, and V in the blood. With severe tissue trauma, clotting can occur in as little as 15 seconds. On the other hand, the intrinsic pathway is much slower to proceed, usually requiring 1 to 6 minutes to cause clotting.

Prevention of Blood Clotting in the Normal Vascular System—The Intravascular Anticoagulants

Endothelial Surface Factors. Probably the most important factors for preventing clotting in the normal vascular system are the *smoothness* of the endothelium and *several proteins* bound to the endothelial cells that prevent activation of the intrinsic clotting system. However, when the endothelial wall is damaged, its smoothness and bound proteins are both lost, which activates both factor XII and the platelets, thus setting off the intrinsic pathway of clotting.

The Antithrombin Action of Fibrin and of Antithrombin III. Among the most important anticoagulants in the blood itself are those that remove thrombin from the blood. The two most powerful of these are the *fibrin threads* formed during the process of clotting and an alpha-globulin called *antithrombin III* or *antithrombin-heparin co-factor.*

While a clot is forming, approximately 85 to 90 per cent of the thrombin formed from the prothrombin becomes adsorbed to the fibrin threads as they develop. This obviously helps prevent the spread of thrombin into the remaining blood and therefore prevents excessive spread of the clot.

The thrombin that does not adsorb to the fibrin threads soon combines with antithrombin III, which inactivates the thrombin during the next 12 to 20 minutes.

Heparin. Heparin is another powerful anticoagulant. Yet its concentration in the blood is normally very slight, so that only under some physiological conditions does it have significant anticoagulant effects. On the other hand, it is used very widely in medical practice to prevent intravascular clotting.

The heparin molecule is a highly negatively charged conjugated polysaccharide. It combines with antithrombin III and increases as much as a hundred- to a thousandfold the effectiveness of antithrombin III in removing thrombin and thus acting as an anticoagulant. Therefore, in the presence of excess heparin, the removal of thrombin from the circulating blood is almost instantaneous.

Heparin is produced by many different cells of the human body, but especially large quantities are formed by the basophilic *mast cells* located in the pericapillary connective tissue throughout the body. These cells continually secrete small quantities of heparin that diffuse into the circulatory system. The *basophil cells* of the blood, which are functionally almost identical with the mast cells, also release small quantities of heparin into the plasma.

Mast cells are extremely abundant in the tissue surrounding the capillaries of the lungs and to a lesser extent the capillaries of the liver. It is easy to understand why large quantities of heparin might be needed in these areas, for the capillaries of the lungs and liver receive many embolic clots formed in the slowly flowing venous blood; sufficient formation of heparin might prevent further growth of the clots.

Lysis of Blood Clots—Plasmin

The plasma proteins contain a euglobulin called *plasminogen* or *profibrinolysin,* which, when activated, becomes a substance called *plasmin* or *fibrinolysin.* Plasmin is a proteolytic enzyme that resembles trypsin, the most important digestive enzyme of pancreatic secretion. It digests the fibrin threads and also digests other clotting factors.

When a clot is formed, a large amount of plasminogen is trapped in the clot along with other plasma proteins. However, this will not become plasmin and will not cause lysis of the clot until it is activated. Fortunately, the injured tissues and vascular endothelium release an activator called *tissue plasminogen activator* that a day or so later, after the clot has stopped the bleeding, eventually converts plasminogen to plasmin and removes the clot. In fact, many small blood vessels in which the blood flow has been stopped by clots are reopened by this mechanism.

CONDITIONS THAT CAUSE EXCESSIVE BLEEDING IN HUMAN BEINGS

Excessive bleeding can result from deficiency of any one of the many different blood clotting factors. Three particular types of bleeding tendencies that have been studied to the greatest extent will be discussed: (1) bleeding caused by vitamin K deficiency, (2) hemophilia, and (3) thrombocytopenia (platelet deficiency).

Decreased Prothrombin, Factor VII, Factor IX, and Factor X Caused by Vitamin K Deficiency

With few exceptions, almost all the blood-clotting factors are formed by the liver. Therefore, diseases of the liver such as *hepatitis, cirrhosis,* and *acute yellow atrophy* all can depress the clotting system so greatly that the patient develops a severe tendency to bleed.

Another cause of depressed formation of clotting factors by the liver is vitamin K deficiency. Vitamin K is necessary for promotion of formation of four of the most important clotting factors, *prothrombin, factor VII, factor IX,* and *factor X.* Therefore, in the absence of vitamin K, insufficiency of these coagulation factors can lead to a serious bleeding tendency.

Fortunately, vitamin K is continually synthesized in the intestinal tract by bacteria so that vitamin K deficiency rarely if ever occurs simply because of its absence from the diet, except in newborn children before they establish their intestinal bacterial flora. However, vitamin K deficiency does often occur as a result of poor absorption of fats from the gastrointestinal tract, because vitamin K is fat soluble and ordinarily is absorbed into the blood along with the fats.

Hemophilia

Hemophilia is a bleeding tendency that occurs almost exclusively in males. In 85 per cent of cases it is caused by *deficiency of factor VIII;* this type of hemophilia is called *hemophilia A* or *classic hemophilia.* About one of every 10,000 males in the United States has classic hemophilia. In the other 15 per cent of the patients, the bleeding tendency is caused by deficiency of factor IX. Both these factors are transmitted genetically by way of the female chromosome as a recessive trait. Therefore, almost never will a woman have hemophilia, because at least one of her two X chromosomes will have the appropriate genes. However, if one of her X chromosomes is deficient, she will be a *hemophilia carrier,* transmitting the disease to half her male offspring and transmitting the carrier state to half her female offspring.

Usually, in hemophilia, bleeding will not occur except after trauma, but the degree of trauma required to cause severe and prolonged bleeding may be so mild that it is hardly noticeable. And bleeding can often last for literally weeks after extraction of a tooth. When a person with classic hemophilia develops severe, prolonged bleeding, almost the only therapy that is truly effective is injection of purified factor VIII.

Thrombocytopenia

Thrombocytopenia means the presence of a very low quantity of platelets in the circulatory system. Persons with thrombocytopenia have a tendency to bleed as do hemophiliacs, except that the bleeding is usually from many small venules or capillaries rather than from larger vessels, as in hemophilia. As a result, small, punctate hemorrhages occur throughout all the body tissues. The skin of such a person displays many small, purplish blotches, giving the disease the name *thrombocytopenic purpura.* It will be remembered that platelets are especially important for repair of minute breaks in capillaries and other small vessels.

Ordinarily, bleeding does not occur until the number of platelets in the blood falls below a value of approximately 50,000 per microliter, rather than the normal 150,000 to 300,000. Levels as low as 10,000 per microliter are frequently lethal.

Most persons with thrombocytopenia have the disease known as *idiopathic thrombocytopenia,* which means simply "thrombocytopenia of unknown cause." However, in the past few years it has been discovered that in most of these persons specific antibodies are destroying the platelets. Usually this results from developing autoimmunity to the person's own platelets, the cause of which, however, is not known.

THROMBOEMBOLIC CONDITIONS IN THE HUMAN BEING

Thrombi and Emboli. An abnormal clot that develops in a blood vessel is called a *thrombus.* Once a clot has developed, continued flow of blood past the clot is likely to break it away from its attachment, and such freely flowing clots are known as *emboli.* Obviously, either can block a vessel such as a coronary artery, a brain artery, or others.

The causes of thromboembolic conditions in the human being are usually twofold: First, any *roughened endothelial surface of a vessel*— as may be caused by arteriosclerosis, infection, or trauma—is likely to initiate the clotting process. Second, blood often clots *when it flows very slowly* through blood vessels, for small quantities of thrombin and other procoagulants are always being formed.

Femoral Thrombosis and Massive Pulmonary Embolism

Because clotting almost always occurs when blood flow is blocked for many hours in any vessel of the body, the immobility of bed patients, plus the practice of propping the knees with underlying pillows, often causes intravascular clotting because of blood stasis in one or more of the leg veins for hours at a time. Then the clot grows, mainly in the direction of the slowly moving blood, sometimes growing the entire length of the leg veins and occasionally even up into the abdomen. Then, about one time out of every ten, a large part of the clot disengages from its attachments to the vessel wall and flows freely with the venous blood into the right side of the heart and thence into the pulmonary arteries to cause *massive pulmonary embolism.* If the clot is large enough to occlude both the pulmonary arteries, immediate death ensues. If only one pulmonary artery or a smaller branch is blocked, death may not occur, or the embolism may lead to death a few hours to several days later because of further growth of the clot within the pulmonary vessels.

ANTICOAGULANTS FOR CLINICAL USE

In some thromboembolic conditions, such as coronary thrombosis or pulmonary embolism, it is desirable to delay the coagulation process. Therefore, various anticoagulants have been developed for treatment of these conditions. The ones most useful clinically are heparin and the coumarins.

Heparin as an Intravenous Anticoagulant

Injection of relatively small quantities of heparin into the blood, approximately 0.5 to 1 mg per kilogram of body weight, causes the blood-clotting time to increase from a normal of approximately 6 minutes to 30 or more minutes. Furthermore, this change in clotting time occurs instantaneously, thereby immediately preventing further development of the thromboembolic condition.

The action of heparin lasts approximately 3 to 4 hours. The injected heparin is destroyed by an enzyme in the blood known as *heparinase.*

Coumarins as Anticoagulants

When a coumarin, such as *warfarin,* is given to a patient, the plasma levels of prothrombin and factors VII, IX, and X, all formed by the liver, begin to fall, indicating that warfarin has a potent depressant effect on liver formation of all these compounds. Warfarin causes this effect by competing with vitamin K for reactive sites in the enzymatic processes for formation of prothrombin and the other three clotting factors, thereby blocking the action of vitamin K.

After administration of an effective dose of warfarin, the coagulant activity of the blood decreases to approximately 50 per cent of normal by the end of 12 hours and to approximately 20 per cent of normal by the end of 24 hours. In other words, the coagulation process is not blocked immediately, but must await the natural destruction of the prothrombin and other factors already present in the plasma. Normal coagulation returns 1 to 3 days after discontinuing therapy.

REFERENCES

Coller, B. S. (ed.): Progress in Hemostasis and Thrombosis, Vol. 9. Philadelphia, W. B. Saunders Co., 1989.

Esmon, C. T.: The regulation of natural anticoagulant pathways. Science, 235:1348, 1987.

Haber, E., et al.: Innovative approaches to plasminogen activator therapy. Science, 243:51, 1989.

Hilgartner, M. W., and Pochedly, C.: Hemophilia in the Child and Adult. 3rd ed. New York, Raven Press, 1989.

Miller, D. R., et al. (eds.): Blood Diseases of Infancy and Childhood. St. Louis, C. V. Mosby Co., 1989.

Renck, H.: Bleeding and Thrombotic Disorders in Surgical Patients. East Norwalk, Conn., Appleton & Lange, 1988.

Rodgers, G. M.: Hemostatic properties of normal and perturbed vascular cells. FASEB J., 2:116, 1988.

Siess, W.: Molecular mechanisms of platelet activation. Physiol. Rev., 69:58, 1989.

Williams, W. J., et al.: Hematology. 4th ed. New York, McGraw-Hill Book Co., 1990.

Zwaal, R. F. A.: Scrambling membrane phospholipids and local control of blood clotting. News Physiol. Sci., 3:57, 1988.

QUESTIONS

1. Explain the role of *vascular spasm* in hemostasis.
2. How do *platelet plugs* contribute to hemostasis?
3. Name the three principal stages of the blood coagulation mechanism.
4. What is the source of *prothrombin,* and what causes it to be converted to thrombin?
5. How does thrombin convert *fibrinogen* into fibrin?
6. What is the role of *platelets* in clot retraction?
7. What are the principal differences between the *extrinsic* and *intrinsic mechanisms* for the formation of *prothrombin activator?*
8. What are the special roles of *factor XII* and *platelets* in the intrinsic mechanism for initiating clotting?
9. What is the relationship of *factor VIII* to *hemophilia?*
10. Explain how tissue trauma leads to clotting.
11. Explain how each of the following factors helps prevent clotting in the normal vascular system: *endothelial surface factors, antithrombin III,* and *heparin.*
12. What is the role of *plasmin* in the lysis of blood clots?
13. Explain the bleeding in each of the following conditions: vitamin K deficiency, hemophilia, and thrombocytopenia.
14. What are the basic causes of *thromboembolic conditions?*
15. Explain the genesis of *pulmonary embolism* and *disseminated intravascular clotting.*

VII

Respiration

27

Pulmonary Ventilation and Pulmonary Circulation

Respiration can be divided into four major functional events: (1) pulmonary ventilation, which means the inflow and outflow of air between the atmosphere and the lung alveoli, (2) diffusion of oxygen and carbon dioxide between the alveoli and the blood, (3) transport of oxygen and carbon dioxide in the blood and body fluids to and from the cells, and (4) regulation of ventilation and other facets of respiration. The present chapter is a discussion of pulmonary ventilation, and the subsequent two chapters cover the other respiratory functions as well as the physiology of special respiratory problems.

MECHANICS OF PULMONARY VENTILATION

The Muscles That Cause Lung Expansion and Contraction

The lungs can be expanded and contracted in two ways: (1) by downward and upward movement of the diaphragm to lengthen or shorten the chest cavity, and (2) by elevation and depression of the ribs to increase and decrease the anteroposterior diameter of the chest cavity. Figure 27–1 illustrates these two methods.

Normal quiet breathing is accomplished almost entirely by the first of the above two methods, that is, by movement of the *diaphragm.* During inspiration, contraction of the diaphragm pulls the lower surfaces of the lungs downward. Then, during expiration, the diaphragm simply relaxes, and the *elastic recoil* of the lungs, chest wall, and abdominal structures compresses the lungs. During heavy breathing, however, the elastic forces are not powerful enough to cause the necessary rapid expiration, so that the extra required force is achieved mainly by contraction of the *abdominal muscles,* which pushes the abdominal contents upward against the bottom of the diaphragm.

The second method for expanding the lungs is to raise the rib cage. This expands the lungs because, in the natural resting position, the ribs slant downward, thus allowing the sternum to fall backward toward the spinal column. But when the rib cage is elevated, the ribs then project almost directly forward so that the sternum now also moves forward, away from the spine, making the anteroposterior thickness of the chest about 20 per cent greater during maximum inspiration than during expiration. Therefore, those muscles that elevate the chest cage can be classified as muscles of inspiration. These especially include the *neck muscles* that pull the upper ribs and sternum upward. Those muscles that depress the chest cage are muscles of expiration. These especially include the *abdominal recti* that pull downward on the sternum and lower ribs.

Movement of Air in and out of the Lungs —and the Pressures That Cause It

The lung is an elastic structure that will collapse like a balloon and expel all its air through the trachea whenever there is no force to keep it inflated. Also, there are no attachments between the lung and the walls of the chest cage except where it is suspended at its hilum from the mediastinum. Instead, the lung literally floats in the thoracic cavity, surrounded by a very thin layer of *pleural fluid* that lubricates the movements of the lungs within the cavity. Further-

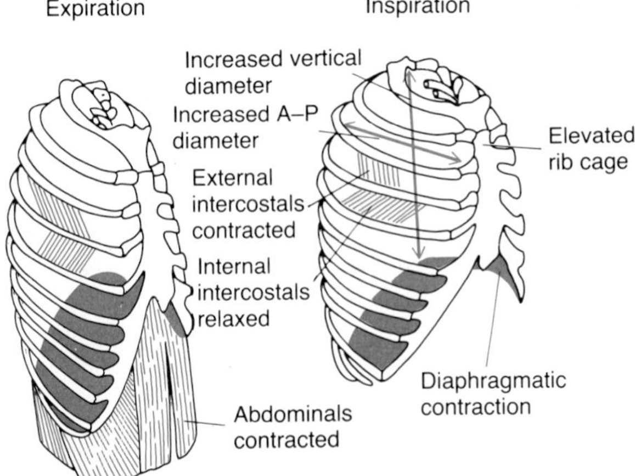

Figure 27-1. Expansion and contraction of the thoracic cage during expiration and inspiration, illustrating especially diaphragmatic contraction, elevation of the rib cage, and function of the intercostals.

more, continual pumping of this fluid into lymphatic channels maintains a slight suction between the visceral surface of the lung pleura and the parietal pleural surface of the thoracic cavity. Therefore, the two lungs are held to the thoracic wall as if glued there, except that they can slide freely, well lubricated, as the chest expands and contracts.

The Pleural Pressure and Its Changes During Respiration

Pleural pressure is the pressure in the narrow space between the lung pleura and the chest wall pleura. As noted, this is normally a slight suction, which means a slightly negative pressure. The normal pleural pressure at the beginning of inspiration is approximately −5 centimeters of water, which is the amount of suction that is required to hold the lungs open to their resting level. Then, during normal inspiration, the expansion of the chest cage pulls the surface of the lungs with still greater force and creates a still more negative pressure down to an average of about −7.5 centimeters of water. These relationships between pleural pressure and changing lung volume are illustrated in Figure 27-2,

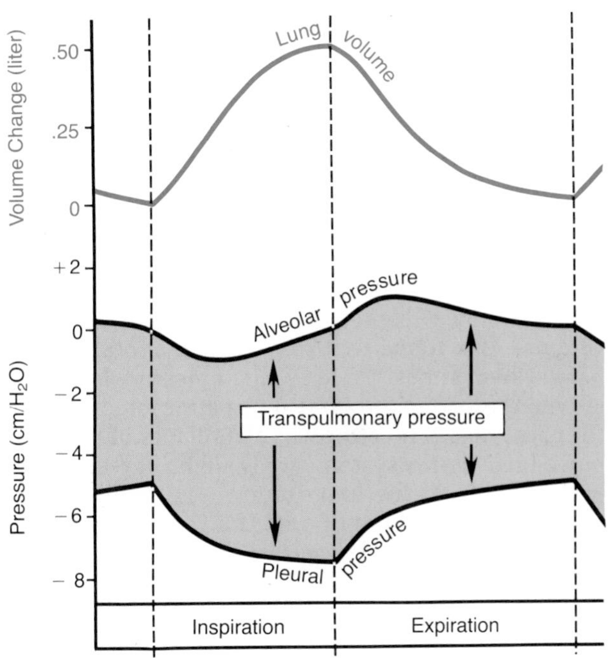

Figure 27-2. Changes in lung volume, alveolar pressure, pleural pressure, and transpulmonary pressure during normal breathing.

Alveolar Pressure

Alveolar pressure is the pressure inside the lung alveoli. When the glottis is open and no air is flowing into or out of the lungs, the pressures in all parts of the respiratory tree, all the way to the alveoli, are exactly equal to atmospheric pressure, which is considered to be 0 centimeter water pressure.

To cause inward flow of air during inspiration, the pressure in the alveoli must fall to a value slightly below atmospheric pressure. Figure 27-2 illustrates in normal inspiration a decrease in alveolar pressure to about −1 centimeter of water. This very slight negative pressure is enough to move about 0.5 liter of air into the lungs in the 2 seconds required for inspiration.

During expiration, opposite changes occur: the alveolar pressure rises to about +1 centimeter of water, and this forces the 0.5 liter of inspired air out of the lungs during the 2 to 3 seconds of expiration.

Compliance of the Lungs

The extent to which the lungs expand for each unit increase in transpulmonary pressure (pleural pressure minus alveolar pressure) is called their *compliance.* The normal total compliance of both lungs together in the average adult human being is approximately 200 ml/cm of water pressure. That is, every time the transpulmonary pressure increases by 1 centimeter of water, the lungs expand 200 milliliters.

The Compliance Diagram of the Lungs. Figure 27-3 is a diagram relating lung volume changes to changes in transpulmonary pressure. Note that the relationship is different for inspiration and expiration. Each curve is recorded by changing the transpulmonary pressure in small steps and allowing the lung volume to come to a steady level between successive steps. The two curves are called the *inspiratory compliance curve* and the *expiratory compliance curve,* and the entire diagram is called the *compliance diagram of the lungs.*

The characteristics of the compliance diagram are determined by the elastic forces of the lungs. These can be divided into two separate parts: (1) the *elastic forces of the lung tissue* itself and (2) the *elastic force caused by surface tension of the fluid that lines the inside walls of the alveoli* and other lung air spaces.

The elastic forces of the lung tissue are determined

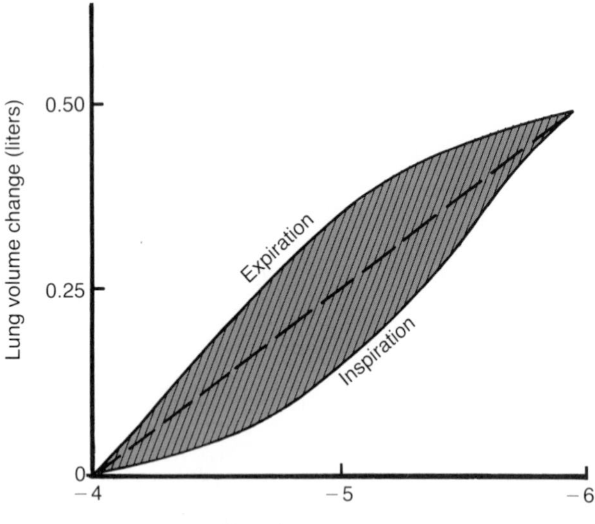

Figure 27-3. Compliance diagram in a normal person. This diagram shows the compliance of the lungs alone.

mainly by the elastin and collagen fibers interwoven among the lung parenchyma. In the deflated lungs, these fibers are in a partially contracted and kinked state, and then when the lungs are expanded, the fibers are partly stretched and partly unkinked, thereby elongating.

The elastic forces caused by surface tension are much more complex. However, surface tension accounts for about two thirds of the total elastic forces in the normal lungs. Furthermore, the surface tension elastic forces of the lungs change tremendously when the substance called "surfactant" is not present in the alveolar fluid. Therefore, let us discuss surfactant and its relationship to the surface tension forces.

"Surfactant," Surface Tension, and Collapse of the Lungs

The Principle of Surface Tension. When water forms a surface with air, the water molecules on the surface of the water have an extra strong attraction for each other. As a result, the water surface is always attempting to contract. This is what holds raindrops together; that is, there is a tight contractile membrane of water molecules around the entire surface of the raindrop. Now let us reverse these principles and see what happens on the inner surfaces of the alveoli and other air spaces. Here, the water surface is also attempting to contract, but this time the surface of the water lining the alveoli surrounds the alveolar air, always attempting to contract like a balloon. Obviously, this attempts to force the air out of the alveoli through the bronchi, and in doing so it causes the alveoli to attempt to collapse. Since this occurs in all of the air spaces of the lungs, the net effect is to cause an elastic contractile force of the entire lungs, which is called the *surface tension elastic force.*

"Surfactant" and Its Effect on Surface Tension. Surfactant is a *surface active agent,* which means that when it spreads over the surface of a fluid it greatly reduces the surface tension. It is secreted by special surfactant-secreting epithelial cells that comprise about 10 per cent of the surface area of the alveoli. These cells are granular in nature, containing lipid inclusions; they are called *type II alveolar epithelial cells.*

Surfactant is a complex mixture of several phospholipids, proteins, and ions. The important component is the phospholipid *dipalmitoyl lecithin,* which is responsible for reducing the surface tension. This will not dissolve in the fluid; instead, it spreads over its surface, because one portion of each phospholipid molecule is hydrophilic and dissolves in the water lining the alveoli, whereas the lipid portion of the molecule is hydrophobic and is oriented toward the air, forming a lipid hydrophobic surface exposed to the air. This surface has from one twelfth to one half the surface tension of a pure water surface.

For the average-sized alveolus with a radius of about 100 micrometers and lined with normal surfactant, the elastic alveolar collapse pressure caused by surface tension calculates to be about 4 centimeters of water pressure (3 mm Hg). However, if the alveoli were lined with pure water, it would calculate to be about 18 centimeters of water pressure. Thus, one sees how important surfactant is in *reducing* the amount of transpulmonary pressure required to keep the lungs expanded.

Effect of the Thoracic Cage on Lung Expansibility

Thus far we have discussed the expansibility of the lungs alone without considering the thoracic cage. However, the thoracic cage also has its own elastic and viscous characteristics, similar to those of the lungs. Even if the lungs were not present in the thorax, considerable muscular effort still would be required to expand the thoracic cage.

Compliance of the Thorax and the Lungs Together

The compliance of the entire pulmonary system (the lungs and the thoracic cage together) is measured while expanding the lungs of a totally relaxed or paralyzed person. To do this, air is forced into the lungs a little at a time while recording the lung pressures and volumes. It is found that to respire this total pulmonary system almost twice as much pressure is needed as when respiring the same lungs after removal from the chest cage. Therefore, the compliance of the combined lung-thorax system is only slightly greater than one half that of the lungs alone—110 milliliters of volume per centimeter of water for the combined system, compared with 200 ml/cm for the lungs alone.

The "Work" of Breathing

We have already pointed out that during normal quiet respiration respiratory muscle contraction occurs only during inspiration, whereas expiration is entirely a passive process caused by elastic recoil of the lung and chest cage structures. Thus, the respiratory muscles normally perform "work" only to cause inspiration and not at all to cause expiration.

The work of inspiration can be divided into three different fractions: (1) that required to expand the lungs against its elastic forces, called *compliance work* or *elastic work;* (2) that required to overcome the viscosity of the lung and chest wall structures, called *tissue resistance work;* and (3) that required to overcome airway resistance during the movement of air into the lungs, called *airway resistance work.*

Work Energy Required for Respiration. During normal quiet respiration, only 3 to 5 per cent of the total work energy expended by the body is required to energize the pulmonary ventilatory process. But during very heavy exercise, the amount of energy required can increase as much as 50-fold, especially if the person has any degree of increased airway resistance or decreased pulmonary compliance. Therefore, one of the major limitations in the intensity of exercise that a person can perform is the ability to provide muscle energy for the respiratory process alone.

THE PULMONARY VOLUMES AND CAPACITIES

Recording Changes in Pulmonary Volume — Spirometry

A simple method for studying pulmonary ventilation is to record the volume movement of air into and out of the lungs, a process called *spirometry.* A typical spirometer is illustrated in Figure 27–4. This consists of a drum inverted over a chamber of water, with the drum counterbalanced by a weight. In the drum is a breathing mixture of gases, usually air or oxygen; a tube connects the mouth with the gas chamber. When one breathes in and out of the chamber the drum rises and falls, and an appropriate recording is made on a moving sheet of paper.

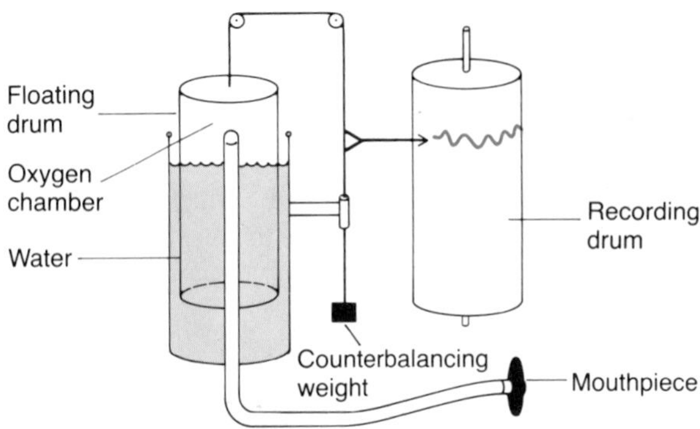

Figure 27–4. A spirometer.

Figure 27–5 illustrates a spirogram showing changes in lung volume under different conditions of breathing. For ease in describing the events of pulmonary ventilation, the air in the lungs has been subdivided at different points on this diagram into four different *volumes* and four different *capacities,* which are the following:

The Pulmonary "Volumes"

To the left in Figure 27–5 are listed four different pulmonary lung "volumes," which, when added together, equal the maximum volume to which the lungs can be expanded. The significance of each of these volumes is the following:

1. The *tidal volume* is the volume of air inspired or expired with each normal breath; it amounts to about 500 milliliters in the average young adult man.
2. The *inspiratory reserve volume* is the extra volume of air that can be inspired over and beyond the normal tidal volume; it is usually equal to approximately 3000 milliliters.

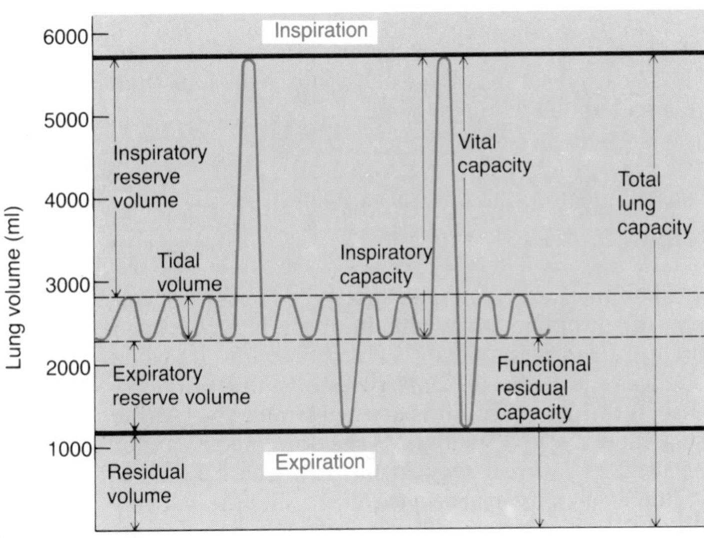

Figure 27–5. Spirogram showing respiratory excursions during normal breathing and during maximum inspiration and maximum expiration.

3. The *expiratory reserve volume* is the extra amount of air that can be expired by forceful expiration after the end of a normal tidal expiration; this normally amounts to about 1100 milliliters.
4. The *residual volume* is the volume of air still remaining in the lungs after the most forceful expiration. This volume averages about 1200 milliliters.

The Pulmonary "Capacities"

In describing events in the pulmonary cycle, it is sometimes desirable to consider two or more of the preceding volumes together. Such combinations are called *pulmonary capacities.* To the right in Figure 27–5 are listed the different pulmonary capacities, which can be described as follows:

1. The *inspiratory capacity* equals the *tidal volume* plus the *inspiratory reserve volume.* This is the amount of air (about 3500 milliliters) that a person can breathe beginning at the normal expiratory level and distending the lungs to the maximum amount.
2. The *functional residual capacity* equals the *expiratory reserve volume* plus the *residual volume.* This is the amount of air remaining in the lungs at the end of normal expiration (about 2300 milliliters).
3. The *vital capacity* equals the *inspiratory reserve volume* plus the *tidal volume* plus the *expiratory reserve volume.* This is the maximum amount of air that a person can expel from the lungs after first filling the lungs to their maximum extent and then expiring to the maximum extent (about 4600 milliliters).
4. The *total lung capacity* is the maximum volume to which the lungs can be expanded with the greatest possible inspiratory effort (about 5800 milliliters); it is equal to the vital capacity plus the residual volume.

All pulmonary volumes and capacities are about 20 to 25 per cent less in women than in men, and they obviously are greater in large and athletic persons than in small and asthenic persons.

Determination of Functional Residual Capacity—the Helium Dilution Method

The functional residual capacity, which is the volume of air that normally remains in the lungs between breaths, is very important to lung function. Its value changes markedly in some types of pulmonary disease, for which reason it is often desirable to measure this capacity. Unfortunately, the spirometer cannot be used in a direct way to measure the functional residual capacity, because the air in the residual volume of the lungs cannot be expired into the spirometer, and this volume comprises about half of the functional residual capacity. Therefore, to measure functional residual capacity, the spirometer must be used in an indirect manner, usually by means of a helium dilution method, as follows:

A spirometer of known volume is filled with air mixed with helium at a known concentration. Before breathing from the spirometer, the person expires normally. At the end of this expiration the remaining volume in the lungs is exactly equal to the functional residual capacity. At this point the subject immediately begins to breathe from the spirometer, and the gases of the spirometer begin to mix with the gases of the lungs. As a result, the helium becomes diluted by the functional residual capacity gases, and the volume of the functional residual capacity can then be calculated from the degree of dilution of the helium with use of the following formula:

$$FRC = \left(\frac{Ci_{He}}{Cf_{He}} - 1\right)Vi_{Spir}$$

in which

FRC is *functional residual capacity*
Ci_{He} is *initial concentration of helium in the spirometer*
Cf_{He} is *final concentration of helium in the spirometer,* and
Vi_{Spir} is *initial volume of the spirometer.*

THE MINUTE RESPIRATORY VOLUME—RESPIRATORY RATE TIMES TIDAL VOLUME

The *minute respiratory volume* is the total amount of new air moved into the respiratory passages each minute; this is equal to the *tidal volume* times the *respiratory rate.* The normal tidal volume of the young adult man is about 500 milliliters, and the normal respiratory rate is approximately 12 breaths per minute. Therefore, the *minute respiratory volume averages about 6 liters per minute.* A person can occasionally live for short periods of time with a minute respiratory volume as low as 1.5 liters per minute and with a respiratory rate as low as two to four breaths per minute.

The respiratory rate occasionally rises to as high as 40 to 50 per minute, and the tidal volume can become as great as the vital capacity, about 4600 milliliters in the young adult man. However, at rapid breathing rates a person usually cannot sustain a tidal volume greater than about one half the vital capacity.

ALVEOLAR VENTILATION

The ultimate importance of the pulmonary ventilatory system is to renew continually the air in the gas exchange areas of the lungs where the air is in close proximity to the pulmonary blood. These areas include the alveoli, the alveolar sacs, the alveolar ducts, and the respiratory bronchioles. The rate at which new air does reach these areas is called *alveolar ventilation.* Strangely, though, during normal quiet respiration the volume of air in the tidal air is only enough to fill the respiratory passageways down as far as the terminal bronchioles, with only a very small portion of the inspired air actually flowing all the way into the alveoli. Therefore, how does new air move this last short distance from the terminal bronchioles into the alveoli? The answer: by *diffusion.* Diffusion is caused by the kinetic motion of molecules, each gas molecule moving at high velocity among the other molecules. Fortunately, the velocity of movement of the molecules in the respiratory air is so great and the distances so short from the terminal bronchioles to the alveoli that the gases move this remaining distance in only a fraction of a second.

The Dead Space and Its Effect on Alveolar Ventilation

Unfortunately, some of the air that a person breathes never reaches the gas exchange areas but instead goes to fill respiratory passages where gas exchange does not occur. This air is called *dead space air* because it is not useful for the gas exchange process; the respiratory passages where no gas exchange takes place is called the *dead space.*

Normal Dead Space Volume. The normal dead space air in the young adult is about 150 milliliters. This increases slightly with age.

Rate of Alveolar Ventilation

Alveolar ventilation per minute is the total volume of new air entering the alveoli (and other adjacent gas exchange areas) each minute. It is equal to the respiratory rate times the amount of new air that enters the alveoli with each breath:

$$\dot{V}_A = \text{Freq} \cdot (V_T - V_D)$$

where $\dot{V}_A$ is the *volume of alveolar ventilation per minute,* Freq is the *frequency of respiration per minute,* V_T is the *tidal volume,* and V_D is the *dead space volume.*

Thus, with a normal tidal volume of 500 milliliters, a normal dead space of 150 milliliters, and a respiratory rate of 12 times per minute, alveolar ventilation equals $12 \times (500 - 150)$, or 4200 ml/min.

Alveolar ventilation is one of the major factors determining the concentrations of oxygen and carbon dioxide in the alveoli. Therefore, almost all discussions of gaseous exchange in the following chapters emphasize alveolar ventilation.

FUNCTIONS OF THE RESPIRATORY PASSAGEWAYS

The Trachea, Bronchi, and Bronchioles

Figure 27–6 illustrates the respiratory system, showing especially the respiratory passageways. The air is distributed to the lungs by way of the trachea, bronchi, and bronchioles.

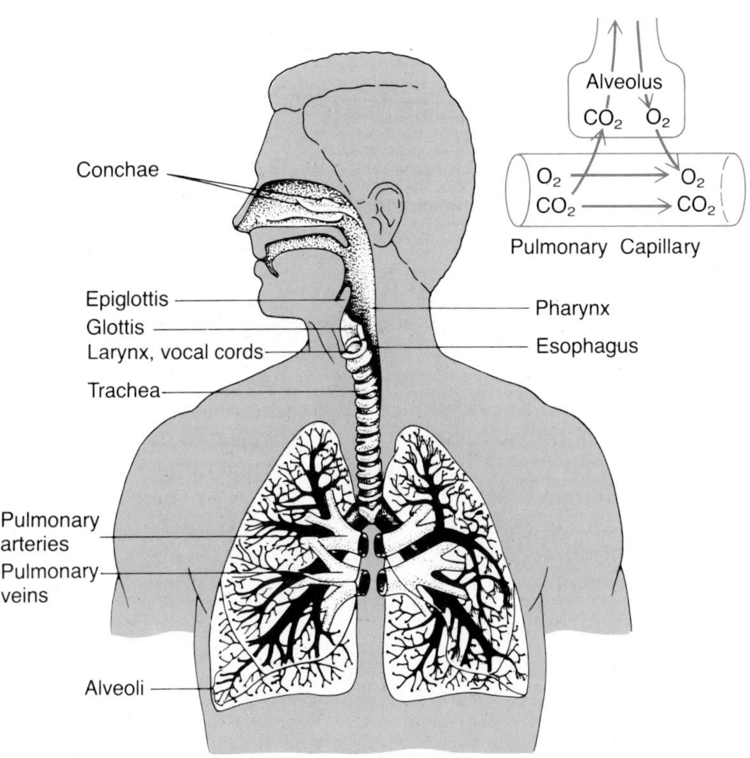

Figure 27–6. The respiratory passages.

One of the most important problems in all the respiratory passageways is to keep them open to allow easy passage of the air to and from the alveoli. To keep the trachea from collapsing, multiple cartilage rings extend about five sixths of the way around the trachea. In the walls of the bronchi are less extensive cartilage plates that also maintain a reasonable amount of rigidity, yet allow sufficient motion for the lungs to expand and contract. These plates become progressively less extensive in the later generations of bronchi and are completely gone in the bronchioles, which have diameters usually less than 1 to 1.5 millimeters.

The Muscular Wall of the Bronchi and Bronchioles and Its Control. In all areas of the trachea and bronchi not occupied by cartilage plates, the walls are composed mainly of smooth muscle. Also, the walls of the bronchioles are almost entirely smooth muscle, with the exception of the most terminal bronchiole, called the *respiratory bronchiole,* which has only a few smooth muscle fibers. Many obstructive diseases of the lung cause narrowing of the smaller bronchi and the bronchioles, often because of excessive contraction of the smooth muscle itself.

Nervous and Local Control of the Bronchiolar Musculature — Sympathetic Control. Direct control of the bronchioles by sympathetic nerve fibers is relatively weak because few of these fibers penetrate to the central portions of the lung. However, the bronchial tree is very much exposed to circulating norepinephrine and epinephrine released into the blood by sympathetic stimulation of the adrenal medullae. Both of these hormones, especially epinephrine, cause dilatation of the bronchial tree.

Parasympathetic Stimulation. A few parasympathetic nerve fibers derived from the vagus nerves also penetrate the lung parenchyma. These nerves secrete acetylcholine and, when activated, cause mild to moderate constriction of the bronchioles. When a disease process such as asthma has already caused some constriction, parasympathetic superimposed nervous stimulation often worsens the condition. When this occurs, administration of drugs that block the effects of acetylcholine, such as *atropine,* can sometimes relax the respiratory passages enough to relieve the obstruction.

Local Factors Affecting Bronchial Contraction. Several different substances formed in the lungs themselves are often quite active in causing bronchiolar constriction. Two of the most important of these are *histamine* and the substance called *slow-reacting substance of anaphylaxis.* Both of these are released in the lung tissues by mast cells during allergic reactions, especially allergic reactions caused by pollen in the air. Therefore, they play key roles in causing the airway obstruction that occurs in allergic asthma; this is especially true of the slow-reacting substance of anaphylaxis.

The Mucous Coat of the Respiratory Passageways, and Action of Cilia to Clear the Passageways

All the respiratory passages, from the nose to the terminal bronchioles, are kept moist by a layer of mucus that coats the entire surface. This mucus is secreted partly by individual goblet cells in the epithelial lining of the passages and partly by small submucosal glands. In addition to keeping the surfaces moist, the mucus also traps small particles out of the inspired air and keeps most of these from ever reaching the alveoli. The mucus itself is removed from the passages in the following manner:

The entire surface of the respiratory passages, both in the nose and in the lower passages down as far as the terminal bronchioles, is lined with ciliated epithelia, with about 200 cilia on each epithelial cell. These beat continually at a rate of 10 to 20 times per second by the mechanism explained in Chapter 2, and the direction of their "power stroke" is always toward the pharynx. That is, the cilia in the lower respiratory passages beat upward while those in the nose beat downward. This continual beating causes the coat of mucus to flow slowly, at a velocity of about 1 cm/min, toward the pharynx. Then the mucus and its entrapped particles are either swallowed or coughed to the exterior.

The Cough Reflex

The bronchi and the trachea are so sensitive to light touch that excessive amounts of any foreign matter or any other cause of irritation initiates the cough reflex. The larynx and carina (the point where the trachea divides into the bronchi) are especially sensitive. Afferent impulses pass from the respiratory passages mainly through the vagus nerves to the medulla. There, an automatic sequence of events is triggered by the neuronal circuits of the medulla, causing the following effects:

First, about 2.5 liters of air is inspired. Second, the epiglottis closes, and the vocal cords shut tightly to entrap the air within the lungs. Third, the abdominal muscles contract forcefully, pushing against the diaphragm while other expiratory muscles, such as the internal intercostals, also contract forcefully. Consequently, the pressure in the lungs rises to as high as 100 mm Hg or more. Fourth, the vocal cords and the epiglottis suddenly open widely so that air under pressure in the lungs *explodes* outward. Indeed, this air is sometimes expelled at velocities as high as 75 to 100 miles an hour. Furthermore, and very important, the strong compression of the lungs also collapses the bronchi and trachea by causing the noncartilaginous parts of these to invaginate inward so that the exploding air actually passes through *bronchial* and *tracheal slits.* The rapidly moving air usually carries with it any foreign matter that is present in the bronchi or trachea.

Respiratory Functions of the Nose

As air passes through the nose, three distinct functions are performed by the nasal cavities: (1) The *air is warmed* by the extensive surfaces of the conchae and septum, a total area of about 160 cm^2, illustrated in Figure 27–6. (2) The *air is almost completely humidi-*

fied even before it passes beyond the nose. (3) The *air is filtered.* These functions together are called the *air conditioning function* of the upper respiratory passageways. Ordinarily, the temperature of the inspired air rises to within 1°F of body temperature and within 2 to 3 per cent of full saturation with water vapor before it reaches the trachea.

Filtration Function of the Nose. The hairs at the entrance to the nostrils are important for removing large particles. Much more important, though, is the removal of particles by *turbulent precipitation.* That is, the air passing through the nasal passageways hits many obstructing vanes: the conchae (also called "turbinates" because they cause turbulence of the air), the septum, and the pharyngeal wall. Each time air hits one of these obstructions it must change its direction of movement; the particles suspended in the air, having far more mass and momentum than air, cannot change their direction of travel as rapidly as can the air. Therefore, they continue forward, striking the surfaces of the obstructions, and are entrapped in the mucous coating and transported by the cilia to the pharynx to be swallowed.

The nasal turbulence mechanism for removing particles from air is so effective that almost no particles larger than 4 to 6 micrometers in diameter enter the lungs through the nose. This size is smaller than the size of red blood cells.

Vocalization

Speech involves not only the respiratory system but also (1) specific speech nervous control centers in the cerebral cortex, which will be discussed in Chapter 39, (2) respiratory control centers of the brain, and (3) the articulation and resonance structures of the mouth and nasal cavities. Basically, speech is composed of two separate mechanical functions: (1) *phonation,* which is achieved by the larynx, and (2) *articulation,* which is achieved by the structures of the mouth.

Phonation. The larynx is especially adapted to act as a vibrator. The vibrating element is the *vocal folds,* commonly called the *vocal cords.* The vocal folds protrude from the lateral walls of the larynx toward the center of the glottis; they are stretched and positioned by several specific muscles of the larynx itself.

Figure 27–7B illustrates the vocal folds as they are seen when looking into the glottis with a laryngoscope. During normal breathing, the folds are wide open to allow easy passage of air. During phonation, the folds close together so that passage of air between them will cause vibration. The pitch of the vibration is determined mainly by the degree of stretch of the folds but also by how tightly the folds are approximated to each other and by the mass of their edges.

Figure 27–7A shows a dissected view of the vocal folds, illustrating the muscles, ligaments, and cartilages responsible for controlling the vocal folds.

Articulation and Resonance. The three major organs of articulation are the *lips,* the *tongue,* and the *soft palate.* These need not be discussed in detail because all of us are familiar with their movements during speech and other vocalizations.

The resonators include the *mouth,* the *nose* and *associated nasal sinuses,* the *pharynx,* and even the *chest cavity* itself. Here again we are all familiar with the resonating qualities of these different structures. For instance, the function of the nasal resonators is illustrated by the change in the quality of the voice when a person has a severe cold that blocks the air passages to these resonators.

THE PULMONARY CIRCULATION

The quantity of blood flowing through the lungs is essentially equal to that flowing through the systemic circulation. However, certain problems related to distribution of blood flow and other hemodynamics are special to the pulmonary circulation and are especially important to the gas exchange function of the lungs.

Physiologic Anatomy of the Pulmonary Circulatory System

The Pulmonary Vessels. The pulmonary artery extends only 5 centimeters beyond the apex of the right ventricle and then divides into the right and left main branches, which supply blood to the two respective lungs. The pulmonary arterial branches are all very short. However, all the pulmonary arteries, even

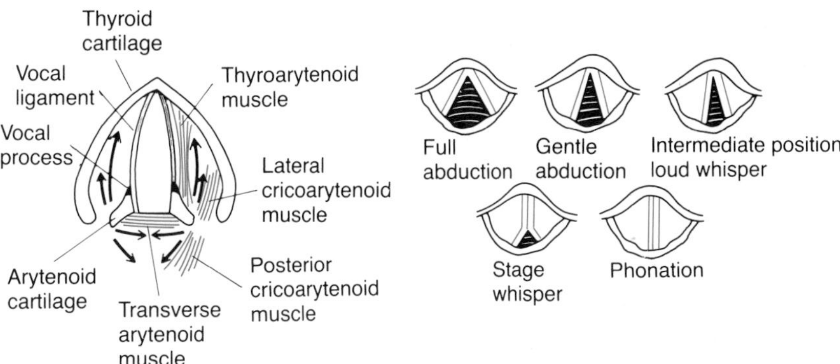

Figure 27–7. Laryngeal function in phonation. (Modified from Greene: The Voice and Its Disorders. 4th ed. Philadelphia, J. B. Lippincott Company, 1980.)

the smaller arteries and arterioles, have much larger diameters than their counterpart systemic arteries. This, combined with the fact that the vessels are very thin and distensible, gives the pulmonary arterial tree a large compliance, averaging almost 3 ml/mm Hg, which is similar to that of the systemic arterial tree. This large compliance allows the pulmonary arteries to accommodate about two thirds of the stroke volume output of the right ventricle each time the heart beats.

The pulmonary veins, like the pulmonary arteries, are also short, but their distensibility characteristics are similar to those of the veins in the systemic circulation.

The Lymphatics. Lymphatics extend from all the supportive tissues of the lung, beginning in the connective tissue spaces surrounding the terminal bronchioles and coursing to the hilum of the lung and thence mainly into the right lymphatic duct. Particulate matter entering the alveoli is partly removed via these channels, and protein is also removed from the lung tissues, thereby helping prevent edema.

Pressures in the Pulmonary System

The Pressure Pulse Curve in the Right Ventricle. The pressure pulse curves of the right ventricle and pulmonary artery are illustrated in the lower portion of Figure 27–8. These are contrasted with the much higher aortic pressure curve shown above. The systolic pressure in the right ventricle of the normal human being averages approximately 25 mm Hg, and the diastolic pressure averages about 0 to 1 mm Hg, values that are only one fifth those for the left ventricle.

Pressures in the Pulmonary Artery. During *systole,* the pressure in the pulmonary artery is essentially equal to the pressure in the right ventricle, as also shown in Figure 27–8. However, after the pulmonary valve closes at the end of systole, the ventricular pressure falls precipitously, whereas the pulmonary arterial pressure falls slowly as blood flows through the capillaries of the lungs.

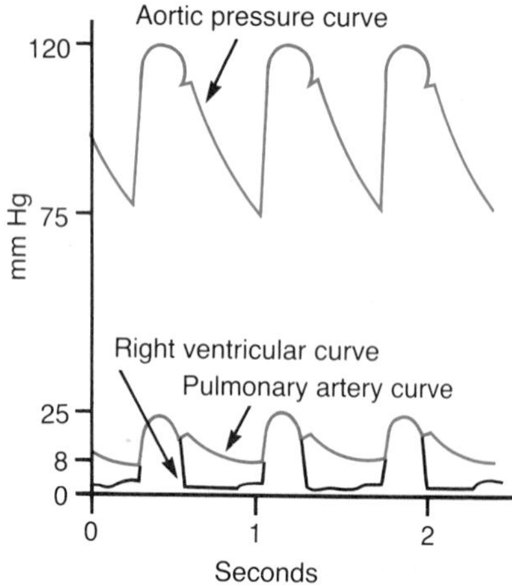

Figure 27–8. Pressure pulse contours in the right ventricle, pulmonary artery, and aorta.

As also shown in Figure 27–8, the *systolic pulmonary arterial pressure* averages approximately 25 mm Hg in the normal human being; the *diastolic pulmonary arterial pressure,* approximately 8 mm Hg; and the *mean pulmonary arterial pressure,* 15 mm Hg.

Pulmonary Capillary Pressure. The mean pulmonary capillary pressure has been estimated by indirect means to be approximately 7 mm Hg. The importance of this low capillary pressure will be discussed in more detail later in the chapter in relation to fluid exchange functions of the capillary.

Left Atrial and Pulmonary Venous Pressure. The mean pressure in the left atrium and in the major pulmonary veins averages approximately 2 mm Hg in the recumbent human being, varying from as low as 1 mm Hg to as high as 5 mm Hg.

BLOOD FLOW THROUGH THE LUNGS AND ITS DISTRIBUTION

The blood flow through the lungs is essentially equal to the cardiac output. Therefore, the factors that control cardiac output—mainly peripheral factors, as discussed in Chapter 17—also control pulmonary blood flow. Under most conditions, the pulmonary vessels act as passive, distensible tubes that enlarge with increasing pressure and narrow with decreasing pressure. However, for adequate aeration of the blood, it is important for the blood to be distributed to those segments of the lungs where the alveoli are best oxygenated. This is achieved by the following mechanism:

Effect of Diminished Alveolar Oxygen on Local Alveolar Blood Flow—Automatic Control of Pulmonary Blood Flow Distribution. When the concentration of oxygen in the alveoli decreases below normal, the adjacent blood vessels slowly constrict during the ensuing 3 to 10 minutes, the vascular resistance increasing as much as fivefold at extremely low oxygen levels. It should be noted specifically that this is *opposite the effect* normally observed in systemic vessels, which dilate, rather than constrict, in response to low oxygen. It is believed that the low oxygen concentration causes some yet undiscovered vasoconstrictor substance to be released from the lung tissue, this substance in turn promoting constriction of the small arteries. It has been suggested that this vasoconstrictor might be secreted by the alveolar epithelial cells when they become hypoxic.

This effect of a low oxygen level on pulmonary vascular resistance has an important function: to distribute blood flow where it is most effective. That is, when some of the alveoli are poorly ventilated so that the oxygen concentration in them becomes low, the local vessels constrict. This in turn causes most of the blood to flow through other areas of the lungs that are better aerated, thus providing an automatic control system for distributing blood flow to the different pulmonary areas in proportion to their degree of ventilation.

EFFECT OF HYDROSTATIC PRESSURE GRADIENTS IN THE LUNGS ON REGIONAL PULMONARY BLOOD FLOW

In Chapter 12 it was pointed out that the pressure in the foot of a standing person can be as much as 90 mm Hg greater than the pressure at the level of the heart. This is caused by *hydrostatic pressure*—that is, by the weight of the blood itself. The same effect, but to a lesser degree, occurs in the lungs. In the normal, upright adult person, the lowest point in the lungs is about 30 cm below the highest point. This represents a 23 mm Hg pressure difference, about 15 mm Hg of which are above the heart and 8 below. That is, the pulmonary arterial pressures in the uppermost portion of the lung of a standing person are about 15 mm Hg less than the pulmonary arterial pressure at the level of the heart, and the pressure in the lowest portion of the lungs is about 8 mm Hg greater. Such pressure differences have profound effects on blood flow through the different areas of the lungs. This is illustrated by the lower curve in Figure 27-9, which plots blood flow per unit of lung tissue against hydrostatic level in the lung. Note that in the standing position, at rest, there is little flow in the top of the lung but about five times this much flow in the lower lung. During exercise, when all pressures are increased, the difference is much less, as illustrated by the top curve of Figure 27-9.

Effect of Increased Cardiac Output on the Pulmonary Circulation During Heavy Exercise

During heavy exercise the blood flow through the lungs increases as much as four- to sevenfold. This extra flow is achieved in two ways: (1) by increasing the number of open capillaries, sometimes as much as

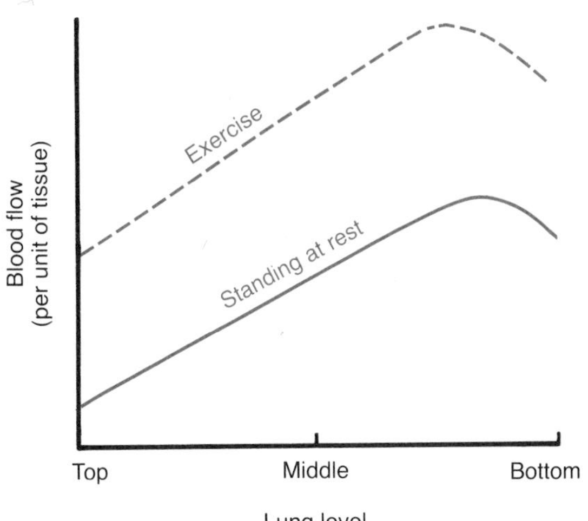

Figure 27-9. Blood flow at different levels in the lung of an upright person, both at rest and during exercise. Note that when the person is at rest, the blood flow is very low at the top of the lungs and most of the flow is through the lower lung.

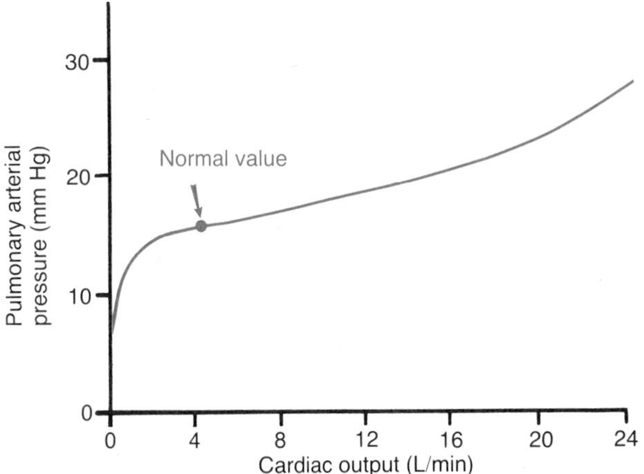

Figure 27-10. Effect on the pulmonary arterial pressure of increasing the cardiac output.

threefold, and (2) by increasing the rate of flow through each capillary, often as much as twofold. Fortunately, in the normal person, these two factors together decrease the pulmonary vascular resistance so much that the pulmonary arterial pressure rises very little even during maximum exercise; this effect is illustrated in Figure 27-10.

This ability of the lungs to accommodate greatly increased blood flow during exercise without large rises in arterial pressure obviously conserves the energy of the right side of the heart, and it also prevents a significant rise in pulmonary capillary pressure and therefore prevents development of pulmonary edema during the increased cardiac output.

Function of the Pulmonary Circulation When the Left Atrial Pressure Rises as a Result of Left Heart Failure

When the left side of the heart fails, blood begins to dam up in the left atrium. As a result, the left atrial pressure can rise on occasion from its normal value of 1 to 5 mm Hg to as high as 40 to 50 mm Hg. The initial pressure rise, up to about 7 mm Hg, has almost no effect on pulmonary circulatory function because this initial rise merely expands the venules and opens up more capillaries so that blood continues to flow with almost equal ease from the pulmonary arteries.

However, when the left atrial pressure rises to greater than 7 or 8 mm Hg, then further increases in left atrial pressure cause almost equally great increases in pulmonary arterial pressure, with concomitant increased work load on the right heart as well.

It is also true that the initial rise in left atrial pressure up to about 7 or 8 mm Hg has virtually no effect on pulmonary capillary pressure either. But any increase in left atrial pressure beyond this increases the capillary pressure almost equally as much. When the left atrial pressure has risen above 25 to 30 mm Hg, causing similar increases in capillary pressure, pulmonary edema is then very likely to develop.

PULMONARY CAPILLARY DYNAMICS

Exchange of gases between the alveolar air and the pulmonary capillary blood will be discussed in the next chapter. However, it is important for us to note here that the alveolar walls are lined with so many capillaries that in most places they almost touch each other. Therefore, it has often been said that the capillary blood flows in the alveolar walls as a "sheet," rather than in individual vessels.

Capillary Exchange of Fluid in the Lungs, and Pulmonary Interstitial Fluid Dynamics

The dynamics of fluid exchange through the lung capillaries are *qualitatively* the same as for peripheral tissues. However, *quantitatively,* there are important differences:

1. The pulmonary capillary pressure is very low, about 7 mm Hg, in comparison with a considerably higher functional capillary pressure in the peripheral tissues, about 17 mm Hg.
2. The interstitial fluid pressure in the lung is slightly more negative than in the peripheral subcutaneous tissue. (This has been measured in two ways: by a pipet inserted into the pulmonary interstitium giving a value of about −5 mm Hg, and by measuring the absorption pressure of fluid from the alveoli giving a value of about −8 mm Hg.)
3. The pulmonary capillaries are relatively leaky to protein molecules, so that the colloid osmotic pressure of the pulmonary interstitial fluids is probably about 14 mm Hg in comparison with less than half this in the peripheral tissues.
4. The alveolar walls are extremely thin, and the alveolar epithelium covering the alveolar surfaces is so weak that it is ruptured by any positive pressure in the interstitial spaces greater than atmospheric pressure (0 mm Hg), which allows dumping of fluid from the interstitial spaces into the alveoli.

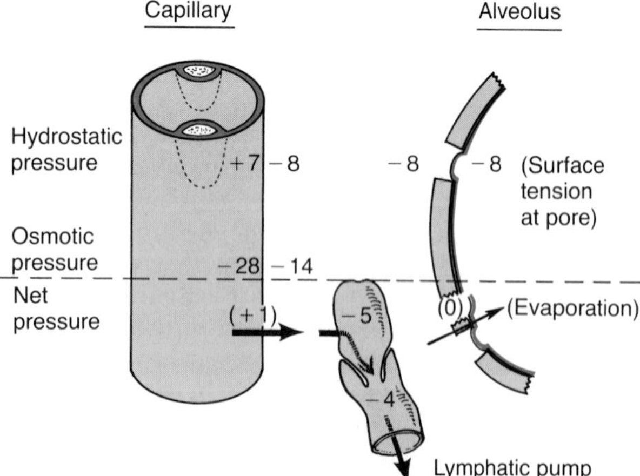

Figure 27–11. Hydrostatic and osmotic forces at the capillary (left) and alveolar membrane (right) of the lungs. Also shown is a lymphatic pump (center) that pumps fluid from the pulmonary interstitial spaces. (Modified from Guyton, Taylor, and Granger: Dynamics and Control of the Body Fluids. Philadelphia, W. B. Saunders Company, 1975.)

Now let us see how these quantitative differences affect pulmonary fluid dynamics.

Interrelationship Between Interstitial Fluid Pressure and Other Pressures in the Lung. Figure 27–11 illustrates a pulmonary capillary, a pulmonary alveolus, and a lymphatic capillary draining the interstitial space between the capillary and the alveolus. Note the approximate balance of forces at the capillary membrane as follows:

	mm Hg
Forces tending to cause movement of fluid outward from the capillaries and into the pulmonary interstitium:	
Capillary pressure	7
Interstitial fluid colloid osmotic pressure	14
Negative interstitial fluid pressure	8
TOTAL OUTWARD FORCE	29
Forces tending to cause absorption of fluid into the capillaries:	
Plasma colloid osmotic pressure	28
TOTAL INWARD FORCE	28

Thus the normal outward forces are slightly greater than the inward forces. The *net mean filtration pressure* at the pulmonary capillary membrane can be calculated as follows:

	mm Hg
Total outward force	+29
Total inward force	−28
NET MEAN FILTRATION PRESSURE	+1

This net filtration pressure causes a slight continual flow of fluid from the pulmonary capillaries into the interstitial spaces; and, except for a small amount that evaporates in the alveoli, this fluid is pumped back to the circulation through the pulmonary lymphatic system.

Negative Interstitial Pressure and the Mechanism for Keeping the Alveoli "Dry." One of the most important problems in lung function is to understand why the alveoli do not fill up with fluid. One's first impulse is to say that the alveolar epithelium keeps fluid from leaking out of the interstitial spaces into the alveoli. However, this is not true, because there are always a small number of openings between the alveolar epithelial cells through which even large protein molecules as well as large quantities of water and electrolytes can pass.

However, if one remembers that the pulmonary capillaries and the pulmonary lymphatic system normally maintain a *negative pressure* in the interstitial spaces, then it is clear that whenever extra fluid appears in the alveoli, it will simply be sucked mechanically, or move by molecular diffusion, into the lung interstitium through the small openings between the alveolar epithelial cells. Then the excess fluid is either carried away in the pulmonary lymphatics or is absorbed into the pulmonary capillaries. Thus, under normal conditions the alveoli are kept in a "dry" state except for a small amount of fluid that seeps from the epithelium onto the lining surfaces of the alveoli to keep them moist.

PULMONARY EDEMA

Pulmonary edema occurs in the same way that it occurs elsewhere in the body. Any factor that causes the pulmonary interstitial fluid pressure to rise from the negative range into the positive range will cause sudden filling of the pulmonary interstitial spaces and, in more severe cases, even of the alveoli with large amounts of free fluid.

The usual causes of pulmonary edema are:

1. Left heart failure or mitral valvular disease with consequent great increase in pulmonary capillary pressure and flooding of the interstitial spaces.
2. Damage to the pulmonary capillary membrane caused by infections such as pneumonia or by breathing noxious substances such as chlorine gas or sulfur dioxide gas, with resultant rapid leakage of both plasma proteins and fluid out of the capillaries.

Pulmonary "Interstitial Fluid" Edema Versus Pulmonary "Alveolar" Edema. The interstitial fluid volume of the lungs usually cannot increase more than about 50 per cent (representing less than 100 milliliters of fluid) before the alveolar epithelial membranes rupture and fluid begins to pour from the interstitial spaces into the alveoli. The cause of this is simply the very slight tensional strength of the pulmonary alveolar epithelium; that is, any positive pressure in the interstitial fluid spaces seems to cause immediate rupture of this epithelium.

Therefore, except in the mildest cases of pulmonary edema, edema fluid always enters the alveoli; if this edema becomes severe enough, it can cause death by suffocation.

Rapidity of Death in Acute Pulmonary Edema. When the pulmonary capillary pressure does rise even slightly above the critical level required to maintain a negative interstitial pressure, lethal pulmonary edema can occur within hours, and even within 20 to 30 minutes if the capillary pressure rises as much as 25 to 30 mm Hg above the safe level. Thus, in acute left heart failure, in which the pulmonary capillary pressure occasionally rises to as high as 50 mm Hg, death frequently ensues in less than one-half hour from acute pulmonary edema.

The Fluids in the Pleural Cavity

When the lungs expand and contract during normal breathing, they slide back and forth within the pleural cavity. To facilitate this, a very thin layer of fluid lies between the parietal and visceral pleurae.

Figure 27-12 illustrates the dynamics of fluid exchange in the pleural space. Each of the two pleurae is a very porous mesenchymal serous membrane through which small amounts of interstitial fluid transude continually into the pleural space. These fluids carry with them tissue proteins, giving the pleural fluid a mucoid characteristic, which is what allows extremely easy slippage of the moving lungs.

The total amount of fluid in each pleural cavity is very slight, only a few milliliters. Yet whenever the quantity becomes more than barely enough to separate the two pleurae, the excess is pumped away by lymphatic vessels opening directly from the pleural cavity into (1) the mediastinum, (2) the superior surface of the diaphragm, and (3) the lateral surfaces of the parietal pleura. Therefore, the *pleural space*— the space between the visceral and parietal pleurae— is called a *potential space* because normally it is so narrow that it is not obviously a physical space at all.

Negative Pressure in the Pleural Fluid. Because the recoil tendency of the lungs causes them to try to collapse, a negative force is always required on the outside of the lungs to keep them expanded. This is provided by a negative pressure in the normal pleural space. The basic cause of this negative pressure is the pumping of fluid from the space by the lymphatics (which is also the basis of the negative pressure found in most tissue spaces of the body). Because the normal collapse tendency of the lungs is about −4 mm Hg (−5 or −6 centimeters of water) the pleural fluid pressure must always be at least as negative as −4 mm Hg simply to keep the lungs expanded. Actual measurements have shown it usually to be about −7 mm Hg, which is a few millimeters of mercury more negative than the collapse pressure of the lungs. Thus, the negativity of the pleural fluid keeps the lungs pulled tightly against the parietal pleura of the chest cavity except for the extremely thin layer of mucoid fluid that acts as a lubricant.

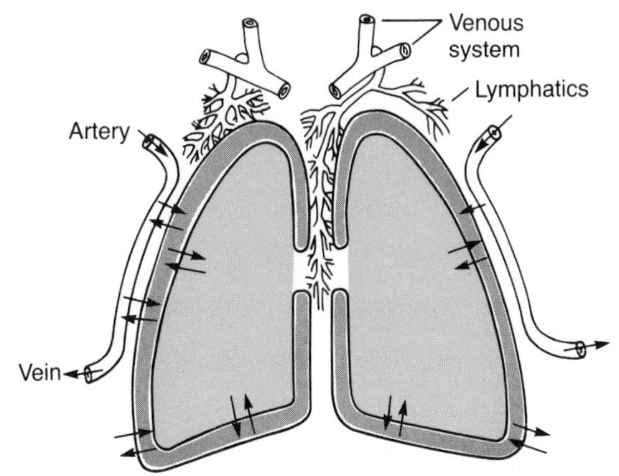

Figure 27-12. Dynamics of fluid exchange in the intrapleural spaces.

REFERENCES

Bourbon, J. R., and Rieutort, M.: Pulmonary surfactant: Biochemistry, physiology, and pathology. News Physiol. Sci., 2:129, 1987.

Deslauriers, J., and Lacquet, L. K.: The Pleural Space. Vol. 6. In Delarue, N. C., and Eschapasse, H. (eds.): International Trends in General Thoracic Surgery Series. St. Louis, C. V. Mosby Co., 1989.

Effros, R. M.: Pulmonary microcirculation and exchange. In Renkin, E. M., and Michel, C. C. (eds.): Handbook of Physiology. Sec. 2, Vol. IV. Bethesda, Md., American Physiology Society, 1984, p. 865.

Fujimura, O.: Vocal Physiology: Voice Production, Mechanisms and Function (Vocal Fold Physiology, Vol. 2). New York, Raven Press, 1988.

Gabella, G.: Innervation of airway smooth muscle: Fine structure. Annu. Rev. Physiol., 49:583, 1987.

Guyton, A. C., and Lindsey, A. W.: Effect of elevated left atrial pressure and decreased plasma protein concentration on the development of pulmonary edema. Circ. Res., 7:649, 1959.

Guyton, A. C., et al.: Forces governing water movement in the lung. In Pulmonary Edema. Washington, D. C., American Physiological Society, 1979, p. 65.

Newman, J. D. (ed.): The Physiological Control of Mammalian Vocalization. New York, Plenum Publishing Corp., 1988.

Staub, N. C.: Pulmonary edema. Physiol. Rev., 54:678, 1974.

Taylor, A. E., et al.: Clinical Respiratory Physiology. Philadelphia, W. B. Saunders Co., 1989.

Van Gold, L. M. G., et al.: The pulmonary surfactant system: Biochemical aspects and functional significance. Physiol. Rev., 68:374, 1988.

West, J. B.: Pulmonary Pathophysiology—The Essentials. 3rd ed. Baltimore, Williams & Wilkins, 1987.

QUESTIONS

1. Explain the roles of the diaphragm and of the elasticity of the chest cage in expansion and contraction of the lungs.
2. Explain the roles of the neck muscles and the abdominal recti in causing expansion and contraction of the lungs.
3. How much does the intra-alveolar pressure change during normal inspiration and expiration?
4. What are the two factors that cause the lungs to collapse when the thoracic cage is opened?
5. Explain the role of *surfactant* in decreasing the tendency of the lungs to collapse.
6. What is meant by the *compliance* of the lungs? How much greater is the compliance of the lungs alone than the compliance of the lungs and thoracic cage together?
7. Define and give normal values for *tidal volume, inspiratory reserve volume, expiratory reserve volume,* and *residual volume.*
8. Define and give normal quantitative values for *inspiratory capacity, functional residual capacity, vital capacity,* and *total lung capacity.*
9. What is the functional significance of the *residual volume?*
10. Give normal values for the *respiratory rate,* the *minute respiratory volume,* and *alveolar ventilation.*
11. Explain the quantitative difference between *minute respiratory volume* and *alveolar ventilation.*
12. What are the air conditioning functions of the nose?
13. Explain the different nervous and humoral factors that control the bronchioles.
14. What are the roles of *mucus* and the *cilia* in the respiratory passageways?
15. Explain the mechanism of the cough reflex.
16. How are the vocal cords controlled for the purpose of changing the frequency and quality of the sounds emitted by the larynx?
17. Explain the important anatomical differences between the pulmonary circulation and the systemic circulation.
18. What are the quantitative differences between the pulmonary vascular pressures and the systemic pressures?
19. What is the importance of the very low pulmonary capillary pressure?
20. Describe the mechanism by which low oxygen concentration in the alveoli controls blood flow through the local pulmonary vessels and explain why this is important to function of the lungs.
21. Explain the important effects of hydrostatic pressure gradients on pulmonary vascular function in both normal and abnormal conditions.
22. Why does the pulmonary arterial pressure not rise markedly in the normal person during heavy exercise?
23. Describe the quantitative differences between pulmonary interstitial fluid dynamics and peripheral interstitial fluid dynamics, beginning with the differences between the forces active at the capillary membrane.
24. What is the mechanism for keeping the alveoli normally "dry"?
25. Why does positive pressure in the pulmonary interstitium usually cause fluid to flood the alveoli?

28

Transport of Oxygen and Carbon Dioxide Between the Alveoli and the Tissue Cells

DIFFUSION OF OXYGEN AND CARBON DIOXIDE

After the alveoli are ventilated with fresh air, the next step in the respiratory process is *diffusion* of oxygen from the alveoli into the pulmonary blood and diffusion of carbon dioxide in the opposite direction.

All the gases that are of concern in respiratory physiology are simple molecules that are free to move among each other, which is the process called diffusion. This is also true of the gases dissolved in the fluids and tissues of the body.

However, for diffusion to occur, there must be a source of energy. This is provided by the kinetic motion of the molecules themselves. That is, except at absolute zero temperature, all molecules of all matter are continually undergoing motion. For free molecules that are not physically attached to others, this means linear movement at high velocity until they strike other molecules. Then they bounce away in new directions and continue again until striking still other molecules. In this way the molecules move rapidly among each other.

Gas Pressures in a Mixture of Gases—Partial Pressures of Individual Gases

Pressure is caused by the constant impact of kinetically moving molecules against a surface. Therefore, the pressure of a gas acting on the surfaces of the respiratory passages and alveoli is proportional to the summated force of impact of all the molecules striking the surface at any given instant.

However, in respiratory physiology, one deals with mixtures of gases, mainly of oxygen, nitrogen, and carbon dioxide. Furthermore, the rate of diffusion of each of these gases is directly proportional to the pressure caused by this gas alone, which is called the *partial pressure* of the gas. Therefore, let us explain the concept of partial pressure.

Consider air, which has an approximate composition of 79 per cent nitrogen and 21 per cent oxygen. The total pressure of this mixture is 760 mm Hg, and it is clear from the above description of the molecular basis of pressure that each gas contributes to the total pressure in direct proportion to its concentration. Therefore, 79 per cent of the 760 mm Hg is caused by nitrogen (about 600 mm Hg) and 21 per cent by oxygen (about 160 mm Hg). Thus, the "partial pressure" of nitrogen in the mixture is 600 mm Hg, and the "partial pressure" of oxygen is 160 mm Hg; the total pressure is 760 mm Hg, the sum of the individual pressures.

The pressures of the individual gases in a mixture are designated by the symbols P_{O_2}, P_{CO_2}, P_{N_2}, P_{H_2O}, P_{He}, and so forth.

Pressures of Gases in Water and Tissues

Gases dissolved in water or in the body tissues also exert pressure, because the dissolved molecules are moving randomly and have kinetic energy, as do the molecules in the gaseous phase. Furthermore, when the molecules of a gas dissolved in fluid encounter a surface like the membrane of a cell, they exert their own pressure in the same way that a gas in the gaseous phase exerts its own individual partial pressure. The pressures of the separate dissolved gases are designated similarly as for the partial pressures of the gases in the gaseous state, i.e., P_{O_2}, P_{CO_2}, P_{N_2}, P_{He}.

The Vapor Pressure of Water

When air enters the respiratory passageways, water immediately evaporates from the surfaces of these passages and humidifies the air. This results from the fact that water molecules, like the different dissolved gas molecules, are continually escaping from the water surface into the gas phase. The pressure that the water molecules exert to escape through the surface is called the *vapor pressure* of the water. At normal body temperature, 37°C, this vapor pressure is 47 mm Hg. Therefore, once the gas mixture has become fully humidified—that is, once it is in "equilibrium" with the surrounding water—the partial pressure of the water vapor in the gas mixture is also 47 mm Hg. This partial pressure, like the other partial pressures, is designated P_{H_2O}.

The vapor pressure of water depends entirely on the temperature of the water. At normal room temperature, the vapor pressure is about 20 mm Hg. But the most important value to remember is the vapor pressure at body temperature, 47 mm Hg; this value will appear in many of our subsequent discussions.

Diffusion of Gases Through Fluids—The Pressure Difference for Diffusion

Now, let us return to the problem of diffusion. From the above discussion it is already clear that when the concentration, or pressure, of a gas is greater in one area than in another area, there will be net diffusion from the high pressure area toward the low pressure area. For instance, in Figure 28-1, one can readily see that the molecules in the area of high pressure at the left end of the chamber, because of their greater number, have a greater statistical chance of moving randomly into the area of low pressure than do molecules attempting to go in the other direction. However, some molecules do bounce randomly from the area of low pressure toward the area of high pressure. Therefore, the *net diffusion* of gas from the area of high pressure to the area of low pressure is equal to the number of molecules bouncing in this direction *minus* the number bouncing in the opposite direction, and this in turn is proportional to the gas pressure difference between the two areas, called simply the *pressure difference for diffusion.*

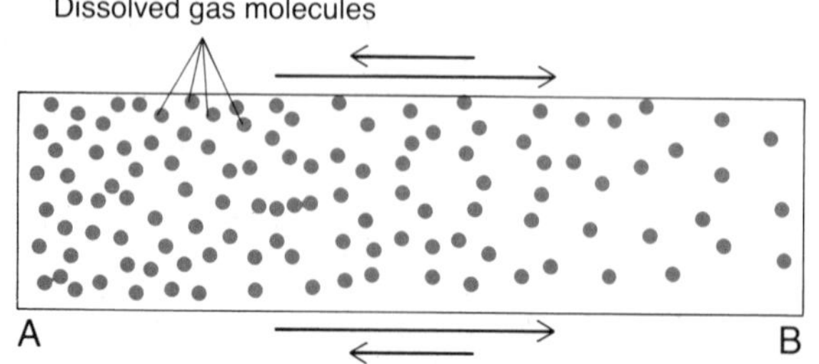

Figure 28-1. Net diffusion of oxygen from one end of a chamber to the other.

Quantifying the Net Rate of Diffusion in Fluids. In addition to the pressure difference, several other factors affect the rate of gas diffusion in a fluid. These are (1) the solubility of the gas in the fluid, (2) the cross-sectional area of the fluid, (3) the distance through which the gas must diffuse, (4) the molecular weight of the gas, and (5) the temperature of the fluid. In the body, the last of these factors, the temperature, remains reasonably constant and usually need not be considered. All of these factors can be expressed in a single formula, as follows:

$$D \propto \frac{\Delta P \times A \times S}{d \times \sqrt{MW}}$$

in which D is the diffusion rate, ΔP is the pressure difference between the two ends of the diffusion pathway, A is the cross-sectional area of the pathway, S is the solubility of the gas, d is the distance of diffusion, and MW is the molecular weight of the gas.

It is obvious from this formula that the characteristics of the gas itself determine two factors of the formula: solubility and molecular weight, and these together are called the *diffusion coefficient* of the gas. That is, the diffusion coefficient equals $S/\sqrt{MW}$; the relative rates at which different gases at the same pressure levels will diffuse are proportional to their diffusion coefficients. Considering the diffusion coefficient for oxygen to be 1, the *relative* diffusion coefficients for different gases of respiratory importance in the body fluids are as follows:

Oxygen	1.0
Carbon dioxide	20.3
Nitrogen	0.53

Diffusion of Gases Through Tissues

The gases that are of respiratory importance are highly soluble in lipids and, consequently, are also highly soluble in cell membranes. Because of this, these gases diffuse through the cell membranes with very little impediment. Instead, the major limitation to the movement of gases in tissues is the rate at which the gases can diffuse through the tissue water instead of through the cell membranes. Therefore, diffusion of gases through the tissues, including through the respiratory membrane, is almost equal to the diffusion of gases through water, as given in the above list. Note especially that carbon dioxide diffuses 20 times as rapidly as oxygen because of its high solubility in tissue fluids.

COMPOSITION OF ALVEOLAR AIR—ITS RELATION TO ATMOSPHERIC AIR

Alveolar air does not have the same concentrations of gases as atmospheric air by any means, which can readily be seen by comparing the alveolar air composition in column 5 of Table 28–1 with the composition of atmospheric air in column 1. There are several reasons for the differences. First, the alveolar air is only partially replaced by atmospheric air with each breath. Second, oxygen is constantly being absorbed from the alveolar air. Third, carbon dioxide is constantly diffusing from the pulmonary blood into the alveoli. And, fourth, dry atmospheric air that enters the respiratory passages is humidified even before it reaches the alveoli.

Humidification of the Air As It Enters the Respiratory Passages. Column 1 of Table 28–1 shows that atmospheric air is composed almost entirely of nitrogen and oxygen; it normally contains almost no carbon dioxide and little water vapor. However, as soon as the atmospheric air enters the respiratory passages, it is exposed to the fluids covering the respiratory surfaces. Even before the air enters the alveoli, it becomes totally humidified. The partial pressure of water vapor at normal body temperature of 37°C is 47 mm Hg, which, therefore, is the partial pressure of water in the alveolar air.

Rate at Which Alveolar Air Is Renewed by Atmospheric Air

In Chapter 27, it was pointed out that the *functional residual capacity* of the lungs, the amount of air remaining in the lungs at the end of normal expiration, measures approximately 2300 milliliters. Yet only 350 milliliters of new air is brought into the alveoli with each normal respiration, and this same amount of old alveolar air is expired. Therefore, the amount of alveolar air replaced by new atmospheric air with each breath is only one seventh of the total, so that many breaths are required to exchange most of the alveolar air. Thus, at normal alveolar ventilation approximately half the gas is exchanged in 17 seconds. This slow replacement of alveolar air is of particular importance in preventing sudden changes in gaseous concentrations in the blood.

Oxygen Concentration and Pressure in the Alveoli

Oxygen is continually being absorbed into the blood of the lungs, and new oxygen is continually being

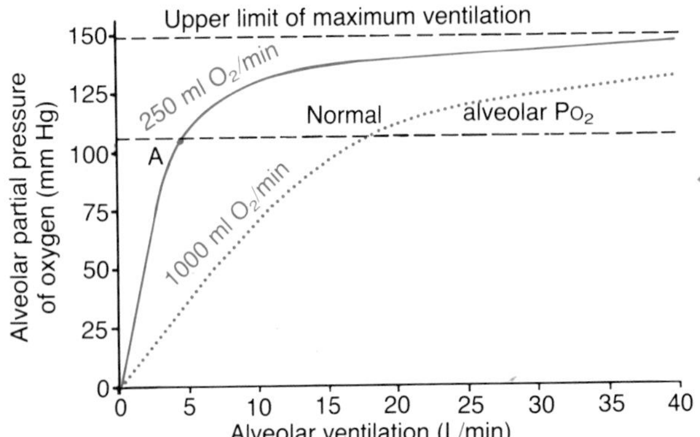

Figure 28–2. Effect of alveolar ventilation and of two rates of oxygen absorption, 250 ml/min and 1000 ml/min, from the alveoli on the alveolar Po_2.

breathed into the alveoli from the atmosphere. The more rapidly oxygen is absorbed, the lower becomes its concentration in the alveoli; on the other hand, the more rapidly new oxygen is breathed into the alveoli from the atmosphere, the higher becomes its concentration. Thus, oxygen concentration in the alveoli, and therefore its pressure as well, is controlled by, first, the rate of absorption of oxygen into the blood and, second, the rate of entry of new oxygen into the lungs by the ventilatory process.

Figure 28–2 illustrates the effect both of alveolar ventilation and of rate of oxygen absorption into the blood on the alveolar pressure of oxygen (PA_{O_2}). The solid curve represents oxygen absorption at a rate of 250 ml/min, and the dotted curve at 1000 ml/min. At a normal ventilatory rate of 4.2 liters/min and an oxygen consumption of 250 ml/min, the normal operating point in Figure 28–2 is point A. The figure also shows that when 1000 milliliters of oxygen is being absorbed each minute, as occurs during moderate exercise, the rate of alveolar ventilation must increase fourfold to maintain the alveolar Po_2 at the normal value of 104 mm Hg.

Another effect illustrated in Figure 28–2 is that an extremely marked increase in alveolar ventilation can never increase the alveolar Po_2 above 149 mm Hg as long as the person is breathing normal atmospheric air, for this is the maximum Po_2 of oxygen in humidified atmospheric air. However, if the person breathes gases containing pressures of oxygen higher than 149 mm Hg, the alveolar Po_2 can approach these higher pressures.

Table 28–1 PARTIAL PRESSURES OF RESPIRATORY GASES AS THEY ENTER AND LEAVE THE LUNGS (AT SEA LEVEL)

	Atmospheric Air* (mm Hg)		Humidified Air (mm Hg)		Alveolar Air (mm Hg)		Expired Air (mm Hg)	
N_2	597.0	(78.62%)	563.4	(74.09%)	569.0	(74.9%)	566.0	(74.5%)
O_2	159.0	(20.84%)	149.3	(19.67%)	104.0	(13.6%)	120.0	(15.7%)
CO_2	0.3	(0.04%)	0.3	(0.04%)	40.0	(5.3%)	27.0	(3.6%)
H_2O	3.7	(0.50%)	47.0	(6.20%)	47.0	(6.2%)	47.0	(6.2%)
TOTAL	760.0	(100.00%)	760.0	(100.00%)	760.0	(100.0%)	760.0	(100.0%)

*On an average cool, clear day.

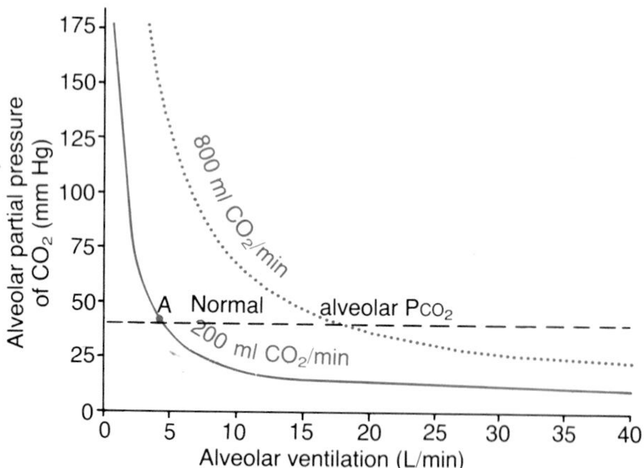

Figure 28-3. Effect on alveolar P_{CO_2} of alveolar ventilation and rate of carbon dioxide excretion from the blood.

CO_2 Concentration and Pressure in the Alveoli

Carbon dioxide is continually being formed in the body, then discharged into the alveoli; and it is continually being removed from the alveoli by ventilation. Figure 28-3 illustrates the effects on the alveolar P_{CO_2} of both alveolar ventilation and two rates of carbon dioxide excretion. The solid curve represents a normal rate of carbon dioxide excretion of 200 ml/min. At the normal rate of alveolar ventilation of 4.2 liters/min, the operating point for alveolar P_{CO_2} is at point A in Figure 28-3—that is, 40 mm Hg.

Two other facts are also evident from Figure 28-3: First, *the alveolar P_{CO_2} increases directly in proportion to the rate of carbon dioxide excretion,* as represented by the elevation of the dotted curve for 800 milliliters CO_2 excretion per minute. Second, *the alveolar P_{CO_2} decreases in inverse proportion to alveolar ventilation.* Therefore, the concentrations and pressures of both oxygen and carbon dioxide in the alveoli are determined by the rates of absorption or excretion of the two gases, and also by the alveolar ventilation.

DIFFUSION OF GASES THROUGH THE RESPIRATORY MEMBRANE

The Respiratory Unit. Figure 28-4 illustrates the respiratory unit, which is composed of a *respiratory bronchiole, alveolar ducts, atria,* and *alveoli* (of which there are about 300 million in the two lungs, each alveolus having an average diameter of about 0.2 millimeter). The alveolar walls are extremely thin, and within them is an almost solid network of interconnecting capillaries, illustrated in Figure 28-5. Indeed, because of the extensiveness of the capillary plexus, gaseous exchange between the alveolar air and the pulmonary blood occurs through the membranes of all the terminal portions of the lungs. These mem-

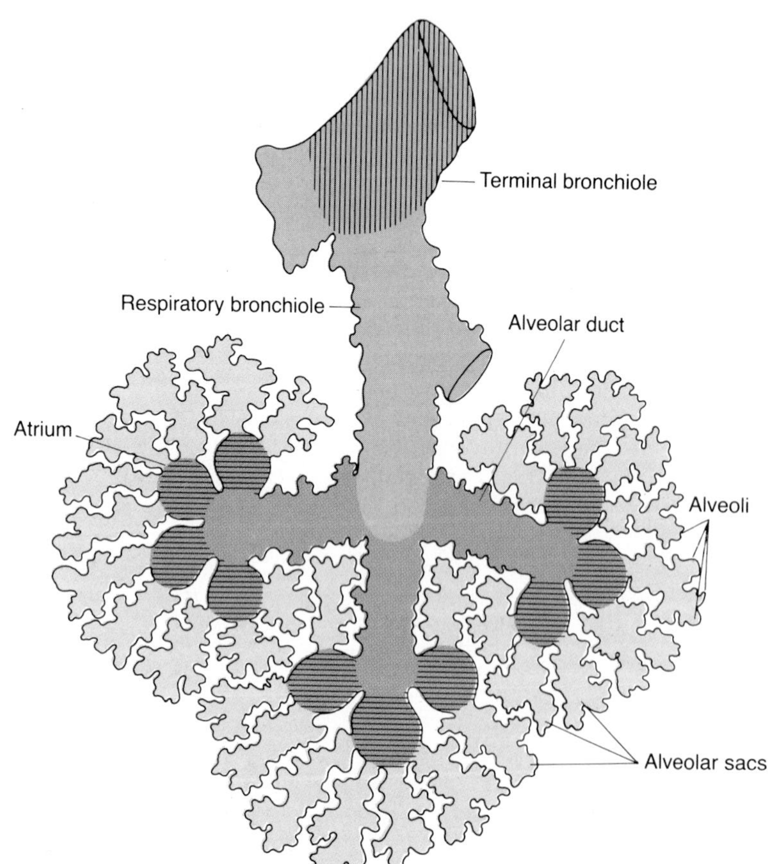

Figure 28-4. The respiratory lobule. (From Miller: The Lung. Springfield, Ill., Charles C Thomas.)

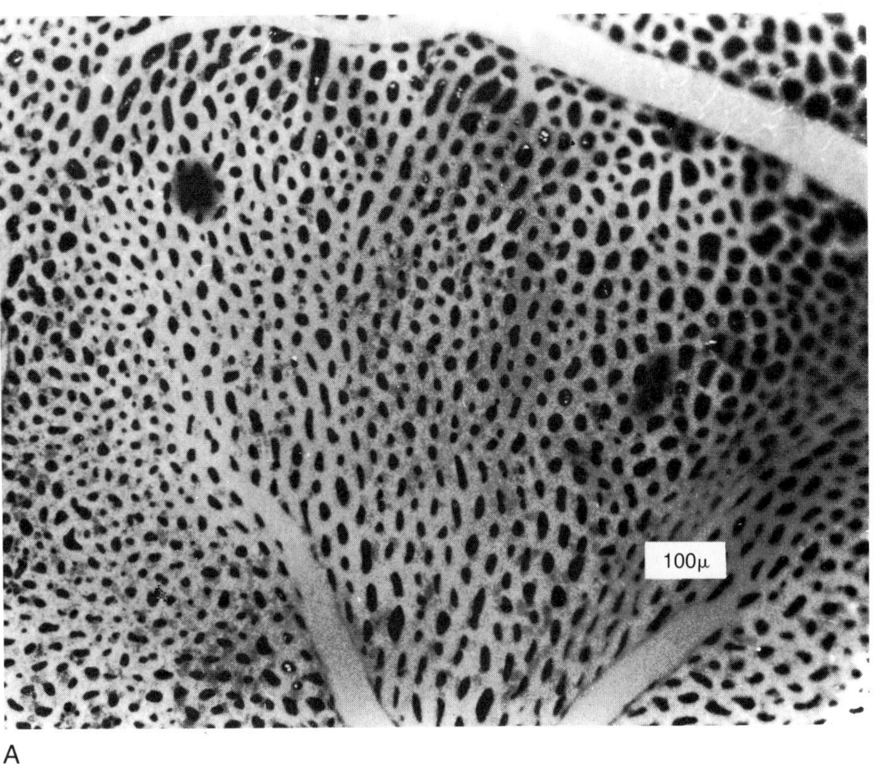

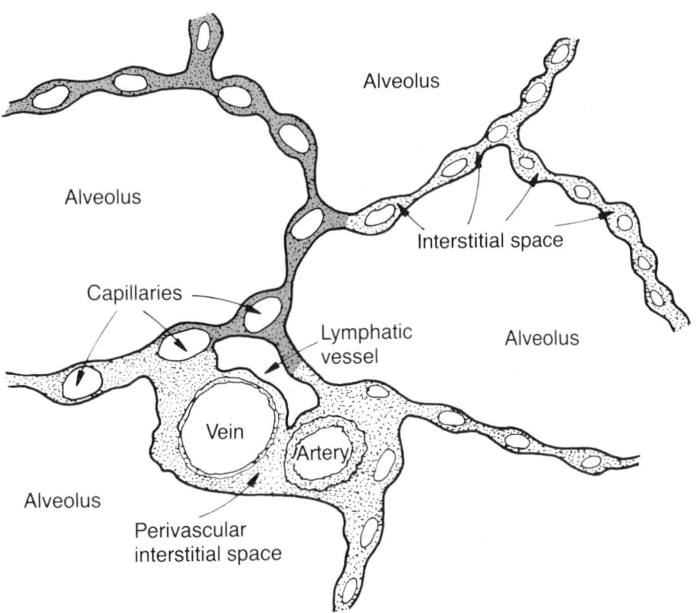

Figure 28–5. *A,* Surface view of capillaries in the alveolar wall. (From Maloney and Castle: *Resp. Physiol.,* 7:150, 1969. Reproduced by permission of ASP Biological and Medical Press. North-Holland Division.) *B,* Cross-sectional view of alveolar walls and their vascular supply.

branes are collectively known as the *respiratory membrane,* also called the *pulmonary membrane.*

The Respiratory Membrane. Figure 28–6 illustrates to the left the ultrastructure of the respiratory membrane shown in cross-section and to the right a red blood cell. It also shows the diffusion of oxygen from the alveolus into the red blood cell and diffusion of carbon dioxide in the opposite direction. Note especially the several different layers of the respiratory membranes.

Despite the large number of layers, the overall thickness of the respiratory membrane in some areas is as little as 0.2 micrometer, and it averages about 0.6 micrometer.

From histologic studies it has been estimated that the total surface area of the respiratory membrane is approximately 50 to 100 square meters in the normal adult. This is equivalent to the floor area of a 25 by 30 foot room. The total quantity of blood in the capillaries of the lung at any given instant is 60 to 140 milliliters. Now imagine this small amount of blood spread over the entire surface of a 25 by 30 foot floor,

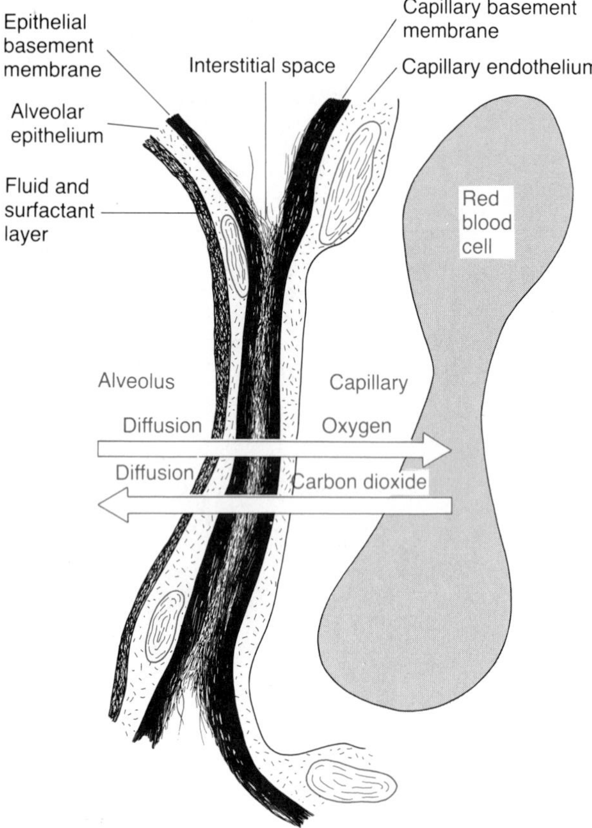

Figure 28-6. Ultrastructure of the respiratory membrane as shown in cross-section.

and it is very easy to understand the rapidity of respiratory exchange of gases.

Factors That Affect the Rate of Gas Diffusion Through the Respiratory Membrane

Referring to the earlier discussion of diffusion through water, one can apply the same principles and same formula to diffusion of gases through the respiratory membrane. Thus, the factors that determine how rapidly a gas will pass through the membrane are (1) the *thickness of the membrane;* (2) the *surface area of the membrane;* (3) the *diffusion coefficient* of the gas in the substance of the membrane—that is, in the water of the membrane; and (4) the *pressure difference* between the two sides of the membrane.

The *thickness of the respiratory membrane* occasionally increases, often as a result of edema fluid in the interstitial space of the membrane and in the alveoli, so that the respiratory gases must then diffuse not only through the membrane but also through this fluid. Also, some pulmonary diseases cause fibrosis of the lungs, which can increase the thickness of some portions of the respiratory membrane. Because the rate of diffusion through the membrane is inversely proportional to the thickness of the membrane, any factor that increases the thickness to more than two to three times normal can interfere significantly with normal respiratory exchange of gases.

The *surface area of the respiratory membrane* can be greatly decreased by many different conditions. For instance, removal of an entire lung decreases the surface area to half normal. Also, in *emphysema* many of the alveoli coalesce, with dissolution of many alveolar walls. Therefore, the new chambers are much larger than the original alveoli, but the total surface area of the respiratory membrane is considerably decreased because of loss of the alveolar walls. When the total surface area is decreased to approximately one third to one fourth normal, exchange of gases through the membrane is impeded to a significant degree *even under resting conditions.* During competitive sports and other strenuous exercise, even the slightest decrease in surface area of the lungs can be a serious detriment to respiratory exchange of gases.

The *diffusion coefficient* for the transfer of each gas through the respiratory membrane depends on its *solubility* in the membrane and inversely on the *square root* of its *molecular weight.* The rate of diffusion in the respiratory membrane is almost exactly the same as that in water, for reasons explained earlier. Therefore, for a given pressure difference, carbon dioxide diffuses through the membrane about 20 times as rapidly as oxygen. Oxygen in turn diffuses about two times as rapidly as nitrogen.

The *pressure difference* across the respiratory membrane is the difference between the pressure of the gas in the alveoli and the pressure of the gas in the blood. The alveolar pressure represents a measure of the total number of molecules of a particular gas striking a unit area of the alveolar surface of the membrane in unit time, and the pressure of the gas in the blood represents the number of molecules attempting to escape from the blood in the opposite direction. Therefore, the difference between these two pressures is a measure of the *net tendency* for the gas to move through the membrane. Obviously, when the pressure of a gas in the alveoli is greater than the pressure of the gas in the blood, as is true for oxygen, net diffusion from the alveoli into the blood occurs; but when the pressure of the gas in the blood is greater than the partial pressure in the alveoli, as is true for carbon dioxide, net diffusion from the blood into the alveoli occurs.

Diffusing Capacity of the Respiratory Membrane

The ability of the respiratory membrane to exchange a gas between the alveoli and the pulmonary blood can be expressed in quantitative terms by its *diffusing capacity,* which is defined as the *volume of a gas that diffuses through the membrane each minute for a pressure difference of 1 mm Hg.*

Obviously, all the factors previously discussed that affect diffusion through the respiratory membrane can affect the diffusing capacity.

The Diffusing Capacity for Oxygen. In the average young male adult the *diffusing capacity for oxygen* under resting conditions averages *21 ml/min/mm Hg.* In functional terms, what does this mean? The mean oxygen pressure difference across the respiratory membrane during normal, quiet breathing is approximately 11 mm Hg. Multiplication of this pressure by the diffusing capacity (11 × 21) gives a total of about 230 milliliters of oxygen diffusing through the respiratory membrane each minute; this is equal to the rate at which the body uses oxygen.

Change in Oxygen-Diffusing Capacity During Exercise. During strenuous exercise, or during other conditions that greatly increase pulmonary blood flow and alveolar ventilation, the diffusing capacity for oxygen increases in young male adults to a maximum of about 65 ml/min/mm Hg, which is three times the diffusing capacity under resting conditions. This increase is caused mainly by opening up of many previously dormant pulmonary capillaries, thereby increasing the surface area of the blood into which the oxygen can diffuse. Therefore, during exercise, the oxygenation of the blood is increased not only by increased alveolar ventilation but also by a greater capacity of the respiratory membrane for transmitting oxygen into the blood.

Diffusing Capacity for Carbon Dioxide. The diffusing capacity for carbon dioxide has never been measured because of the following technical difficulty: Carbon dioxide diffuses through the respiratory membrane so rapidly that the average P_{CO_2} in the pulmonary blood is not far different from the P_{CO_2} in the alveoli—the average difference is less than 1 mm Hg—and with the available techniques, this difference is too small to be measured.

Nevertheless, measurements of diffusion of other gases have shown that the diffusing capacity varies directly with the diffusion coefficient of the particular gas. Since the diffusion coefficient of carbon dioxide is 20 times that of oxygen, one would expect a diffusing capacity for carbon dioxide under resting conditions of about 400 to 450 ml/min/mm Hg and during exercise of about 1200 to 1300 ml/min/mm Hg.

Figure 28–7 compares the measured or calculated diffusing capacities of oxygen, carbon dioxide, and carbon monoxide at rest and during exercise, showing the extreme diffusing capacity of carbon dioxide and also the effect of exercise on the diffusing capacities of all these gases.

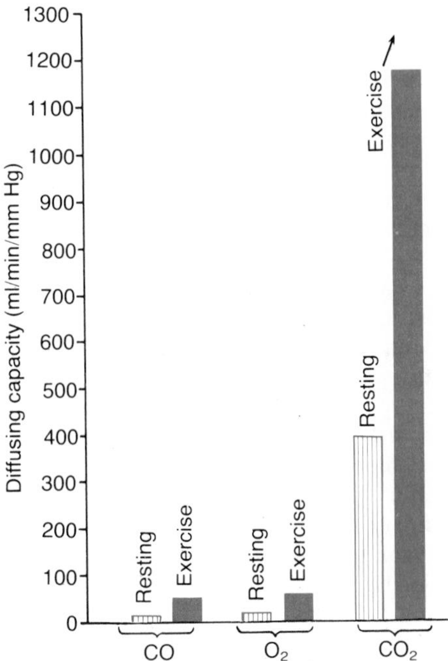

Figure 28–7. Lung diffusing capacities for carbon monoxide, oxygen, and carbon dioxide in the normal lungs.

Uptake of Oxygen from the Alveoli by the Pulmonary Blood

The top part of Figure 28–8 illustrates a pulmonary alveolus adjacent to a pulmonary capillary, showing diffusion of oxygen molecules between the alveolar air and the pulmonary blood. The P_{O_2} of the gaseous oxygen in the alveolus averages 104 mm Hg, whereas the P_{O_2} of the venous blood entering the capillary averages only 40 mm Hg because a large amount of oxygen has been removed from this blood as it has passed through the peripheral tissues. Therefore, the *initial* pressure difference that causes oxygen to diffuse into the pulmonary capillary is 104 − 40, or 64 mm Hg. The curve below the capillary shows the progressive rise in blood P_{O_2} as the blood passes through the capillary, showing that the P_{O_2} rises essentially to equal that of the alveolar air by the time the blood has moved a third of the distance through the capillary, becoming almost 104 mm Hg.

Uptake of Oxygen by the Pulmonary Blood During Exercise. During strenuous exercise, a person's body may require as much as 20 times the normal amount of oxygen. Also, because of the increased

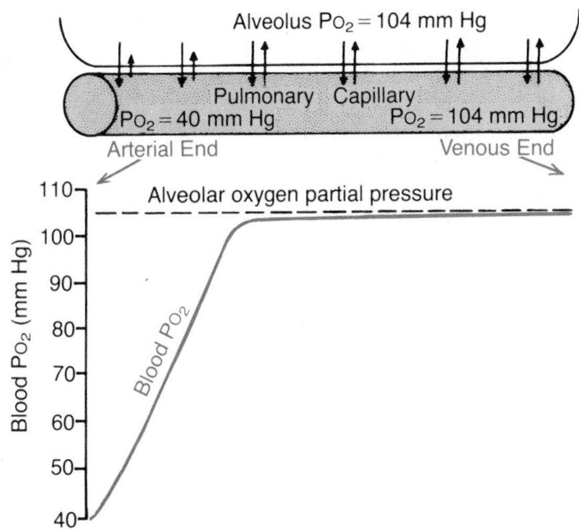

Figure 28–8. Uptake of oxygen by the pulmonary capillary blood. (The curve in this figure was constructed from data in Milhorn and Pulley: *Biophys. J.*, *8*:337, 1968.)

cardiac output, the time that the blood remains in the capillary may be reduced to less than one half normal despite the fact that additional capillaries open up. Therefore, oxygenation of the blood could suffer for two reasons. Yet because of the great *safety factor* for diffusion of oxygen through the pulmonary membrane, the blood is still *almost completely saturated* with oxygen when it leaves the pulmonary capillaries. The reasons for this are as follows:

First, it was pointed out earlier in the chapter that the diffusing capacity for oxygen increases almost threefold during exercise; this results mainly from increased numbers of capillaries participating in the diffusion.

Second, note in Figure 28–8 that during normal pulmonary blood flow the blood becomes almost saturated with oxygen by the time it has passed through one third of the pulmonary capillary, and little additional oxygen enters the blood during the latter two thirds of its transit. That is, the blood normally stays in the lung capillaries about three times as long as necessary to cause full oxygenation. Therefore, even with the shortened time of exposure in exercise, the blood still can become either fully oxygenated or nearly so.

Diffusion of Oxygen from the Capillaries to the Interstitial Fluid

When the arterial blood reaches the peripheral tissues, its Po_2 is still 95 mm Hg. On the other hand, as shown in Figure 28–9, the Po_2 in the interstitial fluid averages only 40 mm Hg. Thus, there is a tremendous initial pressure difference that causes oxygen to diffuse very rapidly from the blood into the tissues, so rapidly that the capillary Po_2 falls almost to equal the 40 mm Hg pressure in the interstitium. Therefore, the Po_2 of the blood entering the veins from the tissue capillaries is also about 40 mm Hg.

Effect of Rate of Blood Flow and Tissue Metabolism on Interstitial Fluid Po_2. If the blood flow through a particular tissue becomes increased, greater quantities of oxygen are transported into the tissue in a given period of time, and the tissue Po_2 becomes correspondingly increased. However, the upper limit to which the Po_2 can rise, even with maximum blood flow, is normally about 95 mm Hg, because this is the oxygen pressure in the arterial blood.

Conversely, if the cells utilize more oxygen for metabolism than normally, this tends to reduce the interstitial fluid Po_2.

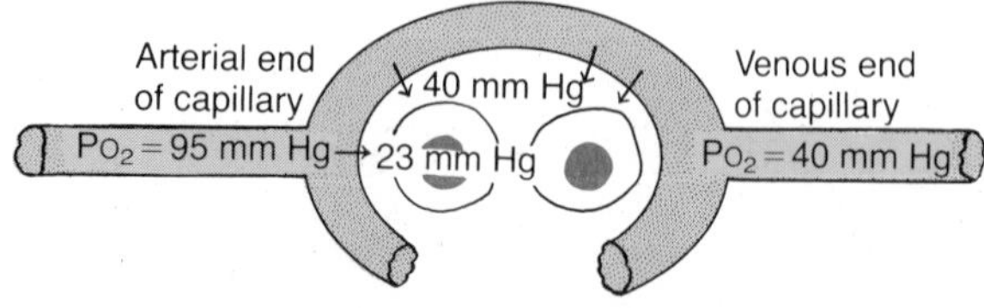

Figure 28–9. Diffusion of oxygen from a tissue capillary to the cells.

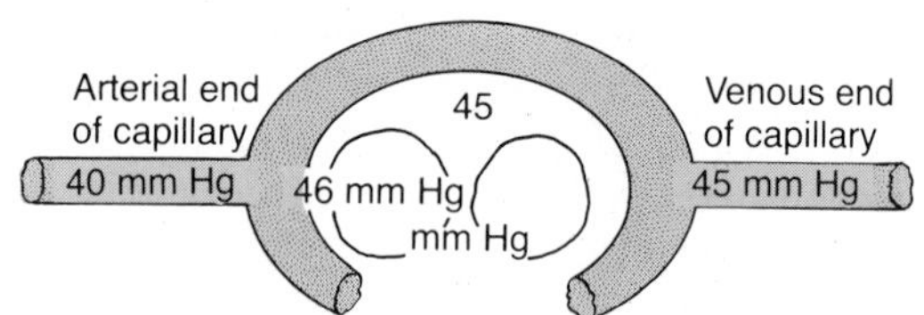

Figure 28–10. Uptake of carbon dioxide by the blood in the capillaries.

In summary, tissue Po_2 is determined by a balance between (1) the rate of oxygen transport to the tissues in the blood and (2) the rate at which the oxygen is utilized by the tissues.

Diffusion of Oxygen from the Capillaries to the Tissue Cells

Oxygen is always being used by the cells. Therefore, the intracellular Po_2 remains lower than the Po_2 in the capillaries. Also, in many instances, there is considerable distance between the capillaries and the cells. Therefore, the normal intracellular Po_2 ranges from as low as 5 mm Hg to as high as 40 mm Hg, averaging (by direct measurement in lower animals) about 23 mm Hg. Because only 1 to 3 mm Hg of oxygen pressure is normally required for full support of the metabolic processes of the cell, one can see that even this low cellular Po_2 of 23 mm Hg is more than adequate and actually provides a considerable safety factor.

Diffusion of Carbon Dioxide from the Cells to the Tissue Capillaries, and from the Pulmonary Capillaries to the Alveoli

When oxygen is used by the cells, most of it becomes carbon dioxide, and this increases the intracellular Pco_2. Therefore, carbon dioxide diffuses from the cells into the tissue capillaries and is then carried by the blood to the lungs, where it diffuses from the pulmonary capillaries into the alveoli. Thus, at each point in the gas transport chain, carbon dioxide diffuses in a direction exactly opposite that of the diffusion of oxygen. Yet there is one major difference between the diffusion of carbon dioxide and that of oxygen: *carbon dioxide diffuses about 20 times as rapidly as oxygen.* Therefore, the pressure differences that cause carbon dioxide diffusion are, in each instance, far less than the pressure differences required to cause oxygen diffusion. These pressures are the following:

1. Intracellular Pco_2, about 46 mm Hg; interstitial Pco_2, about 45 mm Hg; thus, there is only a 1-mm Hg pressure differential, as illustrated in Figure 28–10.
2. Pco_2 of the arterial blood entering the tissues, 40 mm Hg; Pco_2 of the venous blood leaving the tissues, about 45 mm Hg; thus, as also illustrated

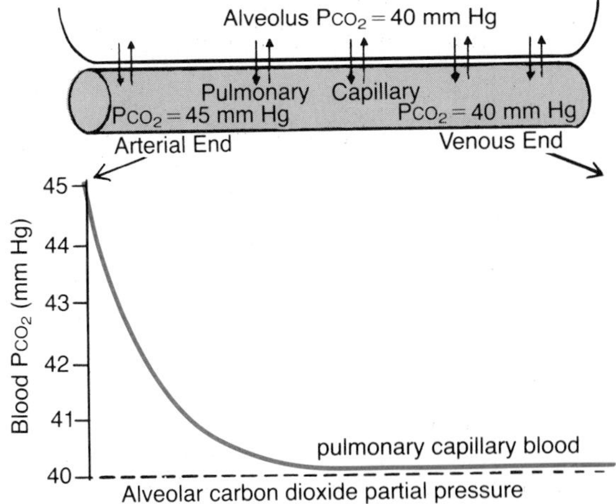

Figure 28-11. Diffusion of carbon dioxide from the pulmonary blood into the alveolus. (This curve was constructed from data in Milhorn and Pulley: *Biophys. J.*, *8*:337, 1968.)

in Figure 28-10, the tissue capillary blood comes almost exactly to equilibrium with the interstitial P_{CO_2}, also 45 mm Hg.

3. P_{CO_2} of the venous blood entering the pulmonary capillaries in the lungs, 45 mm Hg; P_{CO_2} of the alveolar air, 40 mm Hg; thus, only a 5 mm Hg pressure difference causes all the required carbon dioxide diffusion out of the pulmonary capillaries into the alveoli. Furthermore, as illustrated in Figure 28-11, the P_{CO_2} of the pulmonary capillary blood falls almost exactly to equal the alveolar P_{CO_2} of 40 mm Hg before it has passed more than about one third the distance through the capillaries. This is the same effect that was observed earlier for oxygen diffusion.

Effect of Tissue Metabolism and Blood Flow on Interstitial P_{CO_2}. Tissue capillary blood flow and tissue metabolism affect the P_{CO_2} in a way exactly opposite the way in which they affect tissue P_{O_2}. Thus, it is easy to understand that increased tissue metabolism increases the CO_2 in the tissues, but increased blood flow carries more CO_2 away and therefore decreases the concentration.

FUNCTION OF HEMOGLOBIN TO TRANSPORT OXYGEN IN ARTERIAL BLOOD

Normally, about 97 per cent of the oxygen transported from the lungs to the tissues is carried in chemical combination with hemoglobin in the red blood cells, and the remaining 3 per cent is carried in the dissolved state in the water of the plasma and cells. Thus, *under normal conditions* oxygen is carried to the tissues almost entirely by hemoglobin.

The chemistry of hemoglobin was presented in Chapter 24, where it was pointed out that the oxygen molecule combines loosely and reversibly with the heme portion of the hemoglobin. When the P_{O_2} is high, as in the pulmonary capillaries, oxygen binds with the hemoglobin, but when the P_{O_2} is low, as in the tissue capillaries, oxygen is released from the hemoglobin. This is the basis for almost all oxygen transport from the lungs to the tissues.

The Oxygen-Hemoglobin Dissociation Curve. Figure 28-12 illustrates the oxygen-hemoglobin dissociation curve, which shows a progressive increase in the percentage of the hemoglobin that is bound with oxygen as the P_{O_2} increases, which is called the *per cent saturation of the hemoglobin.* Because the blood in the arteries usually has a P_{O_2} of about 95 mm Hg, one can see from the dissociation curve that the *usual oxygen saturation of arterial blood is about 97 per cent.* On the other hand, in normal venous blood returning from the tissues, the P_{O_2} is about 40 mm Hg and *the saturation of the hemoglobin is about 75 per cent.*

Maximum Amount of Oxygen That Can Combine with the Hemoglobin of the Blood. The blood of a normal person contains approximately 15 grams of hemoglobin in each 100 milliliters of blood, and each gram of hemoglobin can bind with a maximum of about 1.34 milliliters of oxygen. Therefore, on the average, the hemoglobin in 100 milliliters of blood can combine with a total of almost exactly 20 milliliters of oxygen when the hemoglobin is 100 per cent saturated. This is usually expressed as 20 *volumes per cent.*

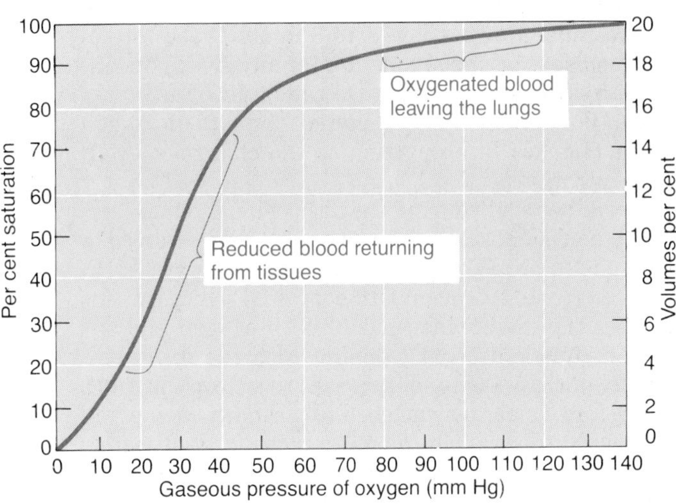

Figure 28-12. The oxygen-hemoglobin dissociation curve.

Amount of Oxygen Released From the Hemoglobin in the Tissues. The total quantity of oxygen *bound with hemoglobin* in normal arterial blood, which is 97 per cent saturated, is approximately 19.4 milliliters per deciliter of blood. On passing through the tissue capillaries, this amount is reduced, on the average, to 14.4 milliliters. Thus, *under normal conditions about 5 milliliters of oxygen is transported to the tissues by each deciliter of blood.*

Transport of Oxygen During Strenuous Exercise. In heavy exercise the muscle cells utilize oxygen at a rapid rate, which causes the interstitial fluid Po_2 to fall to as low as 15 mm Hg. At this pressure only 4.4 milliliters of oxygen remains bound with the hemoglobin in each deciliter of blood, as also shown in Figure 28-12. Thus, 19.4 − 4.4, or 15 milliliters, is the quantity of oxygen then transported by each 100 milliliters of blood. Thus, three times as much oxygen is transported in each volume of blood that passes through the tissues as normally. And when one remembers that the cardiac output can increase to seven times normal in well-trained marathon runners, multiplying these two gives a 20-fold increase in oxygen transport to the tissues: this is about the limit that can be achieved.

Metabolic Use of Oxygen by the Cells

Relationship Between Intracellular Po_2 and Rate of Oxygen Usage. Only a minute level of oxygen pressure is required in the cells for normal intracellular chemical reactions to take place. The reason for this is that the respiratory enzyme systems of the cell, which are discussed in Chapter 47, are geared so that when the cellular Po_2 is more than 1 to 3 mm Hg, oxygen availability is no longer a limiting factor in the rates of the chemical reactions. Instead, the main limiting factor then is the *concentration of adenosine diphosphate* (ADP) in the cells, as was explained in Chapter 3. This effect is illustrated in Figure 28-13, which shows the relationship between intracellular Po_2 and rate of oxygen usage. Note that whenever the intracellular Po_2 is above 1 to 3 mm Hg, the rate of oxygen usage becomes constant for any given concentration of ADP in the cell. On the other hand, when the ADP concentration is altered, the rate of oxygen usage changes in proportion to the change in ADP concentration.

It will be recalled from the discussion in Chapter 3 that when adenosine triphosphate (ATP) is utilized in the cells to provide energy, it is converted into ADP. The increasing concentration of ADP, in turn, increases the metabolic usage of both oxygen and the various nutrients that combine with the oxygen to release energy. This energy is used to reform the ATP. Therefore, *under normal operating conditions the rate of oxygen utilization by the cells is controlled ultimately by the rate of energy expenditure within the cells — that is, by the rate at which ADP is formed from ATP.* Only in abnormal hypoxic states does the availability of oxygen become a limiting condition.

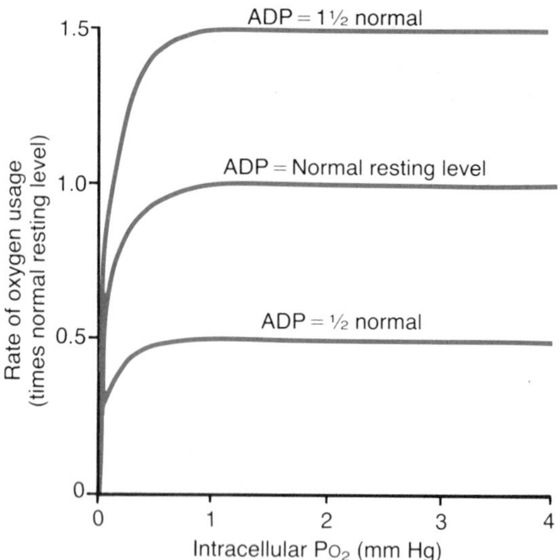

Figure 28-13. Effect of intracellular Po_2 on rate of oxygen usage by the cells. Note that increasing the intracellular concentration of adenosine diphosphate (ADP) increases the rate of oxygen usage.

Transport of Oxygen in the Dissolved State

At the normal arterial Po_2 of 95 mm Hg, approximately 0.29 milliliter of oxygen is dissolved in every deciliter of water in the blood. Then when the Po_2 of the blood falls to 40 mm Hg in the tissue capillaries, only 0.12 milliliter of oxygen remains dissolved. In other words, 0.17 milliliter of oxygen is normally transported in the dissolved state to the tissues by each deciliter of blood water. This compares with almost 5.0 milliliters transported by the hemoglobin. Therefore, the amount of oxygen transported to the tissues in the dissolved state is normally slight, only about 3 per cent of the total, as compared with 97 per cent transported by the hemoglobin. Yet if a person breathes oxygen at very high alveolar Po_2s, the amount then transported in the dissolved state can become much greater, sometimes so much so that serious excesses of oxygen occur in the tissues and "oxygen poisoning" ensues. This often leads to convulsions and even death, as will be discussed in detail in Chapter 30 in relation to high-pressure breathing.

Combination of Hemoglobin with Carbon Monoxide — Displacement of Oxygen

Carbon monoxide combines with hemoglobin at the same point on the hemoglobin molecule as does oxygen and therefore can displace oxygen from the hemoglobin. Furthermore, it binds with about 250 times as much tenacity as oxygen. Therefore, a carbon monoxide pressure of only 0.4 mm Hg in the alveoli, 1/250 that of the alveolar oxygen, allows the carbon monoxide to compete equally with the oxygen for combination with the hemoglobin and causes half the hemoglobin in the blood to become bound with carbon monoxide instead of with oxygen. Therefore, a carbon monoxide pressure only a little greater than 0.4 mm Hg (about 0.7 mm Hg, or a concentration of about 0.1 per cent in the air) can be lethal.

A patient severely poisoned with carbon monoxide can be advantageously treated by administering pure oxygen, for oxygen at high alveolar pressures displaces carbon monoxide from its combination with hemoglobin far more rapidly than can oxygen at the low pressure of atmospheric oxygen.

TRANSPORT OF CARBON DIOXIDE IN THE BLOOD

Transport of carbon dioxide in the blood is not nearly so great a problem as transport of oxygen, because even in the most abnormal conditions carbon dioxide usually can be transported in far greater quantities than can oxygen. However, the amount of carbon dioxide in the blood does have much to do with acid-base balance of the body fluids, which was discussed in Chapter 23.

Under normal resting conditions *an average of 4 milliliters of carbon dioxide is transported from the tissues to the lungs in each deciliter of blood.*

Chemical Forms in Which Carbon Dioxide is Transported

To begin the process of carbon dioxide transport, carbon dioxide diffuses out of the tissue cells in the dissolved molecular CO_2 form. On entering the capillary, the carbon dioxide initiates a host of almost instantaneous physical and chemical reactions, illustrated in Figure 28-14, that are essential for CO_2 transport.

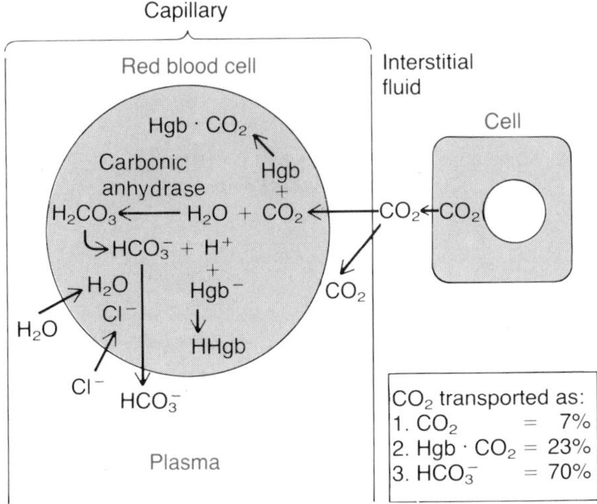

Figure 28-14. Transport of carbon dioxide in the blood.

Transport of Carbon Dioxide in the Dissolved State. A small portion of the carbon dioxide is transported in the dissolved state to the lungs. It will be recalled that the P_{CO_2} of venous blood is 45 mm Hg and that of arterial blood is 40 mm Hg. The amount of carbon dioxide dissolved in the fluid of the blood at 45 mm Hg is about 2.7 ml/dl (2.7 volumes per cent). The amount dissolved at 40 mm Hg is about 2.4 milliliters, or a difference of 0.3 milliliter. Therefore, only about 0.3 milliliter of carbon dioxide is transported in the form of dissolved carbon dioxide by each deciliter of blood. This is about 7 per cent of all the carbon dioxide normally transported.

Transport of Carbon Dioxide in the Form of Bicarbonate Ion. ***Reaction of Carbon Dioxide with Water in the Red Blood Cells—Effect of Carbonic Anhydrase.*** The dissolved carbon dioxide in the blood also reacts with water to form carbonic acid. However, this reaction would occur much too slowly to be of importance were it not for the fact that inside the red blood cells is an enzyme called *carbonic anhydrase,* which catalyzes the reaction between carbon dioxide and water, accelerating its rate about 5000-fold. Therefore, instead of requiring many seconds or minutes to occur, as is true in the plasma, the reaction occurs so rapidly in the red blood cells that it reaches almost complete equilibrium within a small fraction of a second. This allows tremendous amounts of carbon dioxide to react with the red cell water even before the blood leaves the tissue capillaries.

Dissociation of the Carbonic Acid into Bicarbonate and Hydrogen Ions. In another small fraction of a second, the carbonic acid formed in the red cells dissociates into *hydrogen* and *bicarbonate ions.* Most of the hydrogen ions then combine with the hemoglobin in the red blood cells because hemoglobin is a powerful acid-base buffer. In turn, many of the bicarbonate ions diffuse into the plasma while chloride ions diffuse into the red cells to take their place. Thus, the chloride content of venous red blood cells is greater than that of arterial cells, a phenomenon called the *chloride shift.*

The reversible combination of carbon dioxide with water in the red blood cells under the influence of carbonic anhydrase accounts for about 70 per cent of the carbon dioxide transported from the tissues to the lungs. Thus, this means of transporting carbon dioxide is by far the most important of all the methods for transport.

Transport of Carbon Dioxide in Combination with Hemoglobin and Plasma Proteins—Carbaminohemoglobin. In addition to reacting with water, carbon dioxide also reacts directly with hemoglobin to form the compound *carbaminohemoglobin* (CO_2HHb). This combination of carbon dioxide with the hemoglobin is a reversible reaction that occurs with a very loose bond, so that the carbon dioxide is easily released into the alveoli where the P_{CO_2} is lower than in the tissue capillaries. A small amount of carbon dioxide also reacts in this same way with the plasma proteins, but this is much less significant because the quantity of these proteins is only one fourth as great as the quantity of hemoglobin.

The *theoretical* quantity of carbon dioxide that can be carried from the tissues to the lungs in combination with hemoglobin and plasma proteins is approximately 30 per cent of the total quantity transported —that is, about 1.5 milliliters of carbon dioxide in each deciliter of blood. However, this reaction is much slower than the reaction of carbon dioxide with water inside the red blood cells. Therefore, it is doubtful that this mechanism provides transport of more than 15 to 25 per cent of the total quantity of carbon dioxide.

Change in Blood Acidity During Carbon Dioxide Transport

The carbonic acid formed when carbon dioxide enters the blood in the tissues decreases the blood pH. Fortunately, though, the reaction of this acid with the buffers of the blood prevents the hydrogen ion concentration from rising greatly. Ordinarily, arterial blood has a pH of approximately 7.41, and, as the blood acquires carbon dioxide in the tissue capillaries, the pH falls to a venous value of approximately 7.37. In other words, a pH change of 0.04 unit takes place. The reverse occurs when carbon dioxide is released from the blood in the lungs, the pH rising to the arterial value once again. In exercise, or in other conditions of high metabolic activity, or when the blood flow through the tissues is sluggish, the decrease in pH in the tissue blood (and in the tissues themselves) can be as much as 0.50, or on occasion even more than this, thus causing severe tissue acidosis.

THE RESPIRATORY EXCHANGE RATIO

The discerning student will have noted that normal transport of oxygen from the lungs to the tissues by each deciliter of blood is about 5 milliliters, whereas normal transport of carbon dioxide from the tissues to the lungs is about 4 milliliters. Thus, under normal resting conditions only about 80 per cent as much carbon dioxide is expired from the lungs as there is oxygen uptake by the lungs. The ratio of carbon dioxide output to oxygen uptake is called the *respiratory exchange ratio* (R). That is,

$$R = \frac{\text{Rate of carbon dioxide output}}{\text{Rate of oxygen uptake}}$$

The value for R changes under different metabolic conditions. When a person is utilizing entirely carbohydrates for body metabolism, R rises to 1.00. On the other hand, when the person is utilizing fats almost entirely for metabolic energy, the level falls to as low as 0.7. The reason for this difference is that when oxygen is metabolized with carbohydrates, one molecule of carbon dioxide is formed for each molecule of oxygen consumed; whereas when oxygen reacts with fats, a large share of the oxygen combines with hydrogen atoms from the fats to form water instead of carbon dioxide. In other words, the *respiratory quotient of the chemical reactions* in the tissues when fats are metabolized is about 0.70 instead of 1.00, which is the case when carbohydrates are being utilized. The tissue respiratory quotient will be discussed in Chapter 47.

For a person on a normal diet consuming average amounts of carbohydrates, fats, and proteins, the average value for R is considered to be 0.825.

REFERENCES

Bidani, A., and Crandall, E. D.: Velocity of CO_2 exchanges in the lungs. Annu. Rev. Physiol., 50:639, 1988.

Gonzales, N. C., and Fedde, M. R. (eds.): Oxygen Transfer from Atmosphere to Tissues. New York, Plenum Publishing Corp., 1988.

Guyton, A. C., et al.: An arteriovenous oxygen difference recorder. J. Appl. Physiol., 10:158, 1957.

Klocke R. A.: Velocity of CO_2 exchange in blood. Annu. Rev. Physiol., 50:625, 1988.

Konigsberg, W.: Protein structure and molecular dysfunction: Hemoglobin. In Bondy, P. K., and Rosenberg, L. E. (eds.): Metabolic Control and Disease. 8th ed. Philadelphia, W. B. Saunders Co., 1980, p. 27.

Lane, E. E., and Walker, J. F.: Clinical Arterial Blood Gas Analysis. St. Louis, C. V. Mosby Co., 1987.

Mochizuki, M., et al. (eds.): Oxygen Transport to Tissue X. New York, Plenum Publishing Corp., 1988.

Paiva, M., and Engel, L. A.: Theoretical studies of gas mixing and ventilation distribution in the lung. Physiol. Rev., 67:750, 1987.

Perutz, M. F.: Hemoglobin structure and respiratory transport. Sci. Am., 239(6):92, 1987.

Quintanilha, A., (ed.): Oxygen Radicals in Biological Systems. New York, Plenum Publishing Corp., 1988.

Riggs, A. F.: The Bohr effect. Annu. Rev. Physiol., 50:181, 1988.

Tamoru, M., et al.: In vivo study of tissue oxygen metabolism using optical and nuclear magnetic resonance. Annu. Rev. Physiol., 51:813, 1989.

QUESTIONS

1. Explain the concept of *partial presures* of individual gases when they exist in a mixture.
2. Explain why net diffusion of a gas always occurs in the direction of high pressure to low pressure regardless of whether the gas is in the gaseous state, is dissolved in tissues, or is dissolved in the blood.
3. Explain why the *vapor pressure of water* in the alveoli remains very nearly constant under normal conditions at a level of 47 mm Hg.
4. Give the equation for net rate of diffusion of a gas in a fluid or in a tissue, and explain each of the elements of the equation.
5. How much more rapidly does carbon dioxide diffuse through tissues than does oxygen?
6. At normal respiration, approximately how long must a person breathe before half of the alveolar air is exchanged with atmospheric air?
7. State the normal oxygen partial pressure in the alveoli.

At maximum rate of breathing, how high can this rise when the person is breathing normal air at sea level?

8. What is the normal carbon dioxide concentration in the alveoli, and what are the factors that can increase or decrease this?
9. Describe the anatomy of the *respiratory unit.*
10. List and discuss the factors that determine how rapidly a gas will pass through the respiratory membrane.
11. Define the *diffusing capacity* of the respiratory membrane, and give approximate values for the diffusion capacity for oxygen and carbon dioxide at rest and during exercise.
12. Give the approximate quantitative values for Po_2 in the alveoli, in the systemic arterial blood, in the interstitial fluid, and in the cells. Give the approximate quantitative values for Pco_2 in reverse order, from the cells back to the alveoli.
13. Draw the oxygen-hemoglobin dissociation curve, giving exact values for the scales on the abscissa and the ordinate.
14. What minimum intracellular concentration of oxygen is required to allow maximum rates of the oxygen-related metabolic reactions in the cell? When the oxygen Po_2 is above this minimum level, what determines the rate of oxygen utilization?
15. Explain why minute quantities of carbon monoxide can prevent the transport of oxygen to the tissues.
16. List the chemical forms in which carbon dioxide is transported from the cells to the lungs, and give the approximate proportions of the carbon dioxide transported in each form.
17. Define the *respiratory exchange ratio,* and give its value when a person is metabolizing (1) carbohydrates and (2) fats.

29

Regulation of Respiration, and Respiratory Insufficiency

The nervous system adjusts the rate of alveolar ventilation almost exactly to the demands of the body so that the arterial blood oxygen pressure (Po_2) and carbon dioxide pressure (Pco_2) are hardly altered even during strenuous exercise and most other types of stress.

The present chapter describes the operation of this neurogenic system for regulation of respiration and also discusses the different causes of respiratory insufficiency.

THE RESPIRATORY CENTER

The "respiratory center" is composed of several widely dispersed groups of neurons located *bilaterally* in the medulla oblongata and pons, as illustrated in Figure 29–1. It is divided into three major collections of neurons: (1) a *dorsal respiratory group,* located in the dorsal portion of the medulla, which mainly causes inspiration, (2) a *ventral respiratory group,* located in the ventrolateral part of the medulla, which can cause either expiration or inspiration, depending upon which neurons in the group are stimulated, and (3) the *pneumotaxic center,* located dorsally in the superior portion of the pons, which helps control both the rate and pattern of breathing. The dorsal respiratory group of neurons plays the fundamental role in the control of respiration. Therefore, let us discuss its function first.

The Dorsal Respiratory Group of Neurons—Its Inspiratory and Rhythmical Functions

The dorsal respiratory group of neurons extends most of the length of the medulla. Either all or most of its neurons are located within the *nucleus of the tractus solitarius,* though additional neurons in the adjacent reticular substance of the medulla probably also play important roles in respiratory control. The nucleus of the tractus solitarius is also the sensory termination of both the vagal and glossopharyngeal nerves, which transmit sensory signals into the respiratory center from the peripheral chemoreceptors, the baroreceptors, and several different types of receptors in the lung. All the signals from these peripheral areas help in the control of respiration, as we discuss in subsequent sections of this chapter.

Rhythmical Inspiratory Discharges from the Dorsal Respiratory Group. The basic rhythm of respiration is generated mainly in the dorsal respiratory group of neurons. Even when all the peripheral nerves entering the medulla are sectioned and the brain stem is transected both above and below the medulla, this group of neurons still emits repetitive bursts of *inspiratory* action potentials. Unfortunately, though, the basic cause of these repetitive discharges is still unknown. In primitive animals, neural networks have been found in which activity of one set of neurons excites a second set, which in turn inhibits the first. Then after a period of time the mechanism repeats itself, continuing throughout the life of the animal. Therefore, most respiratory physiologists believe that some similar network of neurons located entirely within the medulla, probably involving not only the dorsal respiratory group but adjacent areas of the medulla as well, is responsible for the basic rhythm of respiration.

The Inspiratory "Ramp" Signal. The nervous signal that is transmitted to the inspiratory muscles is not an instantaneous burst of action potentials. Instead, in normal respiration, it begins very weakly at

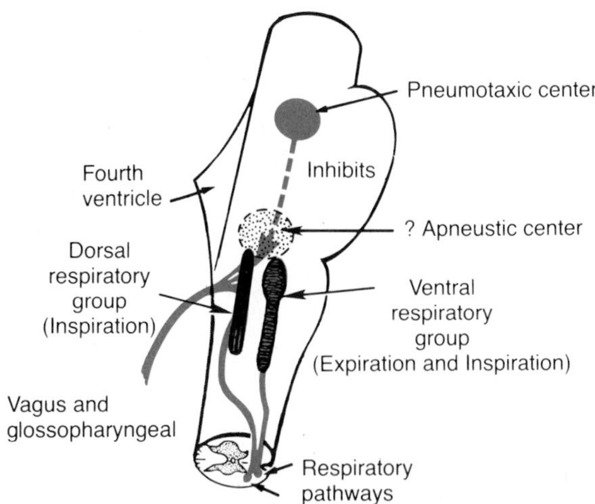

Figure 29-1. Organization of the respiratory center.

first and increases steadily in a ramp fashion for about 2 seconds. It abruptly ceases for approximately the next 3 seconds, then begins again for still another cycle, and again and again. Thus, the inspiratory signal is said to be a *ramp signal.* The obvious advantage of this is that it causes a steady increase in the volume of the lungs during inspiration, rather than inspiratory gasps.

The Pneumotaxic Center—Its Function in Limiting the Duration of Inspiration and Increasing Respiratory Rate

The pneumotaxic center, located dorsally in the upper pons, transmits impulses continuously to the inspiratory area. The primary effect of these is to control the "switch-off" point of the inspiratory ramp, thus controlling the duration of the filling phase of the lung cycle. When the pneumotaxic signals are strong, inspiration might last for as little as 0.5 second; but when weak, for as long as 5 or more seconds, thus filling the lungs with a great excess of air.

Therefore, the function of the pneumotaxic center is primarily to limit inspiration. However, this has a secondary effect of increasing the rate of breathing because limitation of inspiration also shortens expiration and the entire period of respiration. Thus, a strong pneumotaxic signal can increase the rate of breathing up to 30 to 40 breaths per minute.

The Ventral Respiratory Group of Neurons—Its Function in Both Inspiration and Expiration

Located about 5 millimeters anterior and lateral to the dorsal respiratory group of neurons is the ventral respiratory group of neurons. The function of this neuronal group differs from that of the dorsal respiratory group in several important ways:

1. The neurons of the ventral respiratory group remain almost totally *inactive* during normal quiet respiration. Therefore, normal quiet breathing is caused only by repetitive inspiratory signals from the dorsal respiratory group transmitted mainly to the diaphragm, and expiration results from elastic recoil of the lungs and thoracic cage.
2. When the respiratory drive for increased pulmonary ventilation becomes greater than normal, respiratory signals then spill over into the ventral respiratory neurons from the basic oscillating mechanism of the dorsal respiratory area. As a consequence, the ventral respiratory area then does contribute its share to the respiratory drive as well.
3. Electrical stimulation of some of the neurons in the ventral group causes inspiration, whereas stimulation of others causes expiration. Therefore, these neurons contribute to both inspiration and expiration. However, they are especially important in providing the powerful expiratory signals to the abdominal muscles during expiration. Thus, this area operates more or less as an overdrive mechanism when high levels of pulmonary ventilation are required.

Reflex Limitation of Inspiration by Lung Inflation Signals—The Hering-Breuer Inflation Reflex

In addition to the neural mechanisms operating entirely within the brain stem, reflex signals from the periphery also help control respiration. Most important, located in the walls of the bronchi and bronchioles throughout the lungs are *stretch receptors* that transmit signals through the *vagi* into the dorsal respiratory group of neurons when the lungs become overstretched. These signals affect inspiration in much the same way as signals from the pneumotaxic center; that is, when the lungs become overly inflated, the stretch receptors activate an appropriate feedback response that "switches off" the inspiratory ramp and thus stops further inspiration. This is called the *Hering-Breuer inflation reflex.* This reflex also increases the rate of respiration, the same as is true for signals from the pneumotaxic center.

CHEMICAL CONTROL OF RESPIRATION

The ultimate goal of respiration is to maintain proper concentrations of oxygen, carbon dioxide, and hydrogen ions in the tissues. It is fortunate, therefore, that respiratory activity is highly responsive to changes in each of these.

Excess carbon dioxide or hydrogen ions mainly stimulate the respiratory center itself, causing greatly increased strength of both the inspiratory and expiratory signals to the respiratory muscles.

Oxygen, on the other hand, does not have a significant *direct* effect on the respiratory center of the brain in controlling respiration. Instead, it acts almost entirely on peripheral chemoreceptors located in the carotid and aortic bodies, and these in turn transmit appropriate nervous signals to the respiratory center for control of respiration.

Let us discuss first the stimulation of the respiratory center itself by carbon dioxide and hydrogen ions.

Direct Chemical Control Of Respiratory Center Activity By Carbon Dioxide And Hydrogen Ions

The Chemosensitive Area of the Respiratory Center. We have discussed mainly three different areas of the respiratory center: the dorsal respiratory group of neurons, the ventral respiratory group, and the pneumotaxic center. However, it is believed that none of these are affected directly by changes in blood carbon dioxide concentration or hydrogen ion concentration. Instead, an additional neuronal area, a very sensitive *chemosensitive area,* illustrated in Figure 29–2, is located bilaterally and lies less than 1 millimeter beneath the ventral surface of the medulla. This area is highly sensitive to changes in either blood P_{CO_2} or hydrogen ion concentration, and it in turn excites the other portions of the respiratory center.

Response of the Chemosensitive Neurons to Hydrogen Ions — The Primary Stimulus

The sensor neurons in the chemosensitive area are especially excited by hydrogen ions; in fact, it is believed that hydrogen ions are perhaps the only important direct stimulus for these neurons. Unfortunately, though, hydrogen ions do not easily cross either the blood-brain barrier or the blood–cerebrospinal fluid barrier. For this reason, changes in hydrogen ion concentration in the blood actually have considerably less effect in stimulating the chemosensitive neurons than do changes in carbon dioxide, even though carbon dioxide stimulates these neurons indirectly, as is explained next.

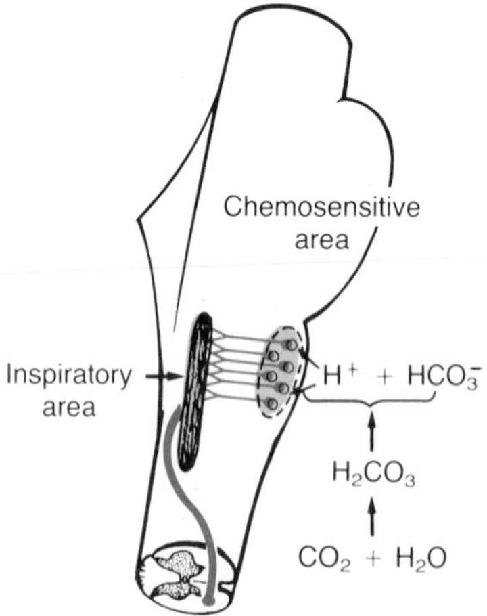

Figure 29–2. Stimulation of the inspiratory area by the *chemosensitive area* located bilaterally in the medulla, lying only a few microns beneath the ventral medullary surface. Note also that hydrogen ions stimulate the chemosensitive area, whereas carbon dioxide in the fluid gives rise to most of the hydrogen ions.

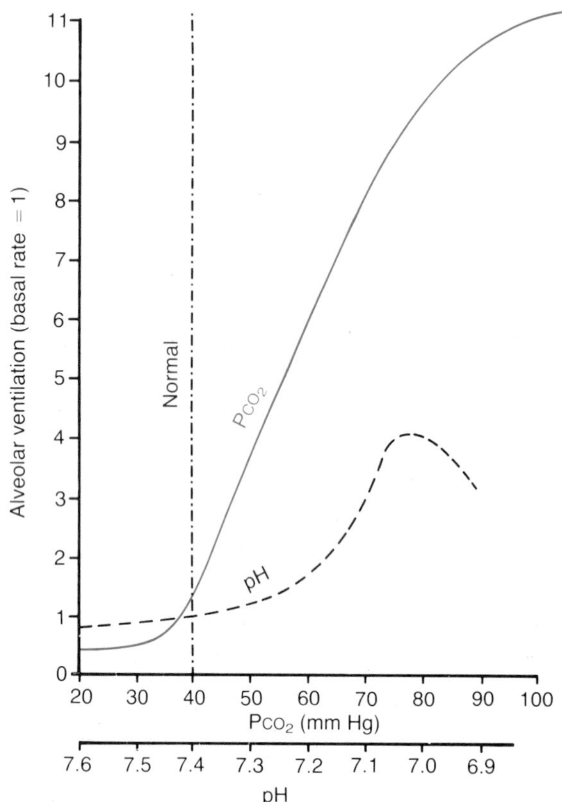

Figure 29–3. Effects of increased arterial P_{CO_2} and decreased arterial pH on the rate of alveolar ventilation.

Effect of Blood Carbon Dioxide on Stimulating the Chemosensitive Area

Though carbon dioxide has very little direct effect in stimulating the neurons in the chemosensitive area, it does have a very potent indirect effect. It does this by reacting with the water of the tissues to form carbonic acid. This in turn dissociates into hydrogen and bicarbonate ions; the hydrogen ions then have a potent direct stimulatory effect. These reactions are illustrated in Figure 29–2.

Why is it that blood carbon dioxide has a more potent effect in stimulating the chemosensitive neurons than do blood hydrogen ions? The answer is that the blood-brain barrier and the blood–cerebrospinal fluid barrier are both almost completely impermeable to hydrogen ions, whereas carbon dioxide passes through both these barriers almost as if they did not exist. Consequently, whenever the blood P_{CO_2} increases, so also does the P_{CO_2} of both the interstitial fluid of the medulla and of the cerebrospinal fluid. In both of these fluids the carbon dioxide immediately reacts with the water to form hydrogen ions. Thus, paradoxically, more hydrogen ions are released into the respiratory chemosensitive sensory area when the blood carbon dioxide concentration increases than when the blood hydrogen ion concentration increases. For this reason, respiratory center activity is affected considerably more by changes in blood carbon dioxide than by changes in blood hydrogen ions, which is discussed quantitatively.

Quantitative Effects of Blood P_{CO_2} and Hydrogen Ion Concentration on Alveolar Ventilation

Figure 29-3 illustrates quantitatively the approximate effects of blood P_{CO_2} and blood pH (which is an inverse logarithmic measure of hydrogen ion concentration) on alveolar ventilation. Note the marked increase in ventilation caused by the increase in P_{CO_2}. But note also the much smaller effect of increased hydrogen ion concentration (that is, decreased pH).

Finally, note the very great change in alveolar ventilation in the normal blood P_{CO_2} range between 35 and 60 mm Hg. This illustrates the tremendous effect that carbon dioxide changes have in controlling respiration.

THE PERIPHERAL CHEMORECEPTOR SYSTEM FOR CONTROL OF RESPIRATORY ACTIVITY—ROLE OF OXYGEN IN RESPIRATORY CONTROL

Aside from the direct control of respiratory activity by the respiratory center itself, still another accessory mechanism is also available for controlling respiration. This is the *peripheral chemoreceptor system,* illustrated in Figure 29-4. Special nervous chemical receptors, called *chemoreceptors,* are located in several areas outside the brain and are especially important for detecting changes in oxygen in the blood, although they respond to changes in carbon dioxide and hydrogen ion concentrations, too. The chemoreceptors in turn transmit nervous signals to the respiratory center to help regulate respiratory activity.

By far the largest number of chemoreceptors is located in the *carotid bodies.* However, a sizable number are in the *aortic bodies,* also illustrated in Figure 29-4. The *carotid bodies* are located bilaterally in the bifurcations of the common carotid arteries, and their afferent nerve fibers pass through Hering's nerves to the *glossopharyngeal nerves* and thence to the dorsal respiratory area of the medulla. The *aortic bodies* are located along the arch of the aorta; their afferent nerve fibers pass through the *vagi* also to the dorsal respiratory area. Each of these chemoreceptor bodies receives a special blood supply through a minute artery directly from the adjacent arterial trunk. Furthermore, the blood flow through these bodies is extreme, 20 times the weight of the bodies themselves each minute. Therefore, the percentage removal of oxygen is virtually zero. This means that *the chemoreceptors are exposed at all times to arterial blood,* not venous blood, and their P_{O_2}s are arterial P_{O_2}s.

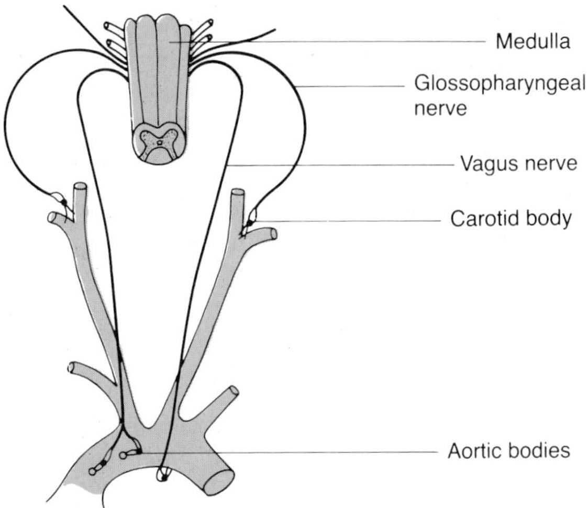

Figure 29-4. Respiratory control by the carotid and aortic bodies.

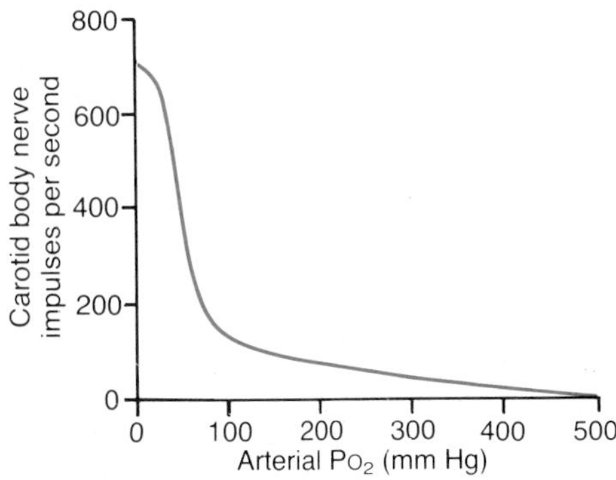

Figure 29-5. Effect of arterial P_{O_2} on impulse rate from the carotid body of a cat. (Curve drawn from data from several sources, but primarily from Von Euler.)

Stimulation of the Chemoreceptors by Decreased Arterial Oxygen. Changes in arterial oxygen concentration have *no* direct stimulatory effect on the respiratory center itself, but when the oxygen concentration in the arterial blood falls below normal, the chemoreceptors become strongly stimulated. This effect is illustrated in Figure 29-5, which shows the effect of different levels of *arterial* P_{O_2} rate of nerve impulse transmission from a carotid body. Note that the impulse rate is particularly sensitive to changes in arterial P_{O_2} in the range between 60 and 30 mm Hg, the range in which the arterial hemoglobin saturation with oxygen decreases rapidly.

Effect of Carbon Dioxide and Hydrogen Ion Concentration on Chemoreceptor Activity. An increase in either carbon dioxide concentration or hydrogen ion concentration also excites the chemoreceptors and in this way indirectly increases respiratory activity. However, the direct effects of both these factors in the respiratory center itself are so much more powerful than their effects mediated through the chemoreceptors (about seven times as powerful) that for most practical purposes the indirect effects through the chemoreceptors do not need to be considered.

Quantitative Effect of Low Arterial P_{O_2} on Alveolar Ventilation

When a person breathes air that has too little oxygen, this obviously will decrease the blood P_{O_2} and excite the carotid and aortic chemoreceptors, thereby increasing respiration. However, the effect usually is much less than one would expect, because the increased respiration will remove carbon dioxide from the lungs and decrease both blood P_{CO_2} and hydrogen ion concentration. Both of these changes then severely depress the respiratory center, as discussed earlier, so that the final effect of the chemoreceptors in increasing respiration in response to low P_{O_2} is mostly suppressed.

Yet the effect of low arterial P_{O_2} on alveolar ventilation is far greater under some other conditions, two of which are (1) low arterial P_{O_2} when arterial carbon dioxide and hydrogen ion concentrations remain normal despite increased respiration and (2) breathing of oxygen at low concentrations for many days.

REGULATION OF RESPIRATION DURING EXERCISE

In strenuous exercise, oxygen consumption and carbon dioxide formation can increase as much as 20-fold. Yet alveolar ventilation ordinarily increases almost exactly in step with the increased level of metabolism, as illustrated by the relationship between oxygen consumption and ventilation in Figure 29–6. Therefore, the arterial P_{O_2}, P_{CO_2}, and pH all remain *almost exactly normal.*

In trying to analyze the factors that cause increased ventilation during exercise, one is tempted immediately to ascribe this to the chemical alterations in the body fluids during exercise, including increase of carbon dioxide, increase of hydrogen ions, and decrease of oxygen. However, this is not valid, for measurements of arterial P_{CO_2}, pH, and P_{O_2} show that none of these usually changes significantly.

Therefore, the question must be asked: What is it during exercise that causes the intense ventilation? This question has not been answered, but at least two different effects seem to be predominantly concerned:

1. The brain, on transmitting impulses to the contracting muscles, is believed to transmit collateral impulses into the brain stem to excite the respiratory center. This is analogous to the stimulatory effect of the higher centers of the brain on the vasomotor center of the brain stem during exercise, causing a rise in arterial pressure as well as an increase in ventilation.
2. During exercise, the body movements, especially of the limbs, are believed to increase pulmonary ventilation by exciting joint proprioceptors that then transmit excitatory impulses to the respiratory center. The reason for believing this is that even passive movements of the limbs often increase pulmonary ventilation severalfold.

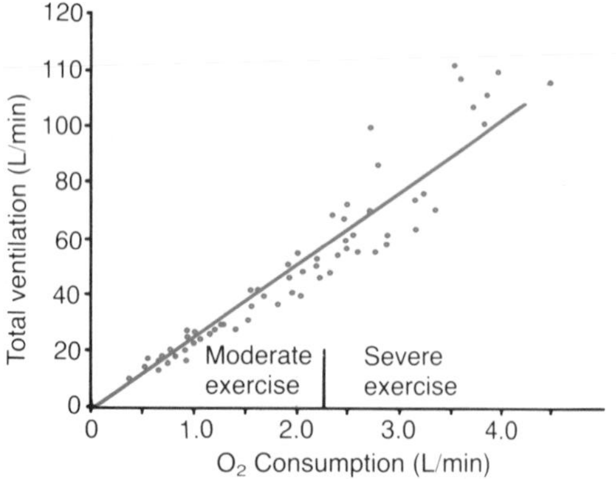

Figure 29–6. Effect of exercise on oxygen consumption and ventilatory rate. (From Gray: Pulmonary Ventilation and Its Physiological Regulation. Springfield, Ill., Charles C Thomas.)

It is possible that still other factors are also important in increasing pulmonary ventilation during exercise. For instance, some experiments even suggest that hypoxia developing in the muscles during exercise elicits afferent nerve signals to the respiratory center to excite respiration. However, because a large share of the total increase in ventilation begins immediately upon the initiation of exercise, most of the increase in respiration probably results from the two neurogenic factors noted above, namely, *stimulatory impulses from the higher centers of the brain and proprioceptive stimulatory reflexes.*

OTHER FACTORS THAT AFFECT RESPIRATION

Anesthesia

Perhaps the most prevalent cause of respiratory depression and respiratory arrest is overdosage of anesthetics or narcotics. For instance, sodium pentobarbital is a poor anesthetic because it depresses the respiratory center considerably more than many other anesthetics such as halothane. At one time, morphine was used as an anesthetic, but this drug is now used only as an adjunct to anesthetics because it greatly depresses the respiratory center while having much less ability to anesthetize the cerebral cortex.

Periodic Breathing

An abnormality of respiration called *periodic breathing* occurs in a number of different disease conditions. The person breathes deeply for a short interval of time and then breathes slightly or not at all for an additional interval, the cycle repeating itself over and over again.

The most common type of periodic breathing, *Cheyne-Stokes breathing,* is characterized by slowly waxing and waning respiration, occurring over and over again approximately every 40 to 60 seconds.

Basic Mechanism of Cheyne-Stokes Breathing. The basic cause of Cheyne-Stokes breathing is the following: When a person overbreathes, thus blowing off too much carbon dioxide from the pulmonary blood and also increasing the blood oxygen, it still takes several seconds before the changed pulmonary blood can be transported to the brain and inhibit ventilation. By this time, the person has already overventilated for an extra few seconds. Therefore, when the respiratory center does eventually respond, it becomes depressed, and now the opposite cycle begins. That is, carbon dioxide builds up and oxygen decreases in the pulmonary blood. Then again it is a few seconds before the brain can respond to the new changes. However, when the brain does respond, the person breathes hard once again. The cycle repeats itself again and again.

Thus, the basic cause of Cheyne-Stokes breathing is present in everyone. However, this mechanism is highly "damped." That is, the fluids of the blood and of the respiratory center have large amounts of stored and chemically bound carbon dioxide and oxygen. Therefore, normally the lungs cannot build up enough extra carbon dioxide or depress the oxygen sufficiently in a few seconds to cause the next cycle of the periodic breathing. Yet under two separate conditions the damping factors are overriden, and Cheyne-Stokes breathing does occur:

1. When there is a long delay in the transport of the blood from the lungs to the brain, as occurs in heart failure, the gas changes in the blood will continue for many more seconds than usual; then the periodic respiratory drive becomes extreme, and Cheyne-Stokes breathing begins.
2. A second cause of Cheyne-Stokes breathing is increased negative feedback gain in the respiratory center. This means that a change in blood carbon dioxide or oxygen now causes far greater change in ventilation than normally. This type of Cheyne-Stokes breathing occurs mainly in patients with brain damage. The brain damage often turns off the respiratory drive entirely for a few seconds; then a very slight increase in blood carbon dioxide turns it back on with great force. Cheyne-Stokes breathing of this type is frequently a prelude to death.

PHYSIOLOGY OF SPECIFIC PULMONARY ABNORMALITIES

Chronic Pulmonary Emphysema

The term *pulmonary emphysema* literally means excess air in the lungs. However, when one speaks of chronic pulmonary emphysema, a complex obstructive and destructive process of the lungs generally is meant, and in most instances it is a consequence of long-term smoking. It results from three major pathophysiological events in the lungs:

1. *Chronic infection* caused by inhaling smoke or other substances that irritate the bronchi and bronchioles.
2. The infection, excess mucus, and inflammatory edema of the bronchiolar epithelium together cause *chronic obstruction* of many of the smaller airways.
3. The obstruction of the airways makes it especially difficult to expire, thus causing *entrapment of air in the alveoli* and overstretching them. This, combined with the lung infection, causes marked destruction of many of the alveolar walls. Therefore, the final picture of the emphysematous lung is that illustrated to the far right in Figure 29-7.

The physiological effects of chronic emphysema are the following:

1. The bronchiolar obstruction greatly *increases airway resistance* and results in greatly increased work of breathing.
2. The marked loss of lung parenchyma greatly *decreases the diffusing capacity* of the lung, which reduces the ability of the lungs to oxygenate the blood and to excrete carbon dioxide.
3. Loss of large portions of the lung parenchyma also decreases the number of pulmonary capillaries through which blood can pass. As a result, the pulmonary vascular resistance increases markedly, causing pulmonary hypertension. This in turn overloads the right side of the heart and frequently causes right-heart failure.

Chronic emphysema usually progresses slowly over many years. The person develops hypoxia and hypercapnia because of hypoventilation of many alveoli and because of loss of lung parenchyma. The net result of all of these effects is severe, prolonged, devastating air hunger that can last for years until the hypoxia and hypercapnia cause death — a very high penalty to pay for smoking.

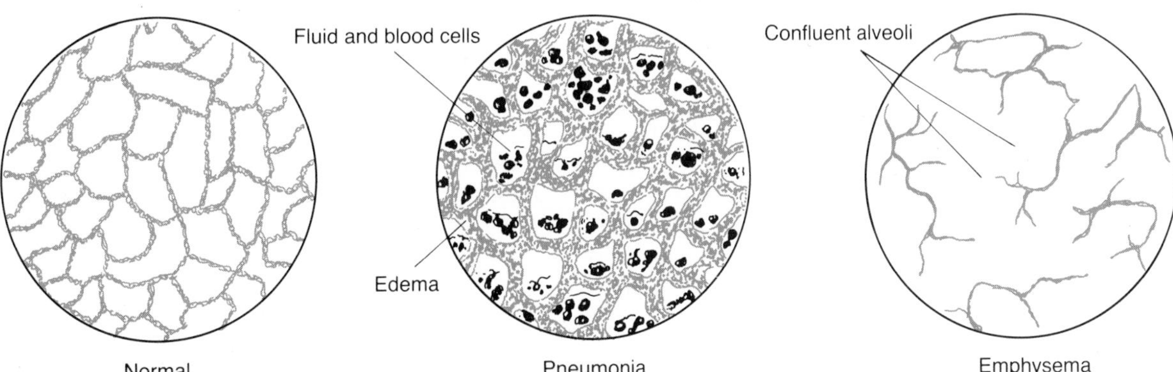

Figure 29-7. Pulmonary changes in pneumonia and emphysema.

Pneumonia

The term *pneumonia* describes any inflammatory condition of the lung in which some or all of the alveoli are filled with fluid and blood cells, as shown in the center panel of Figure 29-7. A common type of pneumonia is *bacterial pneumonia,* caused most frequently by pneumococci. This disease begins with infection in the alveoli; the pulmonary membrane becomes inflamed and highly porous so that fluid and even red and white blood cells pass out of the blood into the alveoli. Thus, the infected alveoli become progressively filled with fluid and cells, and the infection spreads by extension of bacteria from alveolus to alveolus. Eventually, large areas of the lungs, sometimes whole lobes or even a whole lung, become "consolidated," which means that they are filled with fluid and cellular debris.

The pulmonary function of the lungs during pneumonia changes in different stages of the disease. In the early stages, the pneumonia process might well be localized to only one lung, and alveolar ventilation may be reduced even though blood flow through the lung continues normally. This results in two major pulmonary abnormalities: (1) reduction in the total available surface area of the respiratory membrane and (2) no aeration at all of all the blood flowing through the consolidated lung. Both these effects cause reduced diffusing capacity, which results in *hypoxemia* (low blood oxygen) and *hypercapnia* (high blood carbon dioxide).

Figure 29-8 illustrates the effect of the decreased ventilation in pneumonia, showing that the blood passing through the aerated lung becomes 97 per cent saturated, whereas that passing through the unaerated lung remains only 60 per cent saturated, causing the mean saturation of the aortic blood to be about 78 per cent, which is far below normal.

Atelectasis

Atelectasis means collapse of the alveoli. It can occur in a localized area of a lung, in an entire lobe, or in an entire lung. Its most common causes are (1) obstruction of the airway and (2) lack of surfactant in the fluids lining the alveoli.

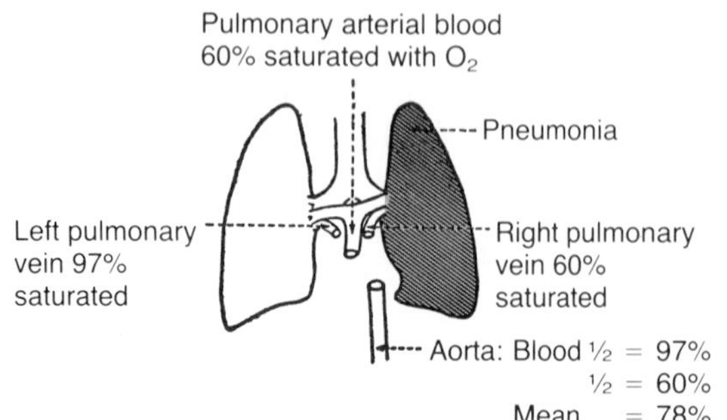

Figure 29-8. Effect of pneumonia on arterial blood oxygen saturation.

Airway Obstruction. The airway obstruction type of atelectasis usually results from (1) blockage of many small bronchi with mucus or (2) obstruction of a major bronchus by either a large mucous plug or some solid object such as cancer. The air entrapped beyond the block is absorbed within minutes to hours by the blood flowing in the pulmonary capillaries. If the lung tissue is pliable enough, this will lead simply to collapse of the alveoli. However, if the lung tissue cannot collapse, absorption of air from the alveoli creates tremendously negative pressures within the alveoli and pulls fluid out of the pulmonary interstitium into the alveoli, thus causing the alveoli to fill completely with edema fluid. This almost always is the effect that occurs when an entire lung becomes atelectatic, a condition called *massive collapse* of the lung.

Lack of Surfactant. The secretion and function of surfactant in the alveoli was discussed in Chapter 27. It was pointed out that the substance surfactant is secreted by the alveolar epithelium into the fluids that line the alveoli. This substance decreases the surface tension in the alveoli twofold to tenfold and plays a major role in preventing alveolar collapse. However, in a number of different conditions, such as in *hyaline membrane disease* (or *respiratory distress syndrome*), which often occurs in newborn premature babies, the quantity of surfactant secreted by the alveoli is greatly depressed. As a result, the surface tension of the alveolar fluid increases so much that it causes a serious tendency for the lungs of these babies to collapse or to become filled with fluid, as explained earlier; many of these infants die of suffocation as increasing portions of the lungs become atelectatic or filled with fluid.

Asthma

Asthma is characterized by spastic contraction of the bronchiolar smooth muscle bronchioles, which causes extremely difficult breathing. It occurs in 3 to 5 per cent of all persons at some time in life. The usual cause is hypersensitivity of the bronchioles to foreign substances in the air. In younger patients, under the age of 30 years, the asthma in about 70 per cent is caused by allergic hypersensitivity, especially sensitivity to plant pollens. In older persons, the cause is almost always hypersensitivity to nonallergic types of irritants in the air, such as irritants in smog.

The allergic reaction that occurs in the allergic type of asthma is believed to occur in the following way: The typically allergic person has a tendency to form abnormally large amounts of IgE antibodies, and these antibodies cause allergic reactions when they react with their complementary antigens, as was explained in Chapter 25. In asthma, these antibodies mainly attach to mast cells that lie in the lung interstitium in close association with the bronchioles and small bronchi. When the person breathes in pollen to which he or she is sensitive (that is, to which the person has developed IgE antibodies), the pollen reacts with the mast cell-attached antibodies and causes these cells to release several different substances. Among them are *histamine, slow-reacting substance of anaphylaxis* (which is a mixture of leukotrienes), *eosinophilic chemotactic factor,* and *bradykinin.* The combined effects of all these factors, especially of the slow-reacting substance of anaphylaxis (SRS-A), are to produce (1) localized edema in the walls of the small bronchioles as well as secretion of thick mucus into the bronchiolar lumens and (2) spasm of the bronchiolar smooth muscle. Obviously, therefore, the airway resistance increases greatly.

In asthma, the bronchiolar diameter becomes more reduced during expiration than during inspiration because the increased intrapulmonary pressure during expiratory effort compresses the outsides of the bronchioles. Because the bronchioles are already partially occluded, further occlusion resulting from the external pressure creates especially severe obstruction during expiration. Therefore, the asthmatic person usually can inspire quite adequately but has great difficulty expiring, and clinical measurements show a greatly reduced maximal expiratory rate. Also, this results in dyspnea, or "air hunger," which is discussed later in the chapter.

Tuberculosis

In tuberculosis, the tubercle bacilli cause a peculiar tissue reaction in the lungs, including (1) invasion of the infected region by macrophages and (2) walling off of the lesion by fibrous tissue to form the so-called tubercle. This walling-off process helps limit further transmission of the tubercle bacilli in the lungs and therefore is part of the protective process against the infection. However, in approximately 3 per cent of all persons who contract tuberculosis, if untreated, the walling-off process fails, and tubercle bacilli spread throughout the lungs, often causing extreme destruction of lung tissue with formation of large abscess cavities. Thus, tuberculosis in its late stages causes many areas of fibrosis throughout the lungs and reduces the total amount of functional lung tissue. These effects cause (1) increased "work" on the part of the respiratory muscles to cause pulmonary ventilation and *reduced vital capacity and breathing capacity,* and (2) *reduced total respiratory membrane surface area* and *increased thickness of the respiratory membrane,* these causing progressively diminished pulmonary diffusing capacity.

Hypoxia

Obviously, almost any of the conditions discussed in the past few sections of this chapter can cause serious degrees of cellular hypoxia. In some of these, oxygen therapy is of great value; in others it is of moderate value; in still others it is of almost no value. Therefore, it is important to classify the different types of hypoxia; then we can readily discuss the physiological principles of therapy. The following is a descriptive classification of different causes of hypoxia:

1. Inadequate oxygenation of the lungs because of extrinsic reasons
   a. Deficiency of oxygen in atmosphere
   b. Hypoventilation (neuromuscular disorders)
2. Pulmonary disease
   a. Hypoventilation due to increased airway resistance or decreased pulmonary compliance
   b. Uneven alveolar ventilation
   c. Diminished respiratory membrane diffusion
3. Inadequate transport and delivery of oxygen
   a. Anemia, abnormal hemoglobin
   b. General circulatory deficiency
   c. Localized circulatory deficiency (peripheral, cerebral, coronary vessels)
   d. Tissue edema
4. Inadequate tissue capability of using oxygen
   a. Poisoning of cellular enzymes
   b. Diminished cellular metabolic capacity because of toxicity, vitamin deficiency, or other factors.

This classification of the different types of hypoxia is mainly self-evident from the discussions earlier in the chapter. Only one of the types of hypoxia in the preceding classification needs further elaboration; this is the hypoxia caused by inadequate capability of the cells to use oxygen.

Inadequate Tissue Capability of Using Oxygen. The classic cause of inability of the tissues to use oxygen is *cyanide poisoning,* in which the action of cytochrome oxidase is completely blocked—to such an extent that the tissues simply cannot utilize the oxygen even though plenty is available.

Also, deficiencies of oxidative enzymes or other elements in the tissue oxidative system can lead to this type of hypoxia. A special example of this occurs in the disease beriberi, in which several important steps in the tissue utilization of oxygen and the formation of carbon dioxide are compromised because of vitamin B deficiency.

Effects of Hypoxia on the Body. Hypoxia, if severe enough, can actually cause death of the cells, but in less severe degrees it results principally in (1) depressed mental activity, sometimes culminating in coma, and (2) reduced work capacity of the muscles.

Oxygen Therapy in the Different Types of Hypoxia

Oxygen can be administered by (1) placing the patient's head in a "tent" that contains air fortified with oxygen, (2) allowing the patient to breathe either pure oxygen or high concentrations of oxygen from a mask, or (3) administering oxygen through an intranasal tube.

Oxygen therapy is of great value in certain types of hypoxia but of almost no value at all in other types. However, recalling the basic physiological principles of the different types of hypoxia, one can readily decide when oxygen therapy is of value and, if so, how valuable. For instance:

In *atmospheric hypoxia,* oxygen therapy can obviously completely correct the depressed oxygen level in the inspired gases and, therefore, provide 100 per cent effective therapy.

In *hypoventilation hypoxia,* a person breathing 100 per cent oxygen can move five times as much oxygen into the alveoli with each breath as when breathing normal air. Therefore, here again oxygen therapy can be extremely beneficial. (However, this provides no benefit for the hypercapnia also caused by the hypoventilation.)

In *hypoxia caused by impaired diffusion,* essentially the same result occurs as in hypoventilation hypoxia, for oxygen therapy can increase the Po_2 in the lungs from a normal value of about 100 mm Hg to as high as 600 mm Hg. This raises the oxygen diffusion gradient between the alveoli and the blood from a normal value of 60 mm Hg to as high as 560 mm Hg, or an increase of more than 800 per cent. This highly beneficial effect of oxygen therapy in diffusion hypoxia is illustrated in Figure 29-9, which shows that the pulmonary blood in this patient with pulmonary edema picks up oxygen four times as rapidly as it would with no therapy.

In *hypoxia caused by anemia, abnormal hemoglobin transport,* or *circulatory deficiency,* oxygen therapy is of much less value because plenty of oxygen is already available in the alveoli. The problem, instead, is that appropriate mechanisms for transporting the oxygen to the tissues are deficient. Even so, a small amount of extra oxygen, between 7 and 30 per cent, can be transported in the dissolved state in the blood even though the amount transported by the hemoglobin is hardly altered. This small amount of extra oxygen may be the difference between life and death.

In the different types of *hypoxia caused by inadequate tissue use of oxygen,* there is abnormality neither of oxygen pickup by the lungs nor of transport to the tissues. Instead, the tissue metabolic system is simply incapable of utilizing the oxygen that is delivered.

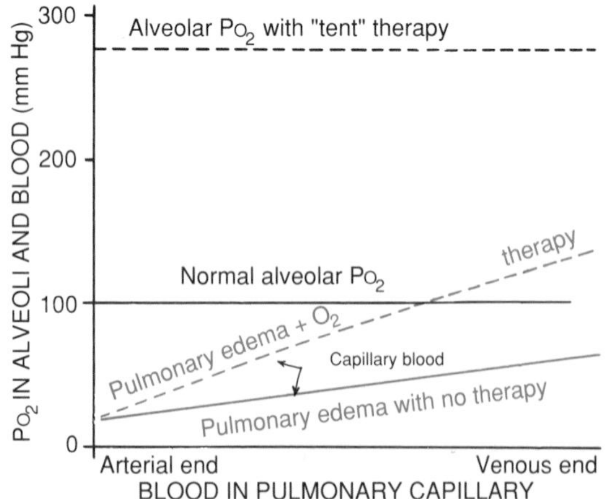

Figure 29-9. Absorption of oxygen into the pulmonary capillary blood in pulmonary edema with and without oxygen therapy.

Therefore, it is doubtful that oxygen therapy is of any benefit at all.

HYPERCAPNIA

Hypercapnia means excess carbon dioxide in the body fluids.

One might suspect on first thought that any respiratory condition that causes hypoxia would also cause hypercapnia. However, hypercapnia usually occurs in association with hypoxia only when the hypoxia is caused by *hypoventilation* or by *circulatory deficiency.* The reasons for this are the following:

Obviously, hypoxia caused by *too little oxygen in the air,* by *too little hemoglobin,* or by *poisoning of the oxidative enzymes* has to do only with the availability of oxygen or use of oxygen by the tissues. Therefore, it is readily understandable that hypercapnia is *not* a concomitant of these types of hypoxia.

Also, in hypoxia resulting from poor diffusion through the pulmonary membrane or through the tissues, serious hypercapnia usually does not occur because carbon dioxide diffuses 20 times as rapidly as oxygen. Also, if hypercapnia does begin to occur this immediately stimulates pulmonary ventilation, which partially corrects the hypercapnia but not necessarily the hypoxia.

However, in hypoxia caused by hypoventilation, carbon dioxide transfer between the alveoli and the atmosphere is affected as much as is oxygen transfer. Therefore, hypercapnia always results along with this type of hypoxia. And in circulatory deficiency, diminished flow of blood decreases the removal of carbon dioxide from the tissues, resulting in tissue hypercapnia. However, the transport capacity of the blood for carbon dioxide is about three times that for oxygen, so that even here the tissue hypercapnia is much less than the tissue hypoxia.

When the alveolar Pco_2 rises above approximately 60 to 75 mm Hg, the person by then is breathing about as rapidly and deeply as possible, and "air hunger," also called *dyspnea,* becomes very severe. As the Pco_2 rises to 80 to 100 mm Hg, the person becomes lethargic and sometimes even semicomatose. Anesthesia and death can result when the Pco_2 rises to 100 to 150 mm Hg.

Dyspnea

Dyspnea means a mental anguish associated with inability to ventilate enough to satisfy the demand for air. A common synonym is "air hunger."

At least three different factors often enter into the development of the sensation of dyspnea. These are (1) abnormality of the respiratory gases in the body fluids, especially hypercapnia (which will be discussed below) and to much less an extent hypoxia, (2) the amount of work that must be performed by the respiratory muscles to provide adequate ventilation, and (3) state of mind.

A person becomes very dyspneic especially from excess buildup of carbon dioxide in body fluids. At times, however, the levels of both carbon dioxide and oxygen in the body fluids are completely normal, but to attain this normality of the respiratory gases, the person has to breathe forcefully. In these instances the forceful activity of the respiratory muscles frequently gives the person a sensation of very severe dyspnea.

Finally, the person's respiratory functions may be completely normal, and still dyspnea may be experienced because of an abnormal state of mind. This is called *neurogenic dyspnea* or, sometimes, *emotional dyspnea.* For instance, almost anyone momentarily thinking about the act of breathing may suddenly start taking breaths a little more deeply than ordinarily because of a feeling of mild dyspnea. This feeling is greatly enhanced in persons who have a psychological fear of not being able to receive a sufficient quantity of air, such as on entering small or crowded rooms.

ARTIFICIAL RESPIRATION

The Resuscitator. Many types of resuscitators are available, and each has its own characteristic principles of operation. Basically, the resuscitator illustrated in Figure 29-10A consists of a supply of oxygen or air; a mechanism for applying intermittent positive pressure and, with some machines, negative pressure as well; and a mask that fits over the face of the patient or a connector for connecting the equipment to an endotracheal tube. This apparatus forces air through the mask into the lungs of the patient during the positive pressure cycle and then usually allows the air to flow passively out of the lungs during the remainder of the cycle.

To prevent damage to the lungs from overexpansion, resuscitators have adjustable positive pressure limits that are commonly set at 12 to 15 cm water pressure for normal lungs but sometimes much higher for very noncompliant lungs.

The Tank Respirator. Figure 29-10B illustrates the tank respirator with a patient's body inside the tank and his head protruding through a flexible but airtight collar. At the end of the tank opposite the patient's head is a motor-driven leather diaphragm that moves back and forth with sufficient excursion to raise and lower the pressure inside the tank. As the leather diaphragm moves inward, positive pressure develops around the body and causes expiration; as the diaphragm moves outward, negative pressure causes inspiration. Check valves on the respirator control the positive and negative pressures. Ordinarily these pressures are adjusted so that the negative pressure that causes inspiration falls to −10 to −20 cm water and the positive pressure rises to 0 to +5 cm water.

Effect of the Resuscitator and the Tank Respirator on Venous Return. When air is forced into the lungs under positive pressure, or when the pressure around the patient's body is greatly reduced but with the trachea exposed to atmospheric pressure through the nose, as in the case of the tank respirator, the pressure inside the chest cavity is greater than the pressure everywhere else in the body. Therefore, the flow of blood into the chest from the peripheral veins becomes impeded. As a result, use of excessive pressures with either the resuscitator or the tank respirator can reduce the cardiac output—sometimes to lethal levels.

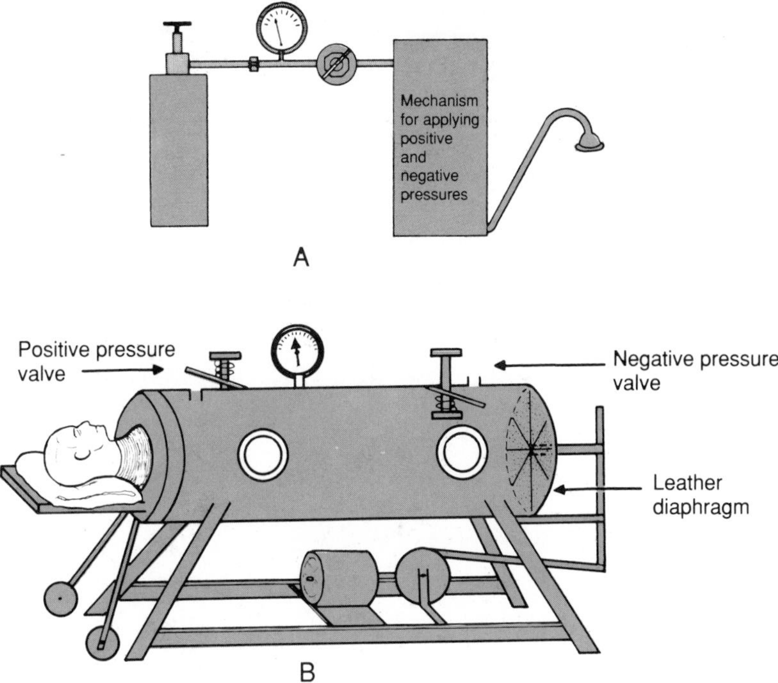

Figure 29-10. *A*, The resuscitator. *B*, Tank respirator.

REFERENCES

Regulation of Respiration

Acker, H.: Po_2 chemoreception in arterial chemoreceptors. Annu. Rev. Physiol., 51:835, 1989.

Feldman, J. L., and Ellenberger, H. H.: Central coordination of respiratory and cardiovascular control in mammals. Annu. Rev. Physiol., 50:593, 1988.

Guyton, A. C., et al.: Basic oscillating mechanism of Cheyne-Stokes breathing. Am. J. Physiol., 187:395, 1956.

Karczewski, W. A., et al.: Control of Breathing During Sleep and Anesthesia. New York, Plenum Publishing Corp., 1988.

Milhorn, H. T., Jr., and Guyton, A. C.: An analog computer analysis of Cheyne-Stokes breathing. J. Appl. Physiol., 20:328, 1965.

Richter, D. W., et al.: How is the respiratory rhythm generated? A model. News Physiol. Sci., 1:109, 1986.

Sinclair, J. D.: Respiratory drive in hypoxia: Carotid body and other mechanisms compared. News Physiol. Sci., 2:57, 1987.

Von Euler, C., and Lagercrantz, H.: Neurobiology of the Control of Breathing. New York, Raven Press, 1987.

Respiratory Insufficiency

Bates, D. V.: Respiratory Function in Disease. 3rd ed. Philadelphia, W. B. Saunders Co., 1989.

Fishman, A. P. (ed.): Pulmonary Diseases and Disorders. 2nd ed. New York, McGraw-Hill Book Co., 1988.

Green, J. F.: Fundamental Cardiovascular and Pulmonary Physiology. 2nd ed. Philadelphia, Lea & Febiger, 1987.

Imlay, J. A., and Linn, S.: DNA damage and oxygen radical toxicity. Science, 240:1302, 1988.

Murray, J. F., and Nadel, J. A.: Textbook of Respiratory Medicine. Philadelphia, W. B. Saunders Co., 1988.

Quintanilha, A. (ed.): Oxygen Radicals in Biological Systems. New York, Plenum Publishing Corp., 1988.

West, J. B.: Pulmonary Pathophysiology—The Essentials. 3rd ed. Baltimore, Williams & Wilkins, 1987.

QUESTIONS

1. Describe the anatomical loci of the various portions of the so-called respiratory center.
2. What part of the respiratory center is responsible for the basic oscillating rhythm of respiration?
3. How does the pneumotaxic center control respiration?
4. What is the function of the Hering-Breuer inflation reflex?
5. What is the role of the ventral respiratory group of neurons in the respiratory center?
6. How powerful is each of the following in directly controlling respiratory center activity: oxygen insufficiency, excess carbon dioxide, excess hydrogen ion concentration?
7. What is the relationship of the chemosensitive area of the respiratory center to the dorsal and ventral groups of respiratory neurons?
8. Approximately how much can excess carbon dioxide in the blood increase alveolar ventilation?
9. How much can excess hydrogen ion concentration in the blood increase ventilation?
10. Describe the relationship of the peripheral chemoreceptors to the respiratory center.
11. What is the importance of the peripheral chemoreceptors in the control of respiration by oxygen lack?
12. Why is oxygen regulation of respiration of minimal importance under normal conditions but very important in pneumonia and at high altitudes?
13. What special mechanisms cause powerful excitation of respiration during exercise?
14. What conditions frequently cause respiratory center depression?
15. Explain *periodic breathing,* especially of the *Cheyne-Stokes* type.
16. Describe the relationship of *pulmonary emphysema* to smoking, its pathological effects on the lungs, and its devastating effects on pulmonary function.
17. Describe the mechanism of *atelectasis* when there is either airway obstruction or lack of surfactant.
18. Why is it often much easier to inspire air than to expire air in asthma and in emphysema?
19. Define *dyspnea* and state its causes.
20. How valuable is oxygen therapy in each of the following types of hypoxia: *atmospheric hypoxia, hypoventilation hypoxia, hypoxia caused by carbon monoxide poinsoning,* and *hypoxia caused by inadequate tissue use of oxygen?*

VIII

Aviation, Space, and Deep Sea Diving Physiology

30

Aviation, Space, and Deep Sea Diving Physiology

As people have ascended to higher and higher altitudes in aviation, in mountain climbing, and in space vehicles, it has become progressively more important to understand the effects of altitude and low gas pressures on the human body. And as divers have gone deeper in the sea, it has become necessary to understand the effects of high gas pressures as well.

The present chapter deals with these problems: first, hypoxia at high altitudes; second, the other physical factors affecting the body at high altitudes; third, the tremendous acceleratory forces that occur in both aviation and space physiology; and, finally, the effects of high pressure gases at the depths of the sea.

EFFECTS OF LOW OXYGEN PRESSURE ON THE BODY

Barometric Pressures at Different Altitudes. Table 30–1 gives the approximate *barometric* and *oxygen pressures* at different altitudes, showing that at sea level the barometric pressure is 760 mm Hg; at 10,000 feet, only 523 mm Hg; and at 50,000 feet, 87 mm Hg. This decrease in barometric pressure is the basic cause of all the hypoxia problems in high altitude physiology, because as the barometric pressure decreases, the oxygen partial pressure decreases proportionately, remaining at all times slightly less than 21 per cent of the total barometric pressure — at sea level approximately 159 mm Hg but at 50,000 feet only 18 mm Hg.

Alveolar Po_2 at Different Elevations

Carbon Dioxide and Water Vapor Decrease the Alveolar Oxygen. Even at high altitudes carbon dioxide is continually excreted from the pulmonary blood into the alveoli. Also, water vaporizes into the inspired air from the respiratory surfaces. Therefore, these two gases dilute the oxygen in the alveoli, thus reducing the oxygen concentration.

Water vapor pressure remains 47 mm Hg as long as the body temperature is normal, regardless of altitude; and during exposure to very high altitudes the pressure of carbon dioxide falls in the acclimatized person, who increases alveolar ventilation about fivefold, from the normal sea level value of 40 mm Hg to about 7 mm Hg, because of increased respiration.

Now let us see how the pressures of these two gases affect the alveolar oxygen. For instance, assume that the barometric pressure falls to 253 mm Hg, which is the measured value at the top of 29,028 foot Mount Everest. Forty-seven millimeters of mercury of this must be water vapor, leaving only 206 mm Hg for all the other gases. In the acclimatized person, 7 mm of the 206 mm Hg must be carbon dioxide, leaving only 199 mm Hg. If there were no use of oxygen by the body, one fifth of this 199 mm Hg would be oxygen and four fifths would be nitrogen; or the Po_2 in the alveoli would be 40 mm Hg. However, some of this remaining alveolar oxygen would be absorbed into the blood, leaving about 35 mm Hg oxygen pressure in the alveoli. Therefore, at the summit of Mount Everest, only the best of acclimatized persons can barely survive when breathing air. But the effect is very differ-

Table 30–1 EFFECTS OF ACUTE EXPOSURE TO LOW ATOMOSPHERIC PRESSURES ON ALVEOLAR GAS CONCENTRATIONS AND ON ARTERIAL OXYGEN SATURATION*

			Breathing Air			Breathing Pure Oxygen		
Altitude (ft)	Barometric Pressure (mm Hg)	Po_2 in Air (mm Hg)	*Pco_2 in Alveoli (mm Hg)*	*Po_2 in Alveoli (mm Hg)*	*Arterial Oxygen Saturation (%)*	*Pco_2 in Alveoli (mm Hg)*	*Po_2 in Alveoli (mm Hg)*	*Arterial Oxygen Saturation (%)*
0	760	159	40 (40)	104 (104)	97 (97)	40	673	100
10,000	523	110	36 (23)	67 (77)	90 (92)	40	436	100
20,000	349	73	24 (10)	40 (53)	73 (85)	40	262	100
30,000	226	47	24 (7)	18 (30)	24 (38)	40	139	99
40,000	141	29				36	58	84
50,000	87	18				24	16	15

* Numbers in parentheses are acclimatized values.

ent when the person is breathing pure oxygen, as we see in the following discussions.

Alveolar Po_2 at Different Altitudes. The fifth column of Table 30–1 shows the Po_2s in the alveoli at different altitudes when one is breathing air, for both the unacclimatized and the acclimatized person. The alveolar Po_2 is 104 mm Hg at sea level; at 20,000 feet altitude it falls to approximately 40 mm Hg in the unacclimatized person but 53 mm Hg in the acclimatized. The difference between these two is that the alveolar ventilation increases only slightly in the unacclimatized but about six times as much in the acclimatized person.

Saturation of Hemoglobin with Oxygen at Different Altitudes. Figure 30–1 illustrates arterial oxygen saturation at different altitudes in breathing air and in breathing oxygen. Up to an altitude of approximately 10,000 feet, even when air is breathed, the arterial oxygen saturation remains at least as high as 90 per cent. However, above 10,000 feet the arterial oxygen saturation falls progressively, as illustrated by the left-hand curve of the figure, until it is only 70 per cent at 20,000 feet and still very much less at higher altitudes.

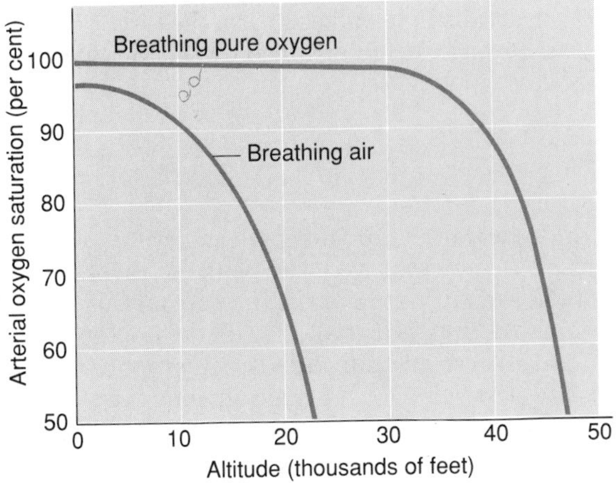

Figure 30–1. Effect of low atmospheric pressure on arterial oxygen saturation when one is breathing air and when one is breathing pure oxygen.

Effect of Breathing Pure Oxygen on the Alveolar Po_2 at Different Altitudes

When a person breathes pure oxygen instead of air, most of the space in the alveoli formerly occupied by nitrogen now becomes occupied by oxygen instead. Therefore, at 30,000 feet the aviator could have an alveolar Po_2 of 139 mm Hg instead of the 18 mm Hg when breathing air.

The second curve of Figure 30–1 illustrates the arterial oxygen saturation at different altitudes when one is breathing pure oxygen. Note that the saturation remains above 90 per cent until the aviator ascends to approximately 39,000 feet; then it falls rapidly to approximately 50 per cent at about 47,000 feet.

The "Ceiling" When Breathing Air and When Breathing Oxygen in an Unpressurized Airplane

Comparing the two arterial oxygen saturation curves in Figure 30–1, one notes that an aviator breathing oxygen can ascend to far higher altitudes than one not breathing oxygen. For instance, the arterial saturation at 47,000 feet when one is breathing oxygen is about 50 per cent and is equivalent to the arterial oxygen saturation at 23,000 feet when one is breathing air. In addition, because an unacclimatized person ordinarily can remain conscious until the arterial oxygen saturation falls to 40 to 50 per cent, the ceiling for an aviator in an unpressurized airplane when breathing air is approximately 23,000 feet and when breathing pure oxygen about 47,000 feet, provided the oxygen-supplying equipment operates perfectly.

Acute Effects of Hypoxia

Some of the important acute effects of hypoxia, beginning at an altitude of approximately 12,000 feet, are drowsiness, lassitude, mental and muscle fatigue, sometimes headache, occasionally nausea, and sometimes euphoria. All these progress to a stage of twitchings or convulsions above 18,000 feet and end, above 23,000 feet in the unacclimatized person, in coma.

One of the most important effects of hypoxia is decreased mental proficiency, which decreases judgment, memory, and the performance of discrete motor movements. For instance, if an aviator stays at 15,000 feet without supplemental oxygen for 1 hour, mental proficiency ordinarily will have fallen to approximately 50 per cent of normal and after 18 hours at this level to approximately 20 per cent of normal.

Acclimatization to Low Po_2

A person remaining at high altitudes for days, weeks, or years becomes more and more acclimatized to the low Po_2, so that it causes fewer deleterious effects on the body and also so that it becomes possible for the person to work harder without hypoxic effects or to ascend to still higher altitudes. The five principal means by which acclimatization comes about are (1) increase in pulmonary ventilation, (2) increased red blood cells, (3) increased diffusing capacity of the lungs, (4) increased vascularity of the tissues, and (5) increased ability of the cells to utilize oxygen despite the low Po_2. All these effects result from the low oxygen in the tissue fluids, for reasons discussed in the previous chapters on respiration.

Natural Acclimatization of Natives Living at High Altitudes

Many natives in the Andes and in the Himalayas live at altitudes above 13,000 feet—one group in the Peruvian Andes actually lives at an altitude of 17,500 feet and works a mine at an altitude of 19,000 feet. Many of these natives are born at these altitudes and live there all their lives. In all the aspects of acclimatization the natives are superior to even the best-acclimatized lowlanders, even though the lowlanders might also have lived at high altitudes for 10 or more years. This process of acclimatization of the natives begins in infancy. The chest size, especially, is greatly increased, whereas the body size is somewhat decreased, giving a high ratio of ventilatory capacity to body mass. In addition, their hearts, particularly the right side of the heart, which provides a high pulmonary arterial pressure to pump blood through a greatly expanded pulmonary capillary system, are considerably larger than the hearts of lowlanders.

The delivery of oxygen by the blood to the tissues is also highly facilitated in these natives. For instance, Figure 30-2 shows the hemoglobin-oxygen dissociation curves for natives who live at sea level and for their counterparts who live at 15,000 feet. Note that the arterial oxygen Po_2 in the natives at high altitude is only 40 mm Hg, but because of the greater quantity of hemoglobin the quantity of oxygen in the arterial blood is actually greater than in the blood of the natives at the lower altitude. Note also that the venous Po_2 in the high altitude natives is only 15 mm Hg less than the venous Po_2 for the lowlanders, despite the very low arterial Po_2, indicating that oxygen transport to the tissues is exceedingly effective in the naturally acclimatized high-altitude natives.

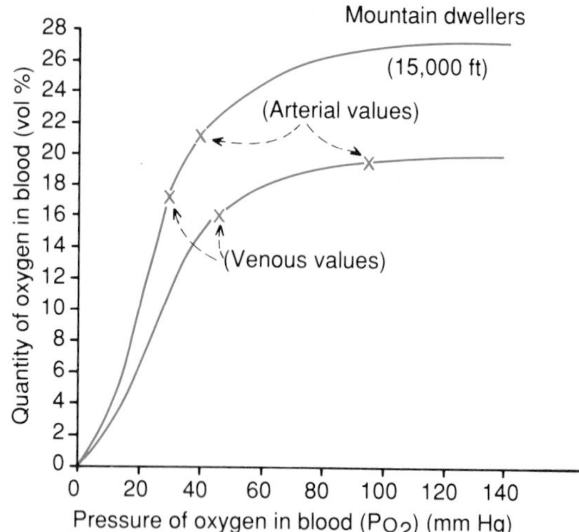

Figure 30-2. Oxygen-dissociation curves for blood of high-altitude and sea-level residents, showing the respective arterial and venous Po_2s and oxygen contents as recorded in their native surroundings. (From Oxygen-dissociation curves for bloods of high-altitude and sea-level residents. PAHO Scientific Publication No. 140, Life at High Altitudes, 1966.)

EFFECTS OF ACCELERATORY FORCES ON THE BODY IN AVIATION AND SPACE PHYSIOLOGY

Because of rapid changes in velocity and direction of motion in airplanes and spacecraft, several types of acceleratory forces often affect the body during flight. At the beginning of flight, simple linear acceleration occurs; at the end of flight, deceleration; and every time the vehicle turns, centrifugal acceleration.

Centrifugal Acceleratory Forces

When an airplane makes a turn, the force of centrifugal acceleration is determined by the following relationship:

$$f = \frac{mv^2}{r}$$

in which f is the centrifugal acceleratory force, m is the mass of the object, v is the velocity of travel, and r is the radius of curvature of the turn. From this formula it is obvious that as the velocity increases, the force of centrifugal acceleration increases in proportion to the *square* of the velocity. It is also obvious that the force of acceleration is directly proportional to the sharpness of the turn (the less the radius).

Measurement of Acceleratory Force—"G." When a person is simply sitting in his or her seat, the force with which he or she is pressing against the seat results from the pull of gravity, and it is equal to body weight. The intensity of this force is said to be +1 G because it is equal to the pull of gravity. If the force with which the person presses against the seat becomes five times the normal weight during pull-out from a dive, the force acting upon the seat is +5 G.

If the airplane goes through an outside loop so that the person is held down by his or her seat belt, *negative G* is applied to the body; and if the force with which the body is thrown against the belt is equal to the weight of the body, the negative force is −1 G.

Effects of Centrifugal Acceleratory Force (Positive G) on the Body. ***Effects on the Circulatory System.*** The most important effect of centrifugal acceleration is on the circulatory system, because blood is mobile and can be translocated by centrifugal forces.

When the aviator is subjected to *positive G,* the blood is centrifuged toward the lower part of the body. Thus, if the centrifugal acceleratory force is +5 G and the person is in an immobilized standing position, the hydrostatic pressure in the veins of the feet is five times normal, or approximately 450 mm Hg; even in the sitting position this pressure is nearly 300 mm Hg. As the pressure in the vessels of the lower part of the body increases, the vessels passively dilate, and a major proportion of the blood from the upper part of the body is translocated into these lower vessels. Because the heart cannot pump unless blood returns to it, the greater the quantity of blood "pooled" in the lower body, the less becomes the cardiac output.

Acceleration greater than 4 to 6 G causes "blackout" of vision within a few seconds and unconsciousness shortly thereafter. If this degree of acceleration is continued, the person will die.

Effects on the Vertebrae. Extremely high acceleratory forces for even a fraction of a second can fracture the vertebrae. The degree of positive acceleration that the average person can withstand in the sitting position before vertebral fracture occurs is approximately 20 G.

Protection of the Body Against Centrifugal Acceleratory Forces. Specific procedures and apparatus have been developed to protect aviators against the circulatory collapse that occurs during positive G. First, if the aviator tightens the abdominal muscles to an extreme degree and leans forward to compress the abdomen, some of the pooling of blood in the large vessels of the abdomen can be prevented, thereby delaying the onset of blackout. Also, special "anti-G" suits have been devised to prevent pooling of blood in the lower abdomen and legs. The simplest of these applies positive pressure to the legs and abdomen by inflating compression bags as the G increases.

Effects of Linear Acceleratory Forces on the Body

Acceleratory Forces in Space Travel. Unlike an airplane, a spacecraft cannot make rapid turns; therefore, centrifugal acceleration is of little importance except when the spacecraft goes into abnormal gyrations. On the other hand, blast-off acceleration and landing deceleration might be tremendous; both of these are types of linear acceleration.

Figure 30–3 illustrates a typical profile of the acceleration during blast-off in a three-stage spacecraft, showing that the first-stage booster causes acceleration as high as 9 G and the second-stage booster, as high as 8 G. In the standing position the human body could not withstand this much acceleration, but in a semi-reclining position *transverse to the axis of acceleration,* this amount of acceleration can be withstood with ease despite the fact that the acceleratory forces continue for as long as 5 minutes at a time. Therefore, we see the reason for the reclining seats used by the astronauts.

Problems also occur during deceleration when the spacecraft re-enters the atmosphere. A person traveling at Mach 1 (the speed of sound and of fast airplanes) can be safely decelerated in a distance of approximately 0.12 mile, whereas a person traveling at a speed of Mach 100 (a speed possible in interplanetary space travel) requires a distance of about 10,000 miles for safe deceleration. The principal reason for this difference is that the total amount of energy that must be dispelled during deceleration is proportional to the *square* of the velocity, which alone increases the distance 10,000-fold. But, in addition to this, a human being can withstand far less deceleration if the period of deceleration lasts for a long time than for a short time. Therefore, deceleration must be accomplished much more slowly from the very high velocities than is necessary at lower velocities.

"Artificial Climate" in the Sealed Spacecraft

Since there is no atmosphere in outer space, an artificial atmosphere and climate must be provided.

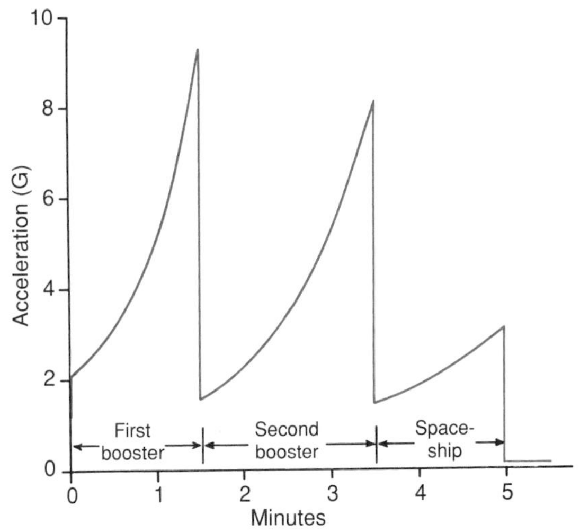

Figure 30–3. Acceleratory forces during the takeoff of a spacecraft.

Most important of all, the oxygen concentration must remain high enough and the carbon dioxide concentration low enough to prevent suffocation. In some of the earlier space missions a capsule atmosphere containing pure oxygen at about 260 mm Hg pressure has been used. In others, a gas mixture of 50 per cent oxygen and 50 per cent nitrogen at a total pressure of about 380 mm Hg has been used. The presence of nitrogen in the mixture greatly diminishes the likelihood of fire and explosion. It also protects against the development of local patches of atelectasis that often occur in breathing pure oxygen, because oxygen is absorbed very rapidly when small bronchi are temporarily blocked by mucous plugs.

For space travel lasting more than several months, it will be impractical to carry along an adequate oxygen supply and enough carbon dioxide absorbent. For this reason, "recycling techniques" have been proposed for use of the same oxygen over and over again. Some recycling processes depend on purely physical procedures, such as electrolysis of water to release oxygen, and so forth. Others depend on biological methods, such as use of algae with their large store of chlorophyll to generate foodstuffs and release oxygen from carbon dioxide at the same time by the process of photosynthesis. Unfortunately, a completely practical system for recycling is yet to be achieved.

Weightlessness in Space

A person in an orbiting satellite or in any nonpropelled spacecraft experiences *weightlessness.* That is, the person is not drawn toward the bottom, sides, or top of the spacecraft but simply floats inside its chambers. The cause of this is not failure of gravity to pull on the body, because gravity from any nearby heavenly body is still active. However, the gravity acts on both the spacecraft and the person at the same time, and since there is no resistance to movement in space, both are pulled with exactly the same acceleratory forces and in the same direction. For this reason, the person simply is not attracted toward any wall of the spacecraft.

Physiological Problems of Weightlessness. Fortunately, the physiological problems of weightlessness have not proved to be severe. Most of the problems that do occur appear to be related to three effects of the weightlessness: (1) motion sickness during the first few days of travel, (2) translocation of fluids within the body because of no gravity to cause hydrostatic pressures, and (3) diminishment of physical activity because no strength of muscle contraction is required to oppose the force of gravity.

The observed effects of prolonged stay in space are the following: (1) decrease in blood volume, (2) decrease in red cell mass, (3) decreased muscle strength and work capacity, (4) decrease in maximum cardiac output, and (5) loss of calcium and phosphate from the bones as well as loss of bone mass. Most of these same effects also occur in persons lying in bed for an extended period of time. For this reason extensive exercise programs are carried out during prolonged Space Laboratory missions, and most of the aforementioned effects are greatly reduced. Therefore, it appears that with an appropriate exercise program the physiological effects of weightlessness will not be a serious problem even during prolonged space voyages.

PHYSIOLOGY OF DEEP SEA DIVING AND OTHER HYPERBARIC CONDITIONS

When human beings descend beneath the sea, the pressure around them increases tremendously. To keep the lungs from collapsing, air must be supplied also under high pressure, which exposes the blood in the lungs to extremely high alveolar gas pressure, a condition called *hyperbarism.* Beyond certain limits these high pressures can cause tremendous alterations in the body physiology.

Relationship of Sea Depth to Pressure. A column of sea water 33 feet deep exerts the same pressure at its bottom as all the atmosphere above the earth. Therefore, a person 33 feet beneath the ocean surface is exposed to a pressure of 2 atmospheres, 1 atmosphere of pressure caused by the air above the water and the second atmosphere by the weight of the water itself. At 66 feet the pressure is 3 atmospheres, and so forth, in accord with the table in Figure 30–4.

Effect of Depth on the Volume of Gases—Boyle's Law. Another important effect of depth is the compression of gases to smaller and smaller volumes. Figure 30–4 also illustrates a bell jar at sea level containing 1 liter of air. At 33 feet beneath the sea where the pressure is 2 atmospheres, the volume has been compressed to only ½ liter, and at 8 atmospheres (233 feet) to ⅛ liter. Thus, the volume to which a given quantity of gas is compressed is inversely proportional to the pressure. This is the physical principle called *Boyle's law,* which is extremely important in diving because increased pressures can collapse air chambers of the diver's body, including the lungs, and often cause serious damage.

Effect of High Partial Pressures of Gases on the Body

The three gases to which a diver breathing air is normally exposed are nitrogen, oxygen, and carbon dioxide, and each of these at times can cause serious physiological effects at high pressures.

Nitrogen Narcosis at High Nitrogen Pressures. Approximately four fifths of the air is nitrogen. At sea level pressure the nitrogen has no known effect on bodily function, but at high pressures it can cause varying degrees of narcosis. When the diver remains beneath the sea for an hour or more and is breathing compressed air, the depth at which the first symptoms of mild narcosis appear is approximately 120 feet, at which level the diver begins to exhibit joviality and to lose many of his cares. At 150 to 200

Depth (feet)	Atmosphere (s)
Sea level	1
33	2
66	3
100	4
133	5
166	6
200	7
300	10
400	13
500	16

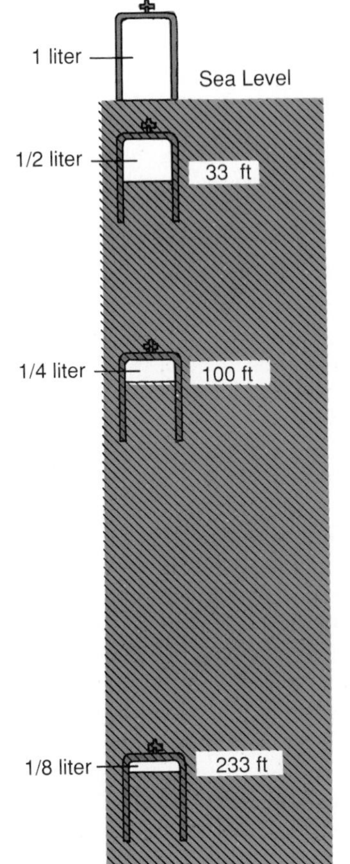

Figure 30-4. Effect of depth on gas volumes.

feet, the diver becomes drowsy. At 200 to 250 feet, his strength wanes considerably, and he often becomes too clumsy to perform the work required of him. Beyond 250 feet (8.5 atmospheres pressure), the diver usually becomes almost useless as a result of nitrogen narcosis if he remains at these depths too long.

Nitrogen narcosis has characteristics very similar to those of alcohol intoxication, and for this reason it has frequently been called "raptures of the depths."

The mechanism of the narcotic effect is believed to be the same as that of essentially all the gas anesthetics. That is, nitrogen dissolves freely in the fats of the body, and it is presumed that it, like most other anesthetic gases, dissolves in the membranes of the neurons and, because of its *physical* effect on altering electrical conductance of the membranes, reduces their excitability.

Oxygen Toxicity at High Pressures. Breathing oxygen under very high partial pressure can be detrimental to the central nervous system, sometimes causing epileptic convulsions followed by coma. Indeed, exposure to 3 atmospheres pressure of oxygen ($Po_2 = 2280$ mm Hg) will cause convulsions and coma in most persons after about 1 hour. These convulsions often occur without any warning, and they obviously are likely to be lethal to a diver submerged in the sea.

The cause or causes of oxygen toxicity are yet unknown, but experiments have shown that excess oxygen in the tissues causes the development of large concentrations of oxidizing free radicals such as superoxide (O_2^-), which can cause oxidative destruction of many essential elements of the cells, thereby damaging the metabolic systems of the cells.

Carbon Dioxide Toxicity at Great Depths. If the diving gear is properly designed and also functions properly, the diver has no problem due to carbon dioxide toxicity, for depth alone does not increase the carbon dioxide partial pressure in the alveoli. This is true because depth does not increase the rate of carbon dioxide production in the body; and as long as the diver continues to breathe a normal tidal volume, he continues to expire the carbon dioxide as it is formed, maintaining his alveolar carbon dioxide partial pressure at a normal value of almost exactly 40 mm Hg.

Unfortunately, though, in certain types of diving gear, such as the diving helmet and the different types of rebreathing apparatuses, carbon dioxide can frequently build up in the dead space air of the apparatus and be rebreathed by the diver. Up to an alveolar carbon dioxide pressure (Pco_2) of about 80 mm Hg, two times that of normal alveoli, the diver tolerates this buildup, his minute respiratory volume increasing up to a maximum of 8-fold to 11-fold to compensate for the increased carbon dioxide. However, beyond the 80 mm Hg level the situation becomes intolerable, and eventually the respiratory center begins to be depressed, rather than excited; the diver's respiration then begins to fail, rather than to compensate. In addition, the diver develops severe respiratory acidosis, and varying degrees of lethargy, narcosis, and finally anesthesia ensue.

Decompression of the Diver After Exposure to High Pressures

When a person breathes air under high pressure for a long time, the amount of nitrogen dissolved in the body fluids becomes great. The reason for this is the following: The blood flowing through the pulmonary capillaries becomes saturated with nitrogen to the same pressure as that in the breathing mixture. Over several hours, enough nitrogen is carried to all the tissues of the body to saturate the tissues also with dissolved nitrogen. Because nitrogen is not metabolized by the body, it remains dissolved until the nitrogen pressure in the lungs decreases, at which time the nitrogen is then removed by the reverse respiratory process.

Volume of Nitrogen Dissolved in the Body Fluids at Different Depths. At sea level almost 1 liter of nitrogen is dissolved in the entire body. A little less than half of this is dissolved in the water of the body and a little more than half in the fat of the body. This is true despite the fact that fat constitutes only 15 per cent of the normal body, because nitrogen is five times as soluble in fat as in water.

After the diver has become totally saturated with nitrogen, the approximate *sea level volume of nitrogen* dissolved in the body fluids at the different depths is:

Feet	*Liters*
33	2
100	4
200	7
300	10

However, several hours are required for the gas pressures of nitrogen in all the body tissues to come to equilibrium with the gas pressure of nitrogen in the alveoli, simply because the blood does not flow rapidly enough and the nitrogen does not diffuse rapidly enough to cause instantaneous equilibrium. For this reason, if a person remains at deep levels for only a few minutes, not much nitrogen dissolves in the fluids and tissues; whereas if the person remains at a deep level for several hours, both the fluids and tissues become almost completely saturated with nitrogen.

Decompression Sickness (Synonyms: Bends, Compressed Air Sickness, Caisson Disease, Diver's Paralysis, Dysbarism). If a diver has been beneath the sea long enough that large amounts of nitrogen have dissolved in his body and then he suddenly comes back to the surface of the sea, significant quantities of nitrogen bubbles can develop in his body fluids either intracellularly or extracellularly, and these can cause minor or serious damage in almost any area of the body, depending on the number of bubbles formed; this is "decompression sickness."

The principles underlying bubble formation are shown in Figure 30–5. To the left, the diver's tissues have become equilibrated to a very high nitrogen pressure. However, as long as the diver remains deep beneath the sea, the pressure against the outside of his body (5000 mm Hg) compresses all the body tissues sufficiently to keep the dissolved gases in solution. But when the diver suddenly rises to sea level, the pressure on the outside of his body becomes only 1 atmosphere (760 mm Hg), whereas the pressure inside the body fluids is the sum of the pressures of water vapor, carbon dioxide, oxygen, and nitrogen, or a total of 4065 mm Hg, which is far greater than the pressure on the outside of the body. Therefore, the gases can escape from the dissolved state and form actual bubbles both in the tissues and especially in the blood, where they plug the small blood vessels.

Symptoms of Decompression Sickness. Most of the symptoms of decompression sickness are caused by gas bubbles blocking blood vessels in the different tissues. At first, only the smallest vessels are blocked by very minute bubbles, but as the bubbles coalesce, progressively larger vessels are affected. Obviously, tissue ischemia and sometimes tissue death are the result.

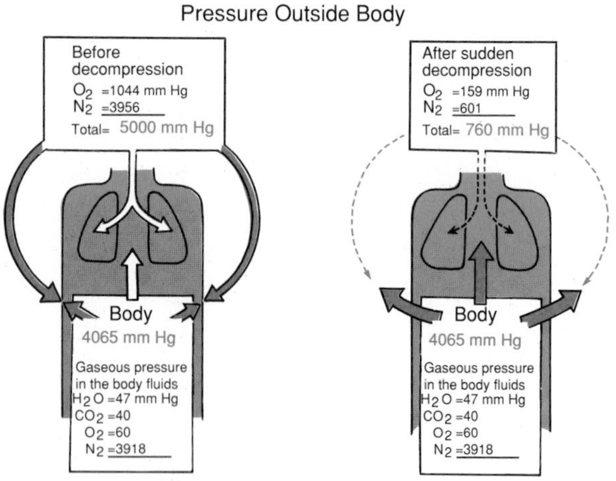

Pressure Outside Body

Before decompression	After sudden decompression
O_2 =1044 mm Hg	O_2 =159 mm Hg
N_2 =3956	N_2 =601
Total= 5000 mm Hg	Total= 760 mm Hg

Body	Body
4065 mm Hg	4065 mm Hg
Gaseous pressure in the body fluids	Gaseous pressure in the body fluids
H_2O =47 mm Hg	H_2O =47 mm Hg
CO_2 =40	CO_2 =40
O_2 =60	O_2 =60
N_2 =3918	N_2 =3918

Figure 30–5. Gaseous pressure both inside and outside the body, showing at right the great excess of intrabody pressure that is responsible for bubble formation in the body tissues.

In most persons with decompression sickness, the symptoms are pain in the joints and muscles of the legs or arms, affecting about 89 per cent of those who develop decompression sickness. The joint pain accounts for the term "bends" that is often applied to this condition.

In 5 to 10 per cent of persons with decompression sickness, nervous system symptoms occur, ranging from dizziness in about 5 per cent to paralysis or collapse and unconsciousness in as many as 3 per cent. The paralysis may be temporary, but in some instances the damage is permanent.

Finally, about 2 per cent of persons with decompression sickness develop "the chokes," caused by massive numbers of microbubbles plugging the capillaries of the lungs; this is characterized by serious shortness of breath, often followed by severe pulmonary edema and occasionally death.

Nitrogen Elimination from the Body; Decompression Tables. Fortunately, if a diver is brought to the surface slowly, the dissolved nitrogen is eliminated through the lungs rapidly enough to prevent decompression sickness. Approximately two thirds of the total nitrogen is liberated in 1 hour and about 90 per cent in 6 hours.

Special decompression tables have been prepared by the U.S. Navy that detail procedures for safe decompression. To give the student an idea of the decompression process, a diver who has been breathing air and has been on the bottom for 60 minutes at a depth of 190 feet is decompressed according to the following schedule:

10 minutes at 50 feet depth
17 minutes at 40 feet depth
19 minutes at 30 feet depth
50 minutes at 20 feet depth
84 minutes at 10 feet depth

Thus, for a work period on the bottom of only 1 hour, the total time for decompression is about 3 hours.

"Saturation Diving" and Use of Helium-Oxygen Mixtures in Deep Dives. When divers must work at very deep levels—between 250 feet and nearly 1000 feet—they frequently live in a large compression tank for weeks at a time, remaining compressed at a pressure level near that at which they will be working. This keeps the tissues and fluids of the body saturated with the gases to which they will be exposed while diving. Then when they work and later return to the same tank after working, there are not significant changes in pressure, and so decompression bubbles do not occur.

In very deep dives, especially during saturation diving, helium is usually used in the gas mixture instead of nitrogen for three different reasons: (1) it has only about one fifth the narcotic effect of nitrogen, (2) only about half as much volume of helium dissolves in the body tissues as nitrogen, and (3) the low density of helium (one seventh the density of nitrogen) keeps the airway resistance for breathing at a minimum, which is extremely important, because highly compressed nitrogen is so dense that airway resistance can become extreme, sometimes making the work of breathing beyond endurance.

Finally, in very deep dives it is important to reduce the oxygen concentration in the gaseous mixture, for otherwise oxygen toxicity would result. For instance, at a depth of 700 feet (22 atmospheres of pressure) a 1 per cent oxygen mixture will provide all the oxygen required by the diver, while a 21 per cent mixture of oxygen (the percentage in air) delivers a Po_2 to the lungs of over 4 atmospheres, a level likely to cause convulsions in as little as 30 minutes.

Scuba Diving (Self-Contained Underwater Breathing Apparatus)

Prior to the 1940s, almost all diving was done using a diving helmet connected to a hose through which air was pumped to the diver from the surface. Then, in 1943, Jacques Cousteau developed and popularized the *self-contained underwater breathing apparatus,* popularly known simply as the scuba apparatus. The type of scuba apparatus used in over 99 per cent of all sports and commercial diving is the *open circuit demand system* illustrated in Figure 30-6. This system consists of the following components: (1) one or more tanks of compressed air or of some other breathing mixture, (2) a first-stage "reducing" valve for reducing the pressure from the tanks to a constant low pressure level, (3) a combination inhalation "demand" valve and exhalation valve that allows air to be pulled into the lungs with very slight negative pressure of breathing and then to be exhausted into the sea at very slight positive pressure, and (4) a mask and tube system with small "dead space."

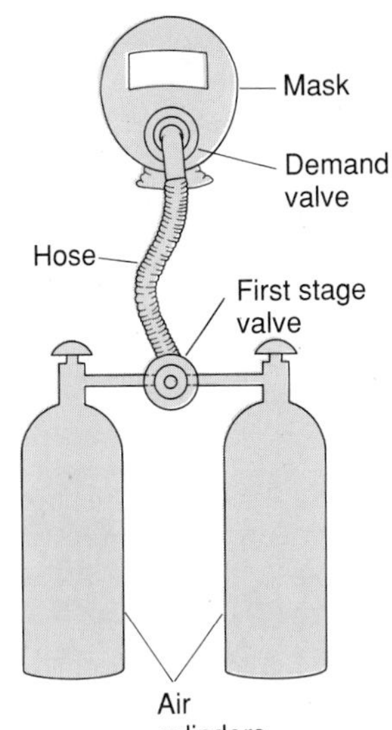

Figure 30-6. The open circuit demand type of scuba apparatus.

Basically, the demand system operates as follows: The first-stage reducing valve reduces the pressure from the tanks usually to a pressure of about 140 pounds per square inch. However, the breathing mixture does not flow continually into the mask. Instead, with each inspiration, slight negative pressure in the mask pulls the diaphragm of the demand valve inward, and this automatically releases air from the hose into the mask and lungs. In this way only the amount of air needed for inhalation enters the system. Then, on expiration, the air cannot go back into the tank, but instead is expired through the expiration valve.

The most important problem in use of the self-contained underwater breathing apparatus is the time limit that one can remain beneath the surface; for instance, only a few minutes are possible at a 200 foot depth. The reason for this is that tremendous airflow from the tanks is required to wash carbon dioxide out of the lungs. That is, the greater the depth, the greater the airflow in terms of *quantity* of air that is required, because the *volume* has been compressed to a small size.

REFERENCES

Aviation and Space Physiology

American Physiological Society: High Altitude and Man. Washington, D.C., American Physiological Society, 1984.

DeHart, R. L. (ed.): Fundamentals of Aerospace Medicine. Philadelphia, Lea & Febiger, 1985.

Life Sciences Report, National Aeronautics and Space Administration, Washington, D.C., December 1987.

McCormack, P. D., et al. (eds.): Terrestrial Space Radiation and Its Biological Effects. New York, Plenum Publishing Corp., 1988.

Nicogossian, A. E., et al. (eds.): Space Physiology and Medicine. 2nd ed. Philadelphia, Lea & Febiger, 1989.

Quintanilha, A. (ed.): Reactive Oxygen Species in Chemistry, Biology, and Medicine. New York, Plenum Publishing Corp., 1988.

West, J. B.: Climbing Mount Everest without oxygen. News Physiol. Sci., 1:25, 1986.

West, J. B.: Man in space. News Physiol. Sci., 1:198, 1986.

Diving Physiology

Brauer, R. W.: Problems of exposure to high pressures. News Physiol. Sci., 1:192, 1986.
Crapo, J. D.: Morphologic changes in pulmonary oxygen toxicity. Annu. Rev. Physiol., 48:721, 1986.
Elsner, R., and de Burgh Daly, M.: Coping with asphyxia: Lessons from seals. News Physiol. Sci., 3:65, 1988.
Fridovich, I.: Superoxide radical: An endogenous toxicant. Annu. Rev. Pharmacol. Toxicol., 23:239, 1983.
Fridovich, I., and Freeman, B.: Antioxidant defenses in the lung. Annu. Rev. Physiol., 48:693, 1986.
Jamieson, D., et al.: The relation of free radical production to hyperoxia. Annu. Rev. Physiol., 48:703, 1986.
Pryor, W. A.: Oxy-radicals and related species. Annu. Rev. Physiol., 48:657, 1986.

QUESTIONS

1. Approximately how much is the atmospheric Po_2 decreased from normal at an altitude of 20,000 feet?
2. Why does water vapor pressure remain approximately constant in the alveoli at 47 mm Hg regardless of the altitude?
3. Why does the Pco_2 not decrease nearly so much in the alveoli at high altitudes as does the Po_2?
4. At what altitude does the saturation of arterial blood with hemoglobin fall below approximately 50 per cent, which is the approximate ceiling at which a person can survive?
5. How does breathing pure oxygen change the Po_2 in the alveoli at 20,000 feet and at 50,000 feet, and what is the approximate ceiling at which a person can survive when breathing pure oxygen?
6. What are the effects of hypoxia on the body, especially the brain?
7. Discuss the different physiological changes that allow a person to become acclimatized to high altitudes.
8. What is the relationship of centrifugal acceleratory force to the velocity of movement and the sharpness of a turn?
9. What is meant by G force?
10. Why are linear acceleratory forces important in space travel?
11. Discuss the problems of artificial climate and weightlessness in space.
12. How deep below sea level must one go for the pressure of gases in the lungs to reach 4 atmospheres?
13. Explain the phenomenon of *nitrogen narcosis,* which occurs at deep levels below the sea surface when breathing air.
14. What are the effects of *oxygen toxicity* at great depths below the sea surface?
15. Explain the cause and the effects of *decompression sickness.*
16. In scuba diving, why is the compressed air mixture that the diver breathes used up far more rapidly at 200 feet than at 50 feet below the sea surface? What is the relationship of carbon dioxide to this difference?

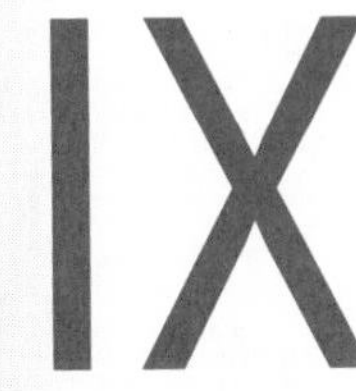

The Nervous System: (A) Basic Organization and Sensory Physiology

31

Organization of the Nervous System; Basic Functions of Synapses and Transmitter Substances

The nervous system, along with the endocrine system, provides most of the control functions for the body. In general, the nervous system controls the rapid activities of the body, such as muscular contractions, rapidly changing visceral events, and even the rates of secretion of some endocrine glands. The endocrine system, by contrast, regulates principally the metabolic functions of the body.

The nervous system is unique in the vast complexity of the control actions that it can perform. It receives literally millions of bits of information from the different sensory organs and then integrates all these to determine the response to be made by the body. The purpose of this chapter is to present a general outline of the overall mechanisms by which the nervous system performs such functions and then to discuss the basic functions of synapses and neuronal circuits. Before beginning this discussion, however, the reader should refer to Chapters 5 and 7, which present, respectively, the principles of membrane potentials and transmission of signals in nerves and through neuromuscular junctions.

GENERAL DESIGN OF THE NERVOUS SYSTEM

The Sensory Division of the Nervous System—Sensory Receptors

Most activities of the nervous system are initiated by sensory experience emanating from *sensory receptors,* whether visual receptors, auditory receptors, tactile receptors on the surface of the body, or other kinds of receptors. This sensory experience can cause an immediate reaction, or its memory can be stored in the brain for minutes, weeks, or years and then can help determine the bodily reactions at some future date.

Figure 31-1 illustrates a portion of the sensory system, the *somatic* portion, which transmits sensory information from the receptors of the entire surface of the body and some deep structures. This information enters the central nervous system through the spinal nerves and is conducted to multiple "primary" sensory areas in (1) the spinal cord at all levels, (2) the reticular substance of the medulla, pons, and mesencephalon, (3) the cerebellum, (4) the thalamus, and (5) the somesthetic areas of the cerebral cortex. But in addition to these primary sensory areas, signals are then relayed to essentially all other parts of the nervous system as well.

The Motor Division—The Effectors

The most important ultimate role of the nervous system is to control the various bodily activities. This is achieved by controlling (1) contraction of skeletal muscles throughout the body, (2) contraction of smooth muscle in the internal organs, and (3) secretion by both exocrine and endocrine glands in many parts of the body. These activities are collectively called *motor functions* of the nervous system, and the muscles and glands are called *effectors,* because they perform the functions dictated by the nerve signals.

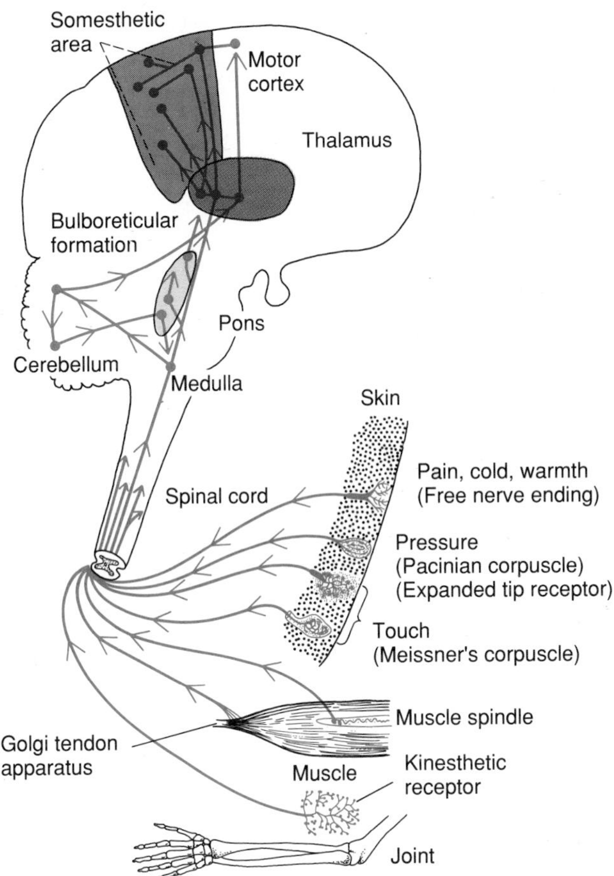

Figure 31–1. The somatic sensory axis of the nervous system.

Figure 31–2 illustrates the *motor axis* of the nervous system for controlling skeletal muscle contraction. Operating parallel to this axis is another similar system for control of the smooth muscles and glands called the *autonomic nervous system,* which is presented in Chapter 41. Note in Figure 31–2 that the skeletal muscles can be controlled from many different levels of the central nervous system, including (1) the spinal cord, (b) the reticular substance of the medulla, pons, and mesencephalon, (3) the basal ganglia, (4) the cerebellum, and (5) the motor cortex. Each of these different areas plays its own specific role in the control of body movements, the lower regions being concerned primarily with automatic, instantaneous responses of the body to sensory stimuli; and the higher regions, with deliberate movements controlled by the thought process of the cerebrum.

Processing of Information— "Integrative" Function of the Nervous System

The major function of the nervous system is to process incoming information in such a way that *appropriate* motor responses occur. More than 99 per cent of all sensory information is discarded by the brain as irrelevant and unimportant. For instance, one is ordinarily totally unaware of the parts of the body that are in contact with clothing and is also unaware of the seat pressure when sitting. Likewise, attention is drawn only to an occasional object in one's field of vision, and even the perpetual noise of our surroundings is usually relegated to the background.

After the important sensory information has been selected, it is then channeled into proper motor regions of the brain to cause the desired responses. This channeling of information is called the *integrative function* of the nervous system. Thus, if a person places a hand on a hot stove, the desired response is to lift the hand. There are other associated responses, too, such as moving the entire body away from the stove and perhaps even shouting with pain. Yet even these responses represent activity by only a small fraction of the total motor system of the body.

Role of Synapses in Processing Information. The synapse is the junction point from one neuron to the next and, therefore, is an advantageous site for control of signal transmission. Later in this chapter we discuss the details of synaptic function. However, it is important to point out here that the synapses determine the directions that the nervous signals spread in the nervous system. That is, the synapses perform a selective action, often blocking the weak signals while allowing the strong signals to pass, often selecting and amplifying certain weak signals, and often channeling the signals in many different directions, rather than simply in one direction.

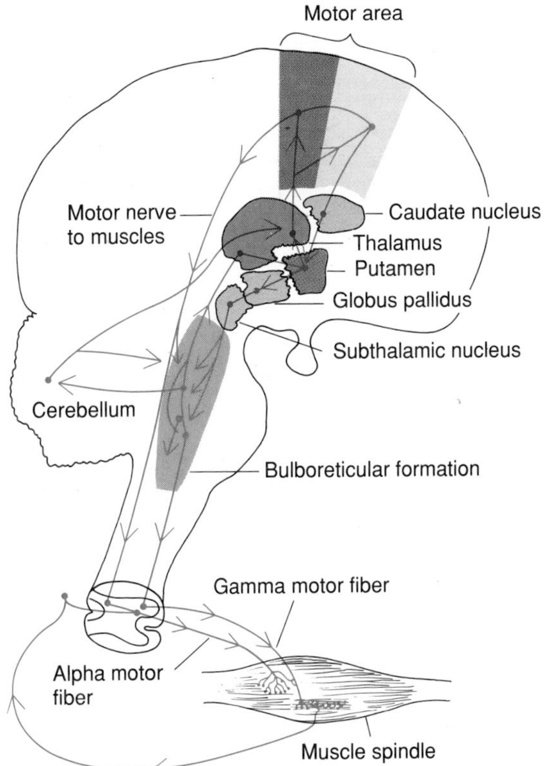

Figure 31–2. The motor axis of the nervous system.

Storage of Information — Memory

Only a small fraction of the important sensory information causes an immediate motor response. Much of the remainder is stored for future control of motor activities and for use in the thinking processes. Most of this storage occurs in the *cerebral cortex,* but not all, for even the basal regions of the brain and perhaps even the spinal cord can store small amounts of information.

The storage of information is the process we call *memory,* and this, too, is a function of the synapses. That is, each time certain types of sensory signals pass through sequences of synapses, these synapses become more capable of transmitting the same signals the next time, which process is called *facilitation.* After the sensory signals have passed through the synapses a large number of times, the synapses become so facilitated that signals generated within the brain itself can also cause transmission of impulses through the same sequences of synapses even though the sensory input has not been excited. This gives the person a perception of experiencing the original sensations, although in effect they are only memories of the sensations.

Once memories have been stored in the nervous system, they become part of the processing mechanism. The thought processes of the brain compare new sensory experiences with the stored memories; the memories help to select the important new sensory information and to channel this into appropriate storage areas for future use or into motor areas to cause bodily responses.

THE THREE MAJOR LEVELS OF CENTRAL NERVOUS SYSTEM FUNCTION

The human nervous system has inherited specific characteristics from each stage of evolutionary development. From this heritage, three major levels of the central nervous system have specific functional attributes: (1) the *spinal cord level,* (2) the *lower brain level,* and (3) the *higher brain,* or *cortical, level.*

The Spinal Cord Level

We often think of the spinal cord as being only a conduit for signals from the periphery of the body to the brain or in the opposite direction from the brain back to the body. However, this is far from the truth. Even after the spinal cord has been cut in the high neck region, many spinal cord functions still occur. For instance, neuronal circuits in the cord can cause (1) walking movements, (2) reflexes that withdraw portions of the body from objects, (3) reflexes that stiffen the legs to support the body against gravity, and (4) reflexes that control local blood vessels, gastrointestinal movements, and so forth, in addition to many other functions.

In fact, the upper levels of the nervous system often operate not by sending signals directly to the periphery of the body but instead by sending signals to the control centers of the cord, simply "commanding" the cord centers to perform their functions.

The Lower Brain Level

Many if not most of what we call subconscious activities of the body are controlled in the lower areas of the brain — in the medulla, pons, mesencephalon, hypothalamus, thalamus, cerebellum, and basal ganglia. Subconscious control of arterial pressure and respiration is achieved mainly in the medulla and pons. Control of equilibrium is a combined function of the older portions of the cerebellum and neuronal centers in the medulla, pons, and mesencephalon. Feeding reflexes, such as salivation in response to the taste of food and the licking of the lips, are controlled by areas in the medulla, pons, mesencephalon, amygdala, and hypothalamus; and many emotional patterns, such as anger, excitement, sexual activities, reaction to pain, or reaction of pleasure, can occur in animals without a cerebral cortex.

The Higher Brain or Cortical Level

After recounting all the nervous system functions that can occur at the cord and lower brain levels, what is left for the cerebral cortex to do? The answer to this begins with the fact that the cerebral cortex is an extremely large memory storehouse. The cortex never functions alone, but always in association with the lower centers of the nervous system.

Without the cerebral cortex, the functions of the lower brain centers are often very imprecise. The vast storehouse of cortical information usually converts these functions to very determinative and precision operations.

Finally, the cerebral cortex is essential for most of our thought processes even though it also cannot function alone in this. In fact, it is the lower centers that cause *wakefulness* in the cerebral cortex, thus opening its bank of memories to the thinking machinery of the brain.

Thus, each portion of the nervous system performs specific functions. Many integrative functions are well developed in the spinal cord, and many of the subconscious functions originate and are executed entirely in the lower regions of the brain. But it is the cortex that opens the world up for one's mind.

THE CENTRAL NERVOUS SYSTEM SYNAPSES

Almost every student is aware that information is transmitted in the central nervous system mainly in the form of nerve impulses through a succession of neurons, one after another. However, it is not immediately apparent that each impulse (a) may be blocked in its transmission from one neuron to the next, (b) may be changed from a single impulse into repetitive impulses, or (c) may be integrated with impulses from other neurons to cause highly intricate patterns of impulses in successive neurons. All these functions are called the *synaptic functions of neurons.*

Almost all the synapses utilized for signal transmission in the central nervous system of the human being are *chemical synapses.* In these, the first neuron secretes a chemical substance called a *neurotransmitter* at the synapse, and this transmitter in turn acts on receptor proteins in the membrane of the next neuron to excite the neuron, to inhibit it, or to modify its sensitivity in some other way. Over 40 different transmitter substances have been discovered thus far. Some of the best known are acetylcholine, norepinephrine, histamine, gamma-aminobutyric acid (GABA), and glutamate.

One-Way Conduction Through the Synapses. Synapses have one exceedingly important characteristic that makes them highly desirable as the form of transmission of nervous system signals: they always transmit the signals in one direction—that is, from the neuron that secretes the transmitter, called the *presynaptic neuron,* to the neuron on which the transmitter acts, called the *postsynaptic neuron.* This is the principle of *one-way conduction* through chemical synapses.

Think for a moment about the extreme importance of the one-way conduction mechanism. It allows signals to be directed toward specific goals. Indeed, it is this specific transmission of signals to discrete and highly focused areas in the nervous system that allows the nervous system to perform its myriad functions of sensation, motor control, memory, and many others.

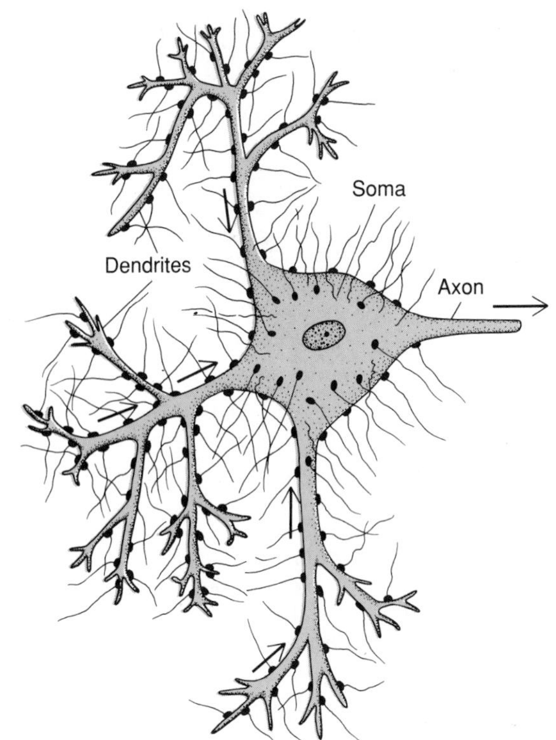

Figure 31-3. A typical motor neuron, showing presynaptic terminals on the neuronal soma and dendrites. Note also the single axon.

Physiological Anatomy of the Synapse

Figure 31-3 illustrates a typical *motor neuron* in the anterior horn of the spinal cord. It is composed of three major parts: the *soma,* which is the main body of the neuron; a single *axon,* which extends from the soma into the peripheral nerve; and the *dendrites,* which are thin projections of the soma that extend up to 1 mm into the surrounding areas of the cord.

Up to as many as 100,000 small knobs called *presynaptic terminals* lie on the surfaces of the dendrites and soma of the motor neuron, approximately 80 to 95 per cent of them on the dendrites and only 5 to 20 per cent on the soma. These terminals are the ends of nerve fibrils that originate in many other neurons; usually not more than a few of the terminals are derived from any single previous neuron. Later it will become evident that many of these presynaptic terminals are *excitatory* and secrete a substance that excites the postsynaptic neuron, but many others are *inhibitory* and secrete a substance that inhibits the neuron.

Neurons in other parts of the cord and brain differ markedly from the motor neuron in (1) the size of the cell body; (2) the length, size, and number of dendrites; ranging in length from almost none at all up to as long as many centimeters; (3) the length and size of the axon, with a few axons having lengths over 1 meter; and (4) the number of presynaptic terminals, which may range from only a few to several hundred thousand. These differences make neurons in different parts of the nervous system react differently to incoming signals and therefore perform different functions.

The Presynaptic Terminals. Electron microscopic studies of the presynaptic terminals show that these have varied anatomical forms, but most resemble small round or oval knobs and therefore are frequently called *terminal knobs, boutons, end-feet,* or *synaptic knobs.*

Figure 31-4 illustrates the basic structure of the presynaptic terminal. It is separated from the neuronal soma by a *synaptic cleft* having a width usually of 200 to 300 angstroms. The terminal has two internal structures important to the excitatory or inhibitory functions of the synapse: the *synaptic vesicles* and the *mitochondria.* The synaptic vesicles contain *transmitter substances* that, when released into the synaptic cleft, either *excite* or *inhibit* the postsynaptic neuron. The mitochondria provide adenosine triphosphate (ATP), which then supplies the energy to synthesize new transmitter substance.

When an action potential spreads over a presynaptic terminal, the membrane depolarization causes a small number of vesicles to empty into the cleft; and the released transmitter in turn causes an immediate

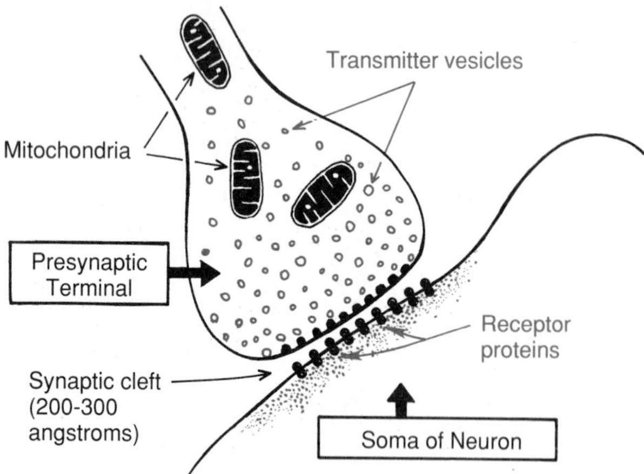

Figure 31-4. Physiologic anatomy of the synapse.

change in the permeability characteristics of the postsynaptic neuronal membrane, which leads to excitation or inhibition of the neuron, depending on its receptor characteristics.

Mechanism by Which Action Potentials Cause Transmitter Release at the Presynaptic Terminals —Role of Calcium Ions

The synaptic membrane of the presynaptic terminals contains large numbers of *voltage-gated calcium channels.* This is quite different from the other areas of the nerve fiber, which contain very few of these channels. When the action potential depolarizes the terminal, large numbers of calcium ions flow into the terminal. The quantity of transmitter substance that is released into the synaptic cleft is directly related to the number of calcium ions that enter the terminal. The precise mechanism by which the calcium ions cause this release is not known but is believed to be the following:

When the calcium ions enter the synaptic terminal, it is believed that they bind with protein molecules on the inner surfaces of the synaptic membrane, called *release sites.* This in turn causes the transmitter vesicles in the local vicinity to bind with the membrane and actually to fuse with it, and finally to open to the exterior by the process called *exocytosis,* which is described in Chapter 2. Usually, a few vesicles release their transmitter into the cleft following each single action potential. For the vesicles that store the neurotransmitter acetylcholine, between 2000 and 10,000 molecules of acetylcholine are present in each vesicle, and there are enough vesicles in the presynaptic terminal to transmit from a few hundred to more than 10,000 action potentials.

Action of the Transmitter Substance on the Postsynaptic Neuron—The Function of Receptors

At the synapse, the membrane of the postsynaptic neuron contains large numbers of *receptor proteins,* also illustrated in Figure 31-4. These receptors have two important components: (1) a *binding component* that protrudes outward from the membrane into the synaptic cleft—it binds with the neurotransmitter from the presynaptic terminal—and (2) an *ionophore component* that passes all the way through the membrane to the interior of the postsynaptic neuron. The ionophore in turn is one of two types: (1) a *chemically activated ion channel* or (2) an *enzyme that activates an internal metabolic change inside the cell.*

The Ion Channels—Excitatory and Inhibitory Receptors. The chemically activated ion channels are usually of three types: (1) *sodium channels* that allow mainly sodium ions to pass through, (2) *potassium channels* that allow mainly potassium ions to pass, and (3) *chloride channels* that allow chloride and a few other anions to pass. We learn later that opening the sodium channels excites the postsynaptic neuron, so that these channels are *excitatory receptors.* Therefore, a transmitter substance that opens the sodium channels is called an *excitatory transmitter.* On the other hand, opening of potassium and chloride channels inhibits the neuron, so that these channels are *inhibitory receptors.* Transmitters that open either or both of them are called *inhibitory transmitters.*

The Enzyme Receptors. Activation of an enzymatic type of receptor causes other effects on the postsynaptic neuron. One effect is to *activate the metabolic machinery of the cell,* such as causing formation of cyclic adenosine monophosphate (AMP), which in turn excites many other intracellular activities. Another is to *activate cellular genes,* which in turn manufacture additional receptors for the postsynaptic membrane. Still a third effect is to *activate protein kinases,* which decrease the numbers of receptors. Changes such as these can alter the reactivity of the synapse for minutes, days, months, or even years. Therefore, transmitter substances that cause such effects are sometimes called synaptic *modulators.* Recent experiments have demonstrated that such modulators are important in at least some of the memory processes, which we discuss in Chapter 39.

Chemical Substances That Function as Synaptic Transmitters

More than 40 different chemical substances have been proved or postulated to function as synaptic transmitters. In general, there are two different groups of synaptic transmitters. One is composed of small molecule, rapidly acting transmitters. The other is a large number of neuropeptides of much larger molecular size and much more slowly acting.

The small molecule, rapidly acting transmitters are the ones that cause most of the acute responses of the nervous system, such as transmission of sensory signals to and inside the brain and motor signals back to the muscles. The neuropeptides, on the other hand, usually cause more prolonged actions, such as long-term changes in numbers of receptors, long-term closure of certain ion channels, and possibly even long-term changes in numbers of synapses.

The Small Molecule, Rapidly Acting Transmitters

The most important of the small molecule transmitters are the following:

Acetylcholine is secreted by neurons in many areas of the brain, but specifically by the large pyramidal cells of the motor cortex, by many different neurons in the basal ganglia, by the motor neurons that innervate the skeletal muscles, by the preganglionic neurons of the autonomic nervous system, by the postganglionic neurons of the parasympathetic nervous system, and by some of the postganglionic neurons of the sympathetic nervous system. In most instances acetylcholine has an excitatory effect; however, it is known to have inhibitory effects at some of the peripheral parasympathetic nerve endings, such as inhibition of the heart by the vagus nerves.

Norepinephrine is secreted by many neurons whose cell bodies are located in the brain stem and hypothalamus. Specifically, norepinephrine-secreting neurons located in the *locus ceruleus* in the pons send nerve fibers to widespread areas of the brain and help control the overall activity and mood of the mind. In most of these areas it probably activates excitatory receptors; but in a few areas, inhibitory receptors instead. Norepinephrine is also secreted by most of the postganglionic neurons of the sympathetic nervous system, where it excites some organs but inhibits others.

Dopamine is secreted by neurons that originate in the substantia nigra. The terminations of these neurons are mainly in the striatal region of the basal ganglia. The effect of dopamine is usually inhibition.

Glycine is secreted mainly at synapses in the spinal cord. It probably always acts as an inhibitory transmitter.

Gamma-aminobutyric acid (GABA) is secreted by nerve terminals in the spinal cord, the cerebellum, the basal ganglia, and many areas of the cortex. It is believed always to cause inhibition.

Glutamate is probably secreted by the presynaptic terminals in many of the sensory pathways as well as in many areas of the cortex. It probably always causes excitation.

Serotonin is secreted by nuclei that originate in the median raphe of the brain stem and project to many brain areas, especially to the dorsal horns of the spinal cord and to the hypothalamus. Serotonin acts as an inhibitor of pain pathways in the cord, and it is also believed to help control the mood of the person, perhaps even to cause sleep.

Recycling of the Small Molecule Types of Vesicles. The vesicles that store and release small molecule transmitters are continually recycled, that is, used over and over again. After they fuse with the synaptic membrane and open to release their transmitters, the vesicle membrane at first simply becomes part of the synaptic membrane. However, within seconds to minutes, the vesicle portion of the membrane invaginates back to the inside of the presynaptic terminal and pinches off to form a new vesicle. It still contains the appropriate transport proteins required for concentrating new transmitter substance inside the vesicle.

Acetylcholine is a typical small molecule transmitter that obeys the above principles of synthesis and release. It is synthesized in the presynaptic terminal from acetyl coenzyme A (acetyl-CoA) and choline in the presence of the enzyme *choline acetyltransferase.* Then it is transported into its specific vesicles. When the vesicles later release the acetylcholine into the synaptic cleft, the acetylcholine, after performing its transmitter function, is rapidly split again to acetate and choline by the enzyme *cholinesterase,* which is bound to the proteoglycan reticulum that fills the space of the synaptic cleft. Then the vesicles are recycled, and choline also is actively transported back into the terminal to be used again for synthesis of new acetylcholine.

The Neuropeptides

The neuropeptide types of transmitter substances are not synthesized in the presynaptic terminals but instead are synthesized along with new vesicles in the soma of the neuron. Then the vesicles are transported all the way to the tips of the nerve fibers by *axonal streaming* of the axon cytoplasm, traveling at the slow rate of only a few centimeters per day. Finally, these vesicles release their transmitter in response to action potentials in the same manner as for small molecule transmitters.

Some of the important neuropeptide transmitters are:

1. Hypothalamic releasing hormones: These are hormones that cause the pituitary gland to release its hormones into the general circulation. For instance, *thyrotropin-releasing hormone* originates in the hypothalamus but eventually is transmitted to the anterior pituitary gland to cause release of thyroid-stimulating hormone, in this way controlling the function of the thyroid gland.
2. Pituitary peptides: These are released into the posterior pituitary gland. An example is *vasopressin,* which is then absorbed into the blood from this gland and carried to the kidneys where it causes the kidneys to retain water in the body, a function called antidiuresis; therefore, vasopressin is also called "antidiuretic hormone" (ADH).
3. Sleep peptides: These small peptides are released into the basal regions of the brain, where they act on other brain neurons to promote sleep.

These are only three of many classes of neuropeptides, most of which will be discussed specifically at different points in this text.

Electrical Events During Neuronal Excitation

The electrical events in neuronal excitation have been studied especially in the large motor neurons of the anterior horns of the spinal cord. Therefore, the events to be described in the following few sections pertain essentially to these neurons. However, except for quantitative differences, they apply to most other neurons of the nervous system as well.

The Resting Membrane Potential of the Neuronal Soma. Figure 31–5 illustrates the soma of a motor neuron, showing the resting membrane potential to be about −65 millivolts. This is somewhat less than the −90 millivolts found in large peripheral nerve fibers and in skeletal muscle fibers; the lower voltage is important, however, because it allows both positive and negative control of the degree of excitability of the neuron. That is, decreasing the voltage to a less negative value makes the membrane of the neuron more excitable, whereas increasing this voltage to a more negative value makes the neuron less excitable. This is the basis of the two modes of function of the neuron—either excitation or inhibition—as is explained in detail in the following sections.

Concentration Differences of Ions Across the Neuronal Somal Membrane. Figure 31–5 also illustrates the concentration differences across the neuronal somal membrane of the three ions that are most important for neuronal function: sodium ions, potassium ions, and chloride ions.

At the top, the sodium ion concentration is shown to be very great in the extracellular fluid but low inside the neuron. This sodium concentration gradient is caused by a strong sodium pump that continually pumps sodium out of the neuron.

The figure also shows that the potassium ion concentration is large inside the neuronal soma but very low in the extracellular fluid. It illustrates that there is also a potassium pump (the other half of the Na^+-K^+ pump, as described in Chapter 4) that pumps potassium to the interior. However, potassium ions leak through the membrane ion channels at a rate sufficient to nullify much of the effectiveness of the potassium pump.

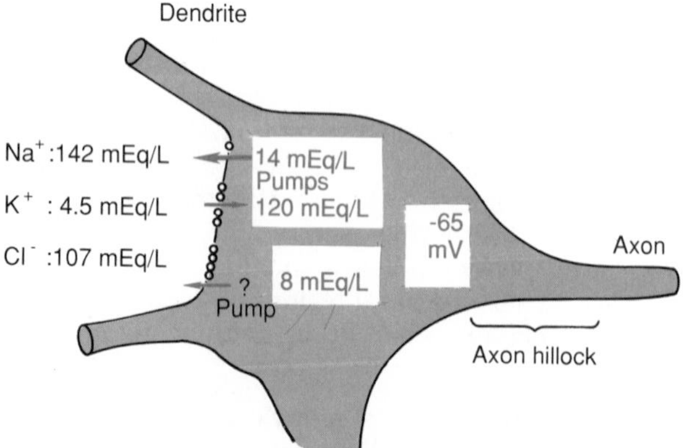

Figure 31–5. Distribution of sodium, potassium, and chloride ions across the neuronal somal membrane; origin of the intrasomal membrane potential.

Finally, Figure 31–5 shows the chloride ion to be of high concentration in the extracellular fluid but low concentration inside the neuron. It also shows that the membrane is quite permeable to chloride ions and that there may be a weak chloride pump. Yet most of the reason for the low concentration of chloride ions inside the neuron is the −65 millivolts in the neuron. That is, this negative voltage repels the negatively charged chloride ions, forcing them outward through the pores until the concentration difference is much greater outside the membrane than inside.

Let us recall at this point what we learned in Chapters 4 and 5 about the relationship of ionic concentration differences to membrane potentials. It will be recalled that an electrical potential across the membrane can exactly oppose the movement of ions through a membrane despite concentration differences between the outside and inside of the membrane if the potential is of the proper polarity and magnitude. Such a potential that exactly opposes movement of each type of ion is called the Nernst potential for that ion; the equation for this is the following:

$$\text{EMF(mV)} = \pm 61 \times \log\left(\frac{\text{Concentration outside}}{\text{Concentration inside}}\right)$$

where EMF is the Nernst potential in millivolts on the *inside of the membrane.* The potential will be positive (+) for a positive ion and negative (−) for a negative ion.

Now, let us calculate the Nernst potential that will exactly oppose the movement of each of the three separate ions: sodium, potassium, and chloride.

For the sodium concentration difference shown in Figure 31–5, 142 mEq/liter on the exterior and 14 mEq/liter on the interior, the membrane potential that would exactly oppose sodium ion movement through the sodium channels would be +61 millivolts. However, the actual membrane potential is −65 millivolts, not +61 millivolts. Therefore, sodium ions normally diffuse inward through the sodium channels; however, not many sodium ions will diffuse because most of the sodium channels are normally closed. Furthermore, those sodium ions that do diffuse to the interior are normally pumped immediately back to the exterior by the sodium pump.

For potassium ions, the concentration gradient is 120 mEq/liter inside the neuron and 4.5 mEq/liter outside. This gives a Nernst potential of −86 millivolts inside the neuron, which is more negative than the −65 that actually exists. Therefore, there is a tendency for potassium ions to diffuse to the outside of the neuron, but this is opposed by the continual pumping of these potassium ions back to the interior.

Finally, the chloride ion gradient, 107 mEq/liter outside and 8 mEq/liter inside, yields a Nernst potential of −70 millivolts inside the neuron, which is slightly more negative than the actual value measured. Therefore, chloride ions tend normally to leak to the interior of the neuron, whereas those that do diffuse are moved back to the exterior, perhaps by an active chloride pump.

Keep these three Nernst potentials in mind and also remember the direction in which the different ions tend to diffuse, for this information will be important in understanding both excitation and inhibition of the neuron by synaptic activation of receptor ion channels.

Origin of the Resting Membrane Potential of the Neuronal Soma. The basic cause of the −65 millivolt resting membrane potential of the neuronal soma is the sodium-potassium pump. This pump causes the extrusion of more positively charged sodium ions to the exterior than potassium to the interior —three sodium ions outward for each two potassium ions inward. Because there are large numbers of negatively charged ions inside the soma that cannot diffuse through the membrane—protein ions, phosphate ions, and many others—extrusion of the excess positive ions to the exterior leaves some of these nondiffusible negative ions inside the cell unbalanced by positive ions. Therefore, the interior of the neuron becomes negatively charged as the result of the sodium-potassium pump. This principle was discussed in more detail in Chapter 5 in relation to the resting membrane potential of nerve fibers.

Uniform Distribution of the Potential Inside the Soma. The interior of the neuronal soma contains a very highly conductive electrolytic solution, the intracellular fluid of the neuron. Furthermore, the diameter of the neuronal soma is very large (from 10 to 80 micrometers in diameter), causing there to be almost no resistance to conduction of electrical current from one part of the somal interior to another part. Therefore, any change in potential in any part of the intrasomal fluid causes an almost exactly equal change in potential at all other points inside the soma. This is an important principle because it plays a major role in the summation of signals entering the neuron from multiple sources, as we shall see in subsequent discussion.

Effect of Synaptic Excitation on the Postsynaptic Membrane—The Excitatory Postsynaptic Potential. Figure 31-6A illustrates the resting neuron with an unexcited presynaptic terminal resting upon its surface. The resting membrane potential everywhere in the soma is −65 millivolts.

Figure 31-6B illustrates a presynaptic terminal that has secreted a transmitter into the cleft between the terminal and the neuronal somal membrane. This transmitter acts on a membrane excitatory receptor *to increase the membrane's permeability to* Na^+. Because of the large electrochemical gradient that tends to move sodium inward, this large increase in membrane conductance for sodium ions allows these ions to rush to the inside of the membrane.

The rapid influx of the positively charged sodium ions to the interior neutralizes part of the negativity of the resting membrane potential. Thus, in Figure 31-6B the resting membrane potential has increased from −65 millivolts to −45 millivolts. This increase in voltage above the normal resting neuronal potential—that is, to a less negative value—is called

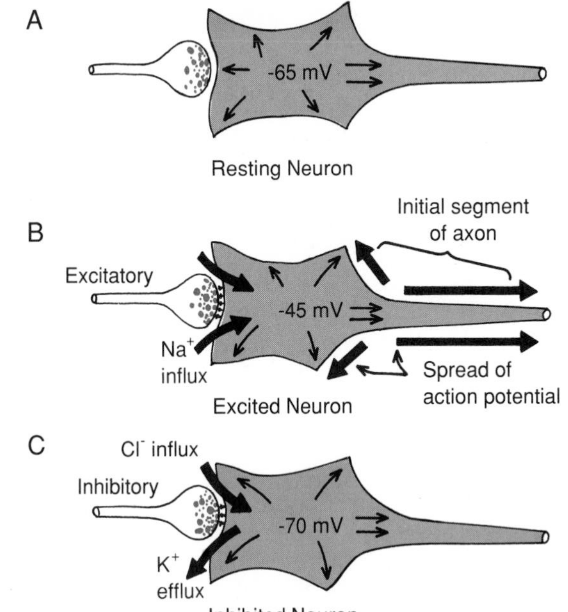

Figure 31-6. Three states of a neuron. *A*, A resting neuron. *B*, A neuron in an excited state, with more positive intraneuronal potential caused by sodium influx. *C*, A neuron in an inhibited state, with more negative intraneuronal membrane potential caused by potassium ion efflux, chloride ion influx, or both.

the *excitatory postsynaptic potential* (or EPSP) because if this potential rises high enough it will elicit an action potential in the neuron, thus exciting it. In this case the EPSP is + 20 millivolts.

However, we must issue a word of warning at this point. Discharge of a single presynaptic terminal can never increase the neuronal potential from −65 millivolts up to −45 millivolts. Instead, an increase of this magnitude requires the simultaneous discharge of many terminals—about 40 to 80 for the usual anterior motor neuron—at the same time or in rapid succession. This occurs by a process called *summation,* which will be discussed in detail in the following sections.

Generation of Action Potentials at the Initial Segment of the Axon Leaving the Neuron—Threshold for Excitation. When the excitatory postsynaptic potential rises high enough, there comes a point at which this initiates an action potential in the neuron. However, the action potential does not begin on the somal membrane adjacent to the excitatory synapses. Instead, it begins in the initial segment of the axon leaving the neuronal soma. The main reason for this point of origin of the action potential is that the soma has relatively few voltage-gated sodium channels in its membrane, which makes it difficult to open the required number of channels to elicit an action potential. On the other hand, the membrane of the initial segment has seven times as great a concentration of voltage-gated sodium channels and therefore can generate an action potential with much greater ease than can the soma. The excitatory postsynaptic potential that will elicit an action potential at the initial segment is between +15 and +20 millivolts. This is in contrast to +30 millivolts or more required on the soma.

Once the action potential begins, it travels both peripherally along the axon and often also backward over the soma. In some instances, it travels backward into the dendrites, too, but not into all of them, because they, like the neuronal soma, also have very few voltage-gated sodium channels and therefore frequently cannot generate action potentials at all.

Thus, in Figure 31-6B, it is shown that under normal conditions the *threshold* for excitation of the neuron is about −45 millivolts, which represents an excitatory postsynaptic potential of +20 millivolts—that is, 20 millivolts more positive than the normal resting neuronal potential of −65 millivolts.

Electrical Events in Neuronal Inhibition

Effect of Inhibitory Synapses on the Postsynaptic Membrane—The Inhibitory Postsynaptic Potential. The inhibitory synapses open the potassium or the chloride channels, or both, instead of sodium channels, allowing easy passage of one or both of these ions. Now, to understand how the inhibitory synapses inhibit the postsynaptic neuron, we must recall what we learned about the Nernst potentials for both the potassium ions and the chloride ions. We calculated this potential for potassium ions to be about −86 millivolts and for chloride ions about −70 millivolts. Both of these potentials are more negative than the −65 millivolts normally present inside the resting neuronal membrane. Therefore, opening the potassium channels will allow positively charged potassium ions to move to the exterior, which will make the membrane potential more negative than normal; and opening the chloride channels will allow negatively charged chloride ions to move to the interior, which also will make the membrane potential more negative than usual. This increases the degree of intracellular negativity, which is called *hyperpolarization*. It obviously inhibits the neuron because the membrane potential is now farther away than ever from the threshold for excitation. Therefore, an increase in negativity beyond the normal resting membrane potential level is called the *inhibitory postsynaptic potential* (IPSP).

Thus, Figure 31-6C illustrates the effect on the membrane potential caused by activation of inhibitory synapses, allowing chloride influx into the cell or potassium efflux from the cell, with the membrane potential decreasing from its normal value of −65 millivolts to the more negative value of −70 millivolts. This membrane potential that is 5 millivolts more negative is the inhibitory postsynaptic potential. Thus the IPSP in this instance is −5 millivolts.

Presynaptic Inhibition

In addition to the inhibition caused by inhibitory synapses operating at the neuronal membrane, which is called *postsynaptic inhibition,* another type of inhibition often occurs in the presynaptic terminals before the signal ever reaches the synapse. This type of inhibition, called *presynaptic inhibition,* is caused by "presynaptic" synapses that lie on the terminal nerve fibrils before they themselves terminate on the following neuron. It is believed that activation of these synapses on the presynaptic terminals decreases the ability of the calcium channels in the terminals to open. Because calcium ions must enter the presynaptic terminals before the vesicles can release transmitter at the neuronal synapse, the obvious result is to reduce neuronal excitation.

The cause of the reduced calcium entry into the presynaptic terminals is still unknown. One theory suggests that the presynaptic synapses release a transmitter that directly blocks calcium channels. Another theory proposes that the transmitter inhibits the opening of sodium channels, thus reducing the action potential in the terminal; because the voltage-activated calcium channels are very highly voltage-sensitive, any decrease in action potential greatly reduces calcium entry.

Presynaptic inhibition occurs in many of the sensory pathways in the nervous system. That is, the adjacent nerve fibers inhibit each other, which minimizes the sideways spread of signals from one fiber to the next. We discuss this phenomenon more fully in subsequent chapters.

Spatial Summation of the Postsynaptic Potentials—The Threshold for Firing

It has already been pointed out that excitation of a single presynaptic terminal on the surface of a neuron will almost never excite the neuron. The reason for this is that sufficient transmitter substance is released by a single terminal to cause an excitatory postsynaptic potential usually no more than 0.5 to 1 millivolt at most, instead of the required 10 to 20 millivolts to reach the usual threshold for excitation. However, during excitation in a neuronal pool of the nervous system, many presynaptic terminals are usually stimulated at the same time; and even though these terminals are spread over wide areas of the neuron, their effects can still summate. The reason for this is the following: It has already been pointed out that a change in the potential at any single point within the soma will cause the potential to change everywhere in the soma almost exactly equally. Therefore, for each excitatory synapse that discharges simultaneously, the intrasomal potential becomes more positive by as much as a fraction of a millivolt up to about 1 millivolt. When the excitatory postsynaptic potential becomes great enough, the *threshold for firing* will be reached, and an action potential will generate in the initial segment of the axon. This effect is illustrated in Figure 31-7, which shows several excitatory postsynaptic potentials. The bottom postsynaptic potential in the figure was caused by simultaneous stimulation of four synapses; the next higher potential was caused by stimulation of two times as many synapses; finally, a still higher excitatory postsynaptic potential was caused by stimulation of four times as many synapses. This time an action potential was generated in the initial axon segment.

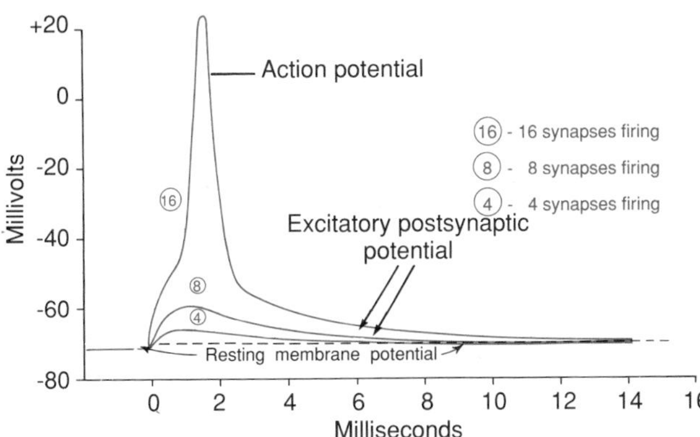

Figure 31-7. Excitatory postsynaptic potentials, showing that simultaneous firing of only a few synapses will not cause sufficient summated potential to elicit an action potential, but the simultaneous firing of many synapses will raise the summated potential to the threshold for excitation and cause a superimposed action potential.

This effect of summing simultaneous postsynaptic potentials by excitation of multiple terminals on widely spaced areas of the membrane is called *spatial summation.*

Temporal Summation

Each time a terminal fires, the released transmitter substance opens the membrane channels for a millisecond or so, but the postsynaptic potential lasts up to 15 milliseconds. Then a second opening of the same channels can increase the postsynaptic potential to a still greater level; therefore, the more rapid the rate of terminal stimulation, the greater the effective postsynaptic potential. Thus, successive postsynaptic potentials, if they occur rapidly enough, can summate in the same way that postsynaptic potentials can summate from widely distributed terminals over the surface of the neuron. This summation is called *temporal summation.*

Facilitation of Neurons. Often the summated postsynaptic potential is excitatory in nature but has not risen high enough to reach the threshold for excitation. When this happens the neuron is said to be *facilitated.* That is, its membrane potential is nearer the threshold for firing than normally but not yet to the firing level. Nevertheless, another signal entering the neuron from some other source can then excite the neuron very easily. Diffuse signals in the nervous system often facilitate large groups of neurons so that they can respond quickly and easily to signals arriving from second sources.

Special Functions of Dendrites in Exciting Neurons

The Large Spatial Field of Excitation of the Dendrites. The dendrites of the anterior motor neurons extend for 500 to 1000 micrometers in all directions from the neuronal soma. Therefore, these dendrites can receive signals from a large spatial area around the motor neuron. This provides vast opportunity for summation of signals from many separate presynaptic neurons.

It is also important that between 80 and 90 per cent of all the presynaptic terminals terminate on the dendrites of the anterior motor neuron, in contrast to only 10 to 20 per cent terminating on the neuronal soma. Therefore, the preponderant share of the excitation is provided by signals transmitted over the dendrites.

Many Dendrites Cannot Transmit Action Potentials—But They Can Transmit Signals by Electrotonic Conduction. Many dendrites fail to transmit action potentials because their membranes have relatively few voltage-gated sodium channels, so that their thresholds for excitation are too high for action potentials ever to occur. Yet they do transmit *electrotonic current* down the dendrites to the soma. Transmission of electrotonic current means the direct spread of current by electrical conduction in the fluids of the dendrites with no generation of action potentials. Stimulation of the neuron by this current has special characteristics, as follows:

Decrement of Electrotonic Conduction in the Dendrites—Greater Excitation by Synapses Near the Soma. In Figure 31-8 a number of excitatory and inhibitory synapses are shown stimulating the dendrites of a neuron. On the two dendrites to the left in the figure are shown excitatory effects near the ends of the dendrites; note the high levels of the excitatory postsynaptic potentials at these ends—that is, the less negative membrane potentials at these points. However, a large share of the excitatory postsynaptic potential is lost before it reaches the soma. The reason for this is that the dendrites are long and thin, and their membranes are also thin and excessively permeable to potassium and chloride ions, making them "leaky" to electrical current. Therefore, before the excitatory potentials can reach the soma, a large share of the potential is lost by leakage through the membrane. This decrease in membrane potential as it

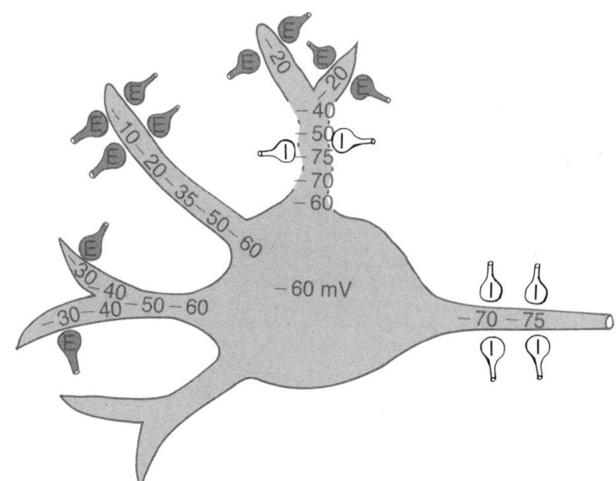

Figure 31-8. Stimulation of a neuron by presynaptic terminals located on dendrites, showing, especially, decremental conduction of excitatory electrotonic potentials in the two dendrites to the left and inhibition of dendritic excitation in the dendrite that is uppermost. A powerful effect of inhibitory synapses at the initial segment is also shown.

spreads electrotonically along dendrites toward the soma is called *decremental conduction.*

It is also obvious that the nearer the excitatory synapse is to the soma of the neuron, the less will be the decrement of conduction. Therefore, those synapses that lie near the soma have far more excitatory effect than those that lie far away from the soma.

Relation of the Rate of Firing of a Neuron to Its Excitatory State

The Excitatory State. The "excitatory state" of a neuron is defined as the degree of excitatory drive to the neuron. If there is a higher degree of excitation than inhibition of the neuron at any given instant, then it is said that there is an *excitatory state.* On the other hand, if there is more inhibition than excitation, then it is said that there is an *inhibitory state.*

When the excitatory state of a neuron rises above the threshold for excitation, then the neuron will fire repetitively as long as the excitatory state remains at this level. However, *the rate at which it will fire is determined by how much* the excitatory state is above threshold.

Response Characteristics of Different Neurons to Increasing Levels of Excitatory State. As would be expected, the ability to respond to stimulation by the synapses varies from one type of neuron to another.

Figure 31–9 illustrates theoretical responses of three different types of neurons to varying levels of the excitatory state. Note that neuron 1 has a low threshold for excitation, whereas neuron 3 has a high threshold. But note also that neuron 2 has the lowest maximum frequency of discharge, whereas neuron 3 has the highest maximum frequency.

Some neurons in the central nervous system fire continuously because even the normal excitatory state is above the threshold level. Their frequency of firing can usually be increased still more by further increasing their excitatory state. Or the frequency may be decreased, or firing even be stopped, by superimposing an inhibitory state on the neuron.

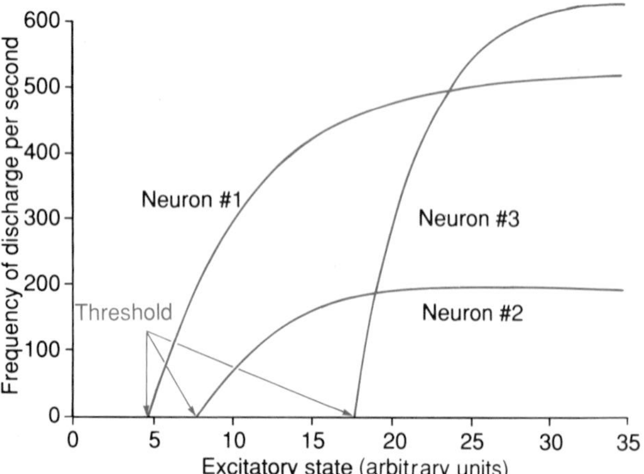

Figure 31–9. Response characteristics of different types of neurons to progressively increasing levels of excitatory state.

Thus, different neurons respond differently, have different thresholds for excitation, and have widely differing maximal frequencies of discharge. With a little imagination one can readily understand the importance of having neurons with many different types of response characteristics to perform the widely varying functions of the nervous system.

SOME SPECIAL CHARACTERISTICS OF SYNAPTIC TRANSMISSION

Fatigue of Synaptic Transmission. When excitatory synapses are repetitively stimulated at a rapid rate, the number of discharges by the postsynaptic neuron is at first very great, but it becomes progressively less in succeeding milliseconds or seconds. This is called *fatigue* of synaptic transmission.

Fatigue is an exceedingly important characteristic of synaptic function, for when areas of the nervous system become overexcited, fatigue causes them to lose this excess excitability after a while. For example, fatigue is probably the most important means by which the excess excitability of the brain during an epileptic convulsion is finally subdued so that the convulsion ceases. Thus, the development of fatigue is a protective mechanism against excess neuronal activity.

The mechanism of fatigue is mainly exhaustion of the stores of transmitter substance in the synaptic terminals, particularly because it has been calculated that the excitatory terminals on most neurons can store enough excitatory transmitter for only 10,000 normal synaptic transmissions, so that the transmitter can be exhausted in only a few seconds to a few minutes of rapid stimulation.

Effect of Drugs on Synaptic Transmission. Many different drugs are known to increase the excitability of synapses, and others are known to decrease the excitability. For instance, caffeine, theophylline, and theobromine, which are found in coffee, tea, and cocoa, respectively, all increase excitability, presumably by reducing the threshold for excitation of the neurons. Also, strychnine is one of the best known of all the agents that increase the excitability of neurons. However, it does not reduce the threshold for excitation of the neurons at all; instead, it *inhibits the action of some of the inhibitory transmitters* on the neurons, especially the inhibitory effect of glycine in the spinal cord. In consequence, the effects of the excitatory transmitters become overwhelming, and the neurons become so excited that they go into rapidly repetitive discharge, resulting in severe tonic muscle spasms.

Most anesthetics increase the membrane threshold for excitation and thereby decrease synaptic transmission at many points in the nervous system. Because most of the anesthetics are lipid-soluble, it has been reasoned that they might change the physical characteristics of the neuronal membranes, making them less responsive to excitatory agents.

REFERENCES

Barchi, R. L.: Probing the molecular structure of the voltage-dependent sodium channel. Annu. Rev. Neurosci., 11:455, 1988.

Bloom, F. E.: Neurotransmitters: Past, present, and future directions. FASEB J., 2:32, 1988.

Grinvald, A., et al.: Optical imaging of neuronal activity. Physiol. Rev., 68:1285, 1988.

Heinemann, S., and Patrick, J. (eds.): Molecular Neurobiology. New York, Plenum Publishing Corp., 1987.

Kito, S., et al. (eds.): Neuroreceptors and Signal Transduction. New York, Plenum Publishing Corp., 1988.

McGeer, P. L., et al.: Molecular Neurobiology of the Mammalian Brain. 2nd ed. New York, Plenum Publishing Corp., 1987.

Millhorn, D. E., and Hokfelt, T.: Chemical messengers and their coexistence in individual neurons. News Physiol. Sci., 3:1, 1988.

Narahashi, T. (ed.): Ion Channels. New York, Plenum Publishing Corp., 1988.

Pickering, P. T., et al. (eds.): Neurosecretion. New York, Plenum Publishing Corp., 1988.

Robinson, M. B., and Coyle, J. T.: Glutamate and related acidic excitatory neurotransmitters: From basic science to clinical application. FASEB J., 1:446, 1987.

Skok, V. I., et al. (eds.): Neuronal Acetylcholine Receptors. New York, Plenum Publishing Corp., 1989.

Williams, R. W., and Herrup, K.: The control of neuron number. Annu. Rev. Neurosci., 11:423, 1988.

QUESTIONS

1. Discuss in general the *sensory and motor divisions* and the *integrative function* of the nervous system.
2. What are the general functions at the three major levels of the central nervous system: the *spinal cord,* the *lower brain,* and the *higher brain,* or *cortical, levels?*
3. Describe the structure of the typical *synapse.*
4. What is the role of calcium ions in the release of *transmitter substance* at a synapse?
5. How is transmitter substance synthesized in the presynaptic terminals?
6. Explain the action of the transmitter substance on the postsynaptic neuron membrane.
7. What determines whether a transmitter substance will be excitatory or inhibitory? Name the specific characteristics of several of the more important neurotransmitter substances.
8. Give the concentrations of the important ions for neuronal function on the two sides of the neuronal cell membrane.
9. Explain what is meant by the *Nernst potential,* and what the mechanism is for developing the resting membrane potential of the neuronal cell membrane.
10. Explain the sequence of events and changes in membrane potential that occur when an excitatory transmitter is released at a synapse.
11. Explain also the events that occur when an inhibitory transmitter is released.
12. Why do the action potentials in the postsynaptic neuron originate in the initial segment of the axon?
13. What is the difference between presynaptic and postsynaptic inhibition?
14. Explain *spatial* and *temporal summation* of postsynaptic potentials; also explain the phenomenon of *facilitation.*
15. What are the special functions of *dendrites* in synaptic transmission?
16. What is the relationship between the excitatory state of a neuron and its rate of firing?
17. What is the mechanism of *synaptic fatigue?*

32

Sensory Receptors; Neuronal Circuits for Processing Information; Tactile and Position Senses

Input to the nervous system is provided by the sensory receptors that detect such sensory stimuli as touch, sound, light, pain, cold, warmth, and so forth. The purpose of this chapter is to discuss the basic mechanisms by which these receptors change sensory stimuli into nerve signals and how the information conveyed in the signals is processed in the nervous system. Also, we will see how these basic principles apply to the tactile and position senses.

TYPES OF SENSORY RECEPTORS AND THE SENSORY STIMULI THEY DETECT

There are basically five different types of sensory receptors: (1) *mechanoreceptors,* which detect mechanical deformation of the receptor or of cells adjacent to the receptor; (2) *thermoreceptors,* which detect changes in temperature, some receptors detecting cold and others warmth; (3) *nociceptors* (pain receptors), which detect damage in the tissues, whether physical damage or chemical damage; (4) *electromagnetic receptors,* which detect light on the retina of the eye; and (5) *chemoreceptors,* which detect taste in the mouth, smell in the nose, oxygen level in the arterial blood, osmolality of the body fluids, carbon dioxide concentration, and perhaps other factors that make up the chemistry of the body.

Figure 32–1 illustrates some of the different types of mechanoreceptors found in the skin or in the deep structures of the body. These are the receptors that are most important for the tactile and position senses, which we will discuss specifically later in the chapter.

Differential Sensitivity of Receptors

The first question that must be answered is, how do different types of sensory receptors detect different types of sensory stimuli? The answer is that each type of receptor is very highly sensitive to the one type of stimulus for which it is designed, and yet is almost nonresponsive to normal intensities of the other types of sensory stimuli. Thus, the rods and cones of the eye are highly responsive to light but are almost completely nonresponsive to heat, cold, pressure on the eyeballs, or chemical changes in the blood. And pain receptors in the skin are almost never stimulated by usual touch or pressure stimuli but do become highly active the moment tactile stimuli become severe enough to damage the tissues.

TRANSDUCTION OF SENSORY STIMULI INTO NERVE IMPULSES

Local Currents at Nerve Endings—Receptor Potentials

All sensory receptors have one feature in common. Whatever the type of stimulus that excites the receptor, its immediate effect is to change the membrane potential of the receptor. This change in potential is called a *receptor potential.*

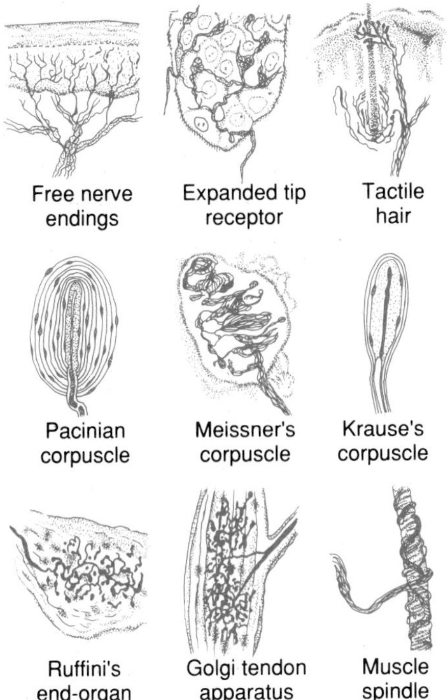

Figure 32-1. Several types of somatic sensory nerve endings.

Mechanisms of Receptor Potentials. Different receptors can be excited in several different ways to cause receptor potentials: (1) by mechanical deformation of the receptor, which stretches the membrane and opens ion channels; (2) by application of a chemical to the membrane, which also opens ion channels; (3) by change of the temperature of the membrane, which alters the permeability of the membrane; and (4) by the effects of electromagnetic radiation such as light on the receptor, which either directly or indirectly changes the membrane characteristics and allows ions to flow through membrane channels. It will be recognized that these four different means of exciting receptors correspond in general with the different types of known sensory receptors. In all instances, the basic cause of the change in membrane potential is a change in receptor membrane permeability, which allows ions to diffuse more or less readily through the membrane and thereby change the transmembrane potential.

Relationship of the Receptor Potential to Action Potentials. When the receptor potential rises above the *threshold* for eliciting action potentials in the nerve fiber attached to the receptor, then action potentials begin to appear. This is illustrated in Figure 32-2. Note also that the more the receptor potential rises above the threshold level, the greater becomes the action potential frequency. Thus, the receptor potential stimulates the sensory nerve fiber in the same way that the excitatory postsynaptic potential in the central nervous system neuron stimulates the neuron's axon.

The Receptor Potential of the Pacinian Corpuscle —An Illustrative Example of Receptor Function

The student should at this point restudy the anatomical structure of the pacinian corpuscle illustrated in Figure 32-1. Note that the corpuscle has a central nerve fiber extending through its core. Surrounding this are multiple concentric capsule layers, so that compression anywhere on the outside of the corpuscle will elongate, indent, or otherwise deform the central fiber.

Now study Figure 32-3, which illustrates only the central fiber of the pacinian corpuscle after all capsule layers have been removed by microdissection. The very tip of the central fiber is unmyelinated, but it becomes myelinated shortly before leaving the corpuscle to enter the peripheral sensory nerve.

The figure also illustrates the mechanism by which the receptor potential is produced in the pacinian corpuscle. Observe the small area of the terminal fiber that has been deformed by compression of the corpuscle, and note that ion channels have opened in the membrane, allowing positively charged sodium ions to diffuse to the interior of the fiber. This in turn creates increased positivity inside the fiber, which is the receptor potential. The receptor potential in turn induces a *local circuit* of current flow, illustrated by the red arrows, that spreads along the nerve fiber. At the first node of Ranvier, which itself lies inside the capsule of the pacinian corpuscle, the local current flow depolarizes the node, and this then sets off typi-

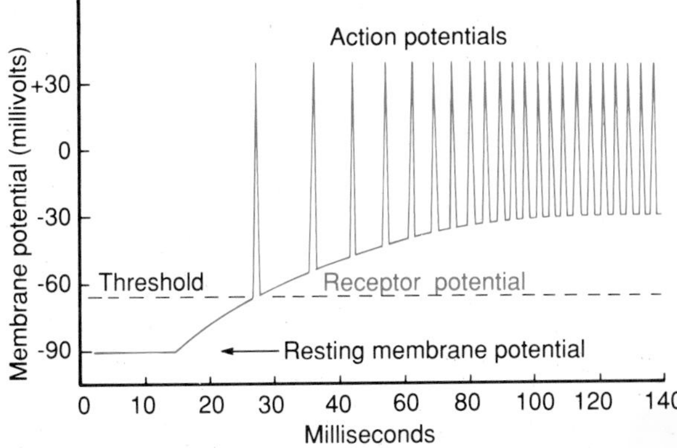

Figure 32-2. Typical relationship between receptor potential and action potentials when the receptor potential rises above the threshold level.

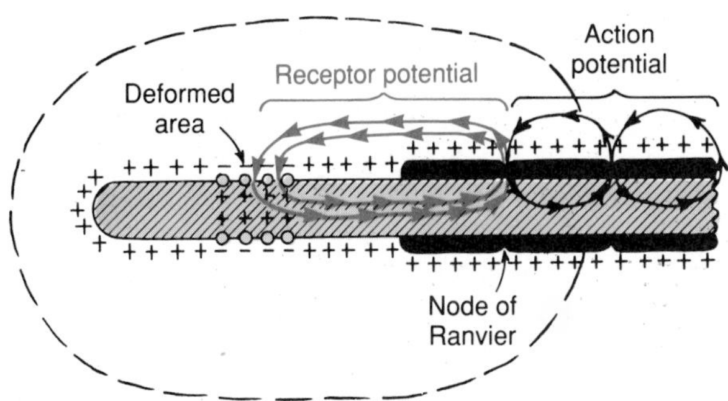

Figure 32-3. Excitation of a sensory nerve fiber by a receptor potential produced in a pacinian corpuscle. (Modified from Loëwenstein: Ann. N.Y. Acad. Sci., 94:510, 1961.)

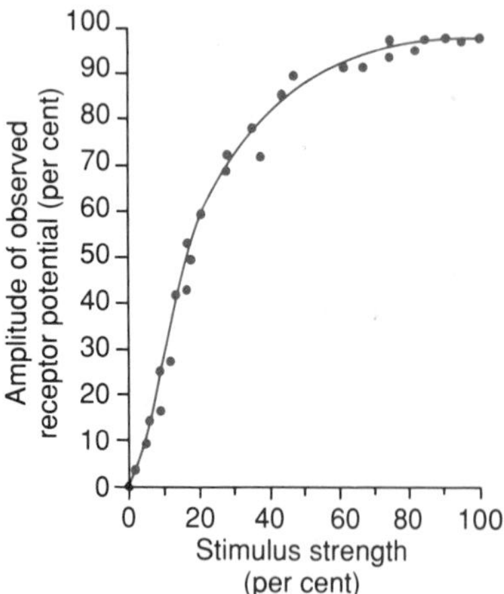

Figure 32-4. Relationship of amplitude of receptor potential to strength of a stimulus applied to a pacinian corpuscle. (From Loëwenstein: Ann. N.Y. Acad. Sci., 94:510, 1961.)

cal action potentials that are transmitted along the nerve fiber toward the central nervous system.

Relationship Between Stimulus Intensity and the Receptor Potential. Figure 32-4 illustrates the changing amplitude of the receptor potential caused by progressively stronger mechanical compression applied experimentally to the central core of a pacinian corpuscle. Note that the amplitude increases rapidly at first but then progressively less rapidly at high stimulus strength. This decreasing sensitivity at higher levels of stimulus is an exceedingly important principle, employed by almost all sensory receptors. It allows the receptor to be very sensitive to weak sensory experience and yet not reach a maximum firing rate until the sensory experience is extreme. Obviously, this allows the receptor to have an extreme range of response, from very weak to very intense.

Adaptation of Receptors

A special characteristic of all sensory receptors is that they *adapt* either partially or completely to their stimuli after a period of time. That is, when a continuous sensory stimulus is applied, the receptors respond at a very high impulse rate at first, then at a progressively lower rate until finally many of them no longer respond at all.

Figure 32-5 illustrates typical adaptation of certain types of receptors. Note that the pacinian corpuscle adapts extremely rapidly and hair receptors adapt within a second or so, whereas joint capsule and muscle spindle receptors adapt very slowly.

Mechanisms by Which Receptors Adapt. Adaptation of receptors is an individual property of each type of receptor in much the same way that development of a receptor potential is an individual property. For instance, in the eye, the rods and cones adapt by changing the concentrations of their light-sensitive chemicals (which is discussed in Chapter 34).

In the case of the mechanoreceptors, the receptor that has been studied for adaptation in greatest detail is again the pacinian corpuscle. Adaptation occurs in this receptor mainly in the following way: The pacinian corpuscle is a viscoelastic structure so that when a distorting force is suddenly applied to one side of the corpuscle, this force is instantly transmitted by the viscous component of the corpuscle directly to the same side of the central core, thus eliciting the receptor potential. However, within a few hundredths of a second the fluid within the corpuscle redistributes, so that the pressure becomes essentially equal all through the corpuscle; this now applies an even pressure on all sides of the central core fiber, so that the receptor potential is no longer elicited. Thus, the receptor potential appears at the onset of compression but then disappears within a small fraction of a second even though the compression continues.

Function of the Rapidly Adapting Receptors in Detecting Change in Stimulus Strength—The "Rate Receptors" or "Movement Receptors." Obviously, receptors that adapt rapidly cannot be used to transmit a continuous signal because these receptors are stimulated only when the stimulus strength changes. Yet they react strongly *while a change is actually taking place.* Furthermore, the number of impulses transmitted is directly related to the *rate at which the change takes place.* Therefore, these receptors are called *rate* receptors or *movement* receptors. Thus, in the case of the pacinian corpuscle, sudden pressure applied to the skin excites this receptor for a few milliseconds, and then its excitation is over even though the pressure continues. But later it transmits a signal again when the pressure is released. In other words, the pacinian corpuscle is exceedingly important for transmitting information about rapid changes in pressure against the body, but it is useless for transmitting information about constant pressure applied to the body.

Importance of the Rate Receptors—Their Predictive Function. If one knows the rate at which some change in bodily status is taking place, one can predict the state of the body a few seconds or even a few minutes later. For instance, the receptors of the semicircular canals in the vestibular apparatus of the ear detect the rate at which the head begins to

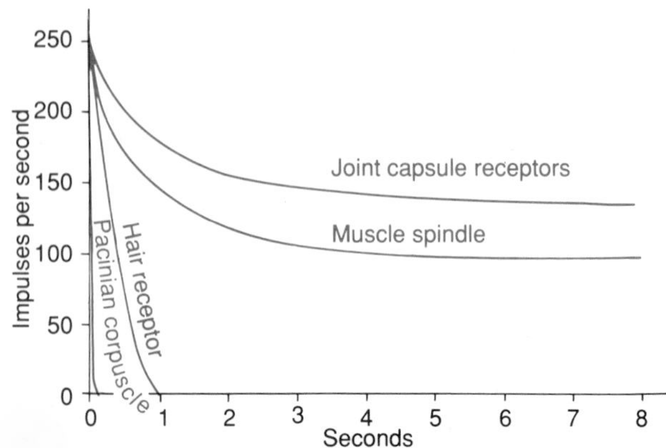

Figure 32-5. Adaptation of different types of receptors, showing rapid adaptation of some receptors and slow adaptation of others.

turn when one runs around a curve. Using this information, a person can predict how much he or she will turn within the next 2 seconds and can adjust the motion of the limbs *ahead of time* to keep from losing balance.

THE NERVE FIBERS THAT TRANSMIT SIGNALS AND THEIR PHYSIOLOGICAL CLASSIFICATION

Some signals need to be transmitted to the central nervous system extremely rapidly; otherwise the information would be useless. An example of this is the sensory signals that apprise the brain of the momentary positions of the limbs at each fraction of a second during running. Another example is the motor signals sent back to the muscles from the brain. At the other extreme, some types of sensory information, such as that depicting prolonged, aching pain, do not need to be transmitted rapidly at all, so that very slowly conducting fibers will suffice. Fortunately, nerve fibers come in all sizes between 0.2 and 20 micrometers in diameter—the larger the diameter, the greater the conducting velocity. The range of conducting velocities is between 0.5 and 120 m/sec.

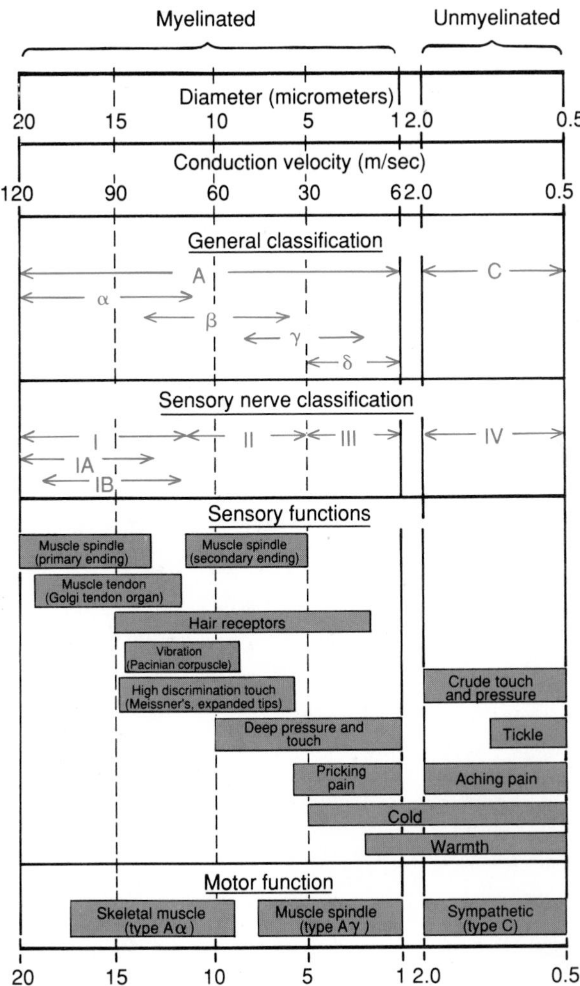

Figure 32-6. Physiological classifications and functions of nerve fibers.

Figure 32-6 gives two different classifications of nerve fibers that are in general use. One of these is a general classification that includes both sensory and motor fibers, including the autonomic nerve fibers as well. The other is a classification of sensory nerve fibers that is used primarily by sensory neurophysiologists.

In the general classification, the fibers are divided into types A and C, and the type A fibers are further subdivided into α, β, γ, and δ fibers.

Type A fibers are the typical myelinated fibers of spinal nerves. Type C fibers are the very small, unmyelinated nerve fibers that conduct impulses at low velocities. These constitute more than half the sensory fibers in most peripheral nerves and also all of the postganglionic autonomic fibers.

The sizes, velocities of conduction, and functions of the different nerve fiber types are given in the figure. Note that a few very large fibers can transmit impulses at velocities as great as 120 m/sec, a distance in 1 second that is longer than a football field. On the other hand, the smallest fibers transmit impulses as slowly as 0.5 m/sec, requiring about 2 seconds to go from the big toe to the spinal cord.

TRANSMISSION OF SIGNALS OF DIFFERENT INTENSITY IN NERVE TRACTS—SPATIAL AND TEMPORAL SUMMATION

One of the characteristics of each signal that always must be conveyed is its intensity, for instance, the intensity of pain. The different gradations of intensity can be transmitted either by utilizing increasing numbers of parallel fibers or by sending more impulses along a single fiber. These two mechanisms are called, respectively, spatial summation and temporal summation.

Figure 32-7 illustrates the phenomenon of *spatial summation,* whereby increasing signal strength is transmitted by using progressively greater numbers of fibers. This figure shows a section of skin innervated by a large number of parallel pain nerve fibers. Each of these arborizes into hundreds of minute *free nerve endings* that serve as pain receptors. The entire cluster of fibers from one pain fiber frequently covers an area of skin as large as 5 centimeters in diameter, and this area is called the *receptor field* of that fiber. The number of endings is large in the center of the field but diminishes toward the periphery. One can also see from the figure that the arborizing nerve fibrils overlap those from other pain fibers. Therefore, a pinprick of the skin usually stimulates endings from many different pain fibers simultaneously. When the pinprick is in the center of the receptive field of a particular pain fiber, however, the degree of stimulation of that fiber is far greater than when it is in the periphery of

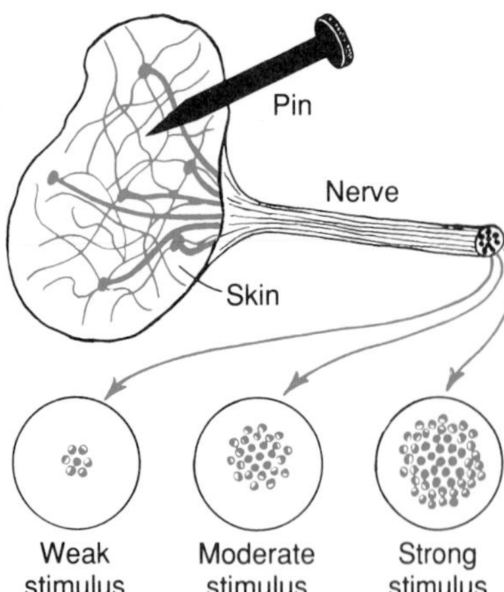

Figure 32–7. Pattern of stimulation of pain fibers in a nerve trunk leading from an area of skin pricked by a pin. This is an example of *spatial summation.*

the field. Thus, in the lower part of Figure 32–7 are shown three separate views of the cross-section of the nerve bundle leading from the skin area. To the left is shown the effect of a weak stimulus, and the other two views show the effect, respectively, of a moderate stimulus and a strong stimulus, with progressively more fibers being stimulated. This is the phenomenon of spatial summation.

A second obvious means for transmitting signals of increasing strength is by increasing the *frequency* of nerve impulses in each fiber, which is called *temporal summation.*

TRANSMISSION AND PROCESSING OF SIGNALS IN NEURONAL POOLS

The central nervous system is made up of literally thousands of separate neuronal pools, some of which contain very few neurons while others hold vast numbers. For instance, the entire cerebral cortex could be considered to be a single large neuronal pool, or it could be considered to be a collection of smaller pools with each observing separate functions. Other neuronal pools include the different basal ganglia, the specific nuclei in the thalamus, and in the cerebellum, mesencephalon, pons, and medulla.

Each pool has its own special characteristics of organization that cause it to process signals in its own special way, thus allowing these special characteristics to achieve the multitude of functions of the nervous system.

Relaying of Signals Through Neuronal Pools

Organization of Neurons for Relaying Signals. Figure 32–8 is a diagram of several neurons in a neuronal pool, showing "input" fibers to the left and "output" fibers to the right. Each input fiber divides hundreds to thousands of times, providing an average of a thousand or more terminal fibrils that spread over a large area in the pool to synapse with the dendrites or cell bodies of the neurons in the pool. The dendrites usually also arborize and spread for hundreds to thousands of micrometers in the pool. Note that large numbers of the terminals from each input fiber lie on the centermost neuron in its area, but progressively fewer terminals lie on the neurons farther from the center.

From the discussion of synaptic function in the previous chapter, it will be recalled that discharge of a single excitatory presynaptic terminal almost never stimulates the postsynaptic neuron. Instead, large numbers of terminals must discharge on the same neuron either simultaneously or in rapid succession to cause excitation. For instance, in Figure 32–8, let us assume that six separate terminals must discharge simultaneously to excite any one of the neurons. If the student will count the number of terminals on each one of the neurons from each input fiber, he or she will see that input *fiber 1* has more than enough terminals to cause *neuron a* to discharge. Therefore, the stimulus from input fiber 1 to this neuron is said to be an *excitatory stimulus.*

Input fiber 1 also contributes terminals to neurons b and c, but not enough to cause excitation. Nevertheless, discharge of these terminals makes both these neurons more excitable to signals arriving through other incoming nerve fibers. Therefore, the neurons are said to be *facilitated.*

It must be recognized that Figure 32–8 represents a highly condensed version of a neuronal pool, for each input nerve fiber usually provides terminals to hundreds or thousands of separate neurons in its distribution "field."

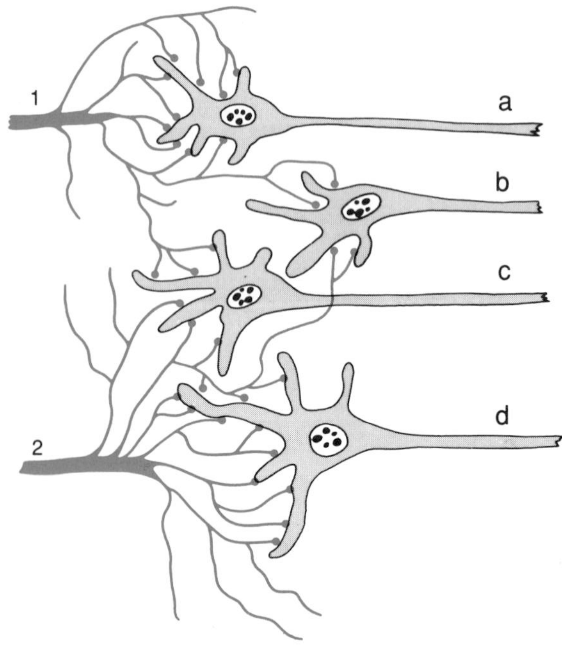

Figure 32–8. Basic organization of a neuronal pool.

Inhibition of a Neuronal Pool. We must also remember that some incoming fibers inhibit neurons, rather than exciting them. This is exactly the opposite of facilitation, and the entire field of the inhibitory branches is called the *inhibitory zone.* The degree of inhibition in the center of this zone obviously is very great because of large numbers of endings in the center; it becomes progressively less toward its edges.

Divergence of Signals Passing Through Neuronal Pools

Often it is important for signals entering a neuronal pool to excite far greater numbers of nerve fibers leaving the pool. This phenomenon is called *divergence.* Two major types of divergence are illustrated in Figure 32–9.

An *amplifying* type of divergence is illustrated in Figure 32–9A. This means simply that an input signal spreads to an increasing number of neurons as it passes through successive orders of neurons in its path. This type of divergence is characteristic of the corticospinal pathway in its control of skeletal muscles, with a single large pyramidal cell in the motor cortex capable, under appropriate conditions, of exciting as many as 10,000 muscle fibers.

The second type of divergence, illustrated in Figure 32–9B, is *divergence into multiple tracts.* In this case, the signal is transmitted in two separate directions from the pool. For instance, in the thalamus almost all sensory information is relayed both into deep structures of the thalamus and to discrete regions of the cerebral cortex.

Convergence of Signals

"Convergence" means signals from multiple inputs converging to excite a single neuron. Figure 32–10A shows *convergence from a single source,* and Figure 32–10B shows *convergence* (excitatory or inhibitory) *from multiple sources.*

Such convergence allows summation of information from different sources, and the resulting response is a summated effect of all the different types of information. Obviously, therefore, convergence is one of the important means by which the central nervous system correlates, summates, and sorts different types of information.

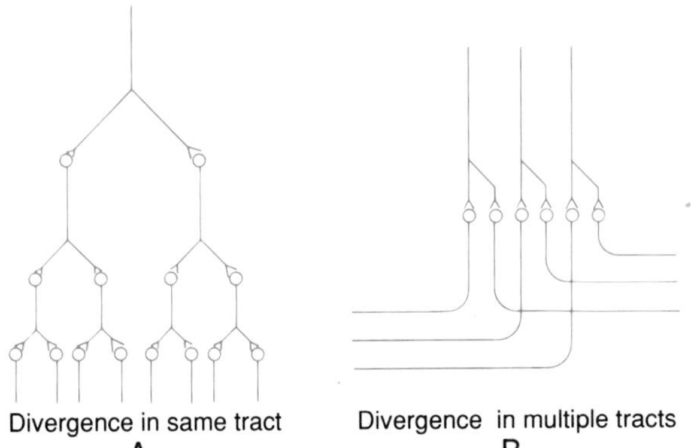

Figure 32–9. "Divergence" in neuronal pathways. *A,* Divergence within a pathway to cause "amplification" of the signal. *B,* Divergence into multiple tracts to transmit the signal to separate areas.

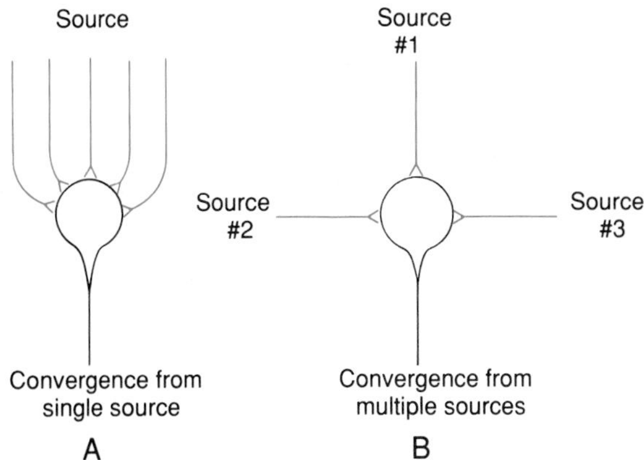

Figure 32–10. "Convergence" of multiple input fibers on a single neuron. *A,* Input fibers from a single source. *B,* Input fibers from multiple sources.

Neuronal Circuit Causing Both Excitatory and Inhibitory Output Signals

Sometimes an incoming signal to a neuronal pool causes an output excitatory signal going in one direction and at the same time an inhibitory signal going elsewhere. For instance, at the same time that an excitatory signal is transmitted by one set of neurons in the spinal cord to cause forward movement of a leg, an inhibitory signal is transmitted simultaneously through a separate set of neurons to inhibit the muscles on the back of the leg so that they will not oppose the forward movement. This type of circuit is characteristic of control of all antagonistic pairs of muscles, and it is called the *reciprocal inhibition circuit.*

Figure 32–11 illustrates the means by which the inhibition is achieved. The input fiber directly excites the excitatory output pathway, but it stimulates an intermediate *inhibitory neuron* (neuron 2) which then inhibits the second output pathway from the pool.

Prolongation of a Signal By a Neuronal Pool—"Afterdischarge"

Thus far, we have considered signals that are merely relayed through neuronal pools. However, in many instances, a signal entering a pool causes a prolonged output discharge, called *afterdischarge,* even

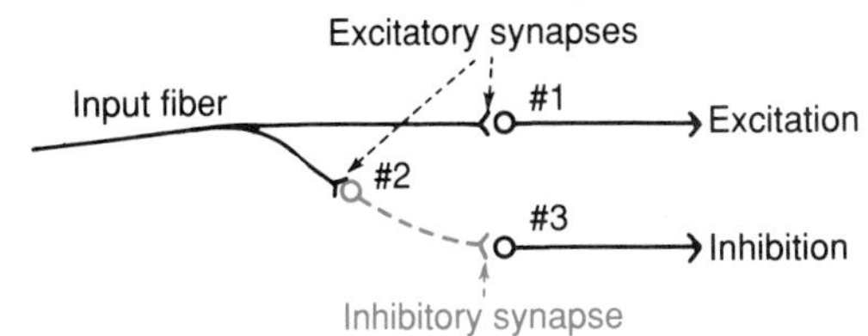

Figure 32–11. Inhibitory circuit. Neuron 2 is an inhibitory neuron.

after the incoming signal is over, and lasting from a few milliseconds to as long as many minutes. The two most important mechanisms by which afterdischarge occurs are the following:

Synaptic Afterdischarge. When excitatory synapses discharge on the surfaces of dendrites or the soma of a neuron, a postsynaptic potential develops in the neuron that lasts for many milliseconds, especially so when some of the long-acting synaptic transmitter substances are involved. As long as this potential lasts, it can continue to excite the neuron, causing it to transmit a continuous train of output impulses. Thus, as a result of this synaptic "afterdischarge" mechanism alone, it is possible for a single instantaneous input to cause a sustained signal output (a series of repetitive discharges) lasting for many milliseconds.

The Reverberatory (Oscillatory) Circuit as a Cause of Signal Prolongation. One of the most important of all circuits in the entire nervous system is the *reverberatory,* or *oscillatory, circuit.* Such circuits are caused by positive feedback within the neuronal network. That is, the output of a neuronal circuit feeds back to re-excite the input of the same circuit. Consequently, once stimulated, the circuit discharges repetitively for a long time.

Several different possible varieties of reverberatory circuits are illustrated in Figure 32-12, the simplest, in Figure 32-12A, involving only a single neuron. In this case, the output neuron simply sends a collateral nerve fiber back to its own dendrites or soma to restimulate itself; therefore, once the neuron discharged, the feedback stimuli could help keep the neuron discharging for a time thereafter.

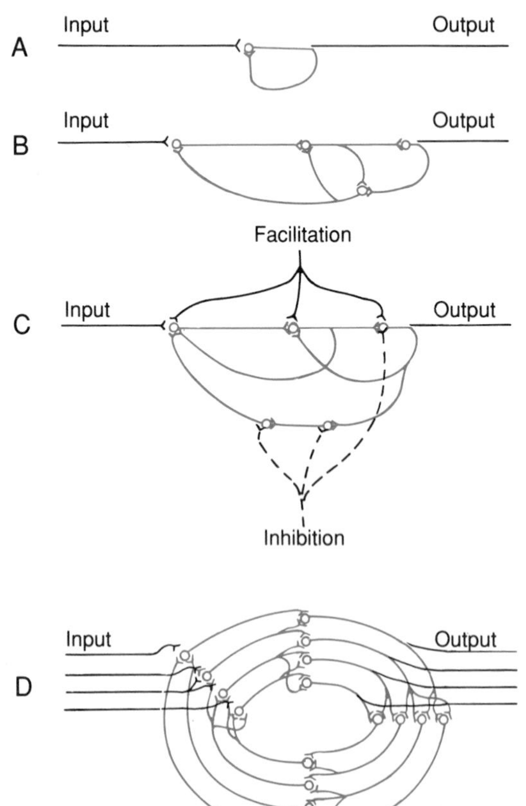

Figure 32-12. Reverberatory circuits of increasing complexity.

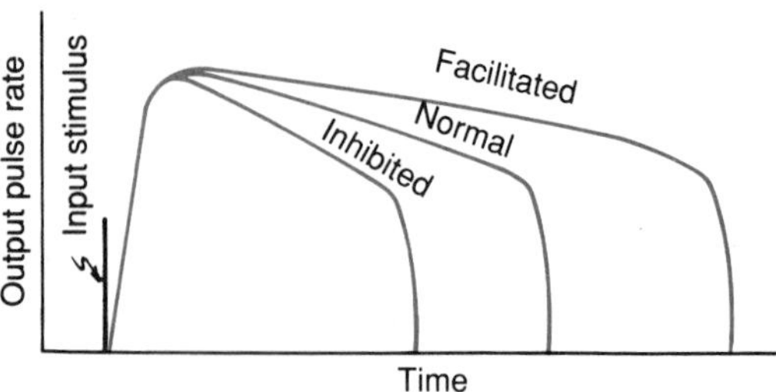

Figure 32-13. Typical pattern of the output signal from a reverberatory circuit following a single input stimulus, showing the effects of facilitation and inhibition.

Figure 32-12B illustrates a few additional neurons in the feedback circuit, which would give a longer period of time between the initial discharge and the feedback signal. Figure 32-12C illustrates a still more complex system in which both facilitatory and inhibitory fibers impinge on the reverberating circuit. A facilitatory signal enhances the intensity and frequency of reverberation, whereas an inhibitory signal depresses or stops the reverberation.

Figure 32-12D illustrates that most reverberating pathways are constituted of many parallel fibers, and at each cell station the terminal fibrils diffuse widely. In such a system the total reverberating signal can be either weak or strong, depending on how many parallel nerve fibers are momentarily involved in the reverberation.

Characteristics of Signal Prolongation From a Reverberatory Circuit. Figure 32-13 illustrates output signals from a typical reverberatory circuit. The input stimulus need last only 1 millisecond or so, and yet the output can last for many milliseconds or even minutes. The figure demonstrates that the intensity of the output signal usually increases to a high value early in the reverberation, then decreases to a critical point, at which it suddenly ceases entirely. The cause of this sudden cessation of reverberation is fatigue of one or more of the synaptic junctions in the circuit, for fatigue beyond a certain critical level lowers the stimulation of the next neuron in the circuit below threshold level so that the circuit is suddenly broken. Obviously, the duration of the signal before cessation can also be controlled by signals from other parts of the brain that inhibit or facilitate the circuit.

Continuous Signal Output From Neuronal Circuits

Some neuronal circuits emit output signals continuously even without excitatory input signals. At least two different mechanisms can cause this effect: (1) intrinsic neuronal discharge and (2) continuous reverberatory signals.

Figure 32-14 illustrates a continual output signal from a pool of neurons, whether a pool emitting impulses because of intrinsic neuronal excitability or as a result of reverberation. Note that an excitatory (or facilitatory) input signal to the pool greatly increases

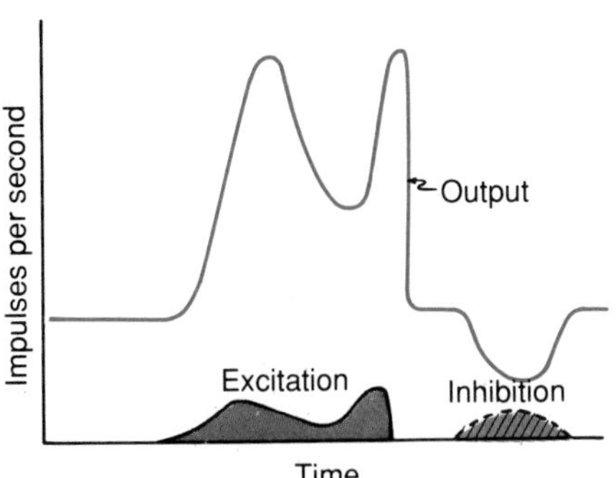

Figure 32-14. Continuous output from either a reverberating circuit or a pool of intrinsically discharging neurons. This figure also shows the effect of excitatory or inhibitory input signals.

the output signal, whereas an inhibitory input signal greatly decreases the output. Those students who are familiar with radio transmitters will recognize this to be a *carrier wave* type of information transmission. That is, the excitatory and inhibitory control signals are not the *cause* of the output signal, but they do *control* it. Note that this carrier wave system allows decrease in signal intensity as well as increase, whereas, up to this point, the types of information transmission that we have discussed have been only positive information. This type of information transmission is used by the autonomic nervous system to control such functions as vascular tone, gut tone, degree of constriction of the iris, heart rate, and others.

Rhythmic Signal Output

Many neuronal circuits emit rhythmic output signals—for instance, the rhythmic respiratory signal originating in the reticular substance of the medulla and pons. This repetitive rhythmic signal continues throughout life, whereas other rhythmic signals, such as those that cause scratching movements by the hind leg of a dog or the walking movements in an animal, require input stimuli into the respective circuits to initiate the signals.

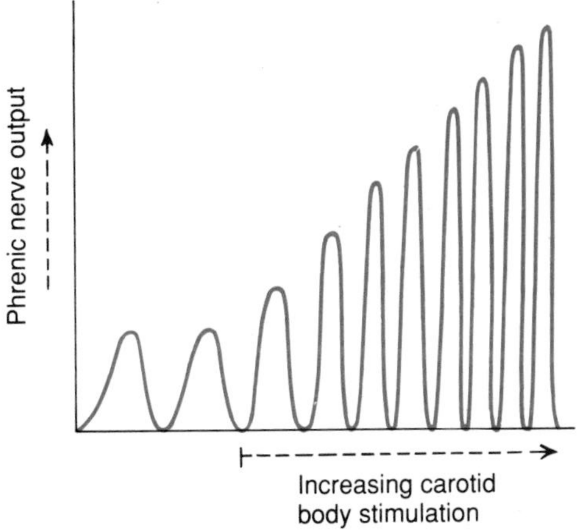

Figure 32-15. The rhythmical output from the respiratory center, showing that progressively increasing stimulation of the carotid body increases both the intensity and frequency of oscillation.

Either all or almost all rhythmic signals that have been studied experimentally have been found to result from reverberating circuits or successive reverberating circuits that feed excitatory or inhibitory signals from one to the next.

Obviously, facilitatory or inhibitory signals can affect rhythmic signal output in the same way that they can affect continuous signal outputs. Figure 32-15, for instance, illustrates the rhythmic respiratory signal in the phrenic nerve. However, when the carotid body is stimulated by arterial oxygen deficiency, the frequency and amplitude of the rhythmic signal pattern increase progressively.

DETECTION AND TRANSMISSION OF TACTILE SENSATIONS

The Tactile Receptors. At least six entirely different types of tactile receptors are known. Some of these receptors were illustrated in Figure 32-1, and their special characteristics are the following:

First, some *free nerve endings,* which are found everywhere in the skin and in many other tissues, can detect touch and pressure. For instance, even light contact with the cornea of the eye, which contains no other type of nerve ending besides free nerve endings, can nevertheless elicit touch and pressure sensations.

Second, a touch receptor of special sensitivity is *Meissner's corpuscle,* an elongated encapsulated nerve ending that excites a large (type Aβ) myelinated sensory nerve fiber. Inside the capsulation are many whorls of terminal nerve filaments. These receptors are present in the nonhairy parts of the skin (called *glabrous skin*) and are particularly abundant in the fingertips, lips, and other areas of the skin where one's ability to discern spatial characteristics of touch sensations is highly developed. Meissner's corpuscles adapt in a fraction of a second after they are stimulated, which means that they are particularly sensitive to movement of very light objects over the surface of the skin and also to low frequency vibration.

Third, the fingertips and some other areas also contain large numbers of *expanded tip tactile receptors,* one type of which is *Merkel's discs,* illustrated in Figure 36-16. These receptors differ from Meissner's corpuscles in that they transmit an initially strong but partially adapting signal and then a continuing weaker signal that adapts only slowly. Therefore, they are responsible for giving steady state signals that allow one to determine continuous touch of objects against the skin. Merkel's discs are often grouped together in a single receptor organ called the *Iggo dome receptor,* as illustrated in Figure 32-16. The epithelium at this point protrudes outward, thus creating a dome and constituting an extremely sensitive receptor. Also note that the entire group of Merkel's discs is innervated by a single large type of myelinated nerve fiber (type Aβ). These receptors, along with Meissner's corpuscles, play extremely important roles in localizing touch sensations to the specific sur-

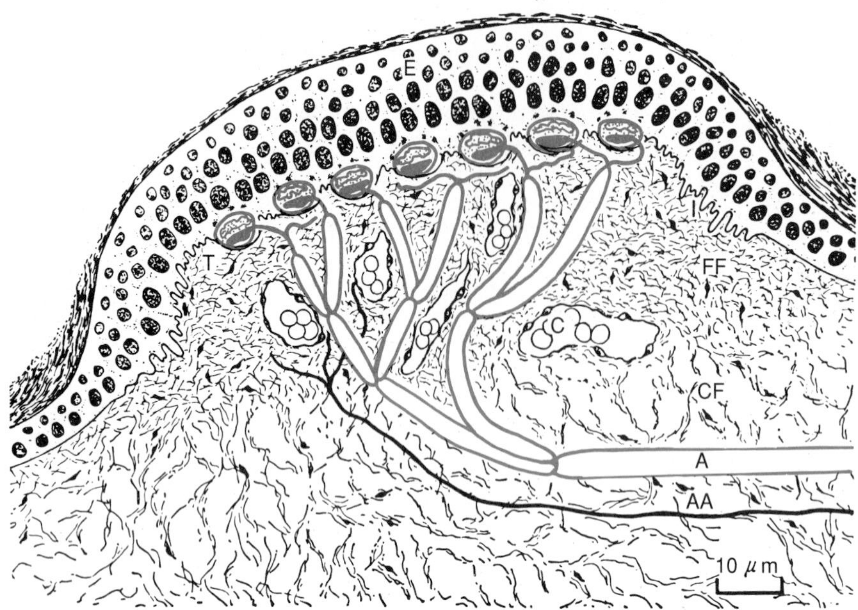

Figure 32-16. The Iggo dome receptor. Note the multiple numbers of Merkel's discs innervated by a single large myelinated fiber and abutting tightly the undersurface of the epithelium. (From Iggo and Muir: J. Physiol., 200:763, 1969.)

face areas of the body and also in determining the texture of what is felt.

Fourth, slight movement of any hair on the body stimulates the nerve fiber entwining its base. Thus, each hair and its basal nerve fiber, called the *hair end-organ,* is also a touch receptor. This receptor adapts readily and, therefore, like Meissner's corpuscles, detects mainly movement of objects on the surface of the body or initial contact with the body.

Fifth, located in the deeper layers of the skin and also in deeper tissues are many *Ruffini's end-organs,* which are multibranched, encapsulated endings, as illustrated in Figure 32-1. These endings adapt very little and, therefore, are important for signaling continuous states of deformation of the skin and deeper tissues, such as heavy and continuous touch signals and pressure signals. They are also found in joint capsules and help signal the degree of joint rotation.

Sixth, *pacinian corpuscles,* which were discussed earlier in the chapter, lie both immediately beneath the skin and also deep in the fascial tissues of the body. These are stimulated only by very rapid movement of the tissues because they adapt in a few hundredths of a second. Therefore, they are particularly important for detecting tissue vibration or other extremely rapid changes in the mechanical state of the tissues.

Transmission of Tactile Sensations in Peripheral Nerve Fibers. Almost all the specialized sensory receptors, such as Meissner's corpuscles, Iggo dome receptors, hair receptors, pacinian corpuscles, and Ruffini's endings, transmit their signals in type Aβ nerve fibers that have transmission velocities of 30 to 70 m/sec. On the other hand, free nerve ending tactile receptors transmit signals mainly via the small type Aδ myelinated fibers that conduct at velocities of 5 to 30 m/sec. Some tactile free nerve endings transmit via type C unmyelinated fibers at velocities of from a fraction of a meter up to 2 m/sec; these send signals into the spinal cord and lower brain stem, probably subserving mainly the sensation of tickle. Thus, the more critical types of sensory signals—those that help determine precise localization on the skin, minute gradations of intensity, or rapid changes in sensory signal intensity—are all transmitted in more rapidly conducting types of sensory nerve fibers. On the other hand, the cruder types of signals, such as crude pressure, poorly localized touch, and especially tickle, are transmitted via much slower nerve fibers that require much less space in the nerve bundle than the faster fibers.

Detection of Vibration

All the different tactile receptors are involved in detection of vibration, though different receptors detect different frequencies of vibration. Pacinian corpuscles can signal vibrations of from 30 to 800 cycles per second, because they respond extremely rapidly to minute and rapid deformations of the tissues, and they also transmit their signals over type Aβ nerve fibers, which can transmit more than 1000 impulses per second.

Low frequency vibrations of up to 80 cycles per second, on the other hand, stimulate other tactile receptors—especially Meissner's corpuscles, which are less rapidly adapting than pacinian corpuscles.

THE TWO SENSORY PATHWAYS FOR TRANSMISSION OF SOMATIC SIGNALS INTO THE CENTRAL NERVOUS SYSTEM

Almost all sensory information from the somatic segments of the body enters the spinal cord through the dorsal roots of the spinal nerves. However, from the entry point of the cord and then to the brain the sensory signals are carried through one of two alternate sensory pathways: (1) the *dorsal column–lemniscal system* and (2) the *anterolateral system.* These two systems again come together partially at the level of the thalamus.

The dorsal column–lemniscal system, as its name implies, carries signals mainly in the *dorsal columns* of the cord and then, after crossing to the opposite side in the medulla, upward through the brain stem to the thalamus by way of the *medial lemniscus.* On the other hand, signals of the anterolateral system, after originating in the dorsal horns of the spinal gray matter, cross to the opposite side of the cord and ascend through the anterior and lateral white columns to terminate at all levels of the brain stem and also in the thalamus.

The dorsal column–lemniscal system is composed of large, myelinated nerve fibers that transmit signals to the brain at velocities of 30 to 110 m/sec, whereas the anterolateral system is composed of much smaller myelinated fibers (averaging 4 micrometers in diameter) that transmit signals at velocities ranging from a few meters per second up to 40 m/sec.

Another difference between the two systems is that the dorsal column–lemniscal system has a very high degree of spatial orientation of the nerve fibers with respect to their origin on the surface of the body, whereas the anterolateral system has a much smaller degree of spatial orientation.

Thus, sensory information that must be transmitted rapidly and with temporal and spatial fidelity is transmitted in the dorsal column–lemniscal system, whereas that which does not need to be transmitted rapidly nor with great spatial fidelity is transmitted mainly in the anterolateral system. On the other hand, the anterolateral system has a special capability that the dorsal system does not have: the ability to transmit a broad spectrum of sensory modalities—pain, warmth, cold, and crude tactile sensations; the dorsal system is limited to the more discrete types of mechanoreceptive sensations alone.

With this differentiation in mind we can now list the types of sensations transmitted in the two systems:

The Dorsal Column–Lemniscal System

1. Touch sensations requiring a high degree of localization of the stimulus.
2. Touch sensations requiring transmission of fine gradations of intensity.
3. Phasic sensations, such as vibratory sensations.
4. Sensations that signal movement against the skin.
5. Position sensations.
6. Pressure sensations having to do with fine degrees of judgment of pressure intensity.

The Anterolateral System

1. Pain.
2. Thermal sensations, including both warm and cold sensations.
3. Crude touch and pressure sensations capable of only crude localizing ability on the surface of the body.
4. Tickle and itch sensations.
5. Sexual sensations.

TRANSMISSION IN THE DORSAL COLUMN–LEMNISCAL SYSTEM

Anatomy of the Dorsal Column–Lemniscal System

On entering the spinal cord from the spinal nerve dorsal roots, the large myelinated fibers from specialized mechanoreceptors pass immediately into the lateral margin of the dorsal white column. However, each fiber then divides to form a *medial branch* and a *lateral branch,* as illustrated by the medial fiber from the dorsal root in Figure 32–17. The medial branch turns upward in the dorsal column and proceeds by way of the dorsal column pathway to the brain.

The lateral branch enters the dorsal horn of the cord gray matter and then divides many times, synapsing with neurons in almost all parts of the intermediate and anterior portions of the cord gray matter. Many of these neurons elicit local spinal cord reflexes, which will be discussed in Chapter 37. Others give rise to the spinocerebellar tracts, which we will discuss in Chapter 38 in relation to the function of the cerebellum.

The Dorsal Column–Medial Lemniscal Pathway. Note in Figure 32–18 that the nerve fibers entering the dorsal columns pass uninterrupted up to the medulla, where they synapse in the *dorsal column nuclei* (the *cuneate* and *gracile nuclei*). From here, *second-order neurons* cross immediately to the opposite side and then continue upward to the thalamus through bilateral pathways called the *medial lemnisci.*

In the thalamus, the medial lemniscal fibers from the dorsal columns terminate in the *ventrobasal complex.* From here, *third-order nerve fibers* project, as

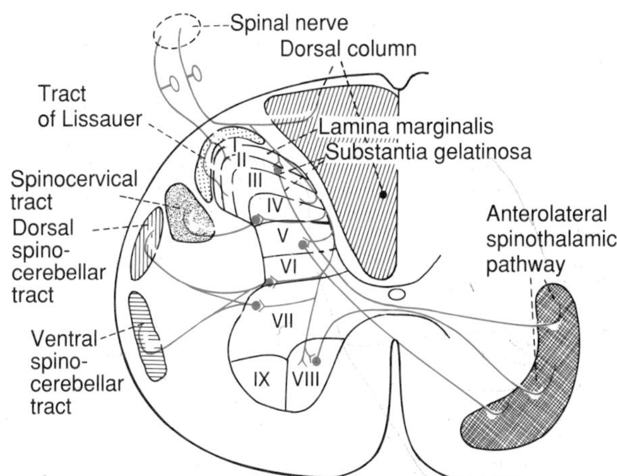

Figure 32–17. Cross-section of the spinal cord, showing the anatomical laminae I through IX of the cord gray matter and the ascending sensory tracts in the white columns of the spinal cord.

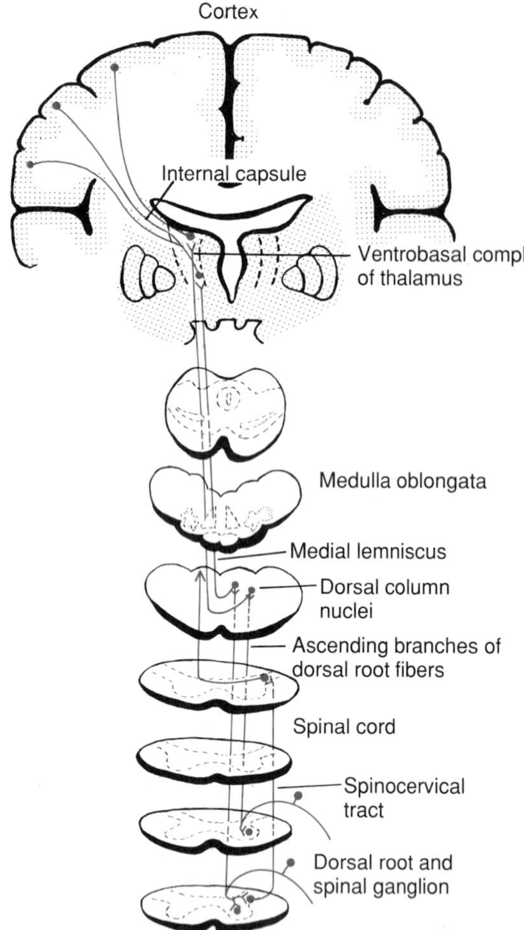

Figure 32-18. The dorsal column and spinocervical pathways for transmitting critical types of tactile signals. (Modified from Ranson, S. W. and Clark, S. L.: Anatomy of the Nervous System. Philadelphia, W. B. Saunders Company, 1959.)

shown in Figure 32-19, mainly to the *postcentral gyrus* of the *cerebral cortex,* which is called *somatic sensory area I.* In addition, a few fibers project to the lowermost lateral portion of each parietal lobe, an area called *somatic sensory area II.*

Spatial Orientation of the Nerve Fibers in the Dorsal Column-Lemniscal System

One of the distinguishing features of the dorsal column-lemniscal system is a distinct spatial orientation of nerve fibers from the individual parts of the body that is maintained throughout. For instance, in the dorsal columns, the fibers from the lower parts of the body lie toward the center, while those that enter the spinal cord at progressively higher segmental levels form successive layers laterally.

In the thalamus, the distinct spatial orientation is still maintained, with the tail end of the body represented by the most lateral portions of the ventrobasal complex and the head and face represented in the medial component of the complex. However, because of the crossing of the medial lemnisci in the medulla, the left side of the body is represented in the right side of the thalamus, and the right side of the body is represented in the left side of the thalamus.

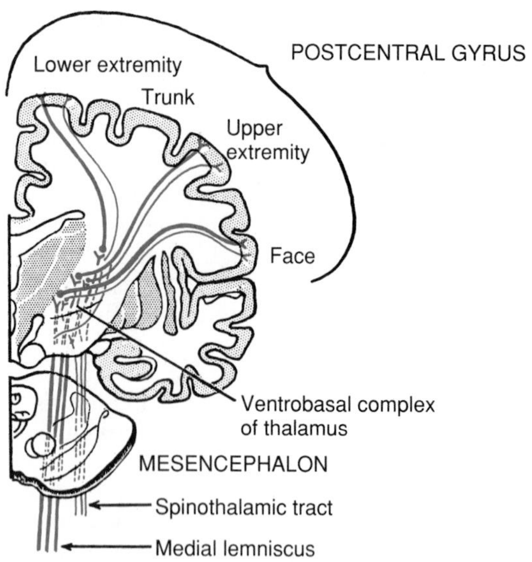

Figure 32-19. Projection of the dorsal column-lemniscal system from the thalamus to the somatic sensory cortex. (Modified from Brodal: Neurological Anatomy in Relation to Clinical Medicine. New York, Oxford University Press, 1969.)

The Somatic Sensory Cortex

Figure 32-20 illustrates the cerebrum of the human brain, but with the temporal lobe pulled downward. On the top of the brain, about midway between the front and the back, is a deep fissure called the *central fissure* that extends horizontally across the brain. In general, sensory signals from all modalities of sensation terminate in the cerebral cortex posterior to the central fissure. Most importantly, the *somatic sensory cortex* lies immediately behind the central fissure, as shown in the figure. This is the area of the cortex called the *parietal lobe.* In addition, visual signals terminate in the occipital lobe, and auditory signals in the temporal lobe.

The portion of the cortex anterior to the central

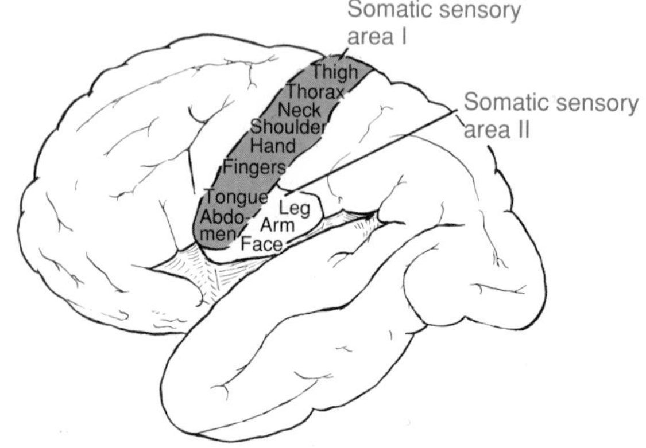

Figure 32-20. The two somatic sensory cortical areas, somatic sensory areas I and II.

fissure is devoted to motor control of the body and to some aspects of analytical thought.

Two distinct and separate areas are known to receive direct afferent nerve fibers from the somesthetic relay nuclei in the ventrobasal complex of the thalamus; these, called *somatic sensory area I* and *somatic sensory area II*, are illustrated in Figure 32–20. However, somatic sensory area I is so much more important to the sensory functions of the body than is somatic sensory area II that in popular usage the term "somatic sensory cortex" most often is used to mean area I.

Projection of the Body in Somatic Sensory Area I. Somatic sensory area I lies in the *postcentral gyrus* of the human cerebral cortex (the gyrus immediately behind the central fissure). A distinct spatial orientation exists in this area for reception of nerve signals from the different areas of the body. Figure 32–21 illustrates a cross-section through the brain at the level of the postcentral gyrus, showing the representations of the different parts of the body in separate regions of somatic sensory area I. Note, however, that each side of the cortex receives sensory information almost exclusively from the opposite side of the body.

Some areas of the body are represented by large areas in the somatic cortex—the lips the greatest of all, followed by the face and thumb—whereas the entire trunk and lower part of the body are represented by relatively small areas. The sizes of these areas are directly proportional to the number of specialized sensory receptors in each respective peripheral area of the body. For instance, a great number of specialized nerve endings are found in the lips and thumb, whereas only a few are present in the skin of the trunk.

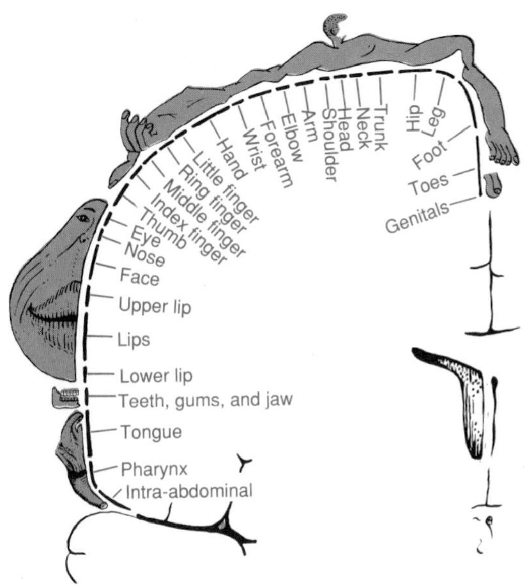

Figure 32–21. Representation of the different areas of the body in the somatic sensory area I of the cortex. (From Penfield and Rasmussen: Cerebral Cortex of Man: A Clinical Study of Localization of Function. New York, Macmillan Company, 1968.)

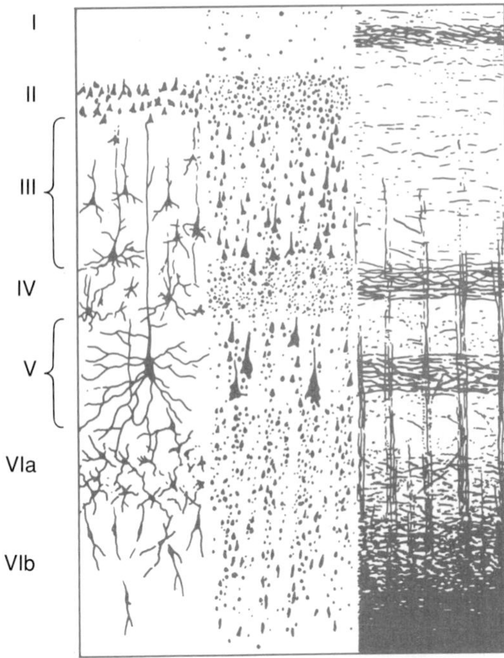

Figure 32–22. Structure of the cerebral cortex, illustrating *I*, molecular layer; *II*, external granular layer; *III*, layer of pyramidal cells; *IV*, internal granular layer; *V*, large pyramidal cell layer; and *VI*, layer of fusiform or polymorphic cells. (From Ranson, S. W., and Clark, S. L. [after Brodmann]: Anatomy of the Nervous System. Philadelphia, W. B. Saunders Company, 1959.)

Note also that the head is represented in the most lateral portion of somatic sensory area I, whereas the lower part of the body is represented medially.

The Layers of the Somatic Sensory Cortex and Their Function

The cerebral cortex contains *six* separate layers of neurons, beginning with layer I next to the surface and extending progressively deeper to layer VI, as illustrated in Figure 32–22. As would be expected, the neurons in each layer perform functions different from those in other layers. Some of these functions are as follows:

1. The incoming sensory signal excites mainly neuronal layer IV first; then the signal spreads both toward the surface of the cortex and also toward the deeper layers.
2. Layers I and II receive a diffuse, nonspecific input from lower brain centers that can facilitate a whole region of the cortex at once; this system will be described in Chapter 40. This input perhaps controls the overall level of excitability of the region stimulated.
3. The neurons in layers II and III send axons to other closely related portions of the cerebral cortex.
4. The neurons in layers V and VI send axons to more distant parts of the nervous system. Those in layer V are generally larger and project to more distant areas. For instance, many of these pass all the way into the brain stem and spinal

cord to provide control signals to these areas. From layer VI, especially large numbers of axons extend to the thalamus, providing feedback signals from the cerebral cortex to the thalamus.

Representation of the Different Sensory Modalities in the Somatic Sensory Cortex — The Vertical Columns of Neurons

Functionally, the neurons of the somatic sensory cortex are arranged in vertical columns extending all the way through the six layers of the cortex, each column having a diameter of 0.3 to 0.5 millimeter and containing perhaps 10,000 neuronal cell bodies. Each of these columns serves a single specific sensory modality, some columns responding to stretch receptors around joints, some to stimulation of tactile hairs, others to discrete localized pressure points on the skin, and so forth. Furthermore, the columns for the different modalities are interspersed among each other. At layer IV, where the signals first enter the cord, the columns of neurons function almost entirely separately from each other. However, at other levels of the columns interactions occur that allow beginning analysis of the meanings of the sensory signals.

In the most anterior portion of the postcentral gyrus, located deep in the central fissure, a disproportionately large share of the vertical columns respond to muscle, tendon, or joint stretch receptors. Many of the signals from these in turn spread directly to the motor cortex located immediately anterior to the central fissure and help control muscle function. As one proceeds more posteriorly in somatic sensory cortex I, more and more of the vertical columns respond to the slowly adapting cutaneous receptors, and then still farther posteriorly greater numbers of the columns are sensitive to deep pressure.

Functions of Somatic Sensory Area I

The functional capabilities of different areas of the somatic sensory cortex have been determined by selective excision of the different portions. Widespread excision of somatic sensory area I causes loss of the following types of sensory judgment:

1. The person is unable to localize discretely the different sensations in the different parts of the body. However, he or she can localize these sensations very crudely, such as to a particular hand, which indicates that the thalamus or parts of the cerebral cortex not normally considered to be concerned with somatic sensations can perform some degree of localization.
2. The person is unable to judge critical degrees of pressure against his body.
3. The person is unable to judge exactly the weights of objects.
4. The person is unable to judge shapes or forms of objects. This is called *astereognosis.*
5. The person is unable to judge texture of materials, for this type of judgment depends on highly critical sensations caused by movement of the skin over the surface to be judged.

Note in the list that nothing has been said about loss of pain and temperature sense. However, in the absence of somatic sensory area I, the appreciation of these sensory modalities may be altered either in quality or in intensity. But more important, the pain and temperature sensations that do occur are poorly localized, indicating that both pain and temperature localization probably depend mainly upon simultaneous stimulation of tactile stimuli that uses the topographical map of the body in somatic sensory area I to localize the source.

Somatic Association Areas

Those areas of the cerebral cortex, located in the parietal cortex behind somatic sensory area I and above somatic sensory area II, play still higher order roles in deciphering the sensory information that enters the somatic sensory areas. Therefore, these areas are called the *somatic association areas.*

Electrical stimulation in the somatic association area can occasionally cause a person to experience a complex somatic sensation, sometimes even the "feeling" of an object such as a knife or a ball. Therefore, it seems clear that the somatic association area combines information from multiple points in the somatic sensory area to decipher its meaning. This also fits with the anatomical arrangement of the neuronal tracts that enter the somatic association area, for it receives signals from (1) somatic sensory area I, (2) the ventrobasal nuclei of the thalamus, (3) other areas of the thalamus, (4) the visual cortex, and (5) the auditory cortex.

Effect of Removing the Somatic Association Area — Amorphosynthesis. When the somatic association area is removed, the person loses the ability to recognize complex objects and complex forms by the process of feeling them. In addition, he or she loses most of the sense of form of his or her own body. Especially interesting, the person is mainly oblivious to the opposite side of the body — that is, forgets that it is there. Therefore, he or she also often forgets to use the other side for motor functions as well. Likewise, when feeling objects, the person will tend to feel only one side of the object and to forget that the other side even exists. This complex sensory deficit is called *amorphosynthesis.*

The Position Senses

The *position senses* can be divided into two subtypes: (1) *static position sense,* which means conscious orientation of the different parts of the body with respect to each other, and (2) *rate of movement sense,* also called *kinesthesia.*

The Position Sensory Receptors. Knowledge of position, both static and dynamic, depends upon knowing the degrees of angulation of all joints in all planes and their rates of change. Therefore, multiple different types of receptors help to determine joint angulation and are used together for position sense. Furthermore, both skin tactile receptors and deep receptors near the joints are also used. In the case of the fingers, where skin receptors are in great abundance, as much as half of position recognition is probably detected through the skin receptors. On the other hand, for most of the larger joints of the body, deep receptors are more important.

For determining joint angulation in midranges of motion, the most important receptors are believed to be the *muscle spindles.* These are also exceedingly important in helping control muscle movement, as we see in Chapter 37. When the angle of a joint is changing, some muscles are being stretched while others are loosened, and the stretch information from the spindles is passed into the computational system of the spinal cord and higher regions of the dorsal column system for deciphering the complex interrelations of joint angulations.

At the extremes of joint angulation, the stretch of the ligaments and deep tissues around the joints is an additional important factor in determining position. Some types of endings used for this are the pacinian corpuscles, Ruffini's endings, and receptors similar to the Golgi tendon receptors found in muscle tendons.

The pacinian corpuscles and muscle spindles are especially adapted for detecting rapid rates of change. Therefore, it is likely that these are the receptors most responsible for detecting rate of movement.

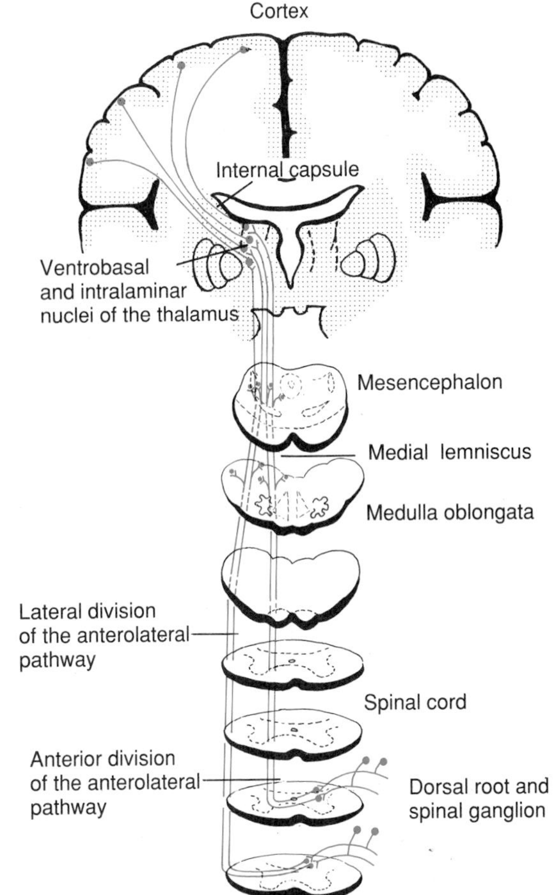

Figure 32-23. The anterior and lateral divisions of the anterolateral pathway.

TRANSMISSION IN THE ANTEROLATERAL SYSTEM

The anterolateral system, in contrast to the dorsal column system, transmits sensory signals that do not require highly discrete localization of the signal source and also that do not require discrimination of fine gradations of intensity. These include pain, heat, cold, crude tactile, tickle and itch, and sexual sensations. In the following chapter pain and temperature sensations are discussed; the present chapter is still concerned principally with transmission of the tactile sensations, but now with the less acute types.

Anatomy of the Anterolateral Pathway

The anterolateral fibers originate mainly in laminae I, IV, V, and VI (see Fig. 32-17) in the dorsal horns of the spinal cord, where many of the dorsal root sensory nerve fibers terminate after entering the cord. Then, as illustrated in Figure 32-23, the fibers cross in the anterior commissure of the cord to the opposite anterior and lateral white columns, where they turn upward toward the brain. These fibers ascend rather diffusely throughout the anterolateral columns. However, anatomical studies suggest a partial differentiation of this pathway into an anterior division, called the *anterior spinothalamic tract,* and a lateral division, called the *lateral spinothalamic tract.*

The upper terminus of the anterolateral pathway is mainly twofold: (1) throughout the *reticular nuclei of the brain stem* and (2) in two different nuclear complexes of the thalamus, the *ventrobasal complex* and the *intralaminar nuclei.* In general, the tactile signals are transmitted mainly into the ventrobasal complex, terminating in the same area as the dorsal column system, and this is probably also true for the temperature signals. From here, the tactile signals are transmitted to the somatosensory cortex along with the signals from the dorsal columns. On the other hand, only part of the pain signals project to this complex. Instead, most of these enter the reticular nuclei of the brain stem and via relay from the brain stem to the intralaminar nuclei of the thalamus, as is discussed in greater detail in the following chapter.

Characteristics of Transmission in the Anterolateral Pathway. In general, the same principles apply to transmission in the anterolateral pathway as in the dorsal column-lemniscal system except for the following differences: (1) the velocities of transmission are only one-third to one-half those in the dorsal column-lemniscal system, ranging between 8 and 40 m/sec; (2) the degree of spatial localization of signals is poor, especially in the pain pathways; (3) the gradations of intensities are also far less accurate, most of the sensations being recognized in 10 to 20 gradations of strength, rather than as many as 100 gradations for the dorsal column system; and (4) the ability to transmit rapidly repetitive signals is poor.

Thus, it is evident that the anterolateral system is a cruder type of transmission system than the dorsal column–lemniscal system. Even so, certain modalities of sensation are transmitted only in this system and not at all in the dorsal column–lemniscal system. These are pain, thermal, tickle and itch, and sexual sensations in addition to crude touch and pressure.

SOME SPECIAL ASPECTS OF SOMATIC SENSORY FUNCTION

Function of the Thalamus in Somatic Sensation

When the somatosensory cortex of a human being is destroyed, that person loses most critical tactile sensibilities, but a slight degree of crude tactile sensibility does return. Therefore, it must be assumed that the thalamus (as well as other lower centers) has a slight ability to discriminate tactile sensation even though the thalamus normally functions mainly to relay this type of information to the cortex.

On the other hand, loss of the somatosensory cortex has little effect on one's perception of pain sensation and only a moderate effect on the perception of temperature. Therefore, there is much reason to believe that the brain stem, the thalamus, and other associated basal regions of the brain play perhaps the dominant role in discrimination of these sensibilities. It is interesting that these sensibilities appeared very early in the phylogenetic development of animalhood, whereas the *critical* tactile sensibilities were a late development.

Cortical Control of Sensory Sensitivity— "Corticofugal" Signals

In addition to somatic sensory signals transmitted from the periphery to the brain, "corticofugal" signals are transmitted in the backward direction from the cerebral cortex to the lower sensory relay stations of the thalamus, medulla, and spinal cord; these control the sensitivity of the sensory input. The corticofugal signals are inhibitory, so that when the input intensity becomes too great, the corticofugal signals automatically decrease the transmission in the relay nuclei. Obviously, this does two things: First, it decreases lateral spread of the sensory signals into adjacent neurons and therefore increases the contrast of the signal pattern. Second, it keeps the sensory system operating in a range of sensitivity that is not so low that the signals are ineffectual nor so high that the system is swamped beyond its capacity to differentiate sensory patterns.

This principle of corticofugal sensory control is utilized by all of the different sensory systems, not only the somatic system.

REFERENCES

See references at end of Chapter 33.

QUESTIONS

1. What are the functions of the following types of sensory receptors: *free nerve endings, Merkel's disks, pacinian corpuscles, Meissner's corpuscles, Ruffini's end-organs,* and *muscle spindles?*
2. What causes receptor potentials in sensory receptors?
3. Which receptors adapt rapidly and which slowly? Why is it important to have some receptors adapt very rapidly?
4. Explain the principal mechanism by which pacinian corpuscles adapt.
5. Explain the differences between A and C types of nerve fibers.
6. Describe the mechanisms of *divergence* and *convergence* in neuronal pools.
7. What is the function of the *reciprocal inhibition* circuit?
8. What are the differences between *synaptic afterdischarge* and afterdischarge caused by a *reverberatory circuit?*
9. Explain the functions of several specific reverberatory neuronal circuits.
10. What is the mechanism of rhythmical signal outputs from neuronal pools?
11. Name the characteristics of the types of sensations that are transmitted in the *dorsal column–lemniscal system.*
12. Give the characteristics of the types of sensations that are transmitted in the *anterolateral system.*
13. Describe the anatomy for signal transmission in the dorsal column–lemniscal system.
14. What is the general difference between the sensations transmitted in the *dorsal columns* and those transmitted in the *anterolateral pathway?*
15. Describe the localization of somatic sensation within *somatic sensory area I.*
16. What are the functions of *somatic sensory area I?*
17. What is the function of the *somatic sensory association area?*
18. Explain how one determines the degrees of rotation of the joints.
19. Explain how the nervous system determines the rate of movement (called kinesthesia) at a joint.
20. Describe the anatomy of the anterolateral sensory pathway.
21. What are the roles of the thalamus in somatic sensation?
22. Explain the mechanisms for cortical control of sensory sensitivity.

33

Pain, Headache, and Thermal Sensations

Many, if not most, ailments of the body cause pain. Furthermore, the ability to diagnose different diseases depends to a great extent on a doctor's knowledge of the different qualities of pain. For these reasons, the present chapter is devoted mainly to pain and to the physiological basis of some of the associated clinical phenomena.

The Purpose of Pain. Pain is a protective mechanism for the body; it occurs whenever any tissues are being damaged, and it causes the individual to react to remove the pain stimulus. Even such simple activities as sitting for a long time on the ischia can cause tissue destruction because of lack of blood flow to the skin where the skin is compressed by the weight of the body. When the skin becomes painful as a result of the ischemia, the person normally shifts weight unconsciously. But a person who has lost the pain sense, such as after spinal cord injury, fails to feel the pain and therefore fails to shift. This very soon results in ulceration at the areas of pressure.

THE TWO TYPES OF PAIN AND THEIR QUALITIES—FAST PAIN AND SLOW PAIN

Pain has been classified into two different major types: *fast pain* and *slow pain.* Fast pain is felt within about 0.1 second when a pain stimulus is applied, whereas slow pain begins only after a second or more and then increases slowly over many seconds and sometimes even minutes.

Fast pain is also described by many alternate names, such as *sharp pain, pricking pain, acute pain, electric pain,* and others. This type of pain is felt when a needle is stuck into the skin or when the skin is cut with a knife, and this pain is also felt when the skin is subjected to electric shock. Fast, sharp pain is not felt in most of the deeper tissues of the body.

Slow pain also goes by multiple additional names such as *burning pain, aching pain, throbbing pain, nauseous pain,* and *chronic pain.* This type of pain is usually associated with *tissue destruction.* It can become excruciating and can lead to prolonged, unbearable suffering. It can occur both in the skin and in almost any deep tissue or organ.

We will learn later that the fast type of pain is transmitted through type Aδ pain fibers, whereas the slow type of pain results from stimulation of the more primitive type C fibers.

THE PAIN RECEPTORS AND THEIR STIMULATION

All Pain Receptors Are Free Nerve Endings. The pain receptors in the skin and other tissues are all free nerve endings. They are widespread in the superficial layers of the *skin* and also in certain internal tissues, such as the *periosteum,* the *arterial walls,* the *joint surfaces,* and the *falx* and *tentorium* of the cranial vault. Most of the other deep tissues are not extensively supplied with pain endings but are weakly supplied; nevertheless, any widespread tissue damage can still summate to cause the slow-chronic-aching type of pain in these areas.

Three Different Types of Stimuli Excite Pain Receptors—Mechanical, Thermal, and Chemical. Most pain fibers can be excited by multiple types of stimuli. However, some fibers are more likely to respond to excessive mechanical stretch, others to extremes of heat or cold, and still others to specific chemicals in the tissues. These are classified respectively as *mechanical, thermal,* and *chemical pain receptors.*

Some of the chemicals that excite the chemical type of pain receptors include *bradykinin, serotonin, histamine, potassium ions, acids, acetylcholine,* and *proteolytic enzymes.* The chemical substances are especially important in stimulating the slow, suffering type of pain that occurs following tissue injury.

Nonadapting Nature of Pain Receptors. In contrast to most other sensory receptors of the body, the pain receptors adapt very little and sometimes not at all. In fact, under some conditions, the excitation of the pain fibers becomes progressively greater as the pain stimulus continues. This increase in sensitivity of the pain receptors is called *hyperalgesia.*

One can readily understand the importance of this failure of pain receptors to adapt, for it allows them to keep the person apprised of a damaging stimulus that causes the pain as long as it persists.

Rate of Tissue Damage as a Cause of Pain

The average person first begins to perceive pain when the skin is heated above 45°C, as illustrated in Figure 33–1. This is also the temperature at which the tissues begin to be damaged by heat; indeed, the tissues are eventually completely destroyed if the temperature remains above this level indefinitely. Therefore, it is immediately apparent that pain resulting from heat is closely correlated with the ability of heat to damage the tissues.

Furthermore, the intensity of pain has also been closely correlated with the rate of tissue damage from causes other than heat—bacterial infection, tissue ischemia, tissue contusion, and so forth.

Special Importance of Chemical Pain Stimuli During Tissue Damage. Extracts from damaged tissues cause intense pain when injected beneath the normal skin. All the chemicals listed above that excite the chemical pain receptors are found in these extracts. However, the chemical that seems to be most painful of all is *bradykinin.* Therefore, many research workers have suggested that bradykinin might be the single agent most responsible for causing the tissue damage type of pain.

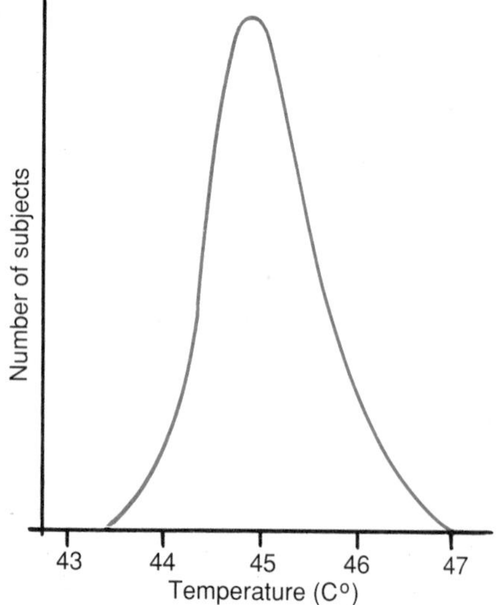

Figure 33–1. Distribution curve obtained from a large number of subjects of the minimal skin temperature that causes pain. (Modified from Hardy: J. Chronic Dis., 4:22, 1956.)

Tissue Ischemia as a Cause of Pain. When blood flow to a tissue is blocked, the tissue becomes very painful within a few minutes. And the greater the rate of metabolism of the tissue, the more rapidly the pain appears. For instance, if a blood pressure cuff is placed around the upper arm and inflated until the arterial blood flow ceases, exercise of the forearm muscles can cause severe muscle pain within 15 to 20 seconds. In the absence of muscle exercise, the pain will not appear for 3 to 4 minutes.

THE DUAL TRANSMISSION OF PAIN SIGNALS INTO THE CENTRAL NERVOUS SYSTEM

Even though all pain endings are free nerve endings, these endings utilize two separate pathways for transmitting pain signals into the central nervous system. The two pathways correspond to the two different types of pain, a *fast-sharp pain pathway,* and a *slow-chronic pain pathway.*

The Peripheral Pain Fibers—"Fast" and "Slow" Fibers. The fast-sharp pain signals are transmitted in the peripheral nerves to the spinal cord by small type Aδ fibers at velocities of between 6 and 30 m/sec. On the other hand, the slow-chronic type of pain is transmitted by type C fibers at velocities of between 0.5 and 2 m/sec. When the type Aδ fibers are blocked without blocking the C fibers by moderate compression of the nerve trunk, the fast-sharp pain disappears. On the other hand, when the type C fibers are blocked without blocking the delta fibers by low concentrations of local anesthetic, the slow-chronic-aching type of pain disappears.

On entering the spinal cord from the dorsal spinal roots, the pain fibers ascend or descend one to three segments in the *tract of Lissauer,* which lies immediately posterior to the dorsal horn of the cord gray matter. Then they terminate on neurons in the dorsal horns. However, here again, there are two systems for processing the pain signals on their way to the brain, as illustrated in Figures 33–2 and 33–3. These are:

Dual Pain Pathways in the Cord and Brain Stem—The Neospinothalamic Tract and the Paleospinothalamic Tract

On entering the spinal cord, the pain signals take two different pathways to the brain, through the *neospinothalamic tract* and through the *paleospinothalamic tract.*

The Neospinothalamic Tract for Fast Pain. The "fast" type Aδ pain fibers transmit mainly mechanical and thermal pain. They terminate mainly in lamina I (lamina marginalis) of the dorsal horns and there excite second-order neurons of the neospino-

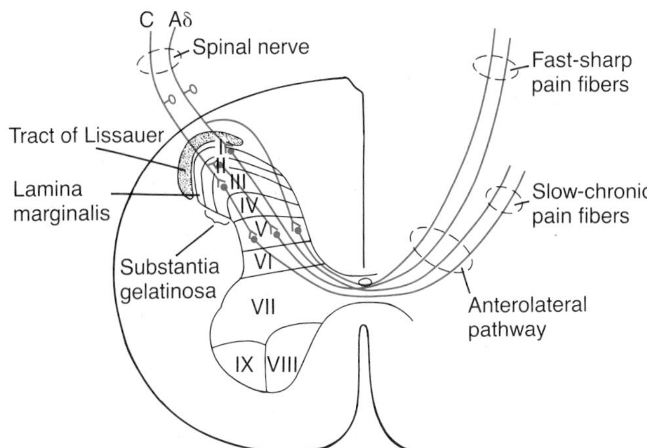

Figure 33-2. Transmission of both "fast-sharp" and "slow-chronic" pain signals into and through the spinal cord on the way to the brain stem.

thalamic tract. These give rise to long fibers that cross immediately to the opposite side of the cord through the anterior commissure and then pass upward to the brain in the anterolateral columns.

Termination of the Neospinothalamic Tract in the Brain Stem and Thalamus. A few fibers of the neospinothalamic tract terminate in the reticular areas of the brain stem, but most pass all the way to the thalamus, terminating mainly in the *ventrobasal complex* along with the dorsal column-medial lemniscal tract discussed in the previous chapter. From this area the signals are transmitted to other basal areas of the brain and to the somatic sensory cortex.

Capability of the Nervous System to Localize Fast Pain in the Body. The fast-sharp type of pain can be localized much more exactly in the different parts of the body than can slow-chronic pain. However, even fast pain, when only pain receptors are stimulated without simultaneously stimulating tactile receptors, is still quite poorly localized, often only within 10 centimeters or so of the stimulated area. Yet when tactile receptors are also stimulated, the localization can be very exact.

The Paleospinothalamic Pathway for Transmitting Slow-Chronic Pain. The paleospinothalamic pathway is a much older system, and transmits pain mainly carried in the peripheral slow-suffering type C pain fibers. In this pathway, the peripheral fibers terminate almost entirely in laminae II and III of the dorsal horns, which together are called the *substantia gelatinosa,* as illustrated by the lateralmost dorsal root fiber in Figure 33-2. Most of the signals then pass through one or more additional short fiber neurons within the dorsal horns themselves before entering mainly lamina V, also in the dorsal horn. Here the last neuron in the series gives rise to long axons that mostly join the fibers from the fast pathway, passing through the anterior commissure to the opposite side of the cord, then upward to the brain in the same anterolateral pathway.

Termination of the Slow-Chronic Pain Signals in the Brain Stem and Thalamus. The slow-chronic pathway terminates very widely in the brain stem, in the large pink-shaded area illustrated in Figure 33-3. Only one tenth to one fourth of the fibers pass all the way to the thalamus. Instead, they terminate principally in multiple areas in the medulla, pons, and mesencephalon. This lower region of the brain appears to be very important in the appreciation of the suffering types of pain, for animals with only their brain stem functioning still evince undeniable evidence of suffering when any part of the body is traumatized.

From the reticular area of the brain stem, multiple short-fiber neurons relay the pain signals upward into the *intralaminar nuclei of the thalamus* and also into certain portions of the hypothalamus and other adjacent regions of the basal brain.

Capability of the Nervous System to Localize Pain Transmitted in the Slow-Chronic Pathway. Localization of pain transmitted in the paleospinothalamic pathway is very poor. In fact, electrophysiological studies suggest that the localization is often only to a major part of the body such as to one

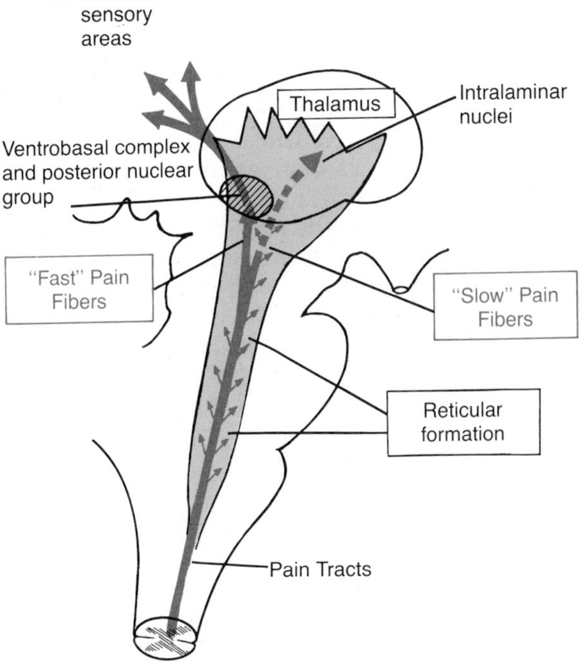

Figure 33-3. Transmission of pain signals into the hindbrain, thalamus, and cortex via the fast "pricking pain" pathway and the slow "burning pain" pathway.

limb but not to a detailed point on the limb. This is in keeping with the multisynaptic, diffuse connectivity to the brain. It also explains why patients often have serious difficulty in localizing the source of some chronic types of pain.

Function of the Reticular Formation, Thalamus, and Cerebral Cortex in the Appreciation of Pain. Complete removal of the somatic sensory areas of the cerebral cortex does not destroy one's ability to perceive pain. Therefore, it is likely that pain impulses entering the reticular formation, thalamus, and other lower centers can cause conscious perception of pain. However, this does not mean that the cerebral cortex has nothing to do with normal pain appreciation; indeed, electrical stimulation of the cortical somatic sensory areas causes a person to perceive mild pain in approximately 3 per cent of the different points stimulated. It is believed that the cortex plays an important role in interpreting the quality of pain even though pain perception might be mainly the function of lower centers.

Special Capability of Pain Signals to Arouse the Nervous System. Electrical stimulation in the reticular areas of the brain stem and also in the intralaminar nuclei of the thalamus, the areas where the slow-suffering type of pain terminates, has a strong arousal effect on nervous activity throughout the brain. In fact, these two areas are parts of the brain's principal arousal system, which is discussed in Chapter 40. This explains why a person with severe pain is frequently strongly aroused, and it also explains why it is almost impossible for a person to sleep when he or she is subjected to pain.

A PAIN CONTROL ("ANALGESIA") SYSTEM IN THE BRAIN AND SPINAL CORD

The degree to which each person reacts to pain varies tremendously. This results partly from the capability of the brain itself to control the degree of input of pain signals to the nervous system by activation of a pain control system, called an *analgesia system.*

The analgesia system is illustrated in Figure 33-4. It consists of three major components (plus other accessory components): (1) The *periaqueductal gray area* of the mesencephalon and upper pons surrounding the aqueduct of Sylvius. Neurons from this area send their signals to (2) the *raphe magnus nucleus,* a thin midline nucleus located in the lower pons and upper medulla. From here the signals are transmitted down the dorsolateral columns in the spinal cord to (3) a *pain inhibitory complex located in the dorsal horns of the spinal cord.* At this point the analgesia signals can block the pain arriving from peripheral nerves before it is relayed on to the brain.

Electrical stimulation either in the periaqueductal gray area or in the raphe magnus nucleus can almost completely suppress many very strong pain signals entering by way of the dorsal spinal roots. Also, stimulation of areas at still higher levels of the brain that in turn excite the periaqueductal gray, especially the *periventricular nuclei in the hypothalamus* lying adjacent to the third ventricle and to a lesser extent the *medial forebrain bundle* also in the hypothalamus, can suppress pain, though perhaps not quite so much so.

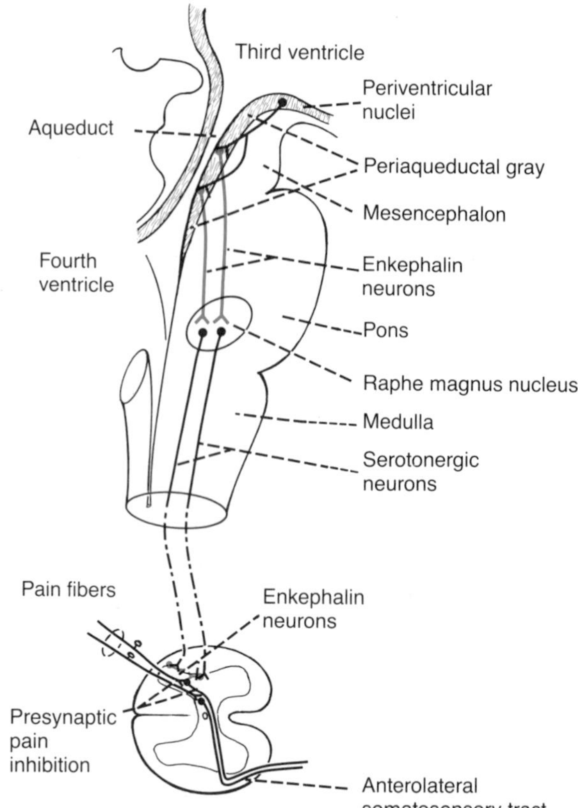

Figure 33-4. The analgesia system of the brain and spinal cord, showing inhibition of incoming pain signals at the cord level.

Several different transmitter substances are involved in the analgesia system; especially involved are *enkephalin* and *serotonin.* Many of the nerve fibers derived from both periventricular nuclei and the periaqueductal gray area secrete enkephalin at their endings. Thus, as shown in Figure 33-4, the endings of many of the fibers in the raphe magnus nucleus release enkephalin. The fibers originating in this nucleus but terminating in the dorsal horns of the spinal cord secrete serotonin at their endings. The eventual result is *inhibition* of both incoming type C and type Aδ pain fibers where they synapse in the dorsal horns.

Thus, the analgesia system can block pain signals at the initial entry point to the spinal cord.

The Brain's Opiate System — The Endorphins and Enkephalins

More than 20 years ago it was discovered that injection of extremely minute quantities of morphine either into the periventricular nucleus around the third ventricle of the diencephalon or into the periaqueductal gray area of the brain stem will cause an extreme degree of analgesia. Therefore, an extensive search was set into motion for a natural opiate of the brain. About a dozen such opiate-like substances have now been found in different points of the nervous system, the most important of which are *β-endorphin, met-enkephalin, leu-enkephalin,* and *dynorphin.*

The two enkephalins are found in the portions of the analgesia system described earlier, and β-endorphin is present both in the hypothalamus and in the pituitary gland.

Thus, although all the fine details of the brain's opiate system are not yet entirely understood, nevertheless activation of the analgesia system either by nervous signals entering the periaqueductal gray area or by morphine-like drugs can totally or almost totally suppress many pain signals entering through the peripheral nerves.

REFERRED PAIN

Often a person feels pain in a part of his or her body that is considerably removed from the tissues causing the pain. This pain is called *referred pain.* Usually the pain is initiated in one of the visceral organs and referred to an area on the body surface.

Mechanism of Referred Pain. Figure 33–5 illustrates the most likely mechanism by which most pain is referred. In the figure, branches of visceral pain fibers are shown to synapse in the spinal cord with some of the same second-order neurons that receive pain fibers from the skin. When the visceral pain fibers are stimulated, pain signals from the viscera are then conducted through at least some of the same neurons that conduct pain signals from the skin, and the person has the feeling that the sensations actually originate in the skin itself.

VISCERAL PAIN

In clinical diagnosis, pain from the different viscera of the abdomen and chest is one of the few criteria that can be used for diagnosing visceral inflammation, disease, and other ailments. In general, the viscera have sensory receptors for no other modalities of sensation besides pain. Also, visceral pain differs from surface pain in several important aspects.

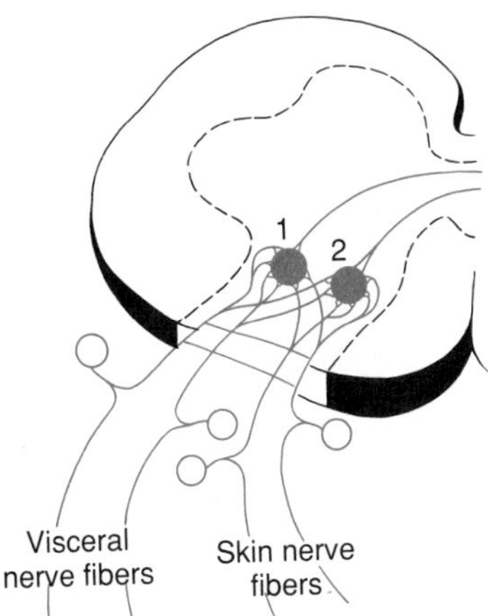

Figure 33–5. Mechanism of referred pain and referred hyperalgesia.

One of the most important differences between surface pain and visceral pain is that highly localized types of damage to the viscera rarely cause severe pain. For instance, a surgeon can cut the gut entirely in two in a patient who is awake without causing significant pain. On the other hand, any stimulus that causes *diffuse stimulation of pain nerve endings* throughout a viscus causes pain that can be extremely severe. For instance, ischemia caused by occluding the blood supply to a large area of gut stimulates many diffuse pain fibers at the same time and can result in extreme pain.

Localization of Visceral Pain—The "Visceral" and the "Parietal" Transmission Pathways

Pain from the different viscera is frequently difficult to localize for a number of reasons. First, the brain does not know from firsthand experience that the different organs exist, and, therefore, any pain that originates internally can be localized only generally. Second, sensations from the abdomen and thorax are transmitted through two separate pathways to the central nervous system—the *true visceral pathway* and the *parietal pathway.* The true visceral pain is transmitted via sensory fibers of the autonomic nervous system (both sympathetic and parasympathetic), and the sensations are *referred* to surface areas of the body often far from the painful organ. On the other hand, parietal sensations are conducted *directly* into the local spinal nerves from the parietal peritoneum, pleura, or pericardium, and the sensations are usually *localized directly over the painful area.*

Localization of Referred Pain Transmitted in the Visceral Pathways. When visceral pain is referred to the surface of the body through the true visceral pathway, the person generally localizes it in the dermatomal segment from which the visceral organ originated in the embryo. For instance the heart originated in the neck and upper thorax, so that the heart's visceral pain fibers pass into the cord between segments C3 and T5. Therefore, as illustrated in Figure 33–6, pain from the heart is referred to the side of the neck, over the shoulder, over the pectoral muscles, down the arm, and into the substernal area of the chest. Most frequently, the pain is on the left side, rather than on the right—because the left side of the heart is much more frequently involved in coronary disease than the right.

The stomach originated approximately from the seventh to the ninth thoracic segments of the embryo. Therefore, stomach pain is referred to the anterior epigastrium above the umbilicus, which is the surface area of the body subserved by the seventh through

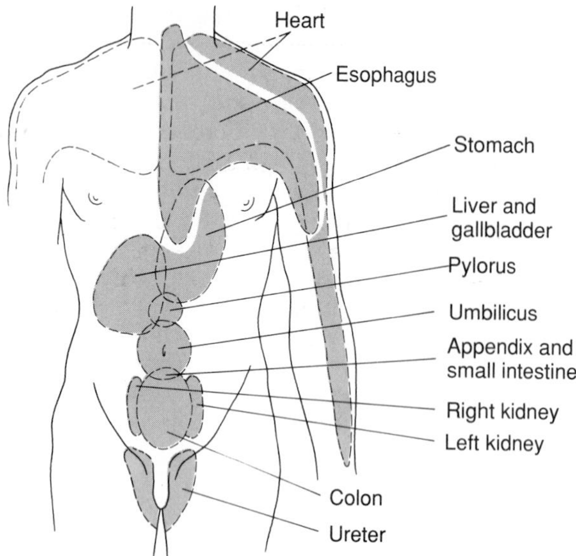

Figure 33–6. Surface areas of referred pain from different visceral organs.

ninth thoracic segments. And Figure 33–6 shows several other surface areas to which visceral pain is referred from other organs, representing in general the areas in the embryo from which the respective organ originated.

SOME CLINICAL ABNORMALITIES OF PAIN AND OTHER SOMATIC SENSATIONS

The Thalamic Syndrome

Occasionally the posterolateral branch of the posterior cerebral artery, a small artery supplying the posteroventral portion of the thalamus, becomes blocked by thrombosis, so that the pain and other sensory nuclei of this area of the thalamus degenerate. The patient suffers a series of abnormalities, as follows: First, loss of almost all sensations from the opposite side of the body occurs because of destruction of the relay nuclei. Second, after a few weeks to a few months some sensory perception in the opposite side of the body returns, but strong stimuli are usually necessary to elicit this. When the sensations do occur, they are poorly—if at all—localized, almost always very painful, sometimes lancinating, regardless of the type of stimulus applied to the body.

The medial nuclei of the thalamus are not destroyed by thrombosis of the artery. Therefore, it is believed that these nuclei become facilitated and give rise to the enhanced sensitivity to pain transmitted through the reticular system.

Headache

Headaches are actually referred pain to the surface of the head from the deep structures. Many headaches result from pain stimuli arising inside the cranium, but others result from pain arising outside the cranium, such as from the nasal sinuses.

Headache of Intracranial Origin

Pain-Sensitive Areas in the Cranial Vault. The brain itself is almost totally insensitive to pain. Even cutting or electrically stimulating the somatic sensory areas of the cortex only occasionally causes pain; instead, it causes pins-and-needles types of paresthesias on the area of the body represented by the portion of the sensory cortex stimulated. Therefore, it is likely that much or most of the pain of headache is not caused by damage within the brain itself.

On the other hand, *tugging on the venous sinuses, damaging the tentorium,* or *stretching the dura at the base of the brain* can all cause intense pain that is recognized as headache. Also, almost any type of traumatizing, crushing, or stretching stimulus to the *blood vessels of the dura* can cause headache. A very sensitive structure is the middle meningeal artery, and neurosurgeons are careful to anesthetize this artery specifically when performing brain operations under local anesthesia.

Areas of the Head to Which Intracranial Headache Is Referred. Stimulation of pain receptors in the intracranial vault above the tentorium, including the upper surface of the tentorium itself, initiates impulses in the fifth nerve and, therefore, causes referred headache to the front half of the head in the area supplied by the fifth cranial nerve, as illustrated in Figure 33–7.

On the other hand, pain impulses from beneath the tentorium enter the central nervous system mainly through the second cervical nerve, which also supplies the scalp behind the ear. Therefore, subtentorial pain stimuli cause "occipital headache" referred to the posterior part of the head as shown in Figure 33–7.

Types of Intracranial Headache. ***Headache of Meningitis.*** One of the most severe headaches of all is that resulting from meningitis, which causes inflammation of all of the meninges, including the sen-

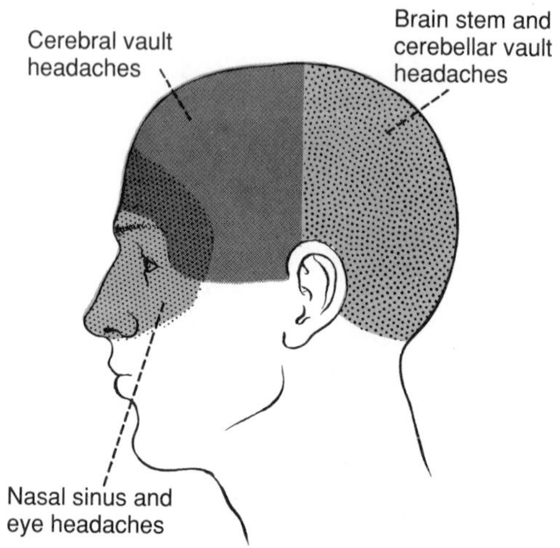

Figure 33–7. Areas of headache resulting from different causes.

sitive areas of the dura and the sensitive areas around the venous sinuses. Such intense damage as this can cause extreme headache pain referred over the entire head.

Migraine Headache. Migraine headache is a special type of headache that is thought to result from abnormal vascular phenomena, though the exact mechanism is unknown.

Migraine headaches often begin with various prodromal sensations, such as nausea, loss of vision in part of the field of vision, visual aura, or other types of sensory hallucinations. Ordinarily, the prodromal symptoms begin half an hour to an hour prior to the beginning of the headache itself. Therefore, any theory that explains migraine headache must also explain these prodromal symptoms.

One of the *theories* of the cause of migraine headaches is that prolonged emotion or tension causes reflex vasospasm of some of the arteries of the head, including arteries that supply the brain itself. The vasospasm theoretically produces ischemia of portions of the brain, and this is responsible for the prodromal symptoms. Then, as a result of the intense ischemia, something happens to the vascular wall to allow it to become flaccid and incapable of maintaining vascular tone for 24 to 48 hours. The blood pressure in the vessels causes them to dilate and pulsate intensely, and it is postulated that the excessive stretching of the walls of the arteries—including some extracranial arteries as well, such as the temporal artery—causes the actual pain of migraine headaches. However, it is possible that diffuse aftereffects of ischemia in the brain itself are at least partially if not mainly responsible for this type of headache.

Alcoholic Headache. As many people have experienced, a headache usually follows an alcoholic binge. It is most likely that alcohol, because it is toxic to tissues, directly irritates the meninges and causes intracranial pain.

Extracranial Types of Headache

Headache Resulting from Muscular Spasm. Emotional tension often causes many of the muscles of the head, including especially those muscles attached to the scalp and the neck muscles attached to the occiput, to become spastic, and it is postulated that this is one of the common causes of headache. The pain of the spastic head muscles supposedly is referred to the overlying areas of the head and gives one the same type of headache as do intracranial lesions.

Headache Caused by Irritation of the Nasal and Accessory Nasal Structures. The mucous membranes of the nose and also of all the nasal sinuses are sensitive to pain, but not intensely so. Nevertheless, infection or other irritative processes in widespread areas of the nasal structures usually cause headache that is referred behind the eyes or, in the case of frontal sinus infection, to the frontal surfaces of the forehead and scalp, as illustrated in Figure 33–7. Also, pain from the lower sinuses—such as the maxillary sinuses—can be felt in the face.

Headache Caused by Eye Disorders. Difficulty in focusing one's eyes clearly may cause excessive contraction of the ciliary muscles in an attempt to gain clear vision. Even though these muscles are extremely small, tonic contraction of them can be the cause of retro-orbital headache. Also, excessive attempts to focus the eyes can result in reflex spasm in various facial and extraocular muscles, which is also a possible cause of headache.

THERMAL SENSATIONS

Thermal Receptors and Their Excitation

The human being can perceive different gradations of cold and heat, progressing from *freezing cold* to *cold* to *cool* to *indifferent* to *warm* to *hot* to *burning hot.*

Thermal gradations are discriminated by at least three different types of sensory receptors: the cold receptors, the warmth receptors, and pain receptors. The pain receptors are stimulated only by extreme degrees of heat or cold and therefore are responsible, along with the cold and warmth receptors, for "freezing cold" and "burning hot" sensations.

The cold and warmth receptors are located immediately under the skin at discrete but separated points, each having a stimulatory diameter of about 1 millimeter. In most areas of the body there are three to ten times as many cold receptors as warmth receptors, and the number in different areas of the body varies from as great as 15 to 25 cold points per square centimeter in the lips, to 3 to 5 cold points per square centimeter in the finger, to less than 1 cold point per square centimeter in some broad surface areas of the trunk. There are correspondingly fewer numbers of warmth points.

Although it is quite certain, on the basis of psychological tests, that there are distinctive warmth nerve endings, these have not yet been identified histologically. They are presumed to be free nerve endings, because warmth signals are transmitted mainly over type C nerve fibers at transmission velocities of only 0.4 to 2 m/sec.

On the other hand, a definitive cold receptor has been identified. It is a special, small, type Aδ myelinated nerve ending that branches a number of times, the tips of which protrude into the bottom surfaces of basal epidermal cells. Signals are transmitted from these receptors via delta nerve fibers at velocities of up to about 20 m/sec. However, some cold sensations are also transmitted in type C nerve fibers, which suggests that some free nerve endings also might function as cold receptors.

Stimulation of Thermal Receptors—Sensations of Cold, Cool, Indifferent, Warm, and Hot. Figure 33–8 illustrates the effects of different temperatures on the responses of four different nerve fibers: (1) a pain fiber stimulated by cold, (2) a cold fiber, (3) a warmth fiber, and (4) a pain fiber stimulated by

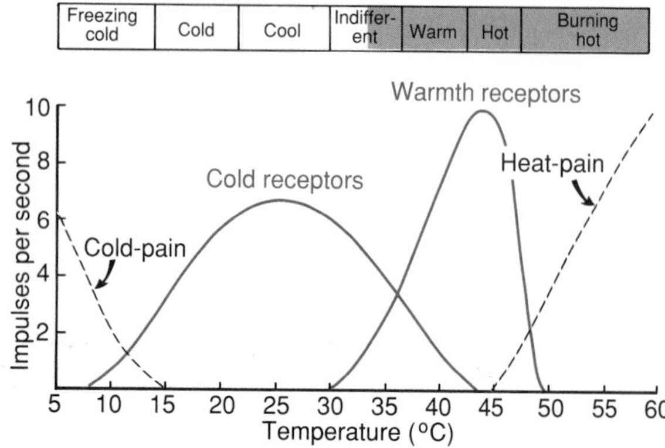

Figure 33-8. Frequencies of discharge of (1) a cold-pain fiber, (2) a cold fiber, (3) a warmth fiber, and (4) a heat-pain fiber. (The responses of these fibers are drawn from original data collected in separate experiments by Zotterman, Hensel, and Kenshalo.)

heat. One can understand from this figure that a person determines the different gradations of thermal sensations by the relative degrees of stimulation of the different types of endings. One can understand also from this figure why extreme degrees of cold or heat can both be painful.

Mechanism of Stimulation of the Thermal Receptors. It is believed that the cold and warmth receptors are stimulated by changes in their metabolic rates, these changes resulting from the fact that temperature alters the rates of intracellular chemical reactions more than twofold for each 10° C change. In other words, thermal detection probably results not from direct physical effects of heat or cold on the nerve endings, but instead from chemical stimulation of the endings as modified by the temperature.

Transmission of Thermal Signals in the Nervous System

In general, thermal signals are transmitted in almost parallel, but not the same, pathways as pain signals. On entering the spinal cord, the signals travel for a few segments upward or downward and then terminate mainly in laminae I, II, and III of the dorsal horns—the same as for pain. After a small amount of processing by one or more cord neurons, the signals enter long, ascending thermal fibers that cross to the opposite anterolateral sensory tract and terminate in (1) the reticular areas of the brain stem and (2) the ventrobasal complex of the thalamus. A few thermal signals are also relayed to the somatic sensory cortex from the ventrobasal complex. Removal of the postcentral gyrus in the human being reduces the ability to distinguish gradations of temperature but does not block the perception of cold or warmth.

REFERENCES

Besson, J. M., and Chaouch, A.: Peripheral and spinal mechanisms of noci+ception. Physiol. Rev., 67:67, 1987.

Darian-Smith, I.: Thermal sensibility. In Darian-Smith, I. (ed.): Handbook of Physiology. Sec. 1, Vol. III. Bethesda, Md., American Physiological Society, 1984, p. 879.

Dumont, J. P. C., and Robertson R. M.: Neuronal circuits: An evolutionary perspective. Science, 233:849, 1986.

Faber, D. S., and Korn, H.: Electrical field effects: Their relevance in central neural networks. Physiol. Rev., 69:821, 1989.

Foreman, R. D., and Blair, R. W.: Central organization of sympathetic cardiovascular response to pain. Annu. Rev. Physiol., 50:607, 1988.

Goldman-Rakic, P. S.: Topography of cognition: Parallel distributed networks in primate association cortex. Annu. Rev. Neurosci., 11:137, 1988.

Hnik, P., et al. (eds.): Mechanoreceptors. Development, Structure and Function. New York, Plenum Publishing Corp., 1988.

Iggo, A., et al. (eds.): Nociception and Pain. New York, Cambridge University Press, 1986.

Llinas, R. R.: The intrinsic electrophysiological properties of mammalian neurons: Insights into central nervous system function. Science, 242:1654, 1988.

Lund, J. S. (ed.): Sensory Processing in the Mammalian Brain. New York, Oxford University Press, 1988.

Price, D. D.: Psychological and Neural Mechanisms of Pain. New York, Raven Press, 1988.

Robinson, D. A.: Integrating with neurons. Annu. Rev. Physiol., 12:33, 1989.

Sejnowski, T. J., et al.: Computational neuroscience. Science, 241:1299, 1988.

Starke, K., et al.: Modulation of neurotransmitter release by presynaptic autoreceptors. Physiol. Rev., 69:864, 1989.

QUESTIONS

1. Discuss the differences between *acute pain* and *slow pain*.
2. What are the different types of pain receptor endings, and what is the relationship between tissue damage and pain?
3. Describe the two separate pathways for transmission of pain signals into the central nervous system and their functional differences.
4. Describe the functions of the reticular formation, the thalamus, and the cerebral cortex in the appreciation of pain.
5. Describe the pain-control (analgesic) system of the brain and spinal cord.
6. What is meant by the brain's *opiate system?*
7. Explain the mechanism of *referred pain.* Why is referred pain from the viscera often localized far from the organ causing the pain?
8. What pain receptor regions within the head are responsible for headache?
9. What is the theoretical mechanism for *migraine headache?*
10. Explain the mechanism by which a person determines the temperature of objects touched by the skin.

34

The Eye: I. Optics of Vision; The Fluids of the Eye; Function of the Retina

THE OPTICS OF THE EYE

The Eye as a Camera

The eye, illustrated in Figure 34–1, is optically equivalent to the usual photographic camera, for it has a lens system, a variable aperture system (the pupil), and a retina that corresponds to the film. The lens system of the eye is composed of four refractive interfaces: (1) the interface between air and the anterior surface of the cornea, (2) the interface between the posterior surface of the cornea and the aqueous humor, (3) the interface between the aqueous humor and the anterior surface of the crystalline lens of the eye, and (4) the interface between the posterior surface of the lens and the vitreous humor.

The Reduced Eye. If all the refractive surfaces of the eye are algebraically added together and then considered to be one single lens, the optics of the normal eye may be simplified and represented schematically as a "reduced eye." This is useful in simple calculations. In the reduced eye, a single refractive surface is considered to exist with its central point 17 mm in front of the retina and to have a total refractive power of approximately 59 diopters when the lens is accommodated for distant vision. (Remember that 1 diopter is the strength of a lens that focuses parallel light rays at a distance of 1 meter.)

Most of the refractive power of the eye is provided not by the crystalline lens but instead by the anterior surface of the cornea. The principal reason for this is that the refractive index of the cornea is markedly different from that of air, as illustrated in Figure 34–1.

On the other hand, the total refractive power of the crystalline lens of the eye, as it normally lies in the eye surrounded by fluid on each side, is only 20 diopters, about one third the total refractive power of the eye's lens system. If this lens were removed from the eye and then surrounded by air, its refractive power would be about six times as great. The reason for this difference is that the fluids surrounding the lens have refractive indices not greatly different from the refractive index of the lens itself, which greatly decreases the amount of light refraction at the lens interfaces. But the importance of the crystalline lens is that its curvature can be increased markedly to provide "accommodation," which will be discussed later in the chapter.

Formation of an Image on the Retina. In exactly the same manner that a glass lens can focus an image on a sheet of paper, the lens system of the eye can focus an image on the retina. The image is inverted and reversed with respect to the object. However, the mind perceives objects in the upright position despite the upside-down orientation on the retina because the brain is trained to consider an inverted image as the normal.

The Mechanism of Accommodation

The refractive power of the crystalline lens of the eye can be voluntarily increased from 20 diopters to approximately 34 diopters in young children; this is a total "accommodation" of 14 diopters. To do this, the shape of the lens is changed from that of a moderately convex lens to that of a very convex lens. The mechanism of this is the following:

In the young person, the lens is composed of a strong elastic capsule filled with viscous, proteinaceous, but transparent fibers. When the lens is in a

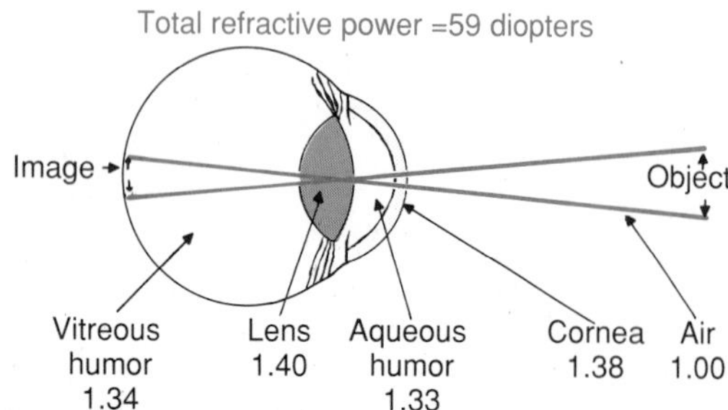

Figure 34–1. The eye as a camera. The numbers are the refractive indices.

relaxed state, with no tension on its capsule, it assumes an almost spherical shape, owing entirely to the elasticity of the lens capsule. However, as illustrated in Figure 34–2, approximately 70 ligaments (called *zonules*) attach radially around the lens, pulling the lens edges toward the anterior edges of the retina. These ligaments are constantly tensed by the elastic pull of their attachments to the ciliary body at the anterior border of the choroid. The tension on the ligaments causes the lens to remain relatively flat under normal resting conditions of the eye. At the insertions of the ligaments in the ciliary body is the *ciliary muscle,* which has two sets of smooth muscle fibers, the *meridional fibers* and the *circular fibers.* The meridional fibers extend to the corneoscleral junction. When these muscle fibers contract, the peripheral insertions of the lens ligaments are pulled forward, thereby releasing a certain amount of tension on the lens. The circular fibers are arranged circularly all the way around the eye so that when they contract, a sphincter-like action occurs, decreasing the diameter of the circle of ligament attachments and also allowing the ligaments to pull less on the lens capsule.

Thus, contraction of both sets of smooth muscle fibers in the ciliary muscle *relaxes* the ligaments to the lens capsule, and the lens assumes a more spherical shape, like that of a balloon, because of the natural elasticity of its capsule. Therefore, when the ciliary muscle is completely relaxed, the dioptric strength of the lens is as weak as it can become. On the other hand, when the ciliary muscle contracts as strongly as possible, the dioptric strength of the lens becomes maximal.

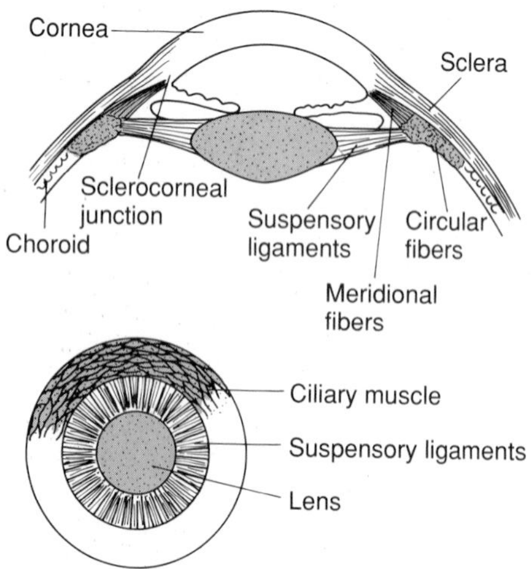

Figure 34–2. Mechanism of accommodation (focusing).

Autonomic Control of Accommodation. The ciliary muscle is controlled almost entirely by the parasympathetic nervous system. Stimulation of the parasympathetic nerves contracts the ciliary muscle, which relaxes the lens ligaments and increases the refractive power. With an increased refractive power, the eye is capable of focusing on objects nearer at hand than when the eye has less refractive power. Consequently, as a distant object moves toward the eye, the number of parasympathetic impulses impinging on the ciliary muscle must be progressively increased for the eye to keep the object constantly in focus.

Presbyopia. As a person grows older, the lens grows larger and thicker, and it also becomes less elastic, partly because of progressive denaturation of the lens proteins. Therefore, the ability of the lens to change shape progressively decreases, and the power of accommodation decreases from approximately 14 diopters in the young child to less than 2 diopters at the age of 45 to 50 years and to about zero at age 70 years. Thereafter, the lens is almost totally nonaccommodating, a condition known as "presbyopia."

Once a person has reached the state of presbyopia, each eye remains focused permanently at an almost constant distance; this distance depends on the physical characteristics of each individual's eyes. Obviously, the eyes can no longer accommodate for both near and far vision. Therefore, to see clearly both in the distance and nearby, an older person must wear bifocal glasses with the upper segment normally focused for far-seeing and the lower segment focused for near-seeing.

The Pupillary Aperture

A major function of the iris is to increase the amount of light that enters the eye during darkness and to decrease the light in bright light. The reflexes for controlling this mechanism will be considered in the discussion of the neurology of the eye in the next chapter. The amount of light that enters the eye through the pupil is proportional to the *area* of the pupil or to the *square of the diameter* of the pupil. The pupil of the human eye can become as small as approximately 1.5 mm and as large as 8 mm in diameter. Therefore, the quantity of light entering the eye may vary approximately 30 times as a result of changes in pupillary aperture.

Errors of Refraction

Emmetropia. As shown in Figure 34–3, the eye is considered to be normal, or "emmetropic," if light rays from distant objects are in sharp focus on the

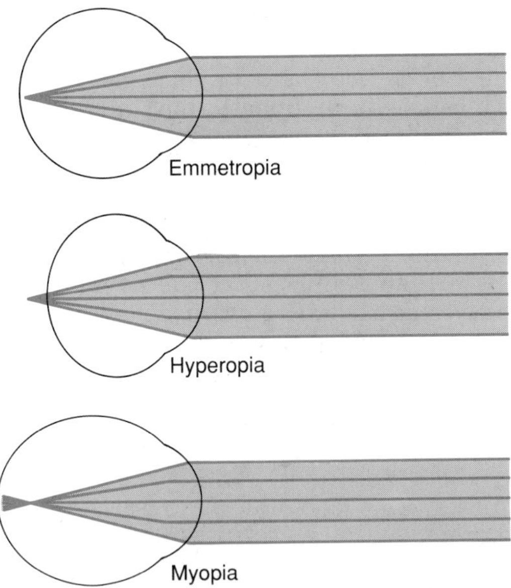

Figure 34-3. Parallel light rays focus on the retina in emmetropia, behind the retina in hyperopia, and in front of the retina in myopia.

retina *when the ciliary muscle is completely relaxed.* This means that the emmetropic eye can see all distant objects clearly, with its ciliary muscle relaxed, but to focus objects at close range it must contract its ciliary muscle and thereby provide various degrees of accommodation.

Hyperopia. Hyperopia, also known as "far-sightedness," is usually due either to an eyeball that is too short or occasionally to a lens system that is too weak when the ciliary muscle is relaxed. In this condition, as seen in the middle panel of Figure 34-3, parallel light rays are not bent sufficiently by the lens system to come to a focus by the time they reach the retina. To overcome this abnormality, the ciliary muscle may contract to increase the strength of the lens. Therefore, the far-sighted person is capable, by using the mechanism of accommodation, of focusing distant objects on the retina. If the person has used only a small amount of strength in the ciliary muscle to accommodate for the distant objects, then he or she still has much accommodative power left, and objects closer and closer to the eye can also be focused sharply until the ciliary muscle has contracted to its limit.

In old age, when the lens becomes presbyopic, the far-sighted person often is not able to accommodate his or her lens sufficiently to focus even distant objects, much less to focus near objects.

Myopia. In myopia, or "near-sightedness," when the ciliary muscle is completely relaxed the light rays coming from distant objects are focused in front of the retina, as shown in the lower panel of Figure 34-3. This is usually due to too long an eyeball, but it can occasionally result from too much refractive power of the lens system of the eye.

No mechanism exists by which the eye can decrease the strength of its lens to less than that which exists when the ciliary muscle is completely relaxed. Therefore, the myopic person has no mechanism by which he or she can ever focus distant objects sharply on the retina. However, as an object comes nearer to the eye, it finally comes near enough that its image will focus. Then, when the object comes still closer to the eye, the person can use the mechanism of accommodation to keep the image focused clearly. Therefore, a myopic person has a definite limiting "far point" for clear vision.

Correction of Myopia and Hyperopia by Use of Lenses. It will be recalled that light rays passing through a concave lens diverge. Therefore, if the refractive surfaces of the eye have too much refractive power, as in *myopia,* some of this excessive refractive power can be neutralized by placing in front of the eye a concave spherical lens, which will diverge rays.

On the other hand, in a person who has *hyperopia*—that is, someone who has too weak a lens system—the abnormal vision can be corrected by adding refractive power with a convex lens in front of the eye. These corrections are illustrated in Figure 34-4.

One usually determines the strength of the concave or convex lens needed for clear vision by "trial and error"—that is, by trying first a strong lens and then a stronger or weaker lens until the one that gives the best visual acuity is found.

Astigmatism

Astigmatism is a refractive error of the lens system, caused usually by an oblong shape of the cornea or, rarely, an oblong shape of the lens. A lens surface like the side of an egg lying sidewise to the incoming light would be an example of an astigmatic lens. The degree of curvature in the plane through the long axis of the egg is not nearly so great as the degree of curvature in the plane through the short axis.

Because the curvature of the astigmatic lens along one plane is less than the curvature along the other plane, light rays striking the peripheral portions of the lens in one plane are not bent nearly so much as are rays striking the peripheral portions of the other plane. This is illustrated in Figure 34-5, which shows rays of light emanating from a point source and pass-

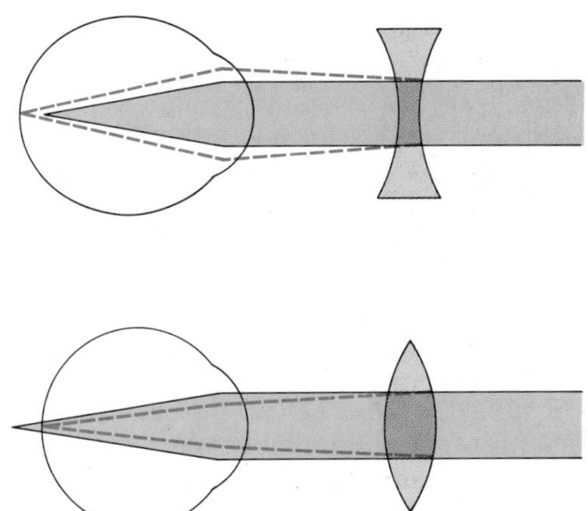

Figure 34-4. Correction of myopia with a concave lens, and correction of hyperopia with a convex lens.

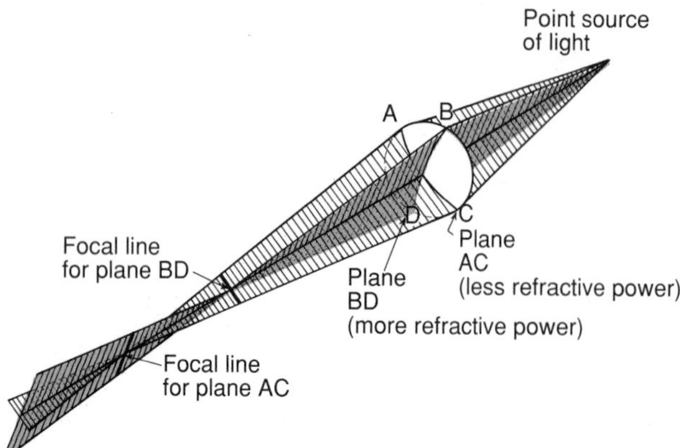

Figure 34-5. Astigmatism, illustrating that light rays focus at one focal distance in one focal plane and at another focal distance in the plane at right angles.

ing through an oblong, astigmatic lens. The light rays in the vertical plane, indicated by plane BD, are refracted greatly by the astigmatic lens because of the greater curvature in the vertical direction than in the horizontal direction. However, the light rays in the horizontal plane, indicated by plane AC, are bent not nearly so much as the light rays in the vertical plane. It is obvious, therefore, that the light rays passing through an astigmatic lens do not all come to a common focal point, because the light rays passing through one plane focus far in front of those passing through the other plane.

The accommodative powers of the eyes can never compensate for astigmatism because, during accommodation, the curvature of the eye lens changes equally in both planes. Therefore, when the accommodation corrects the refractive error in one plane, the error in the other plane is not corrected. That is, each of the two planes requires a different degree of accommodation to be corrected, so that the two planes are never corrected at the same time without the help of glasses. Thus, vision never occurs with a sharp focus.

Correction of Astigmatism with a Cylindrical Lens. One may consider an astigmatic eye as having a lens system made up of two cylindrical lenses of different strengths and placed at right angles to each other. Therefore, to correct for astigmatism the usual procedure is to find a spherical lens by "trial and error" that corrects the focus in one of the two planes of the astigmatic lens. Then an additional cylindrical lens is used to correct the error in the remaining plane. To do this, both the *axis* and the *strength* of the required cylindrical lens must be determined.

There are several methods for determining the axis of the abnormal cylindrical component of the lens system of an eye. One of these methods is based on the use of parallel black bars of the type shown in Figure 34-6. Some of these parallel bars are vertical, some horizontal, and some at various angles to the vertical and horizontal axes. After placing various spherical lenses in front of the astigmatic eye by trial and error, a strength of lens will usually be found that will cause sharp focus of one set of these parallel bars on the retina of the astigmatic eye but will not correct the fuzziness of the set of bars at right angles to the sharp bars. It can be shown from the physical principles of optics that the axis of the *out-of-focus* cylindrical component of the optical system is parallel to the bars that are fuzzy. Once this axis is found, the examiner tries progressively stronger and weaker positive or negative cylindrical lenses, the axes of which are placed parallel to the out-of-focus bars, until the patient sees all the crossed bars with equal clarity. When this has been accomplished, the examiner directs the optician to grind a special lens having the spherical correction as well as the cylindrical correction at the appropriate axis.

Correction of Optical Abnormalities by Use of Contact Lenses

In recent years, either glass or plastic contact lenses have been fitted snugly against the anterior surface of the cornea. These lenses are held in place by a thin layer of tears that fills the space between the contact lens and the anterior eye surface.

A special feature of the contact lens is that it nullifies almost entirely the refraction that normally occurs at the anterior surface of the cornea. The reason for this is that the tears between the contact lens and the cornea have a refractive index almost equal to that of the cornea so that no longer does the anterior surface of the cornea play a significant role in the eye's optical system. Instead, the anterior surface of the contact lens now plays the major role. Thus, the refraction of this lens substitutes for the cornea's usual refraction.

The contact lens has several other advantages as well, including (1) the lens turns with the eye and gives a broader field of clear vision than do usual glasses, and (2) the contact lens has little effect on the size of the object that the person sees through the lens;

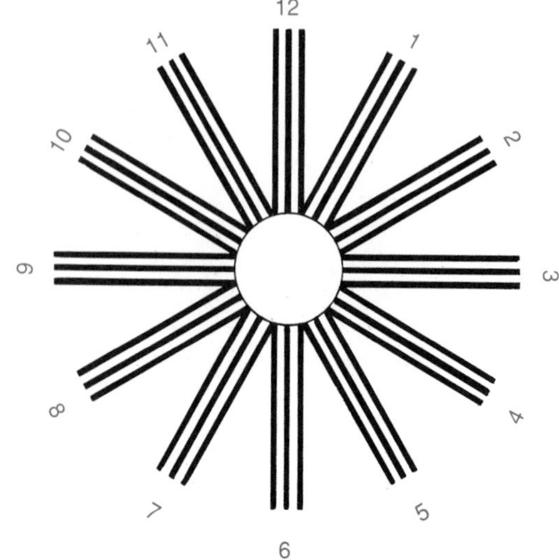

Figure 34-6. Chart composed of parallel black bars for determining the axis of astigmatism.

on the other hand, lenses placed several centimeters in front of the eye do affect the size of the image in addition to correcting the focus.

Cataracts

Cataracts are an especially common eye abnormality that occurs in older people. A cataract is a cloudy or opaque area or areas in the lens. In the early stage of cataract formation the proteins in some of the lens fibers become denatured. Later, these same proteins coagulate to form opaque areas in place of the normal transparent protein fibers.

When a cataract has obscured light transmission so greatly that it seriously impairs vision, the condition can be corrected by surgical removal of the entire lens. When this is done, however, the eye loses a large portion of its refractive power, which must be replaced by a powerful convex lens in front of the eye or an artificial lens of about +20 diopters implanted inside the eye in place of the removed lens.

Visual Acuity

Theoretically, light from a distant point source, when focused on the retina, should be infinitely small. However, since the lens system of the eye is not perfect, such a retinal spot ordinarily has a total diameter of about 11 micrometers even with maximal resolution of the optical system. However, it is brightest in its very center and shades off gradually toward the edges, as illustrated by the two-point images in Figure 34–7.

The average diameter of cones *in the fovea* of the retina, the central part of the retina where vision is most highly developed, is approximately 1.5 micrometers, which is one seventh the diameter of the spot of light. Nevertheless, since the spot of light has a bright center point and shaded edges, a person can distinguish two separate points if their centers lie approximately 2 micrometers apart on the retina, which is slightly greater than the width of a foveal cone. This discrimination between points is also illustrated in Figure 34–7.

The normal visual acuity of the human eye for discriminating between point sources of light is about 45 seconds of arc. This means that a person with normal acuity looking at two bright pinpoint spots of light 10 meters away can barely distinguish the spots as separate entities when they are 1.5 to 2 millimeters apart.

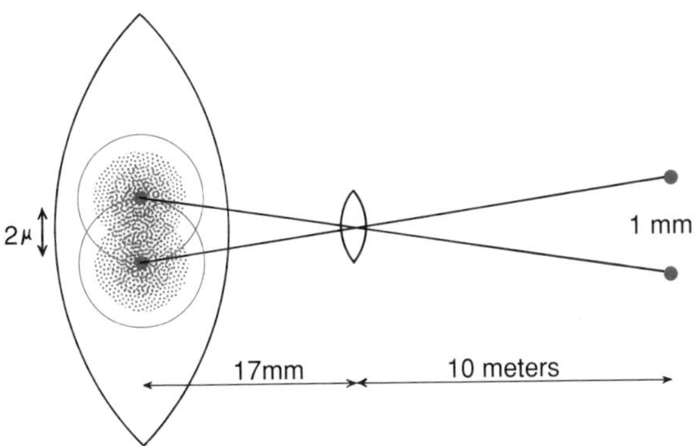

Figure 34–7. Maximal visual acuity for two-point sources of light.

The fovea is less than one half a millimeter (less than 500 micrometers) in diameter, which means that maximal visual acuity occurs in only 3 degrees of the visual field (about 30 centimeters wide at 10 meters distance). Outside this foveal area the visual acuity is reduced five- to tenfold, and it becomes progressively poorer as the periphery is approached. This is caused by the connection of many rods and cones to the same optic nerve fiber in the nonfoveal parts of the retina.

Clinical Method for Stating Visual Acuity. Usually the test chart for testing eyes is placed 20 feet away from the tested person, and if the person can see the letters of the size that he should be able to see at 20 feet, he is said to have 20/20 vision: that is, normal vision. If he can see only letters that he should be able to see at 200 feet, he is said to have 20/200 vision. In other words, the clinical method for expressing visual acuity is to use a mathematical fraction that expresses the ratio of two distances, which is also the ratio of one's visual acuity to that of the normal person.

Determination of Distance of an Object from the Eye — Depth Perception

The visual apparatus normally perceives distance by several different means. This phenomenon is known as *depth perception.* Two of these means are (1) the size of the image of known objects on the retina, and (2) the phenomenon of stereopsis.

Determination of Distance by Sizes of Retinal Images of Known Objects. If one knows that a man whom he is viewing is 6 feet tall, he can determine how far away the man is simply by the size of the man's image on his retina. He does not consciously think about the size, but his brain has learned to calculate automatically from image sizes the distances of objects when the dimensions are known.

Determination of Distance by Stereopsis — Binocular Vision. Another method by which one perceives distance is that of binocular vision. Because one eye is a little more than 2 inches to one side of the other eye, the images on the two retinas are different one from the other — that is, an object that is 1 inch in front of the bridge of the nose forms an image on the temporal portion of the retina of each eye, whereas a small object 20 feet in front of the nose has its image at closely corresponding points in the middle of each retina. This type of effect is illustrated in Figure 34–8, which shows the images of a black spot and a square actually reversed on the two retinas because they are at different distances in front of the eyes. This gives a type of vision that is present all the time when both eyes are being used. It is almost entirely this visual phenomenon (or stereopsis) that gives a person with two eyes far greater ability to judge relative distances

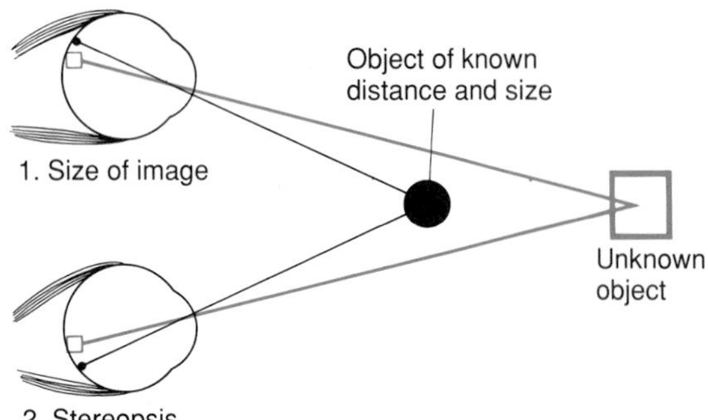

Figure 34-8. Perception of distance (1) by the size of the image on the retina and (2) as a result of stereopsis.

when objects are nearby than a person who has only one eye. However, stereopsis is virtually useless for depth perception at distances beyond 200 feet.

OPTICAL INSTRUMENTS—THE OPHTHALMOSCOPE

The ophthalmoscope is an important instrument used by all doctors to look into another person's eye and see the retina with clarity. Though the ophthalmoscope appears to be a relatively complicated instrument, its principles are simple. The basic components are illustrated in Figure 34-9 and may be explained as follows.

If a bright spot of light is on the retina of an *emmetropic eye,* light rays from this spot diverge toward the lens system of the eye, and, after passing through the lens system, they are parallel with each other because the retina is located exactly one focal length distance behind the lens. Then, when these parallel rays pass into an emmetropic eye of another person, they focus back again to a point focus on the retina of the second person because his retina is also one focal length distance behind the lens. Therefore, any spot of light on the retina of the observed eye comes to a focal spot on the retina of the observing eye. Likewise, when the bright spot of light is moved to different points on the observed retina, the focal spot on the retina of the observer also moves an equal amount. Thus, if the retina of one person is made to emit light, the image of his retina will be focused on the retina of the observer provided the two eyes are simply looking into each other. These principles, of course, apply only to completely emmetropic eyes.

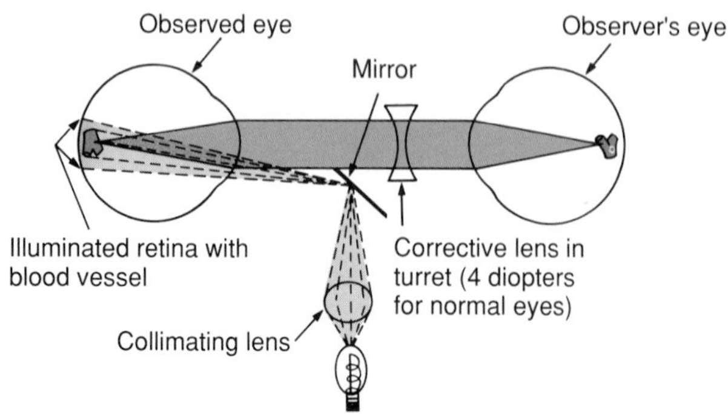

Figure 34-9. The optical system of the ophthalmoscope.

To make an ophthalmoscope, one need only devise a means for illuminating the retina to be examined. Then, the reflected light from that retina can be seen by the observer simply by putting the two eyes close to each other. To illuminate the retina of the observed eye, an angulated mirror or a segment of a prism is placed in front of the observed eye in such a manner, as illustrated in Figure 34-9, that light from a bulb is reflected into the observed eye. Thus, the retina is illuminated through the pupil, and the observer sees into the subject's pupil by looking over the edge of the mirror or prism, or *through* an appropriately designed prism so that the light will not have to enter the pupil at an angle.

It was noted above that these principles apply only to persons with completely emmetropic eyes. If the refractive power of either eye is abnormal, it is necessary to correct this refractive power in order for the observer to see a sharp image of the observed retina. Therefore, the usual ophthalmoscope has a series of lenses mounted on a turret so that the turret can be rotated from one lens to another, and the correction for abnormal refractive power of either or both eyes can be made by selecting a lens of appropriate strength. In normal young adults, when the two eyes come close together, a natural accommodative reflex occurs that causes an approximate +2 diopter increase in the strength of the lens of *each* eye. To correct for this, it is necessary that the lens turret be rotated to an approximate −4 diopter correction.

THE FLUID SYSTEM OF THE EYE—THE INTRAOCULAR FLUID

The eye is filled with *intraocular fluid,* which maintains sufficient pressure in the eyeball to keep it distended. Figure 34-10 illustrates that this fluid can be

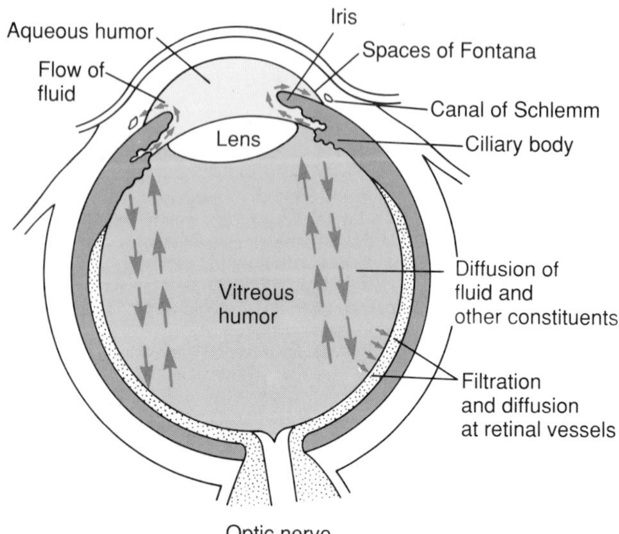

Figure 34-10. Formation and flow of fluid in the eye.

divided into two portions, the *aqueous humor,* which lies in front and to the sides of the lens, and the fluid of the *vitreous humor,* which lies between the lens and the retina. The aqueous humor is a freely flowing fluid, whereas the vitreous humor, sometimes called the *vitreous body,* is a gelatinous mass held together by a fine fibrillar network composed primarily of large proteoglycan molecules. Substances can *diffuse* slowly in the vitreous humor, but there is little *flow* of fluid.

Aqueous humor is continually being formed and reabsorbed. The balance between formation and reabsorption of aqueous humor regulates the total volume and pressure of the intraocular fluid.

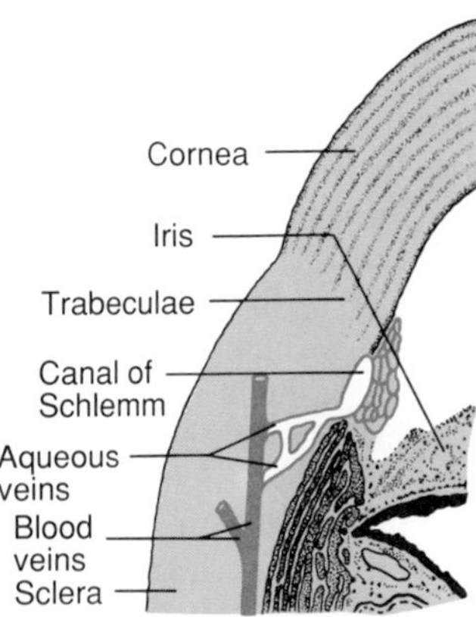

Figure 34-12. Anatomy of the iridocorneal angle, showing the system for outflow of aqueous humor into the conjunctival veins.

Formation of Aqueous Humor by the Ciliary Body

Aqueous humor is formed in the eye *at an average rate of 2 to 3 microliters each minute.* Essentially all of this is secreted by the *ciliary processes,* which are linear folds projecting from the *ciliary body* into the space behind the iris where the lens ligaments also attach to the eyeball. A cross-section of these ciliary processes is illustrated in Figure 34-11, and their relationship to the fluid chambers of the eye can be seen in Figure 34-10. Because of their folded architecture, the total surface area of the ciliary processes is approximately 6 square centimeters in each eye—a large area, considering the small size of the ciliary body. The surfaces of these processes are covered by epithelial cells, and immediately beneath these is a highly vascular area.

Aqueous humor is formed almost entirely as an active secretion of the epithelium lining the ciliary processes. Secretion begins with active transport of sodium ions into the spaces between the epithelial cells. The sodium ions in turn pull chloride and bicarbonate ions along with them to maintain electrical neutrality. Then all these ions together cause osmosis of water from the sublying tissue into the same epithelial intercellular spaces, and the resulting solution washes from the spaces onto the surfaces of the ciliary processes. In addition, several nutrients are transported across the epithelium by active transport or facilitated diffusion; these include amino acids, ascorbic acid, and probably also glucose.

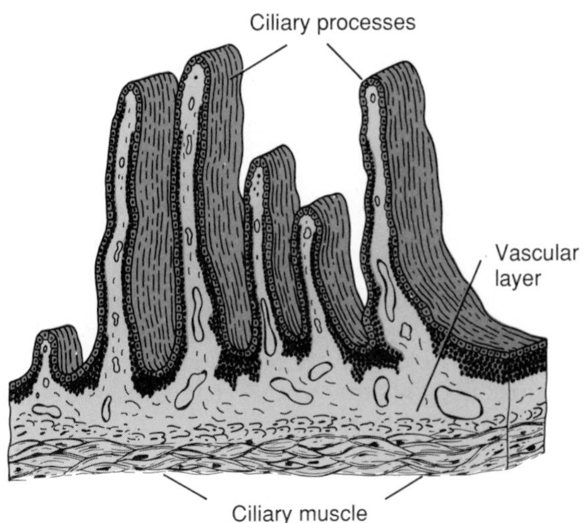

Figure 34-11. Anatomy of the ciliary processes.

Outflow of Aqueous Humor from the Eye

After aqueous humor is formed by the ciliary processes, it flows, as shown in Figure 34-10, *between the ligaments of the lens,* then *through the pupil,* and finally *into the anterior chamber of the eye.* Here, the fluid flows into the *angle between the cornea and the iris* and thence through a meshwork of *trabeculae,* finally entering the *canal of Schlemm,* which empties into extraocular veins. Figure 34-12 illustrates the anatomical structures at the iridocorneal angle, showing that the spaces between the trabeculae extend all the way from the anterior chamber to the canal of Schlemm. The canal of Schlemm in turn is a thin-walled vein that extends circumferentially all the way around the eye. Its endothelial membrane is so porous that even large protein molecules, as well as small particulate matter up to the size of red blood cells, can pass from the anterior chamber into the canal of Schlemm. Even though the canal of Schlemm is actually a venous blood vessel, so much aqueous humor normally flows into it that it is filled only with aqueous humor rather than with blood.

Intraocular Pressure

The average normal intraocular pressure is approximately 15 mm Hg, with a range of from 12 to 20. This pressure remains very constant in the normal eye, normally within about ±2 mm Hg. The level of this pressure is determined mainly by the resistance to outflow of aqueous humor from the anterior chamber into the canal of Schlemm. This outflow resistance results from a meshwork of trabeculae through which the fluid must percolate on its way from the lateral angles of the anterior chamber to the wall of the canal of Schlemm. These trabeculae have minute openings of only 2 to 3 micrometers. Fortunately, though, as the pressure rises above 15 mm Hg, it enlarges these spaces and lets off the excess pressure.

Glaucoma. Glaucoma is one of the most common causes of blindness. It is a disease of the eye in which the intraocular pressure becomes pathologically high, sometimes rising to as high as 60 to 70 mm Hg. Pressures rising above as little as 20 to 30 mm Hg can cause loss of vision when maintained for long periods of time. And extremely high pressures can cause blindness within days or even hours. As the pressure rises, the axons of the optic nerve are compressed where they leave the eyeball at the optic disc. This compression is believed to block axonal flow of cytoplasm from the neuronal cell bodies in the retina to the peripheral optic nerve fibers entering the brain. The result is lack of appropriate nutrition, which eventually causes death of the involved neurons.

In most cases of glaucoma the abnormally high pressure results from increased resistance to fluid outflow through the trabecular spaces into the canal of Schlemm at the iridocorneal junction. For instance, in acute eye inflammation, white blood cells and tissue debris can block these spaces and cause acute increase in intraocular pressure. In chronic conditions, especially in older age, fibrous occlusion of the trabecular spaces appears to be the likely culprit.

Glaucoma can sometimes be treated by placing drops in the eye containing a drug that diffuses into the eyeball and causes reduced secretion or increased absorption of aqueous humor. However, when drug therapy fails, operative techniques to open the spaces of the trabeculae or to make channels directly between the fluid space of the eyeball and the subconjunctival space outside the eyeball can often effectively reduce the pressure.

THE RETINA

The retina is the light-sensitive portion of the eye, containing the cones, which are responsible for color vision, and the rods, which are mainly responsible for vision in the dark. When the rods and cones are excited, signals are transmitted through successive neurons in the retina itself and finally into the optic nerve fibers and cerebral cortex. The purpose of the present chapter is to explain specifically the mechanisms by which the rods and cones detect both white and colored light and then convert the visual image into nerve impulses.

Anatomy and Function of the Structural Elements of the Retina

The Layers of the Retina. Figure 34–13 shows the functional components of the retina arranged in layers from the outside to the inside as follows: (1) pigment layer, (2) layer of rods and cones projecting

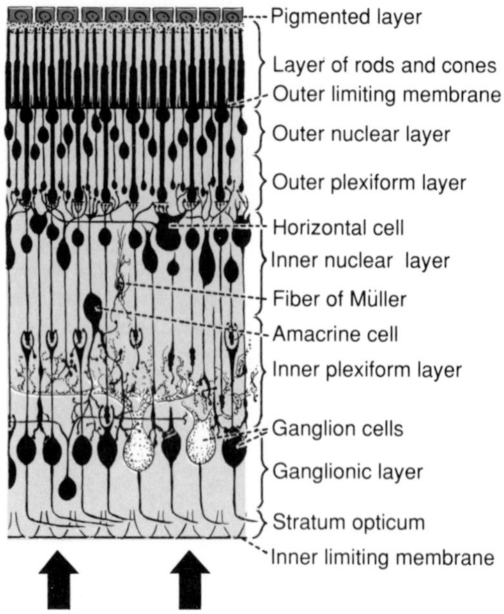

Figure 34–13. Plan of the retinal neurons. (Modified from Polyak: The Retina © 1941 by the University of Chicago. All rights reserved.)

into the pigment, (3) outer limiting membrane, (4) outer nuclear layer containing the cell bodies of the rods and cones, (5) outer plexiform layer, (6) inner nuclear layer, (7) inner plexiform layer, (8) ganglionic layer, (9) layer of optic nerve fibers, and (10) inner limiting membrane.

After light passes through the lens system of the eye and then through the vitreous humor, it enters the retina from the inside (Figure 34–13); that is, it passes through the ganglion cells, the plexiform layers, the nuclear layer, and the limiting membranes before it finally reaches the layer of rods and cones located all the way on the outer side of the retina. This distance is a thickness of several hundred micrometers; visual acuity is obviously decreased by this passage through such nonhomogeneous tissue. However, in the central region of the retina, as will be discussed below, the initial layers are pulled aside for prevention of this loss of acuity.

The Foveal Region of the Retina and Its Importance in Acute Vision. A minute area in the center of the retina, illustrated in Figure 34–14, called the *macula* and occupying a total area of less than 1 square millimeter, is especially capable of acute and detailed vision. The central portion of the macula, only 0.4 millimeter in diameter, is called the *fovea;* this area is composed entirely of cones, and the cones have a special structure that aids their detection of detail in the visual image, especially a long slender body, in contrast to much larger cones located further peripherally in the retina. Also, in this region the blood vessels, the ganglion cells, the inner nuclear layer of cells, and the plexiform layers are all displaced to one side rather than resting directly on top

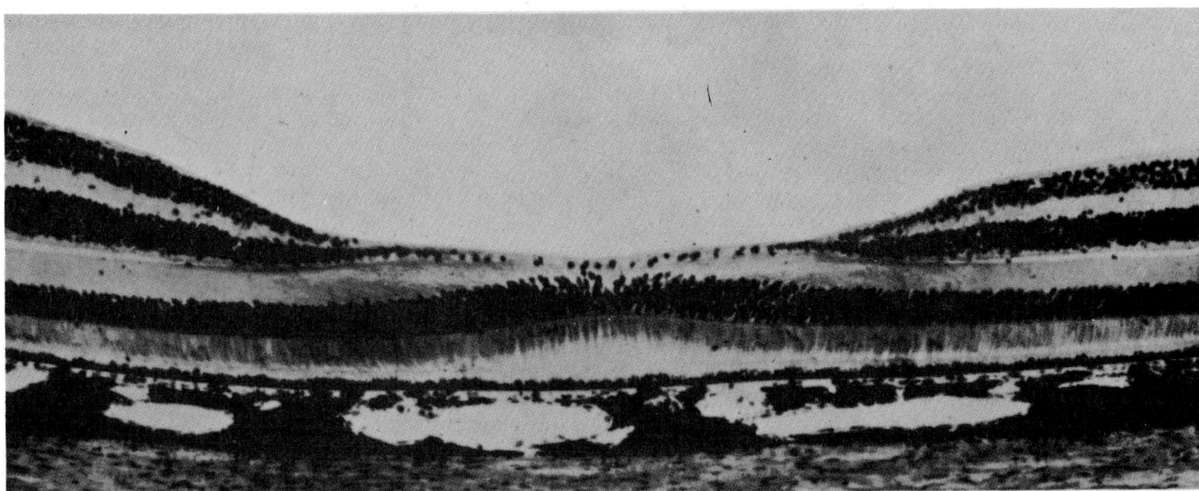

Figure 34-14. Photomicrograph of the macula and of the fovea in its center. Note that the inner layers of the retina are pulled to the side to decrease the interference with light transmission. (From Fawcett, D. W.: Bloom and Fawcett: A Textbook of Histology. 11th ed. Philadelphia, W. B. Saunders Company, 1986; courtesy of H. Mizoguchi.)

of the cones. This allows light to pass unimpeded to the cones.

The Rods and Cones. Figure 34-15 is a diagrammatic representation of a photoreceptor (either a rod or a cone), though the cones are distinguished by having a conical upper end (the outer segment) as shown in Figure 34-16. In general, the rods are narrower and longer than the cones. In the fovea, the cones have a diameter of only 1.5 micrometers.

To the right in Figure 34-15 are labeled the four major functional segments of either a rod or a cone: (1) the *outer segment,* (2) the *inner segment,* (3) the *nucleus,* and (4) the *synaptic body.* In the outer segment the light-sensitive photochemical is found. In the case of the rods, this is *rhodopsin,* and in the cones it is one of several "color" photochemicals that function almost exactly the same as rhodopsin except for differences in spectral sensitivity.

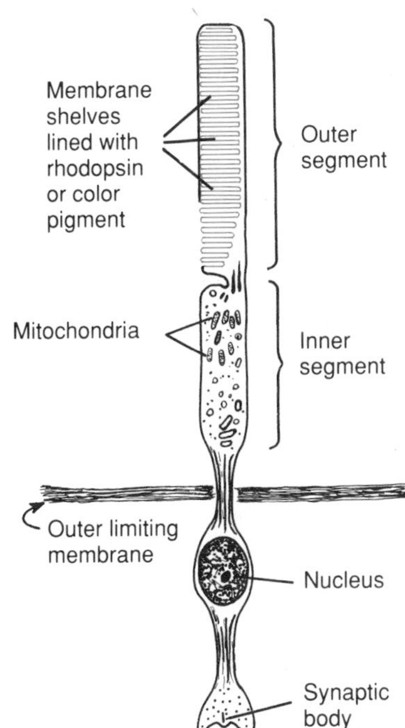

Figure 34-15. The functional parts of the rods and cones.

Note in both Figures 34-15 and 34-16 the large numbers of discs in both the rods and the cones. In the cones, each of the discs is actually an infolded shelf of cell membrane; in the rods this is also true near the base of the rod. However, toward the tip of the rod the discs separate from the membrane and are flat sacs lying totally inside the cell. There are as many as 1000 discs in each rod or cone.

Both rhodopsin and the color photochemicals are conjugated proteins. These are incorporated into the membranes of the discs in the form of transmembrane proteins. The concentrations of these photosensitive pigments in the disc are so great that they constitute approximately 40 per cent of the entire mass of the outer segment.

The inner segment contains the usual cytoplasm of the cell with the usual cytoplasmic organelles. Particularly important are the mitochondria; the mitochondria in this segment play an important role in providing the energy for function of the photoreceptors.

The synaptic body is the portion of the rod and cone that connects with the subsequent neuronal cells, the horizontal and bipolar cells, that represent the next stages in the vision chain.

The Pigment Layer of the Retina. The black pigment *melanin* in the pigment layer prevents light reflection throughout the globe of the eyeball; this is extremely important for clear vision. This pigment performs the same function in the eye as the black coloring inside the bellows of a camera. Without it, light rays would be reflected in all directions within the eyeball and would cause diffuse lighting of the retina rather than the contrast between dark and light spots required for formation of precise images.

The Blood Supply of the Retina — The Arterial System and the Choroid. The nutrient blood

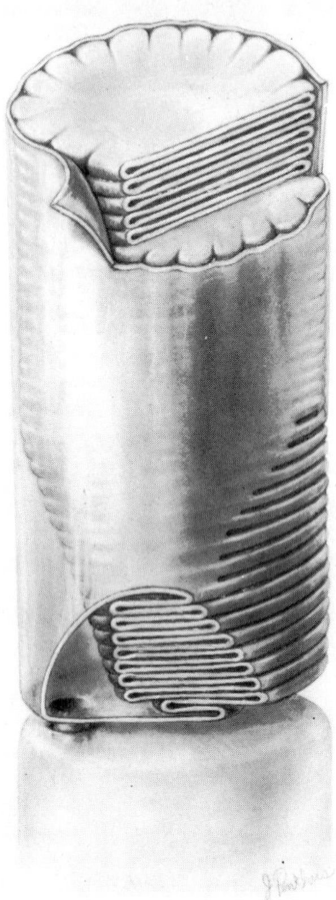

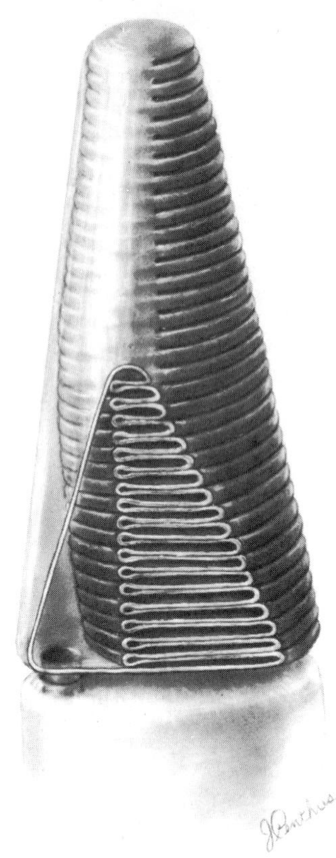

Figure 34–16. Membranous structures of the outer segments of a rod (left) and a cone (right). (Courtesy of Dr. Richard Young.)

supply for the inner layers of the retina is derived from the central retinal artery, which enters the eyeball along with the optic nerve and then divides to supply the entire inner retinal surface. Thus, to a great extent, the retina has its own blood supply independent of the other structures of the eye.

However, the outer surface of the retina is adherent to the *choroid,* which is a highly vascular tissue between the retina and the sclera. The outer layers of the retina, including the outer segments of the rods and cones, depend mainly on diffusion from the choroid vessels for their nutrition, especially for their oxygen.

PHOTOCHEMISTRY OF VISION

Both the rods and cones contain chemicals that decompose on exposure to light and, in the process, excite the nerve fibers leading from the eye. The chemical in the *rods* is called *rhodopsin,* and the light-sensitive chemicals in the *cones* have compositions only slightly different from that of rhodopsin.

In the present section we discuss principally the photochemistry of rhodopsin, but we can apply almost exactly the same principles to the photochemistry of the cones.

The Rhodopsin-Retinal Visual Cycle, and Excitation of the Rods

Rhodopsin and Its Decomposition by Light Energy. The outer segment of the rod that projects into the pigment layer of the retina has a concentration of about 40 per cent of the light-sensitive pigment called *rhodopsin,* or *visual purple.* This substance is a combination of the protein *scotopsin* and the carotenoid pigment *retinal.* Furthermore, the retinal is a particular type called 11-*cis* retinal. This *cis* form of the retinal is important because only this form can bind with scotopsin to synthesize rhodopsin.

When light energy is absorbed by rhodopsin, the rhodopsin begins within trillionths of a second to decompose, as shown at the top of Figure 34–17. The cause of this is photoactivation of electrons in the retinal portion of the rhodopsin, which leads to an instantaneous change (on the order of trillionths of a second) of the *cis* form of retinal into an all-*trans* form, which still has the same chemical structure as the *cis* form but has a different physical structure — a straight molecule rather than a curved molecule. Because the three-dimensional orientation of the reactive sites of the all-*trans* retinal no longer fits with that of the reactive sites on the protein scotopsin, it begins to pull away from the scotopsin. The immediate product is *bathorhodopsin,* which is a partially split combination of the all-*trans* retinal and scotopsin. Bathorhodopsin itself is an extremely unstable compound and decays in nanoseconds to *lumirhodopsin.* This then decays in microseconds to *metarhodopsin I,* then in about a millisecond to *metarhodopsin II,* and, finally, much more slowly (in seconds) into the completely split products: *scotopsin* and *all*-trans *retinal.* It is the metarhodopsin II, also called *activated rhodopsin,* that excites electrical changes in the rods that then transmit the visual image into the central nervous system, as we discuss later.

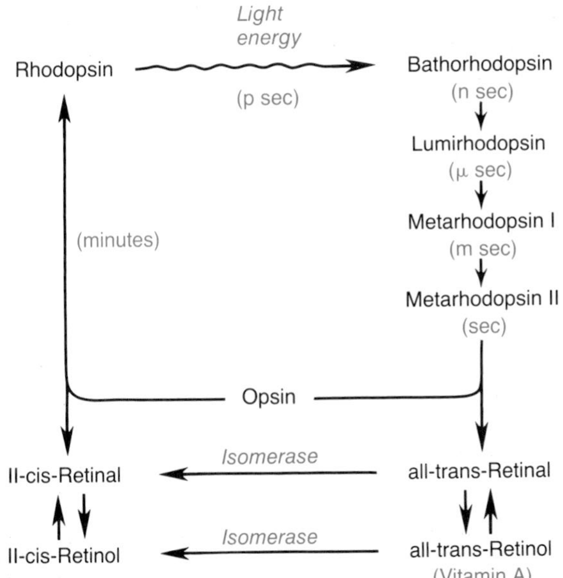

Figure 34–17. The rhodopsin-retinal visual cycle, showing decomposition of rhodopsin during exposure to light and subsequent slow reformation of rhodopsin by the chemical processes of the rod.

Reformation of Rhodopsin. The first stage in reformation of rhodopsin, as shown in Figure 34–17, is to reconvert the all-*trans* retinal into 11-*cis* retinal. In the dark this process is catalyzed by the enzyme *retinal isomerase.* Once the 11-*cis* retinal is formed, it automatically recombines with the scotopsin to re-form rhodopsin, which then remains stable until its decomposition is again triggered by absorption of light energy.

The Role of Vitamin A in the Formation of Rhodopsin. Note in Figure 34–17 that there is a second chemical route by which all-*trans* retinal can be converted into 11-*cis* retinal. This is by conversion of the all-*trans* retinal first into *all*-trans *retinol,* which is one form of vitamin A. Then, the all-*trans* retinol is converted into 11-*cis* retinol under the influence of the enzyme isomerase. And, finally, the 11-*cis* retinol is converted into 11-*cis* retinal.

Vitamin A is present both in the cytoplasm of the rods and in the pigment layer of the retina as well. Therefore, vitamin A is normally always available to form new retinal when needed. On the other hand, when there is excess retinal in the retina, the excess is converted back into vitamin A, thus reducing the amount of light-sensitive pigment in the retina. We shall see later that this interconversion between retinal and vitamin A is especially important in long-term adaptation of the retina to different light intensities.

Night Blindness. Night blindness occurs in severe vitamin A deficiency. The simple reason for this is that not enough vitamin A is then available to form adequate quantities of retinal. Therefore, the amounts of rhodopsin that can be formed in the rods, as well as the amounts of color-photosensitive chemicals in the cones, are all depressed. This condition is called night blindness because the amount of light available at night is then too little to permit adequate vision, though in daylight the cones especially can still be excited despite their reduction in photochemical substances.

Excitation of the Rod When Rhodopsin Is Activated

The Rod Receptor Potential Is Hyperpolarizing, Not Depolarizing. The rod receptor potential is different from the receptor potentials in almost all other sensory receptors. That is, excitation of the rod causes *increased negativity* of the membrane potential, which is a state of *hyperpolarization,* rather than decreased negativity, which is the process of "depolarization" that is characteristic of almost all other sensory receptors.

But how does the activation of rhodopsin cause hyperpolarization? The answer to this is that *when rhodopsin decomposes, it decreases the membrane conductance for sodium ions in the outer segment of the rod.* And this causes hyperpolarization of the entire rod membrane in the following way:

Figure 34–18 illustrates movement of sodium ions in a complete electrical circuit through the inner and outer segments of the rod. The inner segment continually pumps sodium from inside the rod to the outside, thereby creating a negative potential on the inside of the entire cell. However, the membrane of the outer segment, in the *dark* state, is very leaky to sodium. Therefore, sodium continually leaks back to the inside of the rod and thereby neutralizes much of the negativity on the inside of the entire cell. Thus, under normal conditions, when the rod is not excited there is a reduced amount of electronegativity inside the membrane of the rod, normally about −40 millivolts.

When the rhodopsin in the outer segment of the rod is exposed to light and begins to decompose, this de-

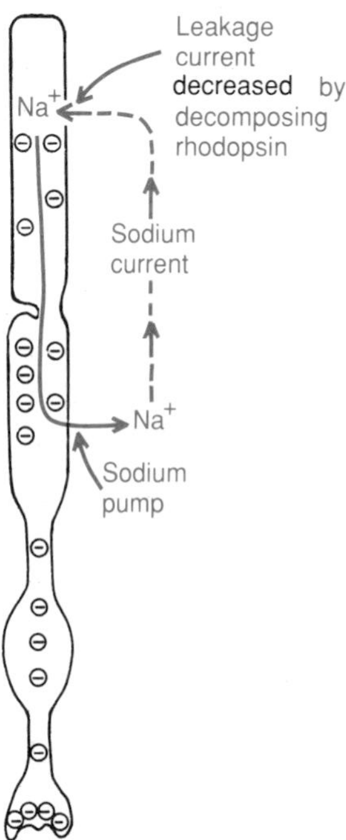

Figure 34–18. Theoretical basis for the generation of a hyperpolarization receptor potential caused by rhodopsin decomposition.

creases the membrane conductance of sodium to the interior of the outer segment even though sodium ions continue to be pumped out of the inner segment. Thus, more sodium ions now leave the rod than leak back in. Because these are positive ions, their loss from inside the rod creates increased negativity inside the membrane; and the greater the amount of light energy striking the rod, the greater the electronegativity—that is, the greater the degree of *hyperpolarization.* At maximal light intensity, the membrane potential approaches −70 to −80 millivolts, which is near the equilibrium potential for potassium ions across the membrane.

Duration of the Receptor Potential and Logarithmic Relationship of the Receptor Potential to Light Intensity. When a sudden pulse of light strikes the retina, the transient hyperpolarization that occurs in rods—that is, the receptor potential that occurs—reaches a peak in about 0.3 second and lasts for more than a second. In cones these changes occur four times as fast. Therefore, a visual image impinged on the retina for only a millionth of a second nevertheless can cause the sensation of seeing the image sometimes for longer than a second.

Another characteristic of the receptor potential is that it is approximately proportional to the logarithm of the light intensity. This is exceedingly important, because it allows the eye to discriminate light intensities through a range many thousand times as great as would be possible otherwise.

Mechanism by Which Rhodopsin Decomposition Decreases Membrane Sodium Conductance—The Excitation "Cascade." Under optimal conditions, a single photon of light, the smallest possible quantal unit of light energy, can cause a receptor potential in a rod of about 1 millivolt. And only 30 photons of light will cause half saturation of the rod. How can such a small amount of light cause such great excitation? The answer is that the photoreceptors have an extremely sensitive chemical cascade that amplifies the stimulatory effects about a millionfold, as follows:

1. The *photon activates an electron* in the *11*-cis *retinal* portion of the rhodopsin; this leads to the formation of *metarhodopsin II,* which is the active form of rhodopsin, as already discussed and illustrated in Figure 34–17.
2. The *activated rhodopsin* functions as an enzyme to activate many molecules of *transducin,* a protein present in an inactive form in the membranes of the discs and cell membrane of the rod.
3. The *activated transducin* in turn activates many more molecules of *phosphodiesterase.*
4. *Activated phosphodiesterase,* which is an enzyme, immediately hydrolyzes many, many molecules of *cyclic* guanosine monophosphate (cGMP), thus destroying it. Before being destroyed, the cGMP had been bound with the sodium channel protein in a way to "splint" it in the open state, allowing continued rapid influx of sodium ions during dark conditions. But in light, when phosphodiesterase hydrolyzes the cGMP, this removes the splinting and causes the sodium channels to close. Several hundred channels close for each originally activated molecule of rhodopsin. Because the sodium flux through each of these channels is extremely rapid, flow of more than a million sodium ions is blocked by the channel closure before the channel opens again. This diminishment of sodium ion flow is what excites the rod, as already discussed.
5. Within a small fraction of a second, another enzyme, *rhodopsin kinase,* that is always present in the rod, inactivates the activated rhodopsin, and the entire cascade reverses back to the normal state with open sodium channels.

Thus, the rods have invented an important chemical cascade that amplifies the effect of a single photon of light to cause movement of millions of sodium ions. This explains the extreme sensitivity of the rods under dark conditions.

The cones are about 300 times less sensitive than the rods, but even this allows color vision in any light greater than very dim twilight.

Photochemistry of Color Vision by the Cones

It was pointed out at the outset of this discussion that the photochemicals in the cones have almost exactly the same chemical composition as that of rhodopsin in the rods. The only difference is that the protein portions, the opsins, called *photopsins* in the cones, are different from the scotopsin of the rods. The retinal portion is exactly the same in the cones as in the rods. The color-sensitive pigments of the cones, therefore, are combinations of retinal and photopsins.

Three different types of photochemicals are present in different cones, thus making these cones selectively sensitive to the different colors of blue, green, and red. These photochemicals are called, respectively, *blue-sensitive pigment, green-sensitive pigment,* and *red-sensitive pigment.* The light absorption characteristics of the pigments in the three types of cones show peak absorbancies at light wavelengths, respectively, of 445, 535, and 570 nanometers. These are also the wavelengths for peak light sensitivity for each type of cone, which begins to explain how the retina differentiates the colors. The approximate absorption curves for these three pigments are shown in Figure 34–19. Also shown is the absorption curve for the rhodopsin of the rods, having a peak at 505 nanometers.

Automatic Regulation of Retinal Sensitivity—Dark and Light Adaptation

If a person has been in bright light for a long time, large proportions of the photochemicals in both the

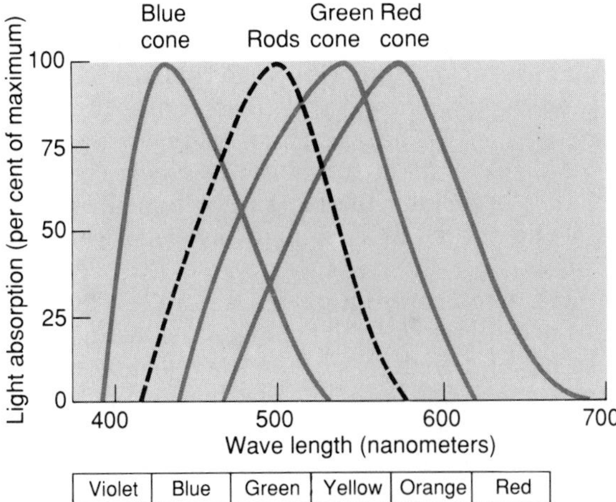

Figure 34–19. Light absorption by the respective pigments of the three color-receptive cones of the human retina. (Drawn from curves recorded by Marks, Dobelle, and MacNichol, Jr.: *Science, 143*:1181, 1964, and by Brown and Wald: *Science, 144*:45, 1964. Copyright 1964 by the American Association for the Advancement of Science.)

rods and cones have been reduced to retinal and opsins. Furthermore, much of the retinal of both the rods and cones has also been converted into vitamin A. Because of these two effects, the concentrations of the photosensitive chemicals are considerably reduced, and the sensitivity of the eye to light is even more reduced. This is called *light adaptation.*

On the other hand, if the person remains in darkness for a long time, the retinal and opsins in the rods and cones are converted back into the light-sensitive pigments. Furthermore, vitamin A is reconverted back into retinal to give still additional light-sensitive pigments, the final limit being determined by the amount of opsins in the rods and cones. This is called *dark adaptation.*

The cones adapt much more rapidly than the rods, because all the chemical events of vision occur about four times as rapidly in cones as in rods. On the other hand, the cones do not achieve anywhere near the same degree of sensitivity as the rods. Therefore, despite rapid adaptation by the cones, they cease adapting after only a few minutes, whereas, the slowly adapting rods continue to adapt for many minutes and even hours, their sensitivity increasing sometimes as much as ½-millionfold.

Since the registration of images by the retina requires detection of both dark and light spots in the image, it is essential that the sensitivity of the retina always be adjusted so that the receptors respond to the lighter areas but not to the darker areas. An example of maladjustment of the retina occurs when a person leaves a movie theater and enters the bright sunlight, for even the dark spots in the images then seem exceedingly bright, and, as a consequence, the entire visual image is bleached, having little contrast between its different parts. Obviously, this is poor vision, and it remains poor until the retina has adapted sufficiently for the darker areas of the image no longer to stimulate the receptors excessively.

Conversely, when a person enters darkness, the sensitivity of the retina is usually so slight that even the light spots in the image cannot excite the retina. After dark adaptation, however, the light spots begin to register.

COLOR VISION

From the preceding sections, we know that different cones are sensitive to different colors of light. The present section is a discussion of the mechanisms by which the retina detects the different gradations of color in the visual spectrum.

The Tricolor Mechanism of Color Detection

All the theories of color vision are based on the well-known observation that the human eye can detect almost all gradations of colors when red, green, and blue monochromatic lights are appropriately mixed in different combinations.

Spectral Sensitivities of the Three Types of Cones. On the basis of color vision tests, the spectral sensitivities of the three different types of cones in human beings have been proved to be essentially the same as the light absorption curves for the three types of pigment found in the respective cones. These were illustrated in Figure 34–19 and are shown again in a different way in Figure 34–20. These curves can explain most of the phenomena of color vision.

Interpretation of Color in the Nervous System. Referring to Figure 34–20, one can see that an orange monochromatic light with a wavelength of 580 nanometers stimulates the red cones to a stimulus value of approximately 99 (99 per cent of the peak stimulation at optimum wavelength), whereas it stimulates the green cones to a stimulus value of approximately 42 and the blue cones not at all. Thus, the ratios of stimulation of the three different types of

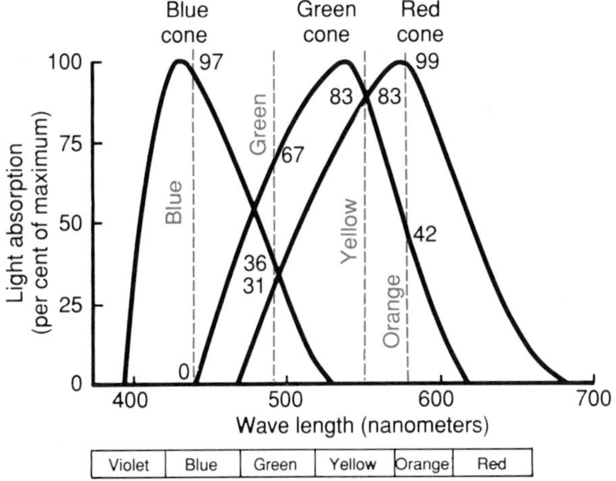

Figure 34–20. Demonstration of the degree of stimulation of the different color-sensitive cones by monochromatic lights of four separate colors: blue, green, yellow, and orange.

cones in this instance are 99:42:0. The nervous system interprets this set of ratios as the sensation of orange. On the other hand, a monochromatic blue light with a wavelength of 450 nanometers stimulates the red cones to a stimulus value of 0, the green cones to a value of 0, and the blue cones to a value of 97. This set of ratios — 0:0:97 — is interpreted by the nervous system as blue. Likewise, ratios of 83:83:0 are interpreted as yellow, and 31:67:36 as green.

Perception of White Light. Approximately equal stimulation of all the red, green, and blue cones gives one the sensation of seeing white. Yet there is no wavelength of light corresponding to white; instead, white is a combination of all the wavelengths of the spectrum. Furthermore, the sensation of white can be achieved by stimulating the retina with a proper combination of only three chosen colors that stimulate the respective types of cones approximately equally.

Color Blindness

Red-Green Color Blindness. When a single group of color receptive cones is missing from the eye, the person is unable to distinguish some colors from others. For instance, one can see in Figure 34–20 that green, yellow, orange, and red colors, which are the colors between the wavelengths of 525 and 675 nanometers, are normally distinguished one from the other entirely by the red and the green cones. If either of these two cones is missing, one no longer can use this mechanism for distinguishing these four colors; the person is especially unable to distinguish red from green and therefore is said to have *red-green color blindness.*

Red-green color blindness is a genetic disease in males that is transmitted through the female. That is, genes in the female X chromosome code for the respective cones. Yet color blindness almost never occurs in the female because at least one of her two X chromosomes will almost always have normal genes for all the cones. But the male has only one X chromosome, so that a missing gene will lead to color blindness in him.

Since the X chromosome in the male is always inherited from the mother, never from the father, color blindness is passed from mother to son, and the mother is said to be a *color blindness* carrier; this is the case for about 8 per cent of all women.

Blue Weakness. Only rarely are blue cones missing, though sometimes they are underrepresented, which is a state also genetically inherited, giving rise to the phenomenon called blue weakness.

REFERENCES

Eye Lens System and Eye Fluids

Apple, D. J., et al.: Intraocular Lenses: Evolution, Design, Complications and Pathology. Baltimore, Williams & Wilkins, 1988.
Caldwell, D. R.: Cataracts. New York, Raven Press, 1988.
Cavanagh, H. D.: The Cornea: Transactions of the World Congress on the Cornea III. New York, Raven Press, 1988.
Koretz, J. F., and Handelman, G. H.: How the human eye focuses. Sci. Am., July, 1988, p. 92.
Michaels, D. D.: Basic Refraction Techniques. New York, Raven Press, 1988.
Ritch, R., et al. (eds.): The Glaucomas. St. Louis, C. V. Mosby Co., 1989.
Shields, M. B.: Textbook of Glaucoma, 2nd Ed. Baltimore, Williams & Wilkins, 1986.
Stenson, S. M.: Contact Lenses: Guide to Selection, Fitting, and Management of Complications. East Norwalk, Conn., Appleton & Lange, 1987.

The Retina

Daw, N. W., et al.: The function of synaptic transmitters in the retina. Annu. Rev. Neurosci., 12:205, 1989.
Gurney, A. M., and Lester, H. A.: Light-flash physiology with synthetic photosensitive compounds. Physiol. Rev., 67:583, 1987.
Hurley, J. G.: Molecular properties of the cGMP cascade of vertebrate photoreceptors. Annu. Rev. Physiol., 49:793, 1987.
Liebman, P. A., et al.: The molecular mechanism of visual excitation and its relation to the structure and composition of the rod outer segment. Annu. Rev. Physiol., 49:765, 1987.
Ryan, S. J., et al. (eds.): Retina. St. Louis, C. V. Mosby Co., 1989.
Saibil, H. R.: From photon to receptor potential: The biochemistry of vision. News Physiol. Sci., 1:122, 1986.
Spaeth, G. L. (ed.): Ophthalmic Surgery: Principles and Practice, 2nd ed. Philadelphia, W. B. Saunders Co., 1989.

QUESTIONS

1. Why is the anterior surface of the cornea the major refractive surface of the eye's lens system?
2. When the ciliary muscle of the eye is completely relaxed, what happens to the tension on the *radial ligaments of the lens*? What happens to the shape of the lens and its focusing strength?
3. What happens to the range of accommmodation of the lens as a person becomes older? What is meant by *presbyopia*?
4. What are the causes of *hypermetropia, myopia,* and *astigmatism*?
5. What type of lens is necessary to correct each of the aforementioned abnormalities of vision?
6. How far apart on the retina must two separate points of light be separated in order for a person to distinguish that there are two points rather than a single point?
7. If a person is said to have 20/50 vision, what is meant?
8. Explain how the visual system determines distance of an object from the eyes by the mechanism of *stereopsis.*
9. Describe the formation, flow, and absorption of fluid in the eyeball.
10. Explain the factors that control the *intraocular pressure.*
11. What is *glaucoma*? Describe its usual cause and its effects on the eye.
12. Give the structure of a typical *rod.* How do *cones* differ from the rods?
13. Describe the *fovea* and its function in high acuity vision.

14. List the major functional segments of a rod or cone. Also describe the *discs* and their relationship to *rhodopsin* or *iodopsin.*
15. What is the relationship of the pigment layer of the retina to the rods and cones, and what is the importance of this relationship?
16. Describe the physical and chemical events that take place after rhodopsin is exposed to an instantaneous bright light.
17. Describe the reformation of rhodopsin after it has been decomposed in bright light.
18. What is the relationship between vitamin A and the visual pigments of the rods and cones?
19. How does generation of the receptor potential in the rods differ from the generation of a receptor potential in most sensory receptors of the body? Explain the mechanism for generating this potential.
20. What are the respective wavelengths for peak absorption by the different types of cones?
21. Why are light and dark adaptation very important in vision?
22. Explain how the brain interprets color by the visual signals received from the retina.
23. What is the cause of color blindness? What types of color blindness are common?

35

The Eye: II. Neurophysiology of Vision

THE NEURAL FUNCTION OF THE RETINA

The Neural Circuitry of the Retina

Figure 34-13 of the previous chapter illustrated the tremendous complexity of neural organization in the retina. To simplify this, Figure 35-1 presents the basic essentials of the retina's neural connections. The different neuronal cell types are:

1. The photoreceptors themselves: the *rods* and *cones*.
2. The *horizontal cells,* which transmit signals horizontally from the rods and cones to the bipolar cell dendrites.
3. The *bipolar cells,* which transmit signals directly from the rods and cones and also from the horizontal cells to either amacrine cells or ganglion cells.
4. The *amacrine cells,* which transmit signals in two directions, either directly from bipolar cells to ganglion cells or horizontally between the axons of the bipolar cells, the dendrites of the ganglion cells, and/or other amacrine cells.
5. The *ganglion cells,* which transmit output signals from the retina through the optic nerve into the brain.

The Direct Visual Pathways from the Receptors to the Ganglion Cells. As is true of many of our sensory systems, the retina has both a very old type of vision based on rod vision and a new type of vision based on cone vision. The neurons and nerve fibers that conduct the visual signals for cone vision are considerably larger than those for rod vision, and the signals are conducted to the brain two to five times as rapidly. Also, the circuitries for the two systems are slightly different, as follows:

To the far right in Figure 35-1 is illustrated the visual pathway from the foveal portion of the retina, representing the new, fast system. This shows three neurons in the direct pathway: (1) cones, (2) bipolar cells, and (3) ganglion cells. In addition, horizontal cells transmit inhibitory signals laterally in the outer plexiform layer, and amacrine cells transmit signals laterally in the inner plexiform layer.

To the left in Figure 35-1 is illustrated the neural connections for the peripheral retina where both rods and cones are present. Three bipolar cells are shown; the middle of these connects only to rods, representing the old visual system. In this case, the output from the bipolar cell passes only to amacrine cells, and these in turn relay the signals to the ganglion cells. Thus, for pure rod vision there are four neurons in the direct visual pathway: (1) rods, (2) bipolar cells, (3) amacrine cells, and (4) ganglion cells. Also, both horizontal and amacrine cells provide lateral connectivity.

The other two bipolar cells illustrated in the peripheral retinal circuitry of Figure 35-1 connect with both rods and cones; the outputs of these bipolar cells pass both directly to ganglion cells and also by way of amacrine cells.

Neurotransmitters Released by Retinal Neurons. The neurotransmitters employed for synaptic transmission in the retina still have not all been delineated clearly. However, it is believed that both the rods and the cones release *glutamate,* an excitatory transmitter, at their synapses with the bipolar and horizontal cells. And histological and pharmacological studies have shown there to be many different types of amacrine cells secreting at least five different types of transmitter substances: *gamma-aminobu-*

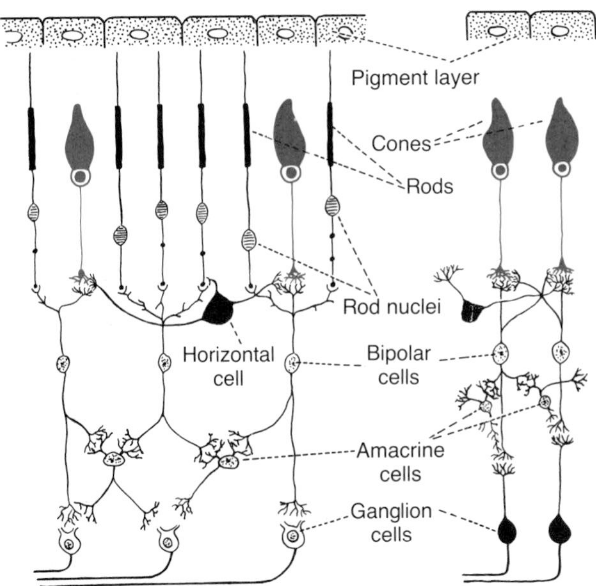

Figure 35-1. Neural organization of the retina: peripheral area to the left, foveal area to the right.

tyric acid (GABA), glycine, dopamine, acetylcholine, and *indolamine,* all of which normally function as inhibitory transmitters. The transmitters of the bipolar and horizontal cells are still unknown.

Transmission of Most Signals Occurs in the Retina by Electrotonic Conduction, Not by Action Potentials. The only retinal neurons that always transmit visual signals by means of action potentials are the ganglion cells; and these send their signals all the way to the brain. Instead , all the other retinal neurons conduct their visual signals almost entirely by *electrotonic conduction,* which can be explained as follows:

Electrotonic conduction means direct flow of electrical current, not action potentials, in the neuronal cytoplasm from the point of excitation all the way to the output synapses. Even in the rods and cones, conduction from their outer segments where the visual signals are generated to the synaptic bodies is by electrotonic conduction. That is, when hyperpolarization occurs in response to light in the outer segment, approximately the same degree of hyperpolarization is conducted by direct electrical current flow to the synaptic body, and no action potential at all occurs. Then, when the transmitter from a rod or cone stimulates a bipolar cell or horizontal cell, once again the signal is transmitted from the input to the output of either of these cells by direct electrical current flow, not by action potentials. Electrotonic conduction is also the means of signal transmission in most, if not all, of the different types of amacrine cells as well.

The importance of electrotonic conduction is that it allows *graded conduction* of signal strength. Thus, for the rods and cones, the hyperpolarizing output signal is directly related to the intensity of illumination; the signal is not all-or-none, as would be the case for action potential conduction.

Lateral Inhibition to Enhance Visual Contrast— Function of the Horizontal Cells

The horizontal cells, illustrated in Figure 35-1, connect laterally between the synaptic bodies of the rods and cones and also with the dendrites of the bipolar cells. The outputs of the horizontal cells are always inhibitory. Therefore, this lateral connection provides the same phenomenon of lateral inhibition that is important in all other sensory systems, that is, to prevent lateral spread of the transmitted visual patterns into the central nervous system. This is an essential mechanism allowing high visual accuracy in transmitting contrast borders in the visual image. It is probable that some of the amacrine cells provide additional lateral inhibition and further enhancement of visual contrast as well.

Excitation of Some Bipolar Cells and Inhibition of Others—The Depolarizing and Hyperpolarizing Bipolar Cells

Two different types of bipolar cells provide opposing excitatory and inhibitory signals in the visual pathway, the *depolarizing bipolar cell* and the *hyperpolarizing bipolar cell.* That is, some bipolar cells depolarize when the rods and cones are excited, and others hyperpolarize. An importance of this reciprocal relationship between depolarizing and hyperpolarizing bipolar cells is that it provides a second mechanism for lateral inhibition in addition to the horizontal cell mechanism. Since depolarizing and hyperpolarizing bipolar cells lie immediately against each other, this gives an extremely acute mechanism for separating contrast borders in the visual image even when the border lies exactly between two adjacent photoreceptors.

The Amacrine Cells and Their Functions

About 30 different types of amacrine cells have been identified by morphological or histochemical means. The functions of a half dozen different types of amacrine cells have been characterized, and all of these are different from each other. It is probable that other amacrine cells have many additional functions yet to be determined.

One type of amacrine cell is part of the direct pathway for rod vision—that is, from rod to bipolar cells to amacrine cells to ganglion cells.

Another type of amacrine cell responds very strongly at the onset of a visual signal, but the response dies out rapidly. Other amacrine cells respond very strongly at the offset of visual signals, but again the response dies quickly. Finally, still other amacrine cells respond when a light is turned on or off, signalling simply a change in illumination irrespective of direction.

Still another type of amacrine cell responds to movement of a spot across the retina in a specific direction; therefore, these amacrine cells are said to be *directional sensitive.*

In a sense, then, amacrine cells are types of interneurons that help in the beginning analysis of visual signals before they ever leave the retina.

Excitation of the Ganglion Cells

Connectivity of the Ganglion Cells with Cones in the Fovea and with Rods and Cones in the Peripheral Retina. Each retina contains about 100,000,000 rods and 3,000,000 cones; yet the number of ganglion cells is only about 1,600,000. Thus, an average of 60 rods and 2 cones converge on each optic nerve fiber.

However, major differences exist between the peripheral retina and the central retina. As one approaches the fovea, fewer rods and cones converge on each optic fiber, and the rods and cones both become slenderer. These two effects progressively increase the acuity of vision toward the central retina. And in the very center, in the *fovea* itself, there are only slender cones, about 35,000 of them, and no rods at all. Also, the number of optic nerve fibers leading from this part of the retina is almost equal to the number of cones, as illustrated to the right in Figure 35–1. This mainly explains the high degree of visual acuity in the central retina in comparison with much poorer acuity peripherally.

Another difference between the peripheral and central portions of the retina is a much greater sensitivity of the peripheral retina to weak light. This results partly from the fact that rods are about 300 times more sensitive to light than are cones, but it is further magnified by the fact that as many as 200 rods converge on the same optic nerve fiber in the more peripheral portions of the retina, so that the signals from the rods summate to give even more intense stimulation of the peripheral ganglion cells.

Three Different Types of Retinal Ganglion Cells and Their Respective Fields

There are three distinct groups of ganglion cells designated as W, X, and Y cells. Each of these serves a different function:

Transmission of Rod Vision by the W Cells. The W cells, constituting about 40 per cent of all the ganglion cells, are small, having a cell body diameter of less than 10 micrometers and transmitting signals in their optic nerve fibers at the slow velocity of only 8 m/sec. These ganglion cells receive most of their excitation from rods, transmitted by way of small bipolar cells and amacrine cells. They have very broad fields in the retina because their dendrites spread widely in the retina.

On the basis of histology as well as physiological experiments, it appears that the W cells are especially sensitive for detecting directional movement anywhere in the field of vision, and they probably also are important for much of our rod vision under dark conditions.

Transmission of the Visual Image and Color by the X Cells. The most numerous of the ganglion cells are the X cells, representing 55 per cent of the total. They are of medium cell body diameter, between 10 and 15 micrometers, and transmit signals in their optic nerve fibers at about 14 m/sec.

The X cells have very small fields because their dendrites do not spread widely in the retina. Because of this, the signals represent rather discrete retinal locations. Therefore, it is through the X cells that the visual image itself is mainly transmitted. Also, because every X cell receives input from at least one cone, X cell transmission is believed to be responsible for all color vision as well.

Function of the Y Cells in Transmitting Instantaneous Changes in the Visual Image. The Y cells are the largest of all, up to 35 micrometers in diameter, and they transmit their signals to the brain faster than 50 m/sec. However, they are also the fewest of all the ganglion cells, representing only 5 per cent of the total. Also, they have very broad dendritic fields, so that signals are picked up by these cells from widespread retinal areas.

The Y ganglion cells respond like many of the amacrine cells to rapid changes in the visual image, either rapid movement or rapid change in light intensity, sending bursts of signals for only a fraction of a second before the signal dies out. Therefore, these ganglion cells undoubtedly apprise the central nervous system almost instantaneously when an abnormal visual event occurs anywhere in the visual field, but without specifying with great accuracy the location of the event other than to give appropriate clues for moving the eyes toward the exciting vision.

Excitation of the Ganglion Cells

Spontaneous, Continuous Action Potentials in the Ganglion Cells. It is from the ganglion cells that the long fibers of the optic nerve lead into the brain. Because of the distance involved, the electrotonic method of conduction is no longer appropriate; and, true enough, ganglion cells transmit their signals by means of action potentials instead. Furthermore, even when unstimulated they still transmit continuous impulses at rates varying between 5 and 40 per second, with the larger nerve fibers, in general, firing more rapidly. The visual signals, in turn, are superimposed onto this background ganglion cell firing.

Transmission of Changes in Light Intensity —The On-Off Response. Many ganglion cells are especially excited by *changes* in light intensity. This is illustrated by the records of nerve impulses in Figure 35–2, showing in the upper panel strong excitation for a fraction of a second when a light was first turned on; then in another fraction of a second the level of excitation diminished. The lower tracing is from a ganglion cell located in the dark area lateral to the spot of light; this cell was markedly inhibited when the light was turned on because of lateral inhibition.

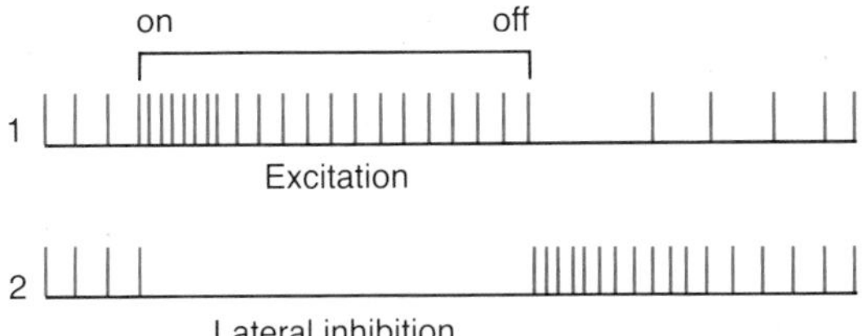

Figure 35-2. Responses of ganglion cells to light in (1) an area excited by a spot of light and (2) an area immediately adjacent to the excited spot; the ganglion cells in this area are inhibited by the mechanism of lateral inhibition. (Modified from Granit: Receptors and Sensory Perception: A Discussion of Aims, Means, and Results of Electrophysiological Research into the Process of Reception. New Haven, Conn., Yale University Press, 1955.)

Then, when the light was turned off, exactly the opposite effects occurred. Thus, these records are called "on-off" and "off-on" responses. The opposite directions of these responses to light are caused, respectively, by the depolarizing and hyperpolarizing bipolar cells, and the transient nature of the responses was probably generated by the amacrine cells, many of which also have similar transient responses themselves.

This capability of the eyes to detect *change* in light intensity is as equally developed in the peripheral retina as in the central retina. For instance, a minute gnat flying across the peripheral field of vision is instantaneously detected. On the other hand, the same gnat sitting quietly remains entirely below the threshold of visual detection.

Transmission of Signals Depicting Contrasts in the Visual Scene—The Role of Lateral Inhibition

Most of the ganglion cells do not respond to the actual level of illumination of the scene; instead they respond mainly to contrast borders in the scene. Since it seems that this is the major means by which the form of the scene is transmitted to the brain, let us explain how this process occurs.

When flat light is applied to the entire retina—that is, when all the photoreceptors are stimulated equally by the incident light—the contrast type of ganglion cell is neither stimulated nor inhibited. The reason for this is that the signals transmitted *directly* from the photoreceptors through the depolarizing bipolar cells are excitatory, whereas the signals transmitted *laterally* through the horizontal cells and hyperpolarizing bipolar cells are inhibitory. Thus, the direct excitatory signal through one pathway is likely to be completely neutralized by the inhibitory signals through the lateral pathways. One circuit for this is illustrated in Figure 35-3, which shows three photoreceptors; the central one of these receptors excites a depolarizing bipolar cell. However, the two receptors on either side are connected to the same bipolar cell through inhibitory horizontal cells that neutralize the direct excitatory signal if the lateral two receptors are also stimulated by light.

Now, let us examine what happens when a contrast border occurs in the visual scene. Referring again to Figure 35-3, let us assume that the central photoreceptor is stimulated by a bright spot of light while one of the two lateral receptors is in the dark. The bright spot of light will excite the direct pathway through the bipolar cell. Then, in addition, the fact that one of the lateral photoreceptors is in the dark causes one of the horizontal cells to be inhibited. In turn, this cell loses its inhibitory effect on the bipolar cell, and this allows still more excitation of the bipolar cell. Thus, when light is everywhere, the excitatory and inhibitory signals to the bipolar cells mainly neutralize each other, but where contrasts occur the signals through the direct and lateral pathways actually accentuate each other.

Thus, the mechanism of lateral inhibition functions in the eye in the same way that it functions in most other sensory systems as well—that is, to provide contrast detection and enhancement.

Transmission of Color Signals by the Ganglion Cells

A single ganglion cell may be stimulated by a number of cones or by only a very few. When all three types of cones—the red, blue, and green types—stimulate the same ganglion cell, the signal transmitted through the ganglion cell is the same for any color of the spectrum.

On the other hand, some of the ganglion cells are excited by only one color type of cone but inhibited by

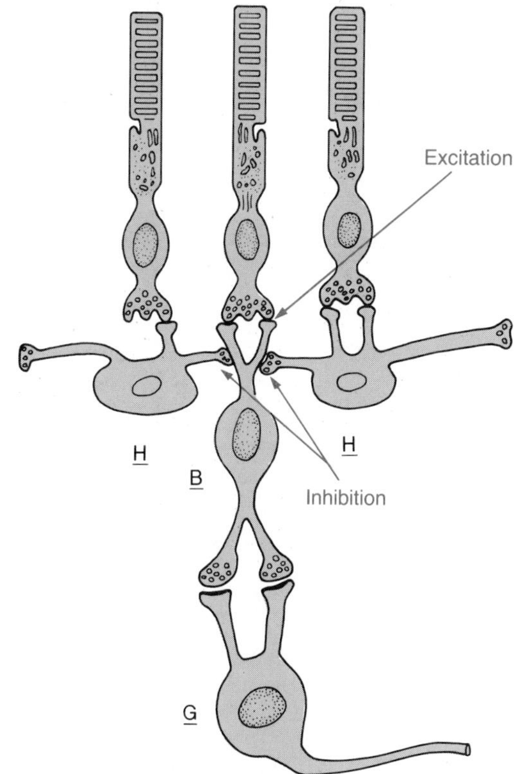

Figure 35-3. Typical arrangement of rods, horizontal cells (H), a bipolar cell (B), and a ganglion cell (G) in the retina, showing excitation at the synapses between the rods and the horizontal cells but inhibition between the horizontal cells and the bipolar cells.

a second type. For instance, this frequently occurs for the red and green cones, red causing excitation and green causing inhibition—or vice versa, with green causing excitation and red, inhibition. The same type of reciprocal effect also occurs between blue cones on the one hand and a combination of red and green cones on the other hand, giving a reciprocal excitation-inhibition relationship between the blue and yellow colors.

The mechanism of this opposing effect of colors is the following: One color-type cone excites the ganglion cell by the direct excitatory route through a depolarizing bipolar cell, while the other color-type cone inhibits the ganglion cell by the indirect inhibitory route through a horizontal cell or a hyperpolarizing bipolar cell.

The importance of these color-contrast mechanisms is that they represent a mechanism by which the retina itself begins to differentiate colors. Thus each color-contrast type of ganglion cell is excited by one color but inhibited by the "opponent color." Therefore, the process of color analysis begins in the retina and is not entirely a function of the brain.

The Visual Pathways into the Brain

Figure 35-4 illustrates the principal visual pathways from the two retinas to the *visual cortex.* After nerve impulses leave the retinas they pass backward through the *optic nerves.* At the *optic chiasm* all the fibers from the nasal halves of the retinas cross to the opposite side, where they join the fibers from the opposite temporal retinas to form the *optic tracts.* The fibers of each optic tract synapse in the *dorsal lateral geniculate nucleus,* and from here the *geniculocalcarine fibers* pass by way of the *optic radiation,* or *geniculocalcarine tract,* to the *primary visual cortex* in the calcarine area of the occipital lobe.

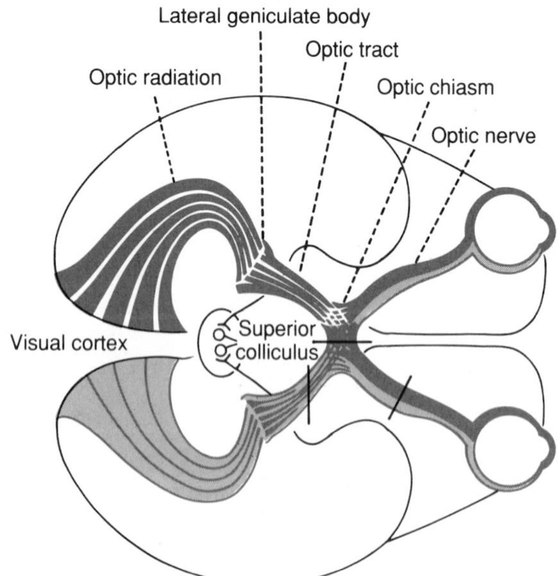

Figure 35-4. The principal visual pathways from the eyes to the visual cortex. (Modified from Polyak: The Retina. ©1941 by The University of Chicago. All rights reserved.)

In addition, visual fibers also pass to older precortical areas of the brain: especially important are fiber pathways (1) from the optic tracts into the *pretectal nuclei,* for eliciting some reflex movements of the eyes focused on objects of importance and also for activating the pupillary light reflex, and (2) into the *superior colliculus,* for control of rapid directional movements of the two eyes.

Thus, the visual pathways can be divided roughly into an *old system* to the midbrain and a *new system* for direct transmission into the visual cortex. The new system is responsible in human beings for the perception of virtually all aspects of visual form, colors, and other conscious vision. On the other hand, in many lower animals, even visual form is detected by the older system, using the superior colliculus in the same manner that the visual cortex is used in mammals.

Function of the Dorsal Lateral Geniculate Nucleus

The optic nerve fibers of the new visual system all terminate in the *dorsal lateral geniculate nucleus,* located at the dorsal end of the thalamus and frequently called simply the *lateral geniculate body.* The dorsal lateral geniculate nucleus serves two principal functions: First, it serves as a relay station to relay visual information from the optic tract to the *visual cortex* by way of the *geniculocalcarine tract.* This relay function is very accurate, so much so that there is exact point-to-point transmission with a high degree of spatial fidelity all the way from the retina to the visual cortex.

It will be recalled that half the fibers in each optic tract, after passing the optic chiasm, are derived from one eye and half from the other eye, representing corresponding points on the two retinas. However, the signals from the two eyes are kept apart in the dorsal lateral geniculate nucleus. This nucleus is composed of six nuclear layers. Layers II, III, and V (from ventral to dorsal) receive signals from the temporal portion of the ipsilateral retina, whereas layers I, IV, and VI receive signals from the nasal retina of the opposite eye. The respective retinal areas of the two eyes connect with neurons that are approximately superimposed over each other in the paired layers, and similar parallel transmission is preserved all the way back to the visual cortex.

The second major function of the dorsal lateral geniculate nucleus is to "gate" the transmission of signals to the visual cortex, that is, to control how much of the signal is allowed to pass to the cortex. The nucleus receives gating control signals from two major sources, (1) *corticofugal fibers* returning in a backward direction from the primary visual cortex to the lateral geniculate nucleus and (2) the reticular areas of the mesencephalon. Both of these are inhibitory and, when stimulated, can either turn off or suppress transmission through selected portions of the dorsal lateral geniculate nucleus.

Finally, the dorsal lateral geniculate nucleus is divided in another way: (1) Layers I and II are called *magnocellular layers* because they contain very large neurons. These receive their usual input almost entirely from the large type Y retinal ganglion cells. This magnocellular system provides a very rapidly conducting pathway to the visual cortex. On the other hand, it is "color blind," transmitting only black and white information. Also, its point-to-point transmission is poor, for there are not so many Y ganglion cells, and their dendrites spread widely in the retina. (2) Layers III through VI are called *parvocellular layers* because they contain large numbers of small to medium-sized neurons. These receive their input almost entirely from the type X retinal ganglion cells that transmit color and also convey accurate point-to-point spatial information but at only a moderate velocity of conduction, rather than high velocity.

ORGANIZATION AND FUNCTION OF THE VISUAL CORTEX

Figures 35-5 and 35-6 show that the *visual cortex* is located primarily in the occipital lobes. Like the cortical representations of the other sensory systems, the visual cortex is divided into a *primary visual cortex* and *secondary visual areas.*

The Primary Visual Cortex. The primary visual cortex (Figure 35-6) lies in the *calcarine fissure area* and extends to the *occipital pole* on the medial aspect of each occipital cortex. This area is the terminus of the most direct visual signals from the eyes. Signals from the macular area of the retina terminate near the occipital pole, while signals from the more peripheral retina terminate in concentric circles anterior to the pole and along the calcarine fissure. Note in the figure the especially large area that represents the macula. The fovea transmits its signals to this region. The fovea is responsible for the highest degree of visual acuity. Based on retinal area, the fovea has several hundred times as much representation in the primary visual cortex as do the peripheral portions of the retina.

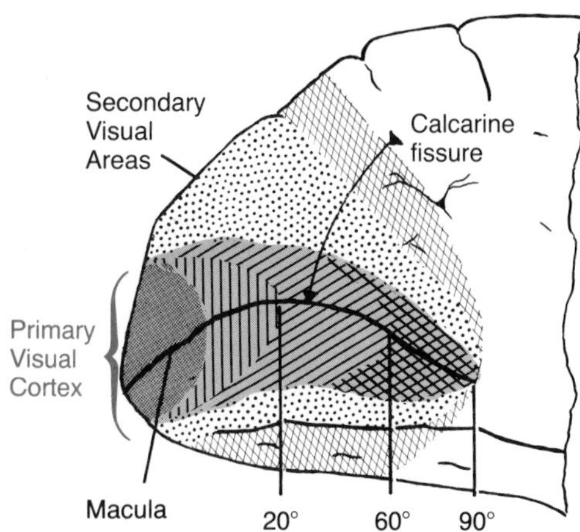

Figure 35-6. The visual cortex.

Still another name for the primary visual cortex is the *striate cortex,* because this area has a grossly striated appearance.

The Secondary Visual Areas. The secondary visual areas, also called *visual association areas,* lie anterior, superior, and inferior to the primary visual cortex. Secondary signals are transmitted to these areas for further analysis of visual meanings. The importance of these areas is that various aspects of the visual image are progressively dissected and analyzed in separate ones.

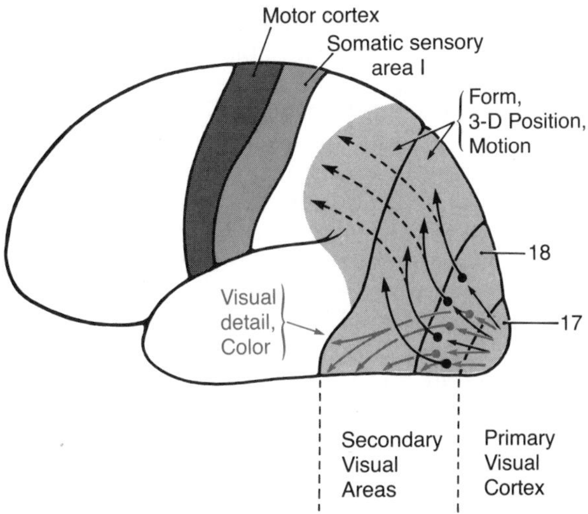

Figure 35-5. Transmission of visual signals from the primary visual cortex into secondary visual areas. Note that the signals representing form, third dimensional position, and motion are transmitted mainly superiorly into the superior portions of the occipital lobe and the posterior parietal lobe. By contrast, the signals for visual detail and color are transmitted mainly into the anteroventral portion of the occipital lobe and ventral portion of the posterior temporal lobe.

The Layered Structure of the Primary Visual Cortex

Like almost all other portions of the cerebral cortex, the primary visual cortex has six distinct layers, as illustrated in Figure 35-7. As is true for the other sensory systems, the geniculocalcarine fibers terminate mainly in layer IV. But this layer, too, is organized in subdivisions. As illustrated to the left, the rapidly conducted signals from the Y retinal ganglion cells terminate in layer 4cα and from here are relayed vertically both outward toward the cortical surface and inward toward deeper levels.

Shown to the right in Figure 35-7, the visual signals from the medium-sized optic nerve fibers, derived from the X ganglion cells in the retina, also terminate in layer 4 but at points different from the Y signals, in layers 4a and 4cβ, the shallowest and deepest portions of layer 4. From here, these signals again are transmitted vertically both toward the surface of the cortex and to deeper layers. These X ganglion pathways transmit the very accurate point-to-point type of vision and also color vision.

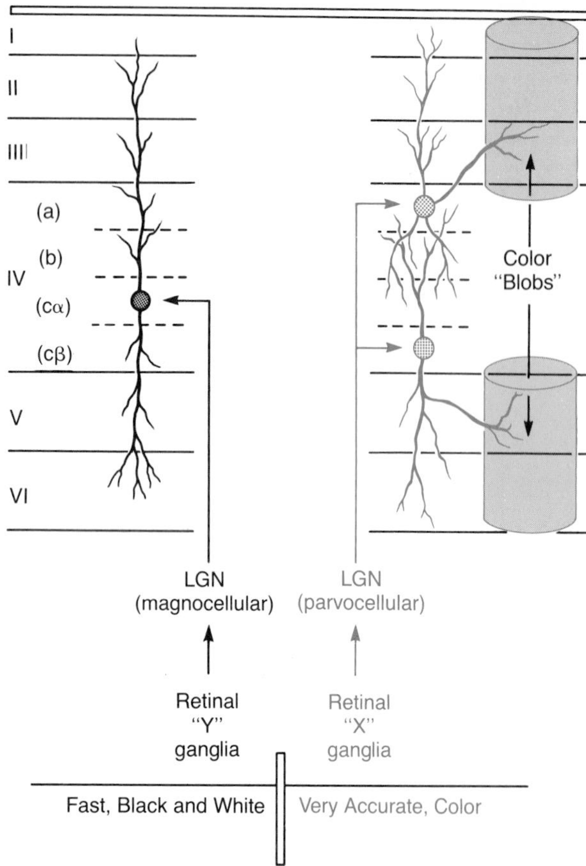

Figure 35-7. The six layers of the primary visual cortex. The connections to the left transmit very rapidly changing black and white visual signals. The pathways to the right transmit signals depicting very accurate detail and also color. Note especially small areas of the visual cortex called "color blobs" that are necessary for detection of color.

The Vertical Neuronal Columns in the Visual Cortex. The visual cortex is organized structurally into several million vertical columns of neuronal cells, each column having a diameter of 30 to 50 micrometers. This same vertical columnar organization is found throughout the cerebral cortex. Each column represents a functional unit. One can calculate from rough data that the number of neurons in each of the visual vertical columns is around 1000.

After the optic signals terminate in layer 4, they are further processed as they spread both outward and inward along each vertical column unit. The signals that pass outward to layers 1, 2, and 3 eventually transmit higher orders of signals for short distances laterally in the cortex. On the other hand, the signals that pass inward to layers 5 and 6 excite neurons that transmit signals much greater distances.

The Color "Blobs" in the Visual Cortex. Interspersed among the primary visual columns are special column-like areas called *color blobs.* These receive lateral signals from the adjacent visual columns and respond specifically to color signals. Therefore, it is presumed that these blobs are the primary areas for deciphering color. Also, in certain secondary visual areas additional color blobs are found, which presumably perform still higher levels of color deciphering.

Interaction of Visual Signals from the Separate Eyes. Recall that the visual signals from the two separate eyes are relayed through separate neuronal layers in the lateral geniculate nucleus. And these signals still remain separated from each other when they arrive in layer 4 of the primary visual cortex. However, as the signals spread vertically into the more superficial or deeper layers of the cortex, this separation is lost because of lateral spread of the visual signals. In the meantime the cortex deciphers whether the respective areas of the two visual images are "in register" with each other, that is, whether corresponding points on the two retinas fit with each other. In turn, this deciphered information is used to control the movements of the eyes so that they will fuse with each other (brought into "register").

Two Major Pathways for Analysis of Visual Information—The Fast "Position" and "Motion" Pathway; The Visual Detail, Color Pathway

Figure 35-5 shows that after leaving the primary visual cortex, the visual information is analyzed in two major pathways in the secondary visual areas.

1. Analysis of Three-Dimensional Position, Gross Form, and Motion of Objects. One of the analytical pathways, illustrated in Figure 35-5 by the broad black arrows, analyzes the third dimensional positions of visual objects in the coordinates of space around the body. From this information, this pathway also analyzes the overall form of the visual scene as well as motion in the scene. In other words, this pathway tells "where" every object is at each instant and whether it is moving. After leaving the primary visual cortex, the signals of this pathway next flow generally into the posterior midtemporal area, and thence upward into the broad occipitoparietal cortex. At the anterior border of this last area, the signals overlap with signals from the posterior somatic association areas that analyze form and three-dimensional aspects of somatic sensory signals. The signals transmitted in this position-form-motion pathway are mainly from the large Y optic nerve fibers of the retinal Y ganglion cells, transmitting rapid signals but only black and white signals.

2. Analysis of Visual Detail and Color. The red arrows in Figure 35-5, passing from the primary visual cortex into the inferior ventral and medial regions of the occipital and temporal cortex, illustrate the principal pathway for analysis of visual detail. Also, separate portions of this pathway specifically dissect out color as well. Therefore, this pathway is concerned with such visual feats as recognizing letters, reading, determining the texture of surfaces, determining detailed colors of objects, and deciphering from all this information "what" the object is and its meaning.

NEURONAL PATTERNS OF STIMULATION DURING ANALYSIS OF THE VISUAL IMAGE

Analysis of Contrasts in the Visual Image. If a person looks at a blank wall, only a few neurons in the primary visual cortex will be stimulated, whether the illumination of the wall is bright or weak. Therefore, the question must be asked, What does the visual cortex detect? To answer this, let us now place on the wall a large solid cross as illustrated to the left in Figure 35-8. To the right is illustrated the spatial pattern of the greater majority of the excited neurons in the visual cortex. *Note that the areas of maximal excitation occur along the sharp borders of the visual pattern.* Thus, the visual signal in the primary visual cortex is concerned mainly with the *contrasts* in the visual scene, rather than with the flat areas. We saw in the previous chapter that this is true of most of the retinal ganglion cells as well, because equally stimulated adjacent retinal receptors mutually inhibit each other. But at any border in the visual scene where there is a change from dark to light or light to dark, mutual inhibition does not occur, and the intensity of stimulation is proportional to the *gradient of contrast* — that is, the greater the sharpness of contrast and the greater the intensity difference between the light and dark areas, the greater the degree of stimulation.

Detection of Orientation of Lines and Borders — The "Simple" Cells. Not only does the visual cortex detect the existence of lines and borders in the different areas of the retinal image, but it also detects the orientation of each line or border — that is, whether it is vertical or horizontal or lies at some degree of inclination. This is believed to result from linear organizations of mutually inhibiting cells that excite second order neurons. Thus, for each such orientation of a line, a specific neuronal cell is stimulated. These neuronal cells are called *simple cells.* They are found mainly in layer 4 of the primary visual cortex.

Detection of Line Orientation When the Line Is Displaced Laterally or Vertically in the Visual Field — "Complex" Cells. As the signal progresses farther away from layer 4, some neurons now respond to lines still oriented in the same direction but not position-specific. That is, the line can be displaced moderate distances laterally or vertically in any direction in the field, and still the neuron will be stimulated if the line has the same direction. These cells are called *complex cells.*

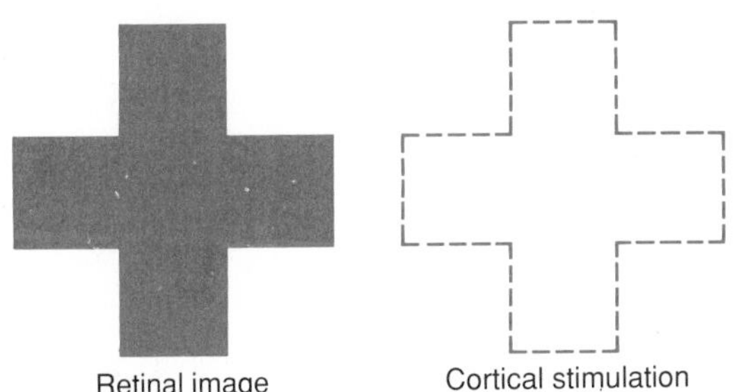

Figure 35-8. Pattern of excitation occurring in the visual cortex in response to a retinal image of a dark cross.

Detection of Lines of Specific Lengths, Angles, or Other Shapes. Many neurons in the outer layers of the primary visual columns, as well as neurons in some secondary visual areas, are stimulated only by lines or borders of specific lengths, or by specific angulated shapes, or by images having other characteristics. Thus, these neurons detect still higher orders of information from the visual scene; therefore, they are called *hypercomplex cells.*

Thus, as one goes farther into the analytical pathway of the visual cortex, progressively more characteristics of each area of the visual scene are deciphered.

Detection of Color

Color is detected by means of color contrast. The contrasts are mainly between cones that lie immediately adjacent to each other. For instance, a red area is often contrasted against a green area, or a blue area against a red, or a green area against a combination of red and green, which is yellow. All these colors can also be contrasted against a white area within the visual scene.

The mechanism of color contrast analysis depends on the fact that contrasting colors, called opponent colors, mutually excite certain of the neuronal cells. It is presumed that the initial details of color contrast are detected by simple cells, whereas more complex contrasts are detected by complex and hypercomplex cells.

EYE MOVEMENTS AND THEIR CONTROL

To make use of the abilities of the eye, almost equally as important as the system for interpretation of the visual signals from the eyes is the cerebral control system for directing the eyes toward the object to be viewed.

Muscular Control of Eye Movements. The eye movements are controlled by three separate pairs of muscles, shown in Figure 35-9: (1) the *medial* and *lateral recti,* (2) the *superior* and *inferior recti,* and (3) the *superior* and *inferior obliques.* The medial and lateral recti contract reciprocally mainly to move the eyes from side to side. The superior and inferior recti contract reciprocally to move the eyes mainly upward or downward. And the oblique muscles function mainly to rotate the eyeballs to keep the visual fields in the upright position.

Neural Pathways for Control of Eye Movements. Figure 35-9 also illustrates the nuclei of the third, fourth, and sixth cranial nerves and their innervation of the ocular muscles. Shown, too, are the

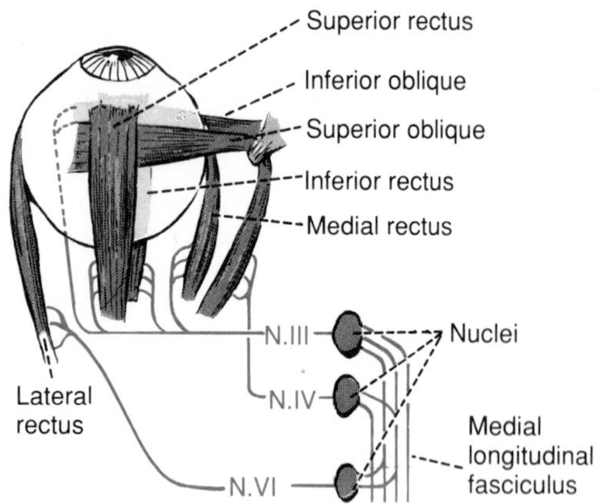

Figure 35-9. The extraocular muscles of the eye and their innervation.

interconnections among these three nuclei through the *medial longitudinal fasciculus.* Either by way of this fasciculus or by way of other closely associated pathways, each of the three sets of muscles to each eye is *reciprocally* innervated so that one muscle of the pair relaxes while the other contracts.

Figure 35-10 illustrates cortical control of the oculomotor apparatus, showing spread of signals from the occipital visual areas through occipitotectal and occipitocollicular tracts into the pretectal and superior colliculus areas of the brain stem. In addition, a frontotectal tract passes from the frontal cortex into the pretectal area. From both the pretectal and the superior colliculus areas, the oculomotor control signals then pass to the nuclei of the oculomotor nerves. Strong signals are also transmitted into the oculomotor system from the vestibular nuclei by way of the medial longitudinal fasciculus.

Fixation Movements of the Eyes

Perhaps the most important movements of the eyes are those that cause the eyes to "fix" on a discrete portion of the field of vision.

The fixation mechanism that causes the eyes to "lock" on the object of attention is controlled by *secondary visual areas of the occipital cortex.* This locking results from a negative feedback that prevents the object of attention from leaving the foveal portion of the retina. When the image of the object drifts away from the middle of the fovea and reaches its edge, a sudden reflex reaction occurs, producing a flicking movement that moves the image back toward the central portion of the fovea. That is, if the drift is to the top, the flicking movement is downward. If the drift is to one side, the flicking movement is in the opposite direction back toward the center of the fovea. Thus, the image is kept on the foveal region of the eye until the eye focuses attention on some other portion of the visual scene.

The neuronal circuit for the fixation movements begins with recognition of the drift in the secondary

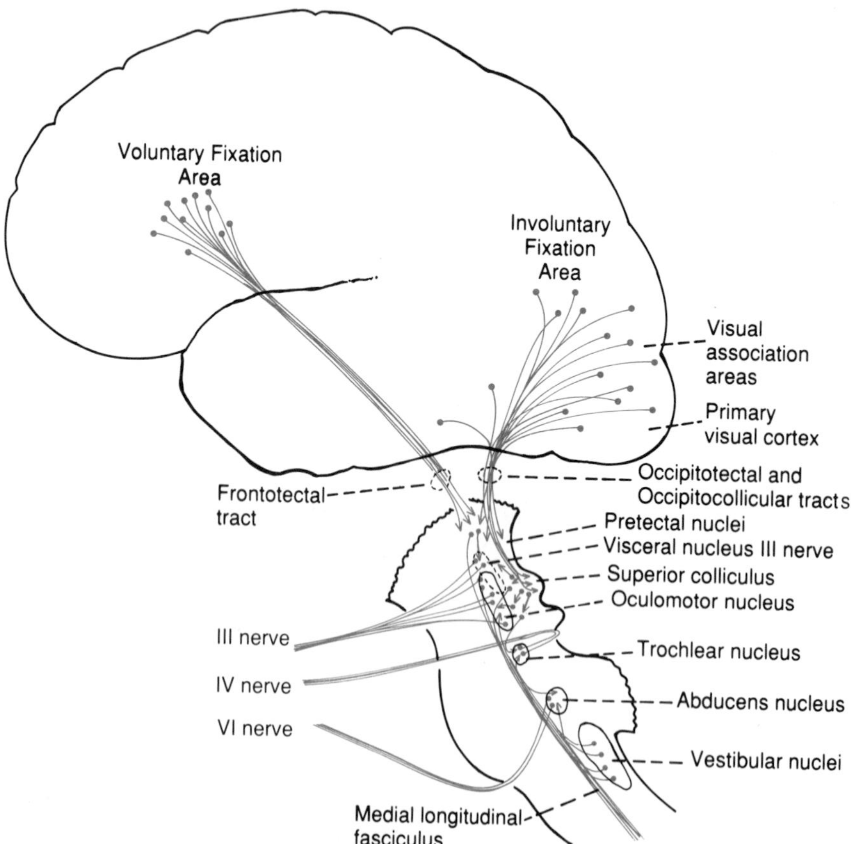

Figure 35-10. Neural pathways for control of conjugate movement of the eyes.

visual areas of the visual cortex. Then, appropriate signals are sent by way of the superior colliculi and eventually the oculomotor nuclei to cause the eye movements.

Fusion of the Visual Images from the Two Eyes

To make the visual perceptions more meaningful, the visual images in the two eyes normally *fuse* with each other on "corresponding points" of the two retinas.

The visual cortex plays a very important role in fusion. It was pointed out earlier in the chapter that corresponding points of the two retinas transmit visual signals to different neuronal layers of the lateral geniculate body, and these signals in turn are relayed to parallel stripes of neurons in the visual cortex. Interactions occur between the stripes of cortical neurons; these cause *interference patterns of excitation* in some of the local neuronal cells when the two visual images are not precisely "in register"—that is, not precisely fused. This excitation presumably provides the signal that is transmitted to the oculomotor apparatus to cause convergence or divergence or rotation of the eyes so that fusion can be reestablished. Once the corresponding points of the retinas are precisely in register with each other, the excitation of the specific cells in the visual cortex is greatly diminished or disappears.

The Neural Mechanism of Stereopsis for Judging Distances of Visual Objects

In the previous chapter, it was pointed out that because the two eyes are more than 2 inches apart the images on the two retinas are not exactly the same. That is, the right eye sees a little more of the right-hand side of the object and the left eye a little more of the left-hand side, and the closer the object the greater the disparity. Therefore, even when the two eyes are fused with each other, it is still impossible for all corresponding points in the two visual images to be absolutely in register at the same time. The degree of nonregister provides the mechanism for *stereopsis,* a very important mechanism for judging distances of visual objects up to about 100 meters.

The neuronal cellular mechanism for stereopsis is based on the fact that some of the fiber pathways from the retinas to the visual cortex stray 1 to 2 degrees on either side of the central pathway. Therefore, some optic pathways from the two eyes will be exactly in register for objects 2 meters away; and still another set of pathways will be in register for objects 75 meters away. Thus, the distance is determined by which set of pathways interact with each other. This phenomenon is called *depth perception,* which is another name for stereopsis.

AUTONOMIC CONTROL OF ACCOMMODATION AND PUPILLARY APERTURE

The Autonomic Nerves to the Eyes. The eye is innervated by both parasympathetic and sympathetic fibers, as illustrated in Figure 35–11. The parasympathetic preganglionic fibers arise in the *Edinger-Westphal nucleus* (the visceral nucleus of the third nerve) and then pass in the *third nerve* to the *ciliary ganglion,* which lies immediately behind the eye. Here the preganglionic fibers synapse with postganglionic parasympathetic neurons that, in turn, excite the ciliary muscle and the sphincter of the iris.

The sympathetic innervation of the eye originates in the *intermediolateral horn cells* of the first thoracic segment of the spinal cord. From here, sympathetic fibers enter the sympathetic chain and pass upward to the *superior cervical ganglion,* where they synapse with postganglionic neurons. Fibers from these spread along the carotid artery and successively smaller arteries until they reach the eye. There the sympathetic fibers innervate the radial fibers of the iris as well as several extraocular structures around the eye.

Control of Accommodation (Focusing the Eyes)

The accommodation mechanism—that is, the mechanism that focuses the lens system of the eye—

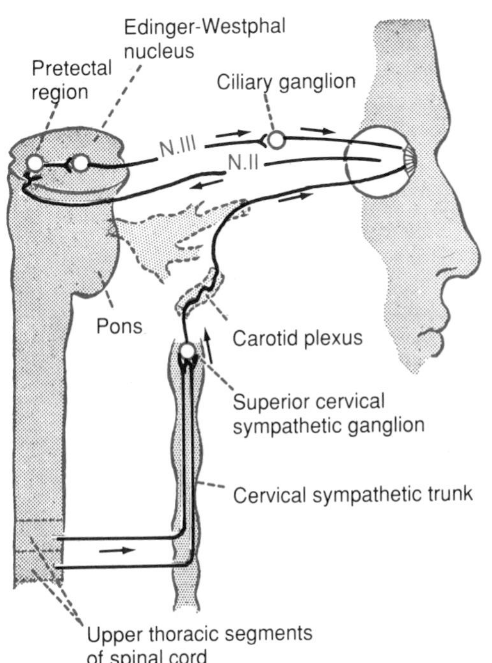

Figure 35–11. Autonomic innervation of the eye, showing also the reflex arc of the light reflex. (Modified from Ranson and Clark: Anatomy of the Nervous System. Philadelphia, W. B. Saunders Company, 1959.)

is essential for a high degree of visual acuity. Accommodation results from contraction or relaxation of the ciliary muscle, contraction causing increased strength of the lens system, as explained in the previous chapter, and relaxation causing decreased strength. The question that must be answered now is, How does a person adjust accommodation to keep the eyes in focus all the time?

Accommodation of the lens is regulated by a negative feedback mechanism that automatically adjusts the focal power of the lens for the highest degree of visual acuity. When the eyes have been fixed on some far object and then suddenly fix on a near object, the lens accommodates for maximal acuity of vision usually within less than 1 second. Though the precise control mechanism that causes this rapid and accurate focusing of the eye is still unclear, some of the different types of clues that help the lens change its strength in the proper direction include the following: (1) When the eyes fixate on a near object they also converge toward each other. The neural mechanisms for *convergence cause a simultaneous signal to strengthen the lens of the eye.* (2) *Because the fovea lies in a hollowed-out depression that is deeper than the remainder of the retina, the clarity of focus in the depth of the fovea versus the clarity of focus on the edges will be different.* It has been suggested that this also gives clues as to which way the strength of the lens needs to be changed. (3) It has been found that *the degree of accommodation of the lens oscillates slightly* all of the time, at a frequency up to two times per second. It has been suggested that the visual image becomes clearer when the oscillation of the lens strength is changing in the appropriate direction and poorer when the lens strength is changing in the wrong direction. This could give a rapid cue as to which way the strength of the lens needs to change to provide appropriate focus.

It is presumed that the cortical areas that control accommodation closely parallel those that control fixation movements of the eyes, with final integration of the visual signals in the occipital cortex and transmission of motor signals to the ciliary muscle through the pretectal area and Edinger-Westphal nucleus.

Control of Pupillary Diameter

Stimulation of the parasympathetic nerves excites the pupillary sphincter muscle, thereby decreasing the pupillary aperture; this is called *miosis.* On the other hand, stimulation of the sympathetic nerves excites the radial fibers of the iris and causes pupillary dilatation, which is called *mydriasis.*

The Pupillary Light Reflex. When light entering the eyes increases, the pupils constrict, a reaction called the *pupillary light reflex.* The neuronal pathway for this reflex is illustrated in Figure 35–11. When light impinges on the retina, the resulting impulses pass through the optic nerves and optic tracts to the pretectal nuclei. From here, impulses pass to the *Edinger-Westphal nucleus* and finally back through the *parasympathetic nerves* to constrict the sphincter of the iris. In darkness, the reflex becomes inhibited, which results in dilatation of the pupil.

The function of the light reflex is to help the eye adapt extremely rapidly to changing light conditions, as explained in the previous chapter. The limits of pupillary diameter are about 1.5 millimeters on the small side and 8 millimeters on the large side. Therefore, the range of light adaptation that can be effected by the pupillary reflex is about 30 to 1.

REFERENCES

Andersen, R. A.: Visual and eye movement functions of the posterior parietal cortex. Annu. Rev. Neurosci., 12:377, 1989.

Bahill, A. T., and Hamm, T. M.: Using open-loop experiments to study physiological systems, with examples from the human eye-movement systems. News Physiol. Sci., 4:104, 1989.

Blasdel, G. G.: Visualization of neuronal activity in monkey striate cortex. Annu. Rev. Physiol., 51:561, 1989.

DeValois, R. L., and DeValois, K. K.: Spatial Vision. New York, Oxford University Press, 1988.

Guyton, D. L.: Sights and Sounds in Ophthalmology: Ocular Motility and Binocular Vision. St. Louis, C. V. Mosby Co., 1989.

Hubel, D. H., and Wiesel, T. N.: Brain mechanisms of vision. Sci. Am., 241(3):150, 1979.

Lennerstrand, G., et al. (eds.): Strabismus and Amblyopia. New York, Plenum Publishing Corp., 1988.

Livingstone, M., and Hubel, D.: Segregation of form, color, movement, and depth: Anatomy, physiology, and perception. Science, 240:740, 1988.

Lund, J. S.: Anatomical organization of Macaque monkey striate visual cortex. Annu. Rev. Neurosci., 11:253, 1988.

Reinecke, R. D., and Parks, M. M.: Strabismus. 3rd ed. East Norwalk, Conn., Appleton & Lange, 1987.

Sparks, D. L.: Translation of sensory signals into commands for control of saccadic eye movements: Role of primate superior colliculus. Physiol. Rev., 66:118, 1986.

Wolfe, J. M. (ed.): The Mind's Eye. New York, W. H. Freeman and Company, 1986.

QUESTIONS

1. Describe the visual pathway.
2. Describe in sequence the stimulation and the functions of the *rods* and *cones,* the *bipolar cells,* the *horizontal cells,* the *amacrine cells,* and the *ganglion cells.*
3. Explain the function of *lateral inhibition* in the retina as a means for highlighting contrasts in the visual scene.
4. Explain the transmission of color signals by ganglion cells.
5. Discuss the relaying of visual signals through the *lateral geniculate body.*
6. Where is the *primary visual cortex* located in the brain?
7. Describe the localization of signals from different parts of the retina in the primary visual cortex.
8. Explain why the visual cortex detects mainly lines and borders rather than flat areas in the visual scene.
9. How does the visual cortex function in the analysis of color?
10. What are the three separate pairs of *extraocular muscles* that control eye movements? Also, give the nervous pathways for control of the eye movements.

11. Explain the feedback mechanism, from the eye to the brain and back to the extraocular muscles, that causes fixation of the eyes on a particular spot in the visual scene.
12. What is the neural mechanism that causes *fusion* of the visual images from the two eyes?
13. Explain the neural mechanism for control of *accommodation.* What are some of the clues in the visual signals that help control accommodation?
14. Describe the neural circuitry for control of the diameter of the pupil.

36

The Sense of Hearing; The Chemical Senses of Taste and Smell

HEARING

The purpose of the first half of this chapter is to describe and explain the mechanism by which the ear receives sound waves, discriminates their frequencies, and finally transmits auditory information into the central nervous system.

The Tympanic Membrane and the Ossicular System

Figure 36–1 illustrates the *tympanic membrane* (commonly called the *eardrum)* and the *ossicular system,* which conducts sound through the middle ear. The tympanic membrane is cone shaped, with its concavity facing downward and outward toward the auditory canal. Attached to the very center of the tympanic membrane is the *handle* of the *malleus.* At its other end the malleus is tightly bound to the *incus* by ligaments so that whenever the malleus moves the incus moves with it. The opposite end of the incus in turn articulates with the stem of the *stapes,* and the *faceplate* of the stapes lies against the membranous labyrinth in the opening of the oval window where sound waves are conducted into the inner ear, the *cochlea.*

The ossicles of the middle ear are suspended by ligaments in such a way that the combined malleus and incus act as a single lever having its fulcrum approximately at the border of the tympanic membrane. The large *head* of the malleus, which is on the opposite side of the fulcrum from the handle, almost exactly balances the other end of the lever.

The articulation of the incus with the stapes causes the stapes to push forward on the cochlear fluid every time the handle of the malleus moves inward and to pull backward on the fluid every time the malleus moves outward, which promotes inward and outward motion of the faceplate at the oval window.

The handle of the malleus is constantly pulled inward by the *tensor tympani muscle,* which keeps the tympanic membrane tensed. This allows sound vibrations on *any* portion of the tympanic membrane to be transmitted to the malleus, which would not be true if the membrane were lax.

The surface area of the tympanic membrane is approximately 55 square millimeters, whereas the surface area of the stapes averages 3.2 square millimeters. This 17-fold difference times a 1.3-fold ratio of the lever system allows energy of a sound wave impinging on the tympanic membrane to be applied to the small faceplate of the stapes, causing approximately 22 times as much *pressure* on the fluid of the cochlea as is exerted by the sound wave against the tympanic membrane. Because fluid has far greater inertia than air, it is easily understood that increased amounts of pressure are needed to cause vibration in the fluid.

In the absence of the ossicular system and tympanum, sound waves can travel directly through the air of the middle ear and can enter the cochlea at the oval window. However, the sensitivity for hearing is then 15 to 20 decibels less than for ossicular transmission—equivalent to a decrease from a medium voice to a barely perceptible voice level.

Attenuation of Sound by Contraction of the Stapedius and Tensor Tympani Muscles. When loud sounds are transmitted through the ossicular system into the central nervous system, a reflex occurs after a latent period of 40 to 80 milliseconds to cause contraction of the *stapedius* and *tensor tympani*

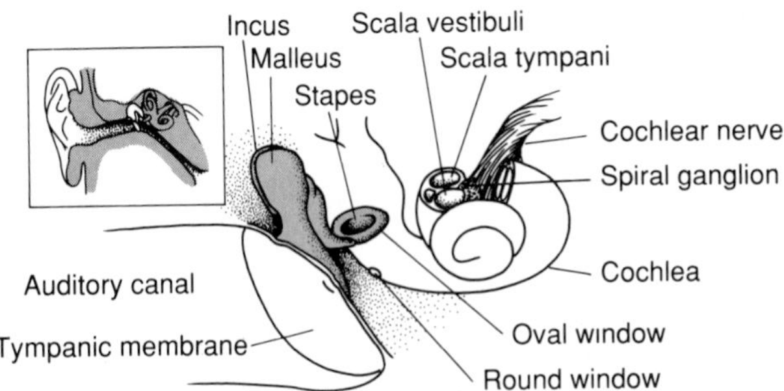

Figure 36-1. The tympanic membrane, the ossicular system of the middle ear, and the inner ear.

muscles. The tensor tympani muscle pulls the handle of the malleus inward while the stapedius muscle pulls the stapes outward. These two forces oppose each other and thereby cause the entire ossicular system to develop a high degree of rigidity, thus greatly reducing the ossicular conduction of low frequency sound, mainly frequencies below 1000 cycles per second.

This *attenuation reflex* can reduce the intensity of sound transmission by as much as 30 to 40 decibels, which is about the same difference as that between a loud voice and the sound of a whisper. The function of this mechanism is probably twofold:

1. To *protect* the cochlea from damaging vibrations caused by excessively loud sound.
2. To *mask* low frequency sounds in loud environments. This usually removes a major share of the background noise and allows a person to concentrate on sounds above 1000 cycles per second, where most of the pertinent information in voice communication is transmitted.

Another function of the tensor tympani and stapedius muscles is to decrease a person's hearing sensitivity to his or her own speech. This effect is activated by collateral signals transmitted to these muscles at the same time that the brain activates the voice mechanism.

Transmission of Sound Through Bone

Because the inner ear, the *cochlea,* is embedded in a bony cavity in the temporal bone called the bony labyrinth, vibrations of the entire skull can cause fluid vibrations in the cochlea itself. Therefore, under appropriate conditions, a tuning fork or an electronic vibrator placed on any bony protuberance of the skull, but especially on the mastoid process, causes the person to hear the sound.

The Cochlea

The cochlea is a system of coiled tubes, shown in Figure 36-1 and in cross section in Figures 36-2 and 36-3. It is composed of three different tubes coiled side by side: the *scala vestibuli,* the *scala media,* and the *scala tympani.* The scala vestibuli and scala media are separated from each other by *Reissner's membrane* (also called the *vestibular membrane*), shown in Figure 36-3; and the scala tympani and scala media are separated from each other by the *basilar membrane.* On the surface of the basilar membrane lies the *organ of Corti,* which contains a series of electromechanically sensitive cells, the *hair cells.* These are the receptive end-organs that generate nerve impulses in response to sound vibrations.

Figure 36-4 diagrams the functional parts of the uncoiled cochlea for conduction of sound vibrations. First, note that Reissner's membrane is missing from this figure. Reissner's membrane is so thin and so easily moved that it does not obstruct the passage of sound vibrations from the scala vestibuli into the scala media at all. Therefore, so far as the conduction of sound is concerned, the scala vestibuli and scala media are considered to be a single chamber. The importance of Reissner's membrane is to maintain a special fluid in the scala media that is required for normal function of the sound-receptive hair cells.

Sound vibrations enter the scala vestibuli from the faceplate of the stapes at the oval window. The faceplate covers this window and is connected with the window's edges by a relatively loose annular ligament so that it can move inward and outward with the sound vibrations. Inward movement causes the fluid to move into the scala vestibuli and scala media, and outward movement causes the fluid to move backward.

The Basilar Membrane and Resonance in the Cochlea. The basilar membrane is a fibrous membrane that separates the scala media and the scala tympani. It contains 20,000 to 30,000 *basilar fibers* that project from the bony center of the cochlea, the *modiolus,* toward the outer wall. These fibers are stiff, elastic, reedlike structures that are fixed at their basal ends in the central bony structure of the cochlea (the modiolus) but not fixed at their distal ends, except that the distal ends are embedded in the loose basilar membrane. Because the fibers are stiff and also free at one end, they can vibrate like reeds of a harmonica.

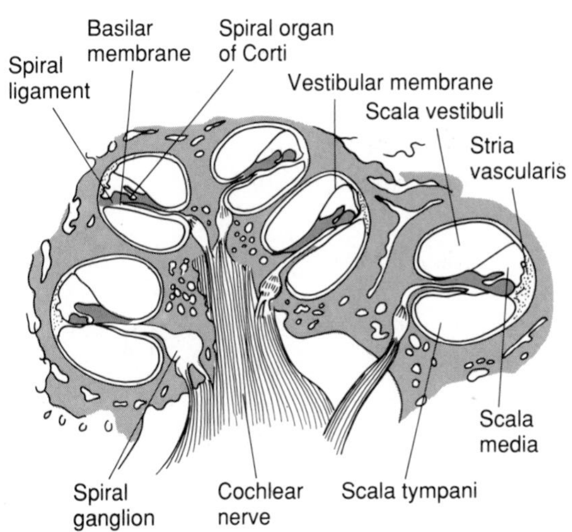

Figure 36-2. The cochlea. (From Goss, C. M. [ed.]: Gray's Anatomy of the Human Body. Philadelphia, Lea & Febiger.)

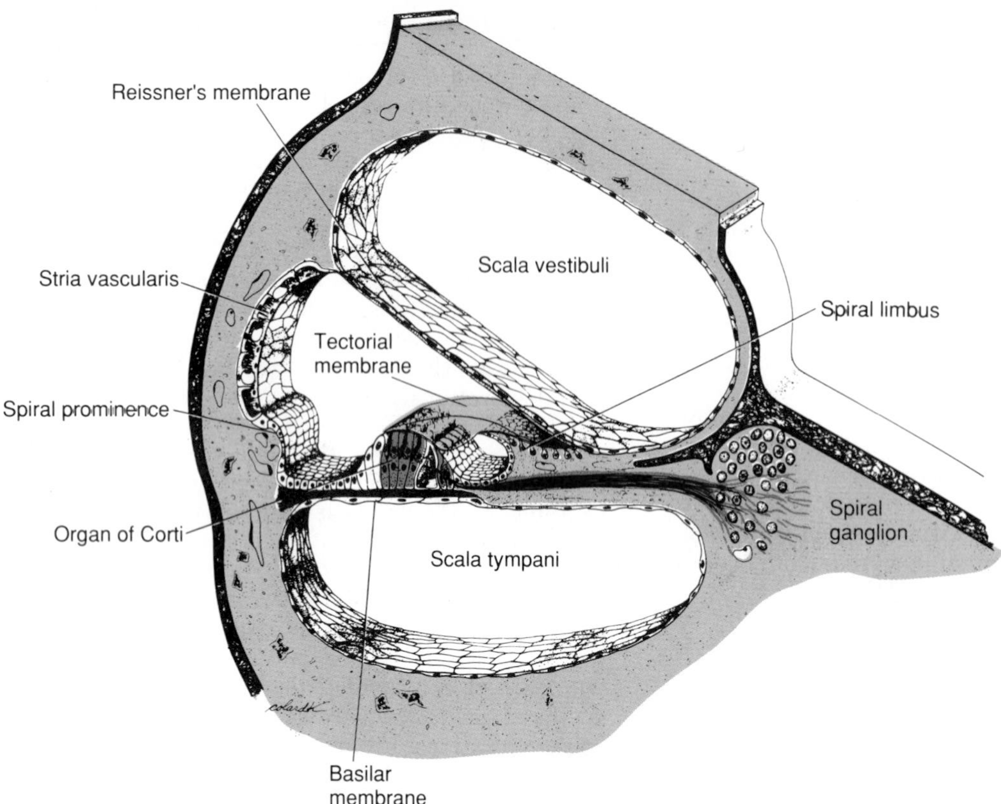

Figure 36-3. A section through one of the turns of the cochlea. (Drawn by Sylvia Colard Keene. From Fawcett: Bloom and Fawcett: A Textbook of Histology. 11th ed. Philadelphia, W. B. Saunders Company, 1986.)

The lengths of the basilar fibers increase progressively as one goes from the base of the cochlea to its apex, from a length of approximately 0.04 millimeter near the oval and round windows to 0.5 millimeter at the tip of the cochlea, a 12-fold increase in length.

The diameters of the fibers, on the other hand, decrease from the base to the helicotrema, so that their overall stiffness decreases more than 100-fold. As a result, the stiff, short fibers near the oval window of the cochlea will vibrate at a high frequency, whereas the long, limber fibers near the tip of the cochlea will vibrate at a low frequency.

Thus, high frequency resonance of the basilar membrane occurs near the base, where the sound waves enter the cochlea through the oval window; and low frequency resonance occurs near the apex mainly because of difference in stiffness of the fibers but also because of increased "loading" of the basilar membrane with extra amounts of fluid that must vibrate with the membrane at the apex.

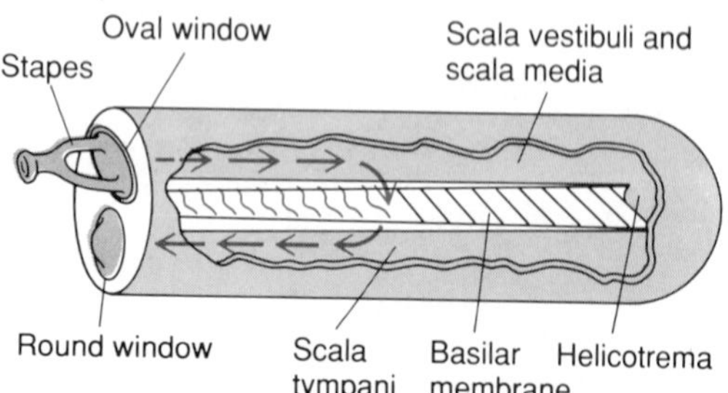

Figure 36-4. Movement of fluid in the cochlea following forward thrust of the stapes.

Transmission of Sound Waves in the Cochlea —The "Traveling Wave"

If the foot of the stapes moves inward instantaneously, the round window must also bulge outward instantaneously because the cochlea is bounded on all other sides by bony walls. Therefore, the initial effect is to cause the basilar membrane at the very base of the cochlea to bulge in the direction of the round window. However, the elastic tension that is built up in the basilar fibers as they bend toward the round window initiates a wave that "travels" along the basilar membrane toward the helicotrema, as illustrated in Figure 36-5. Figure 36-5A shows movement of a high frequency wave down the basilar membrane; Figure 36-5B, a medium frequency wave; and Figure 36-5C, a very low frequency wave. Movement of the wave along the basilar membrane is comparable to the movement of a wave that travels along the surface of a pond.

Pattern of Vibration of the Basilar Membrane for Different Sound Frequencies. Note in Figure 36-5 the different patterns of transmission for sound waves of different frequencies. Each wave is relatively weak at the outset but becomes strong when it reaches that portion of the basilar membrane that has a natural resonant frequency equal to the respec-

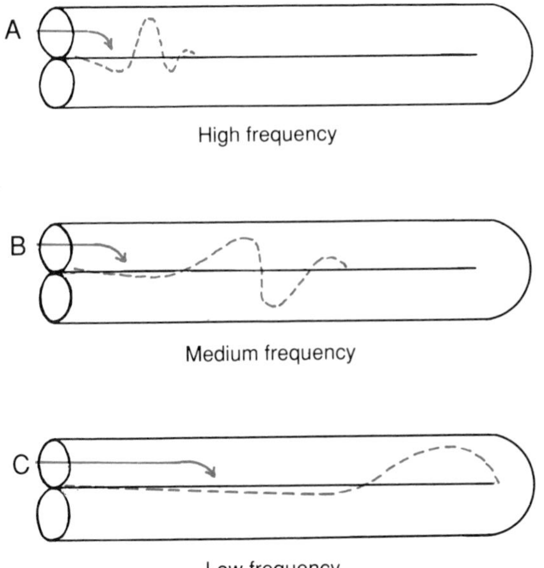

Figure 36-5. "Traveling waves" along the basilar membrane for high, medium, and low frequency sounds.

tive sound frequency. At this point the basilar membrane can vibrate back and forth with such great ease that the energy in the wave is completely dissipated. Consequently, the wave dies out at this point and fails to travel the remaining distance along the basilar membrane. A high frequency sound wave travels only a short distance along the basilar membrane before it reaches its resonant point and dies out; a medium frequency sound wave travels about halfway and then dies out; and finally, a very low frequency sound wave travels the entire distance along the membrane.

Thus, the maximum amplitude for a sound of 8000 cycles per second occurs near the base of the cochlea, whereas that for frequencies of less than 200 cycles per second is all the way at the tip of the basilar membrane near the helicotrema where the scala vestibuli opens into the scala tympani.

Function of the Organ of Corti

The organ of Corti, illustrated in Figures 36-2, 36-3, and 36-6, is the receptor organ that generates

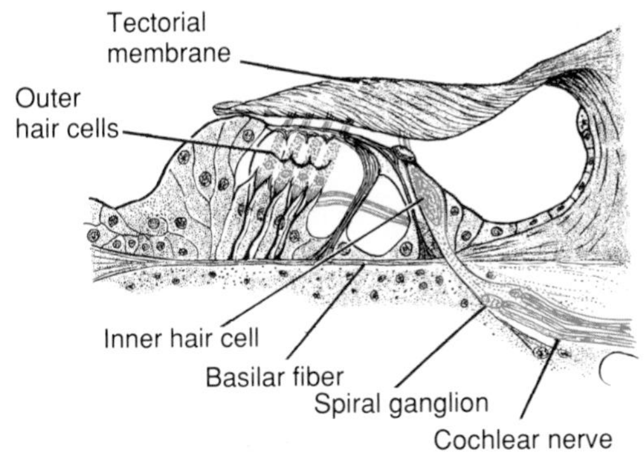

Figure 36-6. The organ of Corti, showing especially the hair cells and the tectorial membrane against the projecting hairs.

nerve impulses in response to vibration of the basilar membrane. Note that the organ of Corti lies on the surface of the basilar fibers and basilar membrane. The actual sensory receptors in the organ of Corti are two types of *hair cells,* a single row of *internal hair cells,* numbering about 3500 and measuring about 12 micrometers in diameter, and three to four rows of *external hair cells,* numbering about 15,000 and having diameters of only about 8 micrometers. The bases and sides of the hair cells synapse with a network of cochlear nerve endings. These lead to the *spiral ganglion of Corti,* which lies in the modiolus (the center) of the cochlea. The spiral ganglion in turn sends axons into the *cochlear nerve* and thence into the central nervous system at the level of the upper medulla.

Excitation of the Hair Cells. Note in Figure 36-6 that minute hairs, or *stereocilia,* project upward from the hair cells and either touch or are embedded in the surface gel coating of the *tectorial membrane,* which lies above the stereocilia in the scala media. Bending of the hairs in one direction depolarizes the hair cells, and bending them in the opposite direction hyperpolarizes them. This in turn excites the nerve fibers synapsing with their bases.

Upward movement of the basilar fibers rocks the hairs upward and *inward.* Then, when the basilar membrane moves downward, the hairs rock downward and *outward.* The inward and outward motion causes the hairs to shear back and forth against the tectorial membrane. Thus, the hair cells are excited whenever the basilar membrane vibrates.

When the basilar fibers bend toward the scala vestibuli, the hair cells depolarize, and in the opposite direction they hyperpolarize, thus generating an alternating hair cell receptor potential. This in turn stimulates the cochlear nerve endings that synapse with the bases of the hair cells. It is believed that a rapidly acting neurotransmitter, possibly glutamate, is released by the hair cells at these synapses during depolarization, but this is not certain.

Determination of Sound Frequency —The "Place" Principle

From earlier discussions in this chapter it is already apparent that low frequency sounds cause maximal activation of the basilar membrane near the apex of the cochlea, sounds of high frequency activate the basilar membrane near the base of the cochlea, and intermediate frequencies activate the membrane at intermediate distances between these two extremes. Furthermore, there is spatial organization of the nerve fibers in the cochlear pathway all the way from the cochlea to the cerebral cortex. And recording of signals from the auditory tracts in the brain stem and from the auditory receptive fields in the cerebral cortex shows that specific neurons are activated by specific sound frequencies. Therefore, the major method used by the nervous system to detect different frequencies is to determine the position along the basilar membrane that is most stimulated. This is called the *place principle* for determination of frequency (or of sound "pitch").

Determination of Loudness

Loudness is determined by the auditory system in at least three different ways: First, as the sound becomes louder, the amplitude of vibration of the basilar membrane and hair cells also increases, so that the hair cells excite the nerve endings at more rapid rates. Second, as the amplitude of vibration increases, it causes more and more of the hair cells on the fringes of the resonating portion of the basilar membrane to become stimulated, thus causing *spatial summation* of impulses — that is, transmission through many nerve fibers, rather than through a few. Third, certain hair cells do not become stimulated until the vibration of the basilar membrane reaches a relatively high intensity, and it is believed that stimulation of these cells in some way apprises the nervous system that the sound is then very loud.

Detection of Changes in Loudness. In the case of sound, the interpreted sensation changes approximately in proportion to the cube root of the actual sound intensity. To express this another way, the ear can discriminate differences in sound intensity from the softest whisper to the loudest possible noise, representing an *approximate 1 trillion times* increase in sound energy or 1 million times increase in amplitude of movement of the basilar membrane. Yet the ear interprets this much difference in sound level as approximately a 10,000-fold change. Thus, the scale of intensity is greatly "compressed" by the sound perception mechanisms of the auditory system. This obviously allows a person to interpret differences in sound intensities over an extremely wide range, a far broader range than would be possible were it not for compression of the scale.

The Decibel Unit. Because of the extreme changes in sound intensities that the ear can detect and discriminate, sound intensities are usually expressed in terms of the logarithm of their actual intensities. A tenfold increase in sound energy is called 1 *bel,* and 0.1 bel is called 1 *decibel.* One decibel represents an actual increase in sound energy of 1.26 times.

Another reason for using the decibel system in expressing changes in loudness is that, in the usual sound intensity range for communication, the ears can barely distinguish an approximate 1 decibel *change* in sound intensity.

Frequency Range of Hearing. The frequencies of sound that a young person can hear, before aging has occurred in the ears, is generally stated to be between 20 and 20,000 cycles per second. However, the sound range depends to a great extent on intensity. If the intensity is very low, the range may be only from 500 to 5000 cycles per second, and only with intense sounds can the complete range of 20 to 20,000 cycles be achieved. In old age, the frequency range falls to 50 to 8000 cycles per second or less.

Central Auditory Mechanisms

The Auditory Pathway

Figure 36–7 illustrates the major auditory pathways. It shows that nerve fibers from the *spiral ganglion of Corti* enter the *dorsal* and *ventral cochlear nuclei* located in the upper part of the medulla. At this point, all the fibers synapse, and second-order neurons pass mainly to the opposite side of the brain stem through the *trapezoid body* to the *superior olivary nucleus.* However, some second-order fibers also pass ipsilaterally to the superior olivary nucleus on the same side. From the superior olivary nucleus the auditory pathway then passes upward through the *lateral lemniscus;* and some, but not all, of the fibers terminate in the *nucleus of the lateral lemniscus.* Many bypass this nucleus and pass on to the inferior colliculus, where either all or almost all of them terminate. From here, the pathway passes to the *medial geniculate nucleus,* where all the fibers again synapse. And, finally, the auditory pathway proceeds by way of the *auditory radiation* to the *auditory cortex,* located mainly in the superior gyrus of the temporal lobe.

Several points of importance in relation to the auditory pathway should be noted. First, signals from both ears are transmitted through the pathways of both sides of the brain with only slight preponderance of transmission in the contralateral pathway. And in at least three different places in the brain stem crossing over occurs between the two pathways.

Second, many collateral fibers from the auditory tracts pass directly into the *reticular activating system of the brain stem.* This system projects diffusely upward into the cerebral cortex and downward into the spinal cord and activates the entire nervous system in response to a loud sound.

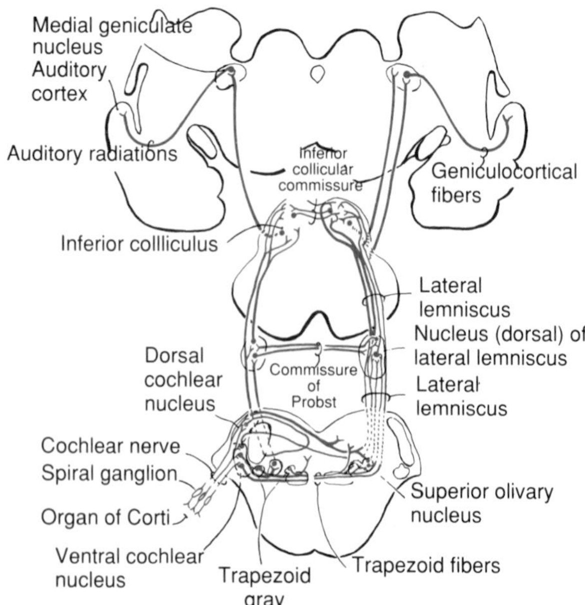

Figure 36–7. The auditory pathway. (Modified from Crosby, Humphrey, and Lauer: Correlative Anatomy of the Nervous System. New York, Macmillan, © 1962. Reprinted with permission.)

Third, a high degree of spatial orientation is maintained in the fiber tracts from the cochlea all the way to the cortex.

Function of the Cerebral Cortex in Hearing

The projection areas of the auditory pathway to the cerebral cortex are illustrated in Figure 36-8, which shows that the auditory cortex lies principally on the *supratemporal plane of the superior temporal gyrus* but also extends over the *lateral border of the temporal lobe,* over much of the *insular cortex,* and even into the most lateral portion of the *parietal operculum.*

Two separate areas are shown in Figure 36-8: the *primary auditory cortex* and the *auditory association cortex* (also called the *secondary auditory cortex*). The primary auditory cortex is directly excited by projections from the medial geniculate body, whereas the auditory association areas are excited secondarily by impulses from the primary auditory cortex and by projections from thalamic association areas adjacent to the medial geniculate body.

Sound Frequency Perception in the Primary Auditory Cortex. At least six different *tonotopic maps* have been found in the primary auditory cortex and auditory association areas. In each of these maps, high frequency sounds excite neurons at one end of the map, whereas low frequency sounds excite the neurons at the opposite end. In most, the low frequency sounds are located anteriorly, as shown in Figure 36-8; and the high frequency sounds, posteriorly. However, this is not true for all the maps. The question that one must ask is why does the auditory cortex have so many different tonotopic maps? The answer is presumably that each of the separate areas dissects out some specific feature of the sounds. For instance, one of the large maps in the primary auditory cortex almost certainly discriminates the sound frequencies themselves and gives the person the psychic sensation of sound pitches. Another one of the maps probably is used to detect the direction from which the sound comes.

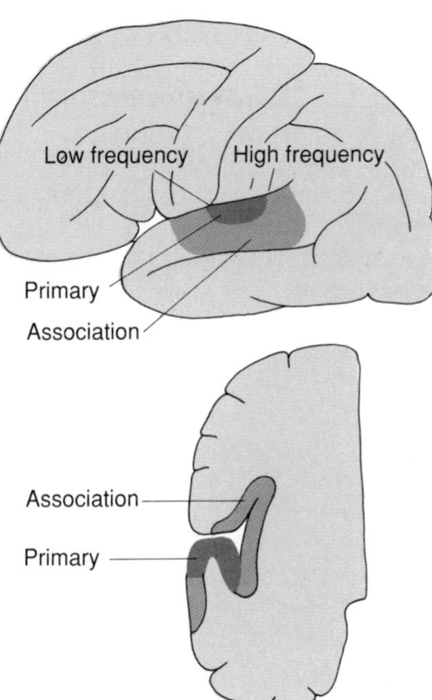

Figure 36-8. The auditory cortex.

Discrimination of Sound "Patterns" by the Auditory Cortex. Complete bilateral removal of the auditory cortex does not prevent a cat or monkey from detecting sounds or reacting in a crude manner to the sounds. However, it does greatly reduce or sometimes even abolish its ability to discriminate different sound pitches and especially *patterns of sound.* For instance, an animal that has been trained to recognize a combination or sequence of tones, one following the other in a particular pattern, loses this ability when the auditory cortex is destroyed; and, furthermore, it cannot relearn this type of response. Therefore, the auditory cortex is important in the discrimination of *tonal* and *sequential sound patterns.*

Total destruction of both primary auditory cortices in the human being is said to greatly reduce sensitivity for hearing, which is quite different from the effect in lower animals. However, this information is not clear. On the other hand, destruction of the primary auditory cortex on only one side in the human being has little effect on hearing because of the many crossover connections from side to side in the neural pathway.

Discrimination of the Direction from Which Sound Emanates

Destruction of the auditory cortex on both sides of the brain, in either human beings or lower mammals, causes loss of almost all ability to detect the direction from which sound comes. Yet the mechanism for this detection process begins in the superior olivary nuclei, even though it requires the neural pathways all the way from these nuclei to the cortex for interpretation of the signals. The mechanism is believed to be the following:

First, the superior olivary nucleus is divided into two sections, (1) the *medial superior olivary nucleus* and (2) the *lateral superior olivary nucleus.* The lateral nucleus is concerned with detecting the direction from which the sound is coming by the *difference in intensities of the sound* reaching the two ears, presumably by simply comparing the two intensities and sending an appropriate signal to the auditory cortex to estimate the direction.

The *medial superior olivary nucleus,* on the other hand, has a very specific mechanism for *detecting the time-lag between acoustic signals entering the two ears.* This nucleus contains large numbers of neurons that have two major dendrites, one projecting to the right and the other to the left. The acoustical signal from the right ear impinges on the right dendrite, and the signal from the left ear impinges on the left dendrite. The intensity of excitation of each of these neurons is highly sensitive to a specific time-lag between the two acoustical signals from the two ears. That is, the neurons near one border of the nucleus respond maximally to a short time-lag; whereas those near the opposite border respond to a very long time-lag; and those between, to intermediate time-lags. Thus, a spatial pattern of the neuronal stimulation develops in the medial superior olivary nucleus, with sound from directly in front of the head stimulating one set of olivary neurons maximally and sounds from different side angles stimulating other sets of neurons on opposite sides of the straight front neurons. This spatial orientation of signals is then transmitted all the way to the auditory cortex, where sound direction is determined by the locus in the cortex that is stimulated maximally.

This mechanism for detection of sound direction indicates again how information in sensory signals is dissected out as the signals pass through different levels of neuronal activity. In this case, the "quality" of sound direction is separated from the other qualities of sound.

Types of Deafness

Deafness is usually divided into two types: first, that caused by impairment of the cochlea or auditory nerve, which is usually classed as "nerve deafness," and, second, that caused by impairment of the mechanisms for transmitting sound into the cochlea, which is usually called "conduction deafness." Obviously, if either the cochlea or the auditory nerve is completely destroyed, the person is permanently deaf. However, if the cochlea and nerve are still intact but the ossicular system has been destroyed, sound waves can still be conducted into the cochlea by means of bone conduction.

The Audiogram in Conduction Deafness. To give a clinical example of one type of deafness, consider the deafness caused by fibrosis of the middle ear following repeated infection in the middle ear. In this instance the sound waves cannot be transmitted easily through the ossicles from the tympanic membrane to the oval window. Figure 36–9 illustrates an audiogram from a person with "middle ear deafness" of this type. In this case the bone conduction is essentially normal at all frequencies, but air conduction is greatly depressed, more so at the low frequencies. In this type of deafness, the faceplate of the stapes frequently becomes "ankylosed" by bony overgrowth to the edges of the oval window. In this case, the person becomes totally deaf for air conduction but can be made to hear again almost normally by surgically removing the stapes and replacing it with a minute Teflon or metal prosthesis that transmits the sound from the incus to the oval window.

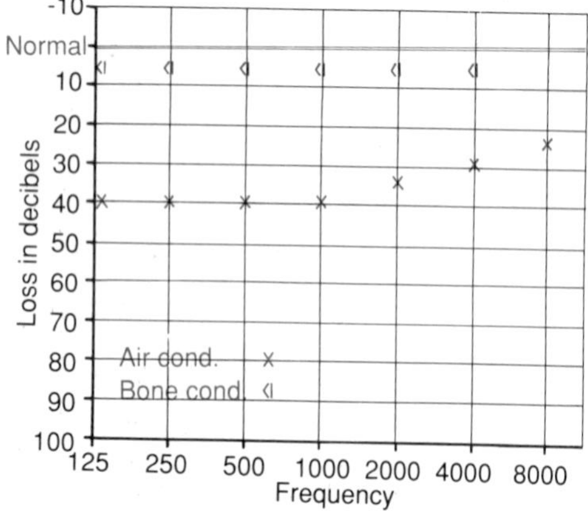

Figure 36–9. Audiogram of deafness resulting from middle ear sclerosis.

THE SENSE OF TASTE

Taste is mainly a function of the *taste buds* in the mouth, but it is common experience that one's sense of smell also contributes strongly to taste perception. Its importance lies in the fact that it allows a person to select food in accord with desires and perhaps also in accord with the needs of the tissues for specific nutritive substances.

The Primary Sensations of Taste

The identities of the specific chemicals that excite different taste receptors are still very incomplete. Even so, psychophysiological and neurophysiological studies have identified at least 13 possible or probable chemical receptors in the different taste cells. However, for practical analysis of taste the receptor capabilities have been collected into four general categories called the *primary sensations of taste.* These are *sour, salty, sweet,* and *bitter.*

The Sour Taste. The sour taste is caused by acids, and the intensity of the taste sensation is approximately proportional to the logarithm of the *hydrogen ion concentration.* That is, the more acidic the acid, the stronger becomes the sensation.

The Salty Taste. The salty taste is elicited by ionized salts. The quality of the taste varies somewhat from one salt to another because the salts also elicit other taste sensations besides saltiness.

The Sweet Taste. The sweet taste is not caused by any single class of chemicals. A list of some of the types of chemicals that cause this taste includes sugars, glycols, alcohols, aldehydes, ketones, amides, esters, amino acids, and others. Note specifically that most of the substances that cause a sweet taste are organic chemicals. It is especially interesting that very slight changes in the chemical structure, such as addition of a simple radical, can often change the substance from sweet to bitter.

The Bitter Taste. The bitter taste, like the sweet taste, is not caused by any single type of chemical agent; but, here again, the substances that give the bitter taste are almost entirely organic substances. Two particular classes of substances are especially likely to cause bitter taste sensations: (1) long chain organic substances containing nitrogen and (2) alkaloids. The alkaloids include many of the drugs used in medicines, such as quinine, caffeine, strychnine, and nicotine.

The bitter taste, when it occurs in high intensity, usually causes the person or animal to reject the food. This is undoubtedly an important purposive function of the bitter taste sensation, because many of the deadly toxins found in poisonous plants are alkaloids, which all cause intensely bitter taste.

The Taste Bud and Its Function

Figure 36-10 illustrates a taste bud, which has a diameter of about 1/30 millimeter and a length of about 1/16 millimeter. The taste bud is composed of about 40 modified epithelial cells, some of which are supporting cells called *sustentacular cells* and others *taste cells.* The taste cells are continually being replaced by mitotic division from the surrounding epithelial cells so that some are young cells and others are mature cells that lie toward the center of the bud and soon break up and dissolve. The life span of each taste cell is about ten days in lower mammals but is unknown for the human being.

The outer tips of the taste cells are arranged around a minute *taste pore,* shown in Figure 36-10. From the tip of each cell, several *microvilli,* or *taste hairs,* protrude outward into the taste pore to approach the cavity of the mouth. These microvilli provide the receptor surface for taste.

Interwoven among the taste cells is a branching terminal network of several *taste nerve fibers* that are stimulated by the taste receptor cells. Many vesicles form beneath the membrane near the fibers, suggesting that these might secrete a neurotransmitter to excite the nerve fibers in response to taste stimulation.

Especially important in relation to taste is the tendency for taste buds subserving particular primary sensations of taste to be located in special areas. The sweet and salty tastes are located *principally* on the tip of the tongue, the sour taste on the two lateral sides of the tongue, and the bitter taste on the posterior tongue and soft palate. The usual adult has about 10,000 buds in all.

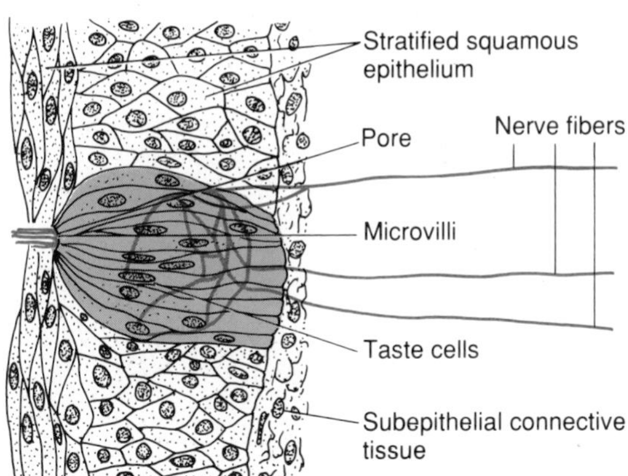

Figure 36-10. The taste bud.

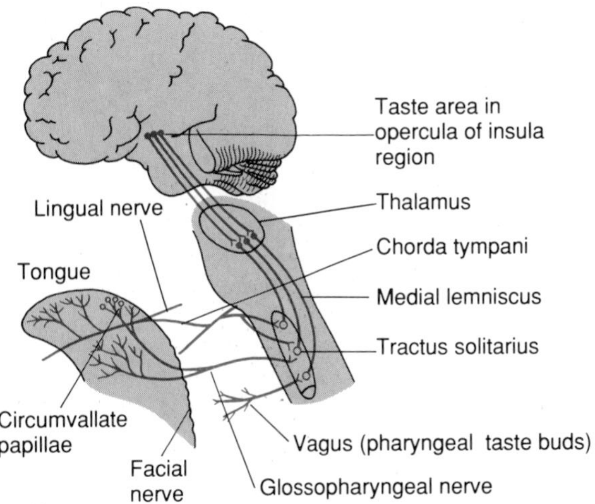

Figure 36-11. Transmission of taste impulses into the central nervous system.

Specificity of Taste Buds for the Primary Taste Stimuli. Microelectrode studies from single taste buds while they are stimulated successively by the four different primary taste stimuli have shown that most of them can be excited by two, three, or even four of the primary taste stimuli as well as by a few other taste stimuli that do not fit into the "primary" categories. Usually, though, one or two of the taste categories will predominate.

Mechanism of Stimulation of Taste Buds. ***The Receptor Potential.*** The membrane of the taste cell, like that of other sensory receptor cells, is negatively charged on the inside with respect to the outside. Application of a taste substance to the taste hairs causes partial loss of this negative potential—that is, the taste cell is *depolarized.* This change in potential is the *receptor potential* for taste.

The mechanism by which the stimulating substance reacts with the taste villi to initiate the receptor potential is believed to be by binding of the taste chemicals to protein receptor molecules that protrude through the villus membrane. This in turn opens ion channels, which allow sodium ions to enter and depolarize the cell.

Transmission of Taste Signals into the Central Nervous System

Figure 36-11 illustrates the neuronal pathways for transmission of taste signals through several of the cranial nerves from the tongue and pharyngeal region into the central nervous system. All the taste fibers first enter the *tractus solitarius* in the brain stem, then synapse in the *nuclei of the tractus solitarius* and send second-order neurons to a small area of the thalamus located slightly medial to the thalamic terminations of the facial regions of the somatic sensory system. From the thalamus, third-order neurons are transmitted to the *lower tip of the postcentral gyrus in the cortex,* terminating near the somatic sensory area for the tongue.

Taste Reflexes Integrated in the Brain Stem. From the tractus solitarius a large number of impulses are transmitted within the brain stem itself directly into the *superior* and *inferior salivatory nuclei,* and these in turn transmit impulses to the submandibular, sublingual, and parotid glands to help control the secretion of saliva during the ingestion of food.

Taste Preference and Control of the Diet

Taste preferences mean simply that an animal will choose certain types of food in preference to others, and it automatically uses this to help control the type of diet it eats. Furthermore, its taste preferences often change in accord with the needs of the body for certain specific substances. For instance, adrenalectomized animals automatically select drinking water with a high concentration of sodium chloride in preference to pure water, and this in many instances is sufficient to supply the needs of the body and prevent death as a result of salt depletion.

The phenomenon of taste preference almost certainly results from some mechanism located in the central nervous system and not from a mechanism in the taste receptors themselves. An important reason for believing taste preference to be mainly a central phenomenon is that previous experience with unpleasant or pleasant tastes plays a major role in determining one's different taste preferences. For instance, if a person becomes sick soon after eating a particular type of food, the person generally develops a negative taste preference, or *taste aversion,* for that particular food thereafter.

THE SENSE OF SMELL

Smell is the least understood of our senses. This results partly from the fact that the sense of smell is a subjective phenomenon that cannot be studied with ease in lower animals. Still another complicating problem is that the sense of smell is almost rudimentary in the human being in comparison with that of some lower animals.

The Olfactory Membrane

The olfactory membrane lies in the superior part of each nostril, as illustrated in Figure 36–12. Medially it folds downward over the surface of the septum, and laterally it folds over the superior turbinate and even over a small portion of the upper surface of the middle turbinate.

The Olfactory Cells. The receptor cells for the smell sensation are the *olfactory cells,* which are actually bipolar nerve cells derived originally from the central nervous system itself. There are about 100 million of these cells in the olfactory epithelium, as shown in Figure 36–13. The mucosal end of the olfactory cell forms a knob from which 6 to 12 *olfactory hairs,* or *cilia,* up to 200 micrometers in length, project into the mucus that coats the inner surface of the nasal cavity. These projecting olfactory cilia form a dense mat in the mucus, and it is these cilia that react to odors in the air and then stimulate the olfactory cells, as discussed later.

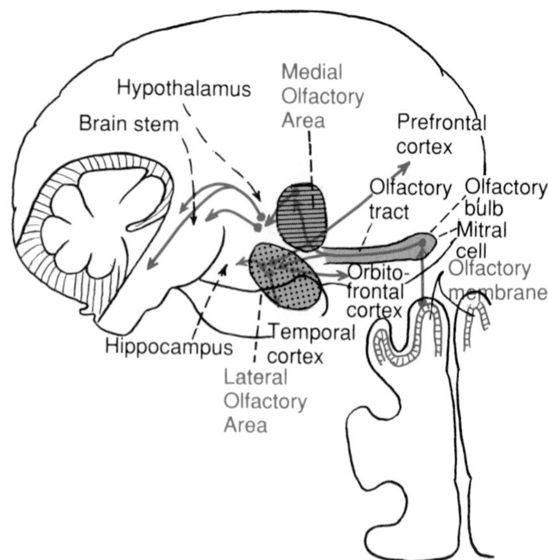

Figure 36–12. Neural connections of the olfactory system.

Stimulation of the Olfactory Cells

The portion of the olfactory cells that responds to the olfactory chemical stimuli is the *cilia.* The membranes of the cilia contain large numbers of protein molecules that protrude all the way through the membrane and that can bind with different odorant sub-

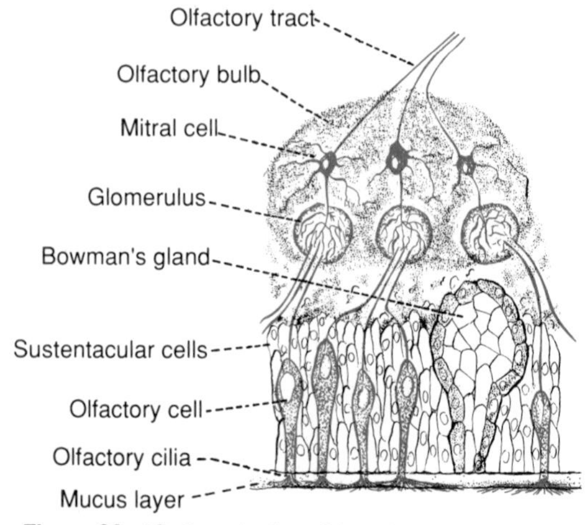

Figure 36–13. Organization of the olfactory membrane.

stances. These proteins are called *odorant-binding proteins.*

Two different theories have been proposed for the mechanism of excitation: The simplest theory suggests that the molecules of the odorant-binding proteins themselves open up to become ion channels when the odorant binds, allowing mainly large numbers of positively charged sodium ions to flow to the interior of the olfactory cell and depolarize it. The second theory proposes that binding of the odorant causes the odorant-binding protein to become an activated adenylate cyclase at its end that protrudes to the interior of the cell. The cyclase in turn catalyzes the formation of cyclic adenosine monophosphate (cAMP), and the cAMP acts on many other membrane proteins to open ion channels through them. This second mechanism would provide an extremely sensitive receptor because of a cascade effect that would occur and allow even the most minute of stimulation to cause a reaction.

Regardless of the basic chemical mechanism by which the olfactory cells are stimulated, several physical factors also affect the degree of stimulation. First, only volatile substances that can be sniffed into the nostrils can be smelled. Second, the stimulating substance must be at least slightly water soluble, so that it can pass through the mucus to reach the olfactory cells. And, third, it must be at least slightly lipid soluble, presumably because the lipid constituents of the cell membrane repel odorants from the membrane receptor proteins.

Search for the Primary Sensations of Smell

Most physiologists are convinced that the many smell sensations are subserved by a few rather discrete primary sensations, in the same way that vision and taste are subserved by a select few sensations. But, thus far, only minor success has been achieved in classifying the primary sensations of smell. Yet, on the basis of psychological tests and action potential studies from various points in the olfactory nerve pathways, it has been postulated that about seven different primary classes of olfactory stimulants preferentially excite separate olfactory cells. These classes of olfactory stimulants are characterized as follows:

1. Camphoraceous.
2. Musky.
3. Floral.
4. Pepperminty.
5. Ethereal.
6. Pungent.
7. Putrid.

However, it is unlikely that this list actually represents the true primary sensations of smell, even though it does illustrate the results of one of the many attempts to classify them.

Gradations of Smell Intensities. The threshold concentrations of substances that evoke smell are often as little as 1 billionth of a gram per liter of air. Even so, concentrations only 10 to 50 times above the threshold values can evoke maximum intensity of smell. This is in contrast to most other sensory systems of the body, in which the ranges of detection are tremendous — for instance, 500,000 to 1 in the case of the eyes and 1 trillion to 1 in the case of the ears. This difference perhaps can be explained by the fact that smell is concerned more with detecting the presence or absence of odors than with quantitative detection of their intensities.

Transmission of Smell Signals into the Central Nervous System

The olfactory portions of the brain are among its oldest structures, and much of the remainder of the brain developed around these olfactory beginnings. In fact, part of the brain that originally subserved olfaction later evolved into the basal brain structures that in the human being control emotions and other aspects of behavior; this is the system we call the *limbic system,* discussed in Chapter 40.

Transmission of Olfactory Signals into the Olfactory Bulb. The olfactory bulb, which is also called cranial nerve I, is illustrated in Figure 36–12. Although it looks like a nerve, in reality it is an anterior outgrowth of brain tissue from the base of the brain; it has a bulbous enlargement, the *olfactory bulb,* at its end that lies over the *cribriform plate* separating the brain cavity from the upper reaches of the nasal cavity. The cribriform plate has multiple small perforations through which an equal number of small nerves enter the olfactory bulb from the olfactory membrane. Figure 36–13 illustrates the close relationship between the *olfactory cells* in the olfactory membrane and the olfactory bulb, showing very short axons terminating in multiple globular structures of the olfactory bulb called *glomeruli.*

Recent research suggests that different glomeruli respond to different odors. Therefore, it is possible that the specific glomeruli that are stimulated are the real clue to the analysis of different odor signals transmitted into the central nervous system.

The Very Old, the Old, and the Newer Olfactory Pathways into the Central Nervous System

The olfactory tract enters the brain at the junction between the mesencephalon and cerebrum; there the tract divides into two pathways, one passing medially into the *medial olfactory area* and the other laterally into the *lateral olfactory area.* The medial olfactory area represents a very old olfactory system, while the lateral olfactory area is the input to both a less old olfactory system and a newer system.

The Very Old Olfactory System — The Medial Olfactory Area. The medial olfactory area consists of a group of nuclei located in the midbasal portions of the brain anterior and superior to the hypothalamus. The importance of this area is best understood by considering what happens in animals when the lateral olfactory areas on both sides of the brain are removed and only the medial system remains. The answer is that this hardly affects the more primitive responses to olfaction, such as licking the lips, salivation, and other feeding responses caused by the smell of food, or such as primitive emotional drives associated with smell. On the other hand, removal of the lateral areas does abolish the more complicated olfactory conditioned reflexes.

The Old Olfactory System — The Lateral Olfactory Area. The lateral olfactory area is composed mainly of the *prepyriform* and *pyriform cortex* plus the *cortical portion of the amygdaloid nuclei.* From these areas, signal pathways pass into almost all portions of the basal brain, which is most important in learning likes and dislikes of foods depending upon experience. For instance, it is this lateral olfactory area and its many connections with the brain's behavioral system that cause a person to develop absolute aversion to foods that have previously caused nausea and vomiting.

The Newer Pathway. A newer olfactory pathway has now been found that does indeed pass through the thalamus, passing to the dorsomedial thalamic nucleus and thence to the lateroposterior quadrant of the orbitofrontal cortex. Based on studies in monkeys, this newer system probably helps especially in the conscious analysis of odor.

Thus, there appears to be a very old olfactory system that subserves the basic olfactory reflexes, an old system that provides automatic but learned control of food intake and aversion to toxic and unhealthy foods, and finally a newer system that is comparable to most of the other cortical sensory systems and is used for conscious perception of olfaction.

REFERENCES

Hearing

Altschuler, R. A., et al.: Neurobiology of Hearing: The Cochlea. New York, Raven Press, 1986.
Borg, E., and Counter, S. A.: The middle-ear muscles. Sci. Am., August, 1989, p. 74.
Green, D. M., and Wier, C. C.: Auditory perception. In Darian-Smith, I. (ed.): Handbook of Physiology. Sec. 1, Vol. III. Bethesda, Md., American Physiological Society, 1984, p. 557.
Hudspeth, A. J.: The cellular basis of hearing: The biophysics of hair cells. Science, 230:745, 1985.
Masterton, R. B., and Imig, T. J.: Neural mechanisms of sound localization. Annu. Rev. Physiol., 46:275, 1984.
Patuzzi, R., and Robertson, D.: Tuning in the mammalian cochlea. Physiol. Rev., 68:1009, 1988.
Rhode, W. S.: Cochlear mechanisms. Annu. Rev. Physiol., 46:231, 1984.
Syka, J., and Masterton, R. B. (eds.): Auditory Pathway; Structure and Function. New York, Plenum Publishing Corp., 1988.
Weiss, T. F.: Relation of receptor potentials of cochlear hair cells to spike discharges of cochlear neurons. Annu. Rev. Physiol., 46:247, 1984.

Taste and Smell

Chanel, J.: The olfactory system as a molecular descriptor. News Physiol. Sci., 2:203, 1987.
Getchell, T. V.: Functional properties of vertebrate olfactory receptor neurons. Physiol. Rev., 66:772, 1986.
Margolis, F. L., and Getchell, T. V. (eds.): Molecular Neurobiology of the Olfactory System. New York, Plenum Publishing Corp., 1988.
Norgren, R.: Central neural mechanisms of taste. In Darian-Smith, I. (ed.): Handbook of Physiology. Sec. 1, Vol. III. Bethesda, Md., American Physiological Society, 1984, p. 1087.
Roper, S. D.: The cell biology of vertebrate taste receptors. Annu. Rev. Neurosci., 12:329, 1989.
Schiffman, S. S.: Taste transduction and modulation. News Physiol. Sci., 3:109, 1988.

QUESTIONS

1. Describe the *tympanic membrane* and the *ossicular system* and their roles in the transmission of sound to the oval window.
2. Explain how the *attenuation reflex* protects the ear from damaging noises.
3. Trace the movement of fluid in the *cochlear* chambers during each phase of a complete sound wave.
4. Explain the role of each of the following in the *resonance* process that occurs in the cochlea: the length of the basilar fibers, the stiffness of the basilar fibers, and the loading effect of the fluid in the scala vestibuli, scala media, and scala tympani.
5. Draw a diagram showing the respective points in the cochlea where the greatest amplitude of vibration occurs on the basilar membrane for low, medium, and high sound frequencies.
6. Describe the anatomy of the *organ of Corti* and the mechanism by which the *hair cells* are excited when sound waves cause them to move.
7. What is meant by the *place principle* for the determination of pitch?
8. Explain how the cochlea determines loudness of a sound and how the ear can operate in a tremendous range of sound intensity.
9. Describe the neural pathway for transmission of sound signals to the cerebral cortex.
10. Describe the function of the *auditory cortex,* including (a) what is meant by *tonotopic maps* in the auditory cortex and (b) the discrimination of sound patterns.
11. How does a person determine the direction from which a sound is coming?
12. Explain the differences between *nerve deafness* and *conduction deafness,* as well as the surgical treatment of conduction deafness.
13. Give the four primary sensations of taste and the types of chemical substances that excite each of these sensations.
14. Describe the *taste bud,* its stimulation, and its specificity for specific types of taste stimuli.
15. Trace the neural circuit for transmission of taste signals into the central nervous system.
16. What role does taste play in the control of the diet?

17. Describe the *olfactory membrane,* the *olfactory cells,* and the sensory portions of the olfactory cells.
18. What are the characteristics of substances that cause smell?
19. What do we know about the primary sensations of smell?
20. Give the theories for the mechanism of excitation of the olfactory cell.
21. Trace the neural pathway for transmission of olfactory signals from the olfactory cells to the brain.
22. What are the differences between the functions of the very old, the old, and the newer olfactory systems of the brain?

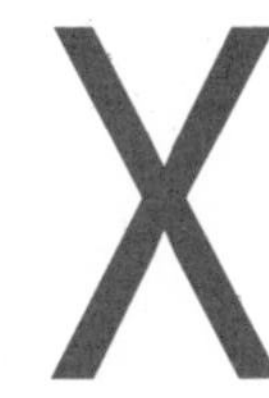

The Nervous System: B. Motor and Integrative Neurophysiology

37

The Spinal Cord and Brain Stem Reflexes, and Function of the Vestibular Apparatus

In the discussion of the nervous system thus far, we have considered principally the input of sensory information. In the following chapters we discuss the origin and output of motor signals, the signals that cause muscle contraction, secretory function, and other motor effects throughout the body.

Sensory information is integrated at all levels of the nervous system and causes appropriate motor responses, beginning in the spinal cord with relatively simple reflexes, extending into the brain stem with still more complicated responses, and finally extending to the cerebrum, where the most complicated responses are controlled. In the present chapter we discuss the control of muscle function by the spinal cord and brain stem.

Organization of the Spinal Cord for Motor Functions

The cord gray matter is the integrative area for the cord reflexes and other motor functions. Figure 37-1 shows the typical organization of the cord gray matter in a single cord segment. Sensory signals enter the cord almost entirely through the sensory (posterior) roots. After entering the cord, every sensory signal travels to two separate destinations. First, one branch of the sensory nerve terminates in the gray matter of the cord and elicits local segmental reflexes and other effects. Second, another branch transmits signals to higher levels of the nervous system — to higher levels in the cord itself, to the brain stem, or even to the cerebral cortex, as described in earlier chapters.

Each segment of the spinal cord has several million neurons in its gray matter. Aside from the sensory relay neurons discussed in Chapters 32 and 33, the remainder of these neurons are of two separate types, the *anterior motor neurons* and the *interneurons.*

The Anterior Motor Neurons. Located in each segment of the anterior horns of the cord gray matter are several thousand neurons that are 50 to 100 per cent larger than most of the others and called *anterior motor neurons.* These give rise to the nerve fibers that leave the cord via the anterior roots and innervate the skeletal muscle fibers. The neurons are of two types, the *alpha motor neurons* and the *gamma motor neurons.*

The Alpha Motor Neurons. The alpha motor neurons give rise to large type A alpha (Aα) nerve fibers ranging from 9 to 20 micrometers in diameter that innervate the large skeletal muscle fibers. Stimulation of a single nerve fiber excites from as few as three to as many as several hundred skeletal muscle fibers, which are collectively called the *motor unit.* Transmission of nerve impulses into skeletal muscles and their stimulation of the muscles were discussed in Chapters 6 and 7.

The Gamma Motor Neurons. In addition to the alpha motor neurons that excite contraction of the skeletal muscle fibers, about one half as many much smaller gamma motor neurons are located along with the alpha motor neurons in the anterior horns. These transmit impulses through type A gamma (Aγ) fibers, averaging 5 micrometers in diameter, to very small, special skeletal muscle fibers called *intrafusal fibers.* These are part of the *muscle spindle,* which helps control muscle contraction and is discussed later in the chapter.

The Interneurons. Interneurons are present in all areas of the cord gray matter — in the dorsal horns, in the anterior horns, and in the intermediate areas between these two. These cells are numerous —

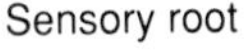

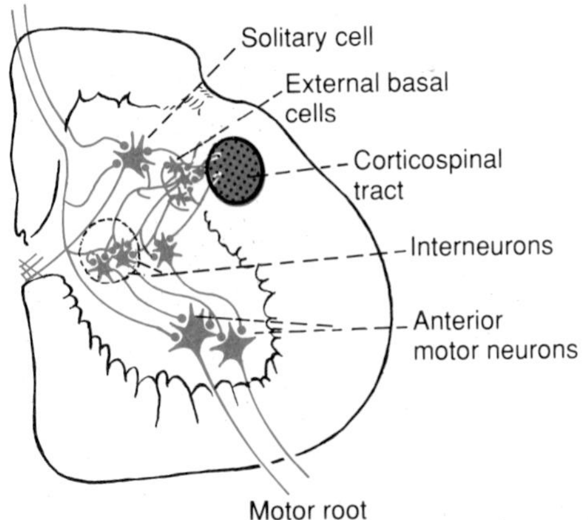

Figure 37-1. Connections of the sensory fibers and corticospinal fibers with the interneurons and anterior motor neurons of the spinal cord.

approximately 30 times as numerous as the anterior motor neurons. They are small and highly excitable, often exhibiting spontaneous activity and capable of firing as rapidly as 1500 times per second. They have many interconnections one with the other, and many of them directly innervate the anterior motor neurons, as illustrated in Figure 37-1. The interconnections among the interneurons and anterior motor neurons are responsible for many of the integrative functions of the spinal cord that are discussed in the remainder of this chapter.

Essentially all the different types of neuronal circuits described in Chapter 31 are found in the interneuron pool of cells of the spinal cord, including the *diverging, converging,* and *repetitive-discharge* circuits. In this chapter we see many applications of these different circuits to the performance of specific reflex acts by the spinal cord.

Only a few incoming sensory signals from the spinal nerves or signals from the brain terminate directly on the anterior motor neurons. Instead, most of them are transmitted first through the interneuron circuits, where they are appropriately processed. Thus, in Figure 37-1, it is shown that the corticospinal tract terminates almost entirely on interneurons, and it is only after the signals from this tract have been integrated in the interneuron pool with signals from other spinal tracts or from the spinal nerves that they finally impinge on the anterior motor neurons to control muscular function.

Multisegmental Connections in the Spinal Cord—The Propriospinal Fibers

More than half of all the nerve fibers ascending and descending in the spinal cord are *propriospinal fibers.* These are fibers that run from one segment of the cord to another. In addition, the sensory fibers as they enter the cord branch both up and down the spinal cord, some of the branches transmitting signals only a segment or two in each direction whereas others transmit signals many segments. These ascending and descending fibers of the cord provide pathways for the multisegmental reflexes that are described later in this chapter, including reflexes that coordinate simultaneous movements in the forelimbs and hindlimbs.

THE MUSCLE RECEPTORS—MUSCLE SPINDLES AND GOLGI TENDON ORGANS—AND THEIR ROLES IN MUSCLE CONTROL

Proper control of muscle function requires not only excitation of the muscle by the anterior motor neurons but also continuous feedback of information from each muscle to the nervous system, giving the status of the muscle at each instant. To provide this information, the muscles and their tendons are supplied abundantly with two special types of sensory receptors: (1) *muscle spindles,* which are distributed throughout the belly of the muscle and send information to the nervous system about either the muscle length or rate of change of its length, and (2) *Golgi tendon organs,* which are located in the muscle tendons and transmit information about tension.

Receptor Function of the Muscle Spindle

Structure and Innervation of the Muscle Spindle. The physiological organization of the muscle spindle is illustrated in Figure 37-2. Each spindle is built around 3 to 12 small *intrafusal muscle fibers* that are pointed at their ends and are attached to the glycocalyx of the surrounding *extrafusal* skeletal muscle fibers. Each intrafusal fiber is a very small skeletal muscle fiber. However, the central region of each of these fibers—that is, the area midway between its two ends—has either no or few actin and myosin filaments. Therefore, this central portion does not contract when the ends do. Instead, it functions as a sensory receptor. The end portions are excited by the small *gamma motor nerve fibers* originating from the gamma motor neurons described earlier. These fibers

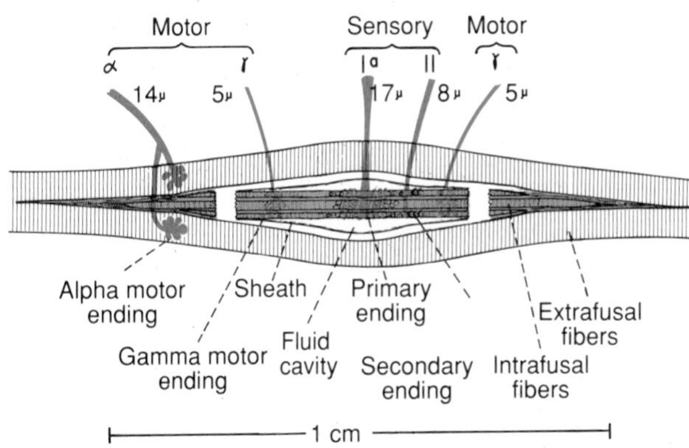

Figure 37-2. The muscle spindle, showing its relationship to the large extrafusal skeletal muscle fibers. Note also both the motor and the sensory innervation of the muscle spindle.

are also called *gamma efferent fibers,* in contradistinction to the *alpha efferent fibers* that innervate the extrafusal skeletal muscle.

The receptor area of the spindle has two types of sensory nerve endings, the *primary ending* and the *secondary ending,* which have slightly different functions.

The Primary Ending. A very large type Ia sensory fiber innervates the center of the spindle receptor. This fiber spirals around the intrafusal fibers, forming the so-called *primary ending,* also called the *annulospiral ending.* When the receptor portion of the spindle is stretched, this ending is stimulated. And, because the innervating fiber is so large, signals are transmitted to the spinal cord at a velocity approaching 100 meters per second, a velocity as great as that in almost any part of the nervous system.

The Secondary Ending. A type II nerve fiber innervates the receptor to one side of the primary ending. This fiber, like the Ia fiber, also spirals around the intrafusal fibers, and when the receptor portion of the intrafusal fibers is stretched, this nerve ending also is stimulated. It is called the *secondary ending.*

Static Response of Both the Primary and the Secondary Endings. When the receptor portion of the muscle spindle is stretched *slowly,* the number of impulses transmitted from both types of endings increases almost directly in proportion to the degree of stretch, and the endings continue to transmit these impulses for many minutes. This effect is called the *static response* of the spindle receptor, meaning simply that the receptor responds to a change in length of the spindle and also continues to transmit its signal for a prolonged period of time.

Dynamic Response of the Primary Ending. In addition to its static response, the primary, but not the secondary, ending also exhibits a very strong *dynamic response,* which means that it responds extremely strongly to sudden *changes* in length. When the length of the spindle receptor area increases only a fraction of a micron, if this increase occurs rapidly, the primary receptor transmits tremendous numbers of impulses into the Ia fiber, but only *while the length is actually increasing.* As soon as the length has stopped increasing, the rate of impulse discharge returns to the much weaker static response level that is still present in the signal.

Conversely, when the spindle receptor area shortens, this change momentarily decreases the impulse output from the primary ending; as soon as the receptor area has reached its new shortened length, the static response impulses reappear in the Ia fiber within a fraction of a second. Thus, the primary ending sends extremely strong signals to the central nervous system to apprise it of any change in length of the spindle receptor area.

Function of the Muscle Spindle in Comparing Intrafusal and Extrafusal Muscle Lengths

From the foregoing description of the muscle spindle, one can see that there are two different ways in which the spindle can be stimulated: (1) *By stretching the whole muscle.* This lengthens the entire spindle and therefore stretches the spindle receptor. (2) *By contracting the intrafusal muscle fibers* while the extrafusal fibers remain at their normal length. Since the intrafusal fibers only contract near their two ends, this stretches the central receptor portion of the intrafusal fibers, obviously exciting the spindle nerve endings.

In effect, the muscle spindle acts as a *comparator* of the lengths of the two types of muscle fibers, the extrafusal and the intrafusal. When the length of the extrafusal fibers is greater than that of the intrafusal fibers, the spindle becomes excited. On the other hand, when the length of the extrafusal fiber is shorter than that of the intrafusal fiber, the spindle is inhibited.

Continuous Discharge of the Muscle Spindles Under Normal Conditions. Normally, particularly when there is a slight amount of intrafusal fiber contraction caused by gamma efferent excitation, the muscle spindles emit sensory nerve impulses all of the time. Stretching the muscle spindles increases the rate of firing, whereas shortening the spindle decreases this rate of firing. Thus, the spindles can operate in both directions; that is, their normal signal output can be either increased or decreased.

The Stretch Reflex (Also Called the Myotatic Reflex)

Sudden stretch of a muscle excites the muscle spindle, and this in turn sends strong signals to the spinal cord, which then transmits signals through the alpha efferent nerve fibers to the extrafusal muscle fibers, causing reflex contraction of the *same* muscle. For obvious reasons, this reflex is frequently simply called a muscle *stretch reflex.* This reflex has a dynamic component and a static component.

The Dynamic Stretch Reflex. The dynamic stretch reflex is caused by the potent dynamic signal from the muscle spindles. That is, when the muscle is suddenly stretched, a very strong signal is transmitted to the spinal cord from the primary endings, but this signal is potent *only while the length of the muscle is increasing.* On entering the spinal cord, most of the signal goes directly to the anterior motor neurons without passing through interneurons, as shown in Figure 37–3, and it causes reflex contraction of the same muscle from which the muscle spindle signals originated. Thus, a sudden stretch of a muscle causes reflex contraction of the same muscle, and *this opposes further stretch of the muscle.*

The Static Stretch Reflex. Though the dynamic stretch reflex is over within a fraction of a second after the muscle has been stretched to its new length, a weaker static stretch reflex continues for a prolonged period of time thereafter. This reflex is elicited by continuous static receptor signals transmitted from

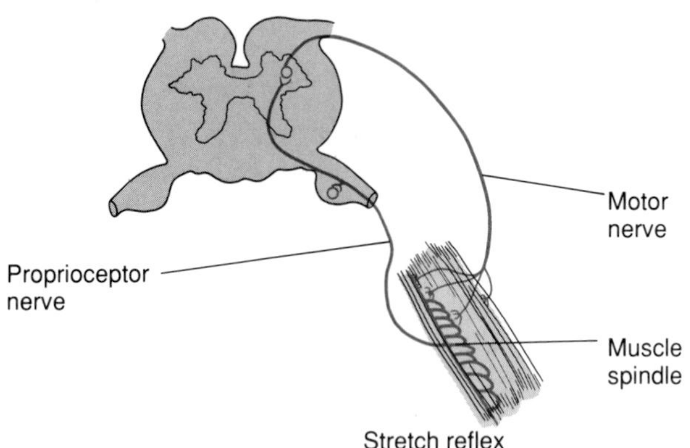

Figure 37-3. Neuronal circuit of the stretch reflex.

both the primary and secondary endings of the muscle spindles. The importance of the static stretch reflex is that it continues to cause muscle contraction as long as the muscle is maintained at an excesssive length (for as long as many minutes or several hours, but not for days). Thus, the muscle contraction opposes the force that is causing the excess length.

The Negative Stretch Reflex. When a muscle is suddenly shortened, exactly opposite effects occur. That is, extrafusal fibers of the muscle lose their stimulation, and the muscle relaxes. Thus, *this negative stretch reflex* opposes the shortening of the muscle in the same way that the positive stretch reflex opposes lengthening of the muscle. Therefore, one can begin to see that the muscle spindle reflex tends to maintain the status quo for the length of a muscle.

Function of the Static Stretch Reflex in Nullifying the Effects of Changes in Load During Muscle Contraction

Let us assume that a person's biceps is contracted so that the forearm is horizontal to the earth. Then assume that a 5-pound weight is put in the hand. The hand will immediately drop. However, the amount that the hand will drop is determined to a great extent by the degree of activity of the static muscle spindle reflex. If the static reflex is very active, even slight lengthening of the biceps, and therefore also of the muscle spindles in the biceps, will cause a strong feedback contraction of the extrafusal skeletal muscle fibers of the biceps. This contraction in turn will limit the degree of fall of the hand, thus automatically maintaining the forearm in a nearly horizontal position despite the increased load. This response is called a *load reflex.*

The Damping Function of the Stretch Reflex. Another extremely important function of the reflex—indeed, probably more important than the load reflex—is the ability of the muscle spindle reflex to prevent oscillation and jerkiness of the body movements. This is a damping, or smoothing, function. An example is the following:

Use of the Damping Mechanism in Smoothing Muscle Contraction. Occasionally, signals from other parts of the nervous system are transmitted to a muscle in an uneven fashion, first increasing in intensity for a few milliseconds, then decreasing in intensity, then changing to another intensity level, and so forth. When the muscle spindle apparatus is not functioning satisfactorily, the muscle contraction can be jerky during the course of such a signal. This effect is illustrated in Figure 37-4, which shows an experiment in which a sensory nerve signal entering one side of the cord is transmitted to a motor nerve on the other side of the cord to excite a muscle. In curve A the muscle spindle reflex of the excited muscle is intact. Note that the contraction is relatively smooth even though the sensory nerve is excited at a slow frequency of 8 per second. Curve B, on the other hand, shows the same experiment in an animal whose muscle spindle sensory nerves had been sectioned 3 months earlier. Note the spasmodic muscle contraction. Thus, curve A illustrates graphically the ability of the damping mechanism of the muscle spindle to make muscle contractions smooth even though the input signals to the muscle motor system are jerky. This effect can also be called a *signal averaging* function of the muscle spindle.

Function of the Gamma Efferent System in Controlling the Intensity of the Stretch Reflex

The gamma efferent system plays a potent role in determining the effectiveness of the load reflex and also the degree of damping. For instance, there are times when a person wishes his or her limbs to move extremely rapidly in respose to rapidly changing input signals. Under such conditions, one would wish less damping and less load reflex. On the other hand, at other times it is important that the muscle contractions be very smooth. Under these conditions one would like a potent stretch reflex. This is achieved by gamma efferent stimulation of the spindle intrafusal muscle fibers, a condition that tenses the intrafusal fibers and therefore greatly enhances the excitability of the muscle spindles.

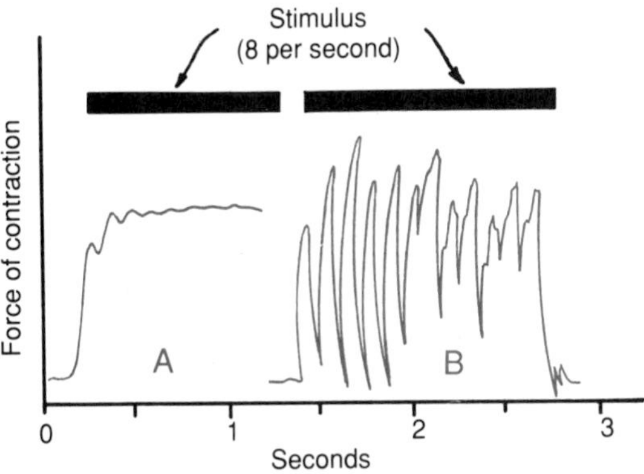

Figure 37-4. Muscle contraction caused by a spinal cord signal under two different conditions: *A*, in a normal muscle, and *B*, in a muscle whose muscle spindles had been denervated by section of the posterior roots of the cord 82 days previously. Note the smoothing effect of the muscle spindle reflex in *A*. (Modified from Creed, R. S., et al.: Reflex Activity of the Spinal Cord. New York, Oxford University Press, 1932.)

Role of the Muscle Spindle in Voluntary Motor Activity

To emphasize the importance of the muscle spindles and the gamma efferent system, one needs only to recognize that 31 per cent of all the motor nerve fibers to the muscles are gamma efferent fibers to the intrafusal muscle fibers of the spindles rather than large type A alpha motor fibers to the extrafusal muscle. Whenever signals are transmitted from the motor cortex or from any other area of the brain to the alpha motor neurons, almost invariably the gamma motor neurons are stimulated simultaneously, a principle called *gamma efferent coactivation.* This dual stimulation causes the intrafusal muscle fibers to contract at the same time that the whole muscle contracts.

The purpose of contracting the muscle spindle fibers at the same time that the large skeletal muscle fibers contract is twofold: First, it keeps the muscle spindle from opposing the muscle contraction. Second, it also maintains proper damping of the muscle regardless of change in muscle length. For instance, if the muscle spindle did not contract and relax along with the large muscle fibers, the receptor portion of the spindle would sometimes be flail and at other times be overstretched, in neither instance operating under optimal conditions for spindle function.

Clinical Application of the Stretch Reflex —The Knee Jerk and Other Muscle Jerks

Clinically, a method used to determine the functional integrity of the stretch reflexes is to elicit the knee jerk and other muscle jerks. The knee jerk can be elicited by simply striking the patellar tendon with a reflex hammer; this stretches the quadriceps muscle and initiates a *dynamic stretch reflex* that causes the lower leg to jerk forward.

Similar reflexes can be obtained from almost any muscle of the body either by striking the tendon of the muscle or by striking the belly of the muscle itself. In other words, sudden stretch of muscle spindles is all that is required to elicit a stretch reflex.

The muscle jerks are used by neurologists to assess the degree of facilitation of spinal cord centers. When large numbers of facilitatory impulses are being transmitted from the upper regions of the central nervous system into the cord, the muscle jerks are greatly exacerbated. On the other hand, if the facilitatory impulses are depressed or abrogated, the muscle jerks are considerably weakened or completely absent. These reflexes are used most frequently to determine the presence or absence of muscle spasticity following lesions in the motor areas of the brain. Ordinarily, diffuse lesions in the motor areas of the opposite side of the cerebral cortex cause greatly exacerbated muscle jerks. This often occurs in patients who have had a stroke, which is damage to the brain resulting from loss of its blood supply.

The Golgi Tendon Reflex

The Golgi Tendon Organ and Its Excitation. The Golgi tendon organ, illustrated in Figure 37–5, is an encapsulated sensory receptor through which a small bundle of muscle tendon fibers pass. An average of 10 to 15 muscle fibers are usually connected in series with each Golgi tendon organ, and the organ is stimulated by the tension produced by this small bundle of muscle fibers. Thus, the major difference between the function of the Golgi tendon organ and the muscle spindle is that the spindle detects changes in muscle length, while the tendon organ detects changes in muscle *tension.*

The tendon organ, like the primary receptor of the muscle spindle, has both a *dynamic response* and a *static response,* responding very intensely when the muscle tension suddenly increases (the dynamic response) but within a small fraction of a second settling down to a lower level of steady-state firing that is almost directly proportional to the muscle tension (the static response).

Inhibitory Nature of the Tendon Reflex and Its Importance

When the Golgi tendon organs of a muscle are stimulated by increased muscle tension, signals are transmitted into the spinal cord to cause reflex inhibition in the respective muscle, the exact opposite of the muscle spindle reflex. Thus, this reflex provides a *negative feedback* mechanism that prevents the development of too much tension on the muscle.

Possible Role of the Tendon Reflex to Equalize Contractile Force Among the Muscle Fibers. A likely function of the Golgi tendon reflex is to equalize the contractile forces of the separate muscle fibers. That is, those fibers that exert excess tension become inhibited by the reflex while those that exert too little tension become more excited because of absence of reflex inhibition. Obviously this would spread the muscle load over all the fibers and especially would prevent local muscle damage where small numbers of fibers would be overloaded.

Function of the Muscle Spindles and Golgi Tendon Organs in Conjunction with Motor Control from Higher Levels of the Brain

Although we have emphasized the function of the muscle spindles and Golgi tendon organs in spinal cord control of motor function, these two sensory organs also apprise the higher motor control centers of instantaneous changes taking place in the muscles. For instance, the dorsal spinocerebellar tracts carry instantaneous information from both the muscle spindles and the Golgi tendon organs directly to the cerebellum at conduction velocities approaching 120

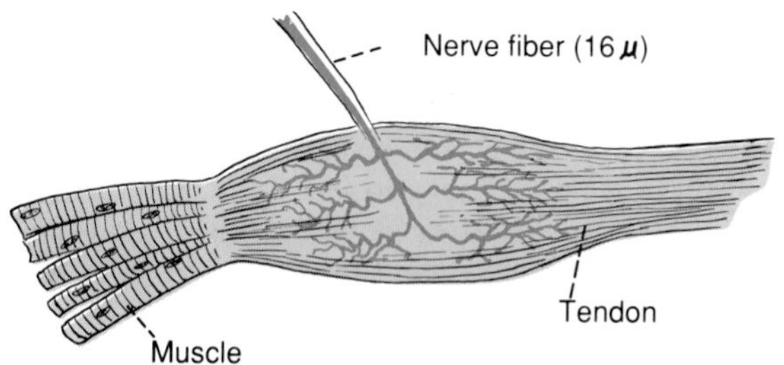

Figure 37-5. Golgi tendon organ.

m/sec. Additional pathways transmit similar information into the reticular regions of the brain stem and also all the way to the motor areas of the cerebral cortex. Information from these receptors is crucial for feedback control of motor signals originating in all of these areas.

THE FLEXOR REFLEX (THE WITHDRAWAL REFLEXES)

In the spinal or decerebrate animal, almost any type of cutaneous sensory stimulus on a limb is likely to cause the flexor muscles of the limb to contract, thereby withdrawing the limb from the stimulus. This is called the *flexor reflex.*

In its classic form the flexor reflex is elicited most powerfully by stimulation of pain endings, such as by a pinprick, heat, or some other painful stimulus, for which reason it is also frequently called a *nociceptive reflex,* or simply *pain reflex.* However, stimulation of the touch receptors can also elicit a weaker and less prolonged flexor reflex.

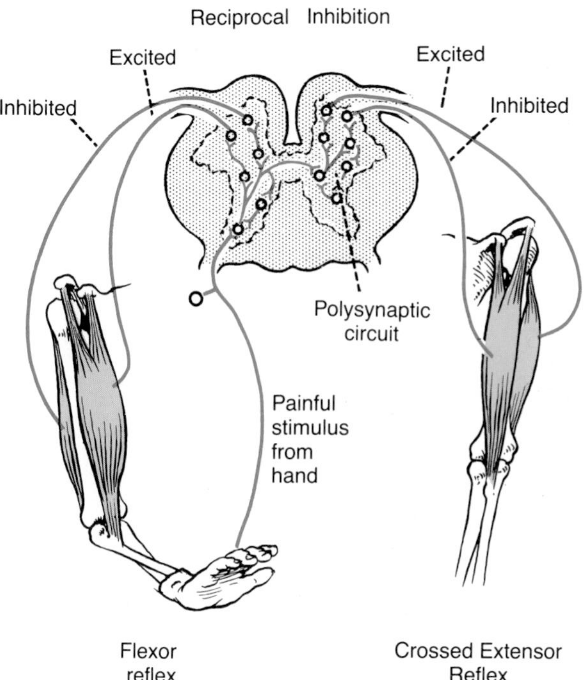

Figure 37-6. The flexor reflex, the crossed extensor reflex, and reciprocal inhibition.

If some part of the body besides one of the limbs is painfully stimulated, this part, in a similar manner, will be *withdrawn from the stimulus,* but the reflex may not be confined entirely to flexor muscles even though it is basically the same type of reflex. Therefore, the many patterns of reflexes of this type in the different areas of the body are called the *withdrawal reflexes.*

Neuronal Mechanism of the Flexor Reflex. The left-hand portion of Figure 37-6 illustrates the neuronal pathways for the flexor reflex. In this instance, a painful stimulus is applied to the hand; as a result, the flexor muscles of the upper arm become reflexly excited, thus withdrawing the hand from the painful stimulus.

The pathways for eliciting the flexor reflex do not pass directly to the anterior motor neurons but, instead, pass first into the interneuron pool of neurons and then to the motor neurons. The shortest possible circuit is a three- or four-neuron arc; however, most of the signals of the reflex traverse many more neurons than this and involve the following basic types of circuits: (1) diverging circuits to spread the reflex to the necessary muscles for withdrawal, (2) circuits to inhibit the antagonist muscles, called *reciprocal inhibition circuits,* and (3) circuits to cause a prolonged repetitive afterdischarge even after the stimulus is over.

Within a few milliseconds after a pain nerve begins to be stimulated, the flexor response appears. Then, soon after the stimulus is over, the contraction of the muscle begins to return toward the base line, but, because of *afterdischarge,* will not return all the way for many milliseconds. The duration of the afterdischarge depends on the intensity of the sensory stimulus that had elicited the reflex; a weak tactile stimulus causes almost no afterdischarge in contrast to an afterdischarge lasting for a second or more following a very strong pain stimulus.

Electrophysiological studies indicate that the immediate afterdischarge, lasting for about 6 to 8 milliseconds, results from repetitive firing of the excited interneurons themselves. However, the prolonged afterdischarge that occurs following strong pain stimuli almost certainly results from recurrent pathways that excite reverberating interneuron circuits, these transmitting impulses to the anterior motor neurons sometimes for several seconds after the incoming sensory signal is completely over.

Thus, the flexor reflex is appropriately organized to withdraw a pained or otherwise irritated part of the body away from the stimulus. Furthermore, because of the afterdischarge, the reflex can still hold the irritated part away from the stimulus for as long as 1 to 3 seconds after the irritation is over.

THE CROSSED EXTENSOR REFLEX

Approximately 0.2 to 0.5 second after a stimulus elicits a flexor reflex in one limb, the opposite limb begins to extend. This is called the *crossed extensor reflex.* Extension of the opposite limb obviously can push the entire body away from the object causing the painful stimulus.

Neuronal Mechanism of the Crossed Extensor Reflex. The right-hand portion of Figure 37–6 illustrates the neuronal circuit responsible for the crossed extensor reflex, showing that signals from the sensory nerves cross to the opposite side of the cord to cause reactions exactly opposite those that cause the flexor reflex. Because the crossed extensor reflex usually does not begin until 200 to 500 milliseconds following the initial pain stimulus, it is certain that many interneurons are involved in the circuit between the incoming sensory neuron and the motor neurons of the opposite side of the cord responsible for the crossed extension. Furthermore, after the painful stimulus is removed, the crossed extensor reflex continues for an even longer period of afterdischarge than that for the flexor reflex. Therefore, again, it is virtually certain that this prolonged afterdischarge results from reverberatory circuits among the internuncial cells.

RECIPROCAL INHIBITION AND RECIPROCAL INNERVATION

In the foregoing paragraphs we have pointed out several times that excitation of one group of muscles is usually associated with inhibition of another group. For instance, when a stretch reflex excites one muscle, it simultaneously inhibits the antagonist muscles. This is the phenomenon of *reciprocal inhibition,* and the neuronal circuit that causes this reciprocal relationship is called *reciprocal innervation.* Likewise, reciprocal relationships exist between the two sides of the cord, as exemplified by the flexor and extensor reflexes described above.

THE REFLEXES OF POSTURE AND LOCOMOTION

The Positive Supportive Reaction. Pressure on the footpad of a decerebrate animal causes the limb to extend against the pressure that is being aplied to the foot. Indeed, this reflex can sometimes be so strong that an animal whose spinal cord was transected several months previously can often be placed on its feet, and the pressure on the footpads will reflexly stiffen the limbs sufficiently to support the weight of the body. This reflex is called the *positive supportive reaction.*

The positive supportive reaction involves a complex circuit in the interneurons similar to those responsible for the flexor and the crossed extensor reflexes. Furthermore, the locus of the pressure on the pad of the foot determines the position to which the limb is extended

The Rhythmical Stepping Reflex. Rhythmical stepping movements are frequently observed in the limbs of spinal animals. Indeed, even when the lower portion is separated from the remainder of the spinal cord and a longitudinal section is made down the center of the cord to block neuronal connections between the two limbs, each hind limb can still perform stepping functions. Forward flexion of the limb is followed a second or so later by backward extension. Then flexion occurs again, and the cycle is repeated over and over.

If the lumbar spinal cord is not sectioned down its center, every time stepping occurs in the forward directions in one limb, the opposite limb ordinarily steps backward. This effect results from reciprocal innervation between the two limbs.

Diagonal Stepping of All Four Limbs—The Mark Time Reflex. Stepping reflexes that involve all four limbs can also be demonstrated in a spinal animal. In general, stepping occurs diagonally between the forelimbs and hindlimbs. That is, the right hindlimb and the left forelimb move backward together while the right forelimb and left hindlimb move forward. This diagonal response is another manifestation of reciprocal innervation, this time occurring the entire distance up and down the cord between the fore- and hind limbs. Such a walking pattern, illustrated in a spinal dog hanging in a sling in Figure 37–7, is often called a *mark time reflex.*

The Galloping Reflex. Another type of reflex that occasionally develops in the spinal animal is the galloping reflex, in which both forelimbs move backward in unison while both hindlimbs move forward. If stretch or pressure stimuli are applied almost exactly equally to opposite limbs at the same time, a galloping reflex is likely to result, whereas unequal stimulation of one side versus the other elicits the diagonal walking reflex. This is in keeping with the normal patterns of walking and galloping, for in walking only one limb at a time is stimulated, which would predispose to continued walking. Conversely, when the animal strikes the ground during galloping, the limbs on both sides are stimulated approximately equally, which obviously would predispose to further galloping and continuation of this pattern of motion in contradistinction to the walking pattern.

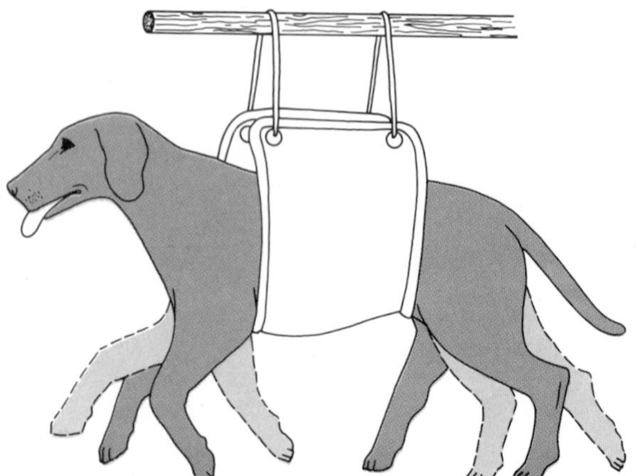

Figure 37–7. Diagonal stepping movements exhibited by a spinal animal.

SPINAL CORD REFLEXES THAT CAUSE MUSCLE SPASM

In human beings, local muscle spasm is often observed. The mechanism of this has not been elucidated to complete satisfaction even in experimental animals, but it is known that pain stimuli can cause reflex spasm of local muscles, which presumably is the cause of much if not most of the muscle spasm observed in localized regions of the human body.

Abdominal Spasm in Peritonitis. A type of local muscle spasm caused by a cord reflex is the abdominal spasm resulting from irritation of the parietal peritoneum by peritonitis. Relief of the pain caused by the peritonitis allows the spastic muscles to relax. Almost the same type of spasm often occurs during surgical operations; pain impulses from the parietal peritoneum cause the abdominal muscles to contract extensively and sometimes actually to squeeze the abdomen and to extrude the intestines through the surgical wound. For this reason deep surgical anesthesia is usually required for intra-abdominal operations.

Muscle Cramps. Another type of local spasm is the typical muscle cramp. Any local irritating factor or metabolic abnormality of a muscle — such as severe cold, lack of blood flow to the muscle, or overexercise of the muscle — can elicit pain or other types of sensory impulses that are transmitted from the muscle to the spinal cord, thus causing reflex muscle contraction. The contraction in turn stimulates the same sensory receptors still more, which causes the spinal cord to increase the intensity of contraction still further. Thus, a positive feedback mechanism occurs, so that a small amount of initial irritation causes more and more contraction until a full-blown muscle cramp ensues.

SPINAL CORD TRANSECTION AND SPINAL SHOCK

When the spinal cord is suddenly transected in the neck, essentially all cord functions, including the cord reflexes, immediately become almost completely blocked, a response called *spinal shock.* The reason for this shock is that normal activity of the cord neurons depends to a great extent on continual *facilitory signals* from higher centers, particularly signals transmitted through the vestibulospinal tract, the reticulospinal tracts, and the corticospinal tracts.

Some of the spinal functions specifically affected during spinal shock are these: (1) The arterial blood pressure falls immediately — sometimes to as low as 40 mm Hg — thus illustrating that activity in the sympathetic nerves to the blood vessels and heart becomes blocked almost to extinction. However, the pressure ordinarily returns to normal within a few hours in lower animals and within a few days in the human being. (2) All skeletal muscle reflexes are completely blocked during the initial stages of spinal shock. In lower animals, a few hours to a week or so are required for the cord reflexes to return to normal, and in human beings several weeks are often required. (3) The sacral reflexes for control of bladder and colon evacuation are completely suppressed in humans for the first few weeks following cord transection, but they eventually return. These effects are discussed in Chapters 23 and 42.

ROLE OF THE BRAIN STEM IN CONTROLLING MOTOR FUNCTION

The brain stem consists of the *medulla, pons,* and *mesencephalon.* In one sense it is an extension of the spinal cord upward into the cranial cavity, because it contains motor and sensory nuclei that perform motor and sensory functions for the face and head regions in the same way that the anterior and posterior gray horns of the spinal cord perform these same functions from the neck down. But in another sense, it is its own master, because it provides many special control functions, such as the following:

1. Control of respiration.
2. Control of the cardiovascular system.
3. Control of gastrointestinal function.
4. Control of many stereotyped movements of the body.
5. Control of equilibrium.
6. Control of eye movement.

Finally, the brain stem serves also as an instrument of higher neural centers that transmit many "command" signals into the brain stem to initiate or modify the brain stem's specific control functions.

In the following sections of this chapter we discuss the role of the brain stem in controlling whole body movement and equilibrium. Especially important for this purpose are the brain stem's *reticular nuclei* and *vestibular nuclei,* plus the *vestibular apparatus* that sends most of the equilibrium control signals to the vestibular nuclei and to a lesser extent to the reticular nuclei as well.

Support of the Body Against Gravity — Roles of the Reticular and Vestibular Nuclei

Excitatory-Inhibitory Antagonism Between Pontine and Medullary Reticular Nuclei

Figure 37–8 illustrates the locations of the reticular and vestibular nuclei. The reticular nuclei are divided into two major groups, (1) the *pontine reticular nuclei,* located mainly in the pons but extending into the mesencephalon as well, lying more laterally in the brain stem, and (2) the *medullary reticular nuclei,* which extend the entire extent of the medulla, lying ventrally and medially near the midline. These two sets of nuclei function mainly antagonistically to each other, the pontine exciting the antigravity muscles

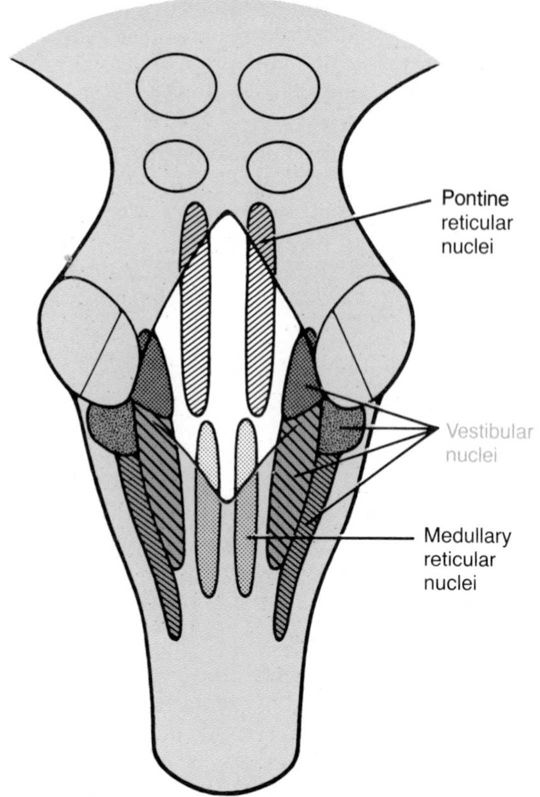

Figure 37–8. Locations of the reticular and vestibular nuclei in the brain stem.

and the medullary inhibiting them. The pontine reticular nuclei transmit excitatory signals downward into the cord through the *pontine* (or *medial*) *reticulospinal tract,* illustrated in Figure 37–9. The fibers of this pathway terminate on the anterior motor neurons that excite the muscles that support the body against gravity, that is, the muscles of the spinal column and the extensor muscles of the limbs.

The pontine reticular nuclei have a high degree of natural excitability. Therefore, when the pontine reticular excitatory system is unopposed by the medullary reticular system, it causes powerful excitation of the antigravity muscles throughout the body, so much so that animals can then stand up against gravity without any signals from the higher levels of the brain.

The Medullary Reticular System. The medullary nuclei, on the other hand, transmit inhibitory signals to the same antigravity anterior motor neurons by way of a different tract, the *medullary* (or *lateral*) *reticulospinal tract,* also illustrated in Figure 37–9. The medullary reticular nuclei receive strong input collaterals from (1) the corticospinal tract, (2) the rubrospinal tract, and (3) other motor pathways. These can activate the medullary reticular inhibitory system to counterbalance the excitatory signals from the pontine reticular system. This allows still higher centers in the brain to elicit other motor activities, which would be impossible if the antigravity muscles opposed the necessary movements.

Therefore, the excitatory and inhibitory reticular nuclei constitute a controllable system that is manipulated by motor signals from the cortex and elsewhere to provide the necessary muscle contractions for standing against gravity and yet to inhibit appropriate groups of muscles as needed so that other functions can be performed as required.

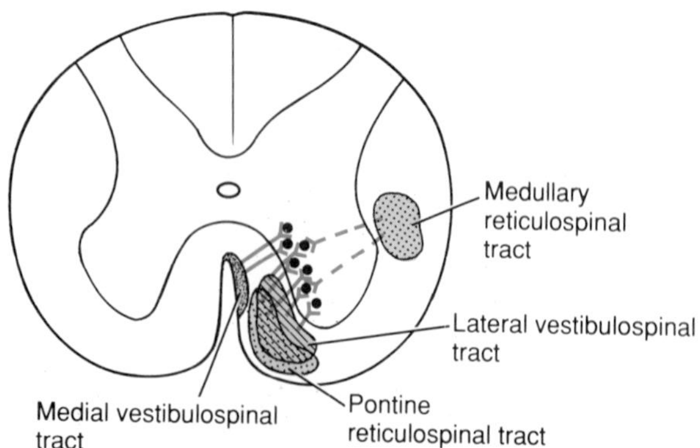

Figure 37–9. The vestibulospinal and reticulospinal tracts descending in the spinal cord to excite (solid lines) or inhibit (dashed lines) the anterior motor neurons that control the body's axial musculature.

Role of the Vestibular Nuclei in Exciting the Antigravity Muscles

The vestibular nuclei, illustrated in Figure 37–8, function also in association with the pontine reticular nuclei to excite the antigravity muscles. The *lateral vestibular nuclei* (indicated by the heavy dots in the figure), especially, transmit strong excitatory signals by way of both the *lateral* and *medial vestibulospinal tracts* in the anterior column of the spinal cord, as illustrated in Figure 37–9. In fact, without the support of the vestibular nuclei, the pontine reticular system loses much of its force. The specific role of the vestibular nuclei, however, is to control selectively the excitatory signals to the different antigravity muscles to maintain equilibrium in response to signals from the vestibular apparatus. We shall discuss this more fully later in the chapter.

VESTIBULAR SENSATIONS AND THE MAINTENANCE OF EQUILIBRIUM

The Vestibular Apparatus

The vestibular apparatus is the organ that detects sensations of equilibrium. It is composed of a system of bony tubes and chambers in the petrous portion of the temporal bone called the *bony labyrinth* and within this a system of membranous tubes and chambers called the *membranous labyrinth,* which is the functional part of the apparatus. The top of Figure 37–10 illustrates the membranous labyrinth; it is composed mainly of the *cochlea,* three *semicircular ducts,* and two large chambers known as the *utricle* and the *saccule.* The cochlea is the major sensory area

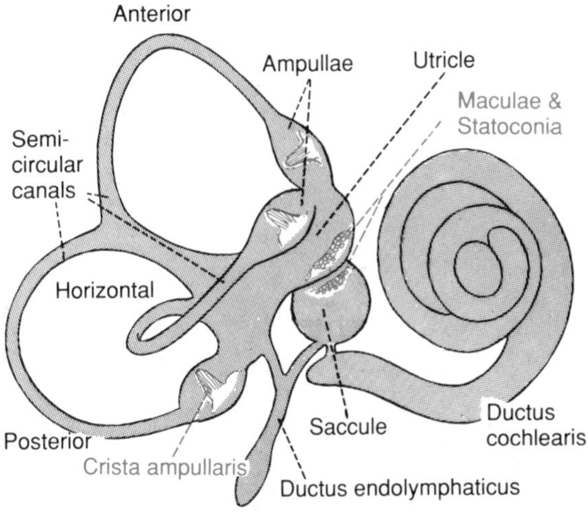

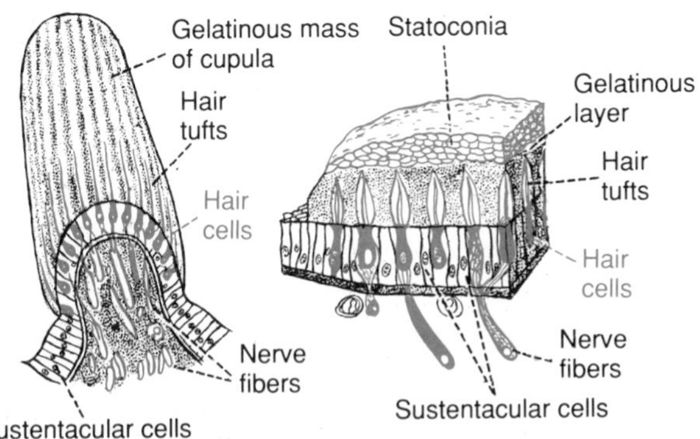

Figure 37-10. The membranous labyrinth and organization of the crista ampullaris and the macula. (Modified from Goss: Gray's Anatomy of the Human Body. Philadelphia, Lea & Febiger; modified from Kolmer by Buchanan: Functional Neuroanatomy. Philadelphia, Lea & Febiger.)

for hearing that was discussed in Chapter 36 and has nothing to do with equilibrium. However, the *utricle,* the *semicircular ducts,* and the *saccule* are all integral parts of the equilibrium mechanism.

The Maculae—The Sensory Organs of the Utricle and the Saccule for Detecting the Orientation of the Head with Respect to Gravity. Located on the inside surface of each utricle and saccule, as shown in Figure 37-10, is a small sensory area slightly over two mm in diameter called a *macula.* Each macula is covered by a gelatinous layer in which many small calcium carbonate crystals called *statoconia* (or *otoliths*) are imbedded. Also in the macula are thousands of *hair cells,* one of which is illustrated in Figure 37-11; these project *cilia* up into the gelatinous layer. The bases and sides of the hair cells synapse with sensory endings of the vestibular nerve.

Directional Sensitivity of the Hair Cells—The Kinocilium. Each hair cell has an average of 50 to 70 small cilia called *stereocilia,* plus one very large cilium, the *kinocilium,* as illustrated in the figure. The kinocilium is located always to one side, and the stereocilia become progressively shorter toward the other side of the cell. Very minute filamentous attachments, almost invisible even to the electron microscope, connect the tip of each stereocilium to the next longer stereocilium and finally to the kinocilium. Because of these attachments, when the brush pile of stereocilia and kinocilium is bent in the direction of the kinocilium, the filamentous attachments tug one after the other on the stereocilia, pulling them away from the cell body. This opens several hundred channels in each cilium membrane for conducting positive sodium ions, and large quantities of these positive ions pour into the cell from the surrounding fluids, causing *depolarization.* Conversely, bending the pile of cilia in the opposite direction (away from the kinocilium) reduces the tension on the attachments, and this closes the ion channels, thus causing *hyperpolarization.*

Under normal resting conditions, the nerve fibers leading from the hair cells transmit continuous nerve

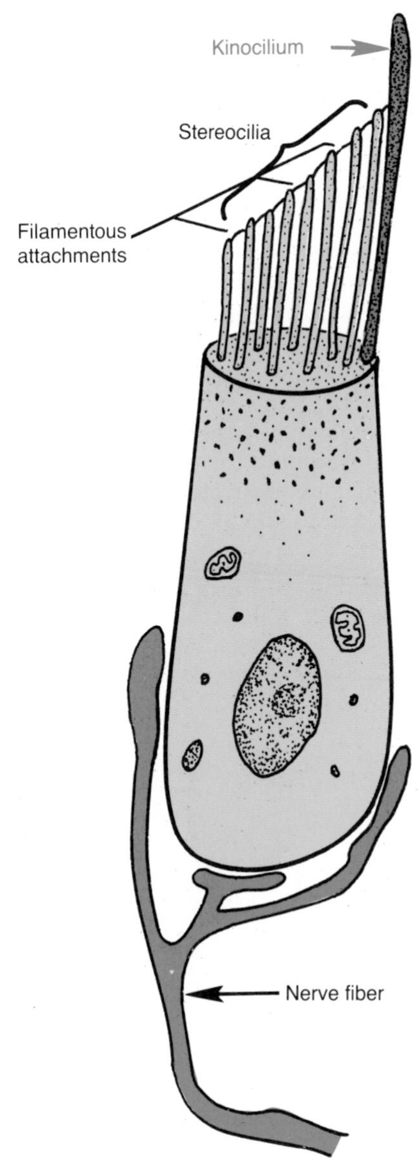

Figure 37-11. A hair cell of the membranous labyrinth of the equilibrium apparatus.

impulses at rates about 100 per second. When the cilia are bent toward the kinocilium, the impulse traffic can increase to several hundred per second; conversely, bending the cilia in the opposite direction decreases the impulse traffic, often turning it off completely. Therefore, as the orientation of the head in space changes and the weight of the statoconia (whose specific gravity is about three times that of the surrounding tissues) bends the cilia, appropriate signals are transmitted to the brain to control equilibrium.

In each macula the different hair cells are oriented in different directions so that some of them are stimulated when the head bends forward, some when it bends backward, others when it bends to one side, and so forth. Therefore, a different pattern of excitation occurs in the nerve fibers from the macula for each position of the head; it is this "pattern" that apprises the brain of the head's orientation.

The Semicircular Ducts. The three semicircular ducts in each vestibular apparatus, known respectively as the *anterior, posterior,* and *horizontal semicircular ducts,* are arranged at right angles to each other so that they represent all three planes in space.

Each semicircular duct has an enlargement at one of its ends called the *ampulla,* and the ducts are filled with a viscous fluid called *endolymph.* Flow of this fluid from one of the ducts into the ampulla excites the sensory organ of the ampulla in the following manner: Figure 37–12 illustrates in each ampulla a small crest called a *crista ampullaris.* On top of this crista is a gelatinous mass, the *cupula.* When the head begins to rotate in any direction, the inertia of the fluid in one or more of the semicircular ducts will cause the fluid to remain stationary while the semicircular duct rotates with the head. This causes fluid flow from the duct into the ampulla, bending the cupula to one side as illustrated by the position of the shaded cupula in Figure 37–12. Rotation of the head in the opposite direction causes the cupula to bend to the opposite side.

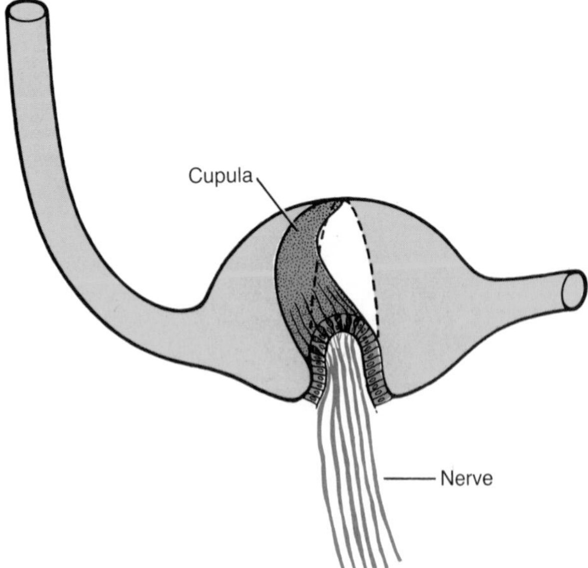

Figure 37–12. Movement of the cupula and its embedded hairs at the onset of rotation.

Into the cupula are projected hundreds of cilia from hair cells located along the ampullary crest. The *kinocilium* of each of these hair cells is always directed toward the same side of the cupula as the others, and bending the cupula in that direction causes depolarization of the hair cells, whereas bending it in the opposite direction will hyperpolarize the cells. From the hair cells, appropriate signals are sent by way of the *vestibular nerve* to apprise the central nervous system of changes in the rate and direction of rotation of the head in the three different planes of space.

Function of the Utricle and Saccule in the Maintenance of Static Equilibrium

It is especially important that the different hair cells are oriented in all different directions in the maculae of the utricles and saccules so that at different positions of the head, different hair cells become stimulated. The "patterns" of stimulation of the different hair cells apprise the nervous system of the position of the head with respect to the pull of gravity. In turn, the vestibular, cerebellar, and reticular motor systems excite by reflex the appropriate muscles to maintain proper equilibrium.

Detection of Linear Acceleration by the Maculae. When the body is suddenly thrust forward—that is, when the body accelerates—the statoconia, which have greater inertia than the surrounding fluids, fall backward on the hair cell cilia, and information of malequilibrium is sent into the nervous centers, causing the individual to feel as though he or she were falling backward. This automatically causes him or her to lean the body forward until the anterior shift of the statoconia caused by leaning exactly equals the tendency for the statoconia to fall backward. At this point, the nervous system detects a state of proper equilibrium and therefore leans the body no farther forward. Thus, the maculae operate to maintain equilibrium during linear acceleration in exactly the same manner as they operate in static equilibrium.

The Semicircular Ducts and Their Detection of Angular Acceleration

When the head suddenly *begins* to rotate in any direction, the endolymph in the membranous semicircular ducts, because of its inertia, tends to remain stationary while the semicircular ducts themselves turn. This causes relative fluid flow in the ducts in a direction opposite to the rotation of the head; this relative flow lasts for a few seconds, thus activating the semicular duct receptors; and the person perceives this onset of rotation, which is called *angular acceleration.*

When the rotation suddenly stops, exactly the opposite effects take place: That is, the endolymph continues to rotate while the semicircular duct itself stops, and the duct receptors are activated in the opposite direction; the person perceives the termination of rotation.

"Predictive" Function of the Semicircular Ducts in the Maintenance of Equilibrium. Because the semicircular ducts do not detect that the body is off balance in the forward direction, in the side direction, or in the backward direction, one might at first ask: What is the function of the semicircular ducts in the maintenance of equilibrium? All they detect is that the person's head is beginning to rotate or stopping rotation in one direction or another. Therefore, the function of the semicircular ducts is not likely to be to maintain static equilibrium or to maintain equilibrium during linear acceleration or when the person is exposed to steady centrifugal forces. Yet loss of function of the semicircular ducts causes a person to have very poor equilibrium when attempting to perform *rapid* and *intricate* body movements.

We can explain the function of the semicircular ducts best by the following illustration. If a person is running forward rapidly, and then suddenly begins to turn to one side, he falls off balance a fraction of a second later unless appropriate corrections are made *ahead of time.* But, unfortunately, the macula of the utricle cannot detect that he is off balance until *after* this has occurred. On the other hand, the semicircular ducts will have already detected that the person is turning, and this information can easily apprise the central nervous system of the fact that the person *will* fall off balance within the next fraction of a second or so unless some correction is made. In other words, the semicircular duct mechanism *predicts ahead of time* that malequilibrium is going to occur even before it does occur and thereby causes the equilibrium centers to make appropriate preventive adjustments. In this way, the person need not fall off balance before he begins to correct the situation.

Other Factors Concerned with Equilibrium

The Neck Proprioceptors. The vestibular apparatus detects the orientation and movements *only of the head.* Therefore, it is essential that the nervous centers also receive appropriate information depicting the orientation of the head with respect to the body. This information is transmitted from the proprioceptors of the neck and body directly into the vestibular and reticular nuclei of the brain. When the head is leaned in one direction by bending the neck, impulses from the neck proprioceptors keep the vestibular apparatus from giving the person a sense of malequilibrium. They do this by transmitting signals that exactly oppose the signals transmitted from the vestibular apparatuses. However, *when the entire body* leans in one direction, the impulses from the vestibular apparatuses *are not opposed* by the neck proprioceptors; therefore, the person in this instance does perceive a change in equilibrium status of the entire body.

Importance of Visual Information in the Maintenance of Equilibrium. After complete destruction of the vestibular apparatus, and even after loss of most proprioceptive information from the body, a person can still use the visual mechanisms effectively for maintaining equilibrium. Even slight linear or rotational movement of the body instantaneously shifts the visual images on the retina, and this information is relayed to the equilibrium centers. Many persons with complete destruction of the vestibular apparatus have almost normal equilibrium as long as their eyes are open and as long as they perform all motions slowly. But when one is moving rapidly or when the eyes are closed, equilibrium is immediately lost.

Neuronal Connections of the Vestibular Apparatus with the Central Nervous System

Figure 37–13 illustrates the central connections of the vestibular nerve. Most of the vestibular nerve fibers end in the vestibular nuclei, which are located approximately at the junction of the medulla and the pons, but some fibers pass without synapsing to the brain stem reticular nuclei and the fastigial nuclei, uvula, and flocculonodular lobes of the cerebellum.

The primary pathway for the reflexes of equilibrium begins in the vestibular nerves and passes next to both the vestibular nuclei and the cerebellum. Then, along with two-way traffic of impulses between these two, signals are also sent into the reticular nuclei of the brain stem as well as down the spinal cord via the vestibulospinal and reticulospinal tracts. In turn, the signals to the cord control the interplay between facilitation and inhibition of the antigravity muscles, thus automatically controlling equilibrium.

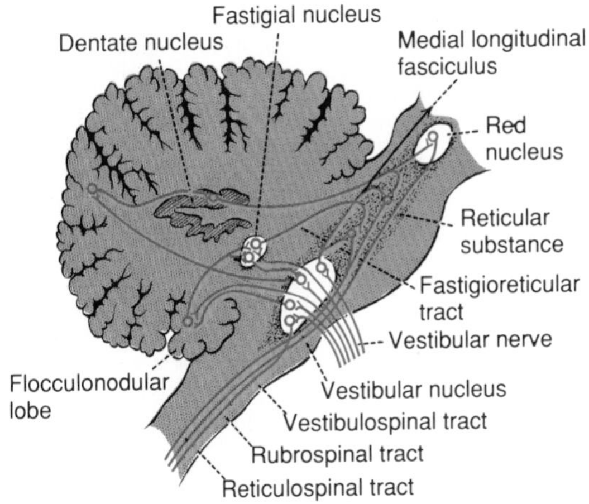

Figure 37–13. Connections of vestibular nerves in the central nervous system.

FUNCTIONS OF SPECIFIC BRAIN STEM NUCLEI IN CONTROLLING SUBCONSCIOUS, STEREOTYPED MOVEMENTS

Rarely, a child is born without brain structures above the mesencephalic region. Some of these children, called *anencephalic monsters,* have been kept alive for many months. They are able to perform essentially all the functions of feeding, such as suckling, extrusion of unpleasant food from the mouth, and moving the hands to the mouth to suck the fingers. In addition, they can yawn and stretch. They can cry and follow objects with movements of the eyes and head. Also, placing pressure on the upper anterior parts of their legs will cause them to pull to the sitting position.

Therefore, it is obvious that many of the stereotyped motor functions of the human being are integrated in the brain stem. Unfortunately, the loci of most of the different motor control systems have not been found except for the following:

Stereotyped Body Movements. Most movements of the trunk and head can be classified into several simple movements, such as forward flexion, extension, rotation, and turning movements of the entire body. These types of movements are controlled by special nuclei located mainly in the mesencephalic and lower diencephalic region. For instance, *rotational movements* of the head and eyes are controlled by the *interstitial nucleus.* This nucleus lies in the mesencephalon in close approximation to the *medial longitudinal fasciculus,* through which it transmits a major portion of its control impulses. The *raising movements* of the head and body are controlled by the *prestitial nucleus,* which is located approximately at the juncture of the diencephalon and mesencephalon. On the other hand, the *flexing movements* of the head and body are controlled by the *nucleus precommissuralis* located at the level of the posterior commissure. Finally, the *turning movements* of the entire body, which are much more complicated, involve both the pontine and mesencephalic reticular nuclei.

SUMMARY OF THE FUNCTIONS OF THE CORD AND BRAIN STEM IN POSTURE AND LOCOMOTION

From the discussions in this chapter, we see that almost all the discrete "patterns" of muscle movements required for posture and locomotion can be elicited by the spinal cord alone. However, coordination of these patterns to provide equilibrium, progression, and purposefulness of movement requires neuronal function at progressively higher levels of the central nervous system. Centers in the brain stem provide most of the nervous energy required to maintain the postural tone for support of the body against gravity. In addition, brain stem centers provide especially the equilibrium adjustments of the body and the control of most stereotyped movements of body as well.

In the following chapter we discuss the functions of still higher centers in the brain to provide the voluntary movements of the body.

REFERENCES

Spinal Cord

Brooks, V. B.: The Neural Basis of Motor Control. New York, Oxford University Press, 1986.

Emonet-Denand, F., et al.: How muscle spindles signal changes of muscle length. News Physiol. Sci., 3:105, 1988.

Hammond, D. L.: New insights regarding organization of spinal cord pain pathways. News Physiol. Sci., 4:98, 1989.

Hasan, Z., and Stuart, D. G.: Animal solutions to problems of movement control: The role of proprioceptors. Annu. Rev. Neurosci., 11:199, 1988.

Hnik, P., et al. (eds.): Mechanoreceptors. Development, Structure, and Function. New York, Plenum Publishing Corp., 1988.

Houk, J. C.: Control strategies in physiological systems. FASEB J., 2:97, 1988.

Janig, W., and McLachlan, E. M.: Organization of lumbar spinal outflow to distal colon and pelvic organs. Physiol. Rev., 67:1332, 1987.

Stein, D. G., and Sabel, B. A. (eds.): Pharmacological Approaches to the Treatment of Brain and Spinal Cord Injury. New York, Plenum Publishing Corp., 1988.

Brain Stem

Bahill, A. T., and Hamm, T. M.: Using open-loop experiments to study physiological systems, with examples from the human eye-movement systems. News Physiol. Sci., 4:104, 1989.

Dutia, M. B.: Mechanisms of head stabilization. News Physiol. Sci., 4:101, 1989.

Evarts, E. V., et al. (eds.): Motor System in Neurobiology. New York, Elsevier Science Publishing Co., 1986.

Fournier, E., and Pierrot-Deseilligny, E.: Changes in transmission in some reflex pathways during movement in humans. News Physiol. Sci., 4:29, 1989.

Hasan, Z., and Stuart, D. G.: Animal solutions to problems of movement control: The role of proprioceptors. Annu. Rev. Neurosci., 11:199, 1988.

Peterson, B. W., and Richmond, F. J. (eds.): Control of Head Movement. New York, Oxford University Press, 1988.

Sherrington, C. S.: Decerebrate rigidity and reflex coordination of movements. J. Physiol. (Lond.), 22:319, 1898.

QUESTIONS

1. Describe the organization of the typical segment of the spinal cord for motor control.
2. Explain the roles of the *alpha motor neurons,* the *gamma motor neurons,* and the *interneurons* in the control of muscle contraction.
3. Describe the *muscle spindle,* its innervation, and the anatomy of its receptor region.
4. What are the functional differences between the *primary* and *secondary sensory endings* of the muscle spindle?

5. Explain the manner in which the spindle receptor is stimulated by (a) stretching the whole muscle or (b) contracting the intrafusal muscle fibers of the spindle. What is meant by the comparator function of the muscle spindle?
6. Explain the difference between the *dynamic stretch reflex* and the *static stretch reflex.*
7. Describe the neuronal circuit of the stretch reflex.
8. How does the stretch reflex help damp jerky muscle movements?
9. How does the stretch reflex prevent large changes in muscle length when different levels of load are applied to the muscle?
10. Describe the *Golgi tendon organ* and the means by which it is excited.
11. Describe the neuronal circuit of the *tendon reflex.*
12. How does the tendon reflex function to equalize tension in the muscle fibers of a contracting muscle?
13. Explain the neuronal circuit of the *flexor reflex* and the function of the flexor reflex. Why is the flexor reflex sometimes called a *withdrawal reflex*?
14. Explain the phenomenon of *reciprocal inhibition* as it applies to the *crossed extensor reflex.*
15. Describe the following reflexes of posture and locomotion; the *positive supportive reaction,* the *rhythmical stepping reflex,* and the *galloping reflex.*
16. Why does peritonitis cause *abdominal spasm*?
17. Describe the brain stem anatomy in relation to its role in the support of the body against gravity.
18. Describe the *macula* of the *utricle* or the *saccule,* including the orientation of hair cells within the macula and function of the macula for detection of equilibrium.
19. Why are the maculae in the utricle and saccule the principal equilibrium sensory receptor organs for both static equilibrium and detection of linear acceleration?
20. Explain the detection of angular acceleration by the *semicircular canals* and the importance of detecting this for the maintenance of balance during rapid movements.
21. Why are the *neck reflexes* of importance in the maintenance of equilibrium?
22. What are some of the stereotyped movements that are controlled by specific nuclei in the brain stem?

38

Control of Muscle Function by the Motor Cortex, the Basal Ganglia, and the Cerebellum

In this chapter we discuss the control of the body's movements by the cerebral cortex, the basal ganglia, and the cerebellum. Virtually all "voluntary" movements involve conscious activity in the cerebral cortex. Yet this does not mean that each contraction of each muscle is willed by the cortex itself. Instead, most control involves patterns of function in lower brain areas—in the cord, in the brain stem, in the basal ganglia, in the cerebellum—and these lower centers in turn send most of the specific activating signals to the muscles. However, for a few types of movements, the cortex does have almost a direct pathway to the anterior motor neurons of the cord, bypassing other motor centers on the way, especially for control of the very fine dexterous movements of our fingers and hands. It is the goal of this chapter to explain the interplay among the different motor areas of the brain and spinal cord that provides this overall synthesis of motor function.

THE MOTOR CORTEX AND THE CORTICOSPINAL TRACT

Figure 38–1 illustrates the functional areas of the cerebral cortex. Anterior to the central sulcus, occupying approximately the posterior third of the frontal lobes, is the *motor cortex.* Posterior to the central sulcus is the *somatic sensory cortex,* an area discussed in detail in earlier chapters that feeds many signals into the motor cortex for control of motor activities.

The motor cortex itself is further divided into three separate subareas, each of which has its own topographical representation of all the muscle groups of the body: (1) the *primary motor cortex,* (2) the *premotor area,* and (3) the *supplemental motor area.*

The Primary Motor Cortex

The primary motor cortex, shown in Figure 38–1, lies in the first convolution of the frontal lobes anterior to the central sulcus. It begins laterally in the sylvian fissure and spreads superiorly to the uppermost portion of the brain, then dips over into the longitudinal fissure.

Figure 38–2 lists the topographical representations of the different muscle areas of the body in the primary motor cortex, beginning with the face and mouth region, near the sylvian fissure; the arm and hand area, in the midportions of the primary motor cortex; the trunk, near the apex of the brain; and the leg and foot areas, in that part of the primary motor cortex that dips into the longitudinal fissure. Note that more than half of the entire primary motor cortex is concerned with controlling the hands and the muscles of speech.

The Premotor Area

The premotor area, also shown in Figure 38–1, lies immediately anterior to the primary motor cortex, projecting 1 to 3 centimeters anteriorly and extending inferiorly into the sylvian fissure and superiorly into the longitudinal fissure, where it abuts the supplemental motor area. Note that the topographical organization of the premotor cortex is roughly the same as that of the primary motor cortex, with the face area located most laterally and then in the upward direction the arm, trunk, and leg areas.

Most nerve signals generated in the premotor area

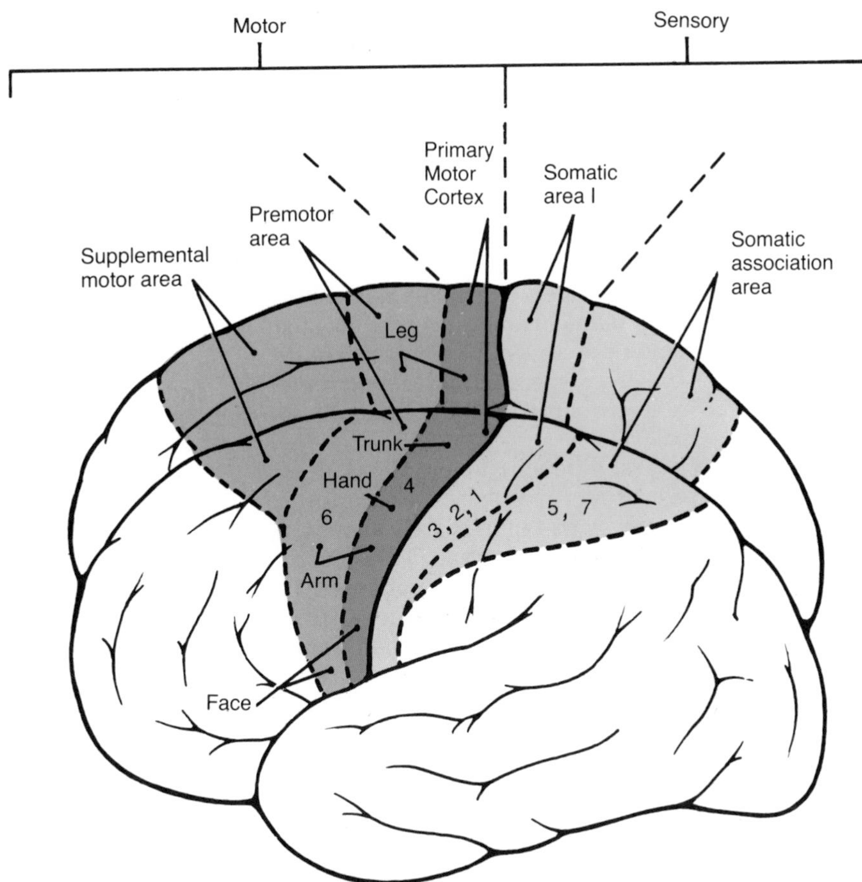

Figure 38-1. The motor and somatic sensory functional areas of the cerebral cortex.

cause patterns of movement involving groups of muscles that perform specific tasks. For instance, the task may be to position the shoulders and arms so that the hands become properly oriented to perform specific tasks. To achieve these results, the premotor area sends its signals either directly into the primary motor cortex to excite multiple groups of muscles or, more likely, by way of the basal ganglia and then back through the thalamus to the primary motor cortex. Thus, the premotor cortex, the basal ganglia, the thalamus, and the primary motor cortex constitute a complex overall system for control of many of the body's more complex patterns of coordinated muscle activity.

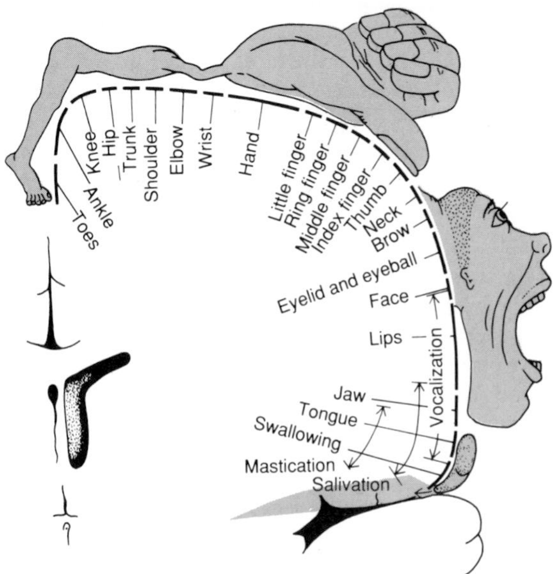

Figure 38-2. Degree of representation of the different muscles of the body in the motor cortex. (From Penfield and Rasmussen: The Cerebral Cortex of Man: A Clinical Study of Localization of Function. New York, Macmillan, 1968.)

The Supplemental Motor Area

The supplemental motor area has still another topographical organization for control of motor function. It lies immediately superior and anterior to the premotor area, lying mainly in the longitudinal fissure but extending a centimeter or so over the edge onto the superiormost portion of the exposed cortex.

Considerably stronger electrical stimuli are required in the supplemental motor area to cause muscle contraction than in the other motor areas. However, when contractions are elicited, they are often bilateral rather than unilateral. And stimulation frequently leads to movements such as unilateral grasping of a hand or at other times bilateral grasping of both hands simultaneously; these movements are perhaps rudiments of the hand functions required for climbing. In general, this area probably functions in concert with the premotor area to provide attitudinal movements, fixation movements of the different segments of the body, positional movements of the head and eyes, and so forth, as background for the finer motor control of the hands and feet by the premotor and primary motor cortex.

Some Specialized Areas of Motor Control Found in the Human Motor Cortex

Neurosurgeons have found a few highly specialized motor regions of the human cerebral cortex, located mainly in the premotor areas as illustrated in Figure 38–3, that control very specific motor functions. Some of the more important of these are the following:

Broca's Area and Speech. Figure 38–3 illustrates a premotor area lying immediately anterior to the primary motor cortex and immediately above the sylvian fissure labeled "word formation." This region is called *Broca's area.* Damage to it does not prevent a person from vocalizing, but it does make it impossible for the person to speak whole words other than simple utterances such as "no" or "yes." A closely associated cortical area also causes appropriate respiratory function so that respiratory activation of vocal cords can occur simultaneously with the movements of the mouth and tongue during speech. Thus, the premotor activities that are related to Broca's area are highly complex.

Head Rotation Area. Slightly higher in the motor association area, electrical stimulation will elicit head rotation. This area is closely associated with an eye movement field as well and is presumably related to directing the head and eyes toward different objects.

Area for Hand Skills. In the premotor area immediately anterior to the primary motor cortex for the hands and fingers is a region neurosurgeons have called an area for hand skills. That is, when tumors or other lesions cause destruction in this area, the hand movements become incoordinate and nonpurposeful, a condition called *motor apraxia.*

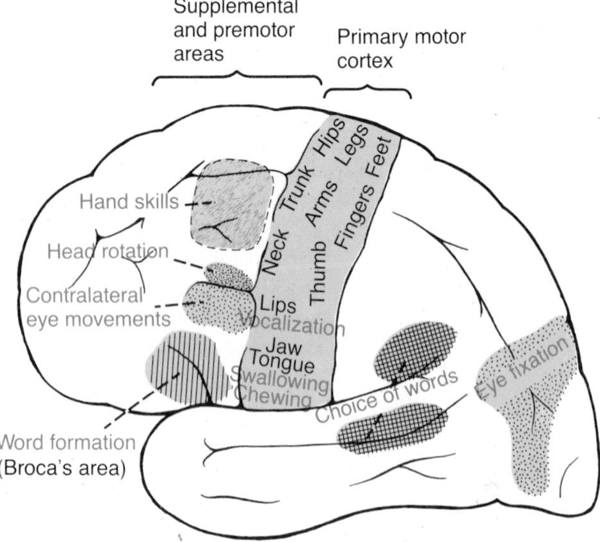

Figure 38–3. Representation of the different muscles of the body in the motor cortex and location of other cortical areas responsible for certain types of motor movements.

Transmission of Signals from the Motor Cortex to the Muscles

Motor signals are transmitted directly from the cortex to the spinal cord through the *corticospinal tract* and indirectly through multiple accessory pathways that involve the *basal ganglia,* the *cerebellum,* and various *nuclei of the brain stem.* In general, the direct pathways are concerned more with discrete and detailed movements, especially of the distal segments of the limbs, such as the hands and the fingers.

The Corticospinal Tract (Pyramidal Tract)

The most important output pathway from the motor cortex is the *corticospinal tract,* also called the *pyramidal tract,* which is illustrated in Figure 38–4.

The corticospinal tract originates about 30 per cent from the primary motor cortex, 30 per cent from the premotor and supplementary motor areas, and 40 per cent from the somatic sensory areas posterior to the central sulcus. After leaving the cortex it passes through the brain stem, forming the *pyramids of the medulla.* By far the majority of the pyramidal fibers then cross to the opposite side and descend in the *lateral corticospinal tracts* of the cord, finally terminating principally on the interneurons in the intermediate regions of the cord gray matter.

The most impressive fibers in the pyramidal tract are a population of large myelinated fibers with mean diameter of 16 micrometers. These originate from the *giant pyramidal cells,* also called *Betz cells,* that are found only in the primary motor cortex. These fibers transmit nerve impulses to the spinal cord at a velocity of about 70 m/sec, the most rapid rate of transmission of any signals from the brain to the cord.

Incoming Fiber Pathways to the Motor Cortex

The functions of the motor cortex are controlled mainly by the somatic sensory system but also to a lesser extent by the other sensory systems such as hearing and vision. Once the sensory information is derived from these sources, the motor cortex operates in association with the basal ganglia and cerebellum to process the information and to determine the appropriate course of motor action. The more important incoming fiber pathways to the motor cortex are as follows:

1. Subcortical fibers from adjacent regions of the cortex.
2. Subcortical fibers that pass through the corpus callosum from the opposite cerebral hemisphere.

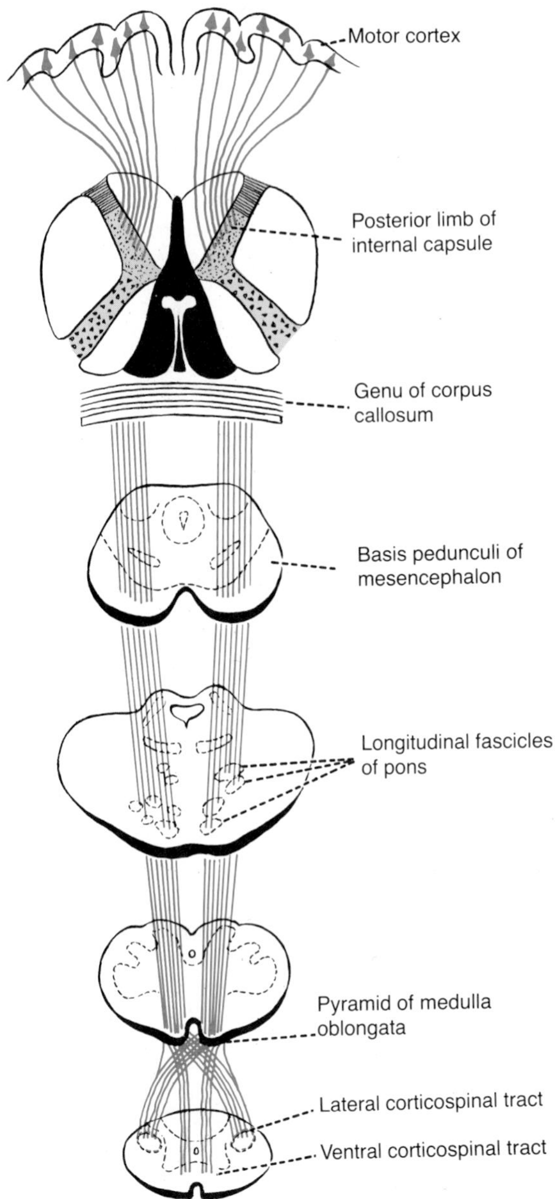

Figure 38-4. The pyramidal tract. (Modified from Ranson and Clark: Anatomy of the Nervous System. Philadelphia, W. B. Saunders Company, 1959.)

3. Somatic sensory fibers derived directly from the ventrobasal complex of the thalamus.
4. Tracts from the ventrolateral and ventroanterior nuclei of the thalamus, which in turn receive tracts from the cerebellum and the basal ganglia. These tracts provide signals that are necessary for coordination between the functions of the motor cortex, the basal ganglia, and the cerebellum.
5. Fibers from the intralaminar nuclei of the thalamus. These fibers control the general level of excitability of the motor cortex in the same manner that they also control the general level of excitability of most other regions of the cerebral cortex.

The Extrapyramidal System

The term *"extrapyramidal motor system"* is widely used in clinical circles to denote all those portions of the brain and brain stem that contribute to motor control that are not part of the direct corticospinal-pyramidal system. This includes pathways through the basal ganglia, the reticular formation of the brain stem, the vestibular nuclei, and the red nuclei. However, this is such an all-inclusive and diverse group of motor control areas that it is difficult to ascribe specific neurophysiological functions to the extrapyramidal system as a whole. For this reason, the term "extrapyramidal" is beginning to have less usage clinically as well as physiologically.

Excitation of the Spinal Cord by the Primary Motor Cortex

Vertical Columnar Arrangement of the Neurons in the Motor Cortex. In previous chapters it is pointed out that the cells in the somatic sensory cortex and visual cortex—and in all other parts of the brain as well—are organized in vertical columns. In a like manner, the cells of the motor cortex are also organized in vertical columns a fraction of a millimeter in diameter and having thousands of neurons in each column.

Each column of cells functions as a unit, stimulating either a single muscle or a group of synergistic muscles. Also, each column is arranged in six distinct layers of cells, like the arrangement throughout almost all the cerebral cortex. The pyramidal cells that give rise to the corticospinal fibers all lie in the fifth layer of cells from the cortical surface, whereas the input signals to the column of cells all enter layers 2 through 4. The sixth layer gives rise mainly to fibers that communicate with other regions of the cerebral cortex itself.

Function of Each Column of Neurons. The neurons of each column operate as an integrative processing system, utilizing information from multiple input sources to determine the output response from the column. In addition, each column can function as an amplifying system to stimulate large numbers of pyramidal fibers to the same muscle or to synergistic muscles simultaneously. This is important because stimulation of a single pyramidal cell can rarely excite a muscle. Instead, as many as 50 to 100 pyramidal cells usually need to be excited simultaneously or in rapid succession to achieve muscle contraction.

Stimulation of the Spinal Motor Neurons

Figure 38-5 shows a segment of the spinal cord, illustrating multiple motor tracts entering the cord from the brain and also showing a representative anterior motor neuron. The corticospinal tract lies in the dorsal portion of the lateral column. At most levels of the cord, its fibers terminate mainly on inter-

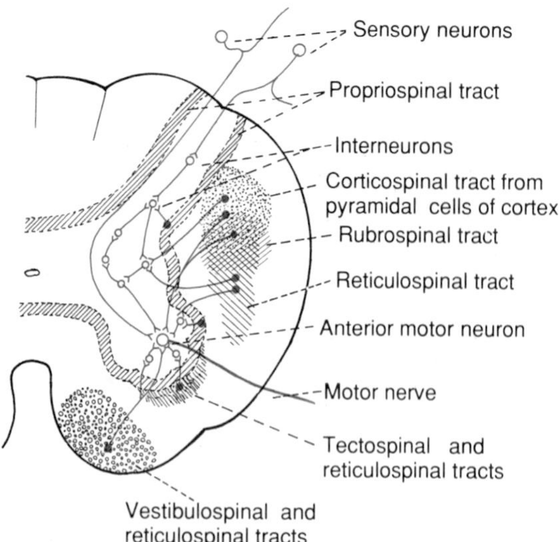

Figure 38-5. Convergence of all the different motor pathways on the anterior motor neurons.

neurons in the intermediate area of the cord gray matter. However, in the cervical enlargement of the cord where the hands and fingers are represented, moderate numbers of corticospinal fibers terminate directly on the anterior motor neurons, thus allowing a direct route from the brain for activating muscle contraction. This is in keeping with the fact that the primary motor cortex has an extremely high degree of representation for fine control of hand, finger, and thumb actions.

Patterns of Movement Elicited by Spinal Cord Centers. From the previous chapter, recall that the spinal cord can provide specific reflex patterns of movement in response to sensory nerve stimulation. Many of these patterns are also important when the anterior motor neurons are excited by signals from the brain. For instance, when a brain signal excites an agonist muscle, it is not necessary to transmit an inverse signal to the antagonist at the same time; this transmission will be achieved by the reciprocal innervation circuit that is always present in the cord for coordinating the functions of antagonist pairs of muscles.

Also, parts of the other reflex mechanisms, such as withdrawal, stepping and walking, scratching, postural mechanisms, and so forth, can be activated by "command" signals from the brain. Thus, very simple signals from the brain can initiate many of our normal motor activities, particularly for such functions as walking and the attainment of different postural attitudes of the body.

Effect of Lesions in the Motor Cortex or Corticospinal Pathway—The "Stroke"

The motor cortex or corticospinal pathway is frequently damaged, especially by the common abnormality called a "stroke." This is caused either by a ruptured blood vessel that allows hemorrhage into the brain or by thrombosis of one of the major arteries supplying the brain, in either case causing loss of blood supply to the cortex, or very frequently to the corticospinal tract, where it passes between the caudate nucleus and the putamen.

Destruction of the Primary Motor Cortex (the Area Pyramidalis). Destruction of a portion of the primary motor cortex—the area that contains the giant Betz pyramidal cells—in a monkey causes varying degrees of paralysis of the represented muscles. If the sublying caudate nucleus and the adjacent premotor area are not damaged, gross postural and limb "fixation" movements can still be performed, but the animal *loses voluntary control of discrete movements of the distal segments of the limbs—especially of the hands and fingers.* This does not mean that the muscles themselves cannot contract, but that the animal's ability to control the fine movements is gone.

From these results one can conclude that the area pyramidalis is essential for voluntary initiation of finely controlled movements, especially of the hands and fingers.

Muscle Spasticity Caused by Lesions That Damage Large Areas Adjacent to the Motor Cortex. Most lesions of the motor cortex, especially those caused by a stroke, involve not only the primary motor cortex but also adjacent cortical areas and deeper structures of the cerebrum as well, especially the basal ganglia. In these instances, muscle spasm almost invariably occurs in the afflicted muscle areas on the opposite side of the body (because all the motor pathways cross to the opposite side in the brain stem). This spasm is believed to result mainly from damage to accessory pathways from the cortex that normally inhibit the brain stem motor nuclei. When these nuclei lose this inhibition (that is, they are said to be "disinhibited"), they become spontaneously active and cause excessive spastic tone in the involved areas of the body. This is the spasticity that normally accompanies a "stroke" in the human being.

THE CEREBELLUM AND ITS MOTOR FUNCTIONS

The cerebellum has long been called a *silent area* of the brain, principally because electrical excitation of this structure does not cause any sensation and rarely any motor movement. However, as we shall see, removal of the cerebellum does cause movement to become highly abnormal. The cerebellum is especially vital to the control of rapid muscular activities such as running, typing, playing the piano, and even talking. Loss of this area of the brain can cause almost total incoordination of these activities even though its loss causes paralysis of no muscles.

But how is it that the cerebellum can be so important when it has no direct ability to cause muscle contraction? The answer to this is that it both helps *sequence the motor activities* and also *monitors and makes corrective adjustments in the motor activities elicited by other parts of the brain.* It receives continuously updated information on the desired program of muscle contractions from the motor control areas of the other parts of the brain; and it receives continuous sensory information from the peripheral parts of the body to determine the sequential changes in the status of each part of the body—its position, its rate of movement, forces acting on it, and so forth. The cerebellum *compares* the actual movements as depicted by the peripheral sensory feedback information with the movements intended by the motor system. If the two do not compare favorably, then appropriate corrective signals are transmitted instantaneously back into the motor system to increase or decrease the levels of activation of the specific muscles.

The Anatomical Functional Areas of the Cerebellum

Anatomically, the cerebellum is divided into three separate lobes by two deep fissures, as shown in Figures 38–6 and 38–7: (1) the *anterior lobe,* (2) the *posterior lobe,* and (3) the *flocculonodular lobe.* The flocculonodular lobe is the oldest of all portions of the cerebellum; it developed along with (and functions with) the vestibular system in controlling equilibrium, as discussed in the previous chapter.

The Longitudinal Functional Divisions of the Anterior and Posterior Lobes. From a functional point of view, the anterior and posterior lobes are organized not by lobes, but instead along the longitudinal axis, as illustrated in Figure 38–7, which shows the human cerebellum after the lower end of the posterior cerebellum has been rolled downward from its normally hidden position. Note down the center of the cerebellum a narrow band separated from the remainder of the cerebellum by shallow grooves. This is the *vermis.* In this area most cerebellar control functions for the muscle movements of the axial body, the neck, and the shoulders and hips are located.

To each side of the vermis is a large, laterally protruding *cerebellar hemisphere,* and each of these hemispheres is divided into an *intermediate zone* and *a lateral zone.*

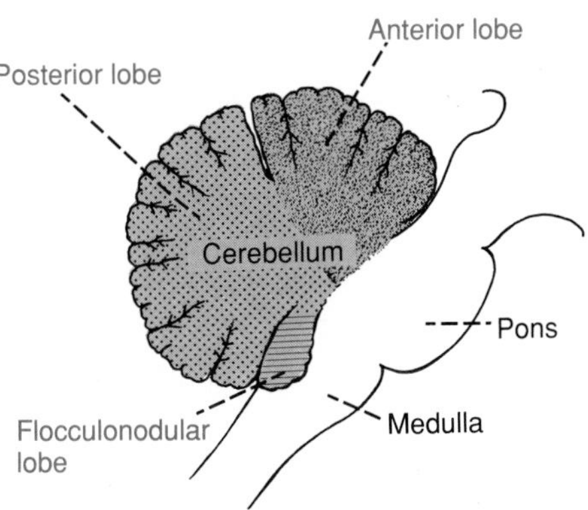

Figure 38–6. The anatomical lobes of the cerebellum as seen from the lateral side.

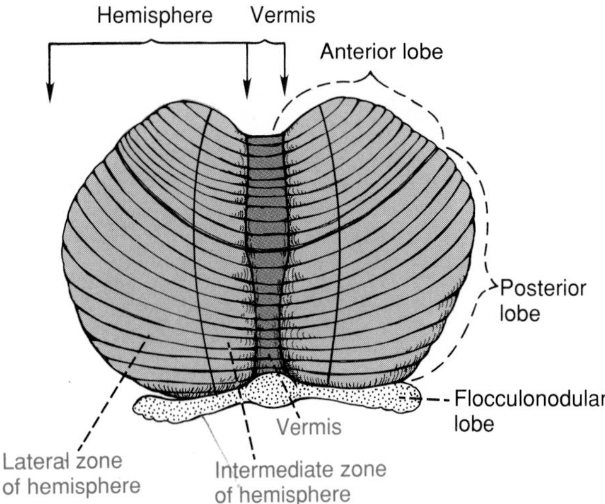

Figure 38–7. The functional parts of the cerebellum as seen from the posteroinferior view, with the inferiormost portion of the cerebellum rolled outward to flatten the surface.

The intermediate zone of the hemisphere is concerned with the control of muscular contractions in the distal portions of the upper and lower limbs, especially of the hands and fingers and feet and toes.

The lateral zone of the hemisphere operates at a much more remote level, for this area joins in the overall planning of sequential motor movements. Without this lateral zone, most motor activities of the body lose their appropriate timing and therefore become incoordinate, as we discuss more fully later.

The Input Pathways to the Cerebellum

Afferent Pathways from the Brain. The basic input pathways to the cerebellum are illustrated in Figure 38–8. An extensive and important afferent pathway is the *corticopontocerebellar pathway,* which originates mainly in the *motor* and *premotor cortices* but to a lesser extent in the sensory cortex as well and then passes by way of the *pontine nuclei* and *pontocerebellar tracts* to the contralateral hemisphere of the cerebellum.

In addition, important afferent tracts originate in multiple nuclei of the brain stem—especially the olivary nuclei and vestibular nuclei—and terminate in widespread areas of the cerebellum.

Afferent Pathways from the Periphery. The cerebellum also receives important sensory signals directly from the peripheral parts of the body. The two most important tracts are illustrated in Figure 38–9: the *dorsal spinocerebellar tract* and the *ventral spinocerebellar tract* (plus similar tracts from the neck and facial regions).

The signals transmitted in the dorsal spinocerebellar tracts come mainly from the muscle spindles and to a lesser extent from other somatic receptors throughout the body, such as from the Golgi tendon organs, the large tactile receptors of the skin, and the joint receptors. All these signals apprise the cerebellum of the momentary status of muscle contraction, degree of tension on the muscle tendons, positions

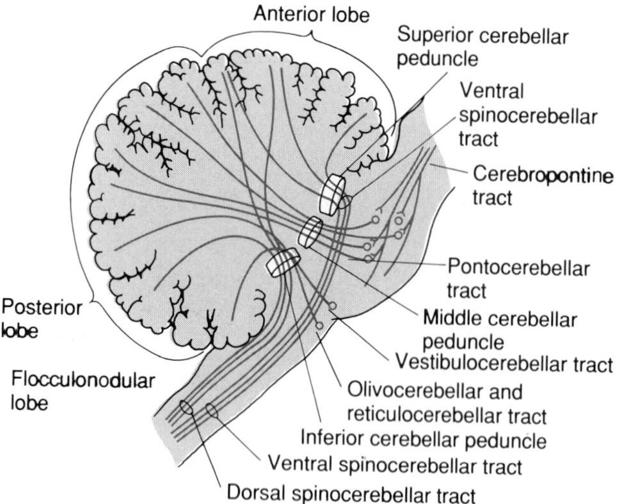

Figure 38–8. The principal afferent tracts to the cerebellum.

and rates of movement of the parts of the body, and forces acting on the surfaces of the body.

On the other hand, the ventral spinocerebellar tracts receive less information from the peripheral receptors. Instead, they are excited mainly by the motor signals arriving in the anterior horns of the spinal cord from the brain through the corticospinal and rubrospinal tracts as well as from the internal motor pattern generators in the cord itself. Thus, this ventral fiber pathway tells the cerebellum what motor signals have arrived at the anterior horns; this feedback is called the *efference copy* of the anterior horn motor drive.

The spinocerebellar pathways can transmit impulses at velocities of up to 120 m/sec, which is the most rapid conduction of any pathway in the entire central nervous system. This extremely rapid conduction is important for the instantaneous apprisal of the cerebellum of the changes that take place in peripheral motor actions.

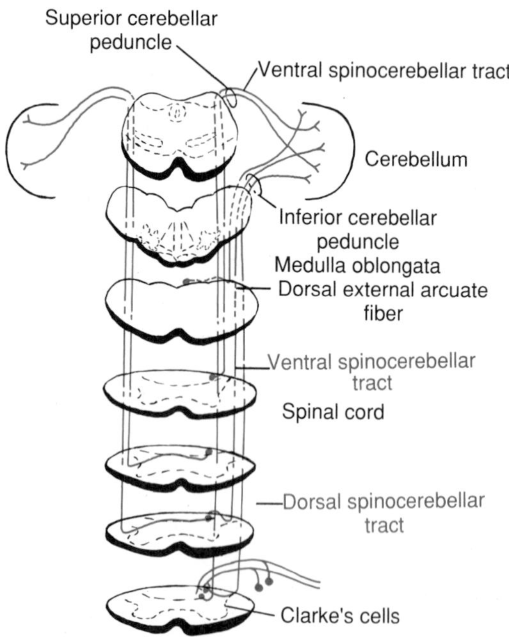

Figure 38–9. The spinocerebellar tracts.

Output Signals from the Cerebellum

The Deep Cerebellar Nuclei and the Efferent Pathways. Located deep in the cerebellar mass are three *deep cerebellar nuclei*—the *dentate, interpositus,* and *fastigial nuclei.* Each time an input signal arrives in the cerebellum, it divides and goes in two directions: (1) directly to one of the deep nuclei and (2) to a corresponding area of the cerebellar cortex overlying the deep nucleus. Then, a short time later, the cerebellar cortex relays its output signals back to the same deep nucleus. Thus, all the input signals that enter the cerebellum eventually end in the deep nuclei, from which output signals are then distributed to other parts of the brain.

Three major efferent pathways lead out of the cerebellum, as illustrated in Figure 38–10:

1. A pathway that originates in the *midline structures of the cerebellum* (the *vermis*) and then passes through the *fastigial nuclei* into the *medullary* and *pontine regions of the brain stem.* This circuit functions in close association with the

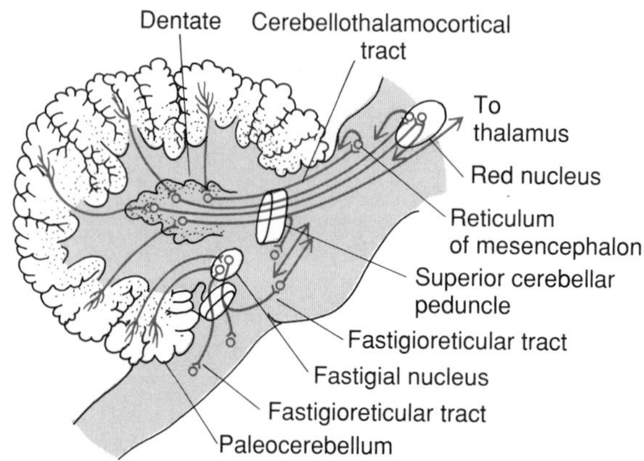

Figure 38–10. Principal efferent tracts from the cerebellum.

equilibrium apparatus to help control equilibrium and also, in association with the reticular formation of the brain stem, to help control the postural attitudes of the body.
2. A pathway that originates in the *intermediate zone of the cerebellar hemisphere,* then passes (a) through the *nucleus interpositus* to the *ventrolateral and ventroanterior nuclei of the thalamus,* and thence to the *cerebral cortex,* (b) to several *midline structures* of the *thalamus* and thence to the *basal ganglia,* and (c) to the *red nucleus* and *reticular formation* of the upper portion of the brain stem. This circuit is believed to coordinate mainly the reciprocal contractions of agonist and antagonist muscles in the peripheral portions of the limbs—especially in the hands, fingers, and thumbs.
3. A pathway that begins in the *cortex of the lateral zone of the cerebellar hemisphere,* then passes to the *dentate nucleus,* next to the *ventrolateral and ventroanterior nuclei of the thalamus,* and finally to the *cerebral cortex.* This pathway plays an important role in helping coordinate sequential motor activities initiated by the cerebral cortex.

The Neuronal Circuit of the Cerebellum

The human cerebellar cortex is actually a large folded sheet, approximately 17 cm wide by 120 cm long, with the folds lying crosswise, as illustrated in Figure 38–7. And lying deep in the folded mass of cortex are the deep nuclei.

The Functional Unit of the Cerebellar Cortex—The Purkinje Cell and the Deep Nuclear Cell. The cerebellum has approximately 30 million nearly identical functional units, one of which is illustrated to the left in Figure 38–11. This functional unit centers on a single, very large *Purkinje cell,* 30 million of which are in the cerebellar cortex.

To the right in Figure 38–11, the three major layers of the cerebellar cortex are illustrated, the *molecular layer,* the *Purkinje cell layer,* and the *granular cell layer.* And far beneath these cortical layers, in the center of the cerebellar mass, are the deep nuclei.

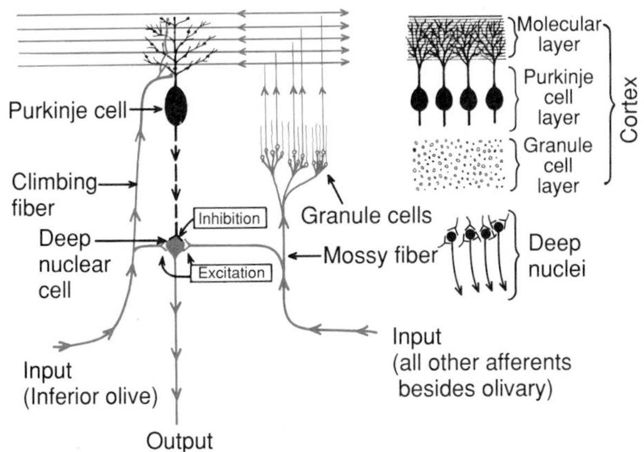

Figure 38–11. The left side of this figure shows the basic neuronal circuit of the cerebellum, with excitatory neurons shown in red. To the right is illustrated the physical relationship of the deep cerebellar nuclei to the cerebellar cortex with its three layers.

The Neuronal Circuit of the Functional Unit. As illustrated in the left half of Figure 38–11, the output from the functional unit is from a deep nuclear cell. However, this cell is continually under the influence of both excitatory and inhibitory influences. The excitatory influences arise from direct connections with the afferent fibers that enter the cerebellum from the brain or the periphery. The inhibitory influences arise entirely from the Purkinje cell in the cortex of the cerebellum.

The afferent inputs to the cerebellum are mainly of two types, one called the *climbing fiber type* and the other called the *mossy fiber type.*

The climbing fibers *all originate from the inferior olivary complex of the medulla.* There is one climbing fiber for about 10 Purkinje cells. After sending branches to several deep nuclear cells, the climbing fiber projects all the way to the molecular layer of the cerebellar cortex, where it makes about 300 synapses with the soma and dendrites of each Purkinje cell. This climbing fiber is distinguished by the fact that a single impulse in it will always cause a single, very prolonged (up to 1 second), peculiar oscillatory type of action potential in each Purkinje cell with which it connects. This action potential is called the *complex spike.*

The mossy fibers are all the other fibers that enter the cerebellum from multiple sources: the higher brain, the brain stem, and the spinal cord. These fibers also send collaterals to excite deep nuclear cells. Then they proceed to the granular layer of the cortex, where they synapse with hundreds of *granule cells.* In turn, the granule cells send very small axons, less than 1 micrometer in diameter, to the outer surface of the cerebellar cortex to enter the molecular layer. Here the axons divide into two branches that extend 1 to 2 millimeters in each direction parallel to the folia. There are literally billions of these *parallel nerve fibers,* for there are some 500 to 1000 granule cells for every Purkinje cell. It is into this molecular layer that the dendrites of the Purkinje cells project, and 80,000 to 200,000 of these parallel fibers synapse with each Purkinje cell.

Yet the mossy fiber input to the Purkinje cell is quite different from the climbing fiber input because their synaptic connections are very weak, so that large numbers of mossy fibers must be stimulated simultaneously to alter the activation of the Purkinje cell. Furthermore, this activation usually takes the form of repetitive Purkinje cell firing of short-duration action potentials called *simple spikes,* rather than the prolonged complex action potential occurring in response to the climbing fiber input.

Continual Firing of the Cerebellum Purkinje Cells and Deep Nuclear Cells Under Normal Resting Conditions. One of the characteristics of both the Purkinje cells and the deep nuclear cells is that normally they fire continually; the Purkinje cell fires at about 50 to 100 action potentials per second and the deep nuclear cells at still much higher rates. Therefore, the output activity of both these cells can be modulated either upward or downward. For instance, a decrease in the firing rate of the deep nuclear cells below the normal level would actually provide an *inhibitory output signal* to the motor system. On the other hand, any factor that should increase the firing rate above normal would provide an *excitatory output signal.* In this way, the cerebellum can provide either excitation or inhibition as the need arises.

Balance Between Excitation and Inhibition of the Deep Cerebellar Nuclei. Referring again to the circuit of Figure 38–11, *one should note that direct stimulation of the deep nuclear cells by both the climbing and the mossy fibers excites them.* By contrast, *the signals arriving from the Purkinje cells inhibit them.* Normally, the balance between these two effects is slightly in favor of excitation, so that the output from the deep nuclear cell remains relatively constant at a moderate level of continuous stimulation. On the other hand, in the execution of rapid motor movements, the *timing* of the two effects on the deep nuclei is such that the excitation appears before the inhibition. Then a few milliseconds later inhibition occurs. In this way, there is first a very rapid excitatory signal fed back into the motor pathway to enhance the motor movement, but this is followed within a few milliseconds by an inhibitory signal. This inhibitory signal is a "delay-line" negative feedback signal that stops the muscle movement from overshooting its mark.

The Purkinje Cells Can "Learn" to Correct Motor Errors — The Role of the Climbing Fibers

Typically, when a person first performs a new motor act, the degree of motor enhancement provided by the cerebellum to the agonist contraction, the degree of inhibition of the antagonist, and the timing of the offset are all amost always incorrect for precise performance of the movement. But after the act has been performed many times, these individual sequential events become progressively more precise in performing the movement exactly as desired, sometimes requiring only a few movements before the desired result is achieved but at other times requiring hundreds of movements.

Yet how do these adjustments come about? The exact answer is not known, although it is known that sensitivity levels of cerebellar circuits themselves progressively adapt during the training process. For instance, the sensitivity of the Purkinje cells to respond to the parallel fibers from the granule cells becomes altered. Furthermore, research studies suggest that this sensitivity change is brought about by signals from the climbing fibers entering the cerebellum from the inferior olivary complex. These signals adjust the long-term sensitivity of the Purkinje cells to stimulation by the parallel fibers.

Under resting conditions, the climbing fibers fire about once per second. But each time they do fire, they cause extreme depolarization of the entire dendritic tree of the Purkinje cell, lasting for up to a second. During this time, the Purkinje cell fires with one initial very strong output spike followed by a series of oscillatory waves in the membrane potential. When a person performs a new movement for the first time and the achieved movement does not match the intended movement, the firing by the climbing fibers changes markedly, either greatly increased or decreased as needed, up to a maximum of about 4 per second or all the way down to zero. These changes in stimulatory rate are believed to alter the long-term sensitivity of the Purkinje cells to the subsequent signals from the mossy fiber circuit. Over a period of time, this change in sensitivity, along with other possible "learning" functions of the cerebellum, is believed to make the timing and other aspects of cerebellar control of movements approach perfection. When this has been achieved, the climbing fibers no longer send their "error" signals to the cerebellum to cause further change.

Finally, we need to answer how the climbing fibers themselves know to alter their own rate of firing when a performed movement is imperfect. What is known about this is that the inferior olivary complex receives full information from the corticospinal tracts as well as from the motor centers of the brain stem detailing the *intent* of each motor movement; and it also receives full information from the sensory nerve endings in the muscles and surrounding tissues detailing the movement that actually occurs. Therefore, it is presumed that the inferior olivary complex then functions as a *comparator* to test how well the actual performance matches the intended performance. If there is a match, no change in firing of the climbing fibers occurs. But if there is a mismatch, then the climbing fibers are stimulated or inhibited as needed in proportion to the degree of mismatch, thus leading to progressive changes in Purkinje cell sensitivity until no further mismatch occurs — or so the theory goes.

Function of the Cerebellum with the Spinal Cord and Brain Stem in Controlling Postural and Equilibrium Movements

The cerebellum originated phylogenetically at about the same time that the vestibular apparatus developed. Furthermore, loss of the flocculonodular lobes and portions of the vermis of the cerebellum causes extreme disturbance of equilibrium.

Yet we still must ask the question, what role does the cerebellum play in equilibrium that cannot be provided by the other neuronal machinery of the brain stem? A clue is the fact that in persons with cerebellar dysfunction equilibrium is far more disturbed during performance of rapid motions than during stasis — especially so when the movements involve changes in direction that stimulate the semicircular ducts. This suggests that the cerebellum is especially important in controlling the balance between agonist and antagonist muscle contractions during *rapid changes* in body positions as dictated by the vestibular apparatus.

One of the major problems in controlling balance is the time required to transmit position signals and velocity of movement signals from the different parts of the body to the brain. Even when the most rapidly conducting sensory pathways, up to 120 m/sec, are used, as by the spinocerebellar system, the delay for transmission from the feet to the brain is still 15 to 20 milliseconds. The feet of a person running rapidly can move as much as 10 inches during this time. Therefore, it is never possible for the return signals from the peripheral parts of the body to reach the brain at the same time that the movements actually occur. How, then, is it possible for the brain to know when to stop a movement in order to perform the next sequential act, especially when the movements are performed very rapidly? The answer is that the signals from the periphery tell the brain not only positions of the different parts of the body but also how rapidly and in what directions they are moving. It is the function of the cerebellum then to *calculate* from these rates and directions where the different parts of the body will be during the next few milliseconds. The results of these calculations are the key to the brain's progression to the next sequential movement.

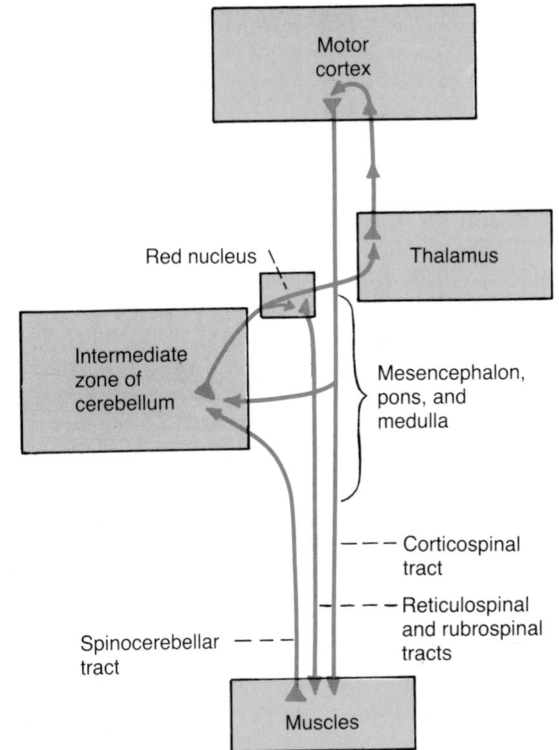

Figure 38-12. Cerebral and cerebellar control of voluntary movements, involving especially the intermediate zone of the cerebellar cortex and its associated nucleus interpositus.

Function of the Cerebellum in Voluntary Muscle Control

In addition to the feedback circuitry between the body periphery and the cerebellum, an almost entirely independent feedback circuitry exists between the motor cortex of the cerebrum and the cerebellum. This circuitry affects only slightly if at all the control of equilibrium and other postural movements of the axial and girdle muscles of the body. Instead, it serves two other principal functions: (1) It helps the cerebral cortex coordinate patterns of movement involving mostly the distal parts of the limbs—especially the hands, fingers, and feet. The part of the cerebellum involved in this function is mainly the *intermediate zone of the cerebellar cortex and its associated nucleus interpositus.* (2) It helps the cerebral cortex plan the timing and sequencing of the next successive movement that will be performed after the present movement is completed. The part of the cerebellum involved in this is the large *lateral zone of the cerebellar hemisphere,* along with its associated *dentate nucleus.* Let us discuss each of these two functions separately.

Cerebellar Feedback Control of Distal Limb Movements by Way of the Intermediate Cerebellar Cortex and the Interpositus Nucleus

As illustrated in Figure 38-12, the intermediate zone of each cerebellar hemisphere receives two types of information when a movement is performed: (1) direct information from the motor cortex and red nucleus, telling the cerebellum the sequential *intended plan of movement* for the next few fractions of a second, and (2) feedback information from the peripheral parts of the body, especially from the distal parts of the limbs, telling the cerebellum what *actual movements* result. After the intermediate zone of the cerebellum has compared the intended movements with the actual movement, the nucleus interpositus sends *corrective* output signals (a) back to the *motor cortex* through relay nuclei in the *thalamus* and (b) to the lower portion *of the red nucleus,* which gives rise to the *rubrospinal tract.* The rubrospinal tract, in turn, joins the corticospinal tract in innervating the lateralmost motor neurons in the anterior horns of the spinal cord gray matter, the neurons that control the distal parts of the limbs, particularly the hands and fingers.

This part of the cerebellar motor control system provides smooth, coordinate movements of the agonist and antagonist muscles of the distal limbs for the performance of acute purposeful patterned movements. The cerebellum seems to compare the "intentions" of the higher levels of the motor control system, as transmitted to the intermediate cerebellar zone through the corticopontocerebellar tract, with the "performance" by the respective parts of the body as transmitted back to the cerebellum from the periphery. If the signals do not compare favorably, the olivary-Purkinje cell system, along with possible other cerebellar learning mechanisms, will eventually correct the motions until they perform the desired function.

Function of the Large Lateral Zone of the Cerebellar Hemisphere—The "Sequencing" and "Timing" Functions

In human beings, the lateral zones of the two cerebellar hemispheres have become very highly developed and greatly enlarged, along with the human ability to perform intricate sequential patterns of movement, especially with the hands and fingers, and along with the ability to speak. Yet, strangely enough, these large lateral portions of the cerebellar hemispheres have no direct input of information from the peripheral parts of the body. Also, almost all the communication between these lateral cerebellar areas and the cortex is not with the primary motor cortex itself but instead with the premotor area and primary and association somatic sensory areas. Even so, destruction of the lateral portions of the cerebellar hemispheres along with their deep nuclei, the dentate nuclei, can lead to extreme incoordination of the purposeful movements of the hands, fingers, feet, and speech apparatus. This has been difficult to understand because of lack of direct communication between this part of the cerebellum and the primary motor cortex. However, recent experimental studies suggest that these portions of the cerebellum are concerned with two other important aspects of motor control: (1) the planning of sequential movements, and (2) the "timing" of the sequential movements.

The Planning of Sequential Movements. The planning of sequential movements seems to be related to the fact that the cerebellar lateral hemispheres communicate with the premotor and sensory portions of the cerebral cortex and that there is also two-way communication between these same areas and corresponding areas of the basal ganglia. It seems that the "plan" of the sequential movements is transmitted from the sensory and premotor areas of the cortex to the lateral zones of the cerebellar hemispheres, and two-way traffic between the cerebellum and the cortex is necessary to provide appropriate transition from one movement to the next. An exceedingly interesting observation that supports this view is that many of the neurons in the dentate nuclei display the activity pattern of the next movement that is yet to follow. Thus, the lateral hemispheres appear to be involved not with what is happening at a given moment, but instead with *what will be happening during the next sequential movement.*

To summarize, one of the most important features of normal motor function is one's ability to progress smoothly from one movement to the next in orderly succession. In the absence of the large lateral cerebellar hemispheres, this capability is seriously disturbed, especially for rapid movements.

The Timing Function. Another important function of the lateral cerebellar hemispheres is to provide appropriate timing for each movement. In the absence of these lateral areas, one loses the subconscious ability to predict ahead of time how far the different parts of the body will move in a given time. And without this timing capability, the person becomes unable to determine when the next movement should begin. As a result, the succeeding movement may begin too early or, more likely, too late. Therefore, cerebellar lesions cause complex movements, such as those required for writing, running, or even talking, to become totally incoordinate, lacking completely in the ability to progress in an orderly sequence from one movement to the next. Such cerebellar lesions are said to cause *failure of smooth progression of movements.*

Clinical Abnormalities of the Cerebellum

Dysmetria and Ataxia. Two of the most important symptoms of cerebellar disease are *dysmetria* and *ataxia.* It was pointed out earlier that in the absence of the cerebellum the subconscious motor control system cannot predict ahead of time how far movements will go. Therefore, the movements ordinarily overshoot their intended mark, and then the conscious portion of the brain overcompensates in the opposite direction for the succeeding movements. This effect is called dysmetria, and it results in incoordinate movements that are called ataxia.

Failure of Progression. *Dysdiadochokinesia.* When the motor control system fails to predict ahead of time where the different parts of the body will be at a given time, it temporarily "loses" the parts during rapid motor movements. As a result, the succeeding movement may begin much too early or much too late, so that no orderly "progression of movement" can occur. One can demonstrate this readily by having a patient with cerebellar damage turn one hand upward and downward at a rapid rate. The patient rapidly "loses" all perception of the instantaneous position of the hand during any portion of the movement. As a result, a series of jumbled movements occurs instead of the normal coordinate upward and downward motions. This is called *dysdiadochokinesia.*

Dysarthria. Another instance in which failure of progression occurs is in talking, for the formation of words depends on rapid and orderly succession of individual muscular movements in the larynx, mouth, and respiratory system. Lack of coordination between these and inability to predict either the intensity of the sound or the duration of each successive sound cause jumbled vocalization, with some syllables loud, some weak, some held long, some held for short intervals, and resultant speech that is almost completely unintelligible. This is called *dysarthria.*

Intention Tremor. When a person who has lost the cerebellum performs a voluntary act, the movements tend to oscillate, especially when they approach the intended mark, first overshooting the mark and then vibrating back and forth several times before settling on the mark. This reaction is called an *intention tremor* or an *action tremor,* and it results from cerebellar overshooting and failure of the cerebellar system to damp the motor movements.

Cerebellar Nystagmus. *Cerebellar nystagmus* is a tremor of the eyeballs that occurs usually when one attempts to fixate the eyes on a scene to one side of the head. This off-center type of fixation results in rapid, tremulous movements of the eyes rather than a steady fixation, and it is another manifestation of the failure of damping by the cerebellum. It occurs especially when the flocculonodular lobes are damaged; in this instance it is associated with loss of equilibrium, presumably because of dysfunction of the pathways through the cerebellum from the semicircular ducts.

THE BASAL GANGLIA—THEIR MOTOR FUNCTIONS

The basal ganglia, like the cerebellum, are another accessory motor system that functions not by itself but always in close association with the cerebral cortex and corticospinal system. In fact, the basal ganglia receive almost all their input signals from the cortex itself and in turn return almost all of their output signals back to the cortex.

Figure 38–13 illustrates the anatomical relationships of the basal ganglia to the other structures of the brain. Note that they are located mainly lateral to the thalamus, occupying a large portion of the deeper regions of both cerebral hemispheres. Note also that almost all the motor and sensory nerve fibers connecting the cerebral cortex and spinal cord pass between the two major masses of the basal ganglia, the *caudate nucleus* and the *putamen.* This mass of nerve fibers is called the *internal capsule* of the brain.

The Neuronal Circuitry of the Basal Ganglia. The anatomical connections between the basal ganglia and the other elements of motor control are very complex, as illustrated in Figures 38–14 and 38–15. However, we try in the next few sections to dissect out the major pathways of action and attempt to describe their functional attributes. We concentrate especially

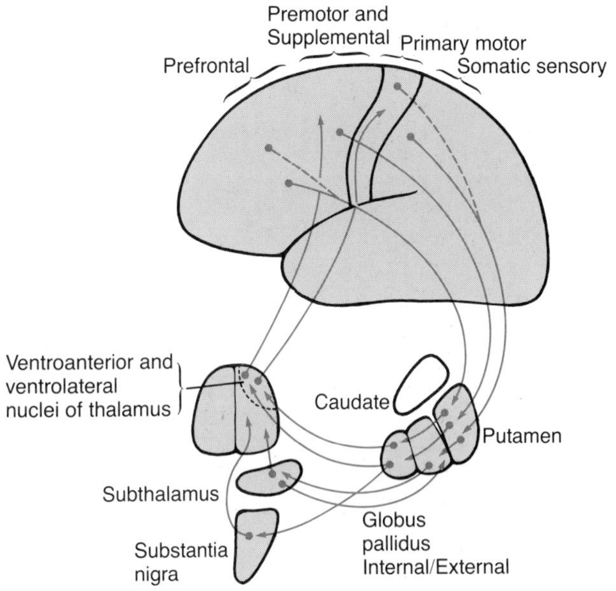

Figure 38–14. The *putamen circuit* through the basal ganglia for subconscious execution of learned patterns of movement.

on two major circuits called, respectively, the *putamen circuit* and the *caudate circuit.*

Function of the Basal Ganglia in Executing Patterns of Motor Activity—The Putamen Circuit

One of the principal roles of the basal ganglia in motor control is to function in association with the corticospinal system to control complex patterns of motor activity. An example is the writing of letters of the alphabet. When there is serious damage to the basal ganglia, the cortical system of motor control can

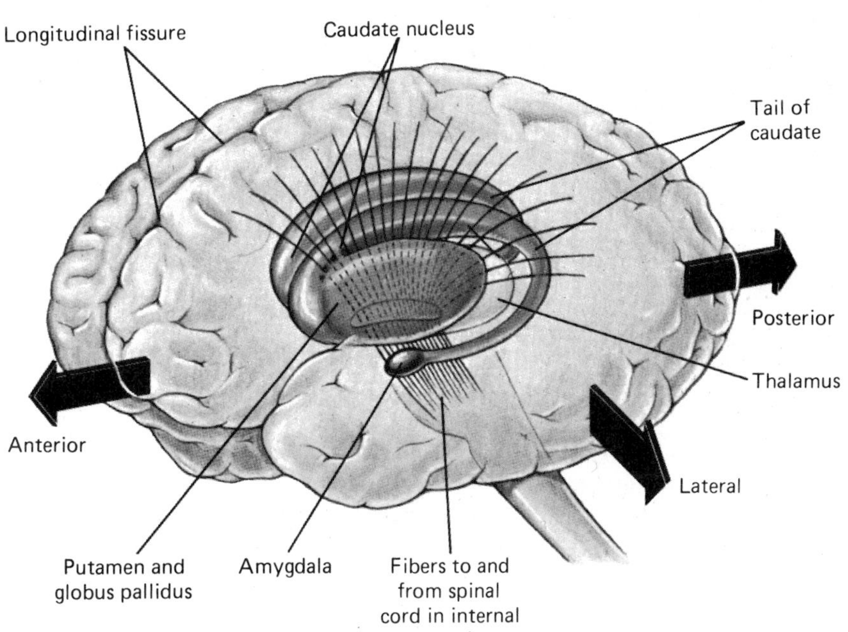

Figure 38–13. Anatomical relationships of the basal ganglia to the cerebral cortex and thalamus, shown in three-dimensional view. (From Guyton: Basic Neuroscience: Anatomy and Physiology. Philadelphia, W. B. Saunders Company, 1987.)

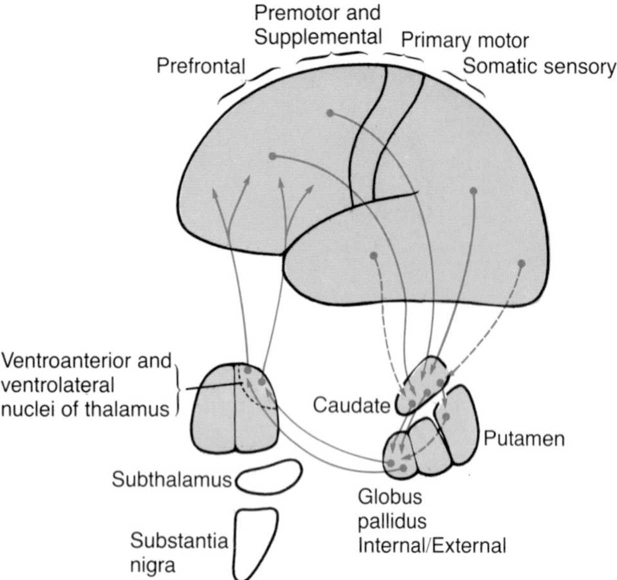

Figure 38–15. The *caudate circuit* through the basal ganglia for cognitive planning of the combinations of sequential and parallel motor patterns to achieve specific conscious goals.

no longer provide these patterns. Instead, one's writing becomes crude, as if one were learning for the first time how to write.

Other patterns requiring the basal ganglia are cutting paper with scissors, hammering nails, shooting basketballs through a hoop, passing a football, throwing a baseball, the movements of shoveling dirt, some aspects of vocalization, and virtually any other of our skilled movements.

The Neural Circuit Through the Putamen for Executing Patterns of Movements. Figure 38–14 illustrates the principal pathways through the basal ganglia for executing learned patterns of movement. These begin mainly in the premotor and supplemental motor areas of the motor cortex and also the primary somatic sensory area of the sensory cortex. Next they pass, as shown in bright red in the figure, to the putamen (mainly bypassing the caudate nucleus), then to the internal portion of the globus pallidus, next to the ventroanterior and ventrolateral nuclei of the thalamus, and then to the primary motor cortex and portions of the premotor and supplemental areas closely associated with the primary motor cortex. In addition, there are side circuits through the substantia nigra and the subthalamus. Thus, this putamen circuit has its inputs mainly from those parts of the brain adjacent to the primary motor cortex, but not much from the primary motor cortex itself. Then its outputs do go mainly back to the *primary* motor cortex.

Athetosis, Hemiballismus, and Chorea. How does the above putamen circuit function in the execution of patterns of movement? The answer is only poorly known. However, when any portion of the circuit is damaged or blocked, certain patterns of movement become severely abnormal. For instance, lesions in the *globus pallidus* frequently lead to spontaneous *writhing movements* of a hand, an arm, the neck, or the face, movements called *athetosis.*

A lesion in the *subthalamus* often leads to sudden *flailing movements* of an entire limb, a condition called *hemiballismus.*

Multiple small lesions in the *putamen* lead to *flicking movements* in the hands, face, and other parts of the body, which is called *chorea.*

And lesions of the *substantia nigra* lead to the common and extremely severe disease of rigidity and tremors known as *Parkinson's disease* that we shall discuss in more detail later.

Role of the Basal Ganglia for Cognitive Control of Sequences of Motor Patterns — The Caudate Circuit

Obviously, most of our motor actions occur as a consequence of thoughts generated in the mind, a process called *cognitive control of motor activity.* The caudate nucleus plays a major role in this cognitive control of motor activity.

The neural connections between the corticospinal motor control system and the caudate nucleus, illustrated in Figure 38–15, are somewhat different from those of the putamen circuit. Part of the reason for this is that the caudate nucleus extends into all lobes of the cerebrum, beginning anteriorly in the frontal lobes, then passing posteriorly through the parietal and occipital lobes, and finally curving forward again like a letter "C" into the temporal lobes. Furthermore, the caudate nucleus receives large amounts of its input from the *association areas* of the cerebral cortex, the areas that integrate the different types of sensory and motor information into usable thought patterns.

After the signals pass from the cerebral cortex to the caudate nucleus, they are transmitted next to the internal globus pallidus, then to the relay nuclei of the ventroanterior and ventrolateral thalamus, and finally back to the prefrontal, premotor, and supplemental motor areas of the cerebral cortex, but with almost none of the returning signals passing directly to the primary motor cortex. Instead, the returning signals go to those accessory motor regions that are concerned with patterns of movement instead of individual muscle movements.

A good example of this would be for a person to see a lion approach and then respond instantaneously and automatically by (1) turning away from the lion, (2) beginning to run, and (3) even attempting to climb a tree. Without the cognitive functions, the person might not have the instinctive knowledge, without thinking for too long a time, to respond quickly and appropriately. Thus, cognitive control of motor activity determines which patterns of movement will be used together and in what sequence to achieve a complex goal.

Function of the Basal Ganglia in Changing the Timing and in Scaling the Intensity of Movements

Two important capabilities of the brain in controlling movement are (1) to determine how rapidly it is to be performed and (2) to control how large the movement will be. For instance, one may write the letter "a" slowly or rapidly. Also, he may write a small "a" or a very large letter "a" on a chalk board. Regardless of the choices, the proportional characteristics of the letter will remain the same. This is also true even though the person might use the fingers for writing the letter in one instance or the whole arm at another time.

In the absence of the basal ganglia, these timing and scaling functions are very poor, in fact almost nonexistent. Of course, here again, the basal ganglia do not function alone; they function in close association with the cerebral cortex as well. One especially important cortical area is the posterior parietal cortex, which is the locus of the spatial coordinates for all parts of the body as well as for the relationship of the body and its parts to all surroundings. Figure 38–16 illustrates the way in which a person lacking a left caudate circuit and posterior parietal cortex might draw the face of another human being, providing proper proportions for the right side of the face, but almost ignoring the left side.

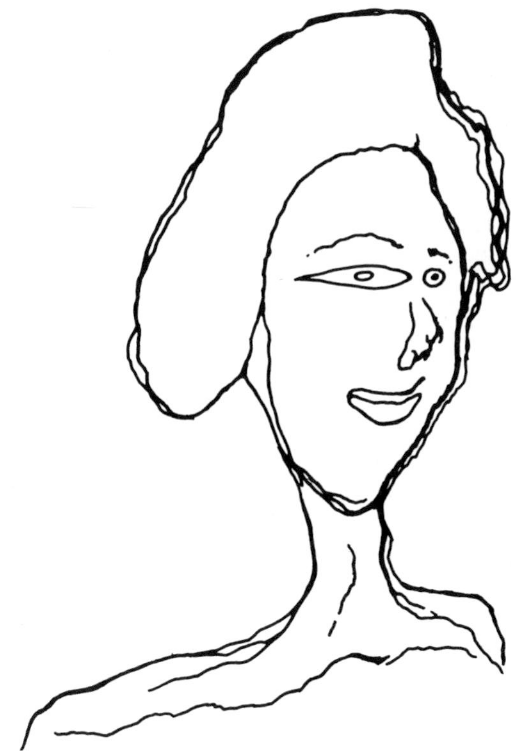

Figure 38–16. A typical drawing made by a person who has severe damage in his or her left parietal cortex, where the spatial coordinates of the right side of the body and right field of vision are calculated.

Functions of Specific Neurotransmitters in the Basal Ganglial System

Figure 38–17 illustrates the interplay of some specific neurotransmitters that are known to function within the basal ganglia, showing (1) a *dopamine* pathway from the substantia nigra to the caudate nucleus and putamen; (2) a *gamma-aminobutyric acid (GABA)* pathway from the caudate nucleus and putamen to the globus pallidus and substantia nigra; (3) *acetylcholine* pathways from the cortex to the caudate nucleus and putamen; and (4) multiple general pathways from the brain stem that secrete *norepinephrine, serotonin, enkephalin,* and several other neurotransmitters in the basal ganglia as well as in other parts of the cerebrum. We will have more to say about some of these hormonal systems in the following sections when we discuss diseases of the basal ganglia as well as in subsequent chapters when we discuss behavior, sleep, wakefulness, and functions of the autonomic nervous system.

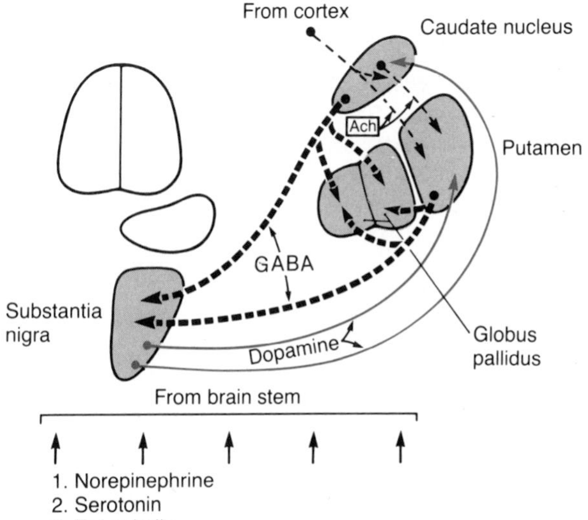

Figure 38–17. Neuronal pathways that secrete different types of neurotransmitter substances in the basal ganglia.

For the present, it should be remembered that the neurotransmitter GABA always functions as an inhibitory agent. Therefore, the GABA neurons in the feedback loops from the cortex through the basal ganglia and then back to the cortex make virtually all these loops *negative feedback loops,* rather than positive feedback loops, thus lending stability to the motor control systems. Dopamine also functions as an inhibitory neurotransmitter in most parts of the brain, so that it too may function as a stabilizer. Acetylcholine, on the other hand, usually functions as an excitatory transmitter and therefore probably provides many of the positive features of motor action.

Clinical Syndromes Resulting from Damage to the Basal Ganglia

Aside from athetosis and hemiballismus, which have already been mentioned in relation to lesions in the globus pallidus and the subthalamus, two other major diseases result from damage in the basal ganglia. These are Parkinson's disease and Huntington's chorea.

Parkinson's Disease

Parkinson's disease, also known as *paralysis agitans,* results from *widespread destruction of that portion of the substantia nigra that sends dopamine-secreting nerve fibers to the caudate nucleus and putamen.* The disease is characterized by (1) *rigidity* of much if not most of the musculature of the body, (2) *involuntary, continuous shaking tremor* of the involved areas even when the person is resting and always at a fixed rate of 3 to 6 cycles per second, and (3) a serious inability to initiate movement called *akinesia.*

The causes of these abnormal motor effects are almost entirely unknown. However, if the dopamine secreted in the caudate nucleus and putamen functions as an inhibitory transmitter, then destruction of the substantia nigra theoretically would allow these structures to become overly active and possibly cause continuous output of excitatory signals to the corticospinal motor control system. These signals could certainly overly excite many or all muscles of the body, thus leading to *rigidity.* And some of the feedback circuits might easily *oscillate* because of high feedback gains after loss of their inhibition, leading to the *tremor* of Parkinson's disease.

The akinesia that occurs in Parkinson's disease is often much more distressing to the patient than are the symptoms of muscle rigidity and tremor, for to perform even the simplest movement in severe Parkinsonism the person must exert the highest degree of concentration. The mental effort, even mental anguish, that is necessary to make the movement "go" is often at the limit of the patient's will power. Then, when the movement does occur, it is stiff and staccato in character instead of occurring smoothly. It is presumed that loss of dopamine secretion in the caudate nucleus and putamen might lead to loss of balance between the excitatory and inhibitory systems. Since *patterns of movement* require sequential changes between excitation and inhibition, any effect that would lock basal ganglia activity always in one direction would obviously prevent the initiation of and progression through sequential patterns, which is exactly what happens in akinesia.

Treatment with L-DOPA. Administration of the drug L-dopa to patients with Parkinson's disease ameliorates many of the symptoms, especially the rigidity and akinesia, in most patients. The reason for this is believed to be that L-dopa is converted in the brain into dopamine, and the dopamine then restores the normal balance between inhibition and excitation in the caudate nucleus and putamen.

Huntington's Chorea

Huntington's chorea is a hereditary disorder that usually begins to cause symptoms in the third or fourth decade of life. It is characterized at first by flicking movements at individual joints and then progressive severe distortional movements of the entire body. In addition, severe dementia also develops along with the motor dysfunctions.

The abnormal movements of Huntington's chorea are *believed to be caused by loss of most of the cell bodies of the GABA-secreting neurons in the caudate nucleus and putamen.* The axon terminals of these neurons normally cause inhibition in the globus pallidus and substantia nigra. This loss of inhibition is believed to allow spontaneous outbursts of globus pallidus and substantia nigra activity that cause the distortional movements.

The dementia in Huntington's chorea probably does not result from the loss of GABA neurons but instead from loss of many acetylcholine-secreting neurons at the same time. This loss occurs not only in the basal ganglia but in much of the cerebral cortex as well.

INTEGRATION OF ALL PARTS OF THE TOTAL MOTOR CONTROL SYSTEM

Finally, we need to summarize as best we can what is known about overall control of movement. To do this, let us first give a synopsis of the different levels of control:

The Spinal Level

Programmed in the spinal cord are local patterns of movement for all muscle areas of the body — for instance, programmed withdrawal reflexes that pull any part of the body away from a source of pain. And the cord is the locus even of complex patterns of rhythmical motions such as to-and-fro movement of the limbs for walking, plus reciprocal activity of opposite sides of the body, or hindlimbs versus forelimbs.

The Hindbrain Level

The hindbrain provides two major functions for general motor control of the body: (1) maintenance of axial tone of the body for the purpose of standing and (2) continuous modification of the different directions of this tone in response to continuous information from the vestibular apparatuses for the purpose of maintaining equilibrium.

The Corticospinal Level

The corticospinal system transmits most of the motor signals from the motor cortex to the spinal cord. It functions partly by issuing commands to set into motion the various cord patterns of motor control. It can also change the intensity of the different patterns or modify their timing or other characteristics. When needed, the corticospinal system can bypass the cord patterns by issuing inhibitory commands and replacing them with higher level patterns from the brain stem or from the cerebral cortex.

The Associated Function of the Cerebellum. The cerebellum functions with all levels of muscle control. It functions with the spinal cord especially to enhance the stretch reflex, so that when a contracting muscle meets an unexpectedly heavy load, a long stretch reflex arc through the cerebellum and back again to the cord strongly facilitates the load-resisting effect of the basic stretch reflex.

At the brain stem level, the cerebellum functions to make the postural movements of the body, especially the rapid movements required by the equilibrium system, smooth and continuous and without abnormal oscillations.

At the cerebral cortex level, the cerebellum functions to provide many accessory motor commands, especially to provide extra motor force to turn on muscle contraction very rapidly and forcefully at the start of movements. And near the end of each movement, the cerebellum turns on antagonist muscles at exactly the right time and with proper force to stop the movement at the intended point.

In addition, the cerebellum functions with the cerebral cortex at still another level of motor planning: it helps program in advance the muscle contractions that are required for smooth progression from the present movement in one direction to the next movement in another direction. The neural circuit for this passes from the cerebral cortex to the large lateral hemispheres of the cerebellum and then back to the cortex.

The Associated Functions of the Basal Ganglia. The basal ganglia are essential to motor control in ways entirely different from those of the cerebellum. Their two most important functions are (1) to help the cortex execute subconscious but *learned* patterns of movement and (2) to help plan multiple parallel and sequential patterns of movement that the mind must put together to accomplish a purposeful task.

The types of motor patterns that require the basal ganglia include those for writing all the different letters of the alphabet, for throwing a ball, for typing, and so forth. Also, the basal ganglia are required to modify these patterns for slow execution, rapid execution, to write small or write very large—thus controlling both timing and dimensions of the patterns.

At still a higher level of control is another cerebral cortex-basal ganglia circuit, beginning in the thinking processes of the brain and providing the overall sequence of action for responding to each new situation —such as planning one's immediate response to an assailant upon being hit in the face or one's sequential response to an unexpectedly fond embrace.

An important part of all these basal ganglial planning processes is not only the motor cortex and basal ganglia but also the somatic sensory cortex of the parietal lobe, especially the posterior portion where the instantaneous spatial coordinates of all parts of one's body are continuously calculated.

REFERENCES

Atkeson, C. G.: Learning arm kinematics and dynamics. Annu. Rev. Neurosci., 12:157, 1989.

Brooks, V. B.: The Neural Basis of Motor Control. New York, Oxford University Press, 1986.

Eckmiller, R.: Neural control of pursuit eye movements. Physiol. Rev., 67:797, 1987.

Evarts, E. V., et al. (eds.): Motor System in Neurobiology. New York, Elsevier Science Publishing Co., 1986.

Georgopoulos, A. P.: Neural integration of movement: role of motor cortex in reaching. FASEB J., 1:2849, 1988.

Glickstein M., and Yeo, C. (eds.): Cerebellum and Neuronal Plasticity. New York, Plenum Publishing Corp., 1987.

Ito, M.: The Cerebellum and Neural Control. New York, Raven Press, 1984.

Lewin, R.: Brain grafts benefit Parkinson's patients. Science, 236:149, 1987.

McCloskey, D. I., et al.: Sensing position and movements of the fingers. News Physiol. Sci., 2:226, 1987.

Palacios, J. M.: Neurotransmitters, their receptors and the degenerative diseases of the aging brain. Triangle, 25:85, 1986.

Peterson, B. W., and Richmond, F. J. (eds.): Control of Head Movement. New York, Oxford University Press, 1988.

Sandler, M., et al. (eds.): Neurotransmitter Interactions in the Basal Ganglia. New York, Raven Press, 1987.

QUESTIONS

1. Describe the *primary motor cortex* and the *pyramidal tract*.
2. What is the difference between the functions of the *premotor cortex* and the primary motor cortex?
3. Describe *Broca's area* for control of speech.
4. What are the functions of the following premotor areas: the voluntary eye movement field, the head rotation area, and the area for hand skills?
5. What type of muscle activity is affected to the greatest extent by ablation of the primary motor cortex?

6. Explain why lesions of the premotor cortex and of the basal ganglia cause spasticity, while lesions limited to the primary motor cortex fail to do so.
7. Describe the putamen and caudate circuits from the cortex to the basal ganglia and then back to the cortex. What are the functions of these circuits?
8. Describe the neuronal circuit between the neostriatum and the substantia nigra. What are some of the possible functions of this pathway?
9. What is a possible cause of the clinical condition called *athetosis*?
10. Give possible physiological explanations for the following three abnormalities found in *Parkinson's disease*: (a) rigidity, (b) tremor at rest, and (c) akinesia.
11. How does the drug L-dopa function in the treatment of Parkinson's disease?
12. Describe both the afferent and efferent nerve tracts of the cerebellum.
13. Describe the spatial localization of signals from the body in the cerebellum.
14. Explain the balance between excitation and inhibition that controls the output from the deep nuclear cells of the cerebellum.
15. How does the cerebellum delay the onset of the inhibitory output signal that occurs at the end of a motor movement?
16. Discuss the principle of error control by the cerebellum.
17. Explain the function of the cerebellum in *prediction* and the phenomena of *dysmetria* and *intention tremor.*
18. Explain the function of the *lateral zone of the cerebellar hemispheres* in planning sequential movements.

39

The Cerebral Cortex and Intellectual Functions of the Brain

It is ironic that of all the parts of the brain, we know least about the mechanisms of the cerebral cortex, even though it is by far the largest portion of the nervous system. Yet we do know the effects of destruction or of specific stimulation of various portions of the cortex. In the early part of the present chapter the facts known about cortical functions are discussed; then some basic theories of the neuronal mechanisms involved in thought processes, memory, analysis of sensory information, and so forth, are presented briefly.

Physiological Anatomy of the Cerebral Cortex

The functional part of the cerebral cortex is composed mainly of a thin layer of neurons 2 to 5 millimeters in thickness, covering the surface of all the convolutions of the cerebrum and having a total area of about one quarter square meter. The total cerebral cortex probably contains 100 billion or more neurons.

Figure 39-1 illustrates the typical structure of the cerebral cortex, showing successive layers of different types of cells. Most of the cells are of three types: *granular*, *fusiform*, and *pyramidal*, the latter named for their characteristic pyramidal shape. The pyramidal cells are very large and give rise to the large fibers that go all the way to the spinal cord.

To the right in Figure 39-1 is illustrated the typical organization of nerve fibers within the different layers of the cortex. Note particularly the large number of *horizontal fibers* extending between adjacent areas of the cortex, but note also the *vertical fibers* that extend to and from the cortex to lower areas of the brain and to the spinal cord or to distant regions of the cerebral cortex through the long association bundles.

Anatomical and Functional Relationships of the Cerebral Cortex to the Thalamus and Other Lower Centers. All areas of the cerebral cortex have extensive to-and-fro efferent and afferent connections with the deeper structures of the brain, but especially so with the thalamus. When the thalamus is damaged along with the cortex, the loss of cerebral function is far greater than when the cortex alone is damaged, for thalamic excitation of the cortex is necessary for almost all cortical activity.

Each area of the cerebral cortex is connected with a specific part of the thalamus. Furthermore, when the thalamic connections are cut, the functions of the corresponding cortical area become entirely abrogated. Also, all pathways from the sensory organs to the cortex pass through the thalamus, with the single exception of most sensory pathways of the olfactory tract.

FUNCTIONS OF SPECIFIC CORTICAL AREAS

Studies in human beings by neurosurgeons, neurologists, and neuropathologists have shown that different cortical areas have their own separate functions, as illustrated in Figure 39-2. This figure shows the major primary and secondary motor areas of the cortex, as well as the major primary and secondary sensory areas for somatic sensation, vision, and hearing, all of which have been discussed in previous chapters. The primary areas have direct connections with specific muscles or specific sensory receptors, for caus-

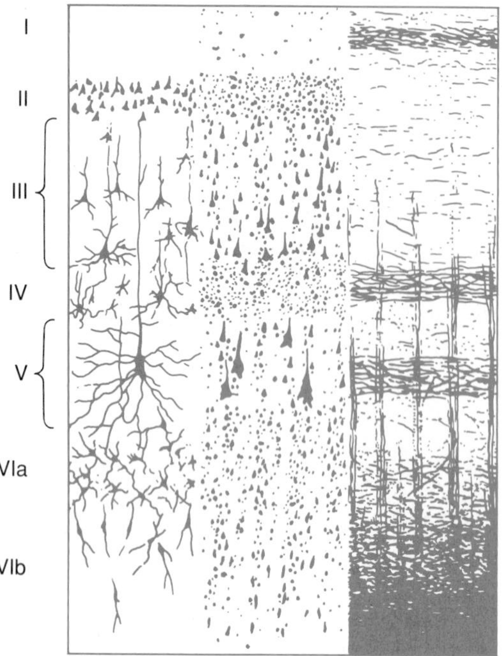

Figure 39–1. Structure of the cerebral cortex, illustrating *I*, molecular layer; *II*, external granular layer; *III*, layer of pyramidal cells: *IV*, internal granular layer: *V*, large pyramidal cell layer; and *VI*, layer of fusiform or polymorphic cells. (From Ranson and Clark (after Brodmann): Anatomy of the Nervous System. Philadelphia, W. B. Saunders Company, 1959.)

ing discrete muscle movements or experiencing a sensation—visual, auditory, or somatic—from a minute receptor area. The secondary areas, on the other hand, make sense out of the functions of the primary areas. For instance, the supplemental and premotor areas function along with the primary motor cortex and basal ganglia to provide highly specific patterns of motor activity. On the sensory side, the secondary sensory areas, which are located within a few centimeters of the primary areas, begin to make sense out of the specific sensory signals, such as interpreting the shape or texture of an object in one's hand; the color, the light intensity, the directions of lines and angles, and other aspects of vision; and the combination of tones, sequence of tones, and beginning interpretation of the meanings of auditory signals.

The Association Areas

Figure 39–2 also shows several large areas of the cerebral cortex that do not fit into the rigid categories of primary or secondary motor and sensory areas. These are called *association areas* because they receive and analyze signals from multiple regions of the cortex and even subcortical structures. Yet even the association areas have their own specializations, as we shall see. The three most important association areas are (1) the *parieto-occipitotemporal association area,* (2) the *prefrontal association area,* and (3) the *limbic association area.* The functions of these are the following:

The Parieto-occipitotemporal Association Area. This association area lies in the large cortical space between the somatic sensory cortex anteriorly, the visual cortex posteriorly, and the auditory cortex laterally. As would be expected, it provides a high level of interpretive meaning for the signals from all the surrounding sensory areas. However, even the parieto-occipitotemporal association area has its own functional subareas, which are illustrated in Figure 39–3:

1. An area beginning in the *posterior parietal cortex and extending into the superior occipital cortex provides continuous analysis of the spatial coordinates of all parts of the body as well as of the surroundings of the body.* This area receives visual information from the posterior occipital cortex and simultaneous somatic information from the anterior parietal cortex; from this it computes the coordinates. But why does a person need to know these spatial coordinates? The answer is that to control the body movements, the brain must know at all times where each part of the body is located and also its relation to the surroundings. The brain also needs this information to analyze incoming somatic sensory signals.
2. The major area for language comprehension, called *Wernicke's area,* lies behind *the primary auditory cortex in the posterior part of the supe-*

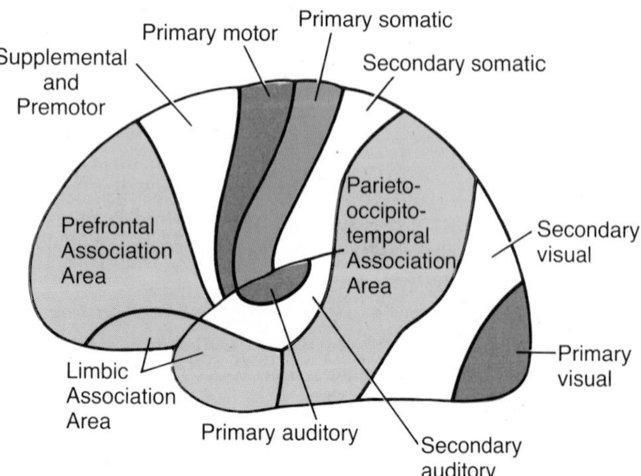

Figure 39–2. Locations of the major association areas of the cerebral cortex, shown in relation to the primary and secondary motor and sensory areas.

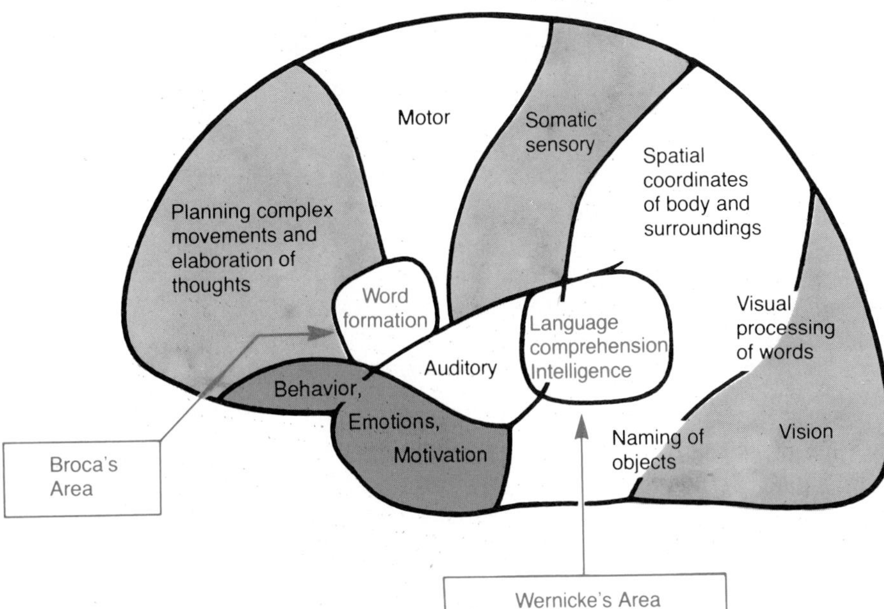

Figure 39–3. Map of specific functional areas in the cerebral cortex, showing especially Wernicke's and Broca's areas for language comprehension and speech production, which in 95 per cent of all persons are located in the left hemisphere.

rior temporal lobe. We discuss this area much more fully later; it is the most important region of the entire brain for higher intellectual functions because almost all intellectual functions are language-based.

3. *Posterior to the language comprehension area, lying mainly in the angular gyrus region of the occipital lobe, is a secondary visual processing area that feeds the visual signals of words read from a page into Wernicke's area, the language comprehension area.* This angular gyrus area is needed to make meaning out of the visually perceived words. In its absence, a person can still have excellent language comprehension through hearing but not through reading.
4. *In the most lateral portions of both the anterior occipital lobe and posterior temporal lobe is an area for naming objects.* The names presumably originate mainly through auditory input, whereas the nature of the objects originates mainly through visual input. In turn, the names are essential for language comprehension and intelligence, functions performed in Wernicke's area, located immediately superior to the "names" region.

The Prefrontal Association Area. In the previous chapter we learned that the prefrontal association area functions in close association with the motor cortex to plan complex patterns and sequences of motor movements. To aid in this function, it receives very strong input through a massive subcortical bundle of fibers connecting the parieto-occipitotemporal association area with the prefrontal association area. Through this bundle the prefrontal cortex receives much preanalyzed sensory information, especially information on the spatial coordinates of the body that is absolutely necessary in the planning of effective movements. Much of the output from the prefrontal area into the motor control system passes through the caudate portion of the basal ganglia-thalamic feedback circuit for motor planning, which provides many of the sequential and parallel components of the movement complex.

The prefrontal association area is also essential to carrying out prolonged thought processes in the mind. This presumably results from some of the same capabilities of the prefrontal cortex that allow it to plan motor activities. That is, it seems to be capable of combining nonmotor information from widespread areas of the brain and therefore to achieve nonmotor types of thinking as well as motor types. In fact, the prefrontal association area is frequently described simply as important for the *elaboration of thoughts.*

A special region in the frontal cortex, called *Broca's area, provides the neural circuitry for word formation.* This area, illustrated in Figure 39–3, is located partly in the posterior lateral prefrontal cortex and partly in the premotor area. It is here that the plans and motor patterns for the expression of individual words or even short phrases are initiated and executed. This area also works in close association with Wernicke's language comprehension center in the temporal association cortex, as we discuss more fully later in the chapter.

The Limbic Association Area. Figure 39–2 illustrates still another association area called the *limbic area.* This is found in the anterior pole of the temporal lobe, in the ventral portions of the frontal lobes, and in the cingulate gyri on the midsurfaces of the cerebral hemispheres. This region is concerned primarily with *behavior, emotions,* and *motivation.* We will learn in the following chapter that the limbic cortex is part of a much more extensive system, the *limbic system,* that includes a complex set of neuronal structures in the midbasal regions of the brain. This limbic system provides most of the drives for setting the other areas of the brain into action and even provides the motivational drive for the process of learning itself.

Interpretative Function of the Posterior Superior Temporal Lobe—Wernicke's Area (A General Interpretative Area)

The somatic, visual, and auditory secondary and association areas, which can actually be called sensory interpretative areas, all meet one another in the posterior part of the superior temporal lobe, as illustrated in Figure 39-4, where the temporal, parietal, and occipital lobes all come together. This area of confluence of the different sensory interpretative areas is especially highly developed in the *dominant* side of the brain—the *left side* in almost all right-handed persons—and it plays the greatest single role of any part of the cerebral cortex in the higher levels of brain function that we call *intelligence*. Therefore, this region has frequently been called by different names suggestive of the area having almost global importance: the *general interpretative area*, the *gnostic area*, the *knowing area*, the *tertiary association area*, and so forth. However, it is best known as *Wernicke's area* in honor of the neurologist who first described its special significance in intellectual processes.

Following severe damage in Wernicke's area, a person might hear perfectly well and even recognize different words but still be unable to arrange these words into a coherent thought. Likewise, the person may be able to read words from the printed page but be unable to recognize the thought that is conveyed.

Electrical stimulation in Wernicke's area of the conscious patient occasionally causes a highly complex thought. This is particularly true when the stimulatory electrode is passed deep enough into the brain to approach the corresponding connecting areas of the thalamus. The types of thoughts that might be experienced include complicated visual scenes that one might remember from childhood, auditory hallucinations such as a specific musical piece, or even a discourse by a specific person. For this reason it is believed that activation of Wernicke's area can call forth complicated memory patterns involving more than one sensory modality even though many of the memory patterns may be stored elsewhere. This belief is in accord with the importance of Wernicke's area in interpretation of the complicated meanings of different sensory experiences.

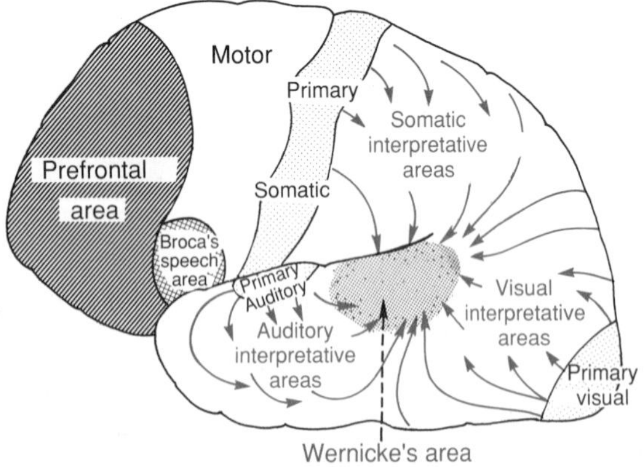

Figure 39-4. Organization of the somatic, auditory, and visual association areas into a general mechanism for interpretation of sensory experience. All these feed also into *Wernicke's area*, located in the posterosuperior portion of the temporal lobe. Note also the prefrontal area and Broca's speech area.

The Angular Gyrus—Interpretation of Visual Information. The angular gyrus is the most inferior portion of the posterior parietal lobe, lying immediately behind Wernicke's area and fusing posteriorly into the visual areas of the occipital lobe as well. If this region is destroyed while Wernicke's area in the temporal lobe is still intact, the person can still interpret auditory experiences as usual, but the stream of visual experiences passing into Wernicke's area from the visual cortex is mainly blocked. Therefore, the person may be able to see words and even know they are words but, nevertheless, not be able to interpret their meanings. This is the condition called *dyslexia*, or *word blindness*.

Let us again emphasize the global importance of Wernicke's area for most intellectual functions of the brain. Loss of this area in an adult usually leads thereafter to a lifetime of almost demented existence.

The Concept of the Dominant Hemisphere

The general interpretative functions of Wernicke's area and of the angular gyrus, and also the functions of the speech and motor control areas, are usually much more highly developed in one cerebral hemisphere than in the other. Therefore, this hemisphere is called the *dominant hemisphere*. In about 95 per cent of all persons the left hemisphere is the dominant one. Even at birth, the area of the cortex that will eventually become Wernicke's area is as much as 50 per cent larger in the left hemisphere than in the right in more than one half of newborn babies. Therefore, it is easy to understand why the left side of the brain might become dominant over the right side. However, if for some reason this left side area is damaged or removed in early childhood, the opposite side of the brain can develop full dominant characteristics.

Functions of the Parieto-occipitotemporal Cortex in the Nondominant Hemisphere

When Wernicke's area in the dominant hemisphere is destroyed, the person normally loses almost all intellectual functions associated with language or verbal symbolism, such as ability to read, ability to perform mathematical operations, and even the ability to think through logical problems. However, many other types of interpretative capabilities, some of which utilize the temporal lobe and angular gyrus regions of the opposite hemisphere, are retained. Psychological studies in patients with damage to their nondominant hemispheres have suggested that this hemisphere may be especially important for understanding and interpreting music, nonverbal visual experiences (especially visual patterns), spatial relationships between the person and the surroundings, the significance of "body language" and intonations of persons' voices, and probably also many somatic experiences related to use of the limbs and hands.

Thus, even though we speak of the "dominant" hemisphere, this dominance is primarily for language-related or verbal symbolism-related intellectual functions; the opposite hemisphere is actually dominant for some other types of intelligence.

The Higher Intellectual Functions of the Prefrontal Association Area

Several decades ago, before the advent of modern drugs for treating psychiatric conditions, it was found that some patients could receive significant relief from severe psychotic depression through severing the neuronal connections between the prefrontal areas of the brain and the remainder of the brain, that is, by a procedure called *prefrontal lobotomy.* Subsequent studies in these patients showed the following mental changes:

1. The patients lost their ability to solve complex problems.
2. They became unable to string together sequential tasks to reach specific goals, and in general lost all ambition.
3. They became unable to learn to do several parallel tasks at the same time.
4. Their level of aggressiveness was decreased, sometimes markedly.
5. Their social responses were often inappropriate for the occasion, including loss of morals and little embarrassment in relation to sex and excretion.
6. The patients could still talk and comprehend language, but they were unable to carry through any long trains of thought, and their moods changed rapidly from sweetness to rage to exhilaration to madness.
7. The patients could also still perform most of the usual patterns of motor function that they had performed throughout life, but often without purpose.

From this information, let us try to piece together a coherent understanding of the function of the prefrontal association areas.

Inability to Progress Toward Goals or to Carry Through with Sequential Thoughts. We learned earlier in the chapter that the prefrontal association areas appear to have the capability of calling forth information from widespread areas of the brain and then using it in deeper thought patterns for attaining goals. If these goals include motor action, so be it. If they do not, then the thought processes attain intellectual analytical goals. Although persons without prefrontal cortices can still think, they show little concerted thinking in logical sequence over any period of time longer than a few seconds or a few minutes at most. One of the results is that persons without prefrontal cortices are *easily distracted from the task* at hand, whereas persons with functioning prefrontal cortices can drive themselves to their goals irrespective of distractions.

Elaboration of Thought, Prognostication, and Performance of Higher Intellectual Functions by the Prefrontal Areas. Another function that has been ascribed to the prefrontal areas by psychologists and neurologists is *elaboration of thought.* This means simply an increase in depth and abstractness of the different thoughts. Psychological tests have shown that prefrontal lobectomized lower animals presented with successive bits of sensory information fail to keep track of these bits even in temporary memory—probably because they are distracted so easily that they cannot hold thoughts long enough for storage to take place. This ability of the prefrontal areas to keep track of many bits of information simultaneously, and then to cause recall of this information bit by bit as it is needed for subsequent thoughts, could well explain the many functions of the brain that we associate with higher intelligence, such as the abilities to (1) prognosticate, (2) plan for the future, (3) delay action in response to incoming sensory signals so that the sensory information can be weighed until the best course of response is decided, (4) consider the consequences of motor actions even before these are performed, (5) solve complicated mathematical, legal, or philosophical problems, (6) correlate all avenues of information in diagnosing rare diseases, and (7) control one's activities in accord with moral laws.

FUNCTION OF THE BRAIN IN COMMUNICATION

One of the most important differences between the human being and lower animals is the facility with which human beings can communicate with one another. Furthermore, because neurological tests can easily assess the ability of a person to communicate with others, we know more about the sensory and motor systems related to communication than about any other segment of cortical function. Therefore, we will review the function of the cortex in communication, and from this one can see immediately how the principles of sensory analysis and motor control apply to this art.

There are two aspects to communication: first, the *sensory aspect,* involving the ears and eyes, and, second, the *motor aspect,* involving vocalization and its control.

Sensory Aspects of Communication

We noted earlier in the chapter that destruction of portions of the *auditory* and *visual association areas* of the cortex can result in inability to understand the spoken word or the written word. These effects are called, respectively, *auditory receptive aphasia* and *visual receptive aphasia* or, more commonly, *word deafness* and *word blindness* (also called *dyslexia*).

Wernicke's Aphasia and Global Aphasia. Some persons are perfectly capable of understanding either the spoken word or the written word but are *unable to interpret the thought* that is expressed. This results most frequently when *Wernicke's area* is damaged or destroyed. Therefore, this type of aphasia is generally called *Wernicke's aphasia.*

When the lesion in Wernicke's area is widespread and extends (1) backward into the angular gyrus region, (2) inferiorly into the lower areas of the temporal lobe, and (3) superiorly into the superior border of the sylvian fissure, the person is likely to be almost totally demented and therefore is said to have *global aphasia.*

Motor Aspects of Communication

The process of speech involves two principal stages of mentation: (1) formation in the mind of thoughts to be expressed and choice of words to be used, then (2) motor control of vocalization and the actual act of vocalization itself.

The formation of thoughts and even most choices of words are the function of the sensory areas of the brain. Again, it is Wernicke's area in the posterior part of the superior temporal gyrus that is most important for this ability. Therefore, persons with either Wernicke's aphasia or global aphasia are unable to formulate the thoughts that are to be communicated. Or, if the lesion is less severe, the person may be able to formulate thoughts but yet be unable to put together the appropriate sequence of words to express the thought. Often, the person is very fluent in words but the words are jumbled.

Motor Aphasia. Often a person is perfectly capable of deciding what he wishes to say, and he is capable of vocalizing, but he simply cannot make his vocal system emit words instead of noises. This effect, called *motor aphasia,* results from damage to *Broca's speech area,* which lies in the *prefrontal* and *premotor* facial region of the cortex—about 95 per cent of the time in the left hemisphere, as illustrated in Figures 39–3 and 39–4. Therefore, we assume that the *skilled motor patterns* for control of the larynx, lips, mouth, respiratory system, and other accessory muscles of articulation are all initiated from this area.

Articulation. Finally, we have the act of articulation itself, which means the muscular movements of the mouth, tongue, larynx, and so forth, that are responsible for the actual emission of sound. The *facial and laryngeal regions of the motor cortex* activate these muscles, and the *cerebellum, basal ganglia,* and *sensory cortex* all help control the muscle contractions by feedback mechanisms described in previous chapters. Destruction of these regions can cause either total or partial inability to speak distinctly.

FUNCTION OF THE CORPUS CALLOSUM AND ANTERIOR COMMISSURE IN TRANSFERING THOUGHTS, MEMORIES, TRAINING, AND OTHER INFORMATION TO THE OPPOSITE HEMISPHERE

Fibers in the *corpus callosum* connect most of the respective cortical areas of the two hemispheres with each other except for the anterior portions of the temporal lobes; these temporal areas, including especially the *amygdala,* are interconnected by fibers that pass through the *anterior commissure.*

One of the functions of the corpus callosum and the anterior commissure is to make information stored in the cortex of one hemisphere available to cortical areas of the opposite hemisphere. Three important examples of such cooperation between the two hemispheres are the following:

1. Cutting of the corpus callosum blocks transfer of information from Wernicke's area of the dominant hemisphere to the motor cortex on the opposite side of the brain. Therefore, the intellectual functions of the brain, located primarily in the dominant hemisphere, lose their control over the right motor cortex and therefore also of the voluntary motor functions of the left hand and arm even though the usual subconscious movements of the left hand and arm are completely normal.
2. Cutting of the corpus callosum prevents transfer of somatic and visual information from the right hemisphere into Wernicke's area of the dominant hemisphere. Therefore, somatic and visual information from the left side of the body frequently fails to reach this general interpretative area of the brain and therefore cannot be used for decision making.
3. Finally, persons whose corpus callosum is completely sectioned are found to have two entirely separate conscious portions of the brain. For example, in a recently studied teen-age boy with a sectioned corpus callosum, only the left half of his brain could understand the spoken word, because it was the dominant hemisphere. On the other hand, the right side of the brain could understand the written word and could elicit a motor response to it without the left side of the brain ever knowing why the response was performed.

Thus, the two halves of the brain have independent capabilities for consciousness, memory storage, communication, and control of motor activities. The corpus callosum is required for the two sides to operate cooperatively, and the anterior commissure plays an important additional role in unifying the emotional responses of the two sides of the basal regions of the brain.

THOUGHTS AND MEMORY

Our most difficult problem in discussing consciousness, thoughts, memory, and learning is that we do not know the neural mechanism of a thought. We know that destruction of large portions of the cerebral cortex does not prevent a person from having thoughts, but it usually does reduce the depth of thought and the degree of awareness.

Each thought almost certainly involves simultaneous signals in many portions of the cerebral cortex, thalamus, limbic system, and reticular formation of the brain stem. Some crude thoughts probably depend almost entirely on lower centers; the thought of pain is probably a good example, for electrical stimulation of the human cortex rarely elicits anything more than the mildest degree of pain, whereas stimulation of certain areas of the hypothalamus and mesencephalon often causes excruciating pain. On the other hand, a type of thought pattern that requires mainly the cerebral cortex is that of vision, because loss of the visual cortex causes complete inability to perceive visual form or color.

Therefore, we might formulate a definition of a thought in terms of neural activity as follows: A thought results from the "pattern" of stimulation of many different parts of the nervous system at the same time and in definite sequence, probably involving most importantly the cerebral cortex, the thalamus, the limbic system, and the upper reticular formation of the brain stem.

Memory—Roles of Synaptic Facilitation and Synaptic Inhibition

Physiologically, memories are caused by changes in the capability of synaptic transmission from one neuron to the next as a result of previous neural activity. These changes in turn cause new pathways to develop for transmission of signals through the neural circuits of the brain. The new pathways are called *memory traces.* They are important because, once established, they can be activated by the thinking mind to reproduce the memories.

Experiments in lower animals have demonstrated that memory traces can occur at all levels of the nervous system. Even spinal cord reflexes can change at least slightly in response to repetitive cord activation, which is part of the memory process. Also, even some long-term memories result from changed synaptic conduction in the lower brain centers. To give an example, the blinking reflex is a learned function involving neuronal circuits in the cerebellum.

Yet there is much reason to believe that most of the memory that we associate with intellectual processes is based on memory traces mainly in the cerebral cortex.

Positive and Negative Memory—"Sensitization" or "Habituation" of Synaptic Transmission. Although we often think of memories as being positive recollections of previous thoughts or experiences, probably the greater share of our memories is negative memories, not positive. That is, our brain is inundated with sensory information from all of our senses. If our minds attempted to remember all of this information, the memory capacity of the brain would be exceeded within minutes. Fortunately, though, the brain has the peculiar capacity to learn to ignore information that is of no consequence. This results from *inhibition* of the synaptic pathways for this type of information, and the resulting effect is called *habituation.* This is, in a sense, a type of negative memory.

On the other hand, for those types of incoming information that cause important consequences, such as pain or pleasure, the brain also has the automatic capability of enhancing and storing the memory traces. Obviously, this is positive memory. It results from *facilitation* of the synaptic pathways, and the process is called *memory sensitization.* We learn later that special areas in the basal limbic regions of the brain determine whether information is important or unimportant and make the subconscious decision whether to store the thought as an enhanced memory trace or to suppress it.

Classification of Memories. We all know that some memories last only a few seconds, and others hours, days, months, or years. For the purpose of discussing these, let us use a common classification of memories that divides memories into (1) *immediate memory,* which includes memories that last for seconds or at most minutes unless they are converted into short-term memories; (2) *short-term memories,* which last for days to weeks but eventually are lost; and (3) *long-term memory,* which, once stored, can be recalled up to years or even a lifetime later.

Immediate Memory

Immediate memory is typified by one's memory of up to seven to ten telephone numbers at a time (or other discrete facts) for a few seconds to a few minutes at a time, but lasting only so long as the person continues to think about the numbers or facts.

Many physiologists have suggested that immediate memory is caused by continual neural activity resulting from nerve signals that travel around and around in a temporary memory trace through a *circuit of reverberating neurons.* Unfortunately, it has not yet been possible to prove this theory.

Another possible explanation is synaptic potentiation, which can enhance synaptic conduction. It can result from the accumulation of large amounts of calcium ions in the presynaptic terminals. That is, when a train of impulses passes through a presynaptic terminal, the amount of calcium ions increases with each impulse. When the amount of calcium ions becomes greater than the mitochondria and endoplasmic reticulum can absorb, the excess calcium then causes prolonged release of transmitter substance at the synapse. Thus, this, too, could be a mechanism for immediate memory.

Short-Term Memory

Now we come to short-term memories that may last for many minutes or even weeks. Yet these will eventually be lost unless the memory traces become more permanent, then are classified as long-term memories. Recent experiments in primitive animals have demonstrated that memories of this type can result from temporary chemical or physical changes, or both, in either the presynaptic terminals or in the postsynaptic membrane, changes that can persist for up to several weeks. These mechanisms are so important that at least one of them deserves special description.

Memory Based on Chemical and Physical Changes in the Presynaptic Terminal or Postsynaptic Neuronal Membrane

Figure 39–5 illustrates a mechanism of memory studied especially by Kandel and his colleagues that can cause memories lasting for up to 3 weeks in the large snail *Aplysia.* In this figure there are two separate presynaptic terminals. One terminal is from a primary input sensory neuron and terminates on the surface of the neuron that is to be stimulated; this is called the *sensory terminal.* The other terminal lies on the surface of the sensory terminal and is called the *facilitator terminal.* When the sensory terminal is stimulated repeatedly but without stimulating the facilitator terminal, signal transmission at first is very great, but this becomes less and less intense with repeated stimulation until transmission almost ceases. This phenomenon is called *habituation.* It is a type of memory that causes the neuronal circuit to lose its response to repeated events that are insignificant.

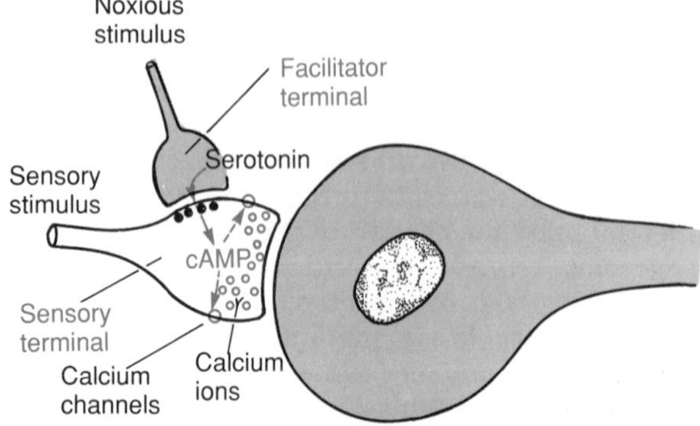

Figure 39–5. A memory system that has been discovered in the snail *Aplysia.*

On the other hand, if a noxious stimulus excites the facilitator terminal at the same time that the sensory terminal is stimulated, then, instead of the transmitted signal becoming progressively weaker, the ease of transmission becomes much stronger and will remain strong for hours, days, or, with more intense training, up to about 3 weeks even without further stimulation of the facilitator terminal. Thus, the noxious stimulus causes the memory pathway to become facilitated for days or weeks thereafter. It is especially interesting that even when habituation has occurred, the pathway can be converted to a facilitated pathway with only a few noxious stimuli.

At the molecular level, the habituation effect in the sensory terminal results from progressive closure of calcium channels of the terminal membrane, although the cause of this is not fully known. Nevertheless, much smaller than normal amounts of calcium can then diffuse into this terminal when action potentials occur, and much less transmitter is therefore released because calcium entry is the stimulus for transmitter release.

In the case of facilitation, the molecular mechanism is believed to be the following:

1. Stimulation of the facilitator neuron at the same time that the sensory neuron is stimulated causes serotonin release at the facilitator synapse on the sensory presynaptic terminal.
2. The serotonin acts on *serotonin receptors* in the sensory terminal membrane, and these activate the enzyme *adenylate cyclase* inside the membrane. This causes the formation of *cyclic adenosine monophosphate (cAMP)* inside the sensory presynaptic terminal.
3. The cAMP activates a *protein kinase* that causes phosphorylation of a protein that is part of the potassium channels in the sensory terminal membrane. This blocks these channels for potassium conductance. This blockage of the potassium channels can last for minutes up to several weeks.
4. Lack of potassium conductance causes a greatly prolonged action potential in the presynaptic terminal because the flow of potassium ions out of the terminal is necessary for recovery from the action potential.
5. The prolonged action potential causes prolonged activation of the calcium pores, allowing tremendous quantities of calcium ions to enter the sensory terminal. These calcium ions then cause greatly increased transmitter release, thereby greatly facilitating synaptic transmission.

Thus, in a very indirect way the associative effect of stimulating the facilitator neuron at the same time that the sensory neuron is stimulated causes a prolonged change in the sensory terminal that produces the memory trace.

Long-Term Memory

There is no real demarcation between the more prolonged types of short-term memory and long-term memory. The distinction is one of degree. However, long-term memory is almost certain to result from actual *structural changes* at the synapses that enhance or suppress signal conduction. Again, let us recall experiments in primitive animals (where the nervous systems are much easier to study) that have aided immensely in understanding possible mechanisms of long-term memory.

Structural and Other Physical Changes in Synapses During the Development of Long-Term Memory

If the reader will refer again to Figure 7–2 in Chapter 7, he or she will see that the vesicles in a presynaptic terminal release their transmitter substance into the synaptic cleft through a special release site. When extra amounts of calcium enter the terminal, those vesicles near the release site attach to receptors at the site; then this attachment causes vesicular exocytosis of the transmitter substance into the synaptic cleft.

Electron microscopic pictures in invertebrate animals have now demonstrated that the total area of this vesicular release site increases in the presynaptic terminal during the development of long-term memory traces. Conversely, during long periods of synaptic inactivity, the release site diminishes and may actually disappear. Furthermore, the growth of the site depends upon activation of specific genetic control mechanisms for synthesizing proteins that are required for assembling the release structures.

An intriguing characteristic of this mechanism for learning is that increased areas of vesicular release sites can be seen experimentally within hours after initiating the training sessions. Thus, it is entirely possible that much of what we now consider to be the longer types of short-term memory are actually early stages of this purely anatomically based long-term memory.

Therefore, at least in these primitive animals, at last we are beginning to understand a physical, structural basis for the development of long-term memory.

Consolidation of Memory

For an immediate memory to be converted into either a more prolonged short-term memory or into a long-term memory that can be recalled weeks or years later, it must become "consolidated." That is, the memory must in some way initiate the chemical, physical, and anatomical changes in the synapses that are responsible for the long-term type of memory. This process requires 5 to 10 minutes for minimal consolidation and an hour or more for maximal consolidation. For instance, if a strong sensory impression is made on the brain but is then followed within a minute or so by an electrically induced brain convulsion, the sensory experience will not be remembered at all. Likewise, brain concussion, sudden application of deep general anesthesia, or any other effect that temporarily blocks the dynamic function of the brain can prevent consolidation.

However, if the strong electrical shock is delayed for more than 5 to 10 minutes, at least part of the memory trace will have become established. If the shock is delayed for an hour, the memory will have become even much more fully consolidated.

The process of consolidation and the time required for consolidation can probably be explained by the phenomenon of *rehearsal* of the immediate memory as follows:

Psychological studies have shown that rehearsal of the same information again and again accelerates and potentiates the degree of transfer of immediate memory into longer-term memory, and therefore also accelerates and potentiates the process of consolidation. The brain has a natural tendency to rehearse newfound information, and especially to rehearse newfound information that catches the mind's attention.

Codifying of Memories During the Process of Consolidation. One of the most important features of the process of consolidation is that memories placed permanently into the longer-term memory storehouse are codified into different classes of information. During this process similar information is recalled from the memory storage bins and is used to help process the new information. The new and old are compared for similarities and for differences, and part of the storage process is to store the information about these similarities and differences, rather than simply to store the information unprocessed. Thus, during the process of consolidation, the new memories are not stored randomly in the brain, but instead are stored in direct association with other memories of the same type. This is obviously necessary if one is to be able to "search" the memory store at a later date to find the required information.

Role of Specific Parts of the Brain in the Memory Process

Role of the Hippocampus for Storage of Memories—Anterograde Amnesia Following Hippocampal Lesions. The hippocampus is the most medial portion of the temporal lobe cortex where it folds underneath the brain and then upward into the lower surface of the lateral ventricle. The two hippocampi have been removed for the treatment of epilepsy in a number of patients. This procedure does not seriously affect the person's memory for information stored in the brain prior to removal of the hippocampi. However, after removal, these persons have very little capacity for storing *verbal and symbolic types* of memories in long-term memory, or even in short-term memory lasting longer than a few minutes. Therefore, these persons are unable to establish new long-term memories of those types of information that are the basis of intelligence. This is called *anterograde amnesia.*

But why is the hippocampus so important in helping the brain store new memories? The probable answer is that the hippocampus is one of the important output pathways from the "reward" and "punishment" areas of the limbic system. These areas are found in many of the basal regions of the brain, and they feed into the hippocampus. Those sensory stimuli, or even thoughts, that cause pain or aversion excite the *punishment centers,* whereas those stimuli that cause pleasure, happiness, or a sense of reward excite the *reward centers.* All of these together provide the background mood and motivations of the person. Among these motivations is the drive in the brain to remember those experiences and thoughts that are either pleasant or unpleasant. The hippocampus especially and to a lesser degree the dorsal medial nuclei of the thalamus, another limbic structure, have proved especially important in making a decision about which of our thoughts are important enough on a basis of reward or punishment to be worthy of memory.

Retrograde Amnesia. *Retrograde amnesia* means inability to recall memories from the past—that is, from the long-term memory storage bins—even though the memories are known to be still there. It has also been claimed that damage in some thalamic areas can lead specifically to retrograde amnesia without causing significant anterograde amnesia. A possible explanation of this is that the thalamus might play a role in helping the person "search" the memory storehouses and thus "read out" the memories. That is, the memory process not only requires the storing of memories but also the ability to search and find the memory at a later date.

REFERENCES

Avoli, M., et al. (eds.): Neurotransmitters and Cortical Function. New York, Plenum Publishing Corp., 1988.

Baddeley, A.: Working Memory. New York, Oxford University Press, 1987.

Bear, M. F., et al.: A physiological basis for a theory of synapse modification. Science, 237:42, 1987.

Brown, T. H., et al.: Long-term synaptic potentiation. Science, 242:724, 1988.

Byrne, J. H.: Cellular analysis of associative learning. Physiol. Rev., 67:329, 1987.

De Wied, D.: Neuroendocrine aspects of learning and memory processes. News Physiol. Sci., 4:32, 1989.

Gold, P. E.: Sweet memories. Am. Sci., 75:151, 1987.

Lieke, E. E., et al.: Optical imaging of cortical activity. Annu. Rev. Physiol., 51:543, 1989.

Peters, A., and Jones, E. G. (eds.): Development and Maturation of Cerebral Cortex. New York, Plenum Publishing Corp., 1988.

Plum, F. (ed.): Language, Communication, and the Brain. New York, Raven Press, 1988.

Rakic, P.: Specification of cerebral cortical areas. Science, 241:170, 1988.

Squire, L. R.: Memory and Brain. New York, Oxford University Press, 1987.

Zucker, R. S.: Short-term synaptic plasticity. Annu. Rev. Neurosci., 12:13, 1989.

QUESTIONS

1. Describe briefly the physiological anatomy of the cerebral cortex.
2. Review the different areas of the cerebral cortex for which specific functions are known.
3. Draw a map of the cerebral cortex showing the *primary sensory areas* and the *sensory association areas.*
4. On the aforementioned map, exactly place *Wernicke's area.* Also show the locus of the *angular gyrus.* What are the functions of Wernicke's area and the angular gyrus?
5. Explain what is meant by the *dominant hemisphere* and explain why it is important to have a single dominant hemisphere.
6. What is the role of language in the function of Wernicke's area?
7. What are some of the important functions of the temporal cortex in the nondominant hemisphere?
8. What are the functions of the *prefrontal areas* of the cerebral cortex, and what happens to a person whose prefrontal areas have been destroyed?
9. Explain the characteristics of immediate memory, short-term memory, and long-term memory.
10. Describe the theories for establishment of short-term and long-term memories.
11. What is meant by *consolidation of memories* and by *codification of memories?*
12. What is the role of the *hippocampus* in the consolidation of memories? How does this relate to *anterograde amnesia?*
13. Explain the differences between *sensory aphasia* and *motor aphasia.*

40

Activation of the Brain; Wakefulness and Sleep; Behavioral Functions of the Brain

One of the remaining great mysteries of the brain is how the brain controls itself. For instance, what sets the overall level of activity? Also, why do we go to sleep or wake up? And perhaps even more mysterious is how behavior is controlled.

Though the answers to these questions are mainly unknown, glimmers of information are beginning to appear that will at least let us construct plausible, even though questionable, theories about activation of the brain, wakefulness, sleep, and behavior.

THE ACTIVATING-DRIVING SYSTEMS OF THE BRAIN

In the absence of continuous transmission of nerve signals from the brain stem into the cerebrum, the brain becomes useless. Normally, nerve signals from the brain stem activate the cerebral part of the brain in two different ways: (1) by directly stimulating the background level of activity in wide areas of the brain and (2) by activating neurohormonal systems that release specific facilitatory or inhibitory hormonal substances into selected areas of the brain. These two activating systems always function together and cannot be distinguished entirely from each other; nevertheless, let us discuss each as a separate entity.

Control of Cerebral Activity by Continuous Excitatory Signals from the Brain Stem

The Reticular Excitatory Area of the Brain Stem

Figure 40-1 illustrates a general system for controlling the level of activity of the brain. The central driving component of this system is an excitatory area called the *bulboreticular facilitatory area.* This lies in the reticular substance of the middle and lateral pons and mesencephalon. Actually, we have already discussed this area earlier, for it is the same brain stem reticular area that transmits facilitatory signals downward to the spinal cord to maintain tone in the antigravity muscles and also to control the level of activity of the spinal cord reflexes. In addition to these downward signals, this area sends a profusion of signals in the upward direction as well. Most of these synapse in the thalamus and are distributed from there to all regions of the cerebral cortex, although others go to most of the other subcortical structures besides the thalamus as well.

The signals passing through the thalamus are of two types. One type is rapidly transmitted action potentials that excite the cerebrum for only a few milliseconds. These originate from very large neuronal cell bodies that lie throughout the reticular area. Their nerve endings release the neurotransmitter substance *acetylcholine,* which serves as the excitatory agent, lasting for only a few milliseconds before it is destroyed.

The second type of excitatory signal originates from large numbers of very small neurons spread throughout the reticular excitatory area. Again, most of these pass to the thalamus, but this time through small, very slowly conducting fibers, and synapsing mainly in the diffuse intralaminar nuclei of the thalamus and reticular nuclei over the surface of the thalamus. From here, additional very small fibers are distributed everywhere in the cerebral cortex. The excitatory effect caused by this system of fibers can build up progressively for many seconds to a minute or more, which suggests that its signals are especially

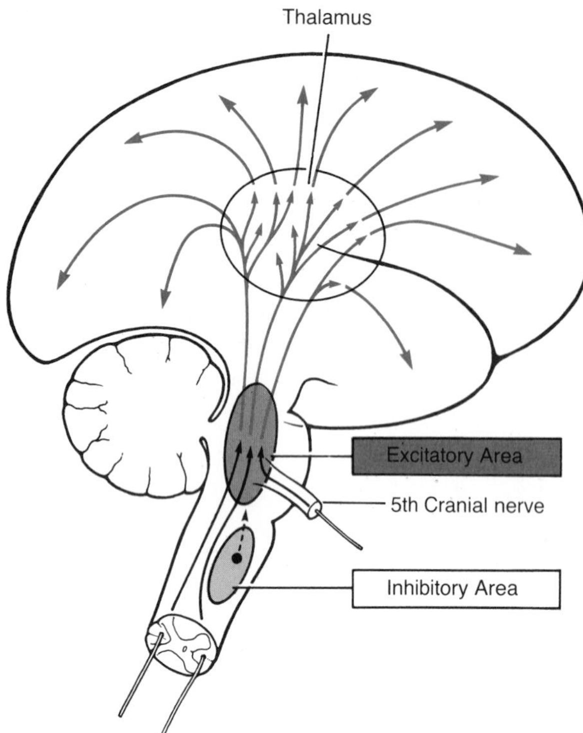

Figure 40-1. The excitatory-activating system of the brain. Also shown is an inhibitory area in the medulla that can inhibit or depress the activating system.

important for controlling the longer-term background excitability level of the brain.

Excitation of the Brain Stem Excitatory Area by Peripheral Sensory Signals. The level of activity of the brain stem excitatory area, and therefore the level of activity of the entire brain, is determined to a great extent by the sensory signals that enter the excitatory area from the periphery. Pain signals, in particular, increase the activity in this area and therefore strongly excite the brain to attention.

Increased Activity of the Brain Stem Excitatory Area Caused by Feedback Signals from the Cerebrum. Not only do excitatory signals pass to the cerebrum from the bulboreticular excitatory area of the brain stem, but signals in turn return from the cerebrum back to the bulbar regions. Therefore, any time the cerebral cortex becomes activated by either thinking or motor processes, reverse signals are sent back to the brain stem excitatory areas; this obviously helps to maintain the level of excitation of the cerebral cortex or even to enhance it. Thus, this is a general mechanism of *positive feedback* that allows any beginning activity in the cerebrum to support still more activity, thus leading to an awake mind.

An Inhibitory Reticular Area Located in the Lower Brain Stem

Figure 40-1 illustrates still another area that is important in controlling brain activity. This is the *reticular inhibitory area* located medially and ventrally in the medulla. In Chapter 37 we saw that this area can inhibit the reticular facilitatory area of the upper brain stem and thereby reduce the tonic nerve signals transmitted through the spinal cord to the antigravity muscles. Likewise, this same inhibitory area, when excited, will decrease activity in the superior portions of the brain as well.

Neurohormonal Control of Brain Activity

Aside from direct control of brain activity by specific transmission of nerve signals from the lower brain areas to the cortical regions of the brain, still another method is also used to control brain activity. This is the release of excitatory or inhibitory neurotransmitter hormonal agents into the substance of the brain. These neurohormones often persist for minutes or even hours and thereby provide long periods of control rather than instantaneous activation or inhibition.

Neurohormonal Systems in the Human Brain. Figure 40-2 illustrates the brain stem areas in the human brain for activating four different neurohormonal systems. Some of the specific functions of these are as follows:

1. *The locus ceruleus and the norepinephrine system.* The *locus ceruleus* is a small area located bilaterally and posteriorly at the juncture between the pons and the mesencephalon. Nerve fibers from this area spread throughout the brain, and they secrete *norepinephrine.* The norepinephrine excites the brain to generalized increased activity. However, it has inhibitory effects in a few areas because of inhibitory receptors at certain neuronal synapses. Later in the chapter we see that this system probably plays a very important role in causing a dreaming type of sleep called REM sleep.

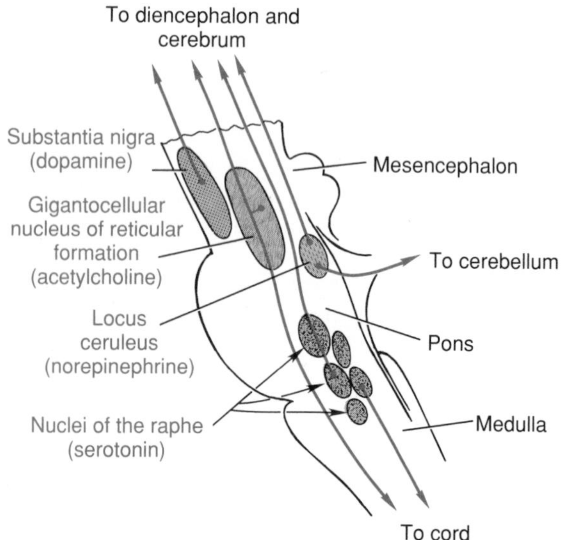

Figure 40-2. Multiple centers in the brain stem, the neurons of which secrete different transmitter substances. These neurons send control signals upward into the diencephalon and cerebrum and downward into the spinal cord.

2. *The substantia nigra and the dopamine system.* The *substantia nigra* is discussed in Chapter 38 in relation to the basal ganglia. It lies anteriorly in the superior mesencephalon, and its neurons send nerve endings mainly to the caudate nucleus and putamen, where they secrete *dopamine.* Other neurons located in adjacent regions also secrete dopamine, but these send their endings into the ventral areas of the cerebrum, especially to the hypothalamus and surrounding areas. The dopamine is believed to act as an inhibitory transmitter in the basal ganglia, but in some of the other areas of the brain it is possibly excitatory. Also, remember from Chapter 38 that destruction of the dopaminergic neurons in the substantia nigra is the basic cause of Parkinson's disease.
3. *The raphe nuclei and the serotonin system.* In the midline of the lower pons and medulla are several very thin nuclei called the *raphe nuclei.* Many of the neurons in these nuclei secrete *serotonin.* They send many fibers into the diencephalon and cerebral cortex; still many others descend to the spinal cord. The cord fibers have the ability to suppress pain, which is discussed in Chapter 33. The serotonin released in the diencephalon and cerebrum almost certainly plays an essential inhibitory role to help cause normal sleep, as we discuss later.
4. *The gigantocellular neurons of the reticular excitatory area and the acetylcholine system.* Earlier, we discussed the gigantocellular neurons (the *giant cells*) in the reticular excitatory area of the pons and mesencephalon. The fibers from these large cells divide immediately into two branches, one passing upward to the higher levels of the brain and the other passing downward through the reticulospinal tracts into the spinal cord. The neurohormone secreted at their terminals is *acetylcholine.* In most places, the acetylcholine functions as an excitatory neurotransmitter at specific synapses.

Other Neurotransmitters and Neurohormonal Substances Secreted in the Brain. Without describing their function, the following is a list of still other neurohormonal substances that, among others, function either at synapses or by release into the fluids of the brain: enkephalins, gamma-aminobutyric acid (GABA), glutamate, vasopressin, adrenocorticotropic hormone, epinephrine, endorphins, angiotensin II, neurotensin.

Thus, there are multiple neurohormonal systems in the brain. The activation of each plays its own role in controlling a different quality of brain function.

THE LIMBIC SYSTEM

The word "limbic" means "border." Originally, the term "limbic" was used to describe the border structures around the basal regions of the cerebrum, but as we have learned more about the functions of the lim-

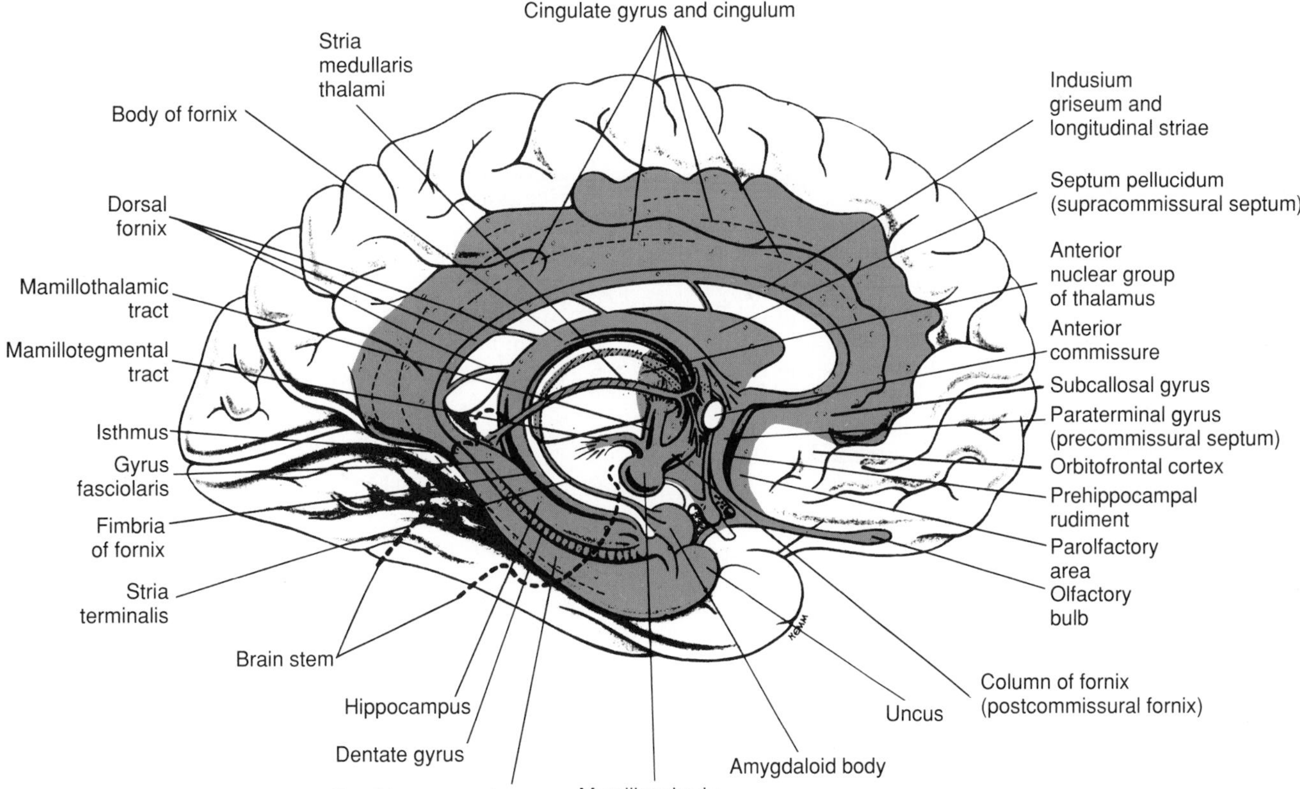

Figure 40-3. Anatomy of the limbic system illustrated by the shaded areas of the figure. (From Williams and Warwick: Gray's Anatomy. 37th Br. ed. New York, Churchill Livingstone, 1989.)

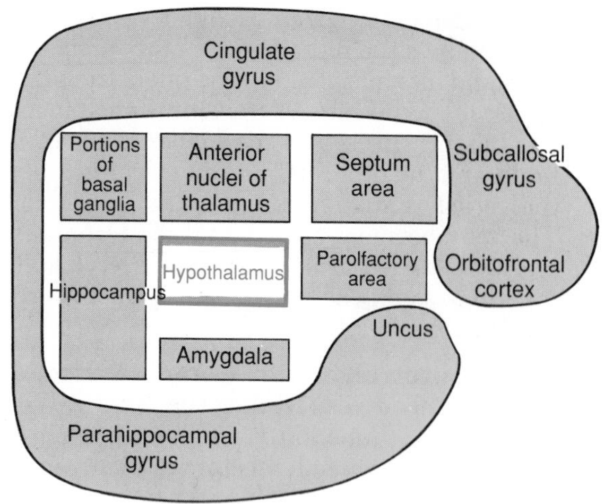

Figure 40-4. The limbic system.

bic system, the term *"limbic system"* has been expanded to mean the entire neuronal circuitry that controls emotional behavior and motivational drives.

FUNCTIONAL ANATOMY OF THE LIMBIC SYSTEM; ITS RELATION ALSO TO THE HYPOTHALAMUS

Figure 40-3 illustrates the anatomical structures of the limbic system, showing these to be an interconnected complex of basal brain elements. Located in the midst of all these is the *hypothalamus.* Figure 40-4 illustrates schematically this key position of the hypothalamus in the limbic system and shows that surrounding it are the other subcortical structures of the limbic system, including the *septum,* the *parolfactory area,* the *epithalamus,* the *anterior nucleus of the thalamus, portions of the basal ganglia,* the *hippocampus,* and the *amygdala.*

Surrounding the subcortical limbic areas is the *limbic cortex,* composed of a ring of cerebral cortex (1) beginning in the *orbitofrontal area* on the ventral surface of the frontal lobes, (2) extending upward beneath the anterior limb of the corpus callosum, (3) over the top of the corpus callosum onto the medial aspect of the cerebral hemisphere in the *cingulate gyrus,* and finally (4) passing behind the corpus callosum and downward onto the ventromedial surface of the temporal lobe to the *parahippocampal gyrus* and *uncus.*

THE HYPOTHALAMUS, A MAJOR OUTPUT PATHWAY OF THE LIMBIC SYSTEM

The hypothalamus has communicating pathways with all levels of the limbic system. In turn, it and its closely allied structures send output signals in three directions: (1) downward to the brain stem, mainly into the reticular areas of the mesencephalon, pons, and medulla; (2) upward toward many higher areas of the diencephalon and cerebrum, especially to the anterior thalamus and the limbic cortex; and (3) into the infundibulum to control most of the secretory functions of the pituitary gland.

Thus, the hypothalamus, which represents less than 1 per cent of the brain mass, nevertheless is one of the most important of the motor output pathways of the limbic system. It controls most of the vegetative and endocrine functions of the body as well as many aspects of emotional behavior.

Vegetative and Endocrine Control Functions of the Hypothalamus

The different hypothalamic mechanisms for controlling the vegetative and endocrine functions of the body are discussed in many different chapters throughout this text. However, to illustrate the organization of the hypothalamus as a functional unit, let us summarize the more important of its vegetative and endocrine functions here as well.

Figure 40-5 illustrates an enlarged sagittal view of the hypothalamus, which represents only a small area in Figure 40-3. Please take a few minutes to study this diagram, especially to read the multiple activities that are excited or inhibited when respective hypothalamic nuclei are stimulated. In addition to those centers illustrated in the figure, a large, *lateral hypothalamic* area overlies the illustrated area on each side of the hypothalamus. The lateral areas are especially important in controlling thirst, hunger, and many of the emotional drives.

A list of the various neurogenic control functions of the hypothalamus includes:

1. Neurogenic control of arterial pressure
2. Regulation of the body temperature
3. Regulation of body water, including especially thirst and excretion of excess water by the kidneys
4. Regulation of uterine contractility
5. Promotion of milk ejection from the breasts
6. Control of many of the emotional drives

Hypothalamic Control of the Anterior Pituitary Gland

Stimulation of certain areas of the hypothalamus also causes the anterior pituitary gland to secrete its hormones that in turn control other bodily functions. This subject is discussed in detail in Chapter 49 in relation to neural control of the endocrine glands. Among the most important effects are the following:

1. Control of growth hormone secretion
2. Control of the secretion of glucocorticoids by the adrenal glands
3. Control of secretion of thyroid hormone by the thyroid gland, and therefore control of much of the body's metabolism

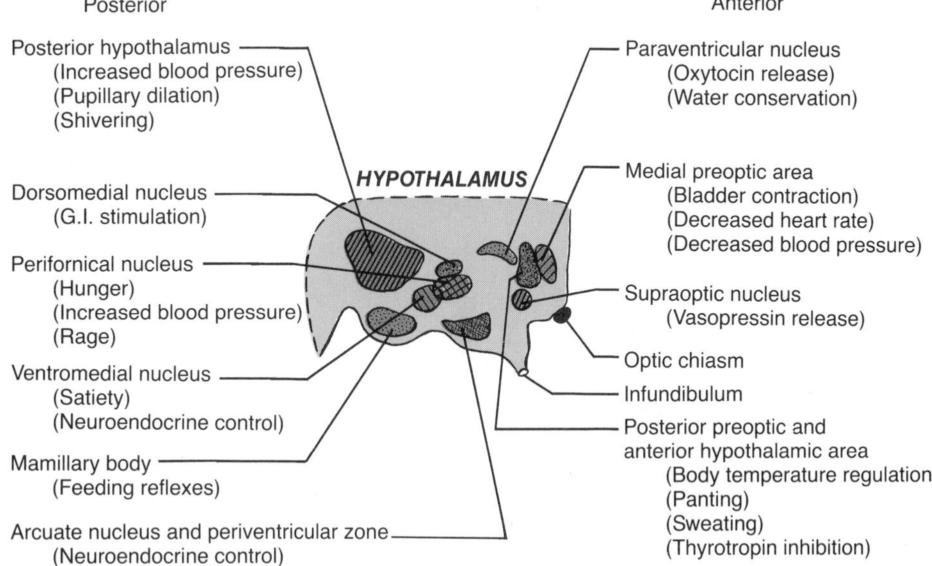

Figure 40-5. Control centers of the hypothalamus.

4. Control of multiple sex hormones that in turn determine the activities of the sexual organs and reproduction

All these various functions of the hypothalamus are discussed in detail at appropriate points throughout this text.

Behavioral Functions of the Hypothalamus and Associated Limbic Structures

Aside from the vegetative and endocrine functions of the hypothalamus, stimulation of or lesions in the hypothalamus often have profound effects on the emotional behavior of animals or human beings.

In animals, some of the behavioral effects of stimulation are the following:

1. Stimulation in the *lateral hypothalamus* not only causes thirst and eating but also increases the general level of activity of the animal, sometimes leading to overt rage and fighting, as is discussed subsequently.
2. Stimulation in the *ventromedial nucleus* and surrounding areas mainly causes effects opposite to those caused by lateral hypothalamic stimulation—that is, a sense of *satiety, decreased eating,* and *tranquility.*
3. Stimulation of a *thin zone of the periventricular nucleus,* located immediately adjacent to the third ventricle (or also stimulation of the central gray area of the brain stem that is continuous with this portion of the hypothalamus) usually leads to *fear* and *punishment reactions.*
4. *Sexual drive* can be stimulated from several areas of the hypothalamus, especially the most anterior and most posterior portions of the hypothalamus.

Lesions in the hypothalamus, in general, cause the opposite effects.

The Reward and Punishment Function of the Limbic System

From the preceding discussion, it is already clear that several limbic structures, including the hypothalamus, are particularly concerned with the *affective* nature of sensory sensations—that is, whether the sensations are *pleasant* or *unpleasant.* These affective qualities are also called *reward* or *punishment,* or *satisfaction* or *aversion.* Electrical stimulation of certain regions pleases or satisfies the animal, whereas electrical stimulation of other regions causes terror, pain, fear, defense, escape reactions, and all the other elements of punishment. Obviously, these two oppositely responding systems greatly affect the behavior of the animal.

Reward Centers

Figure 40-6 illustrates a technique that has been used for localizing specific reward and punishment areas of the brain. In this figure a lever is placed at the side of the animal's cage and is arranged so that depressing the lever makes electrical contact with a stimulator. Electrodes are placed successively at different areas in the brain so that the animal can stimulate the area by pressing the lever. If stimulating the particular area gives the animal a sense of reward, then it will press the lever again and again, sometimes as much as thousands of times per hour. Furthermore, when offered the choice of eating some delectable food

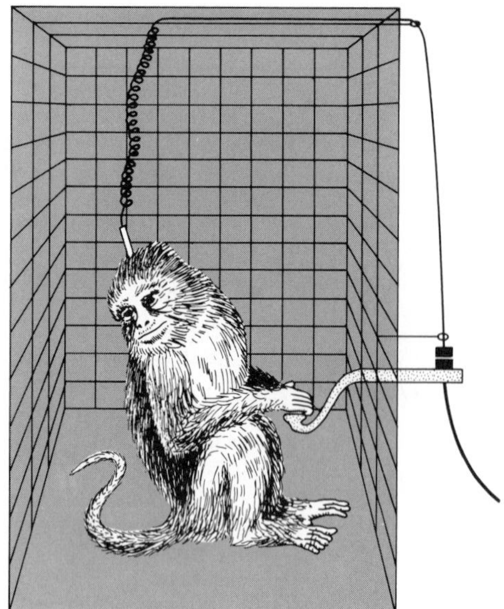

Figure 40-6. Technique for localizing reward and punishment centers in the brain of a monkey.

as opposed to the opportunity to stimulate the reward center, it often chooses the electrical stimulation.

By using this procedure, the major reward centers have been found to be located *along the course of the medial forebrain bundle,* a bundle of nerve fibers that extends from the midlateral region of each side of the hypothalamus, both to the brain stem and to structures anterior to the hypothalamus.

Less potent reward centers, which are perhaps secondary to the major ones in the hypothalamus, are found in the septum, the amygdala, certain areas of the thalamus and basal ganglia, and finally extending downward into the mesencephalon.

Punishment Centers

The apparatus illustrated in Figure 40-6 can also be connected so that pressing the lever turns off, rather than turning on, an electrical stimulus. In this case, the animal will not turn the stimulus off when the electrode is in one of the reward areas; but when it is in certain other areas, it immediately learns to turn it off. Stimulation in these areas causes the animal to show all the signs of displeasure, fear, terror, and punishment. Furthermore, prolonged stimulation for 24 hours or more can cause the animal to become severely sick and actually lead to death.

By means of this technique, the most potent areas for punishment and escape tendencies have been found in the *central gray area surrounding the aqueduct of Sylvius in the mesencephalon* and extending upward into the *periventricular zones of the hypothalamus and thalamus.*

It is particularly interesting that stimulation in the punishment centers can frequently inhibit the reward and pleasure centers completely, illustrating that punishment and fear can take precedence over pleasure and reward.

Importance of Reward and Punishment in Learning and Memory—Habituation or Reinforcement

Animal experiments have shown that a sensory experience causing neither reward nor punishment is remembered hardly at all. Electrical recordings show that new sensory stimuli always excite the cerebral cortex. But repetition of the stimulus over and over leads to almost complete extinction of the cortical response if the sensory experience does not elicit either a sense of reward or punishment. Thus, the animal becomes *habituated* to the sensory stimulus and thereafter ignores it.

However, if the stimulus causes either reward or punishment rather than indifference, the cortical response becomes progressively more and more intense with repeated stimulation instead of fading away, and the response is said to be *reinforced.* Thus, an animal builds up strong memory traces for sensations that are either rewarding or punishing but, on the other hand, develops complete habituation to indifferent sensory stimuli.

Rage

An emotional pattern that involves the hypothalamus and many other limbic structures, and has also been well characterized, is the *rage pattern.* This can be described as follows:

Strong stimulation of the punishment centers of the brain causes the animal to (1) develop a defense posture, (2) extend its claws, (3) lift its tail, (4) hiss, (5) spit, (6) growl, and (7) develop piloerection, wide-open eyes, and dilated pupils. Furthermore, even the slightest provocation causes an immediate savage attack. This is approximately the behavior that one would expect from an animal being severely punished, and it is a pattern of behavior that is called *rage.*

Placidity and Tameness. Exactly the opposite emotional behavior patterns occur when the reward centers are stimulated: placidity and tameness.

SPECIFIC FUNCTIONS OF OTHER PARTS OF THE LIMBIC SYSTEM

Functions of the Amygdala

The amygdala is a complex of nuclei located immediately beneath the cortex of the medial anterior pole of each temporal lobe. It has abundant bidirectional connections with the hypothalamus.

The amygdala receives neuronal signals from all portions of the limbic cortex as well as from the neocortex of the temporal, parietal, and occipital lobes, especially from the olfactory, auditory, and visual association areas. Because of these multiple connections, the amygdala has been called the "window" through which the limbic system sees the place of the person in the world. In turn, the amygdala transmits signals (1) back into these same cortical areas, (2) into the hippocampus, (3) into the septum, (4) into the thalamus, and (5) especially into the hypothalamus.

In general, stimulation in the amygdala can cause almost all the same effects as those elicited by stimulation of the hypothalamus.

Overall Function of the Amygdala. The amygdala seems to be a behavioral awareness area that operates at a semiconscious level. It also seems to project into the limbic system one's present status in relation both to surroundings and thoughts. On the basis of this information, the amygdala is believed to help pattern the person's behavioral response so that it is appropriate for each occasion.

Function of the Hippocampus in Learning

The hippocampus is the elongated, medial portion of the temporal cortex that folds upward and inward to form the ventral surface of the inferior horn of the lateral ventricle.

The hippocampus has numerous but mainly indirect connections with many portions of the cerebral cortex as well as with the basic structures of the limbic system—the amygdala, the hypothalamus, the septum, and the mamillary bodies. Almost any type of sensory experience causes activation of at least some part of the hippocampus. Thus, the hippocampus, like the amygdala, is an additional channel through which incoming sensory signals can lead to appropriate behavioral reactions, but for different purposes.

The hippocampi have been surgically removed bilaterally in a few human beings for the treatment of epilepsy. These persons can recall most previously learned memories satisfactorily. However, they can learn essentially no new information that is based on verbal symbolism. In fact, they cannot even learn the names of persons with whom they come in contact every day. Yet they can remember for a moment or so what transpires during the course of their activities. Thus, they are capable of the type of very short-term memory called "immediate memory" even though their ability to establish secondary memories lasting longer than a few minutes is either completely or almost completely abolished, which is the phenomenon called *anterograde amnesia* discussed in the previous chapter.

Destruction of the hippocampi also causes some deficit in previously learned memories (retrograde amnesia), a little more so for memories in the past year or so than for memories of the distant past.

Theoretical Function of the Hippocampus in Learning. Earlier in this chapter it was pointed out that reward and punishment play a major role in determining whether or not information will be stored in memory. A person rapidly becomes habituated to indifferent stimuli but learns assiduously any sensory experience that causes either pleasure or punishment. It has been suggested that the hippocampus provides the drive that causes translation of immediate memory into secondary memory—that is, it transmits some type of signal or signals that seem to make the mind rehearse over and over the new information until permanent storage takes place.

Whatever the mechanism, without the hippocampi *consolidation* of long-term memories of verbal or symbolic type does not take place.

Function of the Limbic Cortex

Probably the most poorly understood portion of the entire limbic system is the ring of cerebral cortex called the *limbic cortex* that surrounds the subcortical limbic structures. This cortex functions as a transitional zone through which signals are transmitted from the remainder of the cortex into the limbic system. Therefore, it is presumed that the limbic cortex functions as a cerebral *association area for control of behavior.* Essentially all the behavioral patterns that have already been described can also be elicited by stimulation in different portions of the limbic cortex. Likewise, ablation of a few limbic cortical areas can cause persistent changes in an animal's behavior.

SLEEP

Sleep is defined as unconsciousness from which the person can be aroused by sensory or other stimuli. It is to be distinguished from *coma,* which is unconsciousness from which the person cannot be aroused. However, there are multiple stages of sleep, from very light sleep to very deep sleep, and most sleep researchers even divide sleep into two different types of sleep that have different qualities, as follows:

Two Different Types of Sleep—(1) Slow Wave Sleep and (2) REM Sleep. During each night a person goes through stages of two different types of sleep that alternate with each other. These are called (1) *slow wave sleep,* because in this type of sleep the brain waves are very slow, as we discuss later; and (2) *REM sleep,* which stands for *rapid eye movement* sleep, because in this type of sleep the eyes undergo rapid movements despite the fact that the person is still asleep.

Most sleep during each night is of the slow wave variety; this is the deep, restful type of sleep that the person experiences during the first hour of sleep after having been kept awake for many hours. Episodes of REM sleep occur periodically during sleep and occupy about 25 per cent of the sleep time of the young adult; they normally recur about every 90 minutes. This type of sleep is not so restful, and it is usually associated with dreaming, as we discuss later.

Slow Wave Sleep

Most of us can understand the characteristics of deep slow wave sleep by remembering the last time that we were kept awake for more than 24 hours and then remembering the deep sleep that occurred during the first hour after going to sleep. This sleep is exceedingly restful and is associated with a decrease in both peripheral vascular tone and many other vegetative functions of the body as well. In addition, there is a 10 to 30 per cent decrease in blood pressure, respiratory rate, and basal metabolic rate.

Though slow wave sleep is frequently called "dreamless sleep," dreams do occur often during slow wave sleep, and nightmares even occur during this type of sleep. However, the difference between the dreams occurring in slow wave sleep and those in REM sleep is that those of REM sleep are remembered, whereas those of slow wave sleep usually are not. That is, during slow wave sleep the process of consolidation of the dreams in memory does not occur.

REM Sleep (Paradoxical Sleep, Desynchronized Sleep)

In a normal night of sleep, bouts of REM sleep lasting 5 to 30 minutes usually appear on the average every 90 minutes, the first such period occurring 80 to 100 minutes after the person falls asleep. When the person is extremely sleepy, the duration of each bout of REM sleep is very short, and it may even be absent. On the other hand, as the person becomes more rested through the night, the duration of the REM bouts greatly increases.

There are several important characteristics of REM sleep:

1. It is usually associated with active dreaming.
2. The heart rate and respiration usually become irregular, which is characteristic of the dream state.
3. Despite inhibition of the peripheral muscles, a few irregular muscle movements occur. These include, in particular, rapid movements of the eyes; this is the origin of the acronym REM, for "rapid eye movements."
4. The brain is highly active in REM sleep, and the overall brain metabolism may be increased as much as 20 per cent. Also, the electroencephalogram shows a pattern of brain waves similar to those that occur during wakefulness. Therefore, this type of sleep is also frequently called *paradoxical sleep* because it is a paradox that a person can still be asleep despite marked activity in the brain.

In summary, REM sleep is a type of sleep in which the brain is quite active. However, the brain activity is not channeled in the proper direction for persons to be fully aware of their surroundings and therefore to be awake.

Basic Theories of Sleep

The Active Theory of Sleep. An earlier theory of sleep was that the excitatory areas of the upper brain stem, which was called the *reticular activating system,* and other parts of the brain simply became fatigued over the period of a waking day and therefore became inactive as a result. This was called the *passive theory of sleep.* However, an important experiment changed this view to the current belief that *sleep is probably caused by an active inhibitory process.* This was the experiment in which it was discovered that transecting the brain stem in the midpontile region leads to a brain that never goes to sleep. In other words, there seems to be some center or centers located below the midpontile level of the brain stem that actively cause sleep by inhibiting upper parts of the brain. This is called the *active theory* of sleep.

Neuronal Centers, Neurohumoral Substances, and Mechanisms That Can Cause Sleep—A Possible Specific Role for Serotonin

Stimulation of several specific areas of the brain can produce sleep with characteristics very near those of natural sleep. Some of these are the following:

1. The most conspicuous stimulation area for causing almost natural sleep is the raphe nuclei in the lower half of the pons and in the medulla. These are a thin sheet of nuclei located in the midline. Nerve fibers from these nuclei spread widely in the reticular formation and also upward into the thalamus, neocortex, hypothalamus, and most areas of the limbic system. In addition, they extend downward into the spinal cord, terminating in the posterior horns where they can inhibit incoming pain signals, as was discussed in Chapter 33. It is also known that many of the endings of fibers from these raphe neurons secrete *serotonin.* Also, when a drug that blocks the formation of serotonin is administered to an animal, the animal often cannot sleep for the next several days. Therefore, it is assumed that serotonin is the major transmitter substance associated with production of sleep.
2. Stimulation of some areas in the *nucleus of the tractus solitarius,* which is the sensory region of the medulla and pons for the visceral sensory signals entering the brain via the vagus and glossopharyngeal nerves, will also promote sleep. However, this will not occur if the raphe nuclei have been destroyed. Therefore, these regions probably act by exciting the raphe nuclei and the serotonin system.
3. Stimulation of several regions in the diencephalon can also help promote sleep, including (a) parts of the hypothalamus, and (b) an occasional area in the diffuse nuclei of the thalamus.

Effect of Lesions in the Sleep-Promoting Centers. Discrete lesions in the raphe nuclei lead to a high state of wakefulness. This is also true of bilateral lesions in a portion of the anterior hypothalamus. In both instances, the excitatory reticular nuclei of the mesencephalon and upper pons seem to become released from inhibition. Indeed, the lesions of the anterior hypothalamus can sometimes cause such intense wakefulness that the animal actually dies of exhaustion.

Possible Causes of REM Sleep

Why slow wave sleep is broken periodically by REM sleep is not understood. However, a lesion in the *locus ceruleus* on each side of the brain stem can reduce REM sleep, and if the lesion includes other contiguous areas of the brain stem, REM sleep can be prevented altogether. Therefore, it has been postulated that when stimulated, norepinephrine-secreting nerve fibers that originate in the locus ceruleus can activate many portions of the brain. This theoretically causes the excess activity that occurs in certain regions of the brain in REM sleep, but the signals are not channeled appropriately in the brain to cause normal conscious awareness that is characteristic of wakefulness.

The Cycle Between Sleep and Wakefulness

The preceding discussions have merely identified neuronal areas, transmitters, and mechanisms that are related to sleep. However, they have not explained the cyclical, reciprocal operation of the sleep-wakefulness cycle. There is, as yet, no explanation. Therefore, we can let our imaginations run wild and suggest the following possible mechanism for causing the rhythmicity of the sleep-wakefulness cycle:

When the sleep centers are not activated, the release from inhibition of the mesencephalic and upper pontile reticular nuclei allows this region to become spontaneously active. This in turn excites both the cerebral cortex and the peripheral nervous system, both of which then send numerous positive feedback signals back to the same reticular nuclei to activate them still further. Thus, once wakefulness begins, it has a natural tendency to sustain itself because of all this positive feedback activity.

However, after the brain remains activated for many hours, even the neurons within the activating system presumably will become fatigued to some extent, and other factors presumably activate the sleep centers. Consequently, the positive feedback cycle between the mesencephalic reticular nuclei and the cortex will fade, and the inhibitory effects of the sleep centers will take over, leading to rapid transition from the wakefulness state to the sleep state.

Then, one could postulate that during sleep the excitatory neurons of the reticular activating system gradually become more and more excitable because of the prolonged rest, while the inhibitory neurons of the sleep centers become less excitable because of their overactivity, thus leading to a new cycle of wakefulness.

BRAIN WAVES

Electrical recordings from the surface of the brain or even from the outer surface of the head demonstrate continuous electrical activity in the brain. Both the intensity and patterns of this electrical activity are determined to a great extent by the overall level of excitation of the brain resulting from *sleep, wakefulness,* and brain diseases such as *epilepsy* and even some *psychoses.* The undulations in the recorded electrical potentials, shown in Figure 40–7, are called *brain waves,* and the entire record is called an *electroencephalogram* (EEG).

Much of the time, the brain waves are irregular, and no general pattern can be discerned in the EEG. However, at other times, distinct patterns do appear. Some of these are characteristic of specific abnormalities of the brain, such as epilepsy, which is discussed later. Others occur even in normal persons and can be classified as *alpha, beta, theta,* and *delta waves,* which are all illustrated in Figure 40–7.

Alpha waves are rhythmical waves occurring at a frequency of between 8 and 13 per second and are found in the EEGs of almost all normal adult persons when they are awake in a quiet, resting state of cerebration.

Beta waves occur at frequencies of more than 14 cycles per second and as high as 25 and rarely 50 cycles per second. These are most frequently recorded during activation of the central nervous system or during tension.

Theta waves have frequencies of between 4 and 7 cycles per second. These occur mainly in children, but they also occur during emotional stress in some adults and in many brain disorders.

Delta waves include all the waves of the EEG below 3.5 cycles per second and sometimes as low as 1 cycle every 2 to 3 seconds. These occur in very deep sleep, in infancy, and in serious organic brain disease.

Origin of Alpha Waves. Alpha waves will *not* occur in the cortex without connections with the thalamus. Also, stimulation in the nonspecific thalamic nuclei often sets up waves in the generalized thalamocortical system at a frequency of between 8 and 13 per

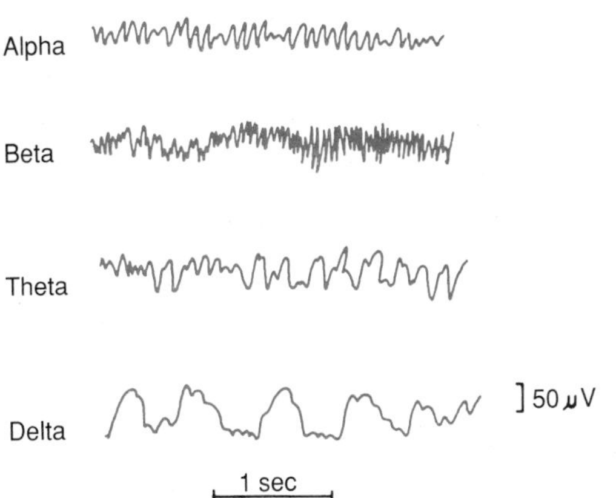

Figure 40–7. Different types of normal electroencephalographic waves.

second, the natural frequency of the alpha waves. Therefore, it is likely that the alpha waves result from spontaneous activity in the nonspecific thalamocortical system, which causes both the periodicity of the alpha waves and the synchronous activation of literally millions of cortical neurons during each wave.

Origin of Delta Waves. Transection of the fiber tracts from the thalamus to the cortex, which blocks the thalamic activation of the cortex and eliminates the alpha waves, nevertheless causes delta waves in the cortex. This indicates that some synchronizing mechanism can occur in the cortical neurons themselves—entirely independently of lower structures in the brain—to cause the delta waves.

Delta waves also occur in very deep slow wave sleep; this suggests that the cortex then might be released from the activating influences of the lower centers.

Electroencephalographic Changes in the Different Stages of Wakefulness and Sleep

Figure 40-8 illustrates the electroencephalogram from a typical person in different stages of wakefulness and sleep. Alert wakefulness is characterized by high frequency *beta waves,* whereas quiet wakefulness is usually associated with *alpha waves,* as illustrated by the first two electroencephalograms of the figure.

Slow wave sleep is generally divided into four stages. In the first stage, a stage of very light sleep, the voltage of the electroencephalographic waves becomes very low; but this is broken by *"sleep spindles,"* that is, short spindle-shaped bursts of alpha waves that occur periodically. In stages 2, 3, and 4 of slow wave sleep the frequency of the electroencephalogram becomes progressively slower until it reaches a frequency of only 2 to 3 waves per second; these are typical *delta waves.*

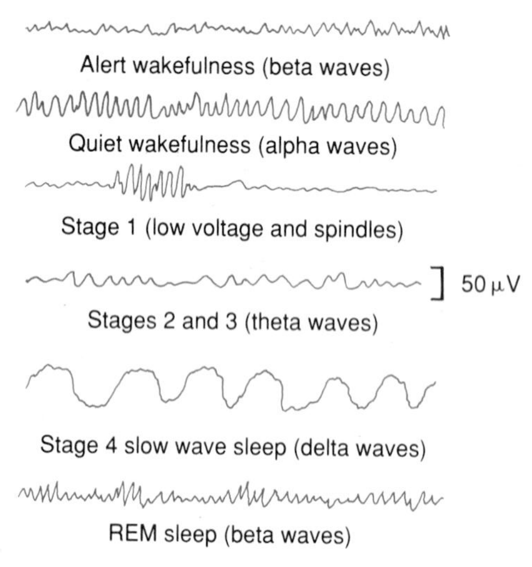

Figure 40-8. Progressive change in the characteristics of the brain waves during different stages of wakefulness and sleep.

Finally, the bottom record in Figure 40-8 illustrates the electroencephalogram during REM sleep. It is often difficult to tell a difference between this brain wave pattern and that of an alert awake person. The voltage of these waves is considerably lower than the voltage in deep stage 4 slow wave sleep, and the waves are themselves irregular high frequency beta waves, which is normally suggestive of excess but desynchronized nervous activity as found in the awake state.

EPILEPSY

Epilepsy is characterized by uncontrolled excessive activity of either a part or all of the central nervous system. A person who is predisposed to epilepsy has attacks when the basal level of excitability of the nervous system (or of the part that is susceptible to the epileptic state) rises above a certain critical threshold. But as long as the degree of excitability is held below this threshold, no attack occurs.

Basically, epilepsy can be classified into three major types: *grand mal epilepsy, petit mal epilepsy,* and *focal epilepsy.*

Grand Mal Epilepsy

Grand mal epilepsy is characterized by extreme neuronal discharges in all areas of the brain—in the cortex, in the deeper parts of the cerebrum, and even in the brain stem and thalamus. Also, discharges into the spinal cord cause generalized *tonic convulsions* of the entire body, followed toward the end of the attack by alternating tonic and then spasmodic muscular contractions called *tonic-clonic convulsions.* Often the person bites or "swallows" the tongue and usually has difficulty in breathing, sometimes to the extent of developing cyanosis. Also, signals to the viscera frequently cause urination and defecation.

The grand mal seizure lasts from a few seconds to as long as 3 to 4 minutes and is characterized by postseizure depression of the entire nervous system; the person remains in stupor for 1 to many minutes after the attack is over and then often remains severely fatigued or even asleep for many hours thereafter.

The top recording of Figure 40-9 illustrates a typical electroencephalogram from almost any region of the cortex during the tonic phase of a grand mal attack. This illustrates that high voltage, synchronous discharges occur over the entire cortex. Furthermore, electrical recordings from the thalamus and also from the reticular formation of the brain stem during the grand mal attack show typical high voltage activity in both these areas similar to that recorded from the cerebral cortex.

Presumably, therefore, a grand mal attack is caused by abnormal activation in the lower portions of the brain-activating system itself.

What Stops the Grand Mal Attack? The cause of the extreme neuronal overactivity during a grand

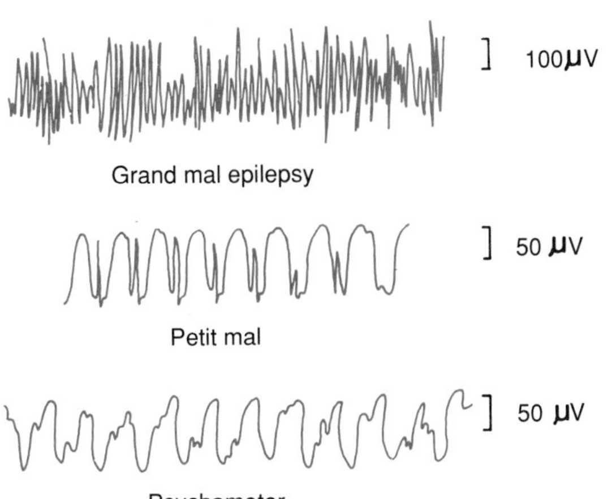

Figure 40-9. Electroencephalograms in different types of epilepsy.

mal attack is presumed to be massive activation of many reverberating pathways throughout the brain. Presumably, also, the major factor, or at least one of the major factors, that stops the attack after a few minutes is the phenomenon of neuronal *fatigue*. The stupor and total body fatigue that occur after a grand mal seizure is over are believed to result from the intense fatigue of the neuronal synapses following their intensive activity during the grand mal attack.

Petit Mal Epilepsy

Petit mal epilepsy is usually characterized by 3 to 30 seconds of unconsciousness during which the person has several twitchlike contractions of the muscles, usually in the head region — especially blinking of the eyes; this is followed by return of consciousness and resumption of previous activities.

The brain wave pattern in petit mal epilepsy is illustrated by the middle record of Figure 40-9, which is typified by a *spike and dome pattern*. The spike portion of this recording is almost identical to the spikes that occur in grand mal epilepsy, but the dome portion is distinctly different. The spike and dome can be recorded over most or all of the cerebral cortex, illustrating that the seizure involves the entire activating system of the brain.

Focal Epilepsy

Focal epilepsy can involve almost any part of the brain, either localized regions of the cerebral cortex or deeper structures of both the cerebrum and brain stem. And almost always, focal epilepsy results from some localized organic lesion or functional abnormality, such as a scar that pulls on the neuronal tissue, a tumor that compresses an area of the brain, a destroyed area of brain tissue, or congenitally deranged local circuitry. Lesions such as these can promote extremely rapid discharges in the local neurons; and when the discharge rate rises above approximately 1000 per second, synchronous waves begin to spread over the adjacent cortical regions. These waves presumably result from *localized reverberating circuits* that gradually recruit adjacent areas of the cortex into the discharge zone.

A focal epileptic attack may remain confined to a single area of the brain, but in many instances the strong signals from the convulsing cortex or other part of the brain excite the mesencephalic portion of the brain-activating system so greatly that a grand mal epileptic attack ensues as well.

PSYCHOTIC BEHAVIOR AND DEMENTIA—ROLES OF SPECIFIC NEUROTRANSMITTER SYSTEMS

Clinical studies of patients with different psychoses and also some types of dementia have suggested that many if not most of these conditions result from diminished function of classes of neurons that secrete specific neurotransmitters. Use of appropriate drugs to counteract the loss of the respective transmitters has been quite successful in treating some patients.

In Chapter 38 we discussed the cause of Parkinson's disease, the loss of the neurons in the substantia nigra whose axons secrete dopamine in the caudate nucleus and putamen. The loss of acetylcholine-secreting neurons in the basal ganglia is associated with the abnormal motor patterns of Huntington's chorea, as well as with the dementia that develops later in the same patients. In the present section, we extend this concept to other abnormalities and other classes of neurons that lead to additional types of psychotic behavior or dementia.

Depression Psychosis—Decreased Activity of the Norepinephrine and Serotonin Neurotransmitter Systems

In the past few years much evidence has accumulated suggesting that the *mental depression psychosis*, which afflicts about 8 million people in the United States at any one time, might be caused by diminished formation of either norepinephrine or serotonin or both. These patients experience symptoms of grief, unhappiness, despair, and misery. In addition, they lose their appetite and sex drive and also have severe insomnia. And associated with all these is often a state of psychomotor agitation despite the depression.

In the previous chapter it was pointed out that large numbers of *norepinephrine-secreting neurons* are located in the brain stem, especially in the *locus ceruleus*, and that these send fibers upward to most parts of the limbic system, the thalamus, and the cerebral cortex. Also, many *serotonin-producing neurons* are located in the *midline raphe nuclei* of the lower pons and medulla and also project fibers to many areas of the limbic system and to some other areas of the brain as well.

A principal reason for believing that depression is

caused by diminished activity of the norepinephrine and serotonin systems is that drugs that block the secretion of norepinephrine and serotonin, such as the drug reserpine, frequently cause depression. Conversely, about 70 per cent of depressive patients can be treated very effectively with one of two types of drugs that increase especially the excitatory effects of norepinephrine at the nerve endings.

Schizophrenia—Depressed Function of Part of the Dopamine System

Schizophrenia comes in many different varieties. One of the most common is the person who hears voices and has delusions of grandeur, or intense fear, or other types of feelings that are unreal. Schizophrenics are often highly paranoid, with a sense of persecution from outside sources; they may develop incoherent speech, dissociation of ideas, and abnormal sequences of thought; and they are often withdrawn, sometimes with abnormal posture and even rigidity.

There is reason to believe that schizophrenia results from excessive functioning of a group of neurons that secretes dopamine. These neurons are located in the ventral tegmentum of the mesencephalon, medial and superior to the substantia nigra. They give rise to the so-called *mesolimbic dopaminergic system,* which projects nerve fibers mainly into the medial and anterior portions of the limbic system, especially into the amygdala, the anterior caudate nucleus, and the anterior cingulate gyrus of the cortex, all of which are powerful behavioral control centers.

A reason for believing the mesolimbic dopaminergic system to be related to schizophrenia is the following: those drugs that are effective in treating schizophrenia, such as chlorpromazine, haloperidol, and thiothixene, all decrease the secretion of dopamine by the dopaminergic nerve endings or decrease the effect of dopamine on the subsequent neurons.

Almost certainly there are other factors in schizophrenia besides excess secretion of dopamine; nevertheless, the symptoms of schizophrenia are similar to the behavioral effects of excessive dopamine.

REFERENCES

Ashton, H.: Brain Systems, Disorders and Psychotropic Drugs. New York, Oxford University Press, 1987.

Avoli, M., et al. (eds.): Neurotransmitters and Cortical Function. New York, Plenum Publishing Corp., 1988.

Borbely, A. A., and Tobler, I.: Endogenous sleep-promoting substances and sleep regulation. Physiol. Rev., 69:605, 1989.

Clynes, M., and Panksepp, J. (eds.): Emotions and Psychopathology. New York, Plenum Publishing Corp., 1988.

Dichter, M. A. (ed.): Mechanisms of Epileptogenesis. New York, Plenum Publishing Corp., 1988.

Doane, B. K., and Livingston, K. E. (eds.): The Limbic System. New York, Raven Press, 1986.

Engel, J., et al. (eds.): Brain Reward Systems and Abuse. New York, Raven Press, 1987.

Georgotas, A., and Cancro, R. (eds.): Depression and Mania. New York, Elsevier Science Publishing Co., 1988.

Jones, E. G., and Peters, A. (eds.): Further Aspects of Cortical Function, Including Hippocampus. New York, Plenum Publishing Corp., 1987.

Kandel, E. R.: Molecular Neurobiology in Neurology and Psychiatry. New York, Raven Press, 1987.

McKinney, W. T.: Models of Mental Disorders. New York, Plenum Publishing Corp., 1988.

Meijer, J. H., and Rietveld, W. J.: Neurophysiology of the suprachiasmatic circadian pacemaker in rodents. Physiol. Rev., 69:671, 1989.

Nerozzi, D., et al. (eds.): Hypothalamic Dysfunction in Neuropsychiatric Disorders. New York, Raven Press, 1987.

Wauquier, A., et al.: Slow Wave Sleep: Physiological, Pathophysiological, and Functional Aspects. New York, Raven Press, 1989.

Wolman, B. B.: Psychosomatic Disorders. New York, Plenum Publishing Corp., 1988.

QUESTIONS

1. Describe the reticular activating system and tell how it causes wakefulness.
2. Explain some of the ways in which the following neurohormones control mental function: (a) norepinephrine, (b) dopamine, (c) serotonin, (d) acetylcholine.
3. What are the four major types of brain waves, and what are the characteristics of each?
4. Describe the successive changes in the brain waves as one passes through all stages of wakefulness and sleep.
5. Characterize *slow wave sleep.*
6. How does *REM sleep* differ from slow wave sleep?
7. Describe the function of the *serotonin-secreting neurons* in causing sleep.
8. What is the role of the *locus ceruleus* and its norepinephrine-secreting nerve fibers in causing REM sleep?
9. Explain, theoretically, the cycling process between wakefulness and sleep.
10. Characterize *grand mal epilepsy,* and explain what stops an epileptic attack.
11. Characterize *petit mal epilepsy.*
12. Explain what is meant by the *limbic system,* and describe, in general, its anatomy.
13. List the control functions of the various hypothalamic nuclei that have to do with behavior.
14. Explain the principle of *reward* and *punishment centers* in the hypothalamus and other portions of the limbic system.
15. What are the roles of reward and punishment in learning and memory? How does the *hippocampus* fit into this scheme?
16. How does the *amygdala* help control the pattern of behavior demanded for each social occasion?
17. Explain the association function of the *limbic cortex* in behavior control.
18. What are the relationships of the norepinephrine and serotonin systems to the *depression psychosis*?
19. What is the possible relationship of the dopamine system to *schizophrenia*?

41

The Autonomic Nervous System; Cerebral Blood Flow and Cerebrospinal Fluid

The portion of the nervous system that controls the visceral functions of the body is called the *autonomic nervous system.* This system helps control arterial pressure, gastrointestinal motility and secretion, urinary bladder emptying, sweating, body temperature, and many other activities, some of which are controlled almost entirely and some only partially by the autonomic nervous system.

GENERAL ORGANIZATION OF THE AUTONOMIC NERVOUS SYSTEM

The autonomic nervous system is activated mainly by centers located in the *spinal cord, brain stem,* and *hypothalamus.* Also, portions of the cerebral cortex, especially of the limbic cortex, can transmit impulses to the lower centers and in this way influence autonomic control. Often the autonomic nervous system also operates by means of *visceral reflexes.* That is, sensory signals entering the autonomic ganglia, cord, brain stem, or hypothalamus can elicit appropriate reflex responses back to the visceral organs to control their activities.

The efferent autonomic signals are transmitted to the body through two major subdivisions called the *sympathetic nervous system* and the *parasympathetic nervous system,* the characteristics and functions of which follow.

Physiological Anatomy of the Sympathetic Nervous System

Figure 41–1 illustrates the general organization of the sympathetic nervous system, showing one of the two *paravertebral sympathetic chains of ganglia* that lie to the two sides of the spinal column, two *prevertebral ganglia* inside the abdomen (the *celiac* and *hypogastric*) inside the abdomen, and nerves extending from the ganglia to the different internal organs. The sympathetic nerves originate in the spinal cord between the segments T-1 and L-2 and pass from here first into the sympathetic chain and thence to the tissues and organs that are stimulated by the sympathetic nerves.

Preganglionic and Postganglionic Sympathetic Neurons

The sympathetic nerves are different from skeletal motor nerves in the following way: Each sympathetic pathway from the cord to the stimulated tissue is composed of two neurons, a *preganglionic neuron* and a *postganglionic neuron,* in contrast to only a single neuron in the skeletal motor pathway. The cell body of each preganglionic neuron lies in the *intermediolateral horn* of the spinal cord; and its fiber passes through an *anterior root* of the cord into the corresponding *spinal nerve.*

Immediately after the spinal nerve leaves the spinal column, the preganglionic sympathetic fibers leave the nerve and pass into one of the *ganglia* of the *sympathetic chain.* Then the course of the fibers can be one of the following three: (1) It can synapse with postganglionic neurons in the ganglion that it enters. (2) It can pass upward or downward in the chain and synapse in one of the other ganglia of the chain. Or (3) it can pass for variable distances through the chain and then through one of the *sympathetic nerves* radiating outward from the chain, finally terminating in one of the *prevertebral ganglia.*

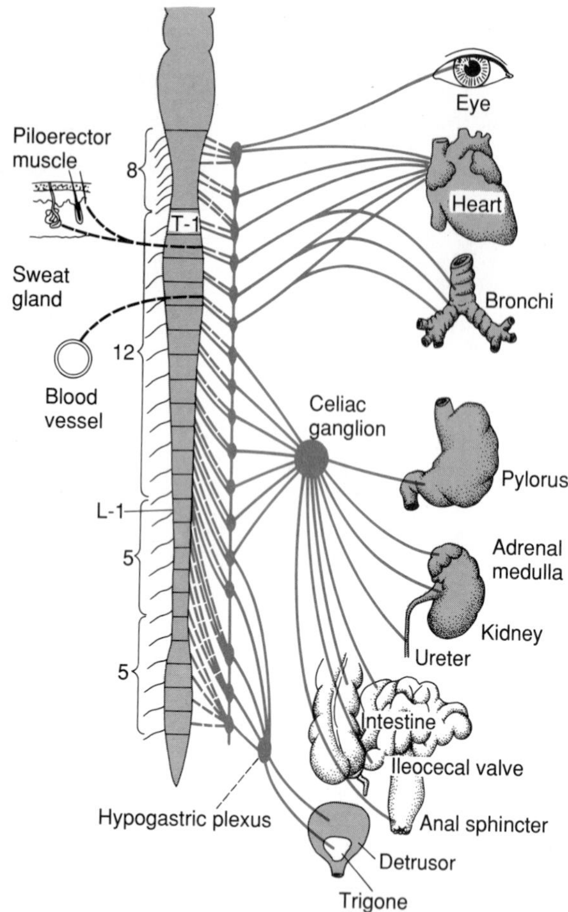

Figure 41-1. The sympathetic nervous system. Dashed lines represent postganglionic fibers in the gray rami leading into the spinal nerves for distribution to blood vessels, sweat glands, and piloerector muscles.

The postganglionic neuron then originates either in one of the sympathetic chain ganglia or in one of the prevertebral ganglia. From either of these two sources, the postganglionic fibers travel to their destinations in the various organs.

Sympathetic Nerve Fibers in the Skeletal Nerves. Some of the postganglionic fibers pass back from the sympathetic chain into the spinal nerves at all levels of the cord. These pathways are made up of very small type C fibers that extend to all parts of the body in the skeletal nerves. They control the blood vessels, sweat glands, and piloerector muscles of the hairs. Approximately 8 per cent of the fibers in the average skeletal nerve are sympathetic fibers, a fact that indicates their importance.

Physiological Anatomy of the Parasympathetic Nervous System

The parasympathetic nervous system is illustrated in Figure 41-2, showing that parasympathetic fibers leave the central nervous system mainly through cranial nerves III, VII, IX, and X and the second and third sacral spinal nerves. About 75 per cent of all parasympathetic nerve fibers are in the vagus nerves, passing to the entire thoracic and abdominal regions of the body. Therefore, a physiologist speaking of the parasympathetic nervous system often thinks mainly of the two vagus nerves. The vagus nerves supply parasympathetic nerves to the heart, the lungs, the esophagus, the stomach, the entire small intestine, the proximal half of the colon, the liver, the gallbladder, the pancreas, and the upper portions of the ureters.

Parasympathetic fibers in the *third nerve* flow to the pupillary sphincters and ciliary muscles of the eye. Fibers from the *seventh nerve* pass to the lacrimal, nasal, and submandibular glands, and fibers from the *ninth nerve* pass to the parotid gland.

The sacral parasympathetic fibers leave the sacral plexus on each side of the cord and distribute to the descending colon, rectum, bladder, and lower portions of the ureters. Also, this sacral group of parasympathetics supplies fibers to the external genitalia to cause sexual stimulation.

Preganglionic and Postganglionic Parasympathetic Neurons. The parasympathetic system, like the sympathetic, has both preganglionic and postganglionic neurons. However, except in the case of a few cranial parasympathetic nerves, the *preganglionic fibers* pass uninterrupted all the way to the organ that is to be controlled. Then, in the wall of the organ are located the *postganglionic neurons.* The preganglionic fibers synapse with these, and short postganglionic fibers, 1 millimeter to several centimeters in length, leave the neurons to spread through the substance of the organ.

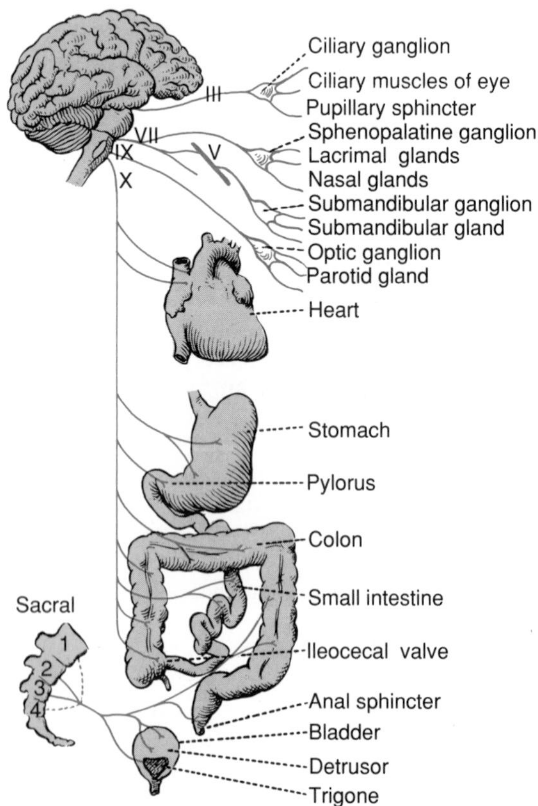

Figure 41-2. The parasympathetic nervous system.

BASIC CHARACTERISTICS OF SYMPATHETIC AND PARASYMPATHETIC FUNCTION

Cholinergic and Adrenergic Fibers—Secretion of Acetylcholine or Norepinephrine

The sympathetic and parasympathetic nerve fibers all secrete one of the two synaptic transmitter substances, *acetylcholine* or *norepinephrine.* Those that secrete acetylcholine are said to be *cholinergic.* Those that secrete norepinephrine are said to be *adrenergic,* a term derived from *adrenaline,* which is the British name for epinephrine.

All *preganglionic neurons* are *cholinergic* in both the sympathetic and parasympathetic nervous systems. Therefore, acetylcholine or acetylcholine-like substances, when applied to the ganglia, will excite both sympathetic and parasympathetic postganglionic neurons.

The *postganglionic neurons of the parasympathetic system are* also *all cholinergic.*

On the other hand, *most of the postganglionic sympathetic neurons are adrenergic,* though this is not entirely true, because the postganglionic sympathetic nerve fibers to the sweat glands, to the piloerector muscles, and to a few blood vessels are cholinergic.

Thus, the terminal nerve endings of the parasympathetic system *all* secrete *acetylcholine,* and *most* of the sympathetic nerve endings secrete *norepinephrine.* These hormones, in turn, act on the different organs to cause the respective parasympathetic and sympathetic effects.

These are the molecular structures of acetylcholine and norepinephrine:

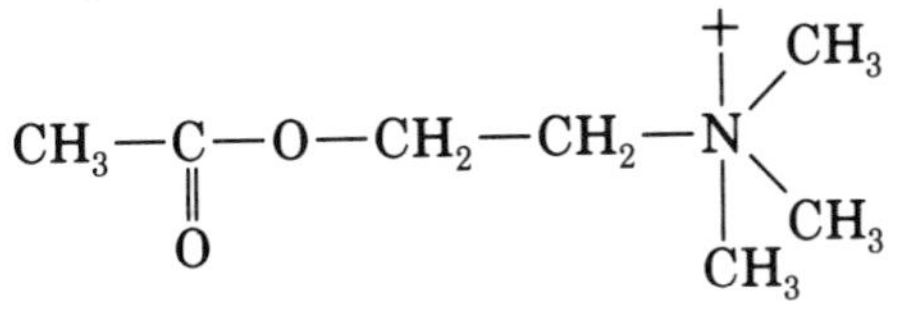

$$CH_3{-}\underset{\substack{\| \\ O}}{C}{-}O{-}CH_2{-}CH_2{-}\overset{+}{N}(CH_3)_3$$

Acetylcholine

$$(HO)_2C_6H_3{-}\underset{\substack{| \\ OH}}{CH}{-}CH_2{-}NH_2$$

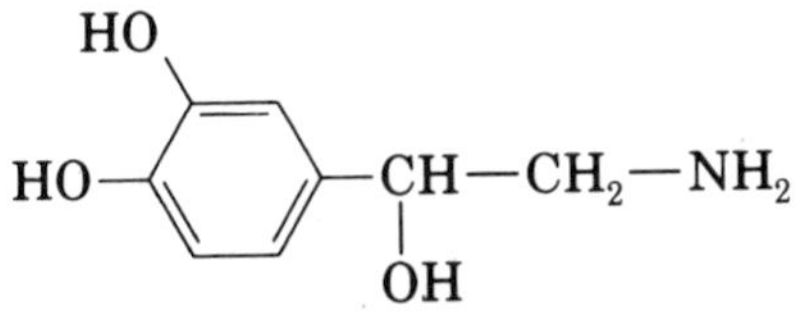

Norepinephrine

Mechanisms of Transmitter Secretion and Removal at the Postganglionic Endings

Secretion of Acetylcholine and Norepinephrine by Postganglionic Nerve Endings. Some of the postganglionic autonomic nerve endings, especially those of the parasympathetic nerves, are similar to but much smaller in size than those of the skeletal neuromuscular junction. However, most of the sympathetic nerve fibers merely touch the effector cells of the organs that they innervate as they pass by; and in some instances they terminate in connective tissue located adjacent to the cells that are to be stimulated. Where these filaments pass over or near the effector cells, they usually have bulbous enlargements called *varicosities;* it is in these varicosities that the transmitter vesicles of acetylcholine or norepinephrine are found. Also in the varicosities are large numbers of mitochondria to supply the adenosine triphosphate (ATP) required to energize acetylcholine or norepinephrine synthesis.

When an action potential spreads over the terminal fibers, the depolarization process increases the permeability of the fiber membrane to calcium ions, allowing these to diffuse into the nerve terminals. There the ions interact with the vesicles that are adjacent to the membrane, causing them to fuse with the membrane and to empty their contents to the exterior. Thus, the transmitter substance is secreted.

Synthesis of Acetylcholine, Its Destruction After Secretion, and Duration of Action. Acetylcholine is synthesized in the terminal endings of cholinergic nerve fibers. Most of this synthesis occurs in the axoplasm outside the vesicles, and then the acetylcholine is transported to the interior of the vesicles, where it is stored in a highly concentrated form until it is released. The basic chemical reaction of this synthesis is the following:

$$\text{Acetyl-CoA} + \text{Choline} \xrightarrow[\textit{transferase}]{\textit{choline acetyl-}} \text{Acetylcholine}$$

Once the acetylcholine has been secreted by the cholinergic nerve ending, it persists in the tissue for a few seconds; then most of it is split into an acetate ion and choline by the enzyme *acetylcholinesterase* bound with collagen and glycosaminoglycans in the local connective tissue. Thus, this is the same mechanism of acetylcholine destruction that occurs at the neuromuscular junctions of skeletal nerve fibers. The choline that is formed is in turn transported back into the terminal nerve ending, where it is used again for synthesis of new acetylcholine.

Synthesis of Norepinephrine, Its Removal, and Duration of Action. Synthesis of norepinephrine begins in the axoplasm of the terminal nerve endings of adrenergic nerve fibers but is completed inside the vesicles. The basic steps are the following:

1. Tyrosine $\xrightarrow{\textit{hydroxylation}}$ DOPA
2. DOPA $\xrightarrow{\textit{decarboxylation}}$ Dopamine
3. Transport of dopamine into the vesicles
4. Dopamine $\xrightarrow{\textit{hydroxylation}}$ Norepinephrine

In the adrenal medulla this reaction goes still one step further to transform about 80 per cent of the norepinephrine into epinephrine, as follows:

5. Norepinephrine $\xrightarrow{methylation}$ Epinephrine

After secretion of norepinephrine by the terminal nerve endings, it is removed from the secretory site in three different ways: (1) reuptake into the adrenergic nerve endings themselves by an active transport process—accounting for removal of 50 to 80 per cent of the secreted norepinephrine; (2) diffusion away from the nerve endings into the surrounding body fluids and thence into the blood—accounting for removal of most of the remainder of the norepinephrine; and (3) destruction by enzymes to a slight extent (one of these enzymes is *monoamine oxidase,* which is found in the nerve endings themselves, and another is *catechol-O-methyl transferase,* which is present diffusely in all tissues).

Ordinarily, the norepinephrine secreted directly into a tissue remains active for only a few seconds, illustrating that its reuptake and diffusion away from the tissue are rapid. However, the norepinephrine and epinephrine secreted into the blood by the adrenal medullae remain active until they diffuse into some tissue where they are destroyed by catechol-O-methyl transferase; this occurs mainly in the liver. Therefore, when secreted into the blood, both norepinephrine and epinephrine remain very active for 10 to 30 seconds and then have additional decreasing activity for 1 to several minutes.

Receptors of the Effector Organs

Before the acetylcholine, norepinephrine, or epinephrine transmitter secreted at the autonomic nerve endings can stimulate the effector organ, it must first bind with highly specific *receptors* of the effector cells. The receptor is usually on the outside of the cell membrane, bound as a prosthetic group to a protein molecule that penetrates all the way through the cell membrane. When the transmitter binds with the receptor, this generally causes a conformational change in the structure of the protein molecule. In turn, the altered protein molecule excites or inhibits the cell, most often by (1) causing a change in the cell membrane permeability to one or more ions or (2) activating or inactivating an enzyme attached to the other end of the receptor protein where it protrudes into the interior of the cell.

Excitation or Inhibition of the Effector Cell by Changing Its Membrane Permeability. Because the receptor protein is an integral part of the cell membrane, a conformational change in the structures of many of these proteins opens or closes *ion channels,* thus altering the permeability of the cell membrane to various ions. For instance, sodium and/or calcium ion channels frequently become opened and allow rapid influx of the respective ions into the cell, usually depolarizing the cell membrane and exciting the cell. At other times, potassium channels are opened, allowing potassium ions to diffuse out of the cell, and this usually inhibits it. Also, in some cells, the ions will cause an internal cell action, such as the direct effect of calcium ions in promoting smooth muscle contraction.

Receptor Action by Altering Intracellular Enzymes. Another way the receptor functions is in activating or inactivating an enzyme (or other intracellular chemical) inside the cell. The enzyme usually is attached to the receptor protein where it protrudes into the interior of the cell. For instance, binding of epinephrine with its receptor on the outside of many cells increases the activity of the enzyme *adenylcyclase* on the inside of the cell, and this then causes the formation of *cyclic adenosine monophosphate (cAMP).* The cAMP in turn can initiate any one of many different intracellular actions, the exact effect depending on the chemical machinery of the effector cell.

The Acetylcholine Receptors—Muscarinic and Nicotinic Receptors

Acetylcholine activates two different types of receptors. These are called *muscarinic* and *nicotinic* receptors. The reason for these names is that muscarine, a poison from toadstools, activates only the muscarinic receptors but will not activate the nicotinic receptors, whereas nicotine will activate only nicotinic receptors; acetylcholine activates both of them.

The muscarinic receptors are found in all effector cells stimulated by the *postganglionic* neurons of the parasympathetic nervous system, as well as those stimulated by the *postganglionic* cholinergic neurons of the sympathetic system.

The nicotinic receptors are found in the synapses between the pre- and postganglionic neurons of both the sympathetic and parasympathetic systems and also in the membranes of skeletal muscle fibers at the neuromuscular junction (discussed in Chapter 7).

An understanding of the two different types of receptors is especially important because specific drugs are frequently used in the practice of medicine to stimulate or to block one or the other of the two types of receptors.

The Adrenergic Receptors—Alpha and Beta Receptors

Research experiments using different drugs that mimic the action of norepinephrine on sympathetic effector organs (called *sympathomimetic drugs*) have shown that there are two major types of adrenergic receptors, *alpha receptors* and *beta receptors.* (The beta receptors in turn are divided into $beta_1$ and $beta_2$ receptors because certain drugs affect some beta receptors but not all. Also, there is a less distinct division of alpha receptors into $alpha_1$ and $alpha_2$ receptors.)

Norepinephrine and epinephrine, both of which are secreted by the adrenal medulla, have somewhat different effects in exciting the alpha and beta receptors.

Norepinephrine excites mainly alpha receptors but excites the beta receptors to a slight extent as well. On the other hand, epinephrine excites both types of receptors approximately equally. Therefore, the relative effects of norepinephrine and epinephrine on different effector organs is determined by the types of receptors in the organs. Obviously, if they are all beta receptors, epinephrine will be the more effective excitant.

Excitatory and Inhibitory Actions of Sympathetic and Parasympathetic Stimulation

Table 41–1 lists the effects on different visceral functions of the body caused by stimulating the parasympathetic and sympathetic nerves. From this table it can be seen again that *sympathetic stimulation causes excitatory effects in some organs but inhibitory effects in others. Likewise, parasympathetic stimulation causes excitation in some but inhibition in others.* Also, when sympathetic stimulation excites a particular organ, parasympathetic stimulation sometimes inhibits it, illustrating that the two systems occasionally act reciprocally. However, most organs are dominantly controlled by one or the other of the two systems.

There is no generalization one can use to explain whether sympathetic or parasympathetic stimulation will cause excitation or inhibition of a particular organ. Therefore, to understand sympathetic and parasympathetic function, one must learn the functions of these two nervous systems as listed in Table 41–1. Some of these functions need to be clarified in still greater detail as follows:

Effects of Sympathetic and Parasympathetic Stimulation on Specific Organs

The Eye. Two functions of the eye are controlled by the autonomic nervous system. These are the pupillary opening and the focus of the lens. Sympathetic stimulation contracts the meridional *fibers of the iris*

Table 41–1 AUTONOMIC EFFECTS ON VARIOUS ORGANS OF THE BODY

Organ	Effect of Sympathetic Stimulation	Effect of Parasympathetic Stimulation
Eye		
Pupil	Dilated	Constricted
Ciliary muscle	Slight relaxation (far vision)	Constricted (near vision)
Glands	Vasoconstriction and slight secretion	Copious secretion (containing many enzymes for enzyme-secreting glands)
Sweat glands	Copious sweating (cholinergic)	Sweating on palms of hands
Heart		
Muscle	Increased rate Increased force of contraction	Slowed rate Decreased force of contraction (especially of atria)
Coronary arteries	Dilated (β_2); constricted (α)	Dilated
Lungs		
Bronchi	Dilated	Constricted
Gut		
Lumen	Decreased peristalsis and tone	Increased peristalsis and tone
Sphincter	Increased tone (most times)	Relaxed (most times)
Liver	Glucose released	Slight glycogen synthesis
Kidney	Decreased output and renin secretion	None
Bladder		
Detrusor	Relaxed (slight)	Contracted
Trigone	Contracted	Relaxed
Penis	Ejaculation	Erection
Systemic arterioles		
Abdominal viscera	Constricted	None
Muscle	Constricted (adrenergic α) Dilated (adrenergic β_2) Dilated (cholinergic)	None
Skin	Constricted	None
Blood		
Coagulation	Increased	None
Glucose	Increased	None
Lipids	Increased	None
Basal metabolism	Increased up to 100%	None
Adrenal medullary secretion	Increased	None
Mental activity	Increased	None

that dilate the pupil, whereas parasympathetic stimulation contracts the *circular muscle of the iris* to constrict the pupil. The parasympathetics that control the pupil are reflexly stimulated when excess light enters the eyes, which is explained in Chapter 35; this reflex reduces the pupillary opening and decreases the amount of light that strikes the retina. On the other hand, the sympathetics become stimulated during periods of excitement and, therefore, increase the pupillary opening at these times.

Focusing of the lens is controlled almost entirely by the parasympathetic nervous system, also discussed in Chapters 34 and 35.

The Glands of the Body. The *nasal, lacrimal, salivary,* and many *gastrointestinal glands* are all strongly stimulated by the parasympathetic nervous system, usually resulting in copious quantities of secretion.

Sympathetic stimulation has a slight direct effect on glandular cells in causing formation of a concentrated secretion. However, it also causes vasoconstriction of the blood vessels supplying the glands and in this way often reduces their rates of secretion.

The *sweat glands* secrete large quantities of sweat when the sympathetic nerves are stimulated, but no effect is caused by stimulating the parasympathetic nerves.

The Gastrointestinal System. The gastrointestinal system has its own intrinsic set of nerves known as the *intramural plexus.* However, both parasympathetic and sympathetic stimulation can affect gastrointestinal activity. Parasympathetic stimulation, in general, increases the overall degree of activity of the gastrointestinal tract by promoting peristalsis and relaxing the sphincters, thus allowing rapid propulsion of contents along the tract. This propulsive effect is associated with simultaneous increases in rates of secretion by many of the gastrointestinal glands, which was described earlier.

Normal function of the gastrointestinal tract is not very dependent on sympathetic stimulation. However, strong sympathetic stimulation inhibits peristalsis and increases the tone of the sphincters. The net result is greatly slowed propulsion of food through the tract and sometimes decreased secretion as well.

The Heart. In general, sympathetic stimulation increases the overall activity of the heart. This is accomplished by increasing both the rate and force of heart contraction. Parasympathetic stimulation causes mainly the opposite effects. To express these effects in another way, sympathetic stimulation increases the effectiveness of the heart as a pump, whereas parasympathetic stimulation decreases its pumping capability.

Systemic Blood Vessels. Most systemic blood vessels, especially those of the abdominal viscera and the skin of the limbs, are constricted by sympathetic stimulation. Parasympathetic stimulation generally has almost no effects on blood vessels but does dilate vessels in certain restricted areas such as in the blush area of the face.

Effect of Sympathetic and Parasympathetic Stimulation on Arterial Pressure. The arterial pressure is determined by two factors, the propulsion of blood by the heart and the resistance to flow of this blood through the blood vessels. Sympathetic stimulation increases both propulsion by the heart and resistance to flow, which usually causes the pressure to increase greatly.

On the other hand, parasympathetic stimulation decreases the pumping by the heart but has virtually no effect on total peripheral resistance. The usual effect is a slight fall in pressure. Yet very strong vagal parasympathetic stimulation can occasionally stop the heart entirely and cause loss of all arterial pressure.

Function of the Adrenal Medullae

Stimulation of the sympathetic nerves to the adrenal medullae causes large quantities of epinephrine and norepinephrine to be released into the circulating blood, and these two hormones in turn are carried in the blood to all tissues of the body. On the average, approximately 80 per cent of the secretion is epinephrine and 20 per cent is norepinephrine.

The circulating epinephrine and norepinephrine have almost the same effects on the different organs as those caused by direct sympathetic stimulation, except that *the effects last five to ten times as long* because these hormones are removed from the blood slowly.

The circulating norepinephrine causes constriction of essentially all the blood vessels of the body; it causes increased activity of the heart, inhibition of the gastrointestinal tract, dilation of the pupils of the eyes, and so forth.

Epinephrine causes almost the same effects as those caused by norepinephrine, but the effects differ in the following respects: First, epinephrine, because of its greater effect in stimulating the beta receptors, has a greater effect on cardiac stimulation than norepinephrine. Second, epinephrine causes only weak constriction of the blood vessels of the muscles, in comparison with the much stronger constriction caused by norepinephrine. Because the muscle vessels represent a major segment of the vessels of the body, this difference is of special importance because norepinephrine greatly increases the total peripheral resistance and thereby greatly elevates arterial pressure, whereas epinephrine raises the arterial pressure to a lesser extent but increases the cardiac output considerably more because of its excitatory effect on the heart.

A third difference between the actions of epinephrine and norepinephrine relates to their effects on tissue metabolism. Epinephrine has up to five to ten times as great a metabolic effect as norepinephrine. Indeed, the epinephrine secreted by the adrenal medullae can increase the metabolic rate of the body often to as much as 100 per cent above normal, in this way increasing the activity and excitability of the whole body. It also increases the rate of other metabolic activities, such as glycogenolysis in the liver and muscle and glucose release into the blood.

Sympathetic and Parasympathetic "Tone"

The sympathetic and parasympathetic systems are continually active, and the basal rates of activity are known, respectively, as *sympathetic tone* and *parasympathetic tone.*

The value of tone is that *it allows a single nervous system to increase or to decrease the activity of a stimulated organ.* For instance, sympathetic tone normally keeps almost all of the systemic arterioles constricted to approximately half their maximum diameter. By increasing the degree of sympathetic stimulation, these vessels can be constricted even more; on the other hand, by inhibiting the normal tone, they can be dilated. If it were not for the continual sympathetic tone, the sympathetic system could cause only vasoconstriction, never vasodilatation.

Another interesting example of tone is that of the parasympathetics in the gastrointestinal tract. Surgical removal of the parasympathetic supply to most of the gut by cutting the vagus nerves can cause serious and prolonged gastric and intestinal "atony" with resulting blockage of gastrointestinal propulsion and consequent serious constipation, thus illustrating that parasympathetic tone to the gut is normally very strong. This tone can be decreased by the brain, thereby inhibiting gastrointestinal motility, or it can be increased, thereby promoting increased gastrointestinal activity.

The Autonomic Reflexes

Many of the visceral functions of the body are regulated by *autonomic reflexes.* Throughout this text the functions of these reflexes are discussed in relation to individual organ systems; but to illustrate their importance, a few are presented here briefly.

Cardiovascular Autonomic Reflexes. Several reflexes in the cardiovascular system help control especially the arterial blood pressure and the heart rate. One of these is the *baroreceptor reflex,* which is described in Chapter 15 along with other cardiovascular reflexes. Briefly, stretch receptors called *baroreceptors* are located in the walls of the major arteries, including the carotid arteries and the aorta. When these become stretched by high pressure, signals are transmitted to the brain stem, where they inhibit the sympathetic impulses to the heart and blood vessels, which allows the arterial pressure to fall back toward normal.

Gastrointestinal Autonomic Reflexes. The uppermost part of the gastrointestinal tract and also the rectum are controlled principally by autonomic reflexes. For instance, the smell of appetizing food or the presence of food in the mouth initiates signals from the nose and mouth to the vagal, glossopharyngeal, and salivary nuclei of the brain stem. These in turn transmit signals through the parasympathetic nerves to the secretory glands of the mouth and stomach, causing secretion of digestive juices even before food enters the mouth. And when fecal matter fills the rectum at the other end of the alimentary canal, sensory impulses initiated by stretching the rectum are sent to the sacral portion of the spinal cord, and a reflex signal is retransmitted through the parasympathetics to the distal parts of the colon; these result in strong peristaltic contractions that empty the bowel.

Other Autonomic Reflexes. Emptying of the bladder is controlled in the same way as emptying the rectum; stretching of the bladder sends impulses to the sacral cord, and this in turn causes contraction of the bladder as well as relaxation of the urinary sphincters, thereby promoting micturition.

Also important are the sexual reflexes, which are initiated both by psychic stimuli from the brain and stimuli from the sexual organs. Impulses from these sources converge on the sacral cord and, in the male, result, first, in erection, mainly a parasympathetic function, and then in ejaculation, a sympathetic function.

Other autonomic reflexes include reflex contributions to the regulation of pancreatic secretion, gallbladder emptying, kidney excretion of urine, sweating, blood glucose concentration, and many other visceral functions, all of which are discussed in detail at other points in this text.

"Stress" Response of the Sympathetic Nervous System

When large portions of the sympathetic nervous system discharge at the same time—that is, a *mass discharge*—this increases in many different ways the ability of the body to perform vigorous muscle activity. Let us quickly summarize these ways:

1. Increased arterial pressure.
2. Increased blood flow to active muscles concurrent with decreased blood flow to organs such as the gastrointestinal tract and the kidneys that are not needed for rapid motor activity.
3. Increased rates of cellular metabolism throughout the body.
4. Increased blood glucose concentration.
5. Increased glycolysis in the liver and in muscle.
6. Increased muscle strength.
7. Increased mental activity.
8. Increased rate of blood coagulation.

The sum of these effects permits the person to perform far more strenuous physical activity than would otherwise be possible. Because it is mental or physical *stress* that usually excites the sympathetic system, it is frequently said that the purpose of the sympathetic system is to provide extra activation of the body in states of stress: this is often called the sympathetic *stress response.*

The sympathetic system is especially strongly activated in many emotional states. For instance, in the state of *rage,* which is elicited mainly by stimulating the hypothalamus, signals are transmitted downward through the reticular formation and spinal cord to cause massive sympathetic discharge, and all of the sympathetic events listed above ensue immediately. This is called the sympathetic *alarm reaction*. It is also frequently called the *fight or flight reaction* because an animal in this state decides almost instantly whether to stand and fight or to run. In either event, the sympathetic alarm reaction makes the animal's subsequent activities vigorous.

Medullary, Pontine, and Mesencephalic Control of the Autonomic Nervous System

Many areas in the reticular substance of the medulla, pons, and mesencephalon, as well as many special nuclei (Fig. 41–3), control different autonomic functions such as arterial pressure, heart rate, glandular secretion in the upper part of the gastrointestinal tract, gastrointestinal peristalsis, the degree of contraction of the urinary bladder, and many others. The control of each of these is discussed at appropriate points in this text. Suffice it to point out here that the most important factors controlled in the lower brain stem are arterial pressure, heart rate, and respiration. Indeed, transection of the brain stem at the midpontine level allows normal basal control of arterial pressure and respiration to continue as before but prevents its modulation by higher nervous centers, particularly the hypothalamus.

Signals from the hypothalamus and even from the cerebrum can affect the activities of almost all the lower brain stem autonomic control centers. For instance, stimulation in appropriate areas of the hypothalamus can activate the medullary cardiovascular control centers strongly enough to increase the arterial pressure to more than double normal. Likewise, other hypothalamic centers can control body temperature, increase or decrease salivation and gastrointestinal activity, or cause bladder emptying. To some extent, therefore, the autonomic centers in the lower brain stem act as relay stations for control activities initiated at higher levels of the brain.

In the previous chapter it is pointed out also that many of our behavioral responses are mediated through the hypothalamus, the reticular areas of the brain stem, and the autonomic nervous system. Indeed, the higher areas of the brain can alter the function of the whole autonomic nervous system or of portions of it strongly enough to cause severe autonomic-induced disease, such as peptic ulcer, constipation, heart palpitation, and even heart attacks.

CEREBRAL BLOOD FLOW

Thus far, we have discussed the function of the brain as if it were independent of its blood flow and its fluids. However, this is far from the truth, for abnormalities of either of these can profoundly affect brain function. For instance, total cessation of blood flow to the brain causes unconsciousness within 5 to 10 seconds. This is true because lack of oxygen delivery to the brain cells shuts down most of their metabolism.

Normal Rate of Cerebral Blood Flow

The normal blood flow through the brain tissue of the adult averages 50 to 55 milliliters per 100 grams of brain per minute. For the entire brain, this is approximately 750 ml/min, or 15 per cent of the total resting cardiac output.

Regulation of Cerebral Blood Flow

Metabolic Control of Flow

As in most other vascular areas of the body, cerebral blood flow is highly related to the metabolism of the cerebral tissue. At least three different metabolic factors have potent effects in controlling cerebral blood flow. These are carbon dioxide concentration, hydrogen ion concentration, and oxygen concentration. An *increase* in either the carbon dioxide or the hydrogen ion concentration increases cerebral blood flow, whereas a *decrease* in oxygen concentration increases the flow.

Regulation of Cerebral Blood Flow in Response to Excess Carbon Dioxide or Hydrogen Ion Concentration. An increase in carbon dioxide concentration in the arterial blood perfusing the brain greatly increases cerebral blood flow. This is illustrated in Figure 41–4, which shows that a 70 per cent increase in arterial P_{CO_2} approximately doubles the blood flow.

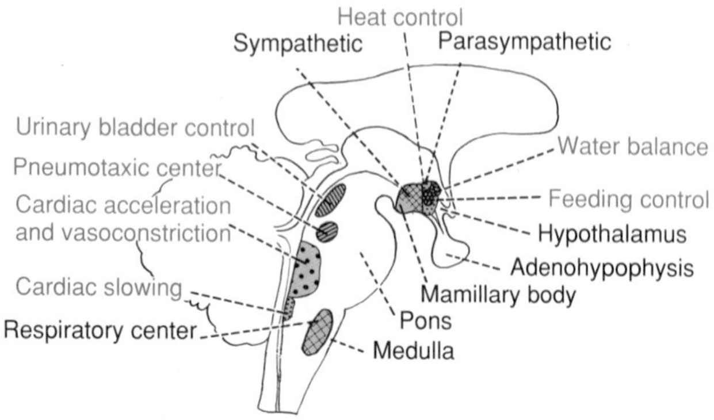

Figure 41–3. Autonomic control areas of the brain stem and hypothalamus.

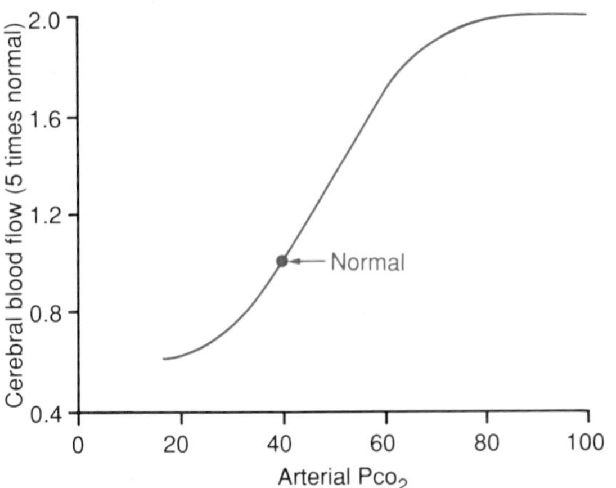

Figure 41-4. Relationship between arterial PCO_2 and cerebral blood flow.

Carbon dioxide is believed to increase cerebral blood flow almost entirely by combining first with water in the body fluids to form carbonic acid, with subsequent dissociation to form hydrogen ions. The hydrogen ions then cause vasodilatation of the cerebral vessels—the dilatation being almost directly proportional to the increase in hydrogen ion concentration.

Importance of the Carbon Dioxide and Hydrogen Control of Cerebral Blood Flow. Increased hydrogen ion concentration greatly depresses neuronal activity. Therefore, it is fortunate that an increase in hydrogen ion concentration causes an increase in blood flow, which in turn carries both carbon dioxide and other acidic substances away from the brain tissues. Thus, this mechanism helps maintain a constant hydrogen ion concentration in the cerebral fluids and thereby helps maintain the normal level of neuronal activity.

Oxygen Deficiency as a Regulator of Cerebral Blood Flow. Except during periods of intense brain activity, the utilization of oxygen by the brain tissue remains within very narrow limits—within a few percentage points of 3.5 milliliters of oxygen per 100 grams of brain tissue per minute. If the blood flow to the brain ever becomes insufficient and cannot supply this needed amount of oxygen, the oxygen deficiency mechanism for causing vasodilatation, discussed in Chapter 14, which functions in essentially all tissues of the body, immediately causes vasodilatation, returning the blood flow and transport of oxygen to the cerebral tissues to near normal. Thus, this local blood flow regulatory mechanism is much the same in the brain as in the coronary and skeletal muscle circulation and in many other circulatory areas of the body.

Experiments have shown that a decrease in cerebral *tissue* Po_2 below approximately 30 mm Hg (normal value is 35 to 40 mm Hg) will begin to increase cerebral blood flow. This is very fortunate, because brain function becomes deranged at not much lower values of Po_2, especially so at Po_2 levels below 20 mm Hg. Even coma can result at these low levels. Thus, the oxygen mechanism for local regulation of cerebral blood flow is also a very important protective response against diminished cerebral neuronal activity and, therefore, against derangement of mental capability.

Role of the Sympathetic Nervous System in Regulating Cerebral Blood Flow

The cerebral circulatory system has a strong sympathetic innervation that passes upward from the superior cervical sympathetic ganglia along with the cerebral arteries. However, neither transection of these sympathetic nerves nor mild to moderate stimulation of them normally causes significant change in the cerebral blood flow. Even so, under rare conditions, cerebral sympathetic stimulation can become activated strongly enough to markedly constrict the cerebral arteries. The reason this usually does not occur is that the local blood flow regulatory mechanisms are so powerful that they normally compensate almost entirely for the effects of the sympathetic stimulation. Yet in those conditions in which the autoregulatory mechanism fails to compensate enough, sympathetic control of cerebral blood flow becomes quite important. For instance, when the arterial pressure rises to a very high level during strenuous exercise and during other states of excessive circulatory activity, the sympathetic nervous system constricts the large and intermediate-sized arteries and prevents the very high pressures from ever reaching the smaller blood vessels. This is important in preventing the occurrence of a vascular hemorrhage into the brain—that is, for preventing the occurrence of cerebral stroke.

The Cerebral Microcirculation

As in almost all other tissues of the body, the density of the blood capillaries in the brain is greatest where the metabolic needs are greatest. The overall metabolic rate of the brain gray matter, where the neuronal cell bodies lie, is about four times as great as that of white matter; correspondingly, the number of capillaries and rate of blood flow are also about four times as great in the gray matter.

Another important structural characteristic of the brain capillaries is that they are much less "leaky" than the capillaries in almost any other tissue of the body. Most importantly, the capillaries are supported on all sides by "glial feet," which are small projections from the surrounding glia that abut against all surfaces of the capillaries and provide physical support to prevent overstretching of the capillaries in case of high pressure. In addition, the walls of the small arterioles leading to the brain capillaries become greatly thickened in persons who develop high blood pressure, and these arterioles remain significantly constricted all of the time to prevent transmission of the high pressure to the capillaries. We shall see later in the chapter that whenever these systems for protecting against transudation of fluid into the brain break down, serious brain edema ensues, which can lead rapidly to coma and death.

THE CEREBROSPINAL FLUID SYSTEM

The entire cavity enclosing the brain and spinal cord has a volume of approximately 1600 milliliters, and about 150 milliliters of this volume is occupied by cerebrospinal fluid. This fluid, as shown in Figure 41–5, is found in the *ventricles of the brain,* in the *cisterns around the brain,* and in the *subarachnoid space around both the brain and the spinal cord.* All these chambers are connected with each other, and the pressure of the fluid is regulated at a constant level.

Cushioning Function of the Cerebrospinal Fluid

A major function of the cerebrospinal fluid is to cushion the brain within its solid vault. Fortunately, the brain and the cerebrospinal fluid have approximately the same specific gravity (only about 4 per cent difference), so that the brain simply floats in the fluid. Therefore, a blow to the head moves the entire brain simultaneously, causing no one portion of the brain to be momentarily contorted by the blow.

Formation, Flow, and Absorption of Cerebrospinal Fluid

Cerebrospinal fluid is formed at a rate of approximately 500 milliliters each day, which is about three times as much as the total volume of fluid in the entire cerebrospinal fluid system. Probably two thirds or more of this fluid originates as a secretion from the choroid plexuses in the four ventricles, mainly in the two lateral ventricles. Additional amounts of fluid are secreted by all the ependymal surfaces of the ventricles and from the arachnoidal membranes, and a small amount comes from the brain itself through the perivascular spaces that surround the blood vessels entering the brain.

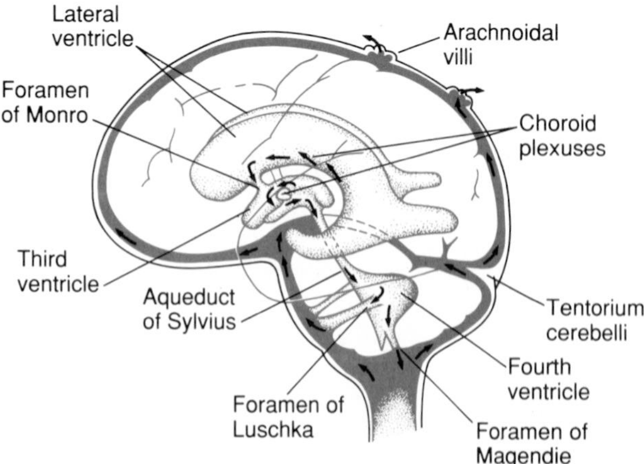

Figure 41–5. Pathway of cerebrospinal fluid flow from the choroid plexuses in the lateral ventricles to the arachnoidal villi protruding into the dural sinuses.

The arrows in Figure 41–5 show the main channel of fluid flow from the choroid plexuses and then through the cerebrospinal fluid system. The fluid secreted in the lateral ventricles and the third ventricle passes along the *aqueduct of Sylvius* into the fourth ventricle, where a small amount of additional fluid is added. It then passes out of the fourth ventricle through three small openings into the *cisterna magna,* a large fluid space that lies behind the medulla and beneath the cerebellum. The cisterna magna is continuous with the *subarachnoid space* that surrounds the entire brain and spinal cord. Almost all the cerebrospinal fluid then flows upward through this space toward the cerebrum. From the cerebral subarachnoid spaces, the fluid flows into multiple *arachnoidal villi* that project into the large sagittal venous sinus and other venous sinuses. Finally, the fluid empties into the venous blood through the surfaces of these villi.

Secretion by the Choroid Plexus. The choroid plexus is a cauliflower-like growth of blood vessels covered by a thin layer of epithelial cells. This plexus projects into (1) the temporal horn of each lateral ventricle, (2) the posterior portion of the third ventricle, and (3) the roof of the fourth ventricle.

The secretion of fluid by the choroid plexus depends mainly on active transport of sodium ions through the epithelial cells that line the outside of the plexus. The sodium ions in turn pull along large amounts of chloride ions as well because the positive charge of the sodium ion attracts the chloride ion's negative charge. The two of these together increase the quantity of osmotically active substances in the cerebrospinal fluid, which then causes almost immediate osmosis of water through the membrane, thus providing the fluid of the secretion.

Absorption of Cerebrospinal Fluid Through the Arachnoidal Villi. The *arachnoidal villi* are microscopic finger-like projections of the arachnoidal membrane through the walls of the venous sinuses. The endothelial cells covering these villi have been shown by electron microscopy to have large vesicular holes directly through the bodies of the cells, and these appear to be large enough to allow relatively free flow of cerebrospinal fluid, protein molecules, and even particles as large as red blood cells into the venous blood.

The Perivascular Spaces and Cerebrospinal Fluid. The blood vessels entering the substance of the brain pass first along the surface of the brain and then penetrate inward, carrying a layer of *pia mater,* the membrane that covers the brain, with them, as shown in Figure 41–6. The pia is only loosely adherent to the vessels, so that a space, the *perivascular space,* exists between it and each vessel. Perivascular spaces follow both the arteries and the veins into the brain as far as the arterioles and venules but not to the capillaries.

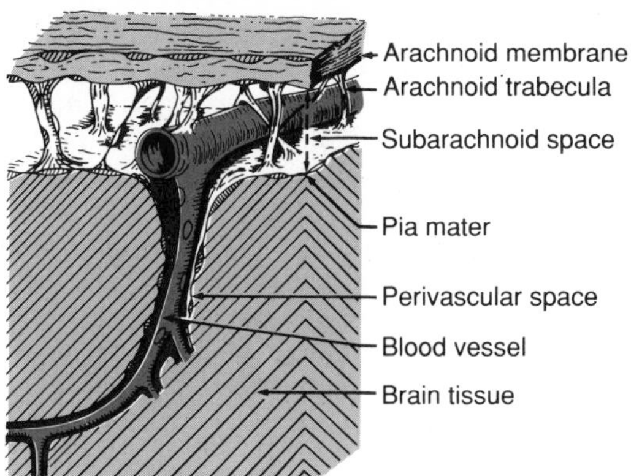

Figure 41-6. Drainage of the perivascular spaces into the subarachnoid space. (From Ranson and Clark: Anatomy of the Nervous System. Philadelphia, W. B. Saunders Company, 1959.)

The Lymphatic Function of the Perivascular Spaces. As is true elsewhere in the body, a small amount of protein leaks out of the parenchymal capillaries into the interstitial spaces of the brain; and because no true lymphatics are present in brain tissue, this protein leaves the tissue mainly through the perivascular spaces but partly also by direct diffusion through the pia mater into the subarachnoid spaces. On reaching the subarachnoid spaces, the protein flows along with the cerebrospinal fluid to be absorbed through the *arachnoidal villi* into the cerebral veins. Therefore, the perivascular spaces, in effect, are a modified lymphatic system for the brain.

Cerebrospinal Fluid Pressure

The normal pressure in the cerebrospinal fluid system when one is lying in a horizontal position averages 130 millimeters of water (10 mm Hg), though this may be as low as 70 millimeters of water or as high as 180 millimeters of water even in the normal person. These values are considerably more positive than the −3 to −5 mm Hg pressure in the interstitial spaces of the subcutaneous tissue.

Regulation of Cerebrospinal Fluid Pressure by the Arachnoidal Villi. The cerebrospinal fluid pressure is regulated almost entirely by absorption of the fluid through the arachnoidal villi. The reason for this is that the rate of cerebrospinal fluid formation is very constant, so that this is rarely a factor in pressure control. On the other hand, the villi function like "valves" that allow the fluid and its contents to flow readily into the venous blood of the sinuses while not allowing the blood to flow backward in the opposite direction. Normally, this valve action of the villi allows cerebrospinal fluid to begin to flow into the blood when its pressure is about 1.5 mm Hg greater than the pressure of the blood in the sinuses. Then, as the cerebrospinal fluid pressure rises still higher, the valves open very widely so that, under normal conditions, the pressure almost never rises more than a few millimeters of mercury over the pressure in the venous sinuses.

On the other hand, in disease states the villi sometimes become blocked by large particulate matter, by fibrosis, or even by excesses of plasma protein molecules that have leaked into the cerebrospinal fluid in brain diseases. Such blockage can cause very high cerebrospinal fluid pressure.

Cerebrospinal Fluid Pressure in Pathological Conditions of the Brain. Often a large *brain tumor* elevates the cerebrospinal fluid pressure by decreasing the rate of absorption of fluid. For instance, if the tumor is above the tentorium and becomes so large that it compresses the brain downward, the upward flow of fluid through the subarachnoid space around the brain stem where it passes through the tentorial opening may become blocked and the absorption of fluid by the cerebral arachnoidal villi greatly curtailed. As a result, the cerebrospinal fluid pressure can rise to as high as 500 millimeters of water (37 mm Hg) or more.

Effect of High Cerebrospinal Fluid Pressure on the Optic Disc—Papilledema. Anatomically, the dura of the brain extends as a sheath around the optic nerve and then connects with the sclera of the eye. When the pressure rises in the cerebrospinal fluid system, it also rises in the optic nerve sheath. The retinal artery and vein pierce this sheath a few millimeters behind the eye and then pass with the optic nerve into the eye itself. The high pressure in the optic sheath pushes fluid along the optic nerve fibers to the interior of the eyeball. Also, the pressure in the sheath impedes the flow of blood in the retinal vein, thereby also increasing the retinal capillary pressure throughout the eye, which results in additional retinal edema. The tissues of the optic disc are much more distensible than those of the remainder of the retina, so that the disc becomes far more edematous than the remainder of the retina and swells into the cavity of the eye. The swelling of the disc, which can be observed with an ophthalmoscope, is called *papilledema,* and neurologists can estimate the cerebrospinal fluid pressure level by assessing the extent to which the optic disc protrudes into the eyeball.

Obstruction to the Flow of Cerebrospinal Fluid

Hydrocephalus. "Hydrocephalus" means excess water in the cranial vault. A common cause of hydrocephalus is blockage of the aqueduct of Sylvius, resulting from *atresia* (closure) before birth in many babies or from a brain tumor at any age. As fluid is formed by the choroid plexuses in the two lateral and the third ventricles, the volumes of these three ventricles increase greatly. This flattens the brain into a thin shell against the skull. In newborn babies the increased pressure also causes the whole head to swell because the skull bones have not yet fused.

The most effective therapy for hydrocephalus is surgical institution of a silicone rubber tube shunt all the way from one of the ventricles to the peritoneal cavity, where the fluid can then be absorbed through the peritoneum.

The Blood-Cerebrospinal Fluid and Blood-Brain Barriers

It has already been pointed out that many large molecular substances hardly pass at all from the blood into the cerebrospinal fluid or into the interstitial fluids of the brain even though these same substances pass readily into the usual interstitial fluids of the body. Therefore, it is said that barriers, called the *blood-cerebrospinal fluid barrier* and the *blood-brain barrier,* exist between the blood and the cerebrospinal fluid and brain fluid, respectively. These barriers exist in essentially all areas of the brain parenchyma *except in some areas of the hypothalamus,* the *pineal gland,* and the *area postrema,* where substances diffuse with ease into the tissue spaces. This ease of diffusion is very important because these areas of the brain have sensory organs that respond to different changes in the body fluids, such as changes in osmolality, glucose concentration, and so forth; these responses provide the signals for feedback regulation of each of the factors.

In general, the blood-cerebrospinal fluid and blood-brain barriers are highly permeable to water, carbon dioxide, oxygen, and most lipid-soluble substances, such as alcohol and most anesthetics; slightly permeable to the electrolytes, such as sodium, chloride, and potassium; and almost totally impermeable to plasma proteins and many large organic molecules. Therefore, the blood-cerebrospinal fluid and blood-brain barriers often make it impossible to achieve effective concentrations of either protein antibodies or some nonlipid-soluble drugs in the cerebrospinal fluid or parenchyma of the brain.

The cause of the low permeability of the blood-cerebrospinal fluid and blood-brain barriers is the manner in which the endothelial cells of the capillaries are joined to each other. They are joined by so-called *tight junctions.* That is, the membranes of the adjacent endothelial cells are almost fused with each other, rather than having slit-pores between them, as is the case in most other capillaries of the body.

Brain Edema

One of the most serious complications of abnormal cerebral hemodynamics and fluid dynamics is the development of brain edema. Because the brain is encased in a solid vault, the accumulation of edema fluid compresses the blood vessels, with rapid depression of blood flow and destruction of brain tissue.

The usual cause of brain edema is either greatly increased capillary pressure or damage to the capillary wall. One cause of excessively high capillary pressure is a sudden increase in the cerebral blood pressure to levels too high for the cerebral blood flow autoregulatory mechanism to cope with. However, the most common cause is brain concussion, in which the brain tissues and capillaries are traumatized and capillary fluid leaks into the traumatized tissues.

Once brain edema has begun, heroic measures must be used to prevent total destruction of the brain. One such measure is to infuse intravenously a concentrated osmotic substance, such as a very concentrated mannitol solution. This pulls fluid by osmosis from the brain tissue and breaks up the vicious circle. Another procedure is to remove fluid quickly from the lateral ventricles of the brain via ventricular puncture, thereby relieving the intracerebral pressure.

REFERENCES

Angerson, W. J., et al. (eds.): Blood Flow in the Brain. New York, Oxford University Press, 1989.

Bannister, R. (ed.): Autonomic Failure. New York, Oxford University Press, 1988.

Bevan, J. A., et al.: Sympathetic control of cerebral arteries: Specialization in receptor type, reserve, affinity, and distribution. FASEB J., 1:193, 1987.

Buckley, J. P., et al. (eds.): Brain Peptides and Catecholamines in Cardiovascular Regulation. New York, Raven Press, 1987.

Burchfield, S. R. (ed.): Stress: Physiological and Psychological Interactions. Washington, D.C., Hemisphere Publishing Corp., 1985.

Finger, S., et al. (eds.): Brain Injury and Recovery. New York, Plenum Publishing Corp., 1988.

Givens, J. R.: The Hypothalamus in Health and Disease. Chicago, Year Book Medical Publishers, 1984.

Goldstein, D. S., and Eisenhofer, G.: Plasma catechols—What do they mean? News Physiol. Sci., 3:138, 1988.

Hirst, G. D. S., and Edwards, F. R.: Sympathetic neuroeffector transmission in arteries and arterioles. Physiol. Rev., 69:546, 1989.

Janig, W.: Pre- and postganglionic vasoconstrictor neurons: Differentiation, types, and discharge properties. Annu. Rev. Physiol., 50:525, 1988.

Mayhan, W. G., et al.: Cerebral microcirculation. News Physiol. Sci., 3:164, 1988.

Rescigno, A., and Boicelli, A.: Cerebral Blood Flow. New York, Plenum Publishing Corp., 1988.

Vanhoutte, P. M.: Vasodilatation: Vascular Smooth Muscle, Peptides, Autonomic Nerves, and Endothelium. New York, Raven Press, 1988.

Wood, J. H. (ed.): Cerebral Blood Flow: Physiologic and Clinical Aspects. New York, McGraw-Hill Book Co., 1987.

QUESTIONS

1. Describe the anatomy of the *sympathetic nervous system,* including the pathways of the *preganglionic* neurons into the sympathetic chain and of the *postganglionic neurons* to the organs that are to be controlled.
2. Describe the *parasympathetic nervous system* as well as its preganglionic and postganglionic neurons.
3. At what points in the sympathetic and parasympathetic nervous systems are *acetylcholine* and *norepinephrine* secreted?

4. What determines whether or not an organ will be excited or inhibited by sympathetic or parasympathetic stimulation?
5. What is meant by *muscarinic* and *nicotinic cholinergic receptors,* and by *alpha* and *beta adrenergic receptors*?
6. Describe briefly the effects of sympathetic and parasympathetic stimulation on (1) the eye, (2) the gastrointestinal system, (3) the heart, (4) the blood vessels, and (5) arterial pressure.
7. Explain the function of the *adrenal medullae* and why this function is important.
8. Explain how sympathetic and parasympathetic tone can allow the sympathetic and parasympathetic systems to cause both excitation and inhibition of an organ.
9. Explain the *mass discharge* response of the sympathetic system and its role in *stress reactions.*
10. How does the stress reaction prepare an animal for increased activity?
11. Explain how carbon dioxide and hydrogen ions interact with each other to control cerebral blood flow.
12. What is the importance of oxygen deficiency as a regulator of cerebral blood flow?
13. Under what conditions can the sympathetic nervous system cause severe constriction of the cerebral blood vessels?
14. Describe the formation, pathway of flow, and absorption of cerebrospinal fluid.
15. Explain how the cerebrospinal fluid pressure is normally controlled. What are some of the serious problems that occur when it becomes too high?
16. What is the "blood-brain barrier," and what is its importance?
17. Why is brain edema such a serious development?

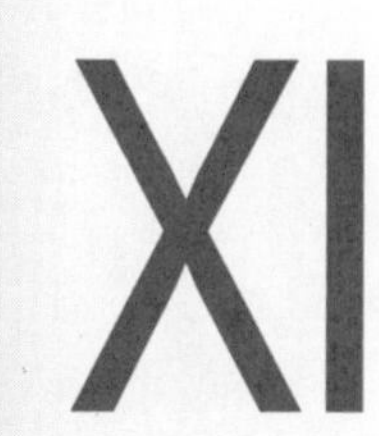

The Gastrointestinal Tract

42

The Gastrointestinal Tract: Nervous Control, Movement of Food Through the Tract, and Blood Flow

The alimentary tract provides the body with a continual supply of water, electrolytes, and nutrients. To achieve this requires (1) movement of food through the alimentary tract; (2) secretion of digestive juices and digestion of the food; (3) absorption of the digestive products, water, and the various electrolytes; (4) circulation of blood through the gastrointestinal organs to carry away the absorbed substances; and (5) control of all these functions by the nervous and hormonal systems.

Figure 42-1 illustrates the entire alimentary tract. Each part is adapted to its specific functions, some to simple passage of food, such as the esophagus; others to storage of food, such as the stomach; and others to digestion and absorption, such as the small intestine. In the present chapter we discuss the basic principles of the function of the entire alimentary tract and movement of food through the tract.

GENERAL PRINCIPLES OF GASTROINTESTINAL MOTILITY

Characteristics of the Gastrointestinal Wall

Figure 42-2 illustrates a typical section of the intestinal wall, showing the following layers from the outer surface inward: (1) the *serosa,* (2) a *longitudinal muscle layer,* (3) a *circular muscle layer,* (4) the *submucosa,* and (5) the *mucosa.* In addition, a sparse layer of smooth muscle fibers, the *muscularis mucosae,* lies in the deeper layers of the mucosa. The motor functions of the gut are performed by the different layers of smooth muscle.

The Gastrointestinal Smooth Muscle—Its Function as a Syncytium. The individual smooth muscle fibers in the gastrointestinal tract are between 200 and 500 micrometers in length and 2 and 10 micrometers in diameter, and they are arranged in bundles of as many as 1000 parallel fibers. In the longitudinal muscle layer, these bundles extend longitudinally down the intestinal tract; in the circular muscle layer they extend around the gut. Within each bundle the muscle fibers are electrically connected with each other through large numbers of *gap junctions* that allow low resistance movement of ions from one cell to the next. Therefore, electrical signals can travel readily from one fiber to the next.

Each bundle of smooth muscle fibers is separated from the next by loose connective tissue, but the bundles fuse with each other at many points so that in reality each muscle layer represents a branching latticework of smooth muscle bundles. Therefore, each muscle layer functions as a *syncytium*—that is, when an action potential is elicited anywhere within the muscle mass, it generally travels in all directions in the muscle. However, the distance that it travels depends upon the excitability of the muscle; sometimes it stops after only a few millimeters and at other times it travels many centimeters or even the entire length of the intestinal tract. Also, a few connections exist between the longitudinal and circular muscle layers so that excitation of one of these layers usually excites the other as well.

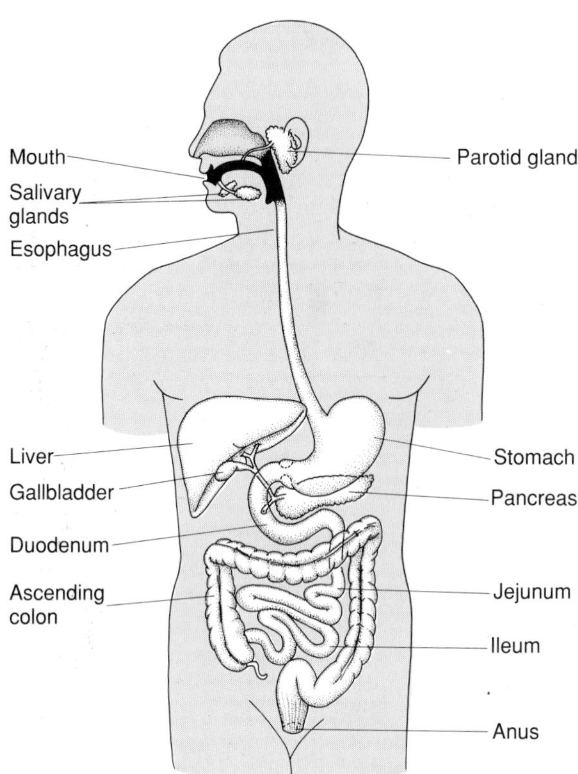

Figure 42-1. The alimentary tract.

Electrical Activity of Gastrointestinal Smooth Muscle

The smooth muscle of the gastrointestinal tract undergoes almost continual but slow electrical activity. This activity tends to have two basic types of electrical waves: (1) *slow waves* and (2) *spikes,* both of which are illustrated in Figure 42-3. In addition, the voltage of the resting membrane potential of the gastrointestinal smooth muscle can change to different levels without the generation of waves, and this too can have important effects in controlling motor activity of the gastrointestinal tract.

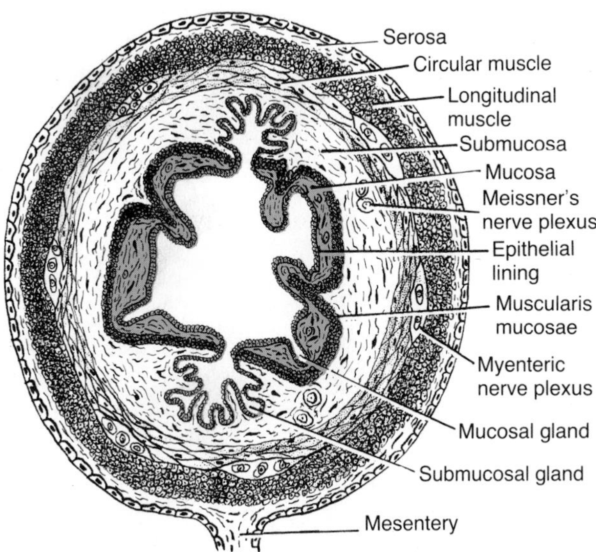

Figure 42-2. Typical cross-section of the gut.

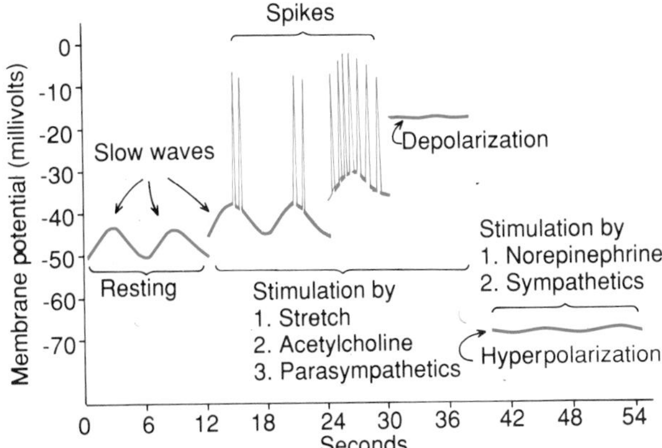

Figure 42-3. Membrane potentials in intestinal smooth muscle. Note the slow waves, the spike potentials, total depolarization, and hyperpolarization, all of which occur under different physiological conditions of the intestine.

The Slow Waves. Most gastrointestinal contractions occur rhythmically, and this rhythm is determined mainly by the frequency of the so-called "slow waves" in the smooth muscle membrane potential. These waves, illustrated in Figure 42-3, are not action potentials. Instead, they are slow, undulating changes in the resting membrane potential of unknown origin. These waves occur as slow as 3 per minute in the stomach and as high as 12 per minute in the small intestine.

The Spike Potentials. The spike potentials are true action potentials. They occur automatically when the resting membrane potential of the gastrointestinal smooth muscle becomes more positive than about −40 millivolts (the normal resting membrane potential is between −50 and −60 millivolts). Thus, note in Figure 42-3 that each time the peaks of the slow waves rise temporarily above the −40 millivolt level—that is, become less negative than −40 millivolts—spike potentials appear on these peaks. And the higher the slow wave potential rises above this level, the greater the frequency of the spike potentials, usually ranging between 1 and 10 spikes per second.

It is the movement of large amounts of calcium ions to the interior of the muscle fiber during the spike potentials that causes the intestinal smooth muscle to contract, as we discuss shortly.

Changes in the Voltage of the Resting Membrane Potential. In addition to the slow waves and spike potentials, the voltage level of the resting membrane potential can also change. Under normal conditions the resting membrane potential averages about −56 millivolts, but multiple factors can change this level, such as (1) stretching of the muscle, (2) stimulation by the parasympathetic nerves that secrete acetylcholine at their endings, and (3) stimulation by the sympathetic nerves that secrete norepinephrine at their endings.

Calcium Ions and Muscle Contraction. Muscle contraction occurs in response to the entry of calcium into the muscle fiber. As was explained in Chapter 7, it is believed that in smooth muscle the calcium ions, acting through a calmodulin control mechanism, activate the myosin filaments in the fiber, causing attractive forces between these and the actin filaments and thereby causing the muscle to contract.

NEURAL CONTROL OF GASTROINTESTINAL FUNCTION

The gastrointestinal tract has a nervous system all its own called the *enteric nervous system.* It lies entirely in the wall of the gut, beginning in the esophagus and extending all the way to the anus. The number of neurons in this enteric system is about 100,000,000, almost exactly equal to the number in the entire spinal cord; this illustrates the importance of the enteric system for controlling gastrointestinal function. It especially controls gastrointestinal movements and secretion.

The enteric system is composed mainly of two plexuses: (1) an outer plexus lying between the longitudinal and circular muscular layers, called the *myenteric plexus* or *Auerbach's plexus;* and (2) an inner plexus, called the *submucosal plexus* or *Meissner's plexus,* that lies in the submucosa. The nervous connections within and between these two plexuses are illustrated in Figure 42–4. The myenteric plexus controls mainly the gastrointestinal movements, and the submucosal plexus controls mainly local gastrointestinal epithelial secretion and local blood flow.

Note in Figure 42–4 the sympathetic and parasympathetic fibers that connect with both the myenteric and submucosal plexuses. Although the enteric nervous system can function on its own, independently of these extrinsic nerves, stimulation of the parasympathetic and sympathetic systems can further activate or inhibit gastrointestinal functions, as we discuss later.

Also shown in Figure 42–4 are sensory nerve endings that originate in the gastrointestinal epithelium or gut wall and then send afferent fibers to both plexuses of the enteric system and also to (1) the prevertebral ganglia of the sympathetic nervous system, (2) the spinal cord, and (3) some fibers traveling in the parasympathetic nerves (the vagi, for instance) all the way to the brain stem. These sensory nerves elicit local reflexes within the gut itself and also reflexes that are relayed back to the gut from either the prevertebral ganglia or the central nervous system.

Types of Neurotransmitters Secreted by the Enteric Neurons

Research workers have recently identified a dozen or more different neurotransmitter substances that are released by the nerve endings of different types of enteric neurons. Two of these with which we are already familiar are (1) *acetylcholine* and (2) *norepinephrine.* Others are (3) *adenosine triphosphate,* (4) *serotonin,* (5) *dopamine,* (6) *cholecystokinin,* (7) *substance P,* (8) *vasoactive intestinal polypeptide,* (9) *somatostatin,* (10) *leu-enkephalin,* (11) *met-enkephalin,* and (12) *bombesin.* The specific functions of most of these are not yet known well enough to justify extensive discussion, other than to point out the following: Acetylcholine most often excites gastrointestinal activity. Norepinephrine, on the other hand, almost always inhibits gastrointestinal activity. This is also true of epinephrine which reaches the gastrointestinal tract by way of the blood after it is secreted by the adrenal medullae into the circulation. The other transmitter substances aforementioned are a mixture of excitatory and inhibitory agents, but their impor-

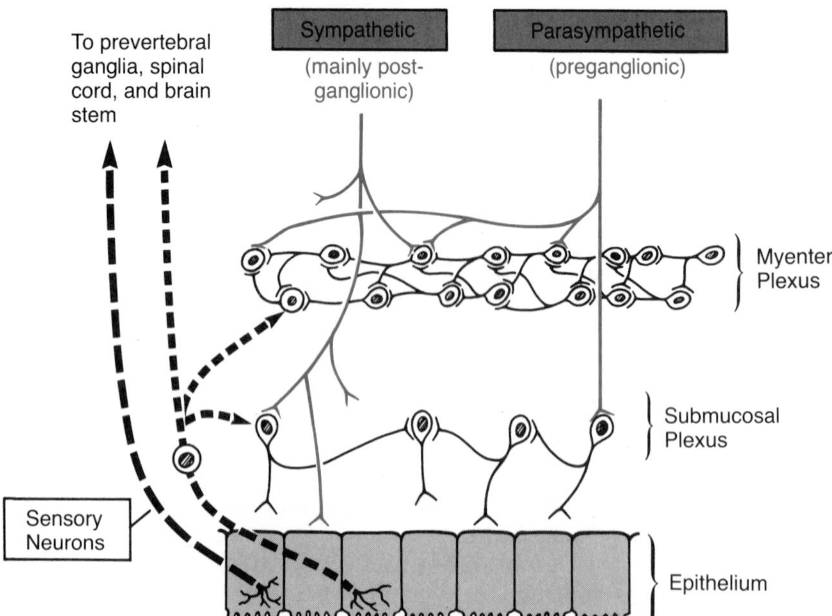

Figure 42–4. Neural control of the gut wall, showing (1) the myenteric and submucosal plexuses; (2) extrinsic control of these plexuses by the sympathetic and parasympathetic nervous systems; and (3) sensory fibers passing from the luminal epithelium and gut wall to the enteric plexuses and from there to the prevertebral ganglia, spinal cord, and brain stem.

tance and even their functions are still mainly to be determined.

Autonomic Control of the Gastrointestinal Tract

Parasympathetic Innervation. Except for a few nerve fibers in the mouth and throat region and others in the distal colon region, almost all the parasympathetic fibers to the gut are carried in the gut. When stimulated, these increase the activity of the entire enteric nervous system. This in turn enhances the activity of most, but not all, gastrointestinal functions, for some of the enteric neurons are inhibitory and therefore inhibit certain of the functions.

Sympathetic Innervation. The sympathetic fibers to the gastrointestinal tract originate in the spinal cord between the segments T-5 and L-2. In general, stimulation of the sympathetic nervous system inhibits activity in the gastrointestinal tract, causing effects essentially opposite to those of the parasympathetic system. It exerts its effects in two different ways: (1) to a slight extent by direct effect of norepinephrine on the smooth muscle to inhibit this, and (2) to a major extent by an inhibitory effect of the norepinephrine on the neurons of the enteric nervous system. Thus, strong stimulation of the sympathetic system can totally block movement of food through the gastrointestinal tract.

FUNCTIONAL TYPES OF MOVEMENTS IN THE GASTROINTESTINAL TRACT

Two basic types of movements occur in the gastrointestinal tract: (1) *propulsive movements,* which cause food to move forward along the tract at an appropriate rate for digestion and absorption, and (2) *mixing movements,* which keep the intestinal contents thoroughly mixed at all times.

The Propulsive Movements — Peristalsis

The basic propulsive movement of the gastrointestinal tract is *peristalsis,* which is illustrated in Figure 42–5. A contractile ring appears around the gut and then moves forward; this is analogous to putting one's fingers around a thin distended tube, then constricting the fingers and sliding them forward along the tube. Obviously, any material in front of the contractile ring is moved forward.

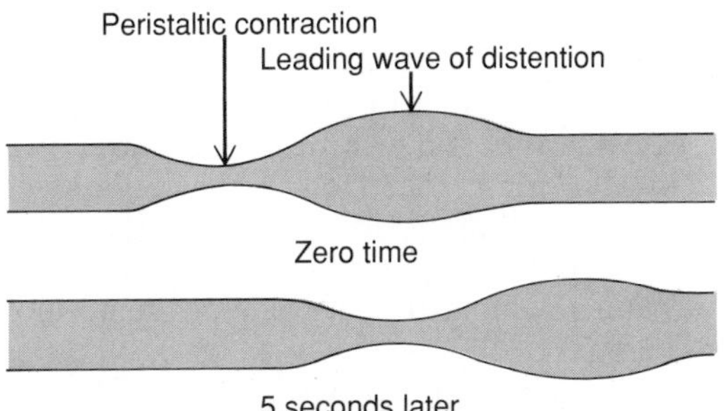

Figure 42–5. Peristalsis.

The usual stimulus for peristalsis is *distention.* That is, if a large amount of food collects at any point in the gut, the stretching of the gut wall stimulates the gut and a contractile ring appears 2 to 3 centimeters above this point that initiates a peristaltic movement.

This complex pattern of peristalsis does not occur in the absence of the myenteric plexus. Therefore, the complex is frequently called the *myenteric reflex,* or it is also called simply the *peristaltic reflex.* And the peristaltic reflex plus the analward direction of movement of the peristalsis is called the "law of the gut."

The Mixing Movements

The mixing movements are quite different in different parts of the alimentary tract. In some areas, the peristaltic contractions themselves cause most of the mixing. This is especially true when forward progression of the intestinal contents is blocked by a sphincter, so that a peristaltic wave can then only churn the intestinal contents, rather than propel them forward. At other times, *local constrictive contractions* occur every few centimeters in the gut wall. These constrictions usually last only a few seconds; then new constrictions occur at other points in the gut, thus "chopping" the contents first here and then there. These peristaltic and constrictive movements are modified in different parts of the gastrointestinal tract for proper propulsion and mixing, and are discussed for each portion of the tract in the following sections.

PROCESSING OF FOOD IN THE MOUTH, PHARYNX, AND ESOPHAGUS

Mastication (Chewing)

The teeth are admirably designed for chewing; the anterior teeth (incisors) providing a strong cutting action and the posterior teeth (molars) a grinding action. All the jaw muscles working together can close the teeth with a force as great as 55 pounds on the incisors and 200 pounds on the molars.

Most of the muscles of chewing are innervated by the motor branch of the fifth cranial nerve, and the chewing process is controlled by nuclei in the brain stem. Stimulation of the reticular formation near the brain stem centers for taste can cause continual rhythmic chewing movements. Also, stimulation of areas in the hypothalamus, amygdala, and even in the cerebral cortex near the sensory areas for taste and smell can cause chewing.

Much of the chewing process is caused by the *chewing reflex,* which may be explained as follows: The presence of a bolus of food in the mouth causes reflex inhibition of the muscles of mastication, which allows the lower jaw to drop. The drop in turn initiates a stretch reflex of the jaw muscles that leads to *rebound* contraction. This automatically raises the jaw to cause closure of the teeth, but it also compresses the bolus again against the linings of the mouth, which inhibits the jaw muscles once again, allowing the jaw to drop and rebound another time; and this is repeated again and again.

Chewing aids in the digestion of food for the following simple reason: Because the *digestive enzymes act only on the surfaces of food particles,* the rate of digestion is highly dependent on the total surface area exposed to the intestinal secretions. Also, grinding the food to a very fine particulate consistency prevents excoriation of the gastrointestinal tract and increases the ease with which food is emptied from the stomach into the small intestine and thence into all succeeding segments of the gut.

Swallowing (Deglutition)

In general, swallowing can be divided into (1) the *voluntary stage,* which initiates the swallowing process, (2) the *pharyngeal stage,* which is involuntary and constitutes the passage of food through the pharynx into the esophagus, and (3) the *esophageal stage,* another involuntary phase that promotes passage of food from the pharynx to the stomach.

Voluntary Stage of Swallowing. When the food is ready for swallowing, it is "voluntarily" squeezed or rolled posteriorly into the pharynx by pressure of the tongue upward and backward against the palate, as shown in Figure 42–6. From here on, the process of swallowing becomes entirely, or almost entirely, automatic and ordinarily cannot be stopped.

Pharyngeal Stage of Swallowing. As the bolus of food enters the pharynx, it stimulates *swallowing receptor areas* all around the opening of the pharynx, especially on the tonsillar pillars, and impulses from these pass to the brain stem to initiate a series of automatic pharyngeal muscular contractions as follows:

1. The soft palate is pulled upward to close the posterior nares.
2. The palatopharyngeal folds on either side of the pharynx are pulled medially to approximate each other. In this way these folds form a sagittal slit through which the food must pass into the posterior pharynx.
3. The vocal cords of the larynx are strongly approximated, and the larynx is pulled upward and anteriorly by the neck muscles. This action, combined with the presence of ligaments that prevent upward movement of the epiglottis, causes the epiglottis to swing backward over the opening of the larynx. Both effects prevent passage of food into the trachea.
4. The upward movement of the larynx also enlarges the opening of the esophagus. At the same time, the upper 3 to 4 centimeters of the esophageal muscular wall, an area called the *upper esophageal sphincter* or the *pharyngoesophageal sphincter,* relaxes, thus allowing food to move easily and freely from the posterior pharynx into the upper esophagus.
5. At the same time that the larynx is raised and the pharyngoesophageal sphincter is relaxed, the entire muscular wall of the pharynx contracts, beginning in the superior part of the pharynx and spreading downward as a rapid peristaltic wave over the middle and inferior pharyngeal muscles and thence into the esophagus, which propels the food into the esophagus.

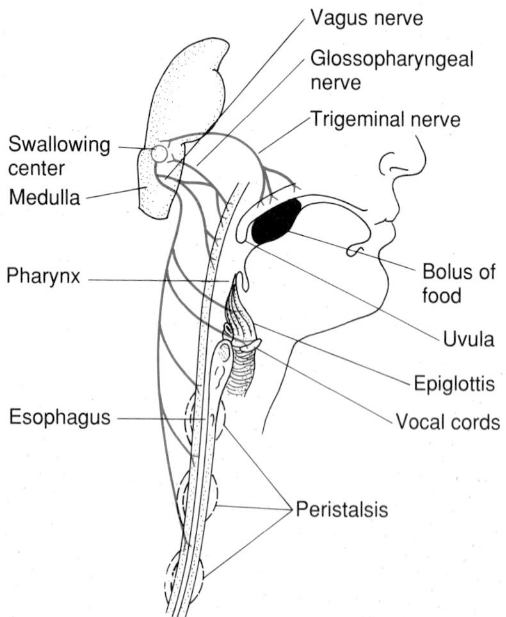

Figure 42–6. The swallowing mechanism.

To summarize the mechanics of the pharyngeal stage of swallowing: the trachea is closed, the esophagus is opened, and a fast peristaltic wave originating in the pharynx forces the bolus of food into the upper esophagus, the entire process occurring in 1 to 2 seconds.

Nervous Control of the Pharyngeal Stage of Swallowing. The successive stages of swallowing are automatically controlled in orderly sequence by neuronal areas distributed throughout the reticular substance of the medulla and lower portion of the pons. The sequence of the swallowing reflex is the same from one swallow to the next, and the timing of the entire cycle also remains constant from one swallow to the next. The areas in the medulla and lower pons that control swallowing are collectively called the *deglutition* or *swallowing center.*

The pharyngeal stage of swallowing is principally a reflex act. It is almost never initiated by direct stimuli to the swallowing center from higher regions of the central nervous system. Instead, it is almost always initiated by voluntary movement of food into the back of the mouth, which, in turn, elicits the swallowing reflex.

Effect of the Pharyngeal Stage of Swallowing on Respiration. The entire pharyngeal stage of swallowing occurs in less than 1 to 2 seconds, thereby interrupting respiration for only a fraction of a usual respiratory cycle. The swallowing center specifically inhibits the respiratory center of the medulla during this time, halting respiration at any point in its cycle to allow swallowing to proceed. Yet even while a person is talking, swallowing interrupts respiration for such a short time that it is hardly noticeable.

Esophageal Stage of Swallowing

The esophagus functions primarily to conduct food from the pharynx to the stomach, and its movements are organized specifically for this function.

Normally the esophagus exhibits two types of peristaltic movements—*primary peristalsis* and *secondary peristalsis.* Primary peristalsis is simply a continuation of the peristaltic wave that begins in the pharynx and spreads into the esophagus during the pharyngeal stage of swallowing. This wave passes all the way from the pharynx to the stomach in approximately 8 to 10 seconds. However, if the primary peristaltic wave fails to move all the food that has entered the esophagus into the stomach, *secondary peristaltic waves* result from distention of the esophagus by the retained food, and they continue until all the food has emptied into the stomach. These secondary waves are initiated partly by intrinsic neural circuits in the esophageal enteric nervous system and partly by reflexes that are transmitted through *vagal afferent fibers* from the esophagus to the medulla and then back again to the esophagus through *vagal efferent fibers.*

Receptive Relaxation of the Stomach. As the esophageal peristaltic wave passes toward the stomach, a wave of relaxation, transmitted through myenteric inhibitory neurons, precedes the constriction. Furthermore, the entire stomach and, to a lesser extent, even the duodenum become relaxed as this wave reaches the lower end of the esophagus and thus they are prepared ahead of time to receive the food propelled down the esophagus during the swallowing act.

Function of the Lower Esophageal Sphincter (Gastroesophageal Sphincter)

At the lower end of the esophagus, extending from about 2 to 5 cm above its juncture with the stomach, the esophageal circular muscle is slightly thickened and functions as a *lower esophageal sphincter* or *gastroesophageal sphincter.* This sphincter remains tonically constricted, in contrast to the mid and upper portions of the esophagus that normally remain completely relaxed. Yet when a peristaltic swallowing wave passes down the esophagus, "receptive relaxation" relaxes the lower esophageal sphincter ahead of the peristaltic wave and allows easy propulsion of the swallowed food into the stomach.

The stomach contents are highly acidic and contain many proteolytic enzymes. The esophageal mucosa, except in the lower eighth of the esophagus, is not capable of resisting for long the digestive action of gastric secretions. Fortunately, the tonic constriction of the lower esophageal sphincter helps to prevent significant reflux of stomach contents into the esophagus except under abnormal conditions.

MOTOR FUNCTIONS OF THE STOMACH

The motor functions of the stomach are threefold: (1) storage of large quantities of food until it can be accommodated in the duodenum, (2) mixing of this food with gastric secretions until it forms a semifluid mixture called *chyme,* and (3) slow emptying of the food from the stomach into the small intestine at a rate suitable for proper digestion and absorption by the small intestine.

Figure 42-7 illustrates the basic anatomy of the stomach. Physiologically, the stomach can be divided into two major parts: (1) the *body* and (2) the *antrum.*

Storage Function of the Stomach

As food enters the stomach, it forms concentric circles in the body of the stomach, the newest food lying closest to the esophageal opening and the oldest food lying nearest the wall of the stomach. Normally, when food enters the stomach, a vagal reflex greatly reduces the tone in the muscular wall of the body of the stomach so that the wall can bulge progressively outward, accommodating greater and greater quantities of food up to a limit of about 1.5 liters. The pressure in the stomach remains low until this limit is approached.

Mixing and Propulsion of Food in the Stomach—The Basic Electrical Rhythm of the Stomach

The digestive juices of the stomach are secreted by the *gastric glands,* which cover almost the entire wall

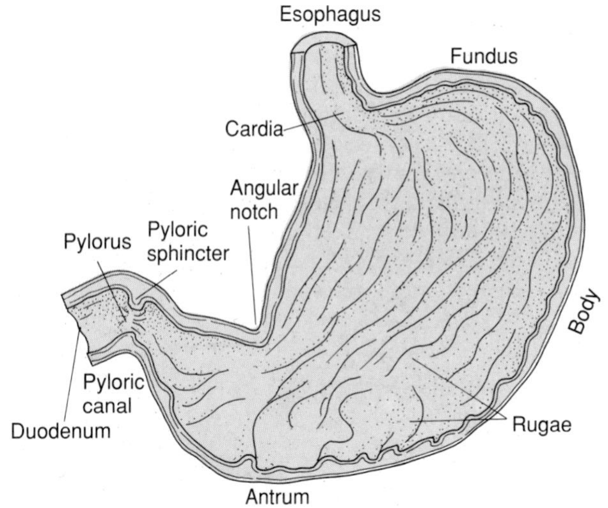

Figure 42-7. Physiological anatomy of the stomach.

of the body of the stomach except along a strip on the lesser curvature of the stomach. These secretions come immediately into contact with that portion of the stored food lying against the mucosal surface of the stomach. At the same time, weak peristaltic *constrictor waves,* also called *mixing waves,* move toward the antrum along the stomach wall approximately once every 20 seconds. These waves are initiated by a *basic electrical rhythm* (called *BER*) consisting of electrical "slow waves" that occur spontaneously in the stomach wall.

As the slow waves move down the stomach, they not only cause the secretions to mix with the outer portions of the stored food but also provide weak propulsion to move the food toward the antrum.

As the constrictor waves progress from the body of the stomach into the antrum, they become more intense, some becoming extremely intense and providing powerful *peristaltic constrictor rings* that force the antral contents under high pressure toward the pylorus. These constrictor rings also play an important role in further mixing of the stomach contents in the following way: Each time a peristaltic wave passes over the antrum toward the pylorus, it digs deeply into the contents of the antrum. Yet the opening of the pylorus is small enough that only a few milliliters of antral contents are expelled into the duodenum with each peristaltic wave. Therefore, most of the antral contents are squirted backward through the peristaltic ring toward the body of the stomach. Thus, the moving peristaltic constrictive ring, combined with this squirting action, called "retropulsion," is an exceedingly important mixing mechanism of the stomach.

Chyme. After the food has become mixed with the stomach secretions, the resulting mixture that passes on down the gut is called *chyme.* The degree of fluidity of chyme depends on the relative amounts of food and stomach secretions and on the degree of digestion that has occurred. The appearance of chyme is that of a murky, milky semifluid or paste.

Hunger Contractions. Besides the peristaltic contractions that occur when food is present in the stomach, another type of intense contractions, called *hunger contractions,* occurs when the stomach has been empty for a long time. These are rhythmical peristaltic contractions in the *body* of the stomach that are usually most intense in young, healthy persons with high degrees of gastrointestinal tonus; and they are greatly increased by a low level of blood sugar.

Hunger contractions are usually associated with a feeling of hunger and therefore are an important means by which the alimentary tract intensifies the animal drive to acquire food.

Emptying of the Stomach

Mainly, stomach emptying is promoted by the intensity of the peristaltic contractions of the stomach antrum. At the same time emptying is opposed by varying degrees of resistance to the passage of chyme at the pylorus.

Intense Antral Peristaltic Contractions During Stomach Emptying. Most of the time the antral peristaltic contractions are weak and function mainly to cause mixing of the food and gastric secretions. However, about 20 per cent of the time while food is in the stomach, the antral contractions become very intense and spread through the antrum no longer as weak mixing contractions but instead as strong peristaltic, ringlike constrictions. As the stomach becomes progressively more and more empty, these constrictions begin farther and farther up the body of the stomach, gradually pinching off the lowermost portions of the stored food and adding this food to the chyme in the antrum. These intense peristaltic contractions often create as much as 50 to 70 centimeters of water pressure, which is about six times as powerful as the usual mixing type of peristaltic waves. Thus, the intensity of this antral peristalsis is the principal factor that determines the rate of stomach emptying.

Role of the Pylorus in Controlling Stomach Emptying. The distal opening of the stomach is the *pylorus.* Here the thickness of the circular muscle becomes 50 to 100 per cent greater than in the earlier portions of the stomach antrum, and it also remains slightly tonically contracted almost all the time. Therefore, the pyloric circular muscle is frequently called the *pyloric sphincter.*

Despite the tonic contraction of the pyloric sphincter, the pylorus usually remains slightly open, large enough for water and other fluids to empty normally from the stomach with ease. On the other hand, the constriction usually prevents passage of most larger food particles until they have become mixed in the chyme to an almost fluid consistency.

However, the degree of constriction of the pylorus can be increased or decreased under the influence of nervous and humoral signals from both the stomach and the duodenum, as is discussed shortly. Thus, the pylorus as well as the stomach's antral contractions also enters into the control of stomach emptying.

Regulation of Stomach Emptying

The rate at which the stomach empties is regulated by signals both from the stomach and from the duodenum, each of which functions for a different purpose.

Gastric Factors That Promote Emptying

Effect of Gastric Food Volume on Rate of Emptying. It is very easy to see how increased food volume in the stomach could promote increased emptying from the stomach. However, it is not increased pressure in the stomach that causes the increased emptying, because in the usual normal range of volume, increasing the volume does not increase the pressure significantly. On the other hand, stretching of the stomach wall does elicit vagal and local myenteric reflexes that both excite the activity of the pyloric pump and at the same time slightly inhibit the pylorus. Thus, these stretch reflexes play an important roll in emptying.

Effect of the Hormone Gastrin on Stomach Emptying. In the following chapter we shall see that stretch, as well as the presence of certain types of foods in the stomach—particularly meat—also elicits release of a hormone called *gastrin* from the antral mucosa, and this has potent effects on causing secretion of highly acidic gastric juice by the stomach fundic glands. Gastrin also has moderate stimulatory effects on motor functions of the stomach. Most important, it enhances the activity of the pyloric pump. Thus, it, too, has an important influence in promoting stomach emptying.

Duodenal Factors That Inhibit Emptying

The Inhibitory Effect of Enterogastric Nervous Reflexes from the Duodenum. When food enters the duodenum, multiple nervous reflexes are initiated from the duodenum wall that pass back to the stomach and slow or even stop stomach emptying when the volume of chyme in the duodenum has become too much. These reflexes are mediated mainly by way of the enteric nervous system in the gut wall. These reflexes have two effects on stomach emptying: first, they strongly inhibit the antral propulsive contractions; and second, they increase slightly to moderately the tone of the pyloric sphincter.

The types of factors that are continually monitored in the duodenum and that can excite the enterogastric reflexes include

1. The degree of distention of the duodenum.
2. The presence of any degree of irritation of the duodenal mucosa.
3. The degree of acidity of the duodenal chyme.
4. The degree of osmolality of the chyme.
5. The presence of certain breakdown products in the chyme, especially breakdown products of proteins and perhaps to a lesser extent of fats.

Hormonal Feedback from the Duodenum in Inhibiting Gastric Emptying—Role of Fats. Not only do nervous reflexes from the duodenum to the stomach inhibit stomach emptying, but hormones released from the upper intestine do so as well. The stimulus for producing the hormones is mainly fats entering the duodenum, though other types of foods can increase the hormones to a lesser degree.

On entering the duodenum, the fats extract several different hormones from the duodenal and jejunal epithelium, either by binding with "receptors" in the epithelial cells or in some other way. In turn, the hormones are carried by way of the blood to the stomach, where they (1) inhibit the activity of the pyloric pump and at the same time (2) increase slightly the strength of contraction of the pyloric sphincter. These effects are important because fats are digested much more slowly than most other foods.

Unfortunately, what the precise hormones are that cause the hormonal feedback inhibition of the stomach is not fully clear. The most potent appears to be *cholecystokinin (CCK),* which is released from the mucosa of the jejunum in response to fatty substances in the chyme. This hormone acts as a competitive inhibitor to block the increased stomach motility caused by gastrin. Another is the hormone *secretin,* which is released mainly from the duodenal mucosa in response to gastric acid released from the stomach through the pylorus. This hormone has a general but weak effect of decreasing gastrointestinal motility.

In summary, several different hormones are known that could serve as hormonal mechanisms for inhibiting gastric emptying when excess quantities of chyme, especially acidic or fatty chyme, enter the duodenum from the stomach. CCK is probably the most important.

Summary of the Control of Stomach Emptying

Emptying of the stomach is controlled to a moderate degree by stomach factors, such as the degree of filling in the stomach and the excitatory effect of gastrin on antral peristalsis. However, probably more important control of stomach emptying resides in feedback signals from the duodenum, including both the enterogastric feedback reflexes and hormonal feedback. These two feedback inhibitory mechanisms work together to slow the rate of emptying when (1) too much chyme is already in the small intestine or (2) the chyme is excessively acid, contains too much unprocessed protein or fat, is hypotonic or hypertonic, or is irritating. In this way the rate of stomach emptying is limited to that amount of chyme that the small intestine can process.

MOVEMENTS OF THE SMALL INTESTINE

The movements of the small intestine, as elsewhere in the gastrointestinal tract, can be divided into *mixing contractions* and *propulsive contractions.* However, to a great extent this separation is artificial because essentially all movements of the small intestine cause at least some degree of both mixing and propulsion. Yet the usual classification of these processes follows.

Mixing Contractions (Segmentation Contractions)

When a portion of the small intestine becomes distended with chyme, the stretch of the intestinal wall elicits localized concentric contractions spaced at intervals along the intestine. The longitudinal length of each one of the contractions is only about 1 cm, so that each set of contractions causes "segmentation" of the small intestine, as illustrated in Figure 42–8,

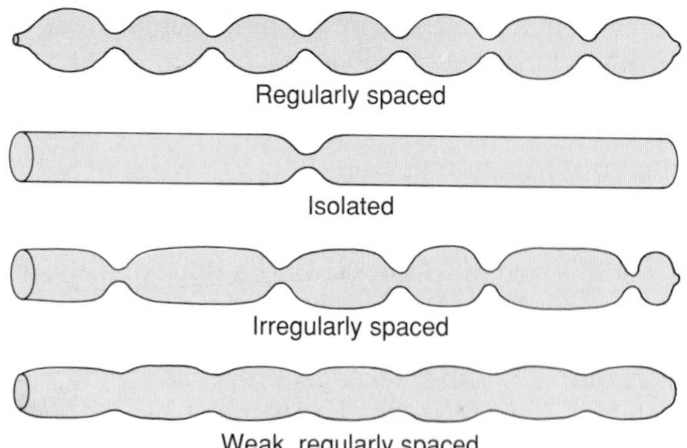

Figure 42-8. Segmentation movements of the small intestine.

dividing the intestine into spaced segments that have the appearance of a chain of sausages. As one set of segmentation contractions relaxes, a new set begins, but the new contractions occur at points between the previous contractions. These segmentation contractions "chop" the chyme as often as 8 to 12 times a minute, in this way promoting progressive mixing of the solid food particles with the secretions of the small intestine.

The maximum frequency of the segmentation contractions in the small intestine is determined by the frequency of the *slow waves* in the intestinal wall, which is the basic electrical rhythm (BER) as explained earlier. Since this frequency is about 12 per minute in the duodenum and proximal jejunum, the maximum frequency of the segmentation contractions in these areas is also about 12 per minute. However, in the terminal ileum, the maximum frequency is usually 8 to 9 contractions per minute.

Propulsive Movements

Peristalsis in the Small Intestine. Chyme is propelled through the small intestine by *peristaltic waves.* These can occur in any part of the small intestine, and they move analward at a velocity of 0.5 to 2 cm/sec, much faster in the proximal intestine and much slower in the terminal intestine. However, they are normally very weak and usually die out after traveling only 3 to 5 centimeters, very rarely farther than 10 centimeters, so that movement of the chyme is also very poor; so poor in fact that the *net* movement of the chyme along the small intestine averages only 1 cm/min. This means that normally 3 to 5 hours are required for passage of chyme from the pylorus to the ileocecal valve.

Control of Peristalsis by Nervous and Hormonal Signals. Peristaltic activity of the small intestine is greatly increased after a meal. This is caused partly by the beginning entry of chyme into the duodenum but also by a so-called *gastroenteric reflex* that is initiated by distention of the stomach and conducted principally through the myenteric plexus from the stomach down along the wall of the small intestine.

In addition to the nervous signals, several hormonal factors also affect peristalsis. These include *gastrin, cholecystokinin, insulin,* and *serotonin,* all of which enhance intestinal motility and are secreted during various phases of food processing. On the other hand, *secretin* and *glucagon* inhibit small intestinal motility. Unfortunately, the quantitative importance of each of these hormonal factors for controlling motility is still questionable.

The Peristaltic Rush. Though peristalsis in the small intestine is normally very weak, intense irritation of the intestinal mucosa, as occurs in some severe cases of infectious diarrhea, can cause very powerful, rapid peristalsis called the *peristaltic rush.* This is initiated partly by extrinsic nervous reflexes to the brain stem and back again to the gut and partly by direct enhancement of the myenteric plexus reflexes. The powerful peristaltic contractions then travel long distances in the small intestine within minutes, sweeping the contents of the intestine into the colon and thereby relieving the small intestine of either irritative chyme or excessive distention.

Function of the Ileocecal Valve

A principal function of the ileocecal valve is to prevent backflow of fecal contents from the colon into the small intestine. As illustrated in Figure 42-9, the lips of the ileocecal valve protrude into the lumen of the cecum and therefore are forcefully closed when any excess pressure builds up in the cecum and tries to push the cecal contents backward against the lips. Usually the valve can resist reverse pressure of as much as 50 to 60 centimeters of water.

In addition, the wall of the ileum for several centimeters immediately preceding the ileocecal valve has a thickened muscular coat called the *ileocecal sphincter.* This normally remains mildly constricted

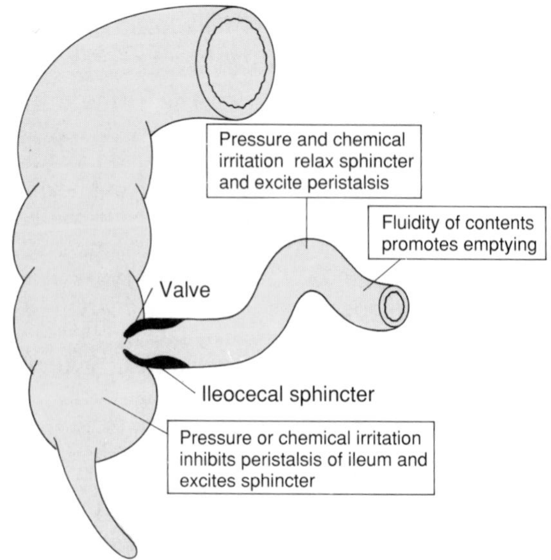

Figure 42-9. Emptying at the ileocecal valve.

and slows the emptying of ileal contents into the cecum except immediately after a meal, when a gastroileal reflex intensifies the peristalsis in the ileum. Also, the hormone *gastrin,* which is liberated from the stomach mucosa in response to food in the stomach, increases ileal contractions and relaxes the ileocecal sphincter.

The resistance to emptying at the ileocecal valve prolongs the stay of chyme in the ileum and, therefore, facilitates absorption. Only about 1500 milliliters of chyme empty into the cecum each day.

Feedback Control of the Ileocecal Sphincter by Reflexes from the Cecum. The degree of contraction of the ileocecal sphincter, as well as the intensity of peristalsis in the terminal ileum, is also controlled strongly by reflexes from the cecum. Whenever the cecum is distended, the contraction of the ileocecal sphincter is intensified while ileal peristalsis is inhibited, which greatly delays emptying of additional chyme from the ileum. Also, any irritant in the cecum delays emptying. For instance, when a person has an inflamed appendix, the irritation of this vestigial remnant of the cecum can cause such intense spasm of the ileocecal sphincter and paralysis of the ileum that this completely blocks emptying of the ileum. These reflexes from the cecum to the ileocecal sphincter and ileum are mediated both by way of the myenteric plexus in the gut wall itself and through extrinsic nerves, especially reflexes of the prevertebral sympathetic ganglia.

MOVEMENTS OF THE COLON

The principal functions of the colon are (1) absorption of water and electrolytes from the chyme and (2) storage of fecal matter until it can be expelled. The proximal half of the colon, illustrated in Figure 42–10, is concerned principally with absorption, and the distal half with storage. Because intense movements are not required for these functions, the movements of the colon are normally sluggish. Yet in a sluggish manner, the movements still have characteristics similar to those of the small intestine and can be divided once again into mixing movements and propulsive movements.

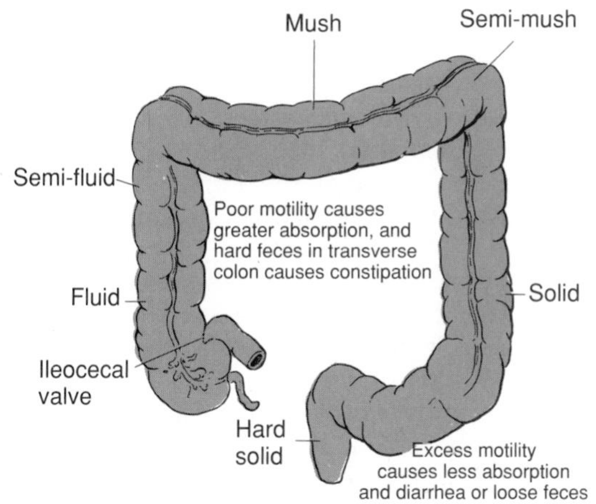

Figure 42–10. Absorptive and storage functions of the large intestine.

Mixing Movements—Haustrations. In the same manner that segmentation movements occur in the small intestine, large circular constrictions also occur in the large intestine. At the same time, the longitudinal muscle of the colon, which is aggregated into three longitudinal strips called the *teneae coli,* contract. These combined contractions of the circular and longitudinal smooth muscle cause the unstimulated portion of the large intestine to bulge outward into baglike sacs called *haustrations.* These contractions, once initiated, usually reach peak intensity in about 30 seconds and then disappear during the next 60 seconds. They also at times move slowly analward during their period of contraction and therefore provide a minor amount of forward propulsion of the colonic contents. After another few minutes, new haustral contractions occur in other areas nearby. Therefore, the fecal material in the large intestine is slowly *dug into and rolled over* in much the same manner that one spades the earth. In this way, all the fecal material is gradually exposed to the surface of the large intestine, and fluid and dissolved substances are progressively absorbed until only 80 to 200 milliliters of the 1500 milliliter daily load of chyme is lost in the feces.

Propulsive Movements—"Mass Movements." Peristaltic waves of the type seen in the small intestine only rarely occur in most parts of the colon. Instead, most propulsion occurs by (1) the slow analward movement of the *haustral contractions* just discussed and (2) *mass movements.*

In the transverse colon and sigmoid, mass movements mainly take over the propulsive role. These movements usually occur only a few times each day, most abundantly for about 15 minutes during the first hour after eating breakfast.

A mass movement is a modified type of peristalsis characterized by the following sequence of events: First, a constrictive ring occurs at a distended or irritated point in the colon, usually in the transverse colon. Then rapidly thereafter 20 or more centimeters of colon *distal* to the constriction contract as a unit, forcing its fecal material *en masse* down the colon. The contraction develops progressively more force for about 30 seconds, and relaxation then occurs during the next 2 to 3 minutes before another mass movement occurs, this time perhaps farther along the colon. But the whole series of mass movements will usually persist for only 10 minutes to half an hour. If defecation does not occur at that time, a new set of mass movements might not recur for another half day or day.

Initiation of Mass Movements by the Gastrocolic and Duodenocolic Reflexes. The appearance of mass movements after meals is facilitated by *gastrocolic* and *duodenocolic reflexes.* These reflexes result from distention of the stomach and duodenum. They can take place only weakly when the extrinsic nerves are removed; therefore, it is probable that reflexes conducted through the extrinsic nerves of the autonomic nervous system probably provide most of the intensity of the gastrocolic and duodenocolic reflexes.

Irritation in the colon can also initiate intense mass movements. For instance, a person who has an ulcerated condition of the colon *(ulcerative colitis)* frequently has mass movements that persist almost all the time.

Also, mass movements can be initiated by intense stimulation of the parasympathetic nervous system.

Defecation

Most of the time, the rectum is empty of feces. This results partly from the fact that a weak functional sphincter exists approximately 20 centimeters from the anus at the juncture between the sigmoid and the rectum. However, when a mass movement forces feces into the rectum, the desire for defecation is normally initiated, including reflex contraction of the rectum and relaxation of the anal sphincters.

Continual dribble of fecal matter through the anus is prevented by tonic constriction of (1) the *internal anal sphincter,* a thickening of the intestinal circular smooth muscle that lies immediately inside the anus, and (2) the *external anal sphincter,* composed of striated voluntary muscle that both surrounds the internal sphincter and also extends distal to it; the external sphincter is controlled by nerve fibers in the pudendal nerve, which is part of the somatic nervous system and therefore is under *voluntary, conscious control.*

The Defecation Reflexes. Ordinarily, defecation is initiated by *defecation reflexes.* One of these reflexes is an *intrinsic reflex* mediated by the local enteric nervous system. That is, when the feces enter the rectum, distention of the rectal wall initiates afferent signals that spread through the *myenteric plexus* to initiate peristaltic waves in the descending colon, sigmoid, and rectum, forcing feces toward the anus. As the peristaltic wave approaches the anus, the internal anal sphincter is relaxed by inhibitory signals from the myenteric plexus; and if the external anal sphincter is voluntarily relaxed at the same time, defecation will occur.

However, the intrinsic defecation reflex itself is weak; and to be effective in causing defecation it usually must be fortified by a *parasympathetic defecation reflex* that involves the sacral segments of the spinal cord, as illustrated in Figure 42–11. When the nerve endings in the rectum are stimulated, signals are transmitted into the spinal cord and thence, reflexly, back to the descending colon, sigmoid, rectum, and anus by way of parasympathetic nerve fibers in the *pelvic nerves.* These parasympathetic signals greatly intensify the peristaltic waves, relax the internal anal sphincter, and thus convert the intrinsic defecation reflex from an ineffectual, weak movement into a powerful process of defecation This is sometimes effective in emptying the large bowel in one movement all the way from the splenic flexure of the colon to the anus. Also, the afferent signals entering the spinal cord initiate other effects, such as taking a deep breath, closing the glottis, contracting the abdominal wall muscles to force the fecal contents of the colon downward, and at the same time causing the pelvic floor to extend downward and pull outward on the anal ring to evaginate the feces.

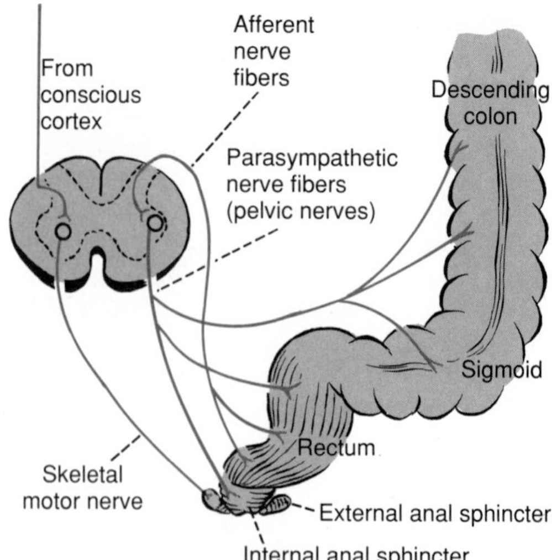

Figure 42–11. The afferent and efferent pathways of the parasympathetic mechanism for enhancing the defecation reflex.

However, despite the defecation reflexes, other effects are also necessary before actual defecation occurs. In the toilet-trained human being, relaxation of the internal sphincter and forward movement of feces toward the anus normally initiate an instantaneous contraction of the external sphincter, which still temporarily prevents defecation. Except in babies and mentally inept persons, the conscious mind then takes over voluntary control of the external sphincter and either relaxes it to allow defecation to occur or further contracts it if the moment is not socially acceptable for defecation.

GASTROINTESTINAL BLOOD FLOW

The blood vessels of the gastrointestinal system are part of a more extensive system called the *splanchnic circulation,* illustrated in Figure 42–12. It includes the blood flow through the alimentary tract itself plus the blood flow through the spleen, the pancreas, and the liver. The design of this system is such that all of the blood that courses through the gut, spleen, and pancreas then flows immediately into the liver by way of the portal vein. In the liver, the blood passes through millions of fine liver sinusoids and finally leaves the liver by way of the hepatic veins that empty into the vena cava of the general circulation. This secondary flow of blood through the liver allows the *reticuloendothelial cells* lining the liver sinusoids to remove bacteria and other particulate matter that

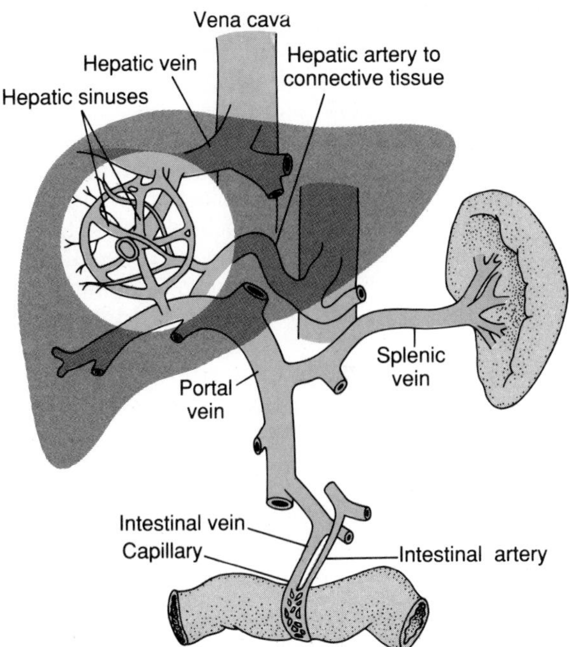

Figure 42-12. The splanchnic circulation.

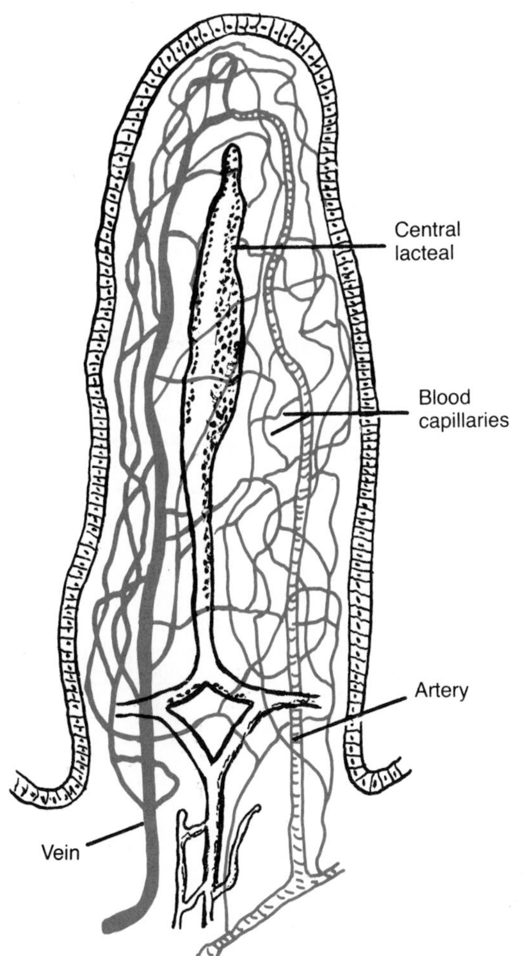

Figure 42-13. Microvasculature of the villus, showing a countercurrent arrangement of blood flow in the arterioles and venules.

might enter the blood from the gastrointestinal tract, thus preventing direct access of potentially harmful agents into the remainder of the body.

Many of the nutrients absorbed from the gut are also transported in the portal venous blood to the same liver sinusoids. Here, both the reticuloendothelial cells and the principal parenchymal cells of the liver, the *hepatic cells,* absorb from the blood and store temporarily from one half to three quarters of all the absorbed nutrients. Much intermediary processing of these nutrients occurs in the liver as well. We discuss these nutritional functions of the liver in later chapters.

Figure 42-13 illustrates the special organization of the blood flow through an intestinal villus, showing a small arteriole and venule that interconnect with a system of multiple looping capillaries. The walls of the arterioles are highly muscular, and they are also highly active in controlling villus blood flow.

Effect of Gut Activity and Metabolic Factors on Gastrointestinal Blood Flow

Under normal conditions the blood flow in each area of the gastrointestinal tract, as well as in each layer of the gut wall, is directly related to the level of local activity. For instance, during active absorption, blood flow in the villi and adjacent regions of the submucosa is greatly increased. Likewise, blood flow in the muscle layers of the intestinal wall increases with increased motor activity in the gut. For instance, after a meal the motor activity, secretory activity, and absorptive activity all increase, and likewise the blood flow increases as much as 100 to 150 per cent, usually lasting for 3 to 6 hours.

Possible Causes of the Increased Blood Flow During Activity. Although the precise cause or causes of the increased blood flow during increased gastrointestinal activity are still unclear, some facts are known.

First, several different vasodilator substances are released from the mucosa of the intestinal tract during the digestive process. Most of these are peptide hormones, including *cholecystokinin, vasoactive intestinal peptide, gastrin,* and *secretin.* These same hormones are also important in controlling certain specific motor and secretory activities of the gut, as discussed earlier in this chapter and in the next chapter.

Second, some of the gastrointestinal glands also release into the gut wall two kinins, *kallidin* and *bradykinin,* at the same time that they secrete their secretions into the lumen. These kinins are powerful vasodilators that are believed by some researchers to cause much of the increased mucosal vasodilatation that occurs along with secretion.

Third, *decreased oxygen concentration* in the gut wall can increase intestinal blood flow by as much as 50 per cent; therefore, the increased metabolic rate during gut activity probably lowers the oxygen concentration enough to cause much of the vasodilatation. Maybe it is the lack of enough oxygen to supply the metabolism of the smooth muscle in the vessel walls that is the cause of this vasodilatation. A lack of oxygen can also lead to the release of *adenosine,* by as much as fourfold, which is a well-known vasodilator that could be responsible for much of the increased flow.

Thus, the answer to the increased blood flow during increased gastrointestinal activity is not clear. It is probably a combination of all or many of the above factors plus still others yet undiscovered.

Nervous Control of Gastrointestinal Blood Flow

Stimulation of the parasympathetic nerves to the *stomach* and *lower colon* increases local blood flow at the same time that it increases glandular secretion. However, this increased flow probably results secondarily from the increased glandular activity and not as a direct effect of nervous stimulation.

Sympathetic stimulation, in contrast, has a direct effect in causing intense vasoconstriction of the arterioles with greatly decreased blood flow. However, after a few minutes of this vasoconstriction, the flow returns almost to normal via a mechanism called "autoregulatory escape." That is, the local metabolic vasodilator mechanisms that are elicited by ischemia become prepotent over the sympathetic vasoconstriction and, therefore, redilate the arterioles, thus causing return of necessary nutrient blood flow to the gastrointestinal glands and muscle.

REFERENCES

Berk, J. E., et al.: Bockus Gastroenterology. 4th ed. Philadelphia, W. B. Saunders Co., 1985.
Costa, M., et al.: Histochemistry of the enteric nervous system. In Johnson, L. R. (ed.) Physiology of the Gastrointestinal Tract, 2nd ed. New York, Raven Press, 1987.
Forte, J. G.: Gastrointestinal physiology. Annu. Rev. Physiol., 48:73, 1986.
Gonella, J., et al.: Extrinsic nervous control of motility of small and large intestines and related sphincters. Physiol. Rev. 67:902, 1987.
Hunt, J. N.: Mechanisms and disorders of gastric emptying. Annu. Rev. Med., 34:219, 1983.
Johnson, L. R., et al.: Physiology of the Gastrointestinal Tract, 2nd ed. New York, Raven Press, 1987.
Kirsner, J. B., and Shorter, R. G. (eds.): Diseases of the Colon, Rectum, and Anal Canal. Baltimore, Williams & Wilkins, 1988.
Mei, N.: Intestinal chemosensitivity. Physiol. Rev., 65:211, 1985.
Murphy, R. A.: Muscle cells of hollow organs. News Physiol. Sci., 3:124, 1988.
Shaffer, E., and Thomson, A. B. R. (eds.): Modern Concepts in Gastroenterology. New York, Plenum Publishing Corp., 1989.
Sternini, C.: Structural and chemical organization of the myenteric plexus. Annu. Rev. Physiol., 50:81, 1988.
Thompson, J. C., et al. (eds.): Gastrointestinal Endocrinology. New York, McGraw-Hill Book Co., 1987.

QUESTIONS

1. Describe the layers of the intestinal wall.
2. Give the characteristics of the smooth muscle in the intestinal wall, describing especially the *gap junctions* and their function.
3. Describe the *enteric nervous system,* and discuss its function in local control of gastrointestinal activity.
4. Explain the relationship of the *parasympathetic* and *sympathetic nervous systems* to the enteric nervous system of the gastrointestinal tract.
5. What are the two basic types of movement in the gastrointestinal tract, and what are their purposes?
6. Describe the mechanics of *mastication* and its control by the nervous system.
7. Describe the mechanics of *swallowing,* giving the sequential steps in the swallowing process.
8. Describe the nervous control of swallowing.
9. What is the role of the esophagus in swallowing, and how does the *lower esophageal sphincter* function?
10. What are the characteristics of the movements in the stomach, and how is *chyme* formed?
11. What are the roles of *pyloric tone* and *antral peristalsis* in stomach emptying?
12. Explain the control of stomach emptying by both *stomach factors* and *intestinal factors.*
13. What are the roles of *gastrin,* the *enterogastric reflex,* and the *intestinal hormones* in the control of stomach emptying?
14. Explain the differences between and the functions of the *segmentation contractions* and the *peristaltic movements* of the small intestine.
15. Describe the function of the *ileocecal valve* and its control.
16. Describe the mixing movements (the *haustrations*) and the propulsive movements (*mass movements*) of the colon.
17. Explain the mechanics of *defecation,* neural control of defecation, and function of the *defecation reflex.*
18. Describe the *splanchnic circulation.*
19. Explain the relationship between gastrointestinal blood flow and secretory and motor activity in the gut.

43

Secretory Functions of the Alimentary Tract

Throughout the gastrointestinal tract secretory glands subserve two primary functions: First, digestive enzymes are secreted in most areas from the mouth to the distal end of the ileum. Second, mucous glands, from the mouth to the anus, provide mucus for lubrication and protection of all parts of the alimentary tract.

Most digestive secretions are formed only in response to the presence of food in the alimentary tract, and the quantity secreted in each segment of the tract is almost exactly the amount needed for proper digestion. Furthermore, in some portions of the gastrointestinal tract even the types of enzymes and other constituents of the secretions are varied in accordance with the types of food present. The purpose of the present chapter, therefore, is to describe the different alimentary secretions, their functions, and regulation of their production.

GENERAL PRINCIPLES OF ALIMENTARY TRACT SECRETION

Anatomical Types of Glands

Several types of glands provide the different types of secretions in the alimentary tract. First, on the surface of the epithelium in most parts of the gastrointestinal tract are literally billions of *single cell mucous glands* called simply *mucous cells* or sometimes *goblet cells.* These function mainly by themselves in response to local stimulation of the epithelium, and they simply extrude their mucus directly onto the epithelial surface to act as a lubricant.

Second, many surface areas of the gastrointestinal tract are lined by pits that represent invaginations of the epithelium into the submucosa. In the small intestine these pits, called *crypts of Lieberkühn,* are deep and contain specialized secretory cells.

Third, in the stomach and upper duodenum are found large numbers of long *tubular glands.*

Fourth, also associated with the alimentary tract are several complex glands — the *salivary glands,* the *pancreas,* and the *liver* — which provide secretions for digestion or emulsification of food. These glands lie completely outside the walls of the alimentary tract and, in this, differ from all other alimentary glands.

Basic Mechanism of Secretion by Glandular Cells

Secretion of Organic Substances. The basic principles of secretion by glandular cells, illustrated in Figure 43-1, are:

1. The nutrient material needed for formation of the secretion must diffuse or be actively transported from the capillary into the base of the glandular cell.
2. Many *mitochondria* located inside the cell near its base utilize oxidative energy for formation of adenosine triphosphate (ATP).
3. Energy from the ATP, along with appropriate substrates, is then used for synthesis of the organic substances; this synthesis occurs almost entirely in the *endoplasmic reticulum* and *Golgi complex.* The *ribosomes* adherent to this reticulum are specifically responsible for formation of the proteins that are to be secreted.
4. The secretory materials are transported through the tubules of the endoplasmic reticulum, passing in about 20 minutes all the way to the vesicles of the Golgi complex that lies near the secretory ends of the cells.
5. In the Golgi complex the materials are modified, added to, concentrated, and discharged into the cytoplasm in the form of *secretory vesicles* that

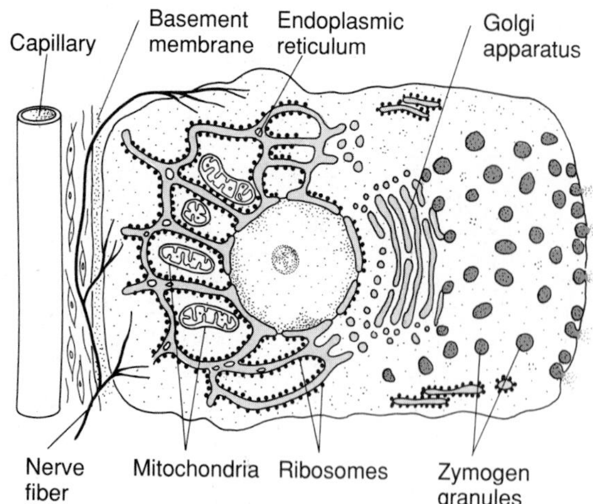

Figure 43-1. Typical function of a glandular cell in formation and secretion of enzymes or other secretory substances.

are stored in the apical ends of the secretory cells.

6. These vesicles remain stored until nervous or hormonal control signals cause them to extrude their contents through the cell's surface. This probably occurs in the following way: The control signal first increases the cell membrane permeability to calcium, and calcium enters the cell. The calcium in turn causes many of the vesicles to fuse with the cell membrane and then to break open on their outer surfaces, thus emptying their contents to the exterior; this process is called *exocytosis.*

Water and Electrolyte Secretion. A second necessity for glandular secretion is sufficient water and electrolytes to be secreted along with the organic substances. The following is a postulated method by which nervous stimulation causes water and salts to pass through the glandular cells in great profusion, which washes the organic substances through the secretory border of the cells at the same time:

1. Nerve stimulation has a specific effect on the *basal* portion of the cell membrane, causing active transport of chloride ions to the interior.
2. The resulting increase in electronegativity inside the cell then causes positive ions also to move to the interior of the cell.
3. The excess of both of these ions inside the cell creates an osmotic force that pulls water to the interior, thereby increasing the hydrostatic pressure inside the cell and causing the cell itself to swell.
4. The pressure in the cell then results in minute ruptures of the secretory border of the cell and causes flushing of water, electrolytes, and organic materials out of the secretory end of the glandular cell and into the lumen of the gland.

Although this mechanism for secretion is still partly theoretical, it does explain how it would be possible for nerve impulses to regulate secretion. Obviously, hormonal effects on the cell membrane could cause similar results.

Lubricating and Protective Properties of Mucus and its Importance in the Gastrointestinal Tract

Mucus is a thick secretion composed mainly of water, electrolytes, and a mixture of several glycoproteins, which themselves are composed of large polysaccharides bound with much smaller quantities of protein. Mucus is both an excellent lubricant and a protectant for the wall of the gut: *First,* mucus has adherent qualities that make it adhere tightly to the food or other particles and also to spread as a thin film over the surfaces. *Second,* it has sufficient *body* that it coats the wall of the gut and prevents actual contact of the food particles with the mucosa. *Third,* mucus has a low resistance for slippage so that the particles can slide along the epithelium with great ease. *Fourth,* mucus causes fecal particles to adhere to each other to form the fecal masses that are expelled during a bowel movement. *Fifth,* mucus is strongly resistant to digestion by the gastrointestinal enzymes. And, *sixth,* the glycoproteins of mucus have amphoteric properties, which means that they are capable of buffering small amounts of either acids or alkalies; also, mucus often contains moderate quantities of bicarbonate ions, which specifically neutralize acids.

In summary, mucus has the ability to allow easy slippage of food along the gastrointestinal tract and also to prevent excoriative or chemical damage to the epithelium.

SECRETION OF SALIVA

The Salivary Glands; Characteristics of Saliva. The principal glands of salivation are the *parotid, submandibular,* and *sublingual* glands; in addition, there are many small *buccal* glands. The daily secretion of saliva normally ranges between about 800 and 1500 milliliters, as shown in Table 43-1.

Saliva contains two major types of protein secretion: (1) a *serous secretion* containing *ptyalin* (an α-amylase), which is an enzyme for digesting starches, and (2) *mucous secretion* containing *mucin* for lubri-

Table 43-1 DAILY SECRETION OF INTESTINAL JUICES

	Daily Volume (ml)	pH
Saliva	1000	6.0–7.0
Gastric secretion	1500	1.0–3.5
Pancreatic secretion	1000	8.0–8.3
Bile	1000	7.8
Small intestinal secretion	1800	7.5–8.0
Brunner's gland secretion	200	8.0–8.9
Large intestinal secretion	200	7.5–8.0
TOTAL	6700	

cating purposes. The parotid glands secrete entirely the serous type, and the submandibular and sublingual glands secrete both the serous type and mucus. The buccal glands secrete only mucus. Saliva has a pH of between 6.0 and 7.4, a favorable range for the digestive action of ptyalin.

Secretion of Ions in the Saliva. Figure 43-2 illustrates secretion by the submaxillary gland, a typical compound gland containing both *acini* and *salivary ducts*. Salivary secretion is a two-stage operation: the first stage involves the acini; and the second, the salivary ducts. The acini secrete a *primary secretion* that contains ptyalin and/or mucin in a solution of ions in concentrations not greatly different from those of typical extracellular fluid. However, as the primary secretion flows through the ducts, two major active transport processes take place that markedly modify the ionic composition of the saliva.

First, *sodium ions* are actively reabsorbed from all of the salivary ducts; and *potassium ions* are actively secreted, in exchange for the sodium. Therefore, the sodium concentration of the saliva becomes greatly reduced, whereas the potassium ion concentration becomes increased. The great excess of sodium reabsorption over potassium secretion creates negativity of about −70 millivolts in the salivary ducts, and this causes chloride ions to be reabsorbed passively; therefore, the chloride ion concentration falls to a very low level along with the decrease in sodium ion concentration.

Second, *bicarbonate ions* are secreted by the ductal epithelium into the lumen of the duct. This is partly caused by exchange of bicarbonate for chloride ions, but it may also result partly from an active secretory process.

The net result of these active transport processes is that *under resting conditions,* the concentrations of sodium and chloride ions in the saliva are only about 15 mEq/liter each, approximately one seventh to one tenth their concentrations in plasma. On the other hand, the concentration of potassium ions is about 30 mEq/liter, seven times as great as the concentration in plasma; and the concentration of bicarbonate ions is 50 to 70 mEq/liter, about two to three times that of plasma.

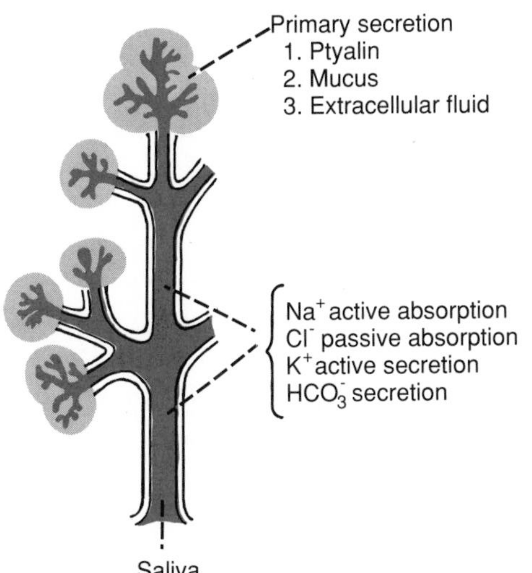

Figure 43-2. Formation and secretion of saliva by a salivary gland.

During maximal salivation, the salivary ionic concentrations change considerably because the rate of formation of primary secretion by the acini can increase as much as 20-fold. As a result, this secretion then flows through the ducts so rapidly that the ductal reconditioning of the secretion is considerably reduced. Therefore, when copious quantities of saliva are secreted, the sodium chloride concentration rises to about one half to two thirds that of plasma, whereas the potassium concentration falls to only four times that of plasma.

Because of the high potassium ion concentration of saliva, in any abnormal state in which the saliva is lost to the exterior of the body for long periods of time, a person can develop serious depletion of potassium ions in the body, leading eventually to serious hypokalemia and paralysis.

Function of Saliva for Oral Hygiene. Under basal conditions, about 0.5 ml/min of saliva, almost entirely of the mucous type, is secreted all the time except during sleep, when the secretion becomes very little. This secretion plays an exceedingly important role in maintaining healthy oral tissues. The mouth is loaded with pathogenic bacteria that can easily destroy tissues and can also cause dental caries. However, saliva helps prevent the deteriorative processes in several ways: *First,* the flow of saliva itself helps wash away the pathogenic bacteria, as well as the food particles that provide their metabolic support. *Second,* the saliva also contains several factors that actually destroy bacteria. One of these is *thiocyanate ions* and another is several *proteolytic enzymes* that (1) attack the bacteria; (2) aid the thiocyanate ions in entering the bacteria, where they in turn become bactericidal; and (3) digest food particles, thus helping further to remove the bacterial metabolic support. And, *third,* saliva often contains significant amounts of protein antibodies that can destroy oral bacteria, including those that cause dental caries.

Therefore, in the absence of salivation, the oral tissues become ulcerated and otherwise infected, and caries of the teeth becomes rampant.

Nervous Regulation of Salivary Secretion. Figure 43-3 illustrates the parasympathetic nervous pathways for regulation of salivation, showing that the salivary glands are controlled mainly by *parasympathetic nervous signals* from the *salivatory nuclei.* The salivatory nuclei are located approximately at the juncture of the medulla and pons and are excited by both taste and tactile stimuli from the tongue and other areas of the mouth. Many taste stimuli, especially the sour taste, elicit copious secretion of saliva —often as much as 5 to 8 ml/min, or 8 to 20 times the basal rate of secretion. Also, certain tactile stimuli, such as the presence of smooth objects in the mouth (a pebble, for instance), cause marked salivation; whereas rough objects cause less salivation and occasionally even inhibit salivation.

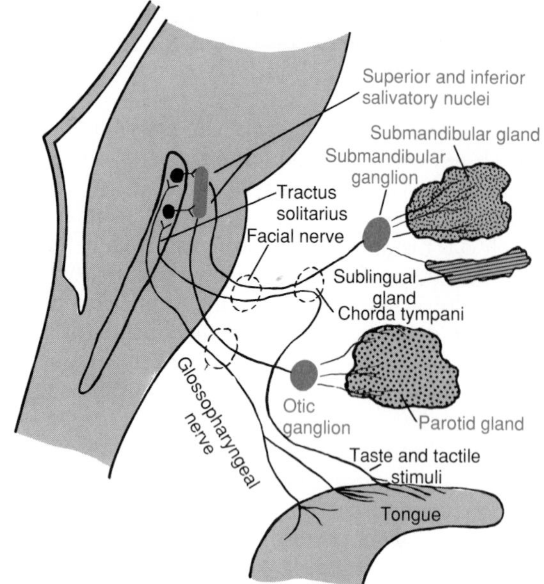

Figure 43-3. Parasympathetic nervous regulation of salivary secretion.

Salivation can also be stimulated or inhibited by impulses arriving in the salivatory nuclei from higher centers of the central nervous system. For instance, when a person smells or eats favorite foods, salivation is greater than when disliked food is smelled or eaten.

Salivation also occurs in response to reflexes originating in the stomach and upper intestines—particularly when very irritating foods are swallowed or when a person is nauseated because of some gastrointestinal abnormality. The swallowed saliva usually helps remove the irritating factor in the gastrointestinal tract by diluting or neutralizing the irritating substances.

ESOPHAGEAL SECRETION

The esophageal secretions are entirely mucoid in character and principally provide lubrication for swallowing. The main body of the esophagus is lined with many *simple mucous glands;* but at the gastric end, and to a lesser extent in the initial portion of the esophagus, there are many *compound mucous glands.* The mucus secreted by the compound glands near the esophagogastric junction protects the esophageal wall from digestion by gastric juices that flow back into the lower esophagus.

GASTRIC SECRETION

Characteristics of the Gastric Secretions

In addition to mucus-secreting cells that line the entire surface of the stomach, the stomach mucosa has two important types of tubular glands: the *oxyntic* (or *gastric*) *glands* and the *pyloric glands.* The oxyntic (acid-forming) glands secrete *hydrochloric acid, pepsinogen, intrinsic factor,* and *mucus,* and the pyloric glands secrete mainly *mucus* for protection of the pyloric mucosa but also some *pepsinogen* and, very important, the hormone *gastrin.* Millions of oxyntic glands are located on the inside surfaces of the body of the stomach, comprising the proximal 80 per cent of the stomach; and the pyloric glands are located in the antral portion of the stomach.

The Secretions from the Oxyntic Glands

A typical oxyntic gland is shown in Figure 43-4. It is composed of three different types of cells: the *mucous neck cells,* which secrete mainly mucus but also some pepsinogen; the *peptic* (or *chief*) *cells,* which secrete large quantities of pepsinogen; and the *parietal* (or *oxyntic*) *cells,* which secrete hydrochloric acid and intrinsic factor.

Basic Mechanism of Hydrochloric Acid Secretion. When stimulated, the parietal cells secrete an acid solution containing about 160 millimoles of hydrochloric acid per liter. The pH of this acid is approximately 0.8, illustrating its extreme acidity. At this pH the hydrogen ion concentration is about 3 million times that of the arterial blood. And to concentrate the hydrogen ions this tremendous amount requires over 1500 calories of energy per liter of gastric juice.

Figure 43-5 illustrates the basic structure of a parietal cell, showing that it contains several large *intracellular canaliculi* that empty directly into the lumen of the oxyntic gland. The hydrochloric acid is formed at the villuslike membranes of these canaliculi and is then conducted to the exterior.

Different suggestions for the precise mechanism of hydrochloric acid formation have been offered. One of these is illustrated in Figure 43-6 and consists of the following steps:

1. Chloride ion is actively transported from the cytoplasm of the parietal cell into the lumen of the canaliculus, and sodium ions are actively transported out of the lumen. These two effects together create a negative potential of −40 to −70 millivolts in the canaliculus, which in turn

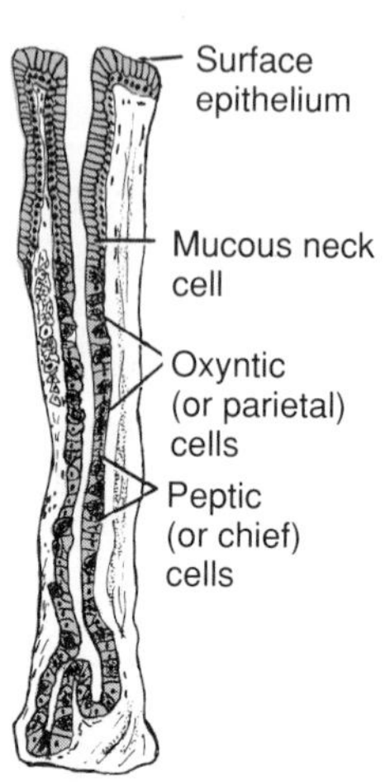

Figure 43-4. An oxyntic gland from the body or fundus of the stomach.

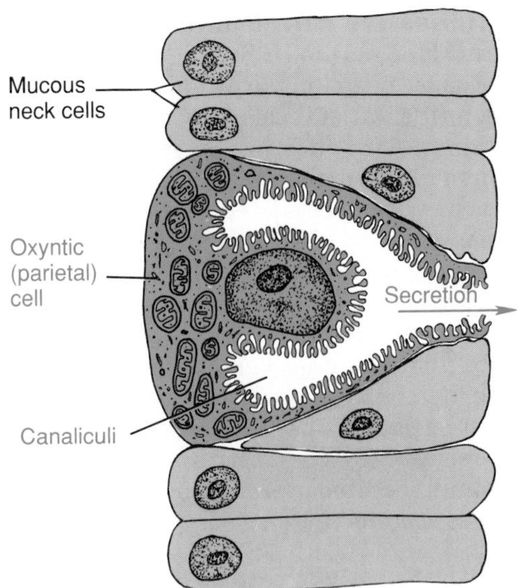

Figure 43-5. Anatomy of the canaliculi in a parietal (oxyntic) cell.

causes passive diffusion of positively charged potassium ions and a small number of sodium ions from the cell cytoplasm also into the canaliculus. Thus, in effect, potassium chloride and much smaller amounts of sodium chloride enter the canaliculus.

2. Water is dissociated into hydrogen ions and hydroxyl ions in the cell cytoplasm. The hydrogen ions are then actively secreted into the canaliculus in exchange for potassium ions; this active exchange process being catalyzed by H^+,K^+-ATPase. In addition, the sodium ions are actively reabsorbed by a separate sodium pump. Thus, most of the potassium and sodium ions that had diffused into the canaliculus are reabsorbed, and hydrogen ions take their place, giving a very strong solution of hydrochloric acid.
3. Water passes through the cell and into the canaliculus by osmosis. Thus the final secretion entering the canaliculus contains hydrochloric acid in a concentration of 155 mEq/liter, potassium chloride in a concentration of 15 mEq/liter, and a very small amount of sodium chloride.

Secretion and Activation of Pepsinogen. Several different types of pepsinogen are secreted by the peptic and mucous cells of the gastric glands. Even so, all the pepsinogens perform essentially the same functions. When the pepsinogens are first secreted, they have no digestive activity. However, as soon as they come in contact with hydrochloric acid, and especially when they come in contact with previously formed pepsin plus the hydrochloric acid, they are immediately activated to form active *pepsin.* In this process, the pepsinogen molecule, having a molecular weight of about 42,500, is split to form the pepsin molecule, having a molecular weight of about 35,000.

Pepsin is an active proteolytic enzyme in a highly acid medium (optimum pH 1.8 to 3.5), but above a pH of about 5 it has little proteolytic activity and even becomes completely inactivated in a short time. Therefore, hydrochloric acid is as necessary as pepsin for protein digestion in the stomach; this is discussed in the following chapter.

Secretion of Intrinsic Factor. The substance *intrinsic factor,* essential for absorption of vitamin B_{12} in the ileum, is secreted by the *parietal cells* along with the secretion of hydrochloric acid. Therefore, when the acid-producing cells of the stomach are destroyed, which frequently occurs in chronic gastritis, the person not only develops *achlorhydria* but also develops *pernicious anemia* because of failure of maturation of the red blood cells in the absence of vitamin B_{12} stimulation of the bone marrow. This was discussed in Chapter 24.

Regulation of Gastric Secretion by Nervous and Hormonal Mechanisms

Stimulation of Acid Secretion

Nervous Stimulation. About half the nerve signals to the stomach that cause gastric secretion origi-

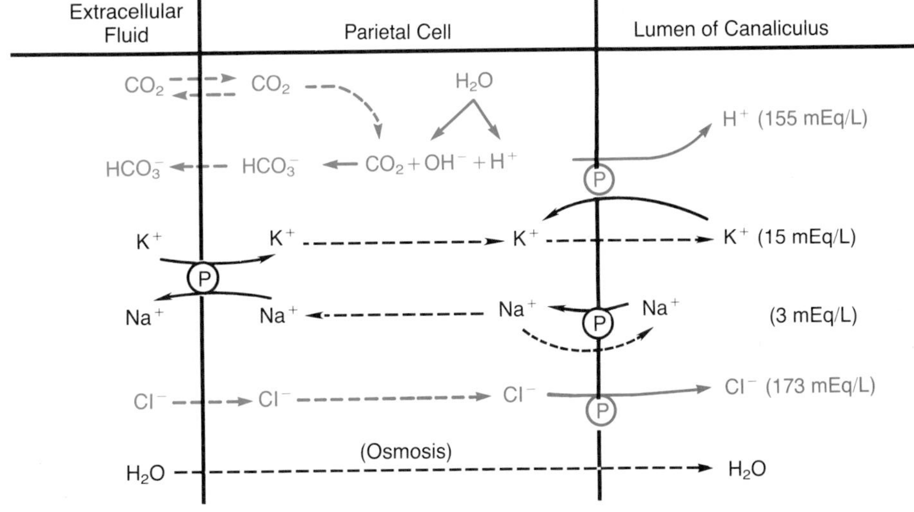

Figure 43-6. Postulated mechanism for the secretion of hydrochloric acid.

nate in the *dorsal motor nuclei of the vagi* and pass via the *vagus nerves* first to the *enteric nervous system* of the stomach wall and then to the gastric glands. The other half of the secretory signals is generated by local reflexes that occur entirely within the enteric nervous system itself. Most of the secretory nerves release *acetylcholine* as the neurotransmitter at their endings on the glandular cells.

Nerve stimulation of gastric secretion can be initiated by signals that originate either in the brain, especially in the limbic system, or in the stomach itself. The types of stimuli that can initiate the intrinsic stomach reflexes are (1) distention of the stomach, (2) tactile stimuli on the surface of the stomach mucosa, and (3) chemical stimuli, including especially *amino acids* derived from protein foods and *acid* that has already been secreted by the gastric glands.

Stimulation of Acid Secretion by Gastrin. Both the nerve signals from the vagus nerves and those from the local enteric reflexes, aside from causing direct stimulation of glandular secretion of stomach juices, also cause the mucosa in the stomach antrum to secrete the hormone *gastrin.* This hormone is a peptide secreted by the *gastrin cells,* in the pyloric glands. It is absorbed into the blood and carried to the *oxyntic glands* in the body of the stomach; there it stimulates the *parietal cells* very strongly and perhaps the peptic cells as well, but to a lesser extent. Thus, the really important effect is to increase the rate of hydrochloric acid secretion, often by as much as eight times.

Role of Histamine in Controlling Gastric Secretion. *Histamine,* an amino acid derivative, also stimulates acid secretion by the *parietal cells.* A small amount of histamine is formed continually in the gastric mucosa, either in response to acid in the stomach or for other reasons. This amount, acting by itself, causes very little acid secretion. However, whenever acetylcholine or gastrin stimulates the parietal cells at the same time, then even the small normal amounts of histamine greatly enhance acid secretion. We know this to be true because when the action of histamine is blocked by an appropriate antihistaminic drug such as cimetidine, neither acetylcholine nor gastrin can then cause significant amounts of acid secretion. Thus, histamine is a necessary *co-factor* for exciting acid secretion.

Multiplicative Effect of Acetylcholine, Gastrin, and Histamine in Stimulating Acid Secretion. Because no one of the primary stimulators of the acid-secreting parietal cells—acetylcholine, gastrin, or histamine—is effective in causing secretion of more than slight amounts of acid when functioning alone, it has been postulated that all three of the receptors to these separate transmitter-hormonal substances must be activated simultaneously to give a truly effective stimulus for gastric acid secretion. The histamine seems to be always present in small amounts under normal conditions. Then when the stomach nerves are stimulated, acetylcholine is released at the parasympathetic nerve endings, and gastrin is released by the gastrin cells. Therefore, all three stimuli become available, and copious amounts of acid are secreted.

Regulation of Pepsinogen Secretion

Regulation of *pepsinogen* secretion is much less complex than that of acid secretion; it occurs in response to two types of signals: (1) stimulation of the *peptic cells* by *acetylcholine* released from the *vagus nerves* or other enteric nerves and (2) stimulation of peptic secretion in response to acid in the stomach. In fact, the rate of secretion of *pepsinogen* is strongly influenced by the amount of acid in the stomach. In persons who have lost the ability to secrete large amounts of acid, the secretion of pepsinogen is very little, even though the peptic cells may still be normal.

Feedback Inhibition of Gastric Secretion by Excess Acid. When the acidity of the gastric juices increases to a pH of 3.0, the gastrin mechanism for stimulating gastric secretion becomes blocked. This obviously protects the stomach against excessive acidity, which would promote peptic ulceration. In addition to this protective effect, the feedback mechanism is also important in maintaining optimal pH for function of the peptic enzymes in the digestive process, which is a pH of about 3.0.

Chemical Composition of Gastrin and Other Gastrointestinal Hormones

Figure 43-7 illustrates the amino acid compositions of *gastrin-17* and also of *cholecystokinin* and *se-*

Gastrin:

Glu- Gly- Pro- Trp- Leu- Glu- Glu- Glu- Glu- Glu- Ala- Tyr- Gly- Trp- Met- Asp- Phe- NH_2
(Tyr: HSO_3)

Cholecystokinin:

Lys- (Ala, Gly, Pro, Ser)- Arg- Val- (Ile, Met, Ser)- Lys- Asn- (Asn, Gln, His, Leu_2,
Pro, Ser_2)- Arg- Ile- (Asp, Ser)- Arg- Asp- Tyr- Met- Gly- Trp- Met- Asp- Phe- NH_2
(Tyr: HSO_3)

Secretin:

His- Ser- Asp- Gly- Thr- Phe- Thr- Ser- Glu- Leu- Ser- Arg- Leu- Arg- Asp- Ser-
Ala- Arg- Leu- Gln- Arg- Leu- Leu- Gln- Gly- Leu- Val- NH_2

Figure 43-7. Amino acid composition of gastrin-17, cholecystokinin, and secretin.

cretin, which will be discussed later in the chapter. Note that all are polypeptides and that the terminal five amino acids in the gastrin and cholecystokinin molecular chains are exactly the same. The activity of gastrin resides in the terminal four amino acids and in the terminal eight amino acids for cholecystokinin; all of the amino acids in the secretin molecule are essential. A synthetic gastrin, composed of the terminal four amino acids of natural gastrins plus the amino acid alanine, has all the same physiological properties as the natural gastrins and is sometimes used clinically to enhance stomach acid secretion. This synthetic product is called *pentagastrin.*

PANCREATIC SECRETION

The pancreas, which lies parallel to and beneath the stomach, is a large compound gland with an internal structure similar to that of the salivary glands. Digestive enzymes are secreted by the pancreatic acini, and large volumes of sodium bicarbonate solution are secreted by both the small ductules and the larger ducts leading from the acini. The combined product then flows through a long pancreatic duct that usually joins the hepatic duct immediately before it empties into the duodenum through the sphincter of Oddi. Pancreatic juice is secreted most abundantly in response to the presence of chyme in the upper portions of the small intestine, and the characteristics of the pancreatic juice are determined to some extent by the types of food in the chyme.

In addition to secreting pancreatic juice into the duodenum, the pancreas is also the focus of many thousands of cellular masses, the *islets of Langerhans,* that secrete insulin into the blood. This will be discussed in Chapter 52.

Secretion of the Pancreatic Digestive Enzymes

Pancreatic juice contains enzymes for digesting all three major types of food: proteins, carbohydrates, and fats. It also contains large quantities of bicarbonate ions, which play an important role in neutralizing the acid chyme emptied by the stomach into the duodenum.

The more important of the proteolytic enzymes are *trypsin, chymotrypsin,* and *carboxypolypeptidase.* By far the most abundant of these is trypsin. The trypsin and chymotrypsin split whole and partially digested proteins into peptides of various sizes, but these do not cause the release of individual amino acids. On the other hand, carboxypolypeptidase splits the peptides into individual amino acids, thus completing the digestion of much of the proteins all the way to the amino acid state.

The digestive enzyme for carbohydrates is *pancreatic amylase,* which hydrolyzes starches, glycogen, and most other carbohydrates (except cellulose) to form disaccharides and a few trisaccharides.

The main enzymes for fat digestion are *pancreatic lipase,* which is capable of hydrolyzing neutral fat into fatty acids and monoglycerides, *cholesterol esterase,* which causes hydrolysis of cholesterol esters, and *phospholipase,* which splits fatty acids from phospholipids.

When synthesized in the pancreatic cells, the proteolytic enzymes are in the inactive forms of *trypsinogen, chymotrypsinogen,* and *procarboxypolypeptidase,* which are all enzymatically inactive. These become activated only after they are secreted into the intestinal tract. Trypsinogen is activated by an enzyme called *enterokinase,* which is secreted by the intestinal mucosa when chyme comes in contact with the mucosa. Then chymotrypsinogen is activated by trypsin to form chymotrypsin, and procarboxypolypeptidase is activated in a similar manner.

Secretion of Trypsin Inhibitor. It is important that the proteolytic enzymes of the pancreatic juice not become activated until they have been secreted into the intestine, for the trypsin and other enzymes would digest the pancreas itself. Fortunately, the same cells that secrete the proteolytic enzymes secrete simultaneously another substance called *trypsin inhibitor.* This substance is stored in the cytoplasm of the glandular cells surrounding the enzyme granules, and it prevents activation of trypsin both inside the secretory cells and in the acini and ducts of the pancreas. Because it is trypsin that activates the other pancreatic proteolytic enzymes, trypsin inhibitor also prevents the subsequent activation of all of these enzymes as well.

However, when the pancreas becomes severely damaged or when a duct becomes blocked, large quantities of pancreatic secretion become pooled in the damaged areas of the pancreas. Under these conditions, the effect of trypsin inhibitor is sometimes overwhelmed, in which case the pancreatic secretions rapidly become activated and literally digest the entire pancreas within a few hours, giving rise to the condition called *acute pancreatitis.* This often is lethal because of accompanying shock; and even if not lethal, it can lead to a lifetime of pancreatic insufficiency.

Secretion of Bicarbonate Ions

Although the enzymes of the pancreatic juice are secreted entirely by the acini of the pancreatic glands, the other two important components of pancreatic juice, bicarbonate ions and water, are secreted in large amounts mainly by the epithelial cells of the ductules and ducts leading from the acini. We shall see later that the stimulatory mechanisms for (1) enzyme production and (2) production of bicarbonate ions and water are also quite different. When the pancreas is stimulated to secrete copious quantities of pancreatic juice, the bicarbonate ion concentration can rise to as high as 145 mEq/liter, a value approximately five times that of bicarbonate ions in the plasma. Obviously, this provides a large quantity of alkali in the pancreatic juice that serves to neutralize acid emptied into the duodenum from the stomach.

Regulation of Pancreatic Secretion

Four basic stimuli are important in causing pancreatic secretion:

1. *Acetylcholine,* which is released from the parasympathetic vagus nerve endings as well as from other cholinergic nerves in the enteric nervous system.
2. *Gastrin,* which is liberated in copious quantities during the gastric phase of stomach secretion.
3. *Cholecystokinin (CCK),* which is secreted by the duodenal and upper jejunal mucosa when food enters the small intestine.
4. *Secretin,* which is secreted by the same duodenal and jejunal mucosa when highly acid food enters the small intestine.

The first three of the above stimuli, acetylcholine, gastrin, and cholecystokinin, all stimulate the acinar cells of the pancreas much more than the ductal cells. Therefore, they cause the production of large quantities of digestive enzymes but relatively small quantities of fluid to go with the enzymes. Without the fluid, most of the enzymes remain temporarily stored in the acini and ducts until more fluid secretion comes along to wash them into the duodenum.

Secretin, in contrast to the other three basic stimuli, mainly stimulates the secretion of large quantities of sodium bicarbonate solution by the ductal epithelium, but there is almost no stimulation of enzyme secretion.

Stimulation of Secretion of Copious Quantities of Bicarbonate by Secretin — Neutralization of the Acidic Chyme. Secretin is a polypeptide containing 27 amino acids that is present in so-called *S cells* in the mucosa of the upper small intestine (duodenum and upper jejunum) in an inactive form called *prosecretin.* When acid enters the intestine from the stomach, it causes the release and activation of secretin, which is subsequently absorbed into the blood.

Secretin causes the pancreas to secrete large quantities of fluid containing a high concentration of bicarbonate ion (up to 145 mEq/liter) but a low concentration of chloride ion. However, this fluid contains very little enzymes when the pancreas is stimulated only by secretin because secretin does not stimulate the acinar cells.

The secretin mechanism is especially important for two reasons: *First,* secretin begins to be released from the mucosa of the small intestine when the pH of the duodenal contents falls below 4.5; then its release increases very greatly as the pH falls to 3.0 and as more and more acid reaches deeper into the duodenum and jejunum. This immediately causes large quantities of pancreatic juice containing abundant amounts of sodium bicarbonate to be secreted, which results in the following reaction with hydrochloric acid in the duodenum:

$$HCl + NaHCO_3 \rightarrow NaCl + H_2CO_3$$

The carbonic acid that is formed immediately dissociates into carbon dioxide and water, and the carbon dioxide is absorbed into the blood and expired through the lungs, thus leaving a neutral solution of sodium chloride in the duodenum. In this way, the acid contents emptied into the duodenum from the stomach become neutralized, and the peptic activity of the gastric juices is immediately blocked. Because the mucosa of the small intestine cannot withstand the digestive action of acid gastric juice, this is a highly important and even essential protective mechanism against the development of duodenal ulcers, discussed in further detail in the following chapter.

Second, bicarbonate secretion by the pancreas provides an appropriate pH for action of the pancreatic enzymes. All of these function optimally in a slightly alkaline or neutral medium. The pH of the sodium bicarbonate secretion averages 8.0.

Cholecystokinin — Control of Enzyme Secretion by the Pancreas. The presence of food in the upper small intestine also causes a second hormone, cholecystokinin, a polypeptide containing 33 amino acids, to be released from a still different group of cells in the mucosa of the duodenum and upper jejunum. This results especially from the presence of *proteoses* and *peptones,* which are products of partial protein digestion, and of *long chain fatty acids.* Cholecystokinin, like secretin, passes by way of the blood to the pancreas but, instead of causing sodium bicarbonate secretion, causes secretion of large quantities of the pancreatic digestive enzymes by the acinar cells, an effect similar to the effects of acetylcholine from the vagus nerves and of gastrin but even more pronounced.

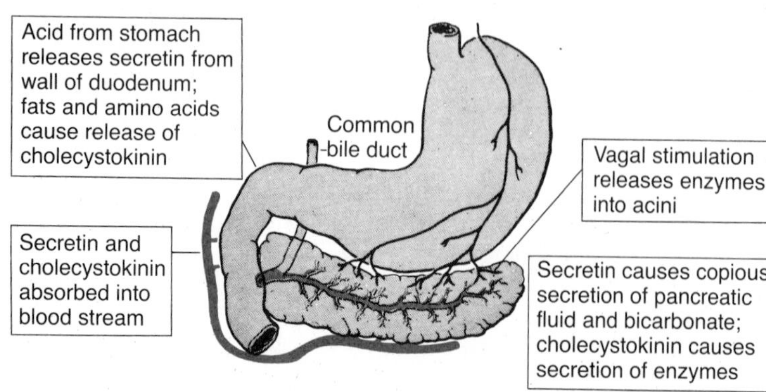

Figure 43-8. Regulation of pancreatic secretion.

Figure 43–8 summarizes the more important factors in the regulation of pancreatic secretion. The total amount secreted each day is about 1000 milliliters.

SECRETION OF BILE AND FUNCTIONS OF THE BILIARY TREE

One of the many functions of the liver is to secrete bile, normally between 600 and 1200 ml/day. Bile serves two important functions: *First,* it plays a very important role in fat digestion and absorption, not because of any enzymes in the bile that cause fat digestion, but instead because bile acids contained in the bile do two things: (1) they help to emulsify the large fat particles of the food into many minute particles that can be attacked by the lipases secreted in pancreatic juice, and (2) they aid in the transport and absorption of the digested fat end-products to and through the intestinal mucosal membrane. *Second,* bile serves as a means for excretion of several important waste products from the blood. These include especially *bilirubin,* an end-product of hemoglobin destruction, and excesses of *cholesterol* synthesized by the liver cells.

Physiological Anatomy of Biliary Secretion

Bile is secreted in two stages by the liver: (1) Initial bile is secreted by the liver hepatocytes; this initial secretion contains large amounts of bile acids and cholesterol secreted into the minute *bile canaliculi* that lie between the hepatic cells in the hepatic plates. (2) Next, the bile flows peripherally toward the interlobular septa, where the canaliculi empty into *terminal bile ducts,* then into progressively larger ducts, finally reaching the *hepatic duct* and *common bile duct,* from which the bile either empties directly into the duodenum or is diverted through the *cystic duct* into the gallbladder, illustrated in Figure 43–9. In its course through these bile ducts, a secondary secretion is added to the initial bile. This additional secretion is a watery solution of sodium and bicarbonate ions, and it sometimes increases the total quantity of bile by as much as an additional 100 per cent. The secondary secretion is stimulated by secretin, thus causing increased quantities of bicarbonate ions that supplement the pancreatic secretions in neutralizing acid from the stomach.

Storage of Bile in the Gallbladder. The bile secreted continually by the liver cells is normally stored in the gallbladder until needed in the duodenum. The maximal volume of the gallbladder is only 20 to 60 milliliters. Nevertheless, as much as 12 hours' bile secretion (usually about 450 milliliters) can be stored in the gallbladder because water, sodium, chloride, and most other small electrolytes are continually absorbed by the gallbladder mucosa, concentrating the other bile constituents, including the bile salts. Most of this absorption is caused by active transport of sodium through the gallbladder epithelium. Bile is normally concentrated about 5-fold, but it can be concentrated up to a maximum of 12- to 20-fold.

By far the most abundant substance secreted in the bile is the *bile salts,* accounting for about half the total solutes of bile, but also secreted or excreted in large

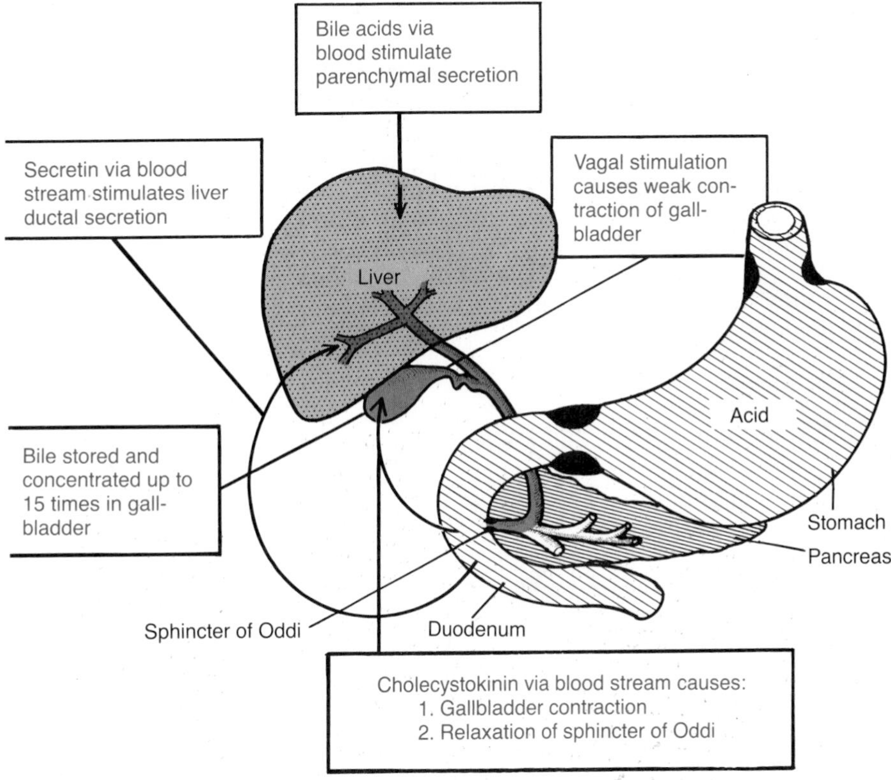

Figure 43–9. Liver secretion and gallbladder emptying.

concentrations are *bilirubin, cholesterol, lecithin,* and the usual *electrolytes* of plasma. In the concentrating process in the gallbladder, water and large portions of the electrolytes (except calcium ions) are reabsorbed by the gallbladder mucosa; but essentially all the other constituents, including especially the bile salts, the lipid substances cholesterol and lecithin, and bilirubin, are not reabsorbed and therefore become highly concentrated in the gallbladder bile.

Emptying of the Gallbladder — Role of Cholecystokinin. When food begins to be digested in the upper gastrointestinal tract, the gallbladder begins to empty, especially as fatty foods enter the duodenum. By far the most potent stimulus for causing the gallbladder contractions is the hormone *cholecystokinin.* This is the same cholecystokinin that causes increased secretion of enzymes by the acinar cells of the pancreas. And the stimulus for its release into the blood from the duodenal mucosa is mainly fatty foods entering the duodenum.

Yet even with relatively strong contractions of the gallbladder, emptying can still be difficult because the sphincter of Oddi normally remains tonically contracted. Therefore, before emptying will occur, it, too, must be relaxed. At least three different factors help in this: First, cholecystokinin itself has a weak relaxing effect; but this effect is usually not sufficient by itself to allow significant emptying. Second, rhythmic contractions of the gallbladder transmit peristaltic waves down the common bile duct to the sphincter of Oddi, causing a leading wave of relaxation that partially inhibits the sphincter in advance of the peristaltic wave. Third, when intestinal peristaltic waves travel over the wall of the duodenum, the relaxation phase of each of these waves strongly relaxes the sphincter of Oddi along with the relaxation of the muscle of the gut wall. As a result, bile usually enters the duodenum in the form of squirts that are synchronized with the duodenal peristaltic contractions.

In summary, the gallbladder empties its store of concentrated bile into the duodenum mainly in response to the cholecystokinin stimulus. When fat is not in the meal, the gallbladder empties poorly; but when adequate quantities of fat are present, the gallbladder empties completely in about 1 hour.

Figure 43-9 summarizes the secretion of bile, its storage in the gallbladder, and its release from the bladder to the gut.

The Bile Salts and Their Function

The liver cells form about 10 grams of *bile salts* daily. The precursor of the bile salts is *cholesterol,* which is either supplied in the diet or synthesized in the liver cells during the course of fat metabolism and then converted to *cholic acid* or *chenodeoxycholic acid* in about equal quantities. These acids then combine principally with glycine and to a lesser extent with taurine to form *glyco-* and *tauro-conjugated bile acids.* The salts of these acids are secreted in the bile.

The bile salts have two important actions in the intestinal tract. First, they have a detergent action on the fat particles in the food, which decreases the surface tension of the particles and allows the agitation in the intestinal tract to break the fat globules into minute sizes. This is called the *emulsifying* or *detergent function* of bile salts. Second, and even more important than the emulsifying function, bile salts help in the absorption of fatty acids, monoglycerides, cholesterol, and other lipids from the intestinal tract. They do this by forming minute complexes with these lipids; the complexes are called *micelles,* and they are highly soluble because of the electrical charges of the bile salts. The lipids are "ferried" in this form to the mucosa, where they are then absorbed; this mechanism is described in detail in the following chapter. Without the presence of bile salts in the intestinal tract, up to 40 per cent of the lipids are lost into the stool, and the person often develops a metabolic deficit due to this nutrient loss.

Secretion of Cholesterol; Gallstone Formation

Bile salts are formed in the hepatic cells from cholesterol, and in the process of secreting the bile salts about one tenth as much cholesterol is also secreted into the bile. This amounts to a total of 1 to 2 grams a day. No specific function is known for the cholesterol in the bile, and it is presumed that it is simply a by-product of bile salt formation and secretion.

Cholesterol is almost insoluble in pure water, but the bile salts and lecithin in bile combine physically with the cholesterol to form ultramicroscopic *micelles* that are soluble, as is explained in more detail in the following chapter.

Nevertheless, under abnormal conditions the cholesterol may precipitate, resulting in the formation of *cholesterol gallstones,* as shown in Figure 43-10. Unfortunately, the stones often block the bile ducts and cause loss of the hepatic secretions to the gut — and

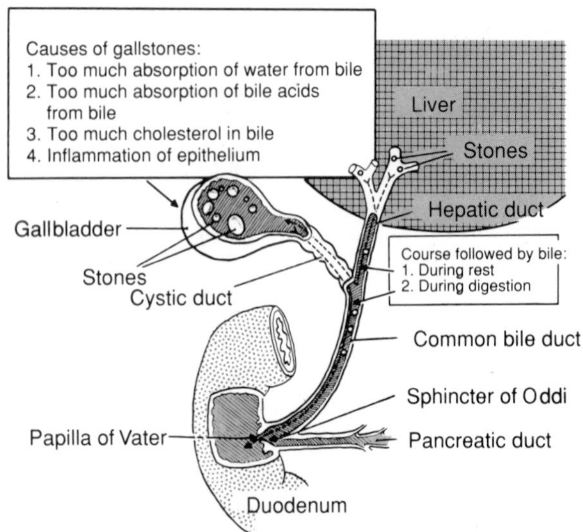

Figure 43-10. Formation of gallstones.

also cause severe pain in the gallbladder region as well. The different conditions that can cause cholesterol precipitation are (1) too much absorption of water from the bile, (2) too much absorption of bile salts and lecithin from the bile, (3) too much secretion of cholesterol in the bile, and (4) inflammation of the epithelium of the gallbladder. The latter two of these require special explanation.

The amount of cholesterol in the bile is determined partly by the quantity of fat that the person eats, for the hepatic cells synthesize cholesterol as one of the products of fat metabolism in the body. For this reason, persons on a high fat diet over a period of many years are prone to the development of gallstones.

Inflammation of the gallbladder epithelium often results from low grade chronic infection; this changes the absorptive characteristics of the gallbladder mucosa, sometimes allowing excessive absorption of water, bile salts, or other substances that are necessary to keep the cholesterol in solution. As a result, cholesterol begins to precipitate, usually forming many small crystals of cholesterol on the surface of the inflamed mucosa. These, in turn, act as nidi for further precipitation of cholesterol, and the crystals grow larger forming stones. Also, calcium ions, which are usually concentrated fivefold or more in the gallbladder, often precipitate in the gallstones, making the stones x-ray-opaque so that they can be seen in x-ray films of the abdomen.

SECRETIONS OF THE SMALL INTESTINE

Secretion of Mucus by Brunner's Glands

An extensive array of compound mucous glands, called *Brunner's glands,* is located in the wall of the first few centimeters of the duodenum, mainly between the pylorus and the papilla of Vater where the pancreatic juices and bile empty into the duodenum. These glands secrete mucus in response to (1) tactile stimuli or irritating stimuli of the overlying mucosa; (2) vagal stimulation, which causes secretion concurrently with increase in stomach secretion; and (3) gastrointestinal hormones, especially secretin. The function of the mucus secreted by Brunner's glands is to protect the duodenal wall from digestion by the gastric juice, and their rapid and intense response to irritating stimuli is especially geared to this purpose.

Secretion of the Intestinal Digestive Juices—The Crypts of Lieberkühn

Located on the entire surface of the small intestine are small pits called *crypts of Lieberkühn,* one of which is illustrated in Figure 43-11. The intestinal secretions are formed by the epithelial cells in these crypts at a rate of about 1800 ml/day. The secretions are almost pure extracellular fluid and have a slightly alkaline pH in the range of 7.5 to 8.0. They are rapidly reabsorbed by the villi. This circulation of fluid from the crypts to the villi obviously supplies a watery vehicle for absorption of substances from the chyme as it comes in contact with the villi, which is one of the primary functions of the small intestine.

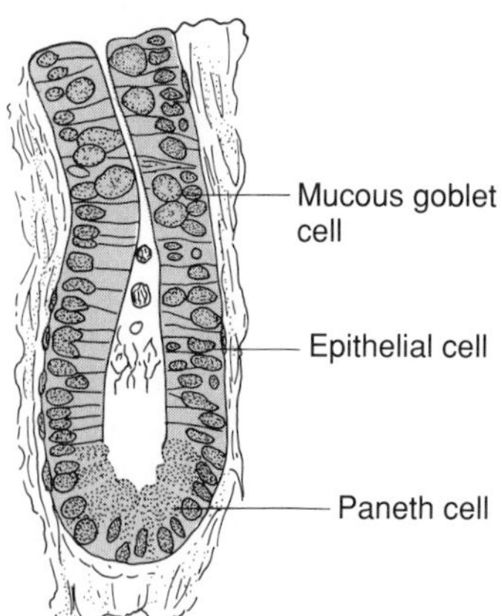

Figure 43-11. A crypt of Lieberkühn, found in all parts of the small intestine between the villi, which secretes almost pure extracellular fluid.

Mechanism of Secretion of the Watery Fluid. The exact mechanism causing the marked secretion of watery fluid by the crypts of Lieberkühn is not known. However, it is believed to involve at least two active secretory processes: (1) active secretion of chloride ions into the crypts and (2) active secretion of bicarbonate ions. The secretion of these ions, especially the chloride ions, causes electrical drag of sodium ions through the membrane as well. Finally, all these ions together cause osmotic movement of water.

Effect of Cholera Toxin on Intestinal Secretion. Cholera toxin causes an extreme rate of fluid secretion into the crypts of Lieberkühn, especially in the jejunal region of the small intestine. During the first day of a cholera infection, as much as 5 to 10 liters of diarrhea fluid can be lost from the bowels, often leading to circulatory shock caused by dehydration, and culminating in death within a few hours. Fortunately, though, most cases of cholera can be treated successfully simply by administering large amounts of saline and glucose solutions, either by mouth or intravenously.

The cholera toxin seems to have a specific effect in increasing active transport of chloride ions into the crypts of Lieberkühn; this in turn leads to the massive loss of fluid into the intestinal tract. Several other bacterial diseases of the intestines can also cause increased chloride transport similar to the effect of cholera and therefore cause severe diarrhea.

Enzymes in the Small Intestinal Secretion. When secretions of the small intestine are collected without cellular debris, they have almost no enzymes. However, the epithelial cells of the mucosa, especially those covering the villi, do contain digestive enzymes that digest some food substances *while* they are being absorbed through the epithelium. These enzymes are the following: (1) several different *peptidases* for splitting small peptides into amino acids, (2) four enzymes for splitting disaccharides into monosaccharides—*sucrase, maltase, isomaltase,* and *lactase,* and (3) small amounts of *intestinal lipase* for splitting neutral fats into glycerol and fatty acids. Most, if not all, of these enzymes are mainly in the brush border of the epithelial cells. They are believed to catalyze hydrolysis of the foods on the outside surfaces of the microvilli prior to absorption of the end products.

The epithelial cells deep in the crypts of Lieberkühn continually undergo mitosis, and the new cells gradually migrate along the basement membrane upward out of the crypts toward the tips of the villi, where they are finally shed into the intestinal secretions. The life cycle of an intestinal epithelial cell is approximately 5 days. This rapid growth of new cells allows rapid repair of excoriations that occur in the mucosa.

Regulation of Small Intestinal Secretion

Local Stimuli. By far the most important means for regulating small intestinal secretion are various local nervous reflexes, especially reflexes initiated by tactile or irritative stimuli. Therefore, for the most part, secretion in the small intestine occurs simply in response to the presence of chyme in the intestine—the greater the amount of chyme, the greater the secretion.

SECRETIONS OF THE LARGE INTESTINE

Mucus Secretion. The mucosa of the large intestine, like that of the small intestine, is lined with crypts of Lieberkühn; but in this mucosa, unlike that of the small intestine, there are no villi. Also, the epithelial cells contain almost no enzymes. Instead, they are lined almost entirely by mucous cells that secrete only mucus. Additionally, on the surface epithelium of the large intestine are large numbers of mucous cells dispersed among the other epithelial cells.

Therefore, the great preponderance of secretion in the large intestine is mucus. This mucus contains large amounts of bicarbonate ions caused by active transport of these ions by the epithelial cells. The rate of secretion of mucus is regulated principally by direct, tactile stimulation of the mucous cells on the surface of the mucosa and by local nervous reflexes to the mucous cells in the crypts of Lieberkühn. However, stimulation of the pelvic nerves, which carry the parasympathetic innervation to the distal one half to two thirds of the large intestine, also causes marked increase in the secretion of mucus. This occurs along with an increase in motility, which was discussed in the preceding chapter. Therefore, during extreme parasympathetic stimulation, often caused by emotional disturbances, so much mucus may be secreted into the large intestine that the person has a bowel movement of ropy mucus as often as every 30 minutes; the mucus contains little or no fecal material.

Mucus in the large intestine obviously protects the wall against excoriation; but, in addition, it provides the adherent medium for holding fecal matter together. Furthermore, it protects the intestinal wall from the great amount of bacterial activity that takes place inside the feces.

Secretion of Water and Electrolytes in Response to Irritation. Whenever a segment of the large intestine becomes intensely irritated, as occurs when bacterial infection becomes rampant during *enteritis,* the mucosa then secretes large quantities of water and electrolytes in addition to the normal viscid solution of alkaline mucus. This acts to dilute the irritating factors and to cause rapid movement of the feces toward the anus. The usual result is *diarrhea,* which promotes earlier recovery from the disease than would otherwise occur.

REFERENCES

Cheli, R., et al.: Gastric Protection. New York, Raven Press, 1988.

Cooke, H. J.: Role of the "little brain" in the gut in water and electrolyte homeostasis. FASEB J., 3:127, 1989.

Daugherty, D., and Yamada, T.: Posttranslational processing of gastrin. Physiol. Rev., 69:482, 1989.

Fushiki, T., and Iwai, K.: Two hypotheses on the feedback regulation of pancreatic enzyme secretion. FASEB J., 3:121, 1989.

Hopfer, U., and Liedtke, C. M.: Proton and bicarbonate transport mechanisms in the intestine. Annu. Rev. Physiol., 49:51, 1987.

Johnson, L. R., et al.: Physiology of the Gastrointestinal Tract. 2nd ed. New York, Raven Press, 1987.

Kuijpers, G. A. J., et al.: Role of proton and bicarbonate transport in pancreatic cell function. Annu. Rev. Physiol., 49:87, 1987.

Machen, T. E., and Paradiso, A. M.: Regulation of intracellular pH in the stomach. Annu. Rev. Physiol., 49:19, 1987.

Muallem, S.: Calcium transport pathways of pancreatic acinar cells. Annu. Rev. Physiol., 51:83, 1989.

Petersen, O. H., and Gallacher, D. V.: Electrophysiology of pancreatic and salivary acinar cells. Annu. Rev. Physiol., 50:65, 1988.

Reuss, L., and Stoddard, J. S.: Role of H^+ and HCO_3^- in salt transport in gallbladder epithelium. Annu. Rev. Physiol., 49:35, 1987.

Streebny, L. M.: The Salivary System. Boca Raton, Fla., CRC Press Inc., 1987.

Thompson, J. C., et al.: Gastrointestinal Endocrinology. New York, McGraw-Hill Book Co., 1987.

Walsh, J. H.: Peptides as regulators of gastric acid secretion. Annu. Rev. Physiol., 50:41, 1988.

QUESTIONS

1. Explain the basic mechanisms by which glandular cells secrete organic substances, and also explain the nervous control of water and electrolyte secretion.
2. What are the special characteristics of *mucus* that make it extremely important for lubrication and protection of the gastrointestinal tract?

3. Describe a salivary gland and explain the secretory processes of the *acini* and the *salivary ducts.*
4. Explain why the electrolytic composition of *saliva* is quite different from the electrolytic composition of plasma.
5. What roles does saliva play in maintaining *oral hygiene?*
6. Describe the nervous regulation of salivary secretion.
7. Explain the mechanism for secretion of hydrochloric acid by the *oxyntic cells* of the *oxyntic glands* in the stomach.
8. How is *pepsin* secreted, how is it activated, and what are its properties?
9. Explain both the *vagal* and the *gastrin mechanisms* for control of gastric secretion.
10. Give general descriptions of the chemical compositions of *gastrin, cholecystokinin,* and *secretin.*
11. What is the role of histamine in controlling gastric secretion, and how does the drug *cimetidine* block the gastrin mechanism for stimulating gastric secretion?
12. What are the roles of *gastric pH* and of different *intestinal factors* in the control of gastric secretion?
13. Describe the types of secretion and the mechanisms for secretion of the different components of pancreatic juice.
14. Describe the regulation of secretion of *water* and *sodium bicarbonate* by the pancreas; also, explain the function of sodium bicarbonate in the duodenum.
15. Explain the control of secretion of *enzymes* by the pancreas.
16. Give the physiological anatomy of the liver, and explain the secretion of bile.
17. Explain the storage and concentration of bile in the *gallbladder,* and explain the control of emptying of the gallbladder.
18. Discuss the ultimate fates of the bile salts, the bilirubin, and the cholesterol that are secreted in the bile. Why and how are gallstones formed?
19. Explain the characteristics of the small intestinal secretions and the manner in which these secretions are regulated.
20. What are the specific characteristics of the large intestinal secretions, and how is large intestinal secretion regulated?

44

Digestion and Absorption in the Gastrointestinal Tract; Gastrointestinal Disorders

The foods on which the body lives, with the exception of small quantities of substances such as vitamins and minerals, can be classified as carbohydrates, fats, and proteins. However, these generally cannot be absorbed in their natural forms through the gastrointestinal mucosa and, for this reason, are useless as nutrients without preliminary digestion. Therefore, this chapter discusses, first, the processes by which carbohydrates, fats, and proteins are digested into compounds small enough for absorption and, second, the mechanisms by which the digestive end-products, as well as water, electrolytes, and other substances, are absorbed.

DIGESTION OF THE VARIOUS FOODS

Hydrolysis as the Basic Process of Digestion. Almost all the carbohydrates of the diet are either *large polysaccharides* or *disaccharides, both of which are combinations of monosaccharides,* bound to each other. The carbohydrates are digested into their constituent monosaccharides; to do this, specific enzymes combine hydrogen and hydroxyl ions, derived from water, with the poly- and disaccharides and thereby separate the monosaccharides from each other. This process, called *hydrolysis,* digests the disaccharide $R'' - R'$ as follows:

$$R'' - R' + H_2O \xrightarrow[\text{enzyme}]{\text{digestive}} R''OH + R'H$$

Almost the entire fat portion of the diet consists of triglycerides (neutral fats), which are combinations of three *fatty acid* molecules with a single *glycerol* molecule. Digestion of the triglycerides consists of fat-digesting enzymes that split fatty acid molecules away from the glycerol. Here again, the process is one of hydrolysis.

Finally, proteins are formed from *amino acids* that are bound together by means of *peptide linkages.* And, again, digestion of proteins also involves the process of hydrolysis, the proteolytic enzymes combining hydroxyl and hydrogen ions derived from water with the protein molecules to split them into their constituent amino acids.

Therefore, the chemistry of digestion is really simple, for in the case of all three major types of food, the same basic process of *hydrolysis* is involved. The only difference is in the enzymes required to promote the reactions for each type of food.

All the digestive enzymes are proteins. Their secretion by the different gastrointestinal glands is discussed in the preceding chapter.

Digestion of Carbohydrates

Only three major sources of carbohydrates exist in the normal human diet. These are sucrose, which is the disaccharide known popularly as cane sugar; lactose, which is a disaccharide in milk; and starches, which are large polysaccharides present in almost all food, particularly in the grains.

Figure 44–1 gives a schema for digestion of the principal carbohydrates. This shows that the starches are first hydrolyzed to maltose, a disaccharide, or

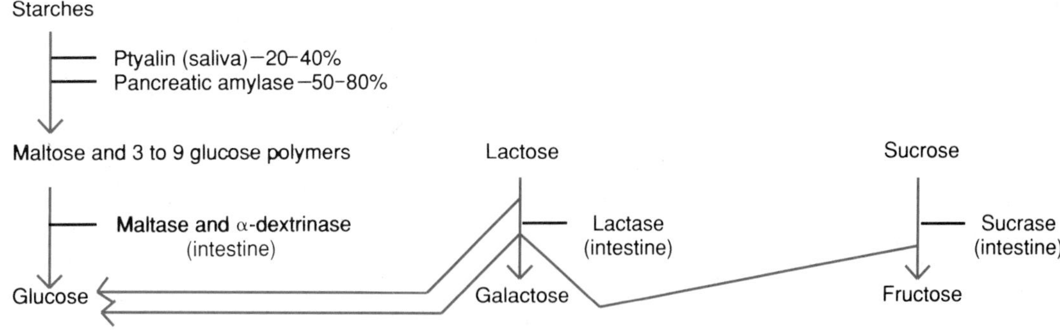

Figure 44-1. Digestion of carbohydrates.

other small glucose polymers. Then these, along with the other major disaccharides, lactose and sucrose, are hydrolyzed into the monosaccharides *glucose, galactose,* and *fructose.*

Hydrolysis of starches begins in the mouth under the influence of the enzyme *ptyalin,* which is secreted mainly in the saliva from the parotid gland. The hydrochloric acid of the stomach provides a slight amount of additional hydrolysis. Finally, the major share of hydrolysis occurs in the upper part of the small intestine under the influence of the enzyme *pancreatic amylase.*

Four enzymes, *lactase, sucrase, maltase,* and *α-dextrinase,* for splitting disaccharides and small glucose polymers are located in the microvilli of the brush border of the epithelial cells. The disaccharides and small polymers are digested into monosaccharides as they come in contact with or diffuse into the microvilli. The digestive products, the monosaccharides *glucose, galactose,* and *fructose,* are then immediately absorbed into the portal blood.

Digestion of Fats

By far the most common fats of the diet are the neutral fats, also known as *triglycerides,* each molecule of which is composed of a glycerol nucleus and three fatty acids.

In the usual diet are also small quantities of *phospholipids, cholesterol,* and *cholesterol esters.* The phospholipids and cholesterol esters contain fatty acid and therefore can be considered fats themselves. Cholesterol, on the other hand, is a sterol compound containing no fatty acid, but it does exhibit some of the physical and chemical characteristics of fats; also it is derived from fats, and it is metabolized similarly to fats. Therefore, cholesterol is considered from a dietary point of view to be a fat.

Though a minute amount of fat can be digested in the stomach under the influence of gastric lipase, 95 to 99 per cent of all fat digestion occurs in the small intestine, mainly under the influence of *pancreatic lipase.*

Emulsification of Fat by Bile Salts. The first step in fat digestion is to break the fat globules into small sizes so that the digestive enzymes, which are not fat soluble, can act on the globule surfaces. This process is called *emulsification* of the fat, and it is achieved under the influence of bile salts that are secreted in the bile by the liver. The bile salts act as a detergent, greatly decreasing the interfacial tension of the fat. With a low interfacial tension, the gastrointestinal mixing movements can break the globules of fat into finer and finer particles, with the total surface area of the fat increasing by a factor of two every time the diameters of the fat globules are decreased by one half.

Digestion of Fat by Pancreatic Lipase and Enteric Lipase. Under the influence of *pancreatic lipase,* most of the fat is split into *monoglycerides* and *fatty acids,* as shown in Figure 44-2. A small portion does not proceed to the monoglyceride stage, but this portion usually is poorly absorbed or not absorbed at all.

The epithelial cells of the small intestine contain a small quantity of lipase, known as *enteric lipase.* This probably causes a very slight additional amount of fat digestion.

Role of Bile Salts in Accelerating Fat Digestion — Formation of Micelles. The hydrolysis of triglycerides is a highly reversible process; therefore, accumulation of monoglycerides and free fatty acids in the vicinity of digesting fats very quickly blocks further digestion. Fortunately, the bile salts play an important role in removing the monosaccharides and the free fatty acids from the vicinity of the digesting fat globules almost as rapidly as these end-products of digestion are formed. This removal occurs in the following way:

Bile salts have the propensity to form *micelles,* which are small, spherical globules 3 to 4 nanometers in diameter and are composed of 20 to 40 molecules of bile salt. The micelles develop because each bile salt molecule is composed of a sterol nucleus that is highly fat-soluble and a polar group that is highly water-soluble. The sterol nuclei of these 20 to 40 bile salt mole-

Fat $\xrightarrow{\text{(Bile + Agitation)}}$ Emulsified fat

Emulsified fat $\xrightarrow{\text{Pancreatic lipase}}$ Fatty acids and 2-monoglycerides

Figure 44-2. Digestion of fats.

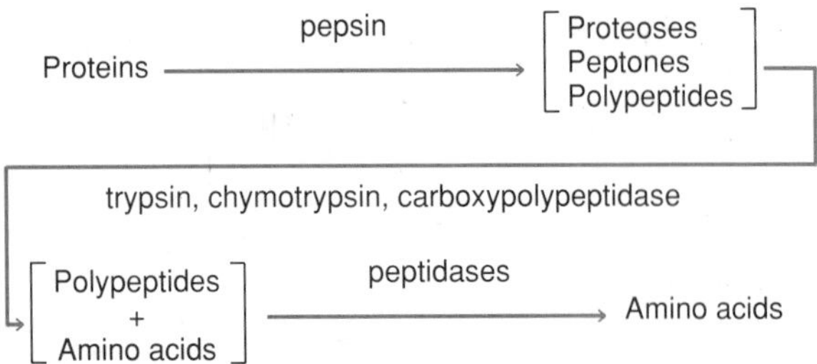

Figure 44-3. Digestion of proteins.

cules of the micelle aggregate to form a small fat globule in the middle of the micelle. This formation causes the polar groups to project outward to cover the surface of the micelle. Since these polar groups are negatively charged and are water soluble, they allow the entire micelle globule to become dissolved in the water of the digestive fluids and to remain in solution despite the very large size of the micelle.

During triglyceride digestion, as rapidly as the monoglycerides and free fatty acids are formed, they become dissolved in the fatty portion of the micelles, which immediately removes these end-products of digestion from the vicinity of the digesting fat globules. Consequently, the digestive process can proceed unabated.

The bile salt micelles also act as a transport medium to carry the monoglycerides and the free fatty acids to the brush borders of the epithelial cells. There the monoglycerides and free fatty acids are absorbed, as will be discussed later. On delivery of these substances to the brush border, the bile salts are released back into the chyme to be used again and again for this "ferrying" process.

Digestion of Proteins

The dietary proteins are derived almost entirely from meats and vegetables, and they are digested primarily in the stomach and upper part of the small intestine.

As illustrated in Figure 44-3, protein digestion begins in the stomach, the enzyme *pepsin* splitting the proteins into *proteoses, peptones,* and large *polypeptides.* This enzyme functions only in a highly acid medium, acting best at a pH of about 2 to 3. Therefore, the hydrochloric acid secreted in the stomach is essential for this digestive process. However, normally only 10 to 20 per cent of the total protein digestion occurs in the stomach, most of it occurring in the upper small intestine.

Pepsin is especially important for its ability to digest collagen, an albuminoid that is little affected by other digestive enzymes. Since collagen is a major constituent of the fibrous tissue in meat, it is essential that this substance be digested so that the remainder of the meat can be attacked by the other digestive enzymes.

The proteins are further digested in the upper part of the small intestine under the influence of the pancreatic enzymes *trypsin, chymotrypsin,* and *carboxypolypeptidases.* The final product of this digestion is mainly *small polypeptides* plus a few *amino acids.*

Finally, the small polypeptides are digested into amino acids when they come in contact with the epithelial cells of the small intestine. These cells contain multiple enzymes (*peptidases*) that convert the remaining protein products into *tripeptides, dipeptides,* and a few *amino acids* that are rapidly absorbed into the epithelial cells. There, the remaining tripeptides and dipeptides are digested into amino acids.

When food has been properly masticated and is not eaten in too large a quantity at any one time, about 98 per cent of the protein finally becomes amino acids, and the remaining 2 per cent is excreted in the feces.

BASIC PRINCIPLES OF GASTROINTESTINAL ABSORPTION

Anatomical Basis of Absorption

The total quantity of fluid that must be absorbed each day is equal to the ingested fluid (about 1.5 liters) plus that secreted in the various gastrointestinal juices (about 7 liters). Together these come to a total of 8 to 9 liters. All but about 1.5 liters is absorbed in the small intestine, leaving only 1.5 liters to pass through the ileocecal valve into the colon each day.

The stomach is a poor absorptive area of the gastrointestinal tract. Only a few highly lipid-soluble substances, such as alcohol and some drugs, can be absorbed in small quantities.

The Absorptive Surface of the Intestinal Mucosa—The Villi. Figure 44-4 illustrates the absorptive surface of the intestinal mucosa, showing many folds called *valvulae conniventes;* these increase

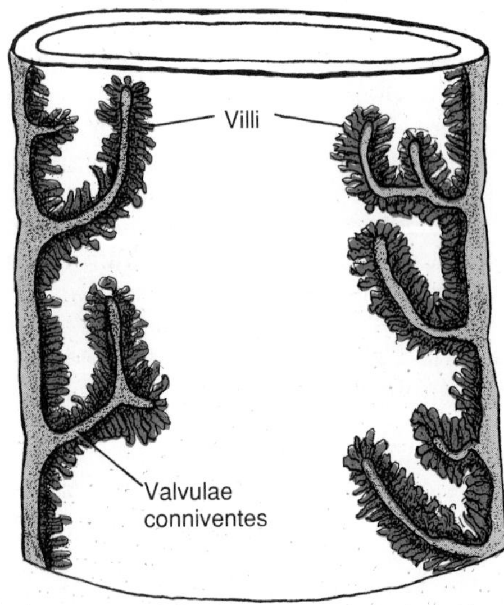

Figure 44-4. A longitudinal section of the small intestine, showing the valvulae conniventes covered by villi.

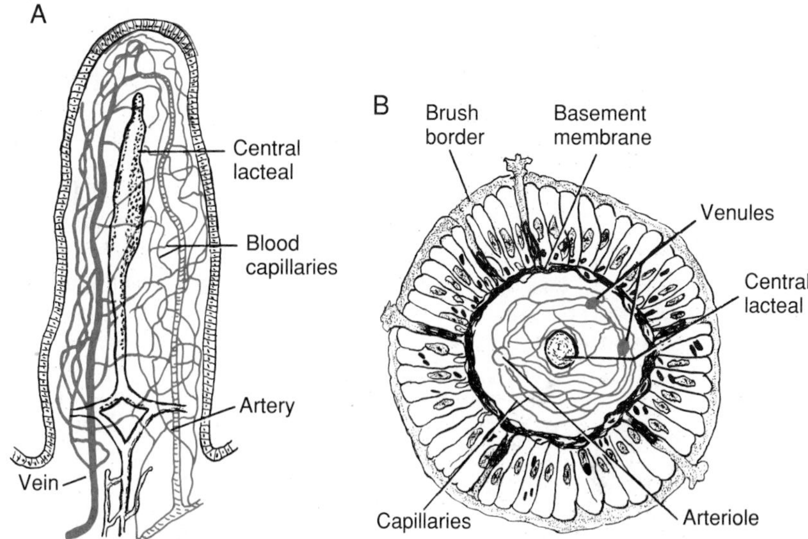

Figure 44-5. Functional organization of the villus. *A,* Logitudinal section. *B,* Cross-section showing the epithelial cells and basement membrane.

the surface area of the absorptive mucosa about threefold.

Also, located over the entire surface of the small intestine, from approximately the point at which the common bile duct empties into the duodenum down to the ileocecal valve, are literally millions of small *villi,* which project about 1 mm from the surface of the mucosa, as shown on the surfaces of the valvulae conniventes in Figure 44-4 and in detail in Figure 44-5. These villi enhance the absorptive area another tenfold.

Finally, the epithelial cells on the surface of the villi are characterized by a brush border, consisting of about *600 microvilli* 1 micrometer in length and 0.1 micrometer in diameter protruding from each cell; these are illustrated in the electron micrograph in Figure 44-6. These microvilli increase the surface area exposed to the intestinal material another 20-fold. Thus, the combination of the valvulae conniventes, the villi, and the microvilli increases the absorptive area of the mucosa about 600-fold, making a very large total area of about 250 square meters for the entire small intestine.

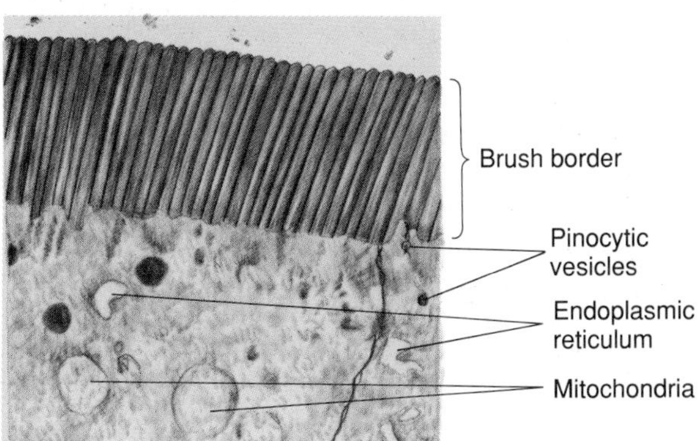

Figure 44-6. Brush border of the gastrointestinal epithelial cell, showing, also, pinocytic vesicles, mitochondria, and endoplasmic reticulum lying immediately beneath the brush border. (Courtesy of Dr. William Lockwood.)

Figure 44-5 illustrates the general organization of a villus, emphasizing especially the advantageous arrangement of the vascular system for absorption of fluid and dissolved material into the portal blood and the arrangement of the *central lacteal* for absorption into the lymphatics.

Basic Mechanisms of Absorption

Absorption through the gastrointestinal mucosa occurs by *active transport* and by *diffusion,* as is also true for other membranes. The physical principles of these processes were explained in Chapter 4.

Briefly, active transport provides energy to move a substance across a membrane. Therefore, the substance can be moved against a concentration gradient or against an electrical potential. On the other hand, the term *diffusion* means simply transport of substances through the membrane as a result of molecular movement *along,* rather than against, an electrochemical gradient.

ABSORPTION IN THE SMALL INTESTINE

Normally, the substances absorbed from the small intestine each day consist of several hundred grams of carbohydrates, 100 or more grams of fat, 50 to 100 grams of amino acids, 50 to 100 grams of ions, and 7 to 8 liters of water. However, the absorptive *capacity* of the normal *small intestine* is far greater than this: as much as several kilograms of carbohydrates per day, 500 to 1000 grams of fat per day, 500 to 700 grams of amino acids per day, and 20 or more liters of water per day. In addition, the *large intestine* can absorb still more water and ions, though almost no nutrients.

Absorption of Water

Isomotic Absorption. Water is transported through the intestinal membrane entirely by the process of *diffusion,* passing mainly through large, 0.7 to 1.5 nanometer pores between the intestinal epithelial cells. Furthermore, this diffusion also obeys the usual laws of osmosis.

As dissolved substances are actively transported from the lumen of the gut into the blood, this decreases the osmotic pressure of the chyme while increasing the osmotic pressure on the other side of the membrane, thus creating an osmotic gradient that moves water through the membrane as well. Water diffuses so readily through the intestinal membrane that it almost instantaneously "follows" the transported substances into the circulation. Therefore, as ions and nutrients are absorbed, an isosmotic equivalent of water is also absorbed. In this way, not only are the ions and nutrients almost entirely absorbed before the chyme passes through the small intestine, but so is about 80 per cent of the water too.

Absorption of the Ions

Active Transport of Sodium. Twenty to thirty grams of sodium are secreted into the intestines with the various secretions each day. Most people eat an additional 5 to 8 grams of sodium daily. Combining these two amounts, the small intestine absorbs 25 to 35 grams of sodium each day, which equals about one seventh of all the sodium that is present in the body.

The basic mechanism of sodium absorption from the intestine is illustrated in Figure 44-7. The principles of this mechanism, which were discussed in Chapter 4, are essentially the same as those for absorption of sodium from the renal tubules, as discussed in Chapter 21. The motive power for the sodium absorption is provided by active transport of sodium from inside the epithelial cells, through the side walls of these cells, into the intercellular spaces. This is illustrated by the heavy black arrows in Figure 44-7. This active transport obeys the usual laws for such transport: It requires a carrier, it requires energy, and it is catalyzed by an appropriate ATPase carrier-enzyme in the cell membrane.

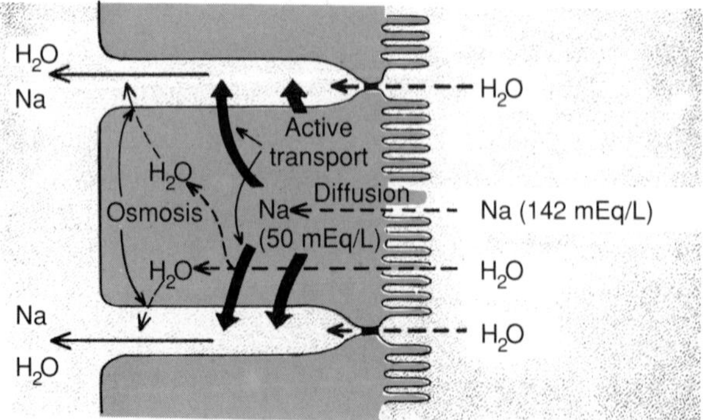

Figure 44-7. Absorption of sodium through the intestinal epithelium. Note also the osmotic absorption of water—that is, the water "follows" the sodium through the epithelial membrane.

The next step in the transport process is osmosis of water into the intercellular spaces. This movement is caused by the osmotic gradient created by the elevated concentration of ions in the intercellular space. Most of this osmosis occurs through the junctions between the apical borders of the epithelial cells, but a smaller proportion occurs through the cells themselves. The osmotic movement of water creates a flow of fluid into the intercellular space and finally into the circulating blood of the villi.

Transport of Chloride. In most parts of the small intestine transport of the positively charged sodium ions through the epithelium creates electronegativity in the chyme and electropositivity on the basal side of the epithelial cells. Then chloride ions move along this electrical gradient to "follow" the sodium ions.

However, the epithelial cells of the distal ileum and of the large intestine have the special capability of actively absorbing chloride ions. This occurs by means of a tightly coupled active transport mechanism in which an equivalent number of bicarbonate ions are secreted. The advantage of this mechanism is that it provides bicarbonate ions for neutralization of acidic products formed by bacteria—especially in the large intestine.

Absorption of Other Ions. Calcium ions are actively absorbed, especially from the duodenum, and calcium ion absorption is exactly controlled in relation to the need of the body for calcium by parathyroid hormone secreted by the parathyroid glands and by vitamin D. These effects are discussed in Chapter 53.

Iron ions are also actively absorbed from the small intestine. The principles of iron absorption and its regulation in proportion to the body's need for iron were discussed in Chapter 24.

Potassium, magnesium, phosphate, and still a few other ions also can be actively absorbed through the muscosa.

Absorption of Nutrients

Absorption of Carbohydrates. Essentially all the carbohydrates are absorbed in the form of monosaccharides, only a small fraction of a per cent being absorbed as disaccharides and almost none as larger carbohydrate compounds. Furthermore, little carbohydrate absorption results from diffusion, for even the monosaccharides have a molecular weight of 180 and the pores of the mucosa through which diffusion occurs are essentially impermeable to water-soluble solutes with molecular weights greater than 100.

Mechanism of Monosaccharide Absorption—Role of Sodium. Most monosaccharide transport becomes blocked whenever sodium transport is blocked. The reason for this is that the energy required for most monosaccharide transport is actually provided by the sodium transport system. Let us explain this process: A large carrier protein for transporting glucose and some other monosaccharides, especially galactose, is present in the brush border of the epithelial cell. However, this carrier will not transport the glucose in the absence of sodium transport. Therefore, it is believed that the carrier has receptor sites for both a glucose molecule and a sodium ion and that the carrier will not transport the glucose to the inside of the cell if the receptor site for sodium is not simultaneously filled. The energy that causes movement of both sodium ion and the glucose molecule from the exterior of the membrane to the interior is derived from the difference in sodium concentration between the outside and inside; the sodium and glucose are coupled in such a way that they must move together. That is, as sodium diffuses to the inside of the cell it "drags" the glucose along with it, thus providing the energy for transport of the glucose. For obvious reasons, this is called the *sodium co-transport theory* for glucose transport.

Absorption of Proteins. As explained earlier in the chapter, most proteins are absorbed through the luminal membranes of the epithelial cells in the form of dipeptides, tripeptides, and a few free amino acids. The energy for most of this transport is supplied by a sodium co-transport mechanism in exactly the same way that sodium co-transport of glucose occurs. That is, most peptide or amino acid molecules bind with a specific transport protein that also requires sodium binding before transport can occur. The sodium ion then moves down its electrochemical gradient to the interior of the cell and pulls the amino acid or peptide along with it. Therefore, this is called *co-transport of the amino acids or peptides.* At least five different types of amino acid and peptide transport proteins have been characterized in the luminal membrane of intestinal epithelial cells. This multiplicity of transport proteins is required because of the diverse binding properties of the different amino acids and peptides.

Absorption of Fats. Earlier in this chapter it was pointed out that when fats are digested to form monoglycerides and free fatty acids, both these digestive end-products become dissolved mainly in the lipid portion of the bile acid micelles. Because of the small dimensions of these micelles and also because of their highly charged exterior, they are soluble in the chyme. In this form the monoglycerides and the fatty acids are transported to the surfaces of the intestinal epithelial cells. On coming in contact with these surfaces, both the monoglycerides and the fatty acids immediately diffuse through the epithelial membrane, leaving the bile acid micelles still in the chyme. The micelles then diffuse back into the chyme and absorb still more monoglycerides and fatty acids, and similarly transport these to the epithelial cells. Thus, the bile acids perform a ferrying function that is highly important for fat absorption. In the presence of an abundance of bile acids, approximately 97 per cent of the fat is absorbed; in the absence of bile acids, only 50 to 60 per cent is normally absorbed.

The mechanism for absorption of the monoglycerides and fatty acids through the brush border is based on the fact that both of these substances are highly lipid-soluble. Therefore, they become dissolved in the membrane and diffuse to the interior of the cell.

After entering the epithelial cell, the fatty acids and monoglycerides are taken up by the smooth endoplasmic reticulum, and here they are mainly recombined to form new triglycerides. However, a few of the monoglycerides are further digested into glycerol and fatty acids by an epithelial cell lipase, and the fatty acids are then combined with newly synthesized glycerol to form entirely new triglycerides rather than simply recombining with absorbed monoglycerides

Once formed, the triglycerides aggregate within the endoplasmic reticulum into globules, along with absorbed cholesterol, absorbed phospholipids, and small amounts of newly synthesized cholesterol and phospholipids. The phospholipids arrange themselves in these globules with the fatty portion of the phospholipid toward the center and the polar portions located on the surface. This arrangement provides an electrically charged surface that makes the globules miscible with the fluids of the cell. In addition, small amounts of *β-lipoprotein,* also synthesized by the endoplasmic reticulum, coat part of the surface of each globule. In this form the globule diffuses to the side of the epithelial cell and is excreted by the process of cellular *exocytosis* into the space between the cells; from there it passes into the lymph in the central lacteal of the villus. These globules are then called *chylomicrons.*

Transport of the Chylomicrons in the Lymph. From the central lacteals of the villi, the chylomicrons are propelled along with the lymph by the lymphatic pump upward through the thoracic duct to be emptied into the great veins of the neck.

ABSORPTION IN THE LARGE INTESTINE; FORMATION OF THE FECES

Approximately 1500 ml of chyme passes through the ileocecal valve into the large intestine each day. Most of the water and electrolytes in the chyme are absorbed in the colon, leaving only 50 to 200 ml of fluid to be excreted in the feces.

Most of the absorption in the large intestine occurs in the proximal half of the colon, giving this portion the name *absorbing colon,* while the distal colon functions principally for storage and is therefore called the *storage colon.*

Absorption and Secretion of Electrolytes and Water. The mucosa of the large intestine, like that of the small intestine, has a very high capacity for active absorption of sodium, and the electrical potential gradient across the epithelium created by the absorption of the sodium causes chloride absorption as well. In addition, as in the distal portion of the small intestine, the mucosa of the large intestine actively secretes bicarbonate ions while it simultaneously absorbs a small amount of chloride ions in exchange for the bicarbonate. The bicarbonate helps neutralize the acidic end-products of bacterial action in the colon.

The absorption of sodium and chloride ions creates an osmotic gradient across the large intestinal mucosa, which in turn causes absorption of water.

Bacterial Action in the Colon. Numerous bacteria, especially colon bacilli, are present in the absorbing colon. Substances formed as a result of bacterial activity are vitamin K, vitamin B_{12}, thiamin, riboflavin, and various gases that contribute to *flatus* in the colon. Vitamin K is especially important, for the amount of this vitamin in the ingested foods is normally insufficient to maintain adequate blood coagulation.

Composition of the Feces. The feces normally are about three fourths water and one fourth solid matter composed of about 30 per cent inorganic matter, 2 to 3 per cent protein, and 30 per cent undigested roughage of the food and dried constituents of digestive juices, such as bile pigment and sloughed epithelial cells.

The brown color of feces is caused by *stercobilin* and *urobilin,* which are derivatives of bilirubin. The odor is caused principally by the products of bacterial action; these vary from one person to another, depending on each person's colonic bacterial flora and on the type of food eaten. The actual odoriferous products include indole, skatole, mercaptans, and *hydrogen sulfide.*

GASTROINTESTINAL DISORDERS

Gastritis

Gastritis means inflammation of the gastric mucosa. This is exceedingly common in the population as a whole, especially in the later years of adult life.

The inflammation of gastritis may be merely superficial and therefore not very harmful, or it may penetrate deeply into the gastric mucosa, and in many longstanding cases it causes almost complete atrophy of the gastric mucosa. In a few cases, gastritis can be very acute and severe, with ulcerative excoriation of the stomach mucosa by the stomach's own peptic secretions.

The cause of gastritis in most instances is not known. In the past it was ascribed mainly to irritant foods, but the present clinical belief is that almost no food can be as irritant to the gastric mucosa as the normal acid-pepsin gastric juices themselves. Therefore, patients with gastritis are usually told to eat almost any food that will not cause nausea or burning epigastric pain. Yet, a few substances can be very damaging to the protective gastric mucosal barrier—that is, to the viscid mucous glands and tight epithelial junctions between the gastric lining cells—often leading to severe acute or chronic gastritis. The two most common of these substances are *alcohol* and *aspirin.*

Gastric Atrophy. In many persons who have chronic gastritis, the mucosa gradually becomes atrophic until little or no gastric gland activity remains. It is also believed that some persons develop autoimmunity against their own gastric mucosa, which leads eventually to gastric atrophy. Loss of the stomach secretions in gastric atrophy leads to *achlorhydria* and, occasionally, to *pernicious anemia.*

Achlorhydria means simply that the stomach fails to secrete hydrochloric acid. Usually, when acid is not secreted, pepsin also is not secreted, and, even if it is, the lack of acid prevents it from functioning because pepsin requires an acid medium for activity. Obviously, then, essentially all digestive function in the stomach is lost when achlorhydria is present.

Pernicious Anemia in Gastric Atrophy. Pernicious anemia, which was discussed in Chapter 24, is a common accompaniment of achlorhydria and gastric atrophy. The normal gastric secretions contain a glycoprotein called *intrinsic factor,* which is secreted by the same parietal cells that secrete hydrochloric acid. Intrinsic factor must be present for adequate absorption of vitamin B_{12}, from the ileum. This factor combines with vitamin B_{12}, and the complex then binds with receptors on the surfaces of the ileal epithelial cells, a necessary step in the absorption of vitamin B_{12}. In the absence of intrinsic factor, an adequate amount of vitamin B_{12} is not made available from the foods. *Maturation failure* then occurs in the formation of red blood cells in the bone marrow, resulting in pernicious anemia.

Pernicious anemia also occurs frequently when most of the stomach has been removed for treatment of either stomach ulcer or stomach cancer or when the ileum, where vitamin B_{12} is absorbed, is removed.

Peptic Ulcer

A peptic ulcer is an excoriated area of the mucosa caused by the digestive action of gastric juice. Figure 44–8 illustrates the points in the gastrointestinal tract at which peptic ulcers frequently occur, showing that by far the most frequent site of peptic ulcers is in the first few centimeters of the duodenum. In addition, peptic ulcers frequently occur along the lesser curvature of the antral end of the stomach or, more

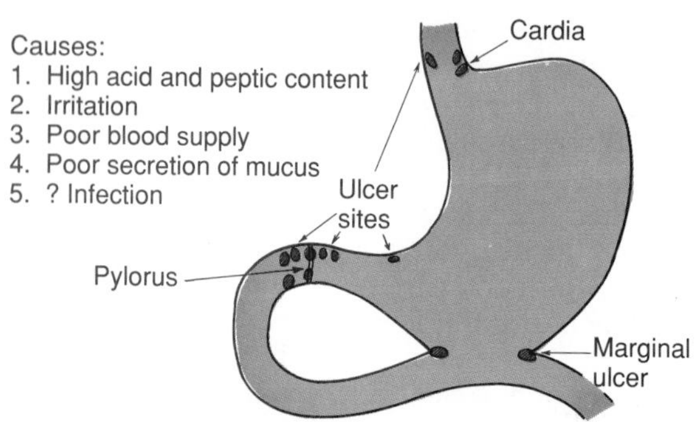

Figure 44–8. Peptic ulcer.

rarely, in the lower end of the esophagus, where there is often reflux of stomach juices.

Basic Cause of Peptic Ulceration. The usual cause of peptic ulceration is too much secretion of gastric juice in relation to the degree of protection afforded by the mucous lining of the stomach and duodenum as well as by neutralization of the gastric acid by duodenal juices. It will be recalled that all areas normally exposed to gastric juices are well supplied with mucous glands, begining with the compound mucous glands of the lower esophagus, then the mucous cell coating of the stomach mucosa, the mucous neck cells of the gastric glands, the deep pyloric glands that secrete mainly mucus, and, finally, the glands of Brunner in the upper duodenum, which secrete a highly alkaline mucus.

In addition to the mucus protection of the mucosa, the duodenum is also protected by the alkalinity of the pancreatic secretion, which contains large quantities of sodium bicarbonate that neutralize the hydrochloric acid of the gastric juice, thus inactivating the pepsin and thereby preventing digestion of the mucosa. Two additional mechanisms insure that this neutralization of gastric juices is complete:

1. When excess acid enters the duodenum, it reflexly inhibits gastric secretion and peristalsis in the stomach, thereby decreasing the rate of gastric emptying. This allows increased time for pancreatic secretion to enter the duodenum to neutralize the acid already present. After neutralization has taken place, the reflex subsides and more stomach contents are emptied.
2. The presence of acid in the small intestine liberates secretin from the intestinal mucosa. The secretin then passes by way of the blood to the pancreas to promote rapid secretion of pancreatic juice, which contains a high concentration of sodium bicarbonate, thus making more sodium bicarbonate available for neutralization of the acid. These mechanisms were discussed in detail in Chapters 42 and 43 in relation to gastrointestinal motility and secretion.

Causes of Peptic Ulcer in the Human Being. About 50 per cent of the patients with peptic ulcer of the *duodenum* secrete up to two times as much gastric acid following injection of a test dose of *pentagastrin* as do normal persons. Therefore, it is believed that the ulcers in these patients are caused by excessive secretion of acid and pepsin by the gastric glands. In the remainder of the patients who secrete normal amounts of acid, it is presumed that one of four other abnormalities is the usual cause: (a) possible secretion of an abnormal mucus that has less than normal protective value, (b) diminished secretion of mucus, (c) failure of the normal duodenal-gastric feedback mechanisms to limit the rate of gastric emptying into the duodenum, or (d) failure of the secretin-pancreatic feedback mechanism to cause the secretion of enough alkaline pancreatic juice to neutralize the gastric juice as it enters the duodenum.

The development of peptic ulcers is strongly hereditary. For instance, like their parents, the offspring of persons who secrete excessive amounts of gastric acid tend to secrete excessive amounts of acid.

Paradoxically, *gastric* ulcers, in contradistinction to duodenal ulcers, often occur in patients who have normal or low secretion of hydrochloric acid. However, these patients almost invariably have an associated gastritis, indicating that ulceration in the stomach almost certainly results from reduced resistance of the stomach mucosa to digestion rather than to excess secretion of gastric juice. Stomach ulceration frequently results in patients who have ingested large quantities of substances that reduce the mucosal resistance, such as aspirin or alcohol.

Physiology of Treatment. The usual medical treatment for peptic ulcer is a combination of (1) reduction of stressful situations that might lead to excessive acid secretion, (2) administration of antacid drugs to neutralize much of the acid in the stomach secretions, (3) administration of the drug *cimetidine* or a similar one, which blocks the action of gastrin in stimulating gastric juice secretion, (4) interdiction against smoking because statistical studies have shown that smokers are several times as prone to have peptic ulcers as are nonsmokers, and (5) removal of such ulcer-causing factors as alcohol, aspirin, or other substances that might irritate the gastroduodenal mucosa.

Surgical treatment of peptic ulceration is usually by one or both of two procedures: (1) *vagotomy* or (2) *removal of a portion of the stomach.* Fortunately, however, since the advent of the drug cimetidine, the more drastic surgical procedures are employed far less frequently than in the past.

Vagotomy means section of the vagus nerves to the stomach; this temporarily blocks almost all secretion of acid and pepsin by the stomach and often cures the ulcer or ulcers within a week after the operation is performed. Unfortunately, though, a large amount of basal stomach secretion returns after a few months, and in many patients the ulcer also returns. Also, *gastric atony* (paralysis of stomach movements) usually follows section of both vagus trunks; this can be very distressing, since stomach motility is often reduced so much that gastric emptying becomes minimal, leading to partial or sometimes almost total pyloric obstruction. To prevent this occurrence, the surgeon often removes the stomach antrum and pylorus, and the body of the stomach is connected directly to the proximal end of the duodenum.

Malabsorption from the Small Intestine —Sprue

Occasionally, nutrients are not adequately absorbed from the small intestine even though the food is well digested. Several different diseases can cause decreased absorbability of the mucosa; these are often classified together under the general heading of *sprue*. Obviously, also, malabsorption can occur when large portions of the small intestine have been removed.

One type of sprue, called variously by the names *idiopathic sprue, celiac disease* (in children), or *gluten enteropathy,* results from the toxic effects of the protein *gluten* present in certain types of grains, especially *wheat* and *rye.* The gluten causes destruction of the villi in some susceptible persons, perhaps as a result of an immunological or allergic reaction. The villi become blunted or disappear altogether, thus greatly reducing the absorptive area of the gut. Removal of wheat and rye flour from the diet, especially in children with this disease, frequently results in an apparently miraculous cure within weeks.

Malabsorption in Sprue. In the early stages of sprue, the absorption of fats is more impaired than the absorption of other digestive products. The fat appears in the stool almost entirely in the form of soaps rather than undigested neutral fat, illustrating that the problem is one of absorption, not of digestion. In this stage of sprue, the condition is frequently called *idiopathic steatorrhea,* which means simply excess fats in the stool as a result of unknown causes.

In more severe cases of sprue, the absorption of proteins, carbohydrates, calcium, vitamin K, folic acid, and vitamin B_{12} as well as many other important substances becomes greatly impaired. As a result, the person suffers (1) severe nutritional deficiency, often developing severe wasting of the tissues, (2) osteomalacia (demineralization of the bones because of calcium lack), (3) inadequate blood coagulation due to lack of vitamin K, and (4) macrocytic anemia of the pernicious anemia type, owing to diminished vitamin B_{12} and folic acid absorption.

Constipation

Constipation means slow movement of feces through the large intestine, and it is often associated with large quantities of dry, hard feces in the descending colon that accumulate because of the long time allowed for absorption of fluid.

A frequent cause of constipation is irregular bowel habits that have developed through a lifetime of inhibition of the normal defecation reflexes. The newborn child is rarely constipated, but part of the training in the early years of life requires that the child learn to control defecation, and this control is effected by inhibiting the natural defecation reflexes. Clinical experience shows that if one fails to allow defecation to occur when the defecation reflexes are excited or if one overuses laxatives to take the place of natural bowel function, the reflexes themselves become progressively less strong over a period of time and the colon often becomes *atonic.* For this reason, if a person establishes regular bowel habits early in life, usually defecating in the morning after breakfast when the gastrocolic and duodenocolic reflexes cause mass movements in the large intestine, the development of constipation can be prevented later in life.

Diarrhea

Diarrhea, the opposite of constipation, results from rapid movement of fecal matter through the large intestine. The major cause of diarrhea is infection in the gastrointestinal tract, which is called *enteritis.*

In usual infectious diarrhea, the infection is most extensive in the large intestine and the distal end of the ileum. Everywhere that the infection is present, the mucosa becomes extensively irritated, and its rate of secretion becomes greatly enhanced. In addition, the motility of the intestinal wall usually increases manifold. As a result, large quantities of fluid are made available for washing the infectious agent toward the anus, and at the same time strong propulsive movements propel this fluid forward. Obviously, this is an important mechanism for ridding the intestinal tract of the debilitating infection.

Of special interest is the diarrhea caused by *cholera.* The cholera toxin directly stimulates excessive secretion of electrolytes and fluid from the crypts of Lieberkühn in the distal ileum and colon, and it specifically enhances the bicarbonate-chloride exchange mechanism, causing extreme quantities of sodium bicarbonate to be secreted into the intestial tract. The loss of fluid and electrolytes can be so debilitating that within a day or so death ensues. Therefore, the most important basis of therapy is simply to replace the fluid and electrolytes as rapidly as they are lost. With proper and simple therapy of this type, almost no cholera patients die, but without treatment, 50 per cent or more succumb.

Vomiting

Vomiting is the means by which the upper gastrointestinal tract rids itself of its contents when the gut becomes excessively irritated, overdistended, or even overexcited. The stimuli that cause vomiting can originate in any part of the gastrointestinal tract, though distention or irritation of the duodenum provides the strongest stimulus. Impulses are transmitted by both vagal and sympathetic afferents to the *vomiting center* of the medulla, which lies near the tractus solitarius at approximately the level of the dorsal motor nucleus of the vagus. Appropriate motor reactions are then instituted to cause the vomiting act, and the motor impulses that cause the actual vomiting are transmitted from the vomiting center through the fifth, seventh, ninth, tenth, and twelfth cranial nerves to the upper gastrointestinal tract and through the spinal nerves to the diaphragm and abdominal muscles.

The Vomiting Act. Once the vomiting center has been sufficiently stimulated and the vomiting act instituted, the first effects are (1) a deep inspiratory breath, (2) raising of the hyoid bone and the larynx to pull the upper esophageal sphincter open, (3) closing of the glottis and (4) lifting of the soft palate to close the posterior nares. Next comes a strong downward contraction of the diaphragm along with simultaneous contraction of all the abdominal muscles. This obviously squeezes the stomach between the two sets of muscles, building the intragastric pressure to a high level. Finally, the lower esophageal sphincter relaxes, allowing expulsion of the gastric contents upward through the esophagus.

Thus, the vomiting act results from a squeezing action of the muscles of the abdomen associated with sudden opening of the esophageal sphincters so that the gastric contents can be expelled.

Gases in the Gastrointestinal Tract (Flatus)

Gases can enter the gastrointestinal tract from three sources: (1) swallowed air, (2) gases released as a result of bacterial action, and (3) diffusion of gases from the blood into the gastrointestinal tract.

Most gases in the stomach are nitrogen and oxygen derived from swallowed air, and a large proportion of these are expelled by belching.

Only small amounts of gas are usually present in the small intestine, and these are composed principally of air that passes from the stomach into the intestinal tract.

In the large intestine, the greater proportion of the gases is derived from bacterial action; these gases include especially *carbon dioxide, methane,* and *hydrogen.* When the methane and hydrogen become suitably mixed with oxygen from swallowed air, an actual explosive mixture is occasionally formed.

Certain foods are known to cause greater amounts of flatus in the large intestine than others—beans, cabbage, onions, cauliflower, corn, and certain highly irritant foods such as vinegar. Some of these foods–beans for instance—serve as a suitable medium for gas-forming bacteria, especially because they contain fermentable types of carbohydrates that are poorly absorbed.

The amount of gases entering or forming in the large intestine each day averages 7 to 10 liters, whereas the average amount expelled is usually only about 0.6 liter. The remainder is absorbed through the intestinal mucosa. Most often, a person expels large quantities of gases not because of excessive bacterial activity but because of excessive motility of the large intestine caused by intestinal irritation. This moves the gases on through the large intestine before they can be absorbed.

REFERENCES

Digestion and Absorption

Buddington, R. K., and Diamond, J. M.: Ontogenetic development of intestinal nutrient transporters. Annu. Rev. Physiol., 51:601, 1989.
Ferraris, R. P., and Diamond, J. M.: Specific regulation of intestinal nutrient transporters by their dietary substrates. Annu. Rev. Physiol., 51:125, 1989.
Horl, W. H., and Heidland, A. (eds.): Proteases. New York, Plenum Publishing Corp., 1988.
Johnson, L. R.: Regulation of gastrointestinal mucosal growth. Physiol. Rev., 68:456, 1988.
Johnson, L., et al.: Physiology of the Gastrointestinal Tract, 2nd ed. New York, Raven Press, 1987.
Liedtke, C. M.: Regulation of chloride transport in epithelia. Annu. Rev. Physiol., 51:143, 1989.
Setchell, K. D. R., et al. (eds.): The Bile Acids. New York, Plenum Publishing Corp., 1988.
Thompson, J. C., et al. (eds.): Gastrointestinal Endocrinology. New York, McGraw-Hill Book Co., 1987.

Gastrointestinal Disorders

Bongiovanni, G. L. (ed.): Essentials of Clinical Gastroenterology. 2nd ed. New York, McGraw-Hill Book Co., 1988.
Gitnick, G. (ed.): Handbook of Gastrointestinal Emergencies. 2nd ed. New York, Elsevier Science Publishing Co., 1988.
Hayworth, M. F., and Jones, A. L.: Immunology of the Gastrointestinal Tract and Liver. New York, Raven Press, 1988.
Kirsner, J. B., and Shorter, R. G. (eds.): Diseases of the Colon, Rectum, and Anal Canal. Baltimore, Williams & Wilkins, 1988.
Rodolfo, C., et al. (eds.): Gastric Protection. New York, Raven Press, 1988.
Shaffer, E., and Thomson, A. B. R.: Modern Concepts in Gastroenterology. New York, Plenum Publishing Corp., 1989.
Snape, W. J., Jr. (ed.): Pathogenesis of Functional Bowel Disease. New York, Plenum Publishing Corp., 1989.

QUESTIONS

1. Explain why *hydrolysis* is the means by which essentially all digestion in the gastrointestinal tract takes place.
2. Give the schema for digestion of *carbohydrates.*
3. Give the schema for digestion of *fats.*
4. What is the role of *bile salts* in fat digestion?
5. Give the schema for digestion of *proteins.*
6. Describe the absorptive surface of the *intestinal mucosa,* including the detailed anatomy of a *villus* and the *microvilli.*
7. What is meant by *isosmotic absorption* of water?
8. Describe the active absorption of sodium ions by the intestinal epithelium. Why does this cause passive absorption of chloride ions?
9. Describe the *co-transport mechanisms* for absorption of glucose and amino acids.
10. Explain the absorption of fats by the intestinal epithelium and the formation of *chylomicrons* that are then transported in the thoracic duct lymph.
11. What are the special characteristics of absorption in the large intestine, and how is this related to the formation of feces?
12. Describe the clinical conditions of *gastritis, gastric atrophy,* and the *pernicious* anemia that occurs in patients with gastric atrophy.
13. What is a *peptic ulcer,* what are its causes, and why do most peptic ulcers occur in the first few centimeters of the duodenum? Explain the medical and surgical treatment of peptic ulcers.
14. What is the cause of *idiopathic sprue,* and what are its effects?
15. What are the causes of *constipation* and *diarrhea?*
16. Give the mechanism of *vomiting,* including its nervous control.
17. Explain the occurrence of gases in the gastrointestinal tract, and how are these different at different levels of the tract?

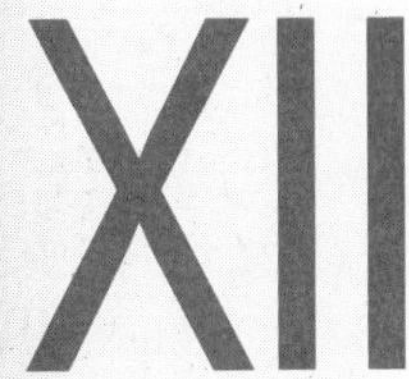

XII

Metabolism and Temperature Regulation

45

Metabolism of Carbohydrates and Formation of Adenosine Triphosphate

The next few chapters deal with metabolism in the body, which means the chemical processes that make it possible for the cells to continue living. It is not the purpose of this textbook, however, to present the chemical details of all the various cellular reactions, for this lies in the discipline of biochemistry. Instead, these chapters are devoted to (1) a review of the principal chemical processes of the cell, and (2) an analysis of their physiological functions, especially in relation to the manner in which they fit into the overall concept of homeostasis.

Role of Adenosine Triphosphate (ATP) in Metabolism

A great proportion of the chemical reactions in the cells is concerned with making the energy in foods available to the various physiological systems of the cell. For instance, energy is required for (1) muscular activity, (2) secretion by the glands, (3) maintenance of membrane potentials in the nerve and muscle fibers, (4) synthesis of substances in the cells, and (5) absorption of foods from the gastrointestinal tract. The substance adenosine triphosphate (ATP) plays a key role in making the energy of the foods available for all these purposes.

ATP, a labile chemical compound present in all cells, has the chemical structure shown in Figure 45–1. From this formula it can be seen that ATP is a combination of adenine, ribose, and three phosphate radicals. The last two phosphate radicals are connected with the remainder of the molecule by so-called *high energy bonds,* which are indicated by the symbol ~. The amount of free energy in each of these high energy bonds per mole of ATP is approximately 7300 calories per mole under standard conditions but 12,000 calories under the conditions of temperature and concentrations of the reactants in the body. Therefore, removal of each phosphate radical liberates 12,000 calories of energy. After loss of one phosphate radical from ATP, the compound becomes *adenosine diphosphate* (ADP), and after loss of the second phosphate radical the compound becomes *adenosine monophosphate* (AMP). The interconversions between ATP, ADP, and AMP are the following:

$$\text{ATP} \underset{+12{,}000\text{ cal.}}{\overset{-12{,}000\text{ cal.}}{\rightleftharpoons}} \left\{ \begin{matrix} \text{ADP} \\ + \\ \text{PO}_4 \end{matrix} \right\} \underset{+12{,}000\text{ cal.}}{\overset{-12{,}000\text{ cal.}}{\rightleftharpoons}} \left\{ \begin{matrix} \text{AMP} \\ + \\ 2\text{PO}_4 \end{matrix} \right\}$$

ATP is present everywhere in the cytoplasm and nucleoplasm of all cells, and essentially all of the physiological mechanisms that require energy for operation obtain it directly from the ATP (or some other similar high-energy compound—guanosine triphosphate, GTP, for example). In turn, the food in the cells is gradually oxidized, and the released energy is used to re-form the ATP, thus always maintaining a supply of this substance.

In summary, ATP is an intermediary compound that has the peculiar ability of entering into many coupled reactions—reactions with the food to extract energy and reactions to many physiological mechanisms to provide energy for their operation. For this reason, ATP has frequently been called the energy *currency* of the body that can be gained and spent again and again.

The principal purpose of the present chapter is to explain how the energy from carbohydrates can be used to form ATP (or GTP) in the cells. At least 99 per

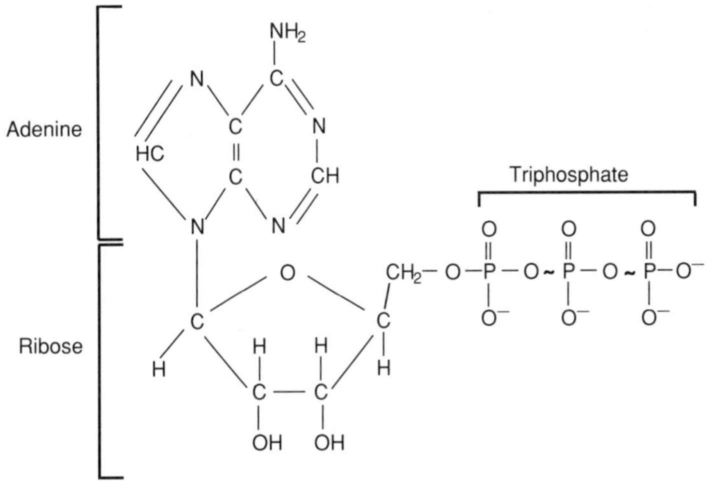

Figure 45-1. Chemical structure of adenosine triphosphate (ATP).

cent of all the carbohydrates utilized by the body is used for this purpose.

TRANSPORT OF MONOSACCHARIDES THROUGH THE CELL MEMBRANE

From the previous chapter it will be recalled that the final products of carbohydrate digestion in the alimentary tract are almost entirely glucose, fructose, and galactose, with glucose representing by far the major amount of these. These three monosaccharides are absorbed into the portal blood and, after passing through the blood sinuses of the liver, are carried everywhere in the body by the circulatory system. But before they can be used by the cells, they must be transported through the cell membrane into the cellular cytoplasm.

Monosaccharides cannot diffuse through the usual pores of the cell membrane, for the maximum molecular weight of substances that can do this is about 100, whereas glucose, fructose, and galactose all have molecular weights of 180. Yet glucose and some of the other monosaccharides combine with a *protein carrier* in the membrane that then allows them to diffuse freely to the inside of the cell. After passing through the membrane they become dissociated from the carrier. The transport mechanism is one of *facilitated diffusion* and not of active transport. These concepts are discussed in more detail in Chapter 4.

Enhancement of Glucose Transport by Insulin

The rate of glucose transport through the cell membrane is greatly increased by insulin. When large amounts of insulin are secreted by the pancreas, the rate of glucose transport into most cells increases to as much as ten times the rate of transport when no insulin at all is secreted. The amounts of glucose that can diffuse to the insides of most cells of the body in the absence of insulin, with the unique exceptions of the liver and the brain, are far too little to supply anywhere near the amount of glucose normally required for energy metabolism. Therefore, in effect, the rate of carbohydrate utilization by the body is controlled mainly by the rate of insulin secretion in the pancreas. The functions of insulin and its control of carbohydrate metabolism will be discussed more fully in Chapter 52.

Phosphorylation of Glucose

Immediately upon entry into the cells, glucose combines with a phosphate radical in accordance with the following reaction:

$$\text{glucose} \xrightarrow[+\text{ATP}]{\text{glucokinase or hexokinase}} \text{glucose 6-phosphate}$$

This phosphorylation is promoted by the enzyme *glucokinase* in the liver or *hexokinase* in most other cells.

The phosphorylation of glucose is almost completely irreversible except in the liver cells, the renal tubular epithelium, and the intestinal epithelial cells in which glucose phosphatase is available for reversing the reaction. Therefore, in most tissues of the body, phosphorylation serves to *capture* the glucose in the cell — once *in* the cell, the glucose will not diffuse back out except from those special cells that have the necessary phosphatase.

Conversion of Fructose and Galactose into Glucose. In liver cells appropriate enzymes are available to promote interconversions between the monosaccharides, and the dynamics of the reactions are such that when the liver releases the monosaccharides back into the blood, the final product of these interconversions is almost entirely glucose. In the case of fructose, much of it is also converted into glucose as it is absorbed through the intestinal epithelial cells into the portal blood. Therefore, essentially all the monosaccharides that circulate in the blood are the final conversion product, glucose.

STORAGE OF GLYCOGEN IN LIVER AND MUSCLE

After absorption into the cells, glucose can be used immediately for release of energy to the cells, or it can be stored in the form of *glycogen,* which is a large polymer of glucose.

All cells of the body are capable of storing at least some glycogen, but certain cells can store large amounts, especially the liver cells, which can store up to 5 to 8 per cent of their weight as glycogen, and muscle cells, which can store up to 1 to 3 per cent of their weight as glycogen. The glycogen molecules can be polymerized to almost any molecular weight, the average molecular weight being five million or more; most of the glycogen precipitates in the form of solid granules.

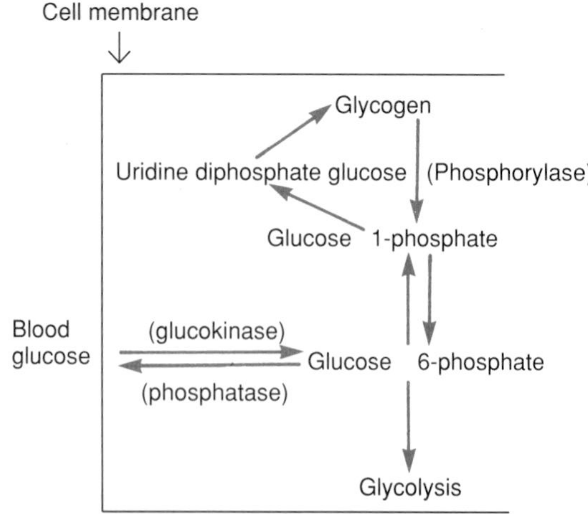

Figure 45-2. The chemical reactions of glycogenesis and glycogenolysis, showing also the interconversions between blood glucose and liver glycogen. (The phosphatase required for release of glucose from the cell is present in liver cells but absent in most other cells.)

Glycogenesis

Glycogenesis is the process of glycogen formation, the chemical reactions of which are illustrated in Figure 45-2. From this figure it can be seen that *glucose 6-phosphate* first becomes *glucose 1-phosphate;* this is then converted to *uridine diphosphate glucose,* which is converted into glycogen. Several specific enzymes are required to cause these conversions. Any monosaccharide that can be converted into glucose obviously can enter into the reactions, and certain smaller compounds, including *lactic acid, glycerol, pyruvic acid,* and some *deaminated amino acids,* can also be converted into glucose or closely allied compounds and thence into glycogen.

Removal of Stored Glycogen—Glycogenolysis

Glycogenolysis means the breakdown of glycogen to re-form glucose in the cells. Glycogenolysis does not occur by reversal of the same chemical reactions that serve to form glycogen; instead, each succeeding glucose molecule on each branch of the glycogen polymer is split away by the process of *phosphorylation* catalyzed by the enzyme *phosphorylase.*

Under resting conditions, the phosphorylase is in an inactive form, so that glycogen can be stored but not reconverted into glucose. When it is required to re-form glucose from glycogen, therefore, the phosphorylase must first be activated. This activation is accomplished in the following ways:

Activation of Phosphorylase by Epinephrine and Glucagon. Two hormones, epinephrine and glucagon, can specifically activate phosphorylase and thereby cause rapid glycogenolysis. The initial effect of each of these hormones is to increase the formation of *cyclic adenosine monophosphate (cAMP)* in the cells. This substance then initiates a cascade of chemical reactions that activate the phosphorylase, a process discussed in more detail in Chapter 52.

Epinephrine is released by the adrenal medullae when the sympathetic nervous system is stimulated. The epinephrine then activates phosphorylase, thus making glucose available for rapid metabolism. This function of epinephrine occurs markedly both in liver cells and in muscle, thereby contributing, along with other effects of sympathetic stimulation, to preparation of the body for action, as discussed in Chapter 41.

Glucagon is a hormone secreted by the *alpha cells* of the pancreas when the blood glucose concentration falls low. It stimulates the formation of cAMP mainly in the liver and thereby activates phosphorylase. Its effect is primarily to dump glucose out of the liver into the blood, thereby raising blood glucose concentration back toward the normal level. The function of glucagon in blood glucose regulation is discussed in Chapter 52.

Transport of Glucose Out of Liver Cells. The cells of the liver contain *phosphatase,* an enzyme that can split phosphate away from glucose 6-phosphate and therefore make the glucose available for retransport out of the cells into the interstitial fluids. Therefore, when glucose is formed in the liver as a result of glycogenolysis, most of it immediately passes into the blood. Thus, liver glycogenolysis causes an immediate rise in blood glucose concentration. Glycogenolysis in most other cells of the body, especially in the muscle cells, simply makes increased amounts of glucose 6-phosphate available inside the cells and increases the local rate of glucose utilization, but it does not release the glucose into the extracellular fluids because the required phosphatase is not available to dephosphorylate the glucose 6-phosphate.

RELEASE OF ENERGY FROM THE GLUCOSE MOLECULE BY THE GLYCOLYTIC PATHWAY

Complete oxidation of 1 mole of glucose releases 686,000 calories of energy, but only 12,000 calories of energy are required to form 1 mole of adenosine triphosphate (ATP). Therefore it would be an extreme waste of energy if glucose decomposed at once into water and carbon dioxide while forming only a single ATP molecule. Fortunately, cells contain an extensive series of different protein enzymes that cause the glucose molecule to split a little at a time in many successive steps, with its energy released in small packets to form one molecule of ATP at a time, forming a total of 38 moles of ATP for each mole of glucose utilized by the cells.

The purpose of the present section is to describe the basic principles by which the glucose molecule is progressively dissected and its energy released to form ATP.

Glycolysis and the Formation of Pyruvic Acid

By far the most important means by which energy is released from the glucose molecule is the process of *glycolysis,* followed by *oxidation of the end-products of glycolysis. Glycolysis* means splitting of the glucose molecule to form two molecules of pyruvic acid. This process occurs by ten successive steps of chemical reactions, illustrated in Figure 45–3. Each step is catalyzed by at least one specific protein enzyme. Note that glucose is first converted into fructose 1,6-phosphate and then split into two three-carbon atom molecules, each of which is then converted through five successive steps into pyruvic acid.

Formation of Adenosine Triphosphate (ATP) During Glycolysis. Despite the many chemical reactions in the glycolytic series, only 2 moles of ATP are formed for each mole of glucose utilized. This amounts to 24,000 calories of energy stored in the form of ATP, but during glycolysis a total of 56,000 calories of energy is lost from the original glucose, giving an overall *efficiency* for ATP formation of 43 per cent. The remaining 57 per cent of the energy is lost in the form of heat.

Conversion of Pyruvic Acid to Acetyl Coenzyme A

The next stage in the degradation of glucose is conversion of its two derivative pyruvic acid molecules into two molecules of *acetyl coenzyme A* (acetyl Co-A) in accordance with the following reaction:

$$\underset{\text{(Pyruvic Acid)}}{2\ CH_3{-}\overset{\overset{\displaystyle O}{\|}}{C}{-}COOH} + \underset{\text{(Coenzyme A)}}{2\ \text{Co-A}{-}SH}$$

$$\longrightarrow \underset{\text{(Acetyl Co-A)}}{2\ CH_3{-}\overset{\overset{\displaystyle O}{\|}}{C}{-}S{-}\text{Co-A}} + 2CO_2 + 4H$$

From this reaction it can be seen that two carbon dioxide molecules and four hydrogen atoms are released, while the remainders of the two pyruvic acid molecules combine with coenzyme A, a derivative of the vitamin pantothenic acid, to form two molecules of acetyl Co-A. In this conversion, no ATP is formed, but six molecules of ATP are produced when the four hydrogen atoms are later oxidized, as is discussed in a later section.

The Citric Acid Cycle

The next stage in the degradation of the glucose molecule is called the *citric acid cycle* (also called the *tricarboxylic acid cycle,* or *the Krebs cycle*). This is a

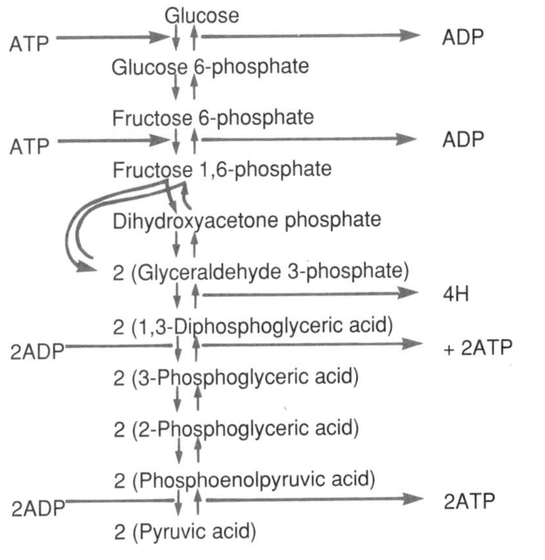

Glucose
ATP → ↓↑ → ADP
Glucose 6-phosphate
↓↑
Fructose 6-phosphate
ATP → ↓↑ → ADP
Fructose 1,6-phosphate
Dihydroxyacetone phosphate
↓↑
2 (Glyceraldehyde 3-phosphate)
↓↑ → 4H
2 (1,3-Diphosphoglyceric acid)
2ADP → ↓↑ → + 2ATP
2 (3-Phosphoglyceric acid)
↓↑
2 (2-Phosphoglyceric acid)
↓↑
2 (Phosphoenolpyruvic acid)
2ADP → ↓↑ → 2ATP
2 (Pyruvic acid)

Net reaction:

Glucose + 2ADP + $2PO_4^{---}$ → 2 Pyruvic acid + 2ATP + 4H

Figure 45–3. The sequence of chemical reactions responsible for glycolysis.

sequence of chemical reactions, illustrated in Figure 45–4, in which the acetyl portion of acetyl Co-A is degraded to carbon dioxide and hydrogen atoms. These reactions all occur *in the matrix of the mitochondrion.* The released hydrogen atoms are subsequently oxidized, as discussed later, releasing tremendous amounts of energy to form ATP.

The substances to the left in Figure 45–4 are added during the chemical reactions, and the products of the chemical reactions are shown to the right. Note at the top of the column that the cycle begins with *oxaloacetic acid,* and then at the bottom of the chain of reactions *oxaloacetic acid* is formed once again. Thus, the cycle can continue indefinitely.

In the initial stage of the citric acid cycle, *acetyl Co-A* combines with *oxaloacetic acid* to form *citric acid.* The coenzyme A portion of the acetyl Co-A is released and can be used again and again for the formation of still more quantities of acetyl Co-A from pyruvic acid. The acetyl portion, however, becomes an integral part of the citric acid molecule. During the successive stages of the citric acid cycle, several molecules of water are added, and *carbon dioxide* and *hydrogen atoms* are released at various stages in the cycle, as shown on the right in the figure.

The net results of the entire citric acid cycle are shown at the bottom of Figure 45–4, illustrating that for each molecule of glucose originally metabolized, two acetyl Co-A molecules enter into the citric acid cycle along with six molecules of water. These molecules are then degraded into four carbon dioxide molecules, 16 hydrogen atoms, and 2 molecules of coenzyme A.

Formation of ATP in the Citric Acid Cycle. No large amount of energy is released during the citric acid cycle itself. However, for each molecule of glucose metabolized, two molecules of ATP are formed.

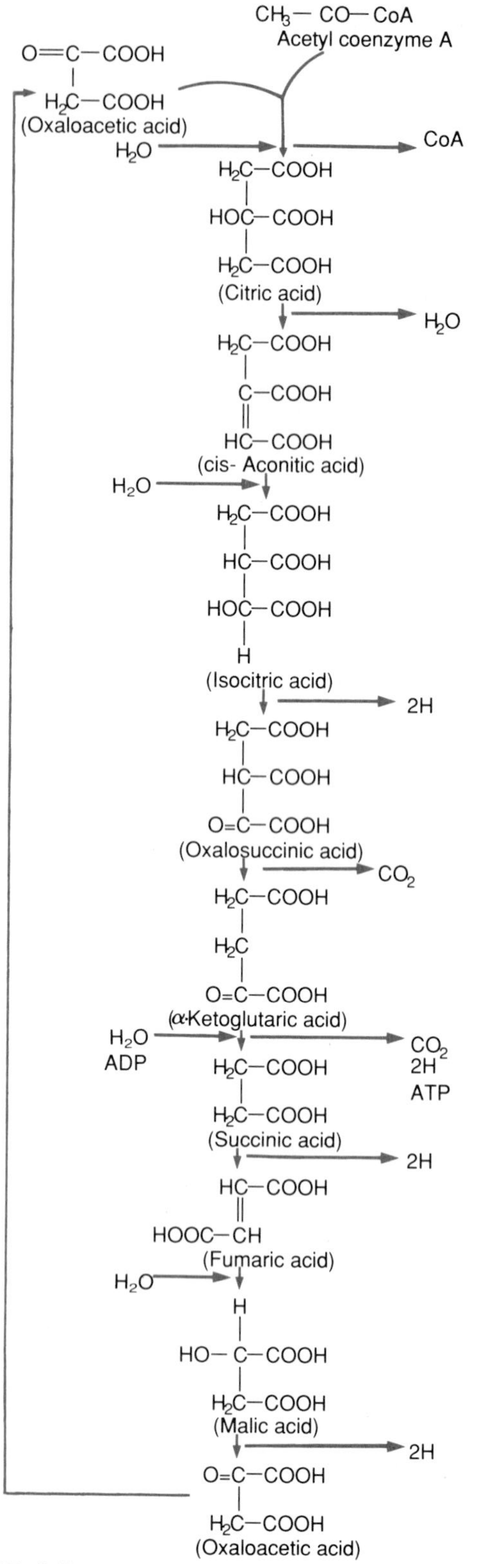

Formation of ATP by Oxidative Phosphorylation of the Hydrogen Atoms

Despite all the complexities of glycolysis and the citric acid cycle, pitifully small amounts of ATP are formed during these processes—only 2 ATP molecules in the glycolysis scheme and another 2 in the citric acid cycle. Instead, almost 95 per cent of the final ATP is formed during subsequent oxidation of the hydrogen atoms that are released during these earlier stages of glucose degradation. Indeed, the principal function of all these earlier stages is to make the hydrogen of the glucose molecule available in a form that can be utilized for oxidation.

Oxidation of hydrogen is accomplished by a series of enzymatically catalyzed reactions that (a) change the hydrogen atoms into hydrogen ions and electrons and (b) use the electrons eventually to change the dissolved oxygen of the fluids into hydroxyl ions. Then the hydrogen and hydroxyl ions combine to form water. During this sequence of oxidative reac-

Figure 45–4. The chemical reactions of the citric acid cycle, showing the release of carbon dioxide and an especially large number of hydrogen atoms during the cycle.

Net reaction per molecule of glucose:

$$2\ \text{Acetyl-CoA} + 6H_2O + 2ADP \rightarrow 4CO_2 + 16H + 2CoA + 2ATP$$

tions, tremendous quantities of energy are released to form ATP. Formation of ATP in this manner is called *oxidative phosphorylation.* It occurs entirely in the mitochondria by a highly specialized process called the chemiosmotic mechanism, illustrated in Figure 45-5.

The Chemiosmotic Mechanism for Forming ATP

Ionization of Hydrogen, the Electron Transport Chain, and Formation of Water. The first step in oxidative phosphorylation is to ionize the hydrogen atoms that are removed from the food substrates. These hydrogen atoms are removed in pairs during glycolysis and during the citric acid cycle; one immediately becomes a hydrogen ion, H^+, and the other combines with NAD^+ to form NADH. The upper portion of Figure 45-5 shows in color the subsequent disposition of the NADH and H^+ in the mitochondrion. The initial effect is to release the other hydrogen atom bound with NAD to form another hydrogen ion, H^+; this process also reconstitutes NAD^+, which will be reused again and again.

During these changes, the electrons that are removed from the hydrogen atoms to cause their ionization immediately enter an *electron transport chain* that is an integral part of the inner membrane (the shelf membrane) of the mitochondrion. This transport chain consists of a series of electron acceptors that can be reversibly reduced or oxidized by accepting or giving up electrons. The important members of this electron transport chain include *flavoprotein, several iron sulfide proteins, ubiquinone,* and *cytochromes*

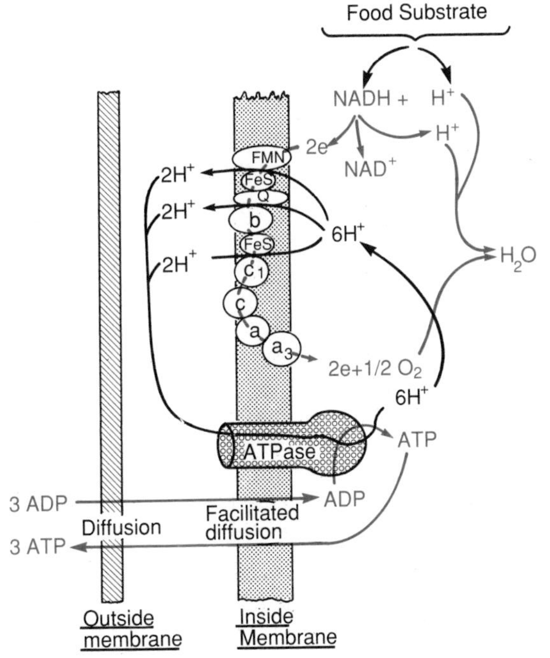

Figure 45-5. The chemiosmotic mechanism of oxidative phosphorylation for forming great quantities of ATP.

B, C_1, C, A, and A_3. Each electron is shuttled from one of these acceptors to the next until it finally reaches cytochrome A_3, which is called *cytochrome oxidase* because it is capable, by giving up two electrons, of causing elemental oxygen to combine with hydrogen ions to form water.

Thus, Figure 45-5 illustrates transport of electrons through the electron chain and their ultimate use by cytochrome oxidase to cause the formation of water molecules. During the transport of these electrons through the electron transport chain, energy is released that is later used to cause synthesis of ATP, as follows:

Pumping of Hydrogen Ions into the Outer Chamber of the Mitochondrion, Caused by the Electron Transport Chain. The energy released as the electrons pass through the electron transport chain is used to pump hydrogen ions from the inner matrix of the mitochondrion into the space between the inner and outer mitochondrial membranes. This creates a high concentration of hydrogen ions in this space, and it also creates a strong negative electrical potential in the inner matrix.

Formation of ATP. The final step in oxidative phosphorylation is to convert ADP into ATP. This conversion occurs in conjunction with a large protein molecule with a knoblike head that protrudes all the way through the inner mitochondrial membrane and into the inner matrix. This molecule is an ATPase, the physical nature of which is illustrated in Figure 45-5. It is called *ATP synthetase.* The high concentration of hydrogen ions in the space between the two mitochondrial membranes and the large electrical potential difference across the inner membrane cause the hydrogen ions to flow into the mitochondrial matrix *through the substance of the ATPase molecule.* In doing so, energy derived from this hydrogen ion flow is utilized by the ATPase to convert ADP into ATP by combining an ADP with a phosphate radical, forming an additional high energy phosphate bond.

For each two hydrogen atoms ionized by the electron transport chain, up to three ATP molecules are synthesized.

Summary of ATP Formation During the Breakdown of Glucose

We can now determine the total number of ATP molecules formed by the energy from one molecule of glucose. The number is

1. Two during glycolysis
2. Two during the citric acid cycle and
3. During oxidative phosphorylation, 34, making a total of *38 ATP molecules* formed for each molecule of glucose degraded to carbon dioxide and water. Thus, 456,000 calories of energy are stored in the form of ATP, while 686,000 calories are released during the complete oxidation of each mole of glucose. This represents an overall *efficiency* of energy transfer of 66

per cent. The remaining 34 per cent of the energy becomes heat and therefore cannot be used by the cells to perform specific functions.

Control of Glycolysis and Glucose Oxidation by Intracellular Adenosine Diphosphate (ADP) Concentration

Continuous release of energy from glucose when the energy is not needed by the cells would be an extremely wasteful process. Fortunately, glycolysis and the subsequent oxidation of hydrogen atoms is continuously controlled in accordance with the needs of the cells for ATP. This control is accomplished mainly in the following manner:

Referring back to the various chemical reactions, we see that at different stages *ADP* is converted into *ATP*. *If ADP is not available, the reactions cannot occur, and the degradation of the glucose molecule is stopped.* Therefore, once all the ADP in the cells has been converted to ATP, the entire glycolytic and oxidative process stops. Then, when more ATP is used to perform different physiological functions in the cell, new ADP is formed, which automatically starts glycolysis and oxidation once more. In this way, essentially a full store of ATP is automatically maintained all the time, except when the activity of the cell becomes so great that ATP is used more rapidly than it can be formed.

Release of Energy in the Absence of Oxygen—"Anaerobic" Glycolysis

Occasionally, oxygen becomes either unavailable or insufficient, so that cellular oxidation of glucose cannot take place. Yet, even under these conditions, a small amount of energy can still be released to the cells by glycolysis, for the chemical reactions in the glycolytic breakdown of glucose to pyruvic acid do not require oxygen. Unfortunately, this process is extremely wasteful of glucose because only 24,000 calories of energy are used to form ATP for each mole of glucose utilized, which represents only a little over 3 per cent of the total energy in the glucose molecule. Nevertheless, this release of glycolytic energy to the cells can be a lifesaving measure for a few minutes when oxygen becomes unavailable.

Formation of Lactic Acid During Anaerobic Glycosis. The *law of mass action* states that as the end-products of a chemical reaction build up in a reacting medium, the rate of the reaction approaches zero. The two end-products of the glycolytic reactions (see Figure 45–3) are (1) pyruvic acid and (2) hydrogen atoms in the forms NADH and H^+. The buildup of excessive amounts of these would stop the glycolytic process and prevent further formation of ATP. Fortunately, when their quantities begin to be excessive, these end-products react with each other to form lactic acid, in accordance with the following equation.

$$\underset{\text{(Pyruvic acid)}}{CH_3{-}\overset{\overset{\displaystyle O}{\|}}{C}{-}COOH} + NADH + H^+ \xrightleftharpoons[]{\text{lactic dehydrogenase}} \underset{\text{(Lactic acid)}}{CH_3{-}\underset{\underset{\displaystyle H}{|}}{\overset{\overset{\displaystyle OH}{|}}{C}}{-}COOH} + NAD^+$$

Thus, under anaerobic conditions, by far the larger portion of the pyruvic acid is converted into lactic acid, which diffuses readily out of the cells into the extracellular fluids and even into the intracellular fluids of other less active cells. Therefore, lactic acid represents a type of "sinkhole" into which the glycolytic end-products can disappear, allowing glycolysis to proceed far longer than would be possible if the pyruvic acid and hydrogen were not removed from the reacting medium. Indeed, glycolysis could proceed for only a few seconds without this conversion. Instead, it can proceed for several minutes, supplying the body with considerable quantities of ATP even in the absence of respiratory oxygen.

When a person begins to breathe oxygen again after a period of anaerobic metabolism, the extra NADH and H^+ as well as the extra pyruvic acid that have built up in the body fluids are rapidly oxidized, mainly in the liver, thereby undergoing great reduction in their concentrations. As a result, the chemical reaction for formation of lactic acid immediately reverses itself, the lactic acid once again becoming pyruvic acid, which is eventually oxidized to supply additional cellular energy.

RELEASE OF ENERGY FROM GLUCOSE BY THE PENTOSE PHOSPHATE PATHWAY

Though essentially all the carbohydrates utilized by the muscles are degraded to pyruvic acid by glycolysis and then converted to carbon dioxide and hydrogen atoms by the citric acid cycle, this glycolytic and citric acid schema is not the only means by which glucose can be degraded to provide energy. A second important schema for glucose breakdown is called the *pentose phosphate pathway.* Though this process is not discussed here, it is responsible for as much as 30 per cent of the glucose breakdown in the liver and for even more than that in fat cells. It is especially important in providing energy and some of the substrates required for conversion of carbohydrates into fat, as will be discussed in the following chapter.

FORMATION OF CARBOHYDRATES FROM PROTEINS AND FATS—"GLUCONEOGENESIS"

When the body's stores of carbohydrates decrease below normal, moderate quantities of glucose can be formed from *amino acids* and from the *glycerol* portion of fat. This process is called *gluconeogenesis*. Approximately 60 per cent of the amino acids in the body proteins can easily be converted into carbohydrates, while the remaining 40 per cent have chemical configurations that make this difficult. Each amino acid is converted into glucose by a slightly different chemical process. For instance, alanine can be converted directly into pyruvic acid simply by deamination; the pyruvic acid then is converted into glucose by the liver.

Regulation of Gluconeogenesis. Diminished carbohydrates in the cells and decreased blood sugar are the basic stimuli that set off an increase in the rate of gluconeogenesis. The diminished carbohydrates can directly cause reversal of many of the glycolytic and phosphogluconate reactions, thus allowing conversion of deaminated amino acids and glycerol into carbohydrates. However, in addition, several of the hormones secreted by the endocrine glands are especially important in this regulation, as follows:

Effect of Corticotropin and Glucocorticoids on Gluconeogenesis. When normal quantities of carbohydrates are not available to the cells, the anterior pituitary gland, for reasons not yet completely understood, begins to secrete increased quantities of corticotropin, which stimulate the adrenal cortex to produce large quantities of *glucocorticoid hormones*, especially *cortisol*. In turn, cortisol mobilizes proteins from essentially all cells of the body, making them available in the form of amino acids in the body fluids. A high proportion of amino acids immediately becomes deaminated in the liver and therefore provides ideal substrates for conversion into glucose. Thus, one of the most important means by which gluconeogenesis is promoted is through the release of glucocorticoids from the adrenal cortex.

BLOOD GLUCOSE

The normal blood glucose concentration in a person who has not eaten a meal within the past 3 to 4 hours is approximately 90 mg per 100 ml of blood, and even after a meal containing large amounts of carbohydrates, this concentration rarely rises above 140 mg per 100 ml of blood unless the person has diabetes mellitus.

The regulation of blood glucose concentration is intimately related to insulin and glucagon; this subject will be discussed fully in relation to the functions of these two hormones in Chapter 52.

REFERENCES

Brazy, P. C., and Mandel, L. J.: Does availability of inorganic phosphate regulate cellular oxidative metabolism? News Physiol. Sci., 1:100, 1986.

Golinick, P. D.: Metabolism of substrates: Energy substrate metabolism during exercise and as modified by training. Fed. Proc., 44:353, 1985.

Jequier, E., and Flatt, J.-P.: Recent advances in human energetics. News Physiol. Sci., 1:112, 1986.

Kraus-Friedmann, N.: Hormonal regulation of hepatic gluconeogenesis. Physiol. Rev., 64:170, 1984.

Lemasters, J. J., et al. (eds.): Integration of Mitochondrial Function. New York, Plenum Publishing Corp., 1988.

Oomura, Y., and Yoshimatsu, H.: Neural network of glucose monitoring system. J. Auton. Nerv. Syst., 10:359, 1984.

Sairam, M. R.: Role of carbohydrates in glycoprotein hormone signal transduction. FASEB J., 3:1915, 1989.

Senior, A. E.: ATP synthesis by oxidative phosphorylation. Physiol. Rev., 68:177, 1988.

Storlien, L. H.: The role of the ventromedial hypothalamic area in periprandial glucoregulation. Life-Sci., 36:505, 1985.

Stryer, L.: Biochemistry, New York. W. H. Freeman Co., 1988.

QUESTIONS

1. Describe the special features of the ATP molecule that allow it to function as an *energy currency*. At body temperature and at the concentrations of ATP found in the body cells, how much energy is present in each high energy phosphate bond per mole of ATP?
2. How is *glucose* transported through the cell membrane, and what is the effect of *insulin* on this transport?
3. How does *phosphorylation of glucose* cause the capture of glucose in the cell?
4. What is the composition of *glycogen*, and what is its role in cells, especially in the liver and in muscle?
5. Explain glycogenolysis and the release of glucose from the liver when glucose is needed elsewhere in the body.
6. Explain, in general, the *glycolytic pathway* for dissolution of the glucose molecule.
7. Describe the conversion of *pyruvic acid* to *acetyl coenzyme A* and the role of the *citric acid cycle* in converting the acetyl portion of the acetyl coenzyme A into carbon dioxide and hydrogen atoms.
8. Explain the *chemiosmotic mechanism* for formation of ATP in the *mitochondria*.
9. What percentage of the ATP normally used by the cell is formed by *oxidative phosphorylation*?
10. How does the concentration of *adenosine diphosphate* in the cells determine the rate of glycolysis?
11. Explain the mechanism and importance of *anaerobic glycolysis;* also explain the formation of *lactic acid* and tell why this is important to anaerobic glycolysis.
12. Explain what is meant by *gluconeogenesis*, how it is controlled, and its importance.
13. What is the normal resting blood glucose concentration, and how high does this rise after meals in the normal person?

46

Lipid and Protein Metabolism

THE BODY LIPIDS

Several different chemical compounds in the food and in the body are classified as *lipids.* These include (1) *neutral fat,* known also as *triglycerides,* (2) *phospholipids,* (3) *cholesterol,* and (4) a few others of less importance. These substances have certain similar physical and chemical properties—especially, they are miscible with each other. Chemically, the basic lipid moiety of both the triglycerides and the phospholipids is *fatty acids,* which are simply long-chain hydrocarbon organic acids. Though cholesterol does not contain fatty acid, its sterol nucleus is synthesized from degradation products of fatty acid molecules, thus giving it many of the physical and chemical properties of other lipid substances.

The triglycerides are used in the body mainly to provide energy for the different metabolic processes; this function they share almost equally with the carbohydrates. However, some lipids, especially cholesterol, the phospholipids, and derivatives of these, are used throughout the body to provide other intracellular functions.

Basic Chemical Structure of Triglycerides (Neutral Fat). Since most of this chapter deals with utilization of triglycerides for energy, the following basic structure of the triglyceride molecule must be understood:

$$\begin{array}{l} CH_3{-}(CH_2)_{16}{-}COO{-}CH_2 \\ \qquad\qquad\qquad\qquad\quad | \\ CH_3{-}(CH_2)_{16}{-}COO{-}CH \\ \qquad\qquad\qquad\qquad\quad | \\ CH_3{-}(CH_2)_{16}{-}COO{-}CH_2 \end{array}$$

Tristearin

Note that three long-chain fatty acid molecules are bound with one molecule of glycerol.

TRANSPORT OF LIPIDS IN THE BLOOD

Transport from the Gastrointestinal Tract—The Chylomicrons

It will be recalled from Chapter 44 that essentially all the fats of the diet are absorbed into the lymph in the form of *chylomicrons,* which have a size averaging 0.4 micron. The chylomicrons are then transported up the thoracic duct and emptied into the venous blood at the juncture of the jugular and subclavian veins.

Removal of the Chylomicrons from the Blood. The chylomicrons are removed from the plasma within an hour or so. Most are removed from the circulating blood as they pass through the capillaries of adipose tissue and the liver. The membranes of the fat cells contain large quantities of an enzyme called *lipoprotein lipase.* This enzyme hydrolyzes the triglycerides of the chylomicrons into fatty acids and glycerol. The fatty acids, being highly miscible with the membranes of the cells, immediately diffuse into the fat cells. Once within these cells, the fatty acids are resynthesized into triglycerides, new glycerol being supplied by the metabolic processes of the fat cells, as will be discussed later in the chapter.

TRANSPORT OF FATTY ACIDS IN COMBINATION WITH ALBUMIN—"FREE FATTY ACID"

When the fat that has been stored in the fat cells is to be used elsewhere in the body, usually for providing energy, it must first be transported to the other tissues. It is transported almost entirely in the form of *free fatty acid,* which is achieved by hydrolysis of the triglycerides stored in the fat cells once again into fatty acids and glycerol. Part of the stimulus for initiating this hydrolysis is reduced glycerol in the cell when glucose is not present in sufficient amounts to form new glycerol. In addition, a cellular lipase called *hormone-sensitive triglyceride lipase* becomes activated by one of several different means, and this activated lipase promotes rapid hydrolysis of the triglycerides.

On leaving the fat cells, the fatty acids ionize strongly in the plasma and immediately combine loosely with albumin of the plasma proteins. The fatty acid bound with proteins in this manner is called *free fatty acid* or *nonesterified fatty acid* (or simply *FFA* or *NEFA*) to distinguish it from other fatty acids in the plasma that exist in the form of esters of glycerol, cholesterol, or other substances.

The concentration of free fatty acid in the plasma under resting conditions is about 15 mg per 100 ml of plasma, which is a total of only 0.45 gram of fatty acids in the entire circulatory system. Yet, strangely enough, even this small amount accounts for almost all of the transport of lipids from one part of the body to another, for the following reasons:

(1) Despite the minute amount of free fatty acid in the blood, its rate of turnover is extremely rapid, *half the plasma fatty acid being replaced by new fatty acid every 2 to 3 minutes.* One can calculate that at this rate over half of all the energy required by the body can be provided by the free fatty acid transported even without increasing the free fatty acid concentration. (2) All conditions that increase the rate of utilization of fat for cellular energy also increase the free fatty acid concentration in the blood; this concentration sometimes increases as much as five- to eightfold. This occurs especially in starvation and in diabetes when a person is not using or cannot use carbohydrates for energy.

The Lipoproteins

In the postabsorptive state — that is, when no chylomicrons are in the blood — over 95 per cent of all the lipids in the plasma (in terms of mass, but *not* in terms of rate of transport) are in the form of lipoproteins, which are particles much smaller than chylomicrons but similar in composition, containing mixtures of *triglycerides, phospholipids, cholesterol,* and *protein.* The protein in the mixture averages about one fourth to one third of the total constituents, and lipids form the remainder. The total concentration of lipoproteins in the plasma averages about 700 mg per 100 ml of plasma and can be broken down into the following average concentrations of the individual constituents:

	mg/100 ml of plasma
Cholesterol	180
Phospholipids	160
Triglycerides	160
Lipoprotein protein	200

Types of Lipoproteins. Chylomicrons sometimes are also classified as lipoproteins because they contain both lipids and protein. In addition to the chylomicrons, however, there are three other major classes of lipoprotein: (1) *very low density lipoproteins,* which contain high concentrations of triglycerides and moderate concentrations of both phospholipids and cholesterol; (2) *low density lipoproteins,* which contain relatively few triglycerides but a very high percentage of cholesterol; and (3) *high density lipoproteins,* which contain about 50 per cent protein with smaller concentrations of the lipids.

Formation of the Lipoproteins. The lipoproteins are formed almost entirely in the liver, which is in keeping with the fact that most plasma phospholipids, cholesterol, and triglycerides (except those in the chylomicrons) are synthesized in the liver.

Function of the Lipoproteins. The principal function of the lipoproteins in the plasma is to transport their special types of lipids throughout the body. The turnover of triglycerides in the lipoproteins is as much as several grams per hour and perhaps half this much turnover of cholesterol and phospholipids.

Triglycerides are synthesized mainly from carbohydrates in the liver and are transported to the adipose tissue and other peripheral tissues in the *very low density lipoproteins.* The *low density lipoproteins* are the residuals of the very low density lipoproteins after they have delivered most of their triglycerides to the adipose tissue, leaving large concentrations of cholesterol and phospholipids in the low density lipoproteins. On the other hand, the *high density lipoproteins* transport cholesterol away from the peripheral tissues and to the liver; therefore, this type of lipoprotein plays a very important role in preventing the development of atherosclerosis, which we shall discuss later in the chapter.

THE FAT DEPOSITS

Adipose Tissue

Large quantities of fat are frequently stored in two major tissues of the body, the adipose tissue and the liver. The adipose tissue is usually called the *fat deposits,* or simply the *fat depots.*

The major function of adipose tissue is storage of triglycerides until these are needed to provide energy elsewhere in the body. However, a subsidiary function is to provide heat insulation for the body, as is discussed in Chapter 47.

The Fat Cells. The fat cells of adipose tissue are modified fibroblasts that are capable of storing almost pure triglycerides in quantities equal to 80 to 95 per cent of their volume.

Fat cells can also synthesize very small quantities of fatty acids and triglycerides from carbohydrates, this function supplementing the synthesis of fat in the liver, as discussed later in the chapter.

Exchange of Fat Between the Adipose Tissue and the Blood — Tissue Lipases. As discussed previously, large quantities of lipases are present in adipose tissue. Some of these enzymes catalyze the deposition of triglycerides derived from the chylomicrons and other lipoproteins. Others, when activated by hormones, cause splitting of the triglycerides of the fat cells to release free fatty acids. Because of rapid exchanges of the fatty acids, the triglycerides in the fat cells are renewed approximately once every two to three weeks, which means that the fat stored in the tissues today is not the same fat that was stored last month, thus emphasizing the dynamic state of the storage fat.

The Liver Lipids

The principal functions of the liver in lipid metabolism are (1) to degrade fatty acids into small compounds that can be used for energy, (2) to synthesize triglycerides mainly from carbohydrates and, to a lesser extent, from proteins, and (3) to synthesize other lipids from fatty acids, especially cholesterol and phospholipids.

The liver cells, in addition to containing triglycerides, contain large quantities of phospholipids and cholesterol, which are continually synthesized by the liver. Also, the liver cells are much more capable than other tissues of desaturating fatty acids, so that the liver triglycerides normally are much more unsaturated than the triglycerides of the adipose tissue. This capability of the liver to desaturate fatty acids is functionally important to all the tissues of the body, because many of the structural members of all cells contain reasonable quantities of desaturated fats, and their principal source is the liver. This desaturation is accomplished by a *dehydrogenase* in the liver cells.

USE OF TRIGLYCERIDES FOR ENERGY AND FORMATION OF ADENOSINE TRIPHOSPHATE (ATP)

Approximately 40 to 45 per cent of the calories in the normal American diet are derived from fats, which amount is about equal to the calories derived from carbohydrates. Therefore, the use of fats by the body for energy is just as important as the use of carbohydrates. In addition, much of the carbohydrates ingested with each meal is converted into triglycerides, then stored, and later utilized as triglycerides for energy.

Entry of Fatty Acids into the Mitochondria. The degradation and oxidation of fatty acids occur only in the mitochondria. Therefore, the first step in the utilization of the fatty acids is their transport into the mitochondria. This is an enzyme-catalyzed process that employs *carnitine* as a carrier substance. Once inside the mitochondria, the fatty acid splits away from the carnitine and is then oxidized.

Degradation of Fatty Acid to Acetyl Coenzyme A by Beta Oxidation. The fatty acid molecule is degraded in the mitochondria by progressive release of 2-carbon segments to form acetyl coenzyme A (acetyl Co-A). This process is illustrated in Figure 46–1; it is called the *beta oxidation* mechanism for degradation of fatty acids. Each time the reactions of this schema go through a complete cycle, beginning at the top left-hand corner of the figure and proceeding to the bottom right-hand corner, a new acetyl Co-A molecule is formed, and the fatty acid chain becomes two carbon atoms shorter. The process is repeated again and again until the entire fatty acid molecule is split into acetyl Co-A. For instance, from each molecule of stearic acid, nine molecules of acetyl Co-A are formed.

Oxidation of Acetyl Co-A. The acetyl Co-A molecules formed by this beta oxidation of fatty acids enter the citric acid cycle, as explained in the preceding chapter regarding the acetyl Co-A derived from glucose, and are degraded into carbon dioxide and hydrogen atoms, the same as the end-stages of carbohydrate metabolism. The hydrogen is subsequently oxidized by the oxidative enzymes of the mitochondria to form ATP, also the same as for carbohydrate metabolism.

Quantity of ATP Formed by Oxidation of Fatty Acid. In Figure 46–1 note that four hydrogen atoms are released each time a molecule of acetyl Co-A is formed from the fatty acid chain. Then additional hydrogen is released in the citric acid cycle. The oxidation of all these hydrogen atoms gives rise to the

(1) $RCH_2CH_2CH_2COOH + CoA + ATP \underset{}{\overset{\text{Thiokinase}}{\rightleftharpoons}} RCH_2CH_2CH_2COCoA + AMP + Pyrophosphate$
(Fatty acid) (Fatty acyl CoA)

(2) $RCH_2CH_2CH_2COCoA + FAD \xrightarrow{\text{Acyl dehydrogenase}} RCH_2CH{=}CHCOCoA + FADH_2$
(Fatty acyl CoA)

(3) $RCH_2CH{=}CHCOCoA + H_2O \overset{\text{Enoyl hydrase}}{\rightleftharpoons} RCH_2CHOHCH_2COCoA$

(4) $RCH_2CHOHCH_2COCoA + NAD^+ \underset{\text{Dehydrogenase}}{\overset{\beta\text{-Hydroxyacyl}}{\rightleftharpoons}} RCH_2COCH_2COCoA + NADH + H^+$

(5) $RCH_2COCH_2COCoA + CoA \overset{\text{Thiolase}}{\rightleftharpoons} RCH_2COCoA + CH_3COCoA$
(Fatty acyl CoA)(Acetyl CoA)

Figure 46–1. Beta oxidation of fatty acids to yield acetylcoenzyme A.

formation of 139 molecules of ATP *for each stearic acid molecule oxidized.* Also, another 7 molecules of ATP are formed in other ways during this entire process, making a total of 146 molecules of ATP.

Formation of Acetoacetic Acid in the Liver — An Accessory Method for Transporting Lipids in the Blood

A large share of the degradation of fatty acids into acetyl Co-A occurs in the liver. However, the liver uses only a small proportion of the acetyl Co-A for its own intrinsic metabolic processes. Instead, pairs of acetyl Co-A condense to form molecules of *acetoacetic acid,* as follows:

$$\underset{\text{Acetyl Co-A}}{2CH_3COCo\text{-}A} + H_2O \underset{\text{other cells}}{\overset{\text{liver cells}}{\rightleftarrows}} \underset{\text{Acetoacetic acid}}{CH_3COCH_2COOH} + 2HCo\text{-}A$$

Then a large part of the acetoacetic acid is converted into *β-hydroxybutyric acid,* and minute quantities to *acetone,* in accordance with the following reactions:

$$\underset{\text{Acetoacetic acid}}{CH_3-\overset{O}{\overset{\|}{C}}-CH_2-\overset{O}{\overset{\|}{C}}-OH}$$

$$\xrightarrow{+2H} \underset{\beta\text{-Hydroxybutyric acid}}{CH_3-\overset{OH}{\overset{|}{C}H}-CH_2-\overset{O}{\overset{\|}{C}}-OH} \qquad \xrightarrow{-CO_2} \underset{\text{Acetone}}{CH_3-\overset{O}{\overset{\|}{C}}-CH_3}$$

The acetoacetic acid and β-hydroxybutyric acid then freely diffuse through the liver cell membranes and are transported by the blood to the peripheral tissues. Here they again diffuse into the cells, where reverse reactions occur and acetyl Co-A molecules are formed. These in turn enter the citric acid cycle of the cell and are oxidized for energy, as explained previously.

Synthesis of Triglycerides from Carbohydrates

Whenever a greater quantity of carbohydrates enters the body than can be used immediately for energy or stored in the form of glycogen, the excess is rapidly converted into triglycerides and is then stored in this form in the adipose tissue. Most triglyceride synthesis occurs in the liver, but a small amount also occurs in the fat cells. The triglycerides that are formed in the liver are mainly transported by the lipoproteins to the fat cells of the adipose tissue to be stored until needed for energy.

Conversion of Carbohydrates into Fatty Acids. The first step in the synthesis of triglycerides from carbohydrates is conversion of the carbohydrates into acetyl Co-A. It will be recalled from the preceding chapter that this conversion occurs during the normal degradation of glucose by the glycolytic system. It will also be remembered from earlier in this chapter that fatty acids are actually large polymers of the acetyl portion of acetyl Co-A. Therefore, without going into the details of the chemical reactions, it is easy to understand how acetyl Co-A can be converted into fatty acids.

Combination of Fatty Acids with α-Glycerophosphate to Form Triglycerides. Once the synthesized fatty acid chains have grown to contain 14 to 18 carbon atoms, they then automatically bind with glycerol to form triglycerides.

The glycerol portion of the triglyceride is furnished by α-glycerophosphate, which is also a product derived from the glycolytic schema of glucose degradation, illustrated in Figure 45-3 (Chapter 45).

The real importance of this mechanism for formation of triglycerides is that the final combination of fatty acids with glycerol is controlled mainly by the concentration of α-glycerophosphate, which in turn is determined by the availability of carbohydrates. When carbohydrates form large quantities of α-glycerophosphate, the equilibrium shifts to promote formation and storage of triglycerides. When carbohydrates are not available, the whole process shifts in the opposite direction, and an excess of fatty acids then becomes available to substitute for lack of carbohydrate metabolism.

Importance of Fat Synthesis and Storage. Fat synthesis from carbohydrates is especially important for two reasons: (1) The ability of the different cells of the body to store carbohydrates in the form of glycogen is generally slight; only a few hundred grams of glycogen are stored in the liver, the skeletal muscles, and all other tissues of the body put together. Therefore, fat synthesis provides a means by which the energy of excess ingested carbohydrates (and proteins, too) can be stored for later use. Indeed, the average person has about 200 times as much energy stored in the form of fat as in the form of carbohydrate. (2) Each gram of fat contains approximately two and one fourth times as many calories of usable energy as each gram of glycogen. Therefore, for a given weight gain, a person can store far more energy in the form of fat than in the form of carbohydrate, which is important when an animal must be highly motile to survive.

Synthesis of Triglycerides from Proteins

Many amino acids can be converted into acetyl Co-A, as will be discussed later in the chapter. Obviously, this acetyl Co-A also can be converted into triglycerides. Therefore, when persons have more proteins in their diet than their tissues can use as proteins or directly for energy, a large share of the excess energy is stored as fat.

Hormonal Regulation of Fat Utilization

At least seven of the hormones secreted by the endocrine glands have marked effects on fat utilization.

Probably the most dramatic increase that occurs in fat utilization is that observed during heavy exercise. This results almost entirely from rapid release of *epinephrine* and *norepinephrine* by the adrenal medullae during exercise, as a result of sympathetic stimulation. These two hormones directly activate *hormone-sensitive triglyceride lipase,* which is present in abundance in the fat cells. This activated hormone then causes very rapid breakdown of triglycerides and mobilization of fatty acids. Sometimes the free fatty acid concentration in the blood rises as much as fivefold to eightfold. Other types of stress that activate the sympathetic nervous system will increase fatty acid mobilization and utilization in a similar manner.

Stress also causes large quantities of *corticotropin* to be released by the anterior pituitary gland, and this release in turn causes the adrenal cortex to secrete excessive quantities of *glucocorticoids* (mainly cortisol). Both the corticotropin and the glucocorticoids activate either the same hormone-sensitive triglyceride lipase as that activated by epinephrine and norepinephrine or a similar lipase, which therefore is still another mechanism for increasing the release of fatty acids from fat tissue.

Growth hormone has an effect similar to but less effective than that of corticotropin and glucocorticoids in activating the hormone-sensitive lipase. Therefore, growth hormone can also have a mild fat-mobilizing effect.

Lack of insulin also activates hormone-sensitive lipase and therefore causes rapid mobilization of fatty acids. When carbohydrates are not available in the diet, insulin secretion diminishes, and this in turn promotes fatty acid metabolism.

Finally, *thyroid hormone* causes rapid mobilization of fat, a process that is believed to result indirectly from an increased rate of energy metabolism in all cells of the body under the influence of this hormone.

The effects of the different hormones on metabolism are discussed further in the chapters dealing with each of them.

PHOSPHOLIPIDS AND CHOLESTEROL

Phospholipids

The three major types of body phospholipids are the *lecithins,* the *cephalins,* and the *sphingomyelins.* A lecithin is shown in Figure 46–2.

$$H_2C-O-\overset{O}{\overset{\|}{C}}-(CH_2)_7-CH{=}CH-(CH_2)_7-CH_3$$
$$HC-O-\overset{O}{\overset{\|}{C}}-(CH_2)_{16}-CH_3$$
$$H_2C-O-\overset{O}{\overset{\|}{\underset{OH}{P}}}-O-CH_2-CH_2-N^{+}(CH_3)_3$$

Figure 46–2. A lecithin.

Phospholipids always contain one or more fatty acid molecules and one phosphoric acid radical, and they usually contain a nitrogenous base. Though the chemical structures of phospholipids vary somewhat, their physical properties are similar, for they are lipid soluble, are transported together in lipoproteins in the blood, and seem to be utilized similarly throughout the body for various structural purposes.

Phospholipids are formed in essentially all cells of the body, though certain cells have a special ability to form them. Probably 90 per cent or more of the phospholipids enter the blood in the lipoproteins that are formed in the liver cells.

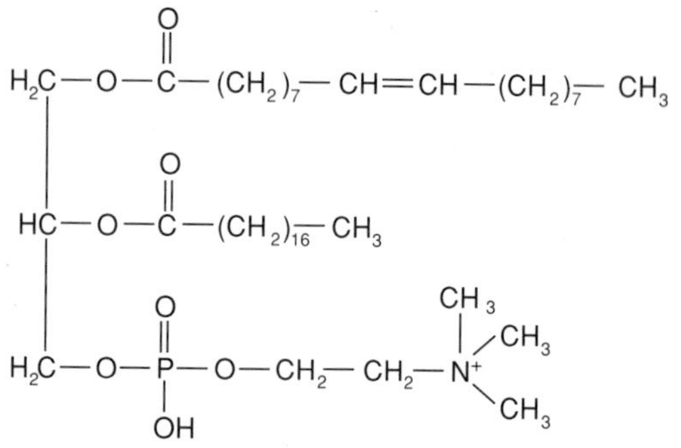

Cholesterol

Cholesterol, the formula of which is illustrated in Figure 46–3, is present in the diet of all persons, and it can be absorbed from the gastrointestinal tract into the intestinal lymph. It is highly fat soluble but only slightly soluble in water, and it is capable of forming esters with fatty acids. Indeed, approximately 70 per cent of the cholesterol of the plasma is in the form of cholesterol esters.

Besides the cholesterol absorbed each day from the gastrointestinal tract, which is called *exogenous cholesterol,* a large quantity, called *endogenous cholesterol,* is formed in the cells of the body. Essentially all the endogenous cholesterol that circulates in the lipoproteins of the plasma is formed by the liver, but all the other cells of the body form at least some cholesterol.

Structural Functions of Phospholipids and Cholesterol

In Chapter 2 it was pointed out that large quantities of phospholipids and cholesterol are present in the cell membrane as well as in the membranes of the internal organelles of all cells.

For membranes to be formed, substances that are not soluble in water must be available, and in general,

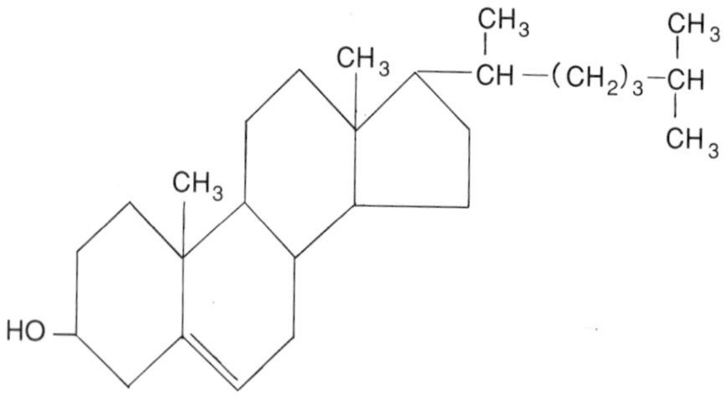

Figure 46–3. Cholesterol.

the only substances in the body that are not soluble in water (besides the inorganic substances of bone) are mainly the lipids and some proteins. Thus, the physical integrity of cells throughout the body is based mainly on phospholipids, triglycerides, cholesterol, and certain insoluble proteins. Some phospholipids are somewhat water soluble as well as lipid soluble, which gives them the important property of helping decrease the interfacial tension between the membranes and the surrounding fluids.

Another fact indicating that phospholipids and cholesterol are mainly concerned with the formation of structural elements of the cells is the slow turnover rate of these substances. For instance, phospholipids formed in the brain remain there for many months or perhaps even for years.

ATHEROSCLEROSIS

Atherosclerosis is principally a disease of the large arteries in which lipid deposits called *atheromatous plaques* appear in the intimal and subintimal layers of the arteries. These plaques contain an especially large amount of cholesterol and often are simply called *cholesterol deposits.* They are also associated with degenerative changes in the arterial wall. In a later stage of the disease, fibroblasts infiltrate the degenerative areas and cause progressive sclerosis of the arteries. In addition, calcium often precipitates with the lipids to develop *calcified plaques.* When these two processes occur, the arteries become extremely hard, and the disease is then called *arteriosclerosis,* or simply "hardening of the arteries."

Obviously, arteriosclerotic arteries lose most of their distensibility, and because of the degenerative areas, they are easily ruptured. Also, the atheromatous plaques often break through the intima and protrude into the flowing blood, and the roughness of their surfaces causes blood clots to develop, with resultant thrombus or embolus formation. Almost half of all human beings die of some complication of arteriosclerosis; approximately two thirds of these deaths are caused by thrombosis of one or more coronary arteries and the remaining one third by thrombosis or hemorrhage of vessels in other organs of the body—especially the brain, kidneys, liver, gastrointestinal tract, limbs, and so forth.

Role of Low Density Lipoproteins in Causing Atherosclerosis. As discussed earlier in the chapter, essentially all the lipoproteins are initially formed in the liver. Furthermore, most of these are formed as *very low density* lipoproteins containing *very* large quantities of triglycerides and cholesterol. However, much of the triglyceride and cholesterol portions of the lipoproteins are released into the tissues, and the lipoproteins change from very low density to simply *low density* lipoproteins. At this stage, many of these are recaptured by the liver, and their constituents are reused to transport more triglycerides and cholesterol. However, the recapture process requires the presence of receptors in the liver cell membranes for attaching the protein portion of the lipoprotein. Many persons have a hereditary deficiency of these receptors so that in them the low density lipoproteins are not captured but instead continue to build up in the blood, causing more cholesterol deposition in the tissues and arterial walls. In fact, when recapture fails to occur, the liver even synthesizes many new lipoproteins, making the situation worse and worse.

The high density lipoproteins are an entirely separate entity from the very low density and low density lipoproteins. They too are formed mainly by the liver, but they have the capability of removing cholesterol from the tissues rather than causing additional deposition. Even though the high density lipoprotein system is still far from being understood, it is known that persons with high blood levels of high density lipoproteins have diminished likelihood of developing atherosclerosis.

THE BODY PROTEINS

About three quarters of the body solids are proteins. These include *structural proteins, enzymes, proteins that transport oxygen, proteins of the muscle that cause contraction,* and many other types that perform specific functions both intracellularly and extracellularly throughout the body.

The basic chemical properties that explain the diverse functions of proteins are so extensive that they constitute a major portion of the entire discipline of biochemistry. For this reason, the present discussion is confined to the general aspects of protein metabolism.

The Amino Acids

The principal constituents of proteins are amino acids, 20 of which are present in the body in significant quantities. Figure 46-4 illustrates the chemical formulas of these 20 amino acids, showing that they all have two features in common: Each amino acid has an acidic group (—COOH) and a nitrogen radical that lies in close association with the acidic radical, usually represented by the amino group ($—NH_2$).

Peptide Linkages and Peptide Chains. In proteins, the amino acids are aggregated into long chains by means of so-called *peptide linkages,* one of which is illustrated by the following reaction:

$$\underset{\substack{|\\ \text{R—CH—COOH}}}{\text{NH}_2} + \underset{\substack{|\\ \text{R}'\text{—CH—COOH}}}{\text{NH}_2} \longrightarrow \begin{array}{c} \text{NH}_2 \\ | \\ \text{R—CH—CO} \\ | \\ \text{NH} \\ | \\ \text{R}'\text{—CH—COOH} \end{array} + H_2O$$

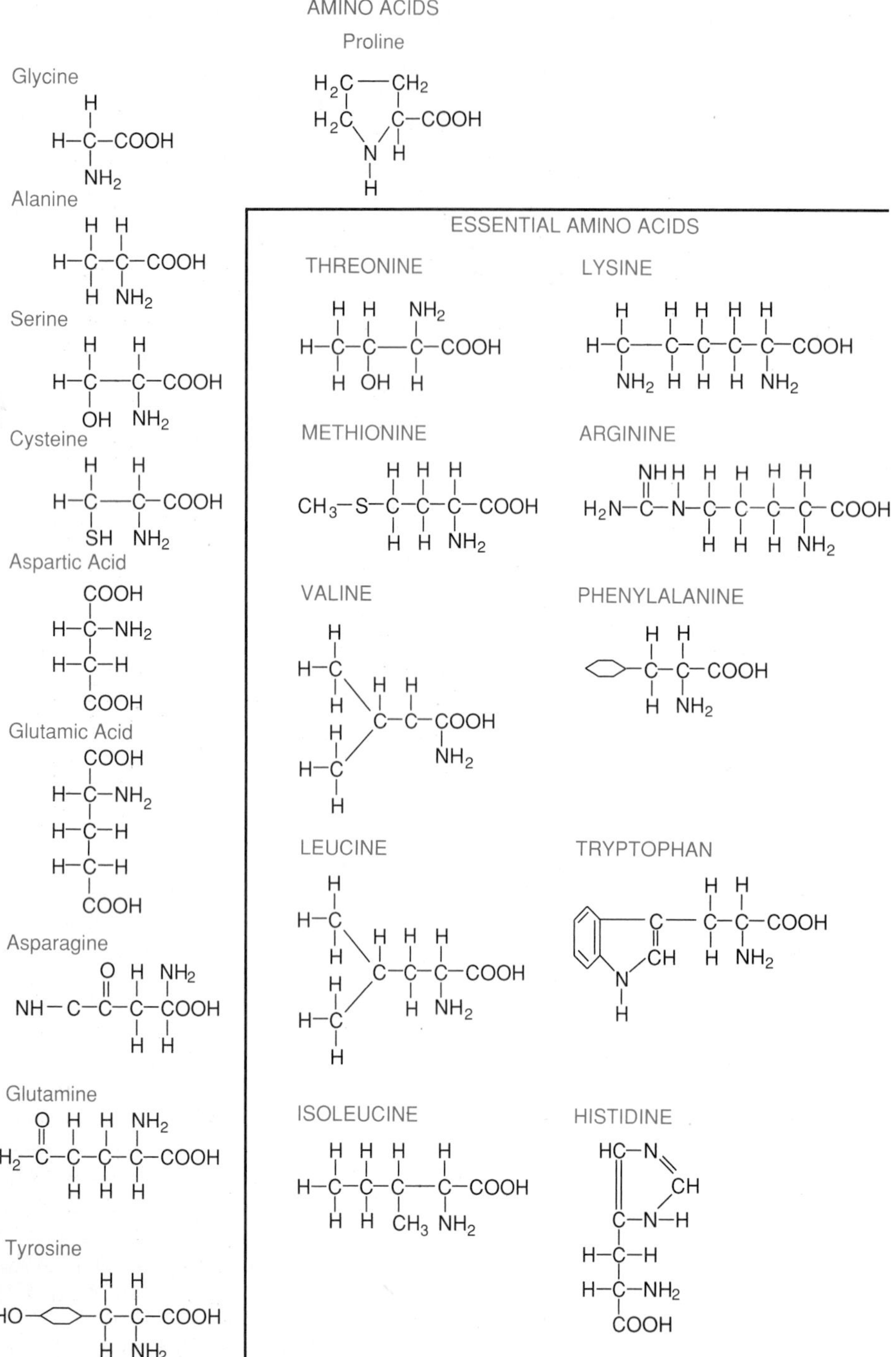

Figure 46-4. The amino acids, showing the 10 essential amino acids that cannot be synthesized at all or in sufficient quantity in the body.

Note that in this reaction the amino radical of one amino acid combines with the carboxyl radical of the other amino acid. A hydrogen atom is released from the amino radical, a hydroxyl radical is released from the carboxyl radical, and these two combine to form a molecule of water. Note that after the peptide linkage has been formed, an amino radical and a carboxyl radical are still in the new molecule, both of which are capable of combining with additional amino acids to form a *peptide chain.* Some complicated protein molecules have as many as a hundred thousand amino acids joined principally by peptide linkages, and even the smallest protein usually has more than 20 amino acids joined by peptide linkages.

Fibrous Proteins

Many of the highly complex proteins are fibrillar and are called fibrous proteins. In these, many separate chains are held together in parallel bundles by cross-linkages. Major types of fibrous proteins are (1) *collagens,* which are the basic structural proteins of connective tissue, tendons, cartilage, and bone; (2)

elastins, which are the elastic fibers of tendons, arteries, and connective tissue; (3) *keratins,* which are the structural proteins of hair and nails; and (4) *actin* and *myosin,* the contractile proteins of muscle.

TRANSPORT AND STORAGE OF AMINO ACIDS

The Blood Amino Acids

The normal concentration of amino acids in the blood is between 35 and 65 mg per 100 ml of plasma. This is an average of about 2 mg per 100 ml for each of the 20 amino acids, though some are present in far greater concentrations than others. Since the amino acids are relatively strong acids, they exist in the blood principally in the ionized state and account for 2 to 3 milliequivalents of the negative ions in the blood.

Fate of Amino Acids Absorbed from the Gastrointestinal Tract. It will be recalled from Chapter 44 that the end-products of protein digestion in the gastrointestinal tract are almost entirely amino acids and that polypeptide or protein molecules are only rarely absorbed into the blood. Immediately after a meal, the amino acid concentration in the blood rises, but the rise is usually only a few milligrams per 100 ml because, after entering the blood, the excess amino acids are absorbed within 5 to 10 minutes by cells throughout the entire body. Therefore, almost never do large concentrations of amino acids accumulate in the blood. Nevertheless, the turnover rate of the amino acids is so rapid that many grams of proteins in the form of amino acids can be carried from one part of the body to another each hour.

Transport of Amino Acids into the Cells. The molecules of essentially all the amino acids are much too large to diffuse through the pores of the cell membranes. Instead, the amino acids are transported through the membrane only by active transport or facilitated diffusion, utilizing carrier mechanisms. The nature of some of the carrier mechanisms is still poorly understood, but some are discussed in Chapter 4.

Storage of Amino Acids as Proteins in the Cells

Almost immediately after entry into the cells, amino acids are conjugated under the influence of intracellular enzymes into cellular proteins, so that the concentration of free amino acids inside the cells almost always remains low. Instead, the amino acids are mainly stored in the form of actual proteins. Yet many intracellular proteins can be rapidly decomposed again into amino acids under the influence of intracellular lysosomal digestive enzymes, and these amino acids in turn can be transported again from the cell into the blood. The proteins that can be thus decomposed include many cellular enzymes as well as some other functioning proteins. However, most of the structural proteins such as collagen and muscle contractile proteins do not participate significantly in this reversible storage of amino acids.

Some tissues of the body participate in the storage of amino acids to a greater extent than others. For instance, the liver, which is a large organ and also has special systems for processing amino acids, stores large quantities of labile proteins.

Release of Amino Acids from the Cells, and Regulation of Plasma Amino Acid Concentration. Whenever the plasma amino acid concentration falls below its normal level, amino acids are transported out of the cells to replenish the supply in the plasma. Simultaneously, intracellular proteins are degraded back into amino acids.

The plasma concentration of each type of amino acid is maintained at a reasonably constant value. Later it will be noted that various hormones secreted by the endocrine glands are able to alter the balance between tissue proteins and circulating amino acids; growth hormone and insulin increase the formation of tissue proteins, while adrenocortical glucocorticoid hormones increase the concentration of circulating amino acids.

The Plasma Proteins

The three major types of protein in the plasma are *albumin, globulin,* and *fibrinogen.* The principal function of albumin is to provide *colloid osmotic pressure,* which in turn prevents plasma loss from the capillaries, as discussed in Chapter 13. The globulins perform a number of enzymatic functions in the plasma itself, but more important than this, they are mainly responsible for *immunity* against invading organisms, a subject discussed in Chapter 20. The fibrinogen polymerizes into long, branching fibrin threads during *blood coagulation,* thereby forming blood clots that help repair leaks in the circulatory system, discussed in Chapter 25.

Formation of the Plasma Proteins. Essentially all the albumin and fibrinogen in the plasma proteins, as well as about one half of the globulins, are formed in the liver. The remainder of the globulins are formed principally in the lymphoid tissues and bone marrow. These are mainly the *gamma globulins* that constitute the antibodies of the immune system.

The rate of plasma protein formation by the liver can be extremely high, as much as 30 grams per day. Certain disease conditions often cause rapid loss of plasma proteins; severe burns that denude large surface areas cause loss of many liters of plasma through the denuded areas each day. The rapid production of plasma proteins by the liver is obviously valuable in preventing death in such states. Furthermore, occasionally, a person with severe renal disease may lose as much as 20 grams of plasma protein in the urine each day for months, and this plasma protein is continuously replaced.

Use of Plasma Proteins by the Tissue as a Source of Amino Acids. When the tissues become depleted of proteins, the plasma proteins can act as a source for rapid replacement of these proteins. Indeed, whole plasma proteins can be imbibed *in toto* by the liver cells and macrophages; then they are split into amino acids that are transported back into the blood and utilized throughout the body to build cellular proteins. In this way, therefore, the plasma proteins function as a labile protein storage medium and represent a rapidly available source of amino acids whenever a particular tissue requires them.

CHEMISTRY OF PROTEIN SYNTHESIS

Proteins are synthesized in all cells of the body, and the functional characteristics of each cell are dependent upon the types of protein that it can form. Basically, the genes of the cells control the protein types and thereby control the functions of the cell. This regulation of cellular function by the genes was discussed in detail in Chapter 3. Chemically, two basic processes must be accomplished for the synthesis of proteins; these are (1) synthesis of the amino acids and (2) appropriate conjugation of the amino acids to form the respective types of whole proteins in each individual cell.

Essential and Nonessential Amino Acids. Ten of the twenty amino acids normally present in animal proteins can be synthesized in the cells, while the other ten either cannot be synthesized at all or are synthesized in quantities too small to supply the body's needs. The first group of amino acids is called *nonessential,* while the second group is called *essential amino acids* because these must be present in the diet if protein formation is to take place in the body. Use of the word *essential* does not mean that the other 10 amino acids are not equally essential in the formation of the proteins, but only that these others are not essential in the diet.

Synthesis of the nonessential amino acids depends on the formation, first, of appropriate α-keto acids, which are the precursors of the respective amino acids. For instance, *pyruvic acid,* which is formed in large quantities during the glycolytic breakdown of glucose, is the keto acid precursor of the amino acid *alanine.* Then, by the simple process of *transamination,* an amino radical is transferred to the α-keto acid to form the alanine molecule while the keto oxygen is transferred to the donor of the amino radical.

Formation of Proteins from Amino Acids. Once the appropriate amino acids are present in a cell, whole proteins are synthesized rapidly. However, each peptide linkage requires from 500 to 4000 calories of energy, and this must be supplied from ATP and GTP (guanosine triphosphate) in the cell. Protein formation proceeds through two steps: (1) "activation" of each amino acid, during which the amino acid is "energized' by energy derived from ATP and GTP, and (2) alignment of the amino acids into the peptide chains, a function that is under control of the DNA-RNA system of each individual cell. Both of these processes were discussed in Chapter 3. Indeed, the formation of cellular proteins is the basis of life itself and is so important that the reader would do well to review Chapter 3.

USE OF PROTEINS FOR ENERGY

There is an upper limit to the amount of protein that can accumulate in each particular type of cell. Once the cells are filled to their limits, the feedback controls of the DNA-RNA system block further protein synthesis, as explained in Chapter 3, and any additional amino acids in the body fluids are degraded and used for energy or stored as fat. This degradation occurs almost entirely in the liver, and it begins with the process known as deamination.

Deamination. Deamination means removal of the amino groups from the amino acids. This can occur by several different means, two of which are especially important: (1) transamination, which means transfer of the amino group to some acceptor substance (as explained earlier in relation to the synthesis of amino acids) and (2) oxidative deamination.

The greatest amount of deamination occurs by the following transamination schema:

$$\alpha\text{-ketoglutaric acid} + \text{amino acid}$$
$$\text{glutamic acid} + \alpha\text{-keto acid}$$
$$+\text{NAD}^+ + H_2O$$
$$\rightarrow \text{NADH} + H^+ + NH_3$$

Note from this schema that the amino group from the amino acid is transferred to α-ketoglutaric acid, which then becomes glutamic acid. The glutamic acid can then transfer the amino group to still other substances or can release it in the form of ammonia. In the process of losing the amino group, the glutamic acid once again becomes α-ketoglutaric acid, so that the cycle can be repeated again and again.

Urea Formation by the Liver. The ammonia released during deamination is removed from the blood almost entirely by conversion into urea, two molecules of ammonia and one molecule of carbon dioxide combining in accordance with the following net reaction:

$$2NH_3 + CO_2 \rightarrow H_2N\text{—}\underset{\underset{\displaystyle O}{\|}}{C}\text{—}NH_2 + H_2O$$

Essentially all urea formed in the human body is synthesized in the liver. In the absence of the liver or in serious liver disease, ammonia accumulates in the blood. This in turn is extremely toxic, especially to the brain, often leading to a state called *hepatic coma.*

The stages in the formation of urea are essentially the following:

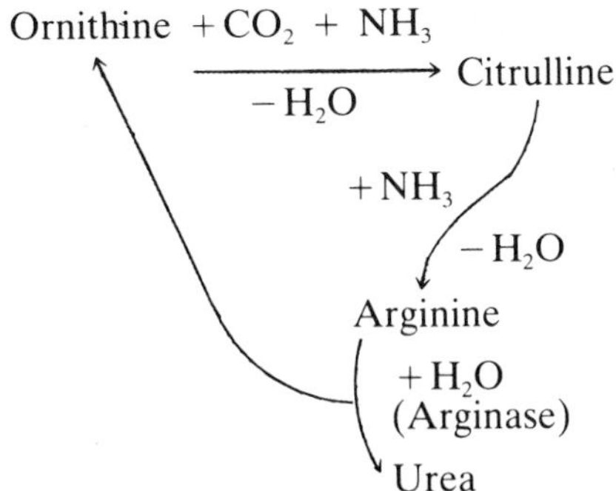

The reaction begins with the amino acid derivative *ornithine,* which combines with one molecule of carbon dioxide and one molecule of ammonia to form a second substane, *citrulline.* This in turn combines with still another molecule of ammonia to form *arginine,* which then splits into *ornithine* and *urea.* The urea diffuses from the liver cells into the body fluids and is excreted by the kidneys, while the ornithine is reused in the cycle again and again.

Oxidation of Deaminated Amino Acids. Once the amino acids have been deaminated, the resulting keto acid products can in most instances be oxidized to release energy for metabolic purposes. This usually involves two processes: (1) The keto acid is changed into an appropriate chemical substance that can enter the citric acid cycle, and (2) this substance is then degraded by this cycle in the same manner that acetyl Co-A derived from carbohydrate and fat metabolism is degraded.

In general, the amount of adenosine triphosphate formed for each gram of protein that is oxidized is slightly less than that formed for each gram of glucose oxidized.

Gluconeogenesis and Ketogenesis. Certain deaminated amino acids are similar to the breakdown products that result from glucose and fatty acid metabolism. For instance, deaminated alanine is pyruvic acid. Obviously, this can be converted into glucose or glycogen; or it can be converted into acetyl Co-A, which can then be polymerized into fatty acids. Also, two molecules of acetyl Co-A can condense to form acetoacetic acid, which is one of the so-called keto acids, as explained earlier in the chapter.

The conversion of amino acids into glucose or glycogen is called *gluconeogenesis,* and the conversion of amino acids into keto acids or fatty acids is called *ketogenesis.* Eighteen of twenty of the deaminated amino acids have chemical structures that allow them to be converted into glucose, and nineteen can be converted into fats — five directly and the other fourteen by becoming carbohydrate first and then becoming fat.

"Obligatory" Degradation of Proteins Even When No Proteins Are in the Diet

When a person eats no proteins, a certain proportion of his or her own body proteins continues to be degraded into amino acids, deaminated, and oxidized. This process involves 20 to 30 grams of protein each day, which is called the *obligatory loss* of proteins. Therefore, to prevent a net loss of protein from the body, one must ingest at least 20 to 30 grams of protein each day, and to be on the safe side a minimum of 60 to 75 grams is usually recommended.

Effect of Starvation on Protein Degradation. Except for the excess protein in the diet or the 20 to 30 grams of obligatory protein degradation each day, the body normally uses almost entirely carbohydrates or fats for energy as long as they are available. However, after several weeks of starvation, when the quantity of stored carbohydrates is completely gone and the stored fats are also beginning to run out, the amino acids of the blood begin to be rapidly deaminated and oxidized for energy. From this point on, the proteins of the tissues degrade rapidly — as much as 125 grams daily — and the cellular functions deteriorate precipitously.

Because use of carbohydrate and fat for energy occurs in preference to protein utilization, carbohydrates and fats are called *protein sparers.*

REFERENCES

Lipid Metabolism

Birdi, K. S.: Lipid and Biopolymer Monolayers at Liquid Interfaces. New York, Plenum Publishing Corp., 1989.

Breslow, J. L.: Apolipoprotein genetic variation and human disease. Physiol. Rev., 68:85, 1988.

Campbell, J. H., and Campbell, G. R.: Potential role of heparinase in atherosclerosis. News Physiol. Sci., 4:9, 1989.

Catapano, A. L., et al.: High-Density Lipoproteins: Physiopathological Aspects and Clinical Significance. New York, Raven Press, 1987.

Gaber, B. P., and Schnur, J. M.: Biotechnological Applications of Lipid Microstructures. New York, Plenum Publishing Corp., 1989.

Levy, R. I., et al.: Lipoproteins and Atherosclerosis. New York, Raven Press, 1988.

Stokes, J. I., and Mancini, M.: Hypercholesterolemia: Clinical and Therapeutic Implications. New York, Raven Press, 1988.

Waite, M.: The Phospholipases. New York, Plenum Publishing Corp., 1987.

Protein Metabolism

DeMartino, G. N., and Croall, D. E.: Calcium-dependent proteases: A prevalent proteolytic system of uncertain function. News Physiol. Sci., 2:82, 1987.

Fasman, G. D. (ed.): Prediction of Protein Structure and the Principles of Protein Conformation. New York. Plenum Publishing Corp., 1989.

Guthrie, H. A.: Introductory Nutrition. 7th ed. St. Louis, C. V. Mosby, Co., 1988.

Stryer, L.: Biochemistry. New York, W. H. Freeman Co., 1988.

Sugden, P. H.: The effects of hormonal factors on cardiac protein turnover. Adv. Myocardiol., 5:105, 1985.

Weinsier, R. L., et al.: Handbook of Clinical Nutrition: Clinician's Manual for the Diagnosis and Management of Nutritional Problems. St. Louis, C. V. Mosby Co., 1988.

Williams, S. R.: Basic Nutrition and Diet Therapy. 8th ed. St. Louis, C. V. Mosby Co., 1989.

QUESTIONS

1. Explain how *fatty acid molecules* combine with *glycerol* to form *triglycerides.*
2. Describe the transport of fats from the digestive tract to the blood and their ultimate storage in the fat tissues of the body.
3. Explain how tremendous quantities of fatty acids can be transported in the "free" fatty acid form by the plasma protein *albumin* even though the concentration of these fatty acids is very slight.
4. Explain what is meant by a *lipoprotein,* and also explain in general the function of lipoproteins in the blood.
5. Describe the storage and release of fats from *adipose tissue,* including the function of *hormone-sensitive lipase.*
6. Explain the general schema for beta oxidation of the fatty acid molecule.
7. What is the role of *acetoacetic acid* in the transport of fat degradation products from the liver to peripheral cells?
8. How are carbohydrates converted into triglycerides, and what controls this process?
9. Explain how the different hormones affect fat utilization.
10. What are the functions of *phospholipids* and *cholesterol* in the body?
11. Describe the development of *atherosclerosis* and *arteriosclerosis* in the arteries of older persons, and explain the effects of heredity and diet on these processes.
12. Explain the *peptide linkage* mechanism for the formation of *peptide chains.*
13. How are amino acids transported in the blood, and how are they stored in cells?
14. Explain how amino acids stored in cells can be released for use elsewhere in the body, and also explain how the plasma proteins can be used to provide amino acids for the body's cells.
15. What is meant by an *essential amino acid*?
16. Explain the processes of *deamination* and *urea formation* as one of the initial steps in the utilization of proteins for energy.
17. What is meant by *gluconeogenesis* and *ketogenesis* in relation to the utilization of amino acids?
18. What is meant by the *"obligatory" loss of proteins*? How great is this loss normally, and how great can protein loss become in starvation?

47

Energetics, Metabolic Rate, and Regulation of Body Temperature

IMPORTANCE OF ADENOSINE TRIPHOSPHATE (ATP) IN METABOLISM

In the last few chapters it has been pointed out that carbohydrates, fats, and proteins can all be used by the cells to synthesize large quantities of ATP and that the ATP in turn can be used as an energy source for many other cellular functions. The attribute of ATP that makes it highly valuable as a means of energy currency is the large quantity of free energy (7300 calories per mole under standard conditions, and 12,000 calories per mole under physiological conditions) vested in each of its two high energy phosphate bonds. The amount of energy in each bond, when liberated by decomposition of one molecule of ATP, is enough to cause almost any step of any chemical reaction in the body to take place if appropriate transfer of the energy is achieved. Some chemical reactions that require ATP energy use only a few hundred of the available 12,000 calories, and the remainder of this energy is then lost in the form of heat. Yet even this inefficiency in the utilization of energy is better than lack of the ability to energize the necessary chemical reactions at all.

Throughout this book we have listed many functions of ATP. So we will review here only its principal functions, which are

1. To energize the synthesis of important cellular components
2. To energize muscle contraction
3. To energize active transport across membranes for (a) absorption from the intestinal tract, (b) absorption from the renal tubules, (c) formation of glandular secretions, and (d) establishment of ionic concentration gradients in nerves, which in turn provide the energy required for nerve impulse transmission.

Phosphocreatine as a Storage Depot for Energy

Despite the paramount importance of ATP as a coupling agent for energy transfer, this substance is not the most abundant store of high energy phosphate bonds in the cells. On the contrary, phosphocreatine, which also contains high energy phosphate bonds, is several times as abundant, at least in muscle. The high energy bond of phosphocreatine contains about 13,000 calories per mole under conditions in the body (37°C and low concentrations of the reactants). This is not greatly different from the 12,000 calories per mole in each of the two high energy phosphate bonds of ATP. The formula for phosphocreatine is the following:

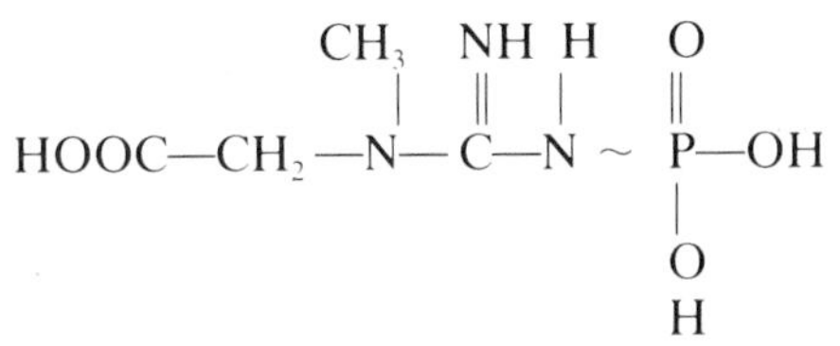

$$
\begin{array}{ccccccc}
 & & CH_3 & & NH & H & O \\
 & & | & & \| & | & \| \\
HOOC—CH_2— & & N— & & C— & N \sim & P—OH \\
 & & & & & & | \\
 & & & & & & O \\
 & & & & & & H
\end{array}
$$

Phosphocreatine, unlike ATP, cannot act as a coupling agent for transfer of energy between the foods and the functional cellular systems. But it can transfer energy interchangeably with ATP. When extra amounts of ATP are available in the cell, much of its energy is utilized to synthesize phosphocreatine, thus building up this storehouse of energy. Then when the ATP begins to be used up, the energy in the phosphocreatine is transferred rapidly back to ATP and then from the ATP to the functional systems of the cells.

The higher energy level of the high energy phosphate bond in phosphocreatine, 13,000 in comparison with 12,000 calories per mole, causes the reaction between phosphocreatine and ATP to proceed very much in favor of ATP. Therefore, the slightest utilization of ATP by the cells calls forth the energy from the phosphocreatine to synthesize new ATP. This effect keeps the concentration of ATP at almost peak level as long as any phosphocreatine remains in the cell. Therefore, one can call phosphocreatine an ATP "buffer" compound.

Summary of Energy Utilization by the Cells

With the background of the past few chapters and the preceding discussion, we can now synthesize a composite picture of overall energy utilization by the cells, as illustrated in Figure 47-1. This figure shows formation of ATP during the initial breakdown of glycogen and glucose, which is called "anaerobic" metabolism because this initial stage does not require oxygen; the figure also shows subsequent aerobic utilization of compounds derived from carbohydrates, fats, proteins, and other substances for the formation of still additional ATP. In turn, ATP is in reversible equilibrium with phosphocreatine in the cells, and since large quantities of phosphocreatine are present in the cell, much of the energy of the cell is stockpiled in this energy storehouse.

Now let us consider the energy used for muscle activity. Much of this energy simply overcomes the viscosity of the muscles themselves or of the surrounding tissues so that the limbs can move. The viscous movement in turn causes friction within the tissues, which generates heat.

We might also consider the energy expended by the heart in pumping blood. The blood distends the arterial system, the distention in itself representing a reservoir of potential energy. However, as the blood flows through the peripheral vessels, the friction of the different layers of blood flowing over each other and the friction of the blood against the walls of the vessels turns this energy into heat.

Therefore, we can say that essentially all the energy expended by the body is eventually converted into heat. The only real exception to this occurs when the muscles are used to perform some form of work outside the body. For instance, when the muscles elevate an object to a height or carry the person's body up steps, a type of potential energy ouside the body is thus created by raising a mass against gravity. But, on the whole, this normally averages no more than 1 per cent of the energy metabolism of the body. Therefore, measuring the body's heat production is an excellent means for studying the body's overall metabolism.

THE METABOLIC RATE

The Calorie. To discuss the rate of energy usage in the body, which is called the "metabolic rate," it is necessary to use some unit for expressing the quantity of energy released from the different foods or expended by the different functional processes of the body. Most often, the *Calorie* is the unit used for this purpose. It will be recalled that 1 *calorie,* spelled with a lower case *c,* is the quantity of heat required to raise the temperature of 1 gram of water 1°C. The calorie is much too small a unit for ease of expression in speaking of energy in the body. Consequently the kilocalorie, or in common parlance the large Calorie, (with a capital C), which is equivalent to 1000 calories, is the unit ordinarily used.

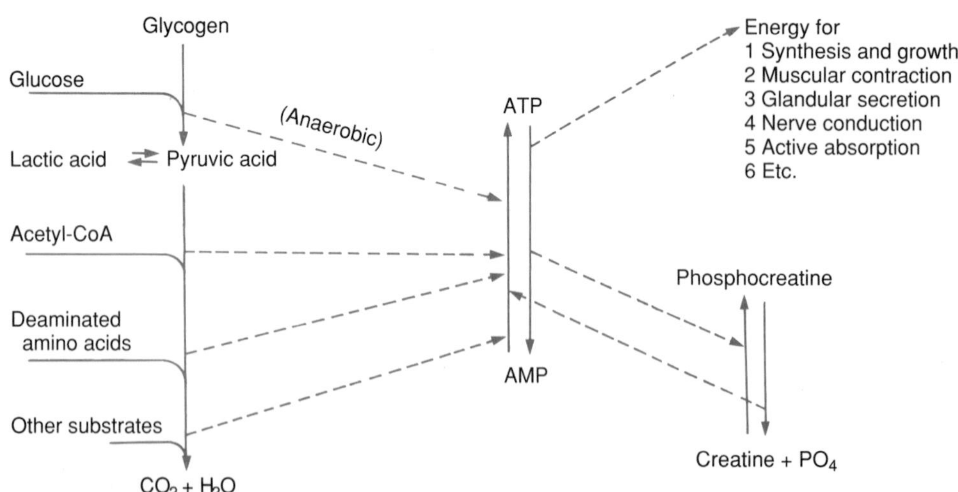

Figure 47-1. Overall scheme of energy transfer from foods to the adenylic acid system and then to the functional elements of the cells. (Modified from Saskin and Levine: Carbohydrate Metabolism. Chicago, University of Chicago Press.

Measurement of the Metabolic Rate—Indirect Calorimetry

Indirect Calorimetry. Since more than 95 per cent of the energy expended in the body is derived from reaction of oxygen with the different foods, the metabolic rate can be calculated with a high degree of accuracy from the rate of oxygen utilization. For the average diet, the *quantity of energy liberated per liter of oxygen utilized in the body averages approximately 4.825 Calories,* and this rarely varies from the average more than plus or minus 3 per cent. Therefore, using this *energy equivalent* of oxygen, one can calculate approximately the rate of heat liberation in the body from the quantity of oxygen utilized in a given period of time. This procedure is called *indirect calorimetry.*

The Metabolator. Figure 47–2 illustrates the metabolator, a device that measures oxygen utilization by the body and is therefore used for indirect calorimetry. This apparatus contains a floating drum, under which here is an oxygen chamber connected to a mouthpiece through two flexible tubes. Valves in these tubes allow air to pass from the oxygen chamber into the mouth through one tube, while the expired air is directed through the second tube. Before this expired air re-enters the oxygen chamber, it flows through a container filled with pellets of soda lime, which combines chemically with the carbon dioxide in the expired air. Therefore, as oxygen is used by the person's body and the carbon dioxide is absorbed by the soda lime, the floating oxygen chamber, which is precisely balanced by a weight, gradually sinks in the water, owing to the oxygen loss. This chamber is coupled to a pen that records on a moving paper drum the rate at which the chamber sinks in the water and thereby records the rate at which the body utilizes oxygen.

Factors That Affect the Metabolic Rate

Factors that increase the chemical activity in the cells also increase the metabolic rate. Some of these are the following.

Exercise. The factor that causes by far the most dramatic effect on metabolic rate is strenuous exercise. Short bursts of maximal muscle contraction in any single muscle liberate as much as a hundred times its normal resting amount of heat for a few seconds at a time. In the entire body, however, maximal muscle exercise can increase the overall heat production of the body for a few seconds to about 50 times normal or can sustain it for several minutes to about 20 times normal in the well-trained athlete, which is an increase in metabolic rate to 2000 per cent of normal.

Energy Requirements for Daily Activities. When an average man weighing 70 kilograms lies in bed all day, he utilizes approximately 1650 Calories of energy in the total 24-hour period. The process of eating increases the amount of energy utilized an additional 200 or more Calories, so that the same man lying in bed and also eating a reasonable diet requires a dietary intake of approximately 1850 Calories per day.

Table 47–1 illustrates the rates of energy utilization while one performs different types of activities. Note that walking up stairs requires approximately 17 times as much energy as lying in bed asleep. In general, over a 24-hour period a laborer can achieve a maximal rate of energy utilization as great as 6000 to 7000 Calories—in other words as much as three and a half times the basal rate of metabolism.

Thyroid Hormone. When the thyroid gland secretes maximal quantities of thyroxine, the metabolic rate sometimes rises to as much as 60 to 100 per cent above normal. On the other hand, total loss of thyroid secretion decreases the metabolic rate to as low as 50 to 60 per cent of normal. These effects can readily be explained by the basic function of thyroxine, which is to increase the rates of activity of almost all the chemical reactions in all cells of the body. This relationship between thyroxine and metabolic rate will be discussed in much greater detail in Chapter 50 in relation to thyroid function, because one of the useful methods for diagnosing abnormal rates of thyroid secretion is to determine the basal metabolic rate of the patient.

Sympathetic Stimulation. Stimulation of the sympathetic nervous system with liberation of nor-

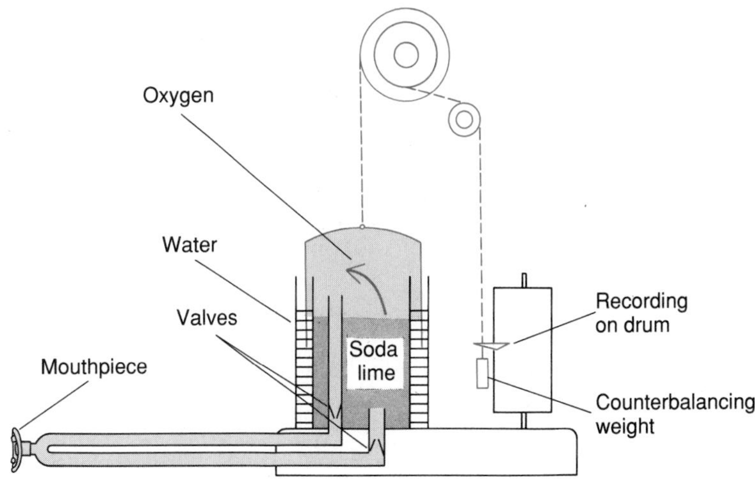

Figure 47–2. The metabolator.

Table 47-1 ENERGY EXPENDITURE PER HOUR DURING DIFFERENT TYPES OF ACTIVITY FOR A 70 KILOGRAM MAN

Form of Activity	Calories per Hour
Sleeping	65
Awake lying still	77
Sitting at rest	100
Standing relaxed	105
Dressing and undressing	118
Tailoring	135
Typewriting rapidly	140
"Light" exercise	170
Walking slowly (2.6 miles per hour)	200
Carpentry, metal working, industrial painting	240
"Active" exercise	290
"Severe" exercise	450
Sawing wood	480
Swimming	500
Running (5.3 miles per hour)	570
"Very severe" exercise	600
Walking very fast (5.3 miles per hour)	650
Walking up stairs	1100

Extracted from data compiled by Professor M. S. Rose.

epinephrine and epinephrine increases the metabolic rates of most tissues of the body. These hormones directly affect cells to cause glycogenolysis, and this, with other intracellular effects of these hormones, increases cellular activity.

Maximal stimulation of the sympathetic nervous system can increase the metabolic rate in some lower animals as much as several hundred per cent, but the magnitude of this effect in human beings is in question. It is probably 15 per cent or less in the adult but as much as 100 per cent in the newborn child.

The Basal Metabolic Rate

The Basal Metabolic Rate as a Method for Comparing Metabolic Rates Between Individuals. It is often important to measure the inherent activity of the tissues independently of exercise and other extraneous factors that would make it impossible to compare one person's metabolic rate with another's. To do so the metabolic rate is measured under so-called *basal conditions*; this rate is called the *basal metabolic rate.* For the normal adult, the average basal metabolic rate is about 70 Calories per hour.

The following basal conditions are necessary for measuring the basal metabolic rate:

1. No food for at least 12 hours
2. A night of restful sleep before determination
3. No strenuous exercise after the night of restful sleep, and complete rest in a reclining position for at least 30 minutes prior to actual determination
4. Elimination of all psychic and physical factors that cause excitement
5. Air temperature comfortable and somewhere between the limits of 20° and 27° C (68° and 80° F).

Constancy of the Basal Metabolic Rate from Person to Person. When the basal metabolic rate is measured in a wide variety of different persons and comparisons are made within single age, weight, and sex groups, 85 per cent of normal persons have been found to have basal metabolic rates within 10 per cent of the mean. Thus, it is obvious that measurements of metabolic rates performed under basal conditions offer an excellent means for comparing the rates of metabolism from one person to another.

THE BODY TEMPERATURE

The temperature of the inside of the body — that is, in the "core" of the body — remains almost exactly constant, within ±0.6° C (1° F), day in and day out except when a person develops a febrile illness. Indeed, a person can be exposed while nude to temperatures as low as 13° C (55° F) or as high as 60° C (140° F) in dry, still air and still maintain an almost constant internal body temperature. Therefore, it is obvious that the mechanisms for control of body temperature represent a beautifully designed control system.

The Normal Body Temperature. No single temperature level can be considered normal, for measurements in many normal persons have shown a *range* of normal temperatures, as illustrated in Figure 47-3, from approximately 36° C (97° F) to over 37.2° C (99° F). When measured by rectum, the values are approximately 0.6° C (1° F) greater than the oral temperatures. The average normal temperature is generally considered to be 98.6° F (37° C). However, when excessive heat is produced in the body by strenuous exercise, the rectal temperature can rise to as high as 38.3° to 40° C (101° to 104° F) for short periods of time.

BALANCE BETWEEN HEAT PRODUCTION AND HEAT LOSS

Heat is continuously being produced in the body as a byproduct of metabolism, and body heat is also continuously being lost to the surroundings. When the

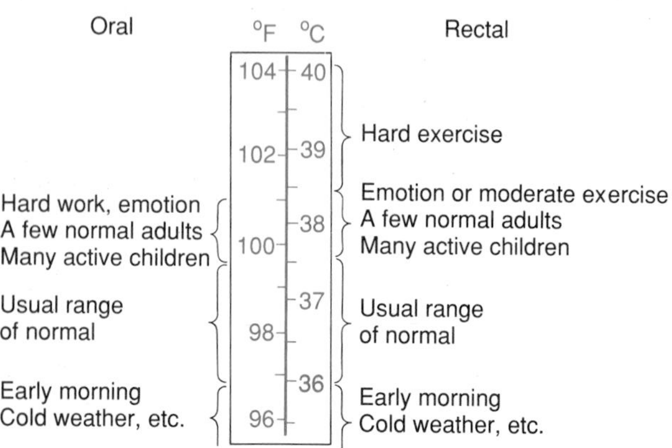

Figure 47-3. Estimated range of body temperature in normal persons. (From DuBois: Fever. Springfield, Ill., Charles C Thomas.)

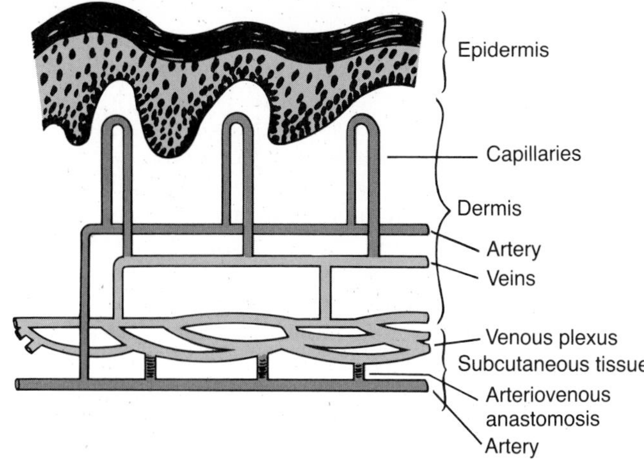

Figure 47-4. The skin circulation.

rate of heat production is exactly equal to the rate of loss, the person is said to be in *heat balance.* But when the two rates are out of equilibrium, body heat, and body temperature as well, will obviously either increase or decrease.

The Insulator System of the Body

The skin, the subcutaneous tissues, and the fat of the subcutaneous tissues are a heat insulator for the internal tissues of the body. The fat is especially important because it conducts heat only *one third* as readily as other tissues. When no blood is flowing from the heated internal organs to the skin, the insulating properties of the normal male body are approximately equal to three quarters the insulating properties of a usual suit of clothes. In women this insulation is still better.

The insulation beneath the skin is an effective means of maintaining normal internal core temperature, even though it allows the temperature of the skin to approach the temperature of the surroundings.

The "Radiator" System of the Body: Flow of Blood to the Skin from the Body Core

Blood vessels penetrate the fatty subcutaneous insulator tissues and are distributed profusely immediately beneath the skin. Especially important is a continuous venous plexus that is supplied by inflow of blood from the skin capillaries, illustrated in Figure 47-4. In the most exposed areas of the body—the hands, feet, and ears—blood is also supplied to the plexus directly from the small arteries through highly muscular venous *arteriovenous anastomoses.* The rate of blood flow into the venous plexus can vary tremendously—from barely above zero to as great as 30 per cent of the total cardiac output. A high rate of blood flow causes heat to be conducted from the core of the body to the skin with great efficiency, whereas reduction in the rate of blood flow to its minimum level decreases the efficiency of heat conduction from the core to as little as one eighth as much.

Obviously, therefore, the skin is an effective "radiator" system, and the flow of blood to the skin is a most effective mechanism of heat transfer from the body core to the skin.

Control of Heat Conduction to the Skin by the Sympathetic Nervous System. Heat conduction to the skin by the blood is controlled by the degree of vasoconstriction of the arterioles and arteriovenous anastomoses that supply blood to the venous plexus of the skin. This vasoconstriction in turn is controlled almost entirely by the sympathetic nervous system in response to changes in the body core temperature and changes in the environmental temperature. This will be discussed later in the chapter in connection with the control of body temperature by the hypothalamus.

Heat Loss

The various methods by which heat is lost from the skin are shown pictorially in Figure 47-5. These include *radiation, conduction,* and *evaporation.* Also, *convection* of the air plays a major role in heat loss by both conduction and evaporation. The amount of heat lost by each of these different mechanisms obviously varies with atmospheric conditions.

Radiation. As illustated in Figure 47-5, a nude person in a room maintained at normal temperature loses about 60 per cent of the total heat loss by radiation.

Loss of heat by radiation means loss in the form of infrared heat rays, electromagnetic waves that radiate from the skin to any surroundings that are colder than the skin itself. This loss increases as the temperature of the surroundings decreases.

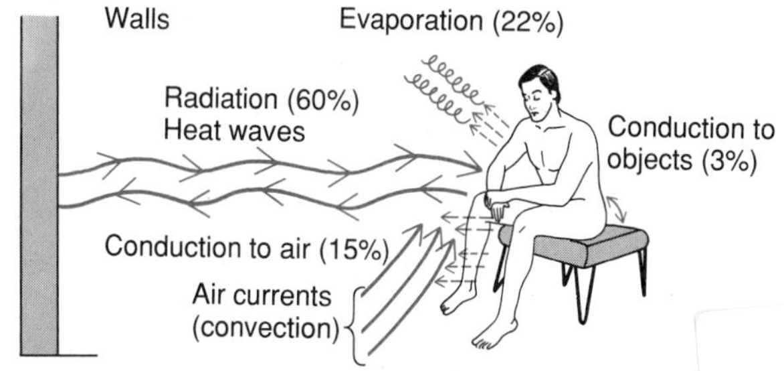

Figure 47-5. Mechanisms of heat loss from the body

Conduction. Usually, only minute quantities of heat — perhaps about 3 per cent of the total — are lost from the body by direct conduction from the body to other objects, such as a chair or a bed. However, loss of heat by *conduction to air* does represent a sizeable proportion of the body's heat loss even under normal conditions. It will be recalled that heat is actually the kinetic energy of molecular motion, and the molecules that compose the skin of the body are continuously undergoing vibratory motion. Thus, the vibratory motion of the skin molecules can cause increased velocity of motion of the air molecules that come into direct contact with the skin. But once the temperature of the air immediately adjacent to the skin approaches the temperature of the skin, additional exchange of heat from the body to the air is self-limited unless the heated air moves away from the skin so that new, unheated air is continuously brought in contact with the skin, a phenomenon called *convection.*

Convection. Movement of air is known as convection, and the removal of heat from the body by convection air currents is commonly called heat loss by convection. Actually, the heat must first be *conducted* to the air and then carried away by the convection currents.

A small amount of convection almost always occurs around the body because of the tendency for the air adjacent to the skin to rise as it becomes heated. Therefore, a nude person seated in a comfortable room loses about 12 per cent of his or her heat by conduction to the air and then by convection away from the body.

Evaporation. When water evaporates from the body surface, 0.58 Calorie of heat is lost for each gram of water that evaporates. Water evaporates *insensibly* from the skin and lungs at a rate of about 600 ml per day. This causes continuous heat loss at a rate of 12 to 16 Calories per hour. Unfortunately, this insensible evaporation of water directly through the skin and lungs cannot be controlled for purposes of temperature regulation because it results from continuous diffusion of water molecules regardless of body temperature. However, additional evaporative loss of heat can be controlled by regulating the rate of sweating, which is discussed later.

Evaporation as a Necessary Refrigeration Mechanism at High Air Temperatures. In the preceding discussions of radiation and conduction, it was noted that as long as the body temperature is greater than that of the surroundings, heat is lost by radiation and conduction; but when the temperature of the surroundings is greater than that of the skin, instead of losing heat, the body gains heat by radiation and conduction from the surroundings. Under these conditions, *the only means by which the body can rid itself of heat is evaporation.* Therefore, any factor that prevents adequate evaporation when the surrounding temperatures are higher than body temperature causes the body temperature to rise to abnormally high levels. This circumstance occurs occasionally in human beings who are born with congenital absence of sweat glands. These persons can withstand cold temperatures as well as a normal person can, but they are likely to die of heat stroke in tropical zones, for without the evaporative refrigeration system, the body temperatures will remain at levels greater than those of the surroundings.

Sweating and Its Regulation by the Autonomic Nervous System

When the body becomes overheated, large quantities of sweat are secreted onto the surface of the skin by the sweat glands to provide rapid *evaporative cooling* of the body. Stimulation of the preoptic area in the anterior part of the hypothelamus excites sweating. The impulses from this area that cause sweating are transmitted in the autonomic pathways to the cord and thence through the sympathetic outflow to the sweat glands in the skin everywhere in the body.

Rate of Sweating. In cold weather the rate of sweat production is essentially zero, but in very hot weather the maximum rate of sweat production is from 0.7 liter per hour in an unacclimatized person to 1.5 to 2 liters per hour in a person maximally acclimatized to heat. Thus, during maximal sweating, a person can lose more than 3 pounds of body weight per hour.

Mechanism of Sweat Secretion. The sweat gland, illustrated in Figure 47–6, is a tubular structure consisting of two parts: (1) a deep *coiled portion* that secretes the sweat and (2) a *duct portion* passing outward to the surface of the skin. As is true of the salivary glands, the secretory portion of the sweat gland emits a fluid called the *precursor secretion*; then the constituents of this fluid are altered as it flows through the duct.

The precursor secretion is an active secretory product of the epithelial cells lining the coiled portion of the sweat gland. Cholinergic sympathetic nerve fibers (fibers that secrete acetylcholine) ending on or near the glandular cells elicit the secretion.

Since large amounts of sodium chloride are lost in the sweat, it is especially important to know how the sweat glands handle sodium and chloride during the secretory process. When the rate of sweat secretion is very low, the sodium and chloride concentrations of the sweat are also very low, because most of these ions are reabsorbed from the precursor secretion before it reaches the surface of the body; their concentrations are sometimes as low as 5 mEq per liter each. On the other hand, when the rate of secretion becomes progressively greater, the rate of sodium chloride reabsorption does not increase commensurately, so that the concentrations in the sweat of the normal unacclimatized person then usually rise to maximum levels of about 60 mEq per liter, or nearly half the levels in plasma.

Effect of Aldosterone on Sodium Loss in the Sweat — Acclimatization to Heat. Aldosterone functions in much the same way in the sweat glands as in the renal tubules: it increases the rate of active reabsorption of sodium by the duct. The reabsorption

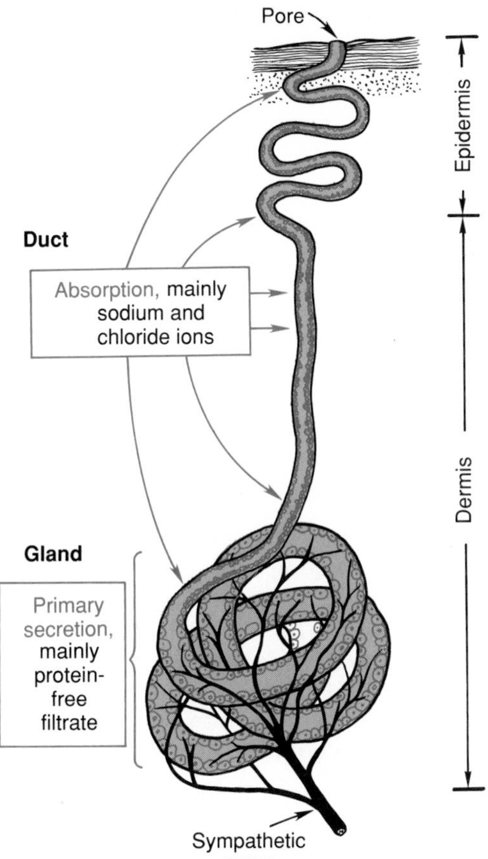

Figure 47-6. A sweat gland innervated by a sympathetic nerve. A *primary secretion* is formed by the glandular portion, but much if not most of the electrolytes are reabsorbed in the duct, leaving a dilute, watery secretion.

of sodium also carries chloride ions along as well, because of the electrical pull that develops across the epithelium when positively charged sodium is reabsorbed. The importance of this aldosterone effect is to minimize loss of sodium chloride in the sweat when the blood sodium chloride concentration is already low.

Extreme sweating, which often occurs in continuously hot surroundings, can deplete the extracellular fluids of electrolytes, particularly of sodium and chloride. A person who sweats profusely may lose as much as 15 to 20 grams of sodium chloride each day until he becomes acclimatized to the heat. On the other hand, after four to six weeks of acclimatization the loss of sodium chloride may be as little as 3 to 5 grams per day. This change occurs because of increased aldosterone secretion resulting from depletion of the salt reserves of the body.

REGULATION OF BODY TEMPERATURE

Figure 47-7 illustrates approximately what happens to the temperature of the nude body after a few hours' exposure to dry, still air ranging from 0° to 68°C (30° to 155° F). Obviously, the precise dimensions of this curve vary, depending on the movement of air, the amount of moisture in the air, and even the nature of the surroundings. However, in general, between approximately 13° and 60° C (55° and 140° F) in dry air, the nude body is capable of maintaining for long periods of time a normal body core temperature somewhere between 36° and 37.8° C (97° and 100° F).

The temperature of the body is regulated almost entirely by nervous feedback control mechanisms, and almost all of them operate through a *temperature-regulating center* located in the *hypothalamus.* However, for these feedback mechanisms to operate, temperature detectors must also exist to determine when the body temperature becomes either too hot or too cold. Some of these receptors are described next.

Temperature Receptors. Probably the most important temperature receptors for control of body temperature are many special *heat-sensitive neurons* located *in the preoptic area of the hypothalamus.* Most of these neurons increase their impulse output as the temperature rises and decrease their output when the temperature decreases, but a few function exactly oppositely. The firing rate sometimes changes as much as tenfold with a change in body temperature of 10° C.

In addition to these heat-sensitive neurons of the preoptic area, other important receptors sensitive to temperature include the following: (1) *skin temperature receptors,* both *warmth* and *cold receptors,* (but four to ten times as many cold as warmth receptors) that transmit nerve impulses into the spinal cord and thence to the hypothalamic region of the brain to help control body temperature; and (2) *receptors in the spinal cord, in the abdomen, and possibly in other internal structures* of the body that also transmit signals—mainly cold signals—to the central nervous system to help control body temperature.

Experiments in recent years have shown that the preoptic receptors play the greatest role in temperature control when the body temperature rises above

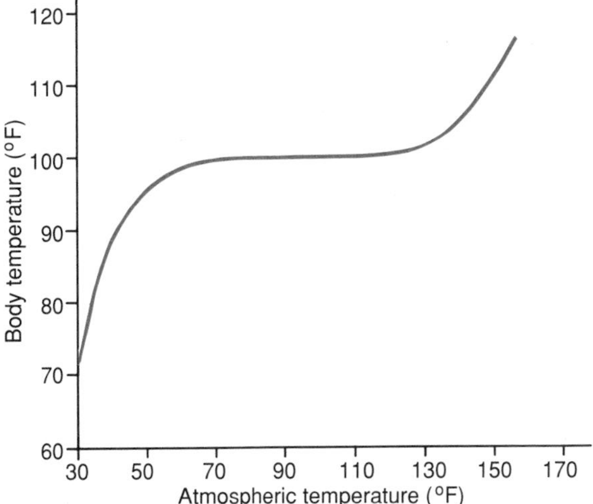

Figure 47-7. Effect of high and low atmospheric temperature for several hours' duration on the internal body temperature, showing that the internal body emperature remains stable despite wide changes in atmospheric temperature.

normal. But at low temperatures, the peripheral cold receptors are probably also of major importance.

Integration of Heat and Cold Thermostatic Signals in the Posterior Hypothalamus—The Hypothalamic Thermostat

The signals that arise in peripheral receptors are transmitted to the *posterior hypothalamus,* where they are integrated with the receptor signals from the preoptic area to give the final efferent signals for controlling heat loss and heat production. Therefore, we generally speak of the overall hypothalamic temperature control mechanism as the *hypothalamic thermostat.*

Figure 47-8 illustrates the effectiveness of the hypothalamic thermostat in initiating temperature regulatory changes when the body temperature rises too high or falls too low. The solid curve shows that as the head temperature increases—almost precisely at 37° C (98.4° F)—sweating begins and then increases rapidly as the temperature rises still higher. On the other hand, sweating ceases at any temperature below this same critical level of 37° C.

Likewise, the hypothalamic thermostat controls the rate of heat production, which is illustrated by the dashed curve. At any temperature above 37.1° C, the heat production remains almost exactly constant, but whenever the temperature falls below this level, the various mechanisms for increasing heat production become markedly activated, especially an increase in muscle excitability, which culminates in shivering.

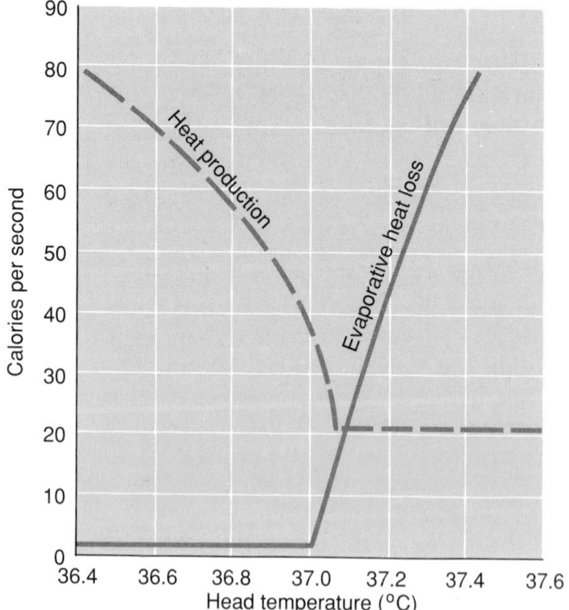

Figure 47-8. Effect of hypothalamic temperature on (1) evaporative heat loss from the body and (2) heat production caused primarily by muscular activity and shivering. This figure demonstrates the extremely critical temperature level at which increased heat loss begins and increased heat production stops. (Drawn from data in Benzinger, Kitzinger, and Pratt, in Hardy [ed.]: Temperature, Part 3, p. 637. Reinhold Publishing Corp.)

Mechanisms of Increased Heat Loss When the Body Becomes Overheated

Overheating the preoptic thermostatic area increases the rate of heat loss from the body in two principal ways: (1) by stimulating the sweat glands to cause evaporative heat loss from the body and (2) by inhibiting sympathetic centers in the posterior hypothalamus that normally constrict the skin vessels; this inhibition allows vasodilatation and, consequently, greatly increased loss of heat from the skin.

Mechanisms of Heat Conservation and Increased Heat Production When the Body Becomes Cooled

When the body core is cooled below approximately 37° C, special mechanisms are set into play to conserve the heat that is already in the body, and still other mechanisms are set into play to increase the rate of heat production, as follows:

Heat Conservation. ***Vasoconstriction in the Skin.*** One of the first effects to cause heat conservation is intense vasoconstriction of the skin vessels over the entire body. The posterior hypothalamus strongly activates the sympathetic nervous signals to the skin vessels, and intense skin vasoconstriction occurs throughout the body. This vasoconstriction obviously prevents the conduction of heat from the internal core of the body to the skin. Consequently, with maximal vasoconstriction the only heat that can leave the body is that which can be conducted directly through the fat insulator layers of the skin. This mechanism can reduce the heat loss from the skin as much as eightfold and therefore conserves the quantity of heat in the body.

Piloerection. A second means by which heat is conserved when the hypothalamus is cooled is piloerection—that is, the hairs "stand on end." Obviously, this effect is not important in the human being because of the paucity of hair, but in lower animals the upright projection of the hairs in cold weather entraps a thick layer of *insulator air* next to the skin so that the transfer of heat to the surroundings is greatly depressed.

Abolition of Sweating. Sweating is completely abolished by cooling the preoptic thermostat below about 37° C (98.6° F). This obviously causes evaporative cooling of the body to cease except for that resulting from insensible evaporation.

Increased Production of Heat. Heat production is increased in three separate ways when the temperature of the body thermostat falls below 37° C.

Hypothalamic Stimulation of Shivering. Located in the dorsomedial portion of the posterior hypothalamus near the wall of the third ventricle is an area called the *primary motor center for shivering.*

This area is normally inhibited by heat signals from the preoptic thermostatic area but is driven by cold signals from the skin and spinal cord. Therefore, in response to cold, this center becomes activated and transmits impulses through bilateral tracts, down the brain stem, into the lateral columns of the spinal cord, and finally to the anterior motoneurons. These impulses are nonrhythmical and do not cause the actual muscle shaking. Instead, they increase the tone of the skeletal muscles throughout the body and also increase the sensitivity of the muscle spindle stretch reflex. When the tone has risen above a certain critical level, shivering begins. This is believed to result from feedback oscillation of the stretch reflex mechanism. During maximal shivering, body heat production can rise to as high as four to five times normal.

Sympathetic Chemical Excitation of Heat Production. Either sympathetic stimulation or circulating epinephrine (and norepinephrine to a slight extent) in the blood can cause an immediate increase in the rate of cellular metabolism; this effect is called *chemical thermogenesis.* However, as discussed earlier in the chapter, in the adult it is rare for chemical thermogenesis to increase the rate of heat production more than 10 to 15 per cent. However, in infants chemical thermogenesis can increase the rate of heat production as much as 100 per cent, which is probably a very important factor in maintaining normal body temperature in the newborn.

Increased Thyroxine Output as a Cause of Increased Heat Production. Cooling the preoptic area of the hypothalamus also increases the production of *thyrotropin-releasing hormone* by the hypothalamus. This hormone is carried by way of the hypothalamic portal veins to the adenohypophysis, where it stimulates the secretion of *thyrotropin.* Thyrotropin, in turn, stimulates increased output of thyroxine by the thyroid gland, as will be explained in Chapter 50. The increased thyroxine increases the rate of cellular metabolism throughout the body. However, this increase in metabolism through the thyroid mechanism does not occur immediately but requires several weeks for the thyroid gland to hypertrophy before it reaches its new level of thyroxine secretion.

Exposure of animals to extreme cold for several weeks can cause their thyroid glands to increase in size as much as 20 to 40 per cent. Unfortunately, however, human beings rarely allow themselves to be exposed to the same degree of cold as that to which animals have been subjected. Therefore, we still do not know, quantitatively, how important the thyroid method of adaptation to cold is in the human being.

Behavioral Control of Body Temperature

Aside from the hypothalamic thermostatic mechanism for body temperature control, the body has still another neural mechanism that is usually even more potent. This mechanism is behavioral control of body temperature, which can be explained as follows: Whenever the internal body temperature becomes too high, signals from the preoptic area of the brain give one a psychic sensation of being overheated. Whenever the body becomes too cold, signals from the skin and perhaps from other peripheral receptors elicit the feeling of cold discomfort. Therefore, one makes appropriate environmental adjustments to reestablish comfort. This is a much more powerful system of body temperature control than most physiologists have recognized in the past; indeed, for human beings it is the only really effective mechanism for body heat control in severely cold environs.

Regulation of Internal Body Temperature After Cutting the Spinal Cord. After cutting of the spinal cord in the neck above the level at which sympathetic nerves leave the cord, automatic regulation of body temperature becomes extremely poor — in fact, almost nonexistent — for the hypothalamus can then no longer control either skin blood flow or the degree of sweating anywhere in the body. Therefore, in persons with this condition, body temperature must be regulated principally by the patient's psychic response to cold and hot sensations in the head region. That is, if the person feels too hot or develops a headache from the heat, he or she knows that cooler surroundings should be selected; and, conversely, cold sensations mean that warmer surroundings are needed.

ABNORMALITIES OF BODY TEMPERATURE REGULATION

Fever

Fever, which means a body temperature above the usual range of normal, may be caused by abnormalities in the brain itself, by toxic substances that affect the temperature regulating centers, by bacterial diseases, by brain tumors, or by dehydration.

Resetting the Hypothalamic Thermostat in Febrile Diseases — Effect of Pyrogens

Many proteins, breakdown products of proteins, and certain other substances, such as lipopolysaccharide toxins secreted by bacteria, can cause the "set point" of the hypothalamic thermostat to rise. Substances that cause this effect are called *pyrogens.* It is pyrogens secreted by toxic bacteria or released from degenerating tissues of the body that cause fever during disease conditions. When the set point of the hypothalamic thermostat becomes increased to a higher level than normal, all the mechanisms for raising the body temperature are brought into play, including heat conservation and increased heat production. Within a few hours after the thermostat has been set to a higher level, the body temperature also approaches this new level.

To give one an idea of the extremely powerful effect of pyrogens in resetting the hypothalamic thermostat, as little as a few nanograms of some purified bacterial pyrogens injected into a person can cause the body temperature to rise as much as 5.6° C (10° F).

Characteristics of Febrile Conditions

Chills. When the thermostat setting is suddenly changed from the normal level to a higher-than-normal level as a result of tissue destruction, pyrogenic substances, or dehydration, the body temperature usually takes several hours to reach the new temperature setting. For instance, the temperature setting of the hypothalamic thermostat, as illustrated in Figure 47–9, might suddenly rise to 103° F. Because the blood temperature is less than the temperature setting of the hypothalamic thermostat, the usual autonomic responses that cause elevation of body temperature occur. During this period chills cause the person to feel extremely cold even though body temperature may already be above normal. Also, the skin is cold because of vasoconstriction, and the body shakes from shivering. The chills continue until body temperature rises to the hypothalamic setting of 103° F. Then, when the temperature of the body reaches this level, the person no longer experiences chills but feels neither cold nor hot. As long as the factor that is causing the hypothalamic thermostat to be set at this high level continues its effect, the body temperature is regulated more or less in the usual manner but at the higher temperature level.

The Crisis, or "Flush." If the factor that is causing the high temperature is suddenly removed, the set-point of the hypothalamic thermostat suddenly returns to the normal lower level, as illustrated in Figure 47–9. In this instance, the blood temperature is still 103° F, but the hypothalamus is now attempting to regulate the body temperature at 98.6° F. This situation is analogous to excessive heating of the normal preoptic area, which causes *intense sweating* and sudden development of a *hot skin* because of vasodilatation everywhere. This sudden change of events in a febrile disease is known as the crisis or, more appropriately, the flush. Before the advent of antibiotics, the doctor always awaited the crisis, for once this occurred he or she knew immediately that the patient's temperature would soon be falling.

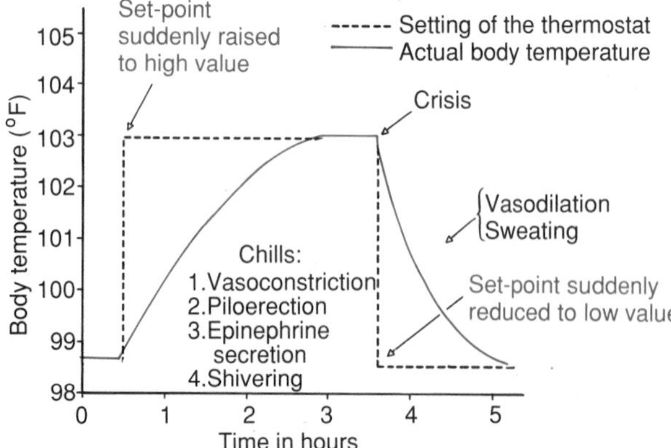

Figure 47–9. Effects of changing the set-point of the "hypothalamic thermostat."

Heat Stroke

The limits of extreme heat that one can stand depend almost entirely on whether the heat is dry or wet. If the air is completely dry and sufficient convection air currents are flowing to promote rapid evaporation from the body, a person can withstand several hours of air temperature at over 54° C (130° F) with no apparent ill effects. On the other hand, if the air is 100 per cent humidified or if the body is in water, the body temperature begins to rise whenever the environmental temperature rises above approximately 34.4° C (94° F). If the person is performing very heavy work, the critical temperature level may fall to 29.4° to 32° C (85° to 90° F) in these humid surroundings.

Unfortunately, there is a limit to the rate at which the body can lose heat even with maximal sweating. Furthermore, when the hypothalamus becomes heated beyond a critical temperature, its heat-regulatory ability then becomes depressed and sweating diminishes. As a result, a high body temperature tends to perpetuate itself unless measures are taken specifically to decrease body heat.

When the body temperature rises into the range of 41° to 42.5° C (106° to 108° F), the person is likely to develop *heat stroke.* The symptoms include dizziness, abdominal distress, sometimes delirium, and, eventually, loss of consciousness if the body temperature is not soon decreased. Many of these symptoms result from a mild degree of *circulatory shock* brought on by excessive loss of fluid and electrolytes in the sweat before the onset of symptoms. However, the hyperpyrexia itself is also exceedingly damaging to the body tissues, especially the brain, and therefore is undoubtedly responsible for many of the effects. In fact, even a few minutes of very high body temperature can sometimes be fatal. For this reason, many authorities recommend immediate treatment of heat stroke by placing the person in an ice-water bath. However, because this often induces uncontrollable shivering with considerable increase in rate of heat production, others have suggested that sponge-cooling of the skin is likely to be more effective for rapidly decreasing the body core temperature.

Harmful Effects of the High Temperature. When the body temperature rises above 41° to 42.5° C (106° to 108° F), the parenchyma of many cells begins to be damaged. The pathological findings in a person who dies of hyperpyrexia are local hemorrhages and parenchymatous degeneration of cells throughout the entire body but especially in the brain. Unfortunately, once neuronal cells are destroyed, they can never be replaced. Damage to the liver, kidneys, and other body organs can also be so great that failure of one or more of these organs eventually causes death, sometimes not till several days after the heat stroke.

Antipyretics. Aspirin, antipyrine, aminopyrine, and a number of other substances known as antipyretics have an effect on the hypothalamic thermostat opposite to that of the pyrogens. In other words, they cause the setting of the thermostat to be lowered, causing the body temperature to fall, though usually not more than a degree or so. Aspirin is especially effective in lowering the hypothalamic setting when pyrogens have raised the setting, but aspirin will not lower the normal temperature. On the other hand, aminopyrine will decrease even the normal body temperature. Obviously, these drugs can be used to prevent damage to the body from excessively high body temperatures in feverish conditions.

Exposure of the Body to Extreme Cold

A person exposed to ice water for approximately 20 to 30 minutes ordinarily dies because of heart standstill or heart fibrillation unless treated immediately. By that time, the internal body temperature has fallen to about 25° C (77° F). Yet if the victim is warmed rapidly by application of external heat, his or her life can often be saved.

Once the body temperature has fallen below 29.4° C (85° F), the ability of the hypothalamus to regulate temperature is completely lost, and it is greatly impaired even when the body temperature falls below approximaely 34.4° C (94° F). Part of the reason for this loss of temperature regulation is that the rate of chemical reactions, and therefore heat production as well, in each cell is greatly depressed by the low temperature. Also, sleepiness and even coma, which depress the activity of the central nervous system heat-control mechanisms and also prevent shivering, are likely to develop. This loss of temperature regulation obviously further accelerates the decrease in body temperature and rapidly leads to death.

REFERENCES

Energetics and Metabolic Rate

Bray, G. A.: Regulation of energy balance. Physiologist, 28:186, 1985.

Calder, W. A. III: Scaling energetics of homeothermic vertebrates: An operational allometry. Annu. Rev. Physiol. 49:107, 1987.

Kim, C. H., et al. (eds.): Advances in Membrane Biochemistry and Bioenergetics. New York, Plenum Publishing Corp., 1989.

Oppenheimer, J. H.: Thyroid hormone action at the nuclear level. Ann. Intern. Med., 102:374, 1985.

Plowman, P. N.: Endocrinology and Metabolic Diseases. New York. Elsevier Science Publishing Co., 1987.

Stryer, L.: Biochemistry. New York. W. H. Freeman Co., 1988.

Van der Laarse, W. J., and Woledge, R. C.: Energetics at the single cell level. News Physiol. Sci., 4:91, 1989.

Body Temperature Regulation

Boulant, J. A., and Dean, J. B.: Temperature receptors in the central nervous system. Anu. Rev. Physiol., 48:639, 1956.

Felig, P., et al. (eds.): Endocrinology and Metabolism. 2nd ed. New York, McGraw-Hill Book Co., 1987.

Gordon, C. J., and Heath, J. E.: Integration and central processing in temperature regulation. Annu. Rev. Physiol., 48:595, 1986.

Harrison, M. H.: Effects of thermal stress and exercise on blood volume in humans. Physiol. Rev. 65:149, 1985.

Hong, S. K., et al.: Humans can acclimatize to cold: A lesson from Korean women divers. News Physiol. Sci., 2:79, 1987.

Kluger, M. J.: Fever: A hot topic. News Physiol. Sci., 1:25, 1986.

Lipton, J. M., and Clark, W. G.: Neurotransmitters in temperature control. Annu. Rev. Physiol., 48:613, 1986.

Simon, E., et al.: Central and peripheral thermal control of effectors in homeothermic temperature regulation. Physiol. Rev., 66:235, 1986.

Spray, D. C.: Cutaneous temperature receptors. Annu. Rev. Physiol., 48:625, 1986.

QUESTIONS

1. Why does the concentration of *ATP* remain almost at the maximal level until all the *phosphocreatine* in a cell has been depleted?
2. What is meant by the function of phosphocreatine to "buffer" the concentration of ATP?
3. Explain the function of the *metabolator* and the physiological principles of *indirect calorimetry.*
4. How do the following factors affect the *metabolic rate:* exercise, thyroid hormone, and sympathetic stimulation?
5. In measuring the *basal metabolic rate,* what are the *basal conditions* that are prerequisite?
6. Explain how each of the following factors contributes to heat loss from the body: *radiation, conduction, convection,* and *evaporation.*
7. Why is evaporation necessary for the maintenance of body temperature when the temperature of the body's surroundings is greater than body temperature? Describe the sweat gland and its formation of sweat.
8. Why is the normal concentration of sodium chloride in the sweat very low and why does this become even lower in heat acclimatization? What is the role of aldosterone in heat acclimatization of the sweating process?
9. Explain the *heat insulator system* of the body and how heat is transferred from the body core to the skin. What regulates the rate at which heat is transferred to the skin?
10. Explain the control of skin temperature by the temperature control center of the hypothalamus.
11. What are the different *temperature receptors* of the body?
12. Describe the organization of the *hypothalamus* for the control of body temperature. What is meant by the *hypothalamic thermostat*?
13. List the mechanisms by which the body conserves heat and increases heat production when the body becomes cooled.
14. Describe the mechanism of *shivering.*
15. What is meant by *chemical excitation of heat production*?
16. How does *behavior* enter into the control of temperature?
17. What is meant by *fever,* and what are pyrogens?
18. Why do chills occur when the set point of the *hypothalamic thermostat* is suddenly increased to a level greater than the present body temperature?
19. Explain the cause of the *crisis,* or flush.
20. What is meant by *heat stroke,* and how does it affect the body?
21. Explain the deleterious effects on the body caused by extreme cold.

48

Dietary Balances, Regulation of Feeding, Obesity, and Vitamins

The intake of food must always be sufficient to supply the metabolic needs of the body and yet not enough to cause obesity. Also, since foods contain different proportions of proteins, carbohydrates, and fats, appropriate balance must be maintained among these different types of food so that all segments of the body's metabolic systems can be supplied with the requisite materials. This chapter therefore discusses especially the problems of balance among the major types of food and the intrinsic homeostatic mechanisms of the body that cause the intake of food to be regulated in accordance with the body's metabolic needs.

DIETARY BALANCES

Energy Available in Foods. The energy liberated from each gram of carbohydrate as it is oxidized to carbon dioxide and water is 4.1 Calories (kilocalories), and that liberated from fat is 9.3 Calories. The energy liberated from metabolism of the average protein in the diet as each gram is oxidized to carbon dioxide, water, and urea is 4.35 Calories. Also, these different substances vary in the average percentage absorbed from the gastrointestinal tract: approximately 98 per cent of the carbohydrate, 95 per cent of the fat, and 92 per cent of the protein. Therefore, in round figures the average *physiologically available energy* in each gram of the three different foodstuffs in the diet is:

	Calories
Carbohydrates	4.0
Fat	9.0
Protein	4.0

Average Composition of the Diet. The average American receives approximately 15 per cent of his or her energy from protein, about 40 per cent from fat, and 45 per cent from carbohydrates. In most other parts of the world the quantity of energy derived from carbohydrates far exceeds that derived from both proteins and fats. Indeed, in some parts of Mongolia, the energy received from fats and proteins combined is said to be no greater than 15 to 20 per cent.

Daily Requirement for Protein. Twenty to thirty grams of body proteins are degraded and used for energy daily. Therefore, all cells must continue to synthesize new proteins to take the place of those that are being destroyed, and a supply of protein is needed in the diet for this purpose. An average man can maintain his normal stores of protein provided his *daily intake is above 30 to 55 grams,* but to be safe another 30 grams is advisable.

Partial Proteins. Another factor that must be considered in analyzing the proteins of the diet is whether the dietary proteins are *complete* or *partial* proteins. Complete proteins have compositions of amino acids *in appropriate proportion to each other* so that all the amino acids can be properly used to form proteins in the cells of the human body. In general, proteins derived from animal food-stuffs are more nearly complete than are proteins derived from vegetable and grain sources. When partial proteins are in the diet, an increased minimal quantity of protein is necessary in the daily rations to maintain normal protein synthesis. A particular example of this occurs in the diet of many African natives who subsist primarily on a corn meal diet. The protein of corn is almost totally lacking in the amino acid tryptophan, which means that this diet in effect is almost completely protein deficient because, if any single amino acid that is needed to make animal proteins is missing, protein synthesis stops entirely, and the remaining amino acids are used for energy instead. As a result, many Africans, especially the children, develop the protein deficiency syndrome called *kwashiorkor,* which consists of failure to grow, lethargy, depressed mentality, and hypoprotein edema.

Study of the Balance Between Fat and Carbohydrate Utilization—The Respiratory Quotient

When glucose is oxidized, the number of molecules of carbon dioxide liberated is exactly equal to the number of oxygen molecules necessary for the oxidative process. This *ratio of carbon dioxide output to oxygen usage* is called the *respiratory quotient.* Thus, for glucose the respiratory quotient is 1.00. On the other hand, oxidation of triolein (the most abundant fat in the body) liberates 57 carbon dioxide molecules while 80 oxygen molecules are being utilized. Consequently, the respiratory quotient in this instance is 0.71. Finally, oxidation of alanine, an amino acid from protein, liberates five carbon dioxide molecules for every six oxygen molecules, giving a respiratory quotient of 0.83.

Because only a small part of one's metabolic energy is derived from protein and because the respiratory quotient of protein is approximately midway between the respiratory quotients of fat and carbohydrate (see preceding paragraph), one can estimate reasonably well the relative quantities of fat and carbohydrate being metabolized by the body by simply measuring the respiratory quotient—that is, by measuring the respiratory intake of oxygen and the output of carbon dioxide. For instance, if the respiratory quotient is approximately 0.71, the body is burning almost entirely fat to the exclusion of carbohydrates. If, on the other hand, the respiratory quotient is 1.00, the body is probably metabolizing almost entirely carbohydrate to the exclusion of fat. Finally, a respiratory quotient of 0.85 indicates approximately equal utilization of carbohydrate and fat.

REGULATION OF FOOD INTAKE

Hunger. The term *hunger* means a craving for food, and it is associated with a number of objective sensations. For instance, in a person who has not had food for many hours, the stomach undergoes intense rhythmic contractions called *hunger contractions.* These cause a tight or gnawing feeling in the pit of the stomach and sometimes actually cause pain called *hunger pangs.* In addition to the hunger pangs, the hungry person also becomes more tense and restless than usual.

Some physiologists actually define hunger as the tonic contractions of the stomach. However, even after the stomach is completely removed, the psychic sensations of hunger still occur, and craving for food still makes the person search for an adequate food supply.

Appetite. The term *appetite* is often used in the same sense as hunger except that it usually implies desire for specific types of food instead of food in general. Therefore, appetite helps determine the quality of food a person eats.

Satiety. Satiety is the opposite of hunger. It means a feeling of fulfillment of the quest for food. Satiety usually results from a filling meal, particularly when the person's nutritional storage depots, the adipose tissue and the glycogen stores, are already filled.

Neural Centers for Regulation of Food Intake

Hunger and Satiety Centers. Stimulation of the *lateral hypothalamus* causes an animal to eat voraciously, while stimulation of the *ventromedial nuclei of the hypothalamus* causes complete satiety, and even in the presence of highly appetizing food an animal will nevertheless refuse to eat if this area is stimulated. Conversely, a destructive lesion of the ventromedial nuclei causes exactly the same effect as stimulation of the lateral hypothalamic nuclei—that is, voracious and continued eating until the animal becomes extremely obese, sometimes as large as four times normal in size. Lesions of the lateral hypothalamic nuclei cause exactly the opposite effects—complete lack of desire for food and progressive inanition of the animal. Therefore, we can label the lateral nuclei of the hypothalamus the *hunger,* or the *feeding, center* and the ventromedial nuclei of the hypothalamus the *satiety center.*

The feeding center operates by directly exciting the emotional drive to search for food. On the other hand, it is believed that the satiety center operates primarily by inhibiting the feeding center.

Other Neural Centers That Enter Into Feeding. If the brain is removed above the mesencephalon, the animal can still perform the basic mechanical features of the feeding process. It can salivate, lick its lips, chew food, and swallow. Therefore, the actual mechanics of feeding are all controlled by centers in the lower brain stem. The function of the hunger center in the hypothalamus, then, is to control the quantity of food intake and to excite the lower centers to activity.

Higher centers than the hypothalamus also play important roles in the control of feeding, particularly in the control of appetite. These centers include especially the *amygdala* and some cortical areas of the limbic system, all of which are closely coupled with the hypothalamus. It will be recalled from the discussion of the sense of smell that the amygdala is one of the major parts of the olfactory nervous system. Destructive lesions in the amygdala have demonstrated that some of its areas greatly increase feeding, while others inhibit feeding. In addition, stimulation of some areas of the amygdala elicits the mechanical act of feeding. However, the most important effect of destruction of the amygdala on both sides of the brain is a "psychic blindness" in the choice of foods. In other words, the animal (and presumably the human being as well) loses or at least partially loses the mechanism of appetite control over the type and quality of food that is eaten.

The cortical regions of the limbic system, including the infraorbital regions, the hippocampal gyrus, and the cingulate gyrus, all have areas that when stimulated can either increase or decrease feeding activities. These areas seem especially to play a role in an animal's drive to search for food when hungry. It is presumed that these centers are also responsible, probably operating in association with the amygdala and hypothalamus, for determining the quality of food that is eaten. For instance, a previous unpleasant experience with almost any type of food often destroys a person's appetite for that food thereafter.

Factors That Regulate Food Intake

We can divide the regulation of food into (1) *nutritional regulation,* which is concerned with maintenance of normal quantities of nutrient stores in the body, and (2) *alimentary regulation,* which is concerned with the immediate effects of feeding on the alimentary tract and is sometimes called *peripheral* or *short-term regulation.*

Nutritional Regulation. An animal that has been starved for a long time and is then presented with unlimited food eats a far greater quantity than does an animal that has been on a regular diet. Conversely, an animal that has been force-fed for several weeks eats little when allowed to eat according to its own desires. Thus, the feeding center in the hypothalamus is geared to the nutritional status of the body. Some of the nutritional factors that control the degree of activity of the feeding center are the following:

Availability of Glucose to the Body Cells—The Glucostatic Theory of Hunger and of Feeding Regulation. It has long been known that a decrease in blood glucose concentration is associated with development of hunger, which has led to the so-called *glucostatic theory of hunger and of feeding regulation,* as follows: When the blood glucose level falls too low, this automatically causes the animal to increase its feeding, which eventually returns the glucose concentration back toward normal. There are two particular observations that also support the glucostatic theory: (1) An increase in blood glucose level increases the measured electrical activity in the satiety center in the ventromedial nuclei of the hypothalamus and simultaneously decreases the electrical activity in the feeding center of the lateral nuclei. (2) Chemical studies show that the ventromedial nuclei (the satiety center) concentrate glucose while other areas of the hypothalamus fail to concentrate glucose; therefore, it is assumed that increased glucose stores in the body limit feeding by increasing the degree of satiety.

Effect of Blood Amino Acid Concentration on Feeding. An increase in amino acid concentration in the blood also reduces feeding, and a decrease enhances feeding. In general, though, this effect is not as powerful as the glucostatic mechanism.

Effect of Fat Metabolites on Feeding—Long-Term Regulation. The overall degree of feeding varies almost inversely with the amount of adipose tissue in the body. That is, as the quantity of adipose tissue increases, the rate of feeding decreases. Therefore, many physiologists believe that *long-term regulation* of feeding is controlled mainly by fat metabolites of an undiscovered nature. This is called the lipostatic theory of feeding regulation. In support of this is the fact that the long-term average concentration of free fatty acids in the blood is directly proportional to the quantity of adipose tissue in the body. Therefore, it is likely that the free fatty acids or some other similar fat metabolites act in the same manner as glucose and amino acids to cause a negative feedback regulatory effect on feeding. It is also possible, if not probable, that this is by far the most important long-term regulatory mechanism of feeding.

Summary of Long-Term Nutritional Regulation. Even though our information on the different feedback factors in long-term feeding regulation is imprecise, we can make the following general statement: When the nutrient stores of the body fall below normal, the feeding center of the hypothalamus becomes highly active and the person exhibits increased hunger; on the other hand, when the nutrient stores are abundant, the person loses hunger and develops a state of satiety.

Alimentary Regulation (Short-Term, Nonmetabolic Regulation). The degree of hunger or satiety can be temporarily increased or decreased by habit. For instance, the normal person has the habit of eating three meals a day, and when one is missed he or she is likely to develop a state of hunger at mealtime despite completely adequate nutritional stores in the tissues. But, in additional to habit, several other short-term physiological stimuli, mainly related to the alimentary tract, can alter one's desire for food for several hours at a time, as follows.

Gastrointestinal Filling. When the gastrointestinal tract becomes distended, especially the stomach or the duodenum, inhibitory signals temporarily suppress the feeding center, thereby reducing the desire for food. This effect probably depends mainly on sensory signals transmitted through the vagi, but part of the effect still persists after the vagi and the sympathetic nerves from the upper gastrointestinal tract have been severed. Therefore, somatic sensory signals from the stretched abdomen may also play a role. And recently it has been found that short-term hormonal feedback also suppresses feeding, for the hormone *cholecystokinin,* which is released mainly in response to fat entering the duodenum, as well as *insulin* that is secreted by the pancreas in response to carbohydrates, both have a strong effect on inhibition of further eating.

Obviously, these mechanisms are of particular importance in bringing one's feeding to a halt during a heavy meal.

Metering of Food by Oral Receptors. When a person with an esophageal fistula is fed large quantities of food, even though this food is immediately lost again to the exterior, the degree of hunger is decreased after a reasonable quantity of food has passed through the mouth. This effect occurs despite the fact that the gastrointestinal tract does not in the least become filled. Therefore, it is postulated that various "oral factors" related to feeding, such as chewing, salivation, swallowing, and tasting, "meter" the food as it passes through the mouth, and after a certain amount has passed through, the hypothalamic feeding center becomes inhibited.

Importance of Having Both Long- and Short-Term Regulatory Systems for Feeding. The long-term regulatory system, especially the lipostatic feedback mechanism, obviously helps an animal maintain constant stores of nutrients in its tissues, preventing them from becoming too little or too great. On the other hand, the short-term regulatory stimuli make the animal feed only when the gastrointestinal tract is receptive to food. Thus, food passes through the gastrointestinal tract fairly continuously, so that its digestive, absorptive, and storage mechanisms can all work at a steady pace rather than only when the animal needs food for energy. Indeed, the digestive, absorptive, and storage mechanisms can increase their rates of activity above normal only four- to five-fold, whereas the rate of usage of stored nutrients for energy sometimes increases to 20 times normal.

It is important, then, that feeding should occur rather continuously (but at a rate that the gastrointestinal tract can accommodate), regulated principally by the short-term mechanisms. However, it is also important that the intensity of the daily rhythmical feeding habits be modulated up or down by the long-term regulatory system, based on the level of nutrient stores in the body.

OBESITY

Energy Input Versus Energy Output. When greater quantities of energy in the form of food enter the body than are expended, the body weight increases. Therefore, obesity is obviously caused by excess energy input over energy output. For each 9.3 Calories excess energy entering the body, 1 gram of fat is stored.

Excess energy input occurs *only during the developing phase of obesity;* once a person has already become obese, all that is required for the person to remain obese is that the energy input equal the energy output. For the person to reduce, the output must be *greater* than the input. Indeed, studies of obese persons, once they have become obese, show that their intake of food is almost exactly the same as that of normal-weight persons.

Effect of Muscular Activity on Energy Output. About one third of the energy used each day by a normal person goes into muscular activity, though in the laborer doing heavy work as much as two thirds and occasionally three fourths is used in this way. Since muscular activity is by far the most important means by which energy is expended in the body, it is frequently said that obesity results from *too high a ratio of food intake to daily exercise.*

Abnormal Feeding Regulation as a Pathological Cause of Obesity

The preceding discussion of the mechanisms that regulate feeding have emphasized that the rate of feeding is normally regulated in proportion to the nutrient stores in the body. When these stores begin to approach an optimal level in a normal person, feeding is automatically reduced to prevent overstorage. However, in most obese persons this is not true, for feeding does not automatically slacken until body weight is far above normal. Therefore, in effect, obesity is often caused by an abnormality of the feeding regulatory mechanism. This can result from either psychogenic factors that affect the regulation or actual abnormalities of the hypothalamus itself.

Psychogenic Obesity. Studies of obese patients show that a large proportion of obesity results from psychogenic factors. Perhaps the most common psychogenic factor contributing to obesity is the prevalent idea that healthy eating habits require three meals a day and that each meal must be filling. Many children are forced into this habit by overly solicitous parents, and these children continue to practice it throughout their lives.

Genetic Factors in Obesity. Obesity definitely runs in families. Furthermore, identical twins usually maintain weight levels within 2 pounds of each other throughout life if they live under similar conditions, or within 5 pounds if their conditions of life differ markedly. This might result partly from eating habits engendered during childhood, but it is generally believed that this close similarity between twins is genetically controlled.

The genes can cause abnormal feeding in several different ways, including (1) a genetic abnormality of the feeding center that sets the level of nutrient storage high or low or (2) abnormal hereditary psychic factors that either whet the appetite or cause a person to eat as a "release" mechanism.

A genetic abnormality in the *chemistry of fat storage* is also known to cause obesity in a certain strain of rats. In these rats, fat is easily stored in the adipose tissue, but the quantity of hormone-sensitive lipase in the adipose tissue is greatly reduced, so that little of the fat can be removed. This obviously results in a one-way path, the fat continuously being deposited but never released. This, too, is another possible mechanism of obesity in some human beings.

Childhood Overnutrition as a Possible Cause of Obesity. The rate of formation of new fat cells is especially rapid in the first few years of life, and the greater the rate of fat storage the greater becomes the number of fat cells. In obese children the number of fat cells is often as much as three times that in normal children. After adolescence, the number of fat cells remains almost identically the same throughout the remainder of life. Therefore, it has been suggested that overfeeding children, especially in infancy, can lead to a lifetime of obesity. The person who has excess fat cells is thought to have a higher setting of the hypothalamic feedback autoregulatory mechanism for control of adipose tissues.

In persons who become obese in middle or old age, most of the obesity results from hypertrophy of already existing fat cells. This type of obesity is far more susceptible to treatment than is the life-long type.

STARVATION

Depletion of Food Stores in the Body Tissues During Starvation. Even though the tissues preferentially use carbohydrate for energy instead of fat and protein, the quantity of carbohydrate stores of the body is only a few hundred grams (mainly glycogen in the liver and muscles), and it can supply the total energy required for body function for only about half a day. Therefore, except for the first few hours of starvation, the major effects are progressive depletion of tissue fat and protein. Since fat is the prime source of energy, its rate of depletion continues unabated, as illustrated in Figure 48–1, until most of the fat stores in the body are gone.

Protein undergoes three different phases of depletion: rapid depletion at first, then greatly slowed depletion, and finally rapid depletion again, shortly before death. The initial rapid depletion is caused by conversion of protein to glucose in the liver by the process of gluconeogenesis. The glucose thus formed (about two thirds of it) is used to supply energy to the brain, which under normal circumstances utilizes almost no metabolic substrate for energy other than glucose. However, after the readily mobilizable protein stores have been depleted during the early phase of starvation, the remaining protein is not so easily removed from the tissues. At this time, the rate of gluconeogenesis decreases to one third to one fifth its previous rate, and the rate of depletion of protein becomes greatly decreased, as illustrated in Figure 48–1. The diminished availability of glucose then initiates a series of events leading to *ketosis,* which means greatly increased formation of ketone bodies, as described in Chapter 46. Fortunately, the ketone bodies (mainly acetoacetic acid and hydroxybutyric acid), like glucose, can cross the blood-brain barrier and can be utilized by the brain cells for energy. Therefore, approximately two thirds of the brain's energy now is derived from these ketone bodies. This sequence of events thus leads to at least partial preservation of the protein stores of the body.

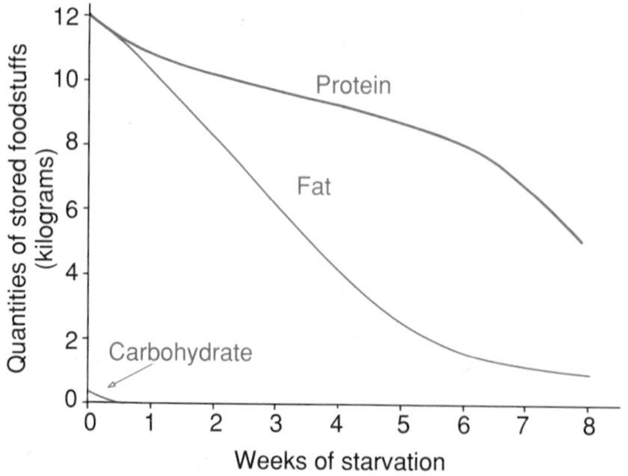

Figure 48–1. Effect of starvation on the food stores of the body.

However, there finally comes a time when the fat stores also are almost totally depleted, and the only remaining source of energy is proteins. At that time, protein stores once again enter a stage of rapid depletion. Since the proteins are essential for maintenance of cellular function, death ordinarily ensues when the proteins of the body have been depleted to approximately one half their normal level.

VITAMINS

Daily Requirements of Vitamins. A vitamin is an organic compound needed in small quantities for operation of normal bodily metabolism and that cannot be manufactured in the cells of the body. When lacking in the diet, vitamins can cause specific metabolic deficits.

Table 48–1 lists the amounts of important vitamins required daily by the average adult. These requirements vary considerably, depending on such factors as (a) body size, (b) rate of growth, (c) amount of exercise, (d) disease and fever, and (e) special need for vitamin D in pregnant or lactating women. Also, a number of metabolic deficits occur pathologically in which the vitamins themselves cannot be utilized properly in the body; in such conditions the requirement for one or more specific vitamins may be extreme.

Vitamin A

Vitamin A precursors occur in abundance in many different vegetable foods. These are the yellow and red *carotenoid pigments,* which, since they have chemical structures similar to that of vitamin A, can be changed into vitamin A in the human body. Vitamin A exists in the body mainly as *retinol.*

The basic function of vitamin A in the metabolism of the body is not known except in relation to its use in formation of the retinal photochemicals (discussed in Chapter 34). Nevertheless, vitamin A is also necessary for normal growth of most cells of the body and especially for normal growth and proliferation of the different types of epithelial cells. When vitamin A is lacking, the epithelial structures of the body tend to become stratified and keratinized. Therefore, vitamin A deficiency manifests itself by (1) scaliness of the skin and sometimes acne, (2) failure of growth of young animals, (3) failure of reproduction in many animals, associated especially with atrophy of the germinal epithelium of the testes and sometimes with

Table 48-1 REQUIRED DAILY AMOUNTS OF THE VITAMINS

A	5000 IU*
Thiamine	1.5 mg
Riboflavin	1.8 mg
Niacin	20 mg
Ascorbic acid	45 mg
D	400 IU*
E	15 IU*
K	none
Folic acid	0.4 mg
B_{12}	3 μg
Pyridoxine	2 mg
Pantothenic acid	unknown

* IU = International units.

interruption of the female sexual cycle, and (4) keratinization of the cornea with resultant corneal opacity and blindness.

Thiamine (Vitamin B_1)

Thiamine operates in the metabolic systems of the body principally as *thiamine pyrophosphate;* this compound functions as a *cocarboxylase,* operating mainly for decarboxylation of pyruvic acid, which was discussed in Chapter 45.

Thiamine deficiency causes decreased utilization of pyruvic acid and some amino acids by the tissues but increased utilization of fats. Thus, thiamine is specifically needed for final metabolism of carbohydrates any many amino acids. Probably the decreased utilization of these nutrients is responsible for the debilities associated with thiamine deficiency.

Thiamine Deficiency and the Nervous System. The central nervous system depends almost entirely on the metabolism of carbohydrates for its energy. In thiamine deficiency the utilization of glucose by nervous tissue may be decreased as much as 50 to 60 per cent. Therefore, it is readily understandable that thiamine deficiency can greatly impair function of the central nervous system. The neuronal cells of the central nervous system frequently show chromatolysis and swelling during thiamine deficiency, changes that are characteristic of neuronal cells with poor nutrition.

Also, thiamine deficiency can cause *degeneration of myelin sheaths* of nerve fibers both in the peripheral nerves and in the central nervous system. The lesions in the peripheral nerves frequently cause these nerves to become extremely irritable, resulting in polyneuritis characterized by pain radiating along the course of one or more peripheral nerves. Also, in severe thiamine deficiency, the peripheral nerve fibers and fiber tracts in the cord can degenerate to such an extent that *paralysis* occasionally results.

Thiamine Deficiency and the Cardiovascular System. Thiamine deficiency also weakens the heart muscle, so that a person with severe thiamine deficiency sometimes develops *cardiac failure. Peripheral edema* and *ascites* also occur to a major extent in some persons with thiamine deficiency, partly because of the cardiac failure but also because thiamine deficiency causes arteriolar dilatation.

Thiamine Deficiency and the Gastrointestinal Tract. Among the gastrointestinal symptoms caused by thiamine deficiency are indigestion, severe constipation, anorexia, gastric atony, and hypochlorhydria. All these effects possibly result from failure of the smooth muscle and glands of the gastrointestinal tract to derive sufficient energy from carbohydrate metabolism.

The overall picture of thiamine deficiency, including polyneuritis, cardiovascular symptoms, and gastrointestinal disorders, is frequently referred to as *beriberi*—especially when the cardiovascular symptoms predominate.

Niacin

Niacin, also called *nicotinic acid,* functions in the body as coenzymes in the forms of nicotinamide adenine dinucleotide (NAD) and nicotinamide adenine dinucleotide phosphate (NADP). These coenzymes are hydrogen acceptors, which combine with hydrogen atoms as they are removed from food substrates by many different types of dehydrogenases. When a deficiency of niacin exists, the normal rate of dehydrogenation cannot be maintained; therefore, oxidation of the hydrogen and consequent delivery of energy from the foodstuffs to the functioning elements of the cells likewise cannot occur at normal rates.

Because NAD and NADP operate in all cells of the body, it is understandable that lack of niacin can cause multiple symptoms. Clinically, niacin deficiency causes mainly gastrointestinal symptoms, neurological symptoms, and a characteristic dermatitis. Pathological lesions appear in many parts of the central nervous system, and permanent dementia or any of many different types of psychoses may result. Also, the skin develops a cracked, pigmented scaliness in areas that are exposed to mechanical irritation or to sun irradiation; thus, the skin is unable to repair the different types of irritative damage. Finally, niacin deficiency causes intense irritation and inflammation of the mucous membranes of the mouth and other portions of the gastrointestinal tract, thus instituting many digestive abnormalities.

The clinical entity called *pellagra* is caused mainly by niacin deficiency. Pellagra is greatly exacerbated in persons on a corn diet (such as in many of the natives of Africa) because corn is deficient in the amino acid tryptophan, which can be converted in limited quantities to niacin in the body.

Riboflavin (Vitamin B_2)

Riboflavin normally combines in the tissues with phosphoric acid to form two coenzymes, *flavin mononucleotide* (FMN), and *flavin adenine dinucleotide* (FAD). These in turn operate as hydrogen carriers in several of the important oxidative systems of the body.

Deficiency of riboflavin in lower animals causes severe *dermatitis; vomiting; diarrhea; muscular spasticity,* which finally becomes muscular weakness; and then *death* preceded by coma and declining body temperature. Thus, severe riboflavin deficiency can cause many of the same effects as lack of niacin in the diet; presumably the debilities that result in each instance are due to generally depressed oxidative processes within the cells.

In the human being, riboflavin is so prevalent in the diet that deficiency has never been known to be severe enough to cause the marked debilities noted in animal experiments, but mild riboflavin deficiency is probably common. Perhaps the most common characteristic lesion of riboflavin deficiency is *cheilosis,* which is inflammation and cracking at the angles of the mouth. In addition, a fine, scaly dermatitis often occurs at the angles of the nares, and keratitis of the cornea may occur, with invasion of the cornea by small blood vessels.

Though its manifestations are usually relatively mild, riboflavin deficiency frequently occurs in association with lack of thiamine or niacin. Therefore, many deficiency syndromes, including pellagra, beriberi, sprue, and kwashiorkor, are probably due to a combined insufficiency of several of the vitamins and also of protein.

Vitamin B_{12}

Several different *cobalamin* compounds exhibit so-called vitamin B_{12} activity.

Vitamin B_{12} performs many metabolic functions, acting as a hydrogen acceptor coenzyme. For instance, it performs this function in the conversion of some amino acids and similar compounds into other substances. Its most important function is to act as a coenzyme for reducing ribonucleotides to deoxyribonucleotides, a step that is important in the formation of genes and that could explain the two major functions of vitamin B_{12}: (1) promotion of growth and (2) red blood cell maturation. This latter function was described in Chapter 24.

A particular effect of vitamin B_{12} deficiency is *pernicious anemia,* in which the red blood cells fail to mature properly and therefore are rapidly destroyed in the circulatory system. In addition, there is often demyelination of the large nerve fibers of the spinal cord, especially of the posterior columns and occasionally of the lateral columns. As a result, persons with pernicious anemia frequently have much simultaneous loss of peripheral sensation and, in severe cases, even become paralyzed.

Folic Acid (Pteroylglutamic Acid)

Several different pteroylglutamic acids exhibit the "folic acid effect." Folic acid functions as a carrier of hydroxymethyl and formyl groups. Perhaps its most important use in the body is in the synthesis of purines and thymine, which are required for formation of deoxyribonucleic acid. Therefore, folic acid is required for reproduction of the cellular genes. This perhaps explains one of the most important functions of folic acid—that is, to promote growth.

Folic acid is an even more potent growth promoter than vitamin B_{12}, and, like vitamin B_{12}, is also important for the maturation of red blood cells, as discussed in Chapter 19. However, vitamin B_{12} and folic acid each perform specific and different functions in promoting growth and maturation of red blood cells.

Pyridoxine (Vitamin B_6)

Pyridoxine exists in the form of *pyridoxal phosphate* in the cells and functions as a coenzyme for many different chemical reactions relating to amino acid and protein metabolism. Its most important role is that of coenzyme in transamination for the synthesis of amino acids. Also, it is believed to act in the transport of some amino acids across cell membranes.

In the human being, pyridoxine deficiency has been known to cause convulsions, dermatitis, and gastrointestinal disturbances such as nausea and vomiting in children. However, this deficiency is rare.

Pantothenic Acid

Pantothenic acid mainly is incorporated in the body into coenzyme A, which has many metabolic roles in the cells. Two of these discussed in Chapters 45 and 46 are (1) acetylation of decarboxylated pyruvic acid to form acetyl Co-A prior to its entry into the citric acid cycle and (2) degradation of fatty acid molecules into multiple molecules of acetyl Co-A by the process of "beta" oxidation. Thus, lack of pantothenic acid can lead to depressed metabolism of both carbohydrates and fats.

However, in the human being, no definite deficiency syndrome has been proved, presumably because of wide occurrence of this vitamin in almost all foods and because small amounts of the vitamin can probably be synthesized in the body. Nevertheless, this does not mean that pantothenic acid is not of value in the metabolic systems of the body; indeed, it is perhaps as necessary as any other vitamin.

Ascorbic Acid (Vitamin C)

Ascorbic acid is essential for activating the enzyme *prolyl hydroxylase* that promotes the hydroxylation step in the formation of hydroxyproline, an integral constituent of collagen. Without ascorbic acid the collagen that is formed is defective and weak. Therefore, this vitamin is essential for growth of subcutaneous tissue, cartilage, bone, and teeth.

Deficiency of ascorbic acid for 20 to 30 weeks, as occurred frequently during long sailing voyages in olden days, causes *scurvy,* some effects of which are the following:

One of the most important effects of scurvy is *failure of wounds to heal.* This is caused by failure of the cells to deposit collagen fibrils and intercellular cement substances. As a result, healing of a wound may require several months instead of the several days ordinarily necessary.

Lack of ascorbic acid causes *cessation of bone growth.* The cells of the growing epiphyses continue to proliferate, but no new collagen matrix is laid down between the cells, and the bones fracture easily at the point of growth because of failure to ossify. Also, when an already ossified bone fractures in a person with ascorbic acid deficiency, the osteoblasts cannot secrete a new matrix for the deposition of new bone. Consequently, the fractured bone does not heal.

The *blood vessel walls become extremely fragile* in scurvy because of failure of the endothelial cells to cement together properly and to form the collagen fibrils normally present in vessel walls. The capillaries especially are likely to rupture, and as a result, many small petechial hemorrhages occur throughout the body. The hemorrhages beneath the skin cause purpuric blotches, sometimes over the entire body.

In extreme scurvy the muscle cells sometimes fragment; lesions of the gums with loosening of the teeth occur; infections of the mouth develop; vomiting of blood, bloody stools, and cerebral hemorrhage all may result; and, finally, high fever often develops before death.

Vitamin D

Vitamin D increases calcium absorption from the gastrointestinal tract and also helps control calcium deposition in the bone. The mechanism by which vitamin D increases calcium absorption is to promote active transport of calcium through the epithelium of the ileum. It increases the formation of a calcium-binding protein in the epithelial cells that aids in calcium absorption. The specific functions of vitamin D in relation to overall body calcium metabolism and to bone formation are presented in detail in Chapter 53.

Vitamin E

Several related compounds exhibit so-called vitamin E activity. Only rare instances of vitamin E deficiency occur in human beings. In lower animals, lack of vitamin E can cause degeneration of the germinal epithelium in the testis and therefore can cause male sterility. Lack of vitamin E can also cause resorption of a fetus after conception in the female. Because of these deficiency effects, vitamin E is sometimes called the antisterility vitamin.

Also, as is true of almost all the vitamins, deficiency of vitamin E prevents normal growth.

Vitamin E is believed to function mainly in relation to unsaturated fatty acids, preventing oxidation of the unsaturated fats. In the absence of vitamin E, the quantity of unsaturated fats in the cells becomes diminished, causing abnormal structure and function of such cellular organelles as the mitochondria, the lysosomes, and even the cell membrane.

Vitamin K

Vitamin K is necessary for the formation by the liver of prothrombin, factor VII (proconvertin), factor IX, and factor X, all of which are important in blood coagulation. Therefore, when vitamin K deficiency occurs, blood clotting is retarded. The function of this vitamin has been presented in greater detail in Chapter 26.

Several different compounds, both natural and synthetic, exhibit vitamin K activity. Because vitamin K is synthesized by bacteria in the colon, a dietary source of this vitamin is not usually necessary; but when the bacteria of the colon are destroyed by administration of large quantities of antibiotic drugs, vitamin K deficiency occurs rapidly because of the paucity of this compound in the normal diet.

REFERENCES

Berger, H.: Vitamins and Minerals in Pregnancy and Lactation. New York, Raven Press, 1988.

Flint, D. J., et al.: Can obesity be controlled? News Physiol. Sci., 2:1, 1987.

Guthrie, H. A.: Introductory Nutrition. 7th ed. St. Louis, C. V. Mosby Co., 1988.

Hanson, L. A.: Biology of Human Milk. New York, Raven Press, 1988.

Katch, F. I., and McArdle, W. D.: Nutrition, Weight Control, and Exercise. Philadelphia, Lea & Febiger, 1988.

Kinney, J. M. et al.: Nutrition and Metabolism in Patient Care. Philadelphia, W. B. Saunders Co., 1988.

Maho, Y. L., et al: Starvation as a treatment for obesity: The need to conserve body protein. News Physiol. Sci., 3:21, 1988.

Muno, H. N., and Danford, D. E.: Nutrition, Aging, and the Elderly. New York, Plenum Publishing Corp., 1989.

Nicolaidis, S.: What determines food intake? The ischymetric theory. News Physiol. Sci., 2:104, 1987.

Oomura, Y.: Regulation of feeding by neural responses to endogenous factors. News Physiol. Sci., 2:199, 1987.

Paige, D. M.: Clinical Nutrition, St. Louis, C. V. Mosby Co., 1988.

Shils, M. E., and Young, V. R.: Modern Nutrition in Health and Disease. 7th ed., Philadelphia, Lea & Febiger, 1988.

Weinsier, R. L., et al.: Handbook of Clinical Nutrition: Clinician's Manual for the Diagnosis and Management of Nutritional Problems. St. Louis, C. V. Mosby Co., 1988.

Williams, S. R., Nutrition and Diet Therapy. 6th ed. St. Louis, C. V. Mosby Co., 1989.

QUESTIONS

1. Approximately how much *physiologically available energy* can be derived from each one of the three foodstuffs in the diet: carbohydrates, fat, and protein?
2. What is meant by a *partial protein,* and why are far greater quantities of protein required to maintain protein balance when partial proteins are eaten?

3. How can one use the *respiratory quotient* to determine the relative utilization of carbohydrates and fat by the metabolic systems of the body?
4. Describe the location of the *hunger* and *satiety centers* in the hypothalamus.
5. How does the *amygdala* contribute to the control of feeding?
6. Explain the roles of blood glucose, blood lipids, and blood amino acids on feeding regulation.
7. Why is it important to have both a *long-term mechanism* for feeding regulation and a *short-term mechanism?* What are the different mechanisms of short-term regulation?
8. In a person who is very obese but has reached a stable weight level, what is the status of this person's energy input-output balance?
9. Explain the role of each of the following factors in *obesity:* psychological status of the person, genetic factors, and childhood overnutrition.
10. In *starvation,* how long do the carbohydrate and fat stores last, and what is the sequence of protein depletion during the starvation period?
11. Describe the functions and the clinical effects of deficits of each of the following vitamins: (a) vitamin A, (b) thiamine, (c) niacin, (d) riboflavin, (e) vitamin B_{12}, (f) folic acid, (g) pyridoxine, (h) pantothenic acid, (i) ascorbic acid, (j) vitamin D, (k) vitamin E, and (l) vitamin K.

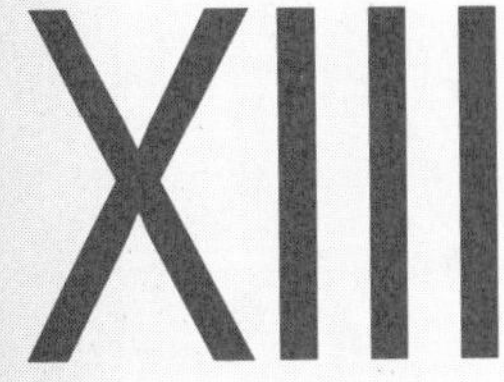

XIII

Endocrinology and Reproduction

49

Introduction to Endocrinology; The Pituitary Hormones

The functions of the body are regulated by two major control systems: (1) the nervous system, which has been discussed, and (2) the hormonal, or endocrine, system. In general, the hormonal system is concerned principally with control of the metabolic functions of the body, controlling the rates of chemical reactions in the cells, the transport of substances through cell membranes, or other aspects of cellular metabolism such as growth and secretion. Some hormonal effects occur in seconds, whereas others require several days simply to start, and then they continue for weeks, months, or even years.

Many interrelationships exist between the hormonal and nervous systems. For instance, at least two glands, the *adrenal medullae* and the *posterior pituitary gland,* secrete their hormones only in response to nerve stimuli, and a few of the anterior pituitary hormones are secreted to a significant extent only in response to nervous and neuroendocrine activity in the hypothalamus (detailed later in this chapter).

Nature of a Hormone

A hormone is a chemical substance that is secreted into the body fluids by one cell or a group of cells and that exerts a physiological *control* effect on other cells of the body.

At many points in this text we have already discussed different hormones, some of which are called *local hormones,* and others, *general hormones.* Examples of local hormones are *acetylcholine,* released at the parasympathetic and skeletal nerve endings; *secretin,* released by the duodenal wall and transported in the blood to the pancreas to cause an alkaline, watery pancreatic secretion; and *cholecystokinin,* released in the small intestine to cause contraction of the gallbladder and to promote enzyme secretion by the pancreas. These hormones obviously have specific local effects, hence the name local hormones.

On the other hand, the general hormones are secreted by specific *endocrine glands* located at different places in the body, as illustrated in Figure 49–1. These hormones are secreted into the blood, and they cause physiological actions in distant tissues. A few of the general hormones affect all, or almost all, cells of the body; examples are *growth hormone* from the adenohypophysis and *thyroid hormone* from the thyroid gland. Other general hormones, however, primarily affect specific tissues; for instance, *corticotropin* from the anterior pituitary gland specifically stimulates the adrenal cortex, and the *ovarian hormones* have specific effects on the uterine endometrium. The tissues affected specifically in this way are called *target tissues.* Many examples of target organs will become apparent in the following chapters on endocrinology.

The following general hormones have proved to be of major significance and are discussed in detail in this and the following chapters:

Anterior Pituitary Hormones

1. *Growth hormone* causes growth of almost all cells and tissues of the body.
2. *Adrenocorticotropin* causes the adrenal cortex to secrete adrenocortical hormones.
3. *Thyroid-stimulating hormone* causes the thyroid gland to secrete thyroxine and triiodothyronine.
4. *Follicle-stimulating hormone* causes growth of follicles in the ovaries prior to ovulation; also promotes the formation of sperm in the testes.

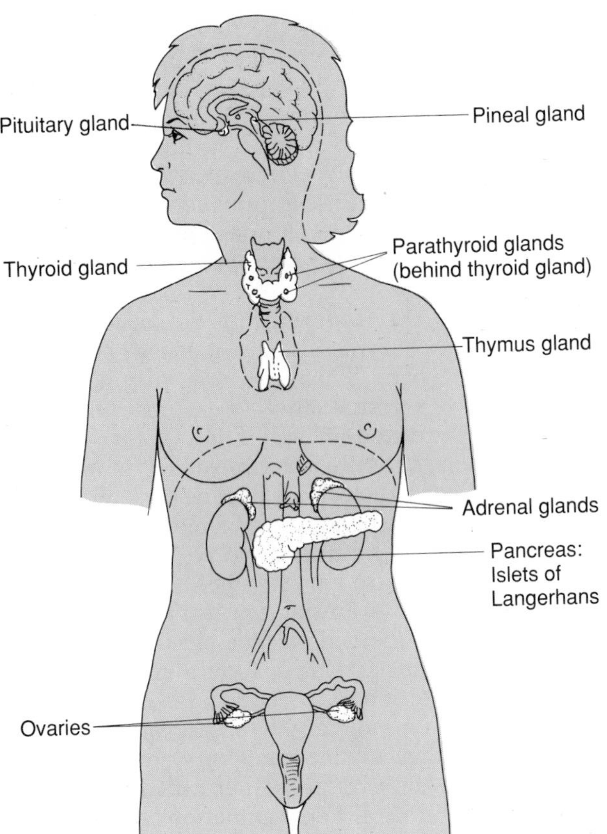

Figure 49–1. The anatomical loci of the principal endocrine glands of the body.

5. *Luteinizing hormone* plays an important role in causing ovulation; also causes secretion of female sex hormones by the ovaries and testosterone by the testes.
6. *Prolactin* promotes development of the breasts and secretion of milk.

Posterior Pituitary Hormones

1. *Antidiuretic hormone* (also called *vasopressin*) causes the kidneys to retain water, also, in higher concentrations, causes constriction of the blood vessels throughout the body and elevates the blood pressure.
2. *Oxytocin* contracts the uterus during the birthing process; it also contracts myoepithelial cells in the breasts, thereby expressing milk from the breasts when the baby suckles.

Adrenal Cortex Hormones

1. *Cortisol* has multiple metabolic functions for control of the metabolism of proteins, carbohydrates, and fats.
2. *Aldosterone* reduces sodium excretion by the kidneys and increases potassium excretion, thus increasing sodium in the body while decreasing the amount of potassium.

Thyroid Gland Hormones

(1, 2). *Thyroxine and triiodothyronine* increase the rates of chemical reactions in almost all cells of the body, thus increasing the general level of body metabolism.

3. *Calcitonin* promotes the deposition of calcium in the bones and thereby decreases calcium concentration in the extracellular fluid.

Hormones of the Islets of Langerhans in the Pancreas

1. *Insulin* promotes glucose entry into most cells of the body, in this way controlling the rate of metabolism of most carbohydrates.
2. *Glucagon* increases the release of glucose from the liver into the circulating body fluids.

Hormones of the Ovaries

1. *Estrogens* stimulate the development of the female sex organs, the breasts, and various secondary sexual characteristics.
2. *Progesterone* stimulates secretion of "uterine milk" by the uterine endometral glands; also helps promote development of the secretory apparatus of the breasts.

Hormone of the Testes

1. *Testosterone* stimulates growth of the male sex organs; also promotes the development of male secondary sex characteristics.

Parathyroid Gland Hormone

1. *Parathormone* controls the calcium ion concentration of the body by controlling (a) absorption of calcium from the gut, (b) excretion of calcium by the kidneys, and (c) release of calcium from the bones.

Placental Hormones

1. *Human chorionic gonadotropin* promotes growth of the corpus luteum and secretion of estrogens and progesterone by the corpus luteum.
2. *Estrogens* promote growth of the mother's sex organs and of some of the tissues of the fetus.
3. *Progesterone* promotes special development of the uterine endometrium in advance of implantation of the fertilized ovum; probably promotes development of some of the fetal tissues and organs; helps promote development of the secretory apparatus of the mother's breasts.
4. *Human somatomammotropin* probably promotes growth of some fetal tissues as well as mother's breasts.

MECHANISMS OF HORMONAL ACTION

Hormone Receptors and Their Activation

The endocrine hormones almost invariably first combine with *hormone receptors* on the membrane surfaces of the cells or inside the cells. The combination of hormone and receptor then usually initiates a cascade of reactions in the cell.

Either all or almost all hormonal receptors are very large proteins, and each receptor is almost always highly specific for a single hormone.

Activation of the Receptors. The receptors in their unbound state usually are inactive, and the intracellular mechanisms that are associated with them are also inactive. However, in a few instances the unbound receptors are in the active form, and when bound with the hormone they become inhibited.

Activation of a receptor occurs in different ways for different types of receptors. For instance, in Chapter 31 we discussed the many types of receptors located in the postsynaptic membranes of neurons and activated by the synaptic hormones called transmitter substances. The transmitter substance combines with the receptor and causes a conformational change of the receptor molecule; this in turn alters the membrane permeability to one or more ions, especially sodium, chloride, potassium, and calcium ions. A few of the general endocrine hormones also function in this same way—for instance, epinephrine and norepinephrine change the membrane permeability in certain of their target tissues.

In addition to this direct effect of some hormone receptors to change cell membrane permeability, there are also two very important general mechanisms by which a large share of the hormones function: (1) by *activating the cyclic AMP system of the cells,* which in turn activates multiple other intracellular functions, or (2) by *activating the genes of the cell,* which causes the formation of intracellular proteins that in turn initiate specific cellular functions. These two general mechanisms are described as follows:

The Cyclic AMP Mechanism for Controlling Cell Function—A "Second Messenger" for Hormone Mediation

Many hormones exert their effects on cells by causing the substance *cyclic 3′,5′-adenosine monophosphate* (cyclic AMP) to be formed in the cell. Once formed, it is then the cyclic AMP that causes the hormonal effects inside the cell. Thus, *cyclic AMP is an intracellular hormonal mediator.* It is also frequently called a "second messenger" for hormone mediation—the "first messenger" being the original stimulating hormone.

The cyclic AMP mechanism has been shown to be a way in which all the following hormones (and many more) can stimulate their target tissues:

1. Adrenocorticotropin
2. Thyroid-stimulating hormone
3. Luteinizing hormone
4. Follicle-stimulating hormone
5. Vasopressin
6. Parathyroid hormone
7. Glucagon
8. Catecholamines
9. Secretin
10. The hypothalamic-releasing hormones

Figure 49–2 illustrates the function of the cyclic AMP mechanism in more detail. The stimulating hormone first binds with a specific "receptor" for that hormone on the membrane surface of the target cell. Then this combination of hormone and receptor activates the enzyme *adenyl cyclase,* which is the portion of the receptor protein that protrudes into the cytoplasm inside the cell membrane. This in turn causes immediate *conversion of much of the cytoplasmic ATP into cyclic AMP.*

Once cyclic AMP is formed inside the cell, it activates still other enzymes. In fact, it usually activates a *cascade of enzymes.* That is, a first enzyme is activated, and this activates another enzyme, which activates still a third, and so forth. The importance of this mechanism is that only a few molecules of activated adenyl cyclase in the cell membrane can cause many more molecules of the second enzyme to be activated, and these can cause still many times that number of molecules of the third enzyme to be activated, and so forth. In this way, even the slightest amount of hormone acting on the cell surface can initiate a very powerful cascading activating force for the entire cell.

The specific action that occurs in response to cyclic AMP in each type of target cell depends upon the nature of the intracellular machinery, some cells having one set of enzymes and other cells having other enzymes. Therefore, different functions are elicited in different target cells—such functions as

1. initiating synthesis of specific intracellular chemicals
2. causing muscle contraction or relaxation
3. initiating secretion by the cells
4. altering the cell permeability
5. and many other possible effects.

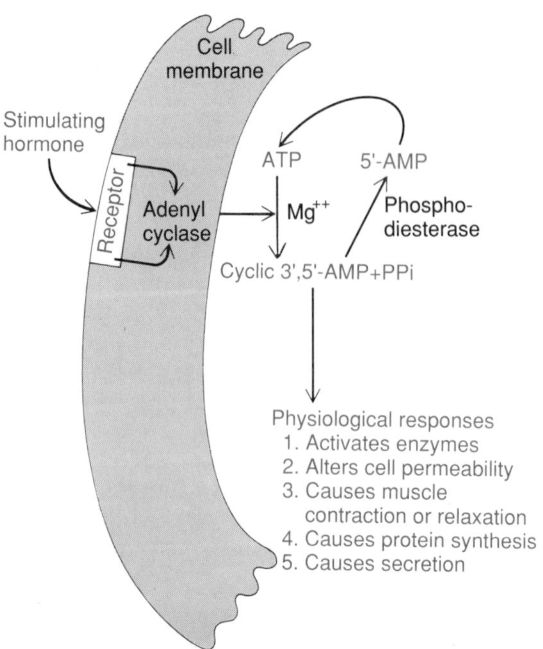

Figure 49–2. The cyclic AMP mechanism by which many hormones exert their control of cell function.

Thus, a thyroid cell stimulated by cyclic AMP forms the metabolic hormones thyroxine and triiodothyronine, whereas the same cyclic AMP in an adrenocortical cell causes secretion of the adrenocortical steroid hormones. On the other hand, cyclic AMP affects epithelial cells of the renal tubules by increasing their permeability to water.

Role of Calcium Ions and Calmodulin as Another Second Messenger System. Another second messenger system operates in response to the entry of calcium ions into cells caused by a hormone that acts on membrane receptors that open calcium channels. On entering the cell, the calcium ions bind with a protein called *calmodulin.* A conformational change occurs that activates the calmodulin, causing multiple effects inside the cell in the same way that cyclic AMP functions. For instance, calmodulin activates many other enzymes in addition to those activated by cyclic AMP, thus causing an additional set of intracellular metabolic reactions. One of the specific functions of calmodulin is to activate myosin kinase that then acts directly on the myosin of smooth muscle to cause smooth muscle contraction.

Action of Steroid Hormones on the Genes to Cause Protein Synthesis

A second major means by which some hormones act—specifically, the steroid hormones secreted by the adrenal cortex, the ovaries, and the testes—is to cause synthesis of proteins in target cells; some of these proteins are enzymes that in turn activate other functions of the cells.

The sequence of events in steroid function is the following:

1. The steroid hormone enters the cytoplasm of the cell, where it binds with a specific *receptor protein.*
2. The combined receptor protein–hormone then diffuses, or is transported, into the nucleus.
3. The combination then activates specific genes to form messenger RNA.
4. The messenger RNA diffuses into the cytoplasm, where it promotes the translation process at the ribosomes to form new proteins.

To give an example, aldosterone, one of the hormones secreted by the adrenal cortex, enters the cytoplasm of renal tubular cells, which contain a specific aldosterone receptor protein. Then the outlined sequence of events ensues. After about 45 minutes, proteins that promote sodium reabsorption from the tubules and potassium secretion into the tubules begin to appear in the renal tubular cells. Thus, there is a characteristic delay in the final action of the steroid hormone of 45 minutes to several hours, which is in marked contrast to the almost instantaneous action of some of the peptide and peptide-derived hormones that stimulate cells by the cyclic AMP mechanism.

Action of the Thyroid Hormones in the Cell Nucleus. The thyroid hormones thyroxine and triiodothyronine also activate the genetic mechanisms for formation of many different types of intracellular proteins—probably a hundred or more. Many of these are enzymes that promote enhanced intracellular metabolic activity, as we shall discuss more fully in Chapter 50.

MEASUREMENT OF HORMONE CONCENTRATIONS IN THE BLOOD—RADIOIMMUNOASSAY

Most hormones are present in the blood in extremely minute quantities, some in concentrations as low as one millionth of a milligram (1 picogram) per milliliter. Therefore, except in a few instances, it has been almost impossible to measure these concentrations by usual chemical means. Fortunately, though, an extremely sensitive method was developed about twenty-five years ago that revolutionized the measurement of hormones, their precursors, and their metabolic end-products. This is the method of *radioimmunoassay.*

The principle of radioimmunoassay is as follows:

First, an antibody is developed that is highly specific for the hormone to be measured.

Second, a small quantity of this antibody is simultaneously mixed with (a) a quantity of fluid (from the person) containing the hormone to be measured and (b) an appropriate amount of purified standard hormone of the same type that has been tagged with a radioactive isotope. However, one specific condition must be met: there must be too little antibody to bind completely both the tagged hormone and the hormone in the fluid to be assayed. Therefore, the natural hormone in the assay fluid and the radioactive standard hormone *compete for the binding sites* on the antibody. In the process of competing, the quantity of each of the two hormones that binds is proportional to its concentration.

Third, after binding has reached equilibrium, the antibody-hormone complex is separated from the remainder of the solution, and the quantity of radioactive hormone bound with antibody is measured by radioactive counting techniques. If a *large amount of radioactive hormone* has bound with the antibody, then it is clear that there was only a *small amount of natural hormone* to compete with the radioactive hormone, and therefore the concentration of the natural hormone in the assayed fluid was small. Conversely, if only a small amount of radioactive hormone was bound, it is clear that there was a very large amount of natural hormone to complete for the binding sites.

Fourth, to make the assay highly quantitative, the radioimmunoassay procedure is performed also for standard solutions of untagged hormone at several different concentration levels. Then, a standard curve is plotted as illustrated in Figure 49–3. By comparing the radioactive counts recorded from the original assay procedure with the standard curve, one can determine within an error of ± 10 to 15 per cent the concentration of the hormone in the assayed fluid. As

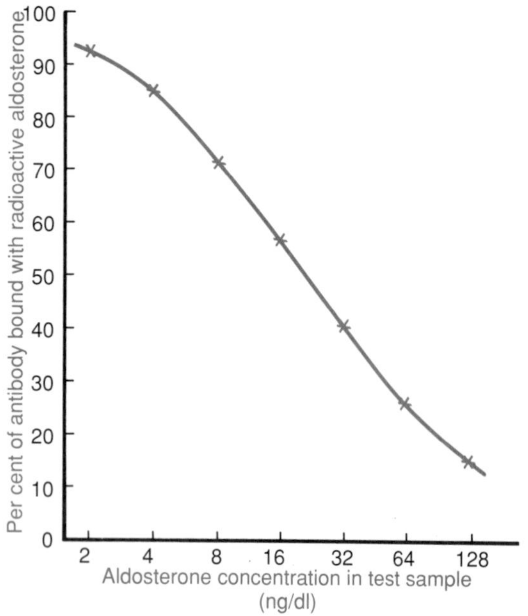

Figure 49-3. A "standard curve" for radioimmunoassay of aldosterone. (Courtesy of Dr. Manis Smith.)

little as one trillionth of a gram of hormone is often assayed in this way.

THE PITUITARY GLAND, ITS MULTIPLE CONTROL FUNCTIONS, AND ITS RELATIONSHIP TO THE HYPOTHALAMUS

The *pituitary gland* Fig. 49-4, also called the *hypophysis,* is a small gland — less than 1 cm in diameter and about 0.5 to 1 gram in weight — that lies in the *sella turcica* at the base of the brain and is connected with the hypothalamus by the *pituitary* (or *hypophysial*) *stalk.* Physiologically, the pituitary gland is divisible into two distinct portions: the *anterior pituitary,* also known as the *adenohypophysis,* and the posterior pituitary, also known as the *neurohypophysis.*

Six very important hormones plus several less important ones are secreted by the *anterior* pituitary, and two important hormones are secreted by the *posterior* pituitary. The hormones of the anterior pituitary play major roles in the control of metabolic functions throughout the body, as shown in Figure 49-5; thus: (1) *Growth hormone* promotes growth by enhancing protein formation, cell multiplication, and cell differentiation. (2) *Adrenocorticotropin* controls the secretion of some of the adrenocortical hormones, which in turn affect the metabolism of glucose, proteins, and fats. (3) *Thyroid-stimulating hormone* controls the rate of secretion of thyroxine by the thyroid gland, and thyroxine in turn controls the rates of most chemical reactions of the entire body. (4) *Prolactin* promotes mammary gland development and milk production. And two separate gonadotropic hormones, (5) *follicle-stimulating hormone* and (6) *luteinizing hormone,* control growth of the gonads as well as their reproductive activities.

The anterior pituitary gland contains at least five different types of secretory cells. Usually, there is one cell type for each major hormone formed in this gland. Using special stains attached to high affinity antibodies that bind with the distinctive hormones, these various cell types can be differentiated one from another. The only major exception to this general rule is that the same cell type seems to secrete both luteinizing hormone and follicle-stimulating hormone.

The two hormones secreted by the posterior pituitary play other roles: (1) *Antidiuretic hormone* controls the rate of water excretion into the urine and in this way helps to control the concentration of water in the body fluids. (2) *Oxytocin* (a) contracts the alveoli of the breasts, thereby helping to deliver milk from

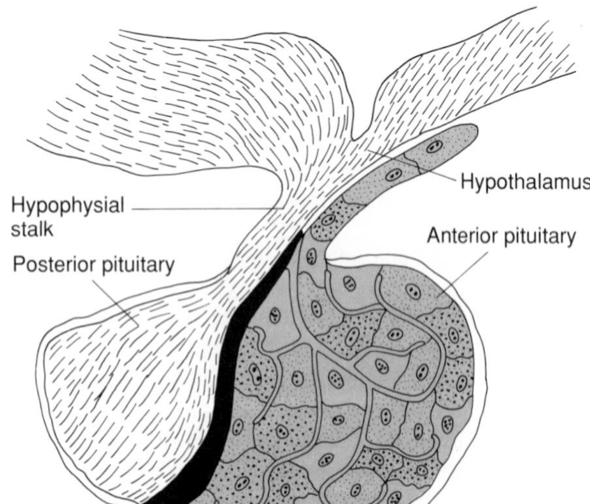

Figure 49-4. The pituitary gland

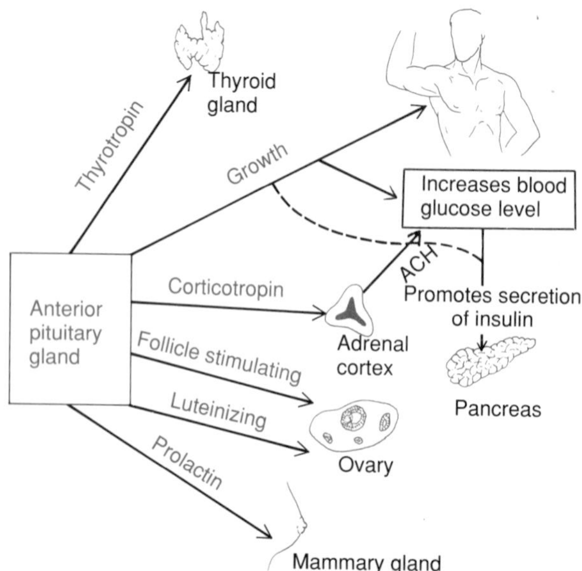

Figure 49-5. Metabolic functions of the anterior pituitary hormones.

the glands of the breast to the nipples during suckling, and (b) contracts the uterus, thus helping in delivery of the baby at the end of gestation.

Control of Anterior Pituitary Secretion by the Hypothalamus—Hypothalamic-Releasing and Inhibitory Hormones

Secretion by the anterior pituitary is controlled by hormones called *hypothalamic-releasing* and *inhibitory hormones* (or *factors*) secreted within the hypothalamus itself and then conducted to the anterior pituitary through minute blood vessels called *hypothalamic-hypophysial portal vessels.* In the anterior pituitary, these releasing and inhibitory hormones act on the glandular cells to control their secretion. This system of control will be discussed in detail later in the chapter.

The hypothalamus receives signals from almost all possible sources in the nervous system. Thus, when a person is exposed to pain, a portion of the pain signal is transmitted into the hypothalamus. Likewise, when a person experiences some powerful depressing or exciting thought, a portion of the signal is transmitted into the hypothalamus. Olfactory stimuli denoting pleasant or unpleasant smells transmit strong signal components through the amygdaloid nuclei into the hypothalamus. *Even the concentrations of nutrients, electrolytes, water, and various hormones* in the blood excite or inhibit various portions of the hypothalamus. Thus, the hypothalamus is a collecting center for information concerned with the well-being of the body, and in turn much of this information is used to control secretion by the pituitary gland.

The Hypothalamic-Hypophysial Portal System

The anterior pituitary is a highly vascular gland with extensive capillary sinuses among the glandular cells. Almost all the blood that enters these sinuses passes first through a capillary bed in the tissue of the lower hypothalamus and then through small *hypothalamic-hypophysial portal vessels* that pass downward along the pituitary stalk into the anterior pituitary sinuses. Thus, Figure 49–6 illustrates a small artery supplying the lowermost portion of the hypothalamus, called the *median eminence.* Small vascular tufts project into the substance of the median eminence and then return to its surface, coalescing to form the hypothalamic-hypophysial portal vessels. These in turn pass downward along the pituitary stalk to supply the anterior pituitary sinuses.

Secretion of Hypothalamic-Releasing and Inhibitory Hormones in the Median Eminence. Special neurons in the hypothalamus synthesize and secrete the *hypothalamic-releasing* and *inhibitory hormones.* These neurons originate in various parts of the hypothalamus and send their nerve fibers into the median eminence. The endings of these fibers are different from most endings in the central nervous system in that their function is not to transmit signals from one neuron to another but merely to secrete the hypothalamic-releasing and inhibitory hormones into the tissue fluids. These hormones are immediately absorbed into the hypothalamic-hypophysial portal capillaries and carried directly to the sinuses of the anterior pituitary gland.

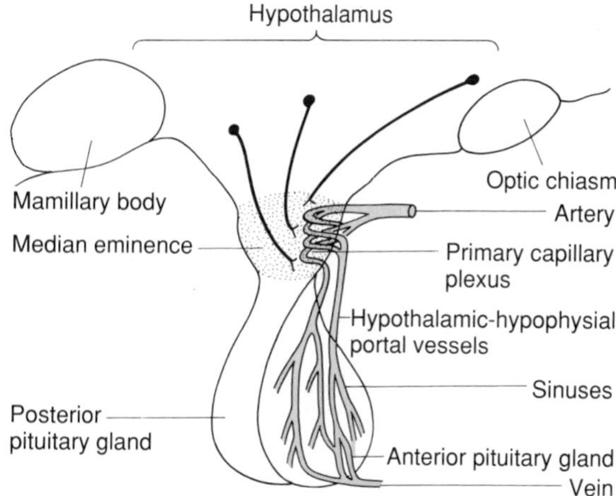

Figure 49–6. The hypothalamic-hypophysial portal system.

Function of the Releasing and Inhibitory Hormones. The function of the releasing and inhibitory hormones is to control the secretion of the anterior pituitary hormones. For each type of anterior pituitary hormone there is usually a corresponding hypothalamic-releasing hormone; for some of the anterior pituitary hormones there is also a corresponding hypothalamic inhibitory hormone. For most of the anterior pituitary hormones, it is the releasing hormones that are important; but for prolactin, the inhibitory hormone probably exerts most control. The hypothalamic-releasing and inhibitory hormones that are of major importance are

1. *Thyroid-stimulating hormone-releasing hormone* (TRH), which causes release by the anterior pituitary gland of thyroid-stimulating hormone
2. *Corticotropin-releasing hormone* (CRH), which causes release of adrenocorticotropin
3. *Growth hormone-releasing hormone* (GHRH), which causes release of growth hormone
4. *Gonadotropin-releasing hormone* (GnRH), which causes release of both luteinizing hormone and follicle-stimulating hormone
5. *Prolactin inhibitory factor* (PIF), which causes inhibition of prolactin secretion.

PHYSIOLOGICAL FUNCTIONS OF THE ANTERIOR PITUITARY HORMONES

All the major anterior pituitary hormones besides growth hormone exert their effects by stimulating "target glands"—the thyroid gland, the adrenal cortex, the ovaries, the testicles, and the mammary glands. The functions of each of the anterior pituitary hormones, except for growth hormone, are so intimately concerned with the functions of the respective target glands that their functions will be discussed in subsequent chapters along with the functions of these target glands. Growth hormone, in contrast to other hormones, does not function through a target gland but instead exerts effects on all or almost all tissues of the body.

PHYSIOLOGICAL FUNCTIONS OF GROWTH HORMONE

Growth hormone (GH), also called *somatotropic hormone* (SH) or *somatotropin,* is a small protein molecule containing 191 amino acids in a single chain and having a molecular weight of 22,005. It causes growth of all tissues of the body that are capable of growing. It promotes both increased sizes of the cells and increased mitosis with development of increased numbers of cells. As an example, Figure 49-7 illustrates weight charts of two growing rats, one of which received daily injections of growth hormone, compared with a litter-mate that did not receive growth hormone.

Metabolic Effects of Growth Hormone

Aside from its general effect of causing growth, growth hormone has many specific metabolic effects as well, including especially:

1. Increased rate of protein synthesis in all cells of the body
2. Increased mobilization of fatty acids from adipose tissue, and increased use of the fatty acids for energy
3. Decreased rate of glucose utilization throughout the body

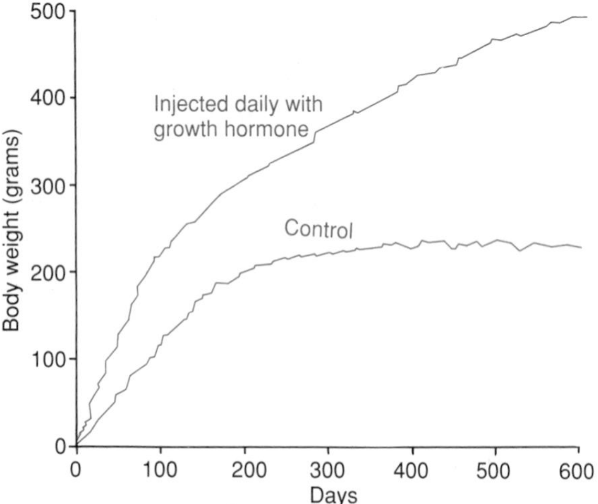

Figure 49-7. Comparison of weight gain of a rat injected daily with growth hormone with that of a normal rat.

Thus, in effect, growth hormone enhances the body protein, uses up the fat stores, and conserves carbohydrate.

Role of Growth Hormone in Promoting Protein Deposition

Although the most important basis for the increased protein deposition caused by growth hormone is not known, a series of different effects are known, all of which can lead to enhanced protein. These effects are

1. Enhancement of Amino Acid Transport Through the Cell Membranes. Growth hormone directly enhances transport of at least some and perhaps most amino acids through the cell membranes to the interior of the cells. This increases the concentrations of the amino acids in the cells and is presumed to be at least partly responsible for the increased protein synthesis.

2. Enhancement of Protein Synthesis by the Ribosomes. Even when the amino acids are not increased, growth hormone still causes protein to be synthesized in increased amounts in the cells. This is believed to be partly due to a direct effect of the hormone on the ribosomal machinery, making it produce greater numbers of protein molecules.

3. Increased Formation of RNA. Over more prolonged periods of time, growth hormone also stimulates the transcription process in the nucleus, causing formation of increased quantities of RNA. This in turn promotes protein synthesis.

4. Decreased Catabolism of Protein and Amino Acids. In addition to the increase in protein synthesis, there is a decrease in the breakdown of intracellular protein and in the utilization of protein and amino acids for energy. A probable reason for this effect is that growth hormone also mobilizes large quantities of free fatty acids from the adipose tissue, and these in turn are used to supply most of the energy for the body cells; thus growth hormone acts as a potent "protein sparer."

Summary. Growth hormone enhances almost all facets of amino acid uptake and protein synthesis by cells while at the same time reducing the breakdown of proteins.

Effect of Growth Hormone in Enhancing Fat Utilization for Energy

Growth hormone has a specific effect in causing release of fatty acids from adipose tissue and therefore increasing the fatty acid concentration in the body fluids. In addition, in the tissues it enhances the conversion of fatty acids to acetyl-CoA, with subsequent utilization of this product for energy. Therefore, under the influence of growth hormone, fat is utilized for energy in preference to both carbohydrates and proteins.

Effect of Growth Hormone on Carbohydrate Metabolism

Growth hormone has three major effects on cellular metabolism of glucose. These effects are (1) decreased utilization of glucose for energy, (2) marked enhancement of glycogen deposition in the cells, and (3) diminished uptake of glucose by the cells.

Decreased Glucose Utilization for Energy. Unfortunately, we do not know the precise mechanism by which growth hormone decreases glucose utilization by the cells. However, the decrease probably results partially from the increased mobilization and utilization of fatty acids for energy caused by growth hormone. That is, the fatty acids form large quantities of acetyl Co-A, which in turn initiate feedback effects that block the glycolytic breakdown of glucose and glycogen.

Enhancement of Glycogen Deposition. Since glucose and glycogen cannot be utilized for energy, the glucose that does enter the cells is rapidly polymerized into glycogen and deposited. Therefore, the cells rapidly become saturated with glycogen and can store no more.

Diminished Uptake of Glucose by the Cells and Increased Blood Glucose Concentration. When growth hormone is first administered to an animal, the cellular uptake of glucose is enhanced and the blood glucose concentration falls slightly. However, as the cells become saturated with glycogen and their utilization of glucose for energy decreases, further uptake of glucose then becomes greatly diminished. Without normal cellular uptake, the blood concentration of glucose increases, sometimes to as high as 50 to 100 per cent above normal.

Stimulation of Cartilage and Bone Growth — Role of the Somatomedins

Though we have discussed at length the role of growth hormone in causing growth, growth hormone does not have a significant *direct* effect on the growth of the skeletal elements cartilage and bone. For instance, when growth hormone is applied directly to cartilage chondrocytes cultured outside the body, no discernible proliferation or enlargement of the chondrocytes occurs, even though growth hormone injected into the intact animal does cause such proliferation and growth. To make a long story short, it has been found that growth hormone acts indirectly on cartilage and bone by causing the liver to form several small proteins called *somatomedins,* with molecular weights varying between 4500 and 7500. These somatomedins, especially *somatomedin-C,* then act on the cartilage and bone to promote their growth. Their basic function is to cause secretion by the chondrocytes of chondroitin sulfate and collagen, both of which are necessary for cartilage and bone growth.

Other Metabolic and Growth Functions of the Somatomedins. Though growth hormone, when added directly to tissues removed from the body, can cause all the metabolic effects that we have discussed thus far except cartilage and bone growth, the concentrations of growth hormone that are required to cause these actions are often many times as great as those known to exist in the body. On the other hand, the different somatomedins in very small concentrations can cause essentially all the same effects as the direct actions of growth hormone. Therefore, it is probable that most of the metabolic functions of growth hormone are caused not by its direct effects on the tissues, but indirectly through the somatomedins.

Regulation of Growth Hormone Secretion

For many years it was believed that growth hormone was secreted primarily during the period of growth but then disappeared from the blood at adolescence. However, this belief has proved to be very far from the truth, because after adolescence secretion continues at a rate almost as great as that in childhood. Furthermore, the rate of growth hormone secretion can increase within minutes in relation to the person's state of nutrition or stress — during starvation, hypoglycemia, exercise, excitement, and trauma.

The normal concentration of growth hormone in the plasma of an adult is about 3 nanograms per milliliter and in the child about 5 nanograms per milliliter. However, these values often increase to as high as 50 nanograms per milliliter after depletion of the body stores of proteins or carbohydrates. Under acute conditions, hypoglycemia is a far more potent stimulator of growth hormone secretion than is a decrease in the amino acid concentration in the blood. On the other hand, in chronic conditions the degree of cellular protein depletion seems to be more correlated with the level of growth hormone secretion than is the availability of glucose. For instance, the extremely high levels of growth hormone that occur during starvation are very closely related to the amount of protein depletion.

Thus, it is almost certain that growth hormone secretion is controlled moment by moment by the nutritional and stress status of the body, and it seems that the most important factor in the control of growth hormone secretion is the level of cell protein, though changes in blood glucose concentration can also cause extremely rapid and dramatic alterations in growth hormone secretion. Consequently, it can be postulated that growth hormone operates in a feedback control system as follows: When the tissues begin to suffer from malnutrition, especially from poor protein nutrition, large quantities of growth hormone are secreted. Growth hormone, in turn, promotes the synthesis of new proteins, while at the same time conserving the protein already present in the cells.

Role of the Hypothalamus and Growth Hormone–Releasing Hormone (GHRH). All the feedback effects that control growth hormone secretion are believed to be mediated through the hypothalamus. Most important, the hypothalamus secretes *growth hormone-releasing hormone* (GHRH), which in turn causes the anterior pituitary to secrete the growth hormone. The hypothalamic center that causes growth hormone-releasing hormone secretion is the *ventromedial nucleus,* the same nucleus that helps control other aspects of metabolism, such as the level of hunger and feeding.

Abnormalities of Growth Hormone Secretion

Dwarfism. Most instances of dwarfism result from deficiency of anterior pituitary secretion of growth hormone during childhood. In general, the features of the body develop in appropriate proportion to each other, but the rate of development is greatly decreased. A child who has reached the age of 10 years may have the bodily development of a child of 4 to 5 years, whereas the same person on reaching the age of 20 years may have the bodily development of a child of 7 to 10 years.

Two thirds of the pituitary dwarfs do not pass through puberty and do not secrete a sufficient quantity of gonadotropic hormones to develop adult sexual functions. In one third, however, the deficiency is of growth hormone alone; these individuals do mature sexually and occasionally reproduce.

Giantism. Occasionally, the growth hormone-producing cells of the anterior pituitary become excessively active, and often growth hormone cell (acidophilic cell) tumors occur in the gland. As a result, large quantities of growth hormone are produced. All body tissues grow rapidly, including the bones, and if the epiphyses of the long bones have not already become fused with the shafts—that is, if this occurs before adolescence—height increases, so that the person becomes a giant with a height of up to 8 to 9 feet.

Most giants, unfortunately, eventually develop hypopituitarism if they remain untreated, because the tumor of the pituitary gland grows until the gland itself is destroyed. This general deficiency of pituitary hormones, if untreated, usually causes death in early adulthood. However, once giantism is diagnosed, further development of the disease can usually be blocked by microsurgical removal of the tumor from the pituitary gland or by irradiation of the gland.

Acromegaly. If a growth hormone cell tumor occurs after adolescence—that is, after the epiphyses of the long bones have fused with the shafts—the person cannot grow taller; but his soft tissues can continue to grow, and the bones can grow in thickness. This condition is known as *acromegaly.* Enlargement is especially marked in the small bones of the hands and feet and in the *membranous bones,* including the cranium, the nose, the bosses on the forehead, the supraorbital ridges, the lower jawbone, and portions of the vertebrae, for their growth does not cease at adolescence anyway. Consequently, as illustrated in Figure 49-8 (a typical acromegalic), the jaw protrudes forward, sometimes as much as a half inch; the forehead slants forward because of excess development of the supraorbital ridges; and the nose increases to as much as twice normal size. Also, the foot requires a

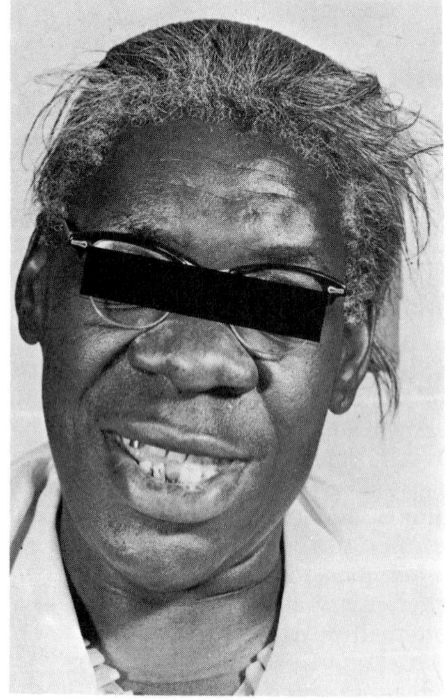

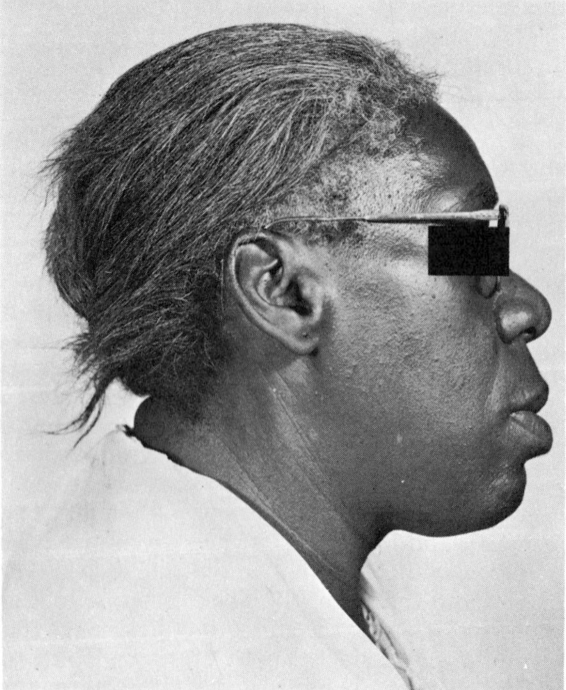

Figure 49-8. An acromegalic patient. (Courtesy of Dr. Herbert Langford.)

size 14 or larger shoe, and the fingers become extremely thickened, so that the hand develops a size almost twice normal. In addition to these effects, changes in the vertebrae ordinarily cause a hunched back. Finally, many soft tissue organs, such as the tongue, the liver, and especially the kidneys, become greatly enlarged.

THE POSTERIOR PITUITARY GLAND AND ITS RELATION TO THE HYPOTHALAMUS

The *posterior pituitary gland,* also called the *neurohypophysis,* is composed mainly of glia-like cells called *pituicytes.* However, the pituicytes do not secrete hormones; they act simply as a supporting structure for large numbers of *terminal nerve fibers* and *terminal nerve endings* from nerve tracts that originate in the *supraoptic* and *paraventricular nuclei* of the hypothalamus, as shown in Figure 49-9. These tracts pass to the neurohypophysis through the *pituitary stalk* (hypophysial stalk). The nerve endings are bulbous knobs that lie on the surfaces of capillaries onto which they secrete the two posterior pituitary hormones: (1) *antidiuretic hormone* (ADH), also called *vasopressin,* and (2) *oxytocin.* Both of these hormones are small polypeptides, each containing nine amino acids. They are identical with each other except for two of the amino acids.

If the pituitary stalk is cut near the pituitary gland, leaving the entire hypothalamus intact, the posterior pituitary hormones continue, after a transient decrease for a few days, to be secreted almost normally, but they are then secreted by the cut ends of the fibers within the hypothalamus and not by the nerve endings in the posterior pituitary. The reason for this is that the hormones are initially synthesized in the cell bodies of the neurons in the supraoptic and paraventricular nuclei and are then transported to the nerve endings in the posterior pituitary gland, requiring several days to reach the gland.

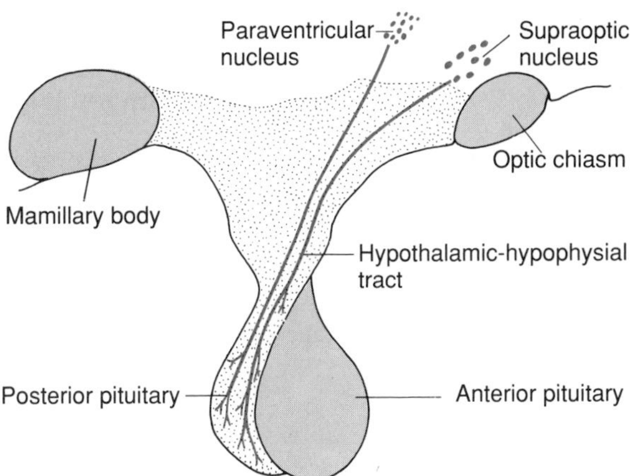

Figure 49-9. Hypothalamic control of the posterior pituitary.

ADH is formed primarily in the supraoptic nuclei, while *oxytocin is formed primarily in the paraventricular nuclei.* However, each of these two nuclei can synthesize approximately one sixth as much of the second hormone as the primary hormone.

Under resting conditions, large quantities of both ADH and oxytocin accumulate in the nerve endings of the posterior pituitary gland. Then, when nerve impulses are transmitted downward along the fibers from the supraoptic and paraventricular nuclei, the hormones are immediately released from the nerve endings and are absorbed into the adjacent capillaries.

Physiological Functions of Antidiuretic Hormone (Vasopressin)

Extremely minute quantities of antidiuretic hormone (ADH) — as little as 2 nanograms — when injected into a person can cause antidiuresis, that is, decreased excretion of water by the kidneys. This antidiuretic effect was discussed in detail in Chapter 22. Briefly, in the absence of ADH, the collecting ducts and collecting tubules are almost totally impermeable to water, which prevents significant reabsorption of water and therefore allows extreme loss of water into the urine. On the other hand, in the presence of ADH, the permeability of these ducts to water increases greatly and allows most of the water in the tubular fluid to be reabsorbed, thereby conserving water in the body.

Regulation of ADH Production

Osmotic Regulation. When the body fluids become highly concentrated, the supraoptic nuclei become excited, impulses are transmitted to the posterior pituitary, and ADH is secreted. This hormone then passes by way of the blood to the kidneys, where it increases the permeability of the collecting tubules and ducts to water. As a result, most of the water is reabsorbed from the tubular fluid, while electrolytes continue to be lost into the urine. This effect dilutes the extracellular fluids, returning them to a normal osmotic composition. The details of this mechanism were also discussed in Chapter 22 in relation to body fluid electrolyte control.

Stimulation of ADH Secretion When the Blood Volume Decreases — Pressor Effect of ADH. ADH in moderate and high concentrations has a very potent effect of constricting the arterioles and therefore of increasing the arterial pressure. Also, one of the most powerful stimuli of all for increasing the secretion of ADH is severe loss of blood volume. As little as a 10 per cent loss of blood will promote a moderate increase in ADH secretion, and a blood loss of 25 per cent or more can cause as much as 20 to 50 times normal rates of secretion.

The increased secretion is believed to result mainly from the low pressure caused in the atria of the heart by the low blood volume. The relaxation of the atrial stretch receptors supposedly sends signals by way of sensory pathways to the hypothalamus to elicit the increase in ADH secretion. However, the baroreceptors of the carotid, aortic, and pulmonary regions also participate in this control of ADH secretion.

The marked secretion of ADH following severe hemorrhage perhaps plays a very important role in the homeostasis of arterial pressure. Because ADH has this potent pressor effect, it is also called *vasopressin.*

Oxytocic Hormone

Effect on the Uterus. An oxytocic substance is one that causes contraction of the pregnant uterus. The hormone *oxytocin,* in accordance with its name, powerfully stimulates the pregnant uterus, especially toward the end of gestation. Therefore, this hormone is believed to be at least partially responsible for effecting the birth of the baby. This will be discussed in Chapter 56 in relation to reproduction and pregnancy.

Effect of Oxytocin on Milk Ejection. Oxytocin also has an especially important function in the process of lactation, for this hormone causes milk to be expressed from the alveoli into the ducts so that the baby can obtain it by suckling. This, too, will be discussed in Chapter 56.

REFERENCES

General Endocrinology

Blalock, J. E.: A molecular basis for bidirectional communication between the immune and neuroendocrine systems. Physiol. Rev., 69:1, 1989.
Conn, P. M. (ed.): Neuroendocrine Peptide Methodology. San Diego, Cal., Academic Press, 1988.
DeGroot, L. J., et al.: Endocrinology. 2nd ed. Philadelphia, W. B. Saunders Co., 1989.
Evans, R. M.: The steroid and thyroid hormone receptor superfamily. Science, 240:889, 1988.
Goodman, H. M.: Basic Medical Endocrinology. New York, Raven Press, 1988.
Greengard, P., and Alan, R. G.: Advances in Second Messenger and Phosphoprotein Research. New York, Raven Press, 1988.
Martini, L., and Ganong, W. F., (eds.): Frontiers in Neuroendocrinology. New York, Raven Press, 1988.
Sowers, J. R., and Felicetta, J. V.: Endocrinology of Aging, New York, Raven Press, 1988.

Pituitary Hormones

Bercu, B. B. (ed.): Basic and Clinical Aspects of Growth Hormone. New York, Plenum Publishing Corp., 1988.
Campion, D. R., et al. (eds.): Animal Growth Regulation. New York, Plenum Publishing Corp., 1989.
Collu, R., et al.: Pediatric Endocrinology. 2nd ed. New York, Raven Press, 1989.
Felig, P., et al. (eds.): Endocrinology and Metabolism. 2nd ed. New York, McGraw-Hill Book Co., 1987.
Gash, D. M., and Boer, G. J. (eds.): Vasopressin, New York, Plenum Publishing Corp., 1987.
Kannan, C. R.: The Pituitary Gland. New York, Plenum Publishing Corp., 1987.
Kudlow, J. E., et al. (eds.): Biology of Growth Factors. New York, Plenum Publishing Corp., 1988.
Muller, E. E.: Neural control of somatotropic function. Physiol. Rev., 67:962, 1987.
Nishimoto, I., and Kojima I.: Calcium signalling system triggered by insulin-like growth factor II. News Physiol. Sci. 4:94, 1989.
Robbins, R. J., and Melmed, S. (eds.): Acromegaly. New York, Plenum Publishing Corp., 1987.

QUESTIONS

1. Explain the role of *membrane receptors* in the activation of tissue cells by hormones.
2. Describe the *cyclic AMP mechanism* as a second messenger system for controlling cell function.
3. Explain the role of *calmodulin* as a second messenger system.
4. Explain how steroid hormones and thyroid hormone act on the *cell genes* to cause their hormonal effects.
5. Describe the relationship of the pituitary gland to the hypothalamus, especially the *hypothalamic-hypophysial portal system.*
6. What are the important *releasing* and *inhibitory hormones* secreted by the hypothalamus, and what are their functions?
7. How does growth hormone promote *protein deposition?*
8. What is the effect of growth hormone on *fat mobilization* and utilization for energy?
9. What are the effects of growth hormone on *carbohydrate metabolism?*
10. Explain the role of the *somatomedins* in promoting bone and cartilage growth as well as other possible functions of growth hormone.
11. What are the principal metabolic and nervous factors that can cause increased growth hormone secretion? How do the hypothalamus and *growth hormone-releasing hormone* function in the control of growth hormone secretion?
12. Explain the causes of pituitary *dwarfism, giantism,* and *acromegaly.*
13. Describe the secretion and the release of the posterior pituitary hormones.
14. What are the principal functions of *antidiuretic hormone?*
15. What are the principal functions of *oxytocic* hormone?

50

The Thyroid Metabolic Hormones

The thyroid gland, which is located immediately below the larynx on either side of and anterior to the trachea, secretes large amounts of two hormones, *thyroxine* and *triiodothyronine,* that have a profound effect on the metabolic rate of the body. It also secretes *calcitonin,* a hormone that is important for calcium metabolism and which will be considered in Chapter 53. Complete lack of thyroid secretion usually causes the basal metabolic rate to fall to about 40 per cent below normal, and extreme excesses of thyroid secretion can cause the basal metabolic rate to rise as high as 60 to 100 per cent above normal. Thyroid secretion is controlled primarily by thyroid-stimulating hormone secreted by the anterior pituitary gland.

The purpose of this chapter is to discuss the formation and secretion of the thyroid metabolic hormones, their functions in the metabolic schema of the body, and the regulation of their secretion.

FORMATION AND SECRETION OF THE THYROID HORMONES

The most abundant of the hormones secreted by the thyroid gland is *thyroxine.* However, moderate amounts of *thiiodothyronine* are also secreted. The functions of these two hormones are qualitatively the same, but they differ in rapidity and intensity of action. Triiodothyronine is about four times as potent as thyroxine, but it is present in the blood in smaller quantities and persists for a much shorter time than does thyroxine.

Physiological Anatomy of the Thyroid Gland. The thyroid gland is composed, as shown in Figure 50-1, of large numbers of closed *follicles* filled with a secretory substance called *colloid* and lined with *cuboidal epitheloid cells* that secrete into the interior of the follicles. The major constituent of colloid is a large glycoprotein, *thyroglobulin,* which contains the thyroid hormones as part of its molecule. Once the secretion has entered the follicles, the thyroid hormones must be absorbed back through the follicular epithelium into the blood before they can function in the body, which is a very slow process.

Requirements of Iodine for Formation of Thyroxine and Triiodothyronine

To form normal quantities of thyroxine and triiodothyronine, approximately 50 mg of ingested iodine are required *each year,* or approximately *1 mg per week.* To prevent iodine deficiency, common table salt is iodized with one part of sodium iodide to every 100,000 parts of sodium chloride.

The Iodide Pump (Iodide Trapping)

The first stage in the formation of thyroid hormones, shown in Figure 50-2, is the transfer of iodides from the extracellular fluid into the thyroid glandular cells and thence into the follicle. The basal membrane of the thyroid cell has a specific ability to transport iodides actively to the interior of the cell; this is called the *iodide pump,* or *iodide trapping.* In a normal gland, the iodide pump concentrates the iodide ion to about 30 times its concentration in the blood. However, when the thyroid gland becomes maximally active, the concentration ratio can rise to as high as 250 times.

Thyroglobulin and the Chemistry of Thyroxine and Triiodothyronine Formation

Formation and Secretion of Thyroglobulin by the Thyroid Cells. The thyroid cells are typical pro-

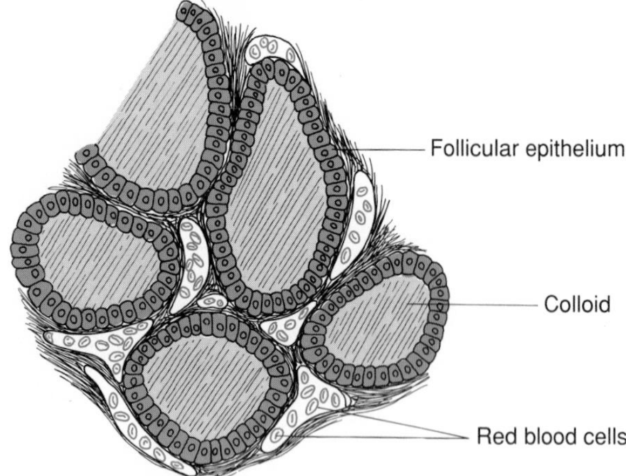

Figure 50-1. Microscopic appearance of the thyroid gland, showing the secretion of thyroglobulin into the follicles.

tein-secreting glandular cells, as illustrated in Figure 50-2. The endoplasmic reticulum and the Golgi complex synthesize and secrete into the follicles a large glycoprotein molecule, with a molecular weight of 670,000, called *thyroglobulin.*

Each molecule of thyroglobulin contains 140 tyrosine amino acids, and these are the major substrates that combine with iodine to form the thyroid hormones. These hormones form *within* the thyroglobulin molecule. That is, the tyrosine amino acid residues, as well as the thyroxine and triiodothyronine hormones formed from them, remain a part of the thyroglobulin molecule during the entire synthesis of the thyroid hormones.

In addition to secreting the thyroglobulin, the glandular cells also provide the iodine, the enzymes, and the other substances necessary for thyroid hormone synthesis.

Oxidation of the Iodide Ion. An essential step in the formation of the thyroid hormones is conversion of the iodide ions to an *oxidized form of iodine* that is then capable of combining directly with the amino acid tyrosine. This oxidation of iodine is promoted by the enzyme *peroxidase* and the accompanying *hydrogen peroxide,* which together provide a potent system capable of oxidizing iodides. The peroxidase is located either in the apical membrane of the cell or in the cytoplasm immediately adjacent to this membrane, thus providing the oxidized iodine at exactly the point in the cell where the thyroglobulin molecule first issues from the Golgi apparatus.

Iodination of Tyrosine and Formation of the Thyroid Hormones. Oxidized iodine even in the molecular form will bind directly but slowly with the amino acid tyrosine, but in the thyroid cell, the oxidized iodine is associated with an *iodinase* enzyme that causes the process to occur in seconds or minutes. Therefore, almost as rapidly as the thyroglobulin molecule is released from the Golgi apparatus or as it is secreted through the apical cell membrane into the follicle, iodine binds with about one sixth of the tyrosine residues within the thyroglobulin molecule.

Figure 50-3 illustrates the successive stages of iodination of tyrosine and the final formation of the two important thyroid hormones, thyroxine and triiodothyronine. Tyrosine is first iodized to form *monoiodotyrosine* and then to form *diiodotyrosine.* Then during the next few minutes, hours, and days, more and more of the diiodotyrosine residues become *coupled* with each other. The product of the coupling reaction is the molecule *thyroxine,* which also remains part of the thyroglobulin molecule. Or, one molecule of monoiodotyrosine couples with one molecule of diiodotyrosine to form *triiodothyronine.*

Storage of Thyroglobulin. After synthesis of the thyroid hormones has run its course, each thyroglobulin molecule contains one to three thyroxine molecules and an average of one triiodothyronine molecule for every ten molecules of thyroxine. In this form the thyroid hormones are often stored in the follicles for several months. In fact, the total amount stored is sufficient to supply the body with its normal requirements of thyroid hormones for 2 to 3 months. Therefore, even when synthesis of thyroid hormone ceases entirely, the effects of deficiency will not be observed for several months.

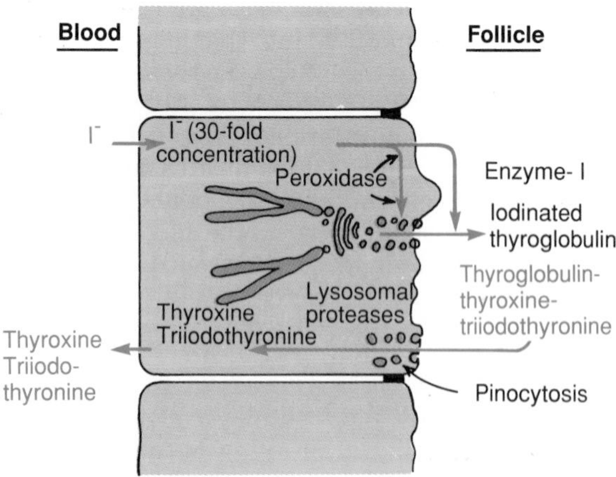

Figure 50-2. Thyroid cellular mechanisms for iodine transport, thyroxine (and triiodothyronine) formation, and thyroxine (and triiodothyronine) release into the blood.

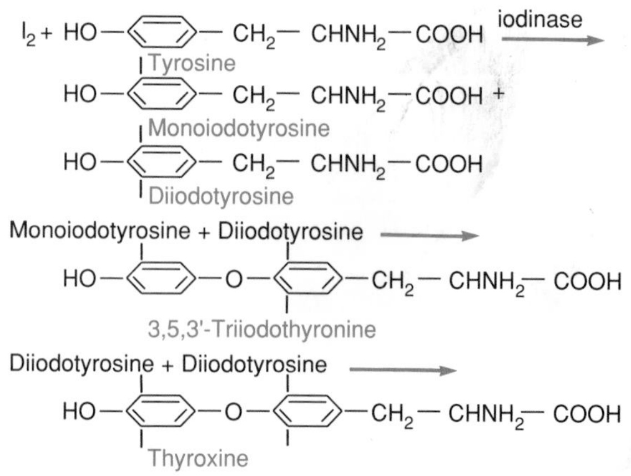

I_2 + HO—⟨ring⟩— CH_2— $CHNH_2$—COOH —iodinase→

Tyrosine

HO—⟨ring⟩— CH_2— $CHNH_2$—COOH +

Monoiodotyrosine

HO—⟨ring⟩— CH_2— $CHNH_2$—COOH

Diiodotyrosine

Monoiodotyrosine + Diiodotyrosine ⟶

HO—⟨ring⟩—O—⟨ring⟩— CH_2— $CHNH_2$— COOH

3,5,3′-Triiodothyronine

Diiodotyrosine + Diiodotyrosine ⟶

HO—⟨ring⟩—O—⟨ring⟩— CH_2— $CHNH_2$— COOH

Thyroxine

Figure 50-3. Chemistry of thyroxine and triiodothyronine formation.

Release of Thyroxine and Triiodothyronine from the Thyroid Gland

Thyroglobulin itself is not released into the circulating blood; instead, the thyroxine and triiodothyronine are first cleaved from the thyroglobulin molecule, and then these free hormones are released. This process occurs as follows: The apical surface of the thyroid cells continually sends out pseudopod extensions into the colloid cavity of the follicle, and these pseudopods close around small portions of the colloid to form pinocytic vesicles inside the thyroid cells. Then lysosomes immediately fuse with these vesicles to form digestive vesicles containing the digestive enzymes from the lysosomes mixed with the colloid. The *proteinases* among these enzymes digest the thyroglobulin molecules and release the thyroxine and triiodothyronine, which then diffuse through the base of the thyroid cell into the surrounding capillaries. In this way, the thyroid hormones are released into the blood.

Transport of Thyroxine and Triiodothyronine to the Tissues

Binding of Thyroxine and Triiodothyronine with the Plasma Proteins. On entering the blood, all but minute portions of the thyroxine and triiodothyronine combine immediately with several of the plasma proteins, especially with *thyroxine-binding globulin,* which is a glycoprotein. Then, half the thyroxine bound with the proteins is released to the tissue cells approximately every 6 days, whereas half the triiodothyronine—because of its lower affinity for the proteins—is released to the cells in approximately 1 day.

On entering the tissue cells, both these hormones again bind with intracellular proteins, the thyroxine once again binding more strongly than the triiodothyronine. They therefore are again stored, but this time in the functional cells themselves, and they are used slowly over a period of days or weeks.

Latency and Duration of Action of the Thyroid Hormones. After injection of a large quantity of thyroxine into a human being, essentially no effect on the metabolic rate can be discerned for 2 to 3 days, thereby illustrating that there is a *long latent period* before thyroxine activity begins. Once activity does begin, it increases progressively and reaches a maximum in 10 to 12 days, as shown in Figure 50-4. Thereafter, activity decreases, with a half-time of about 15 days. Some of the activity still persists as long as 6 weeks to 2 months later.

The actions of triiodothyronine occur about four times as rapidly as those of thyroxine, with a latent period as short as 6 to 12 hours and maximum cellular activity occurring within 2 to 3 days.

A large part of the latency and prolonged period of action of these hormones is caused by their binding with proteins both in the plasma and in the tissue cells, followed by their slow release. However, we shall see in subsequent discussions that part of the latent period also results from the manner in which these hormones perform their functions in the cells themselves.

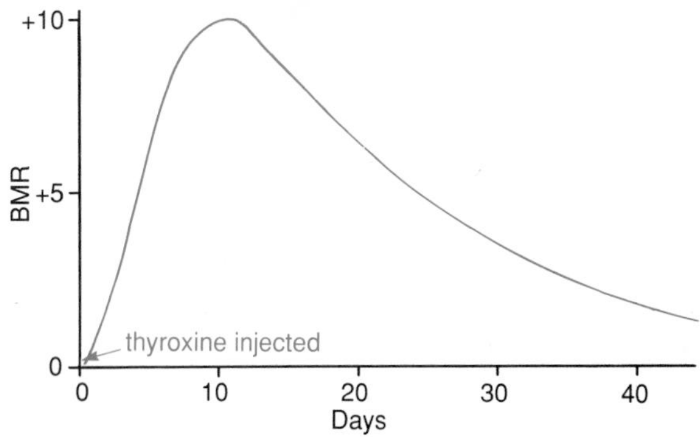

Figure 50-4. Approximate prolonged effect on the basal metabolic rate caused by administering a single large dose of thyroxine.

FUNCTIONS OF THE THYROID HORMONES IN THE TISSUES

Effect of Thyroid Hormones in Increasing the Transcription of Large Numbers of Genes

The general effect of thyroid hormone is to cause wholesale nuclear transcription of large numbers of genes. Therefore, in virtually all cells of the body great numbers of protein enzymes, structural proteins, transport proteins, and other substances increase. The net result of all this is a generalized increase in functional activity throughout the body.

Conversion of Thyroxine (T_4) into Triiodothyronine (T_3), and Activation of Nuclear Receptors. Before acting on the genes to increase genetic transcription, almost all the thyroxine is deiodinated by one iodide ion, thus forming triiodothyronine. This in turn has a very high binding affinity to the cellular thyroid hormone receptors.

The thyroid hormone receptors are either attached to the DNA genetic strands or are in close proximity to them. Upon binding with thyroid hormone, they become activated and initiate the transcription process. Then large numbers of different types of messenger RNA are formed, followed within another few minutes and hours by RNA translation on the cytoplasmic ribosomes to form hundreds of new types of proteins. However, not all proteins are increased by similar percentages—some only slightly and others at least as much as sixfold. It is believed that most, if not all, of the actions of thyroid hormone result from the enzymatic and other functions of these new proteins.

Important Types of Increased Cellular Metabolic Activity

The thyroid hormones increase the metabolic activities of all or almost all the tissues of the body. The basal metabolic rate can increase to as much as 60 to 100 per cent above normal when large quantities of the hormones are secreted. The rate of utilization of foods for energy is greatly accelerated. Although the rate of protein synthesis is increased, at the same time the rate of protein catabolism is also increased. The growth rate of young persons is greatly accelerated. The mental processes are excited, and the activity of most of the endocrine glands is increased.

Effect of Thyroid Hormones on Mitochondria. When thyroxine or triiodothyronine is given to an animal, the mitochondria in most cells of the body increase in size and also in number. Furthermore, the total membrane surface area of the mitochondria increases almost directly in proportion to the increased metabolic rate of the whole animal. Therefore, it seems almost to be an obvious deduction that one of the principal functions of thyroxine might be simply to increase the number and activity of mitochondria, and these in turn increase the rate of formation of adenosine triphosphate (ATP) to energize cellular function. Unfortunately, though, the increase in the number and activity of mitochondria could be the *result* of increased activity of the cells as well as the cause of the increase.

Effect of Thyroid Hormone in Increasing Active Transport of Ions Through Cell Membranes. One of the enzymes that becomes increased in response to thyroid hormone is *Na,K-ATPase.* This in turn increases the rate of transport of both sodium and potassium through the cell membranes of some tissues. Because this process utilizes energy and also increases the amount of heat produced in the body, it has also been suggested that this might be one of the mechanisms by which thyroid hormone increases the body's metabolic rate. In fact, thyroid hormone also causes the cell membranes of most cells to become leaky to sodium ions, therefore further activating the sodium pump and further increasing heat production.

Effect of Thyroid Hormone on Growth

Thyroid hormone has both general and specific effects on growth. For instance, it has long been known that thyroid hormone is essential for the metamorphic change of the tadpole into the frog. In the human being, the effect of thyroid hormone on growth is manifest mainly in growing children. In those who are hypothyroid, the rate of growth is greatly retarded. In those who are hyperthyroid, excessive skeletal growth often occurs, causing the child to become considerably taller at an earlier age. However, the bones also mature more rapidly, and the epiphyses close at an early age so that the duration of growth, and the eventual height of the adult, may actually be shortened.

An important effect of thyroid hormone is to promote growth and development of the brain during fetal life and for the first few years of postnatal life. If the fetus does not secrete sufficient quantities of thyroid hormone, growth and maturation of the brain both before birth and afterward are greatly retarded. Without specific thyroid therapy within days or weeks after birth, the child without a thyroid gland will remain mentally deficient throughout life. This is discussed more fully later in the chapter.

Effects of Thyroid Hormone on Specific Bodily Mechanisms

Effect on Carbohydrate Metabolism. Thyroid hormone stimulates almost all aspects of carbohydrate metabolism, including rapid uptake of glucose by the cells, enhanced glycolysis, enhanced gluconeogenesis, increased rate of absorption from the gastrointestinal tract, and even increased insulin secretion with its resultant secondary effects on carbohydrate metabolism. All these effects probably result from the overall increase in enzymes caused by thyroid hormone.

Effect of Fat Metabolism. Essentially all aspects of fat metabolism are also enhanced under the influence of thyroid hormone. However, because fats are the major source of long-term energy supplies, the fat stores of the body are depleted to a greater extent than are most of the other tissue elements. In particular, lipids are mobilized from the fat tissue, which increases the free fatty acid concentration in the plasma; and thyroid hormone also greatly accelerates the oxidation of free fatty acids by the cells.

Effect on Plasma and Liver Fats. Increased thyroid hormone *decreases* the quantity of cholesterol, phospholipids, and triglycerides in the plasma, even though it *increases* the free fatty acids. On the other hand, decreased thyroid secretion greatly increases the concentrations of cholesterol, phospholipids, and triglycerides and almost always causes excessive deposition of fat in the liver. The large increase in circulating plasma cholesterol in prolonged hypothyroidism is often associated with severe arteriosclerosis, discussed in Chapter 46.

Effect on Basal Metabolic Rate. Because thyroid hormone increases metabolism in almost all cells of the body, excessive quantities of the hormone can occasionally increase the basal metabolic rate to as much as 60 to 100 per cent above normal. On the other hand, when no thyroid hormone is produced, the basal metabolic rate falls almost to half normal; that is, the basal metabolic rate becomes −30 to −50.

Effect on Body Weight. Greatly increased thyroid hormone production almost always decreases the body weight, and greatly decreased production almost always increases the body weight; but these effects do not always occur, because thyroid hormone increases the appetite, and this may overbalance the change in the metabolic rate.

Effect on the Cardiovascular System ***Blood Flow and Cardiac Output.*** Increased metabolism in the tissues causes more rapid utilization of oxygen than normal and causes greater than normal quantities of metabolic end products to be released from the tissues. These effects cause vasodilatation in most of the body tissues, thus increasing blood flow. The rate of blood flow in the skin especially increases because of the increased need for heat elimination.

As a consequence of the increased blood flow, the cardiac output also increases, sometimes rising to 60 per cent or more above normal when excessive thyroid hormone is present, and falling to only 50 per cent of normal in severe hypothyroidism.

Heart Rate. The heart rate increases considerably more under the influence of thyroid hormone than would be expected from the increase in cardiac output. This effect is of particular importance because the heart rate is one of the sensitive physical signs that the clinician uses in determining whether a patient has excessive or diminished thyroid hormone production.

Effect on Respiration. The increased rate of metabolism increases the utilization of oxygen and the formation of carbon dioxide; these effects activate all the mechanisms that increase the rate and depth of respiration.

Effect on the Gastrointestinal Tract. In addition to increased appetite and food intake, which has been discussed, thyroid hormone increases both the rate of secretion of the digestive juices and the motility of the gastrointestinal tract. Often, diarrhea results. Lack of thyroid hormone causes constipation.

Effect on the Central Nervous System. In general, thyroid hormone increases the rapidity of cerebration but also often dissociates this; on the other hand, lack of thyroid hormone decreases this function. The hyperthyroid individual is likely to have extreme nervousness and many psychoneurotic tendencies, such as anxiety complexes, extreme worry, or paranoia.

Effect on the Function of the Muscles. Slight increase in thyroid hormone usually makes the muscles react with vigor, but when the quantity of hormone becomes excessive, the muscles become weakened because of excess protein catabolism. On the other hand, lack of thyroid hormone causes the muscles to become extremely sluggish, and they relax slowly after a contraction.

Muscle Tremor. One of the most characteristic signs of hyperthyroidism is a fine muscle tremor. This occurs at the rapid frequency of 10 to 15 times per second. The tremor can be observed easily by placing a sheet of paper on the extended fingers and noting the degree of vibration of the paper. This tremor is believed to be caused by increased reactivity of the neuronal synapses in the areas of the cord that control muscle tone. The tremor is an important means for assessing the degree of thyroid hormone effect on the central nervous system.

Effect on Sleep. Because of the exhausting effect of thyroid hormone on the musculature and on the central nervous system, the hyperthyroid subject often has a feeling of constant tiredness; but because of the excitable effects of thyroid hormone on the synapses, it is difficult to sleep. On the other hand, extreme somnolence is characteristic of hypothyroidism.

REGULATION OF THYROID HORMONE SECRETION

To maintain normal metabolic activity in the body, precisely the right amount of thyroid hormone must be secreted all the time, and to provide this, specific feedback mechanisms operate through the hypothalamus and anterior pituitary gland to control the rate of thyroid secretion. This system is illustrated in Figure 50-5 and can be explained as follows:

Effects of Thyroid-Stimulating Hormone on Thyroid Secretion. Thyroid-stimulating hormone (TSH), also known as *thyrotropin,* is an anterior pituitary hormone, a glycoprotein with a molecular weight of about 28,000; it increases the secretion of thyroxine and triiodothyronine by the thyroid gland. Its specific effect on the thyroid gland are (1) increased proteolysis of the thyroglobulin in the follicles, with resultant release of thyroid hormone into the circulating blood and diminishment of the follicular substance itself; (2) increased activity of the iodide pump, which increases the rate of iodide trapping in the glandular cells, increasing the ratio of intracellular to extracellular iodide concentration severalfold; (3) increased iodination of tyrosine and increased coupling to form the thyroid hormones; (4) both increased size and secretory activity of the thyroid cells; and (5) increased number of thyroid cells, plus a change from cuboidal to columnar cells with much infolding of the thyroid epithelium into the follicles. In summary, thyroid-stimulating hormone *increases all the known activities of the thyroid glandular cells.*

Role of Cyclic AMP in the Stimulatory Effects of TSH. In an attempt to explain the many and varied effects of thyroid-stimulating hormone on the thy-

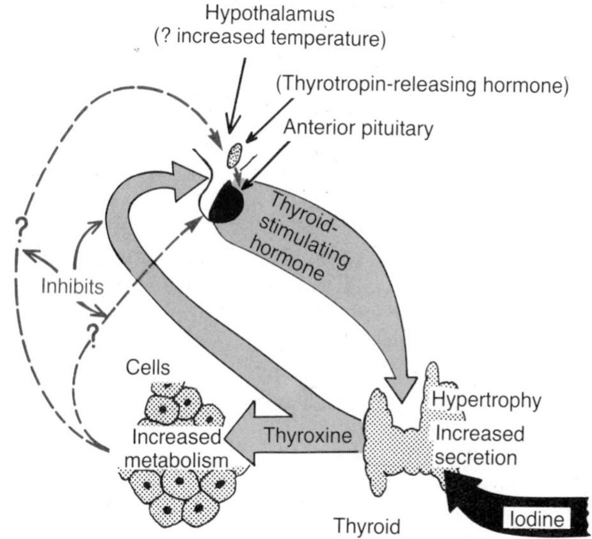

Figure 50-5. Regulation of thyroid secretion.

roid cell, a single primary action of this hormone has been sought for years. Recent experiments have shown that the hormone almost certainly does have such a single primary effect, which is to activate *adenyl cyclase* in the membrane of the thyroid cell. This in turn causes formation in the cell of *cyclic AMP*, which then acts as a *second messenger* to activate almost all systems of the thyroid cell. The result is both an immediate increase in release of the thyroid hormones followed by prolonged growth of the thyroid glandular tissue itself. This method of controlling thyroid cell activity is similar to the function of cyclic AMP in many other target tissues of the body.

Hypothalamic Regulation of TSH Secretion by the Anterior Pituitary — Thyrotropin-Releasing Hormone (TRH)

Electrical stimulation of several areas of the hypothalamus, but most particularly of the paraventricular nuclei, increases the anterior pituitary secretion of TSH and correspondingly increases the activity of the thyroid gland. This control of anterior pituitary secretion is exerted by a hypothalamic hormone, *thyrotropin-releasing hormone* (TRH), which is secreted by nerve endings in the median eminence of the hypothalamus and then is transported from there to the anterior pituitary in the hypothalamic-hypophysial portal blood, as explained in Chapter 49. TRH has been obtained in pure form, and it has proved to be a very simple substance, a tripeptide amide — *pyroglutamyl-histidyl-proline-amide.*

TRH has the direct effect on the anterior pituitary gland cells of increasing their output of thyroid-stimulating hormone. When the portal system from the hypothalamus to the anterior pituitary gland is completely blocked, so that TRH cannot reach the anterior pituitary gland, the rate of secretion of TSH by the anterior pituitary is greatly decreased but not reduced to zero.

Effects of Cold and Other Neurogenic Stimuli on TSH Secretion. One of the best-known stimuli for increasing the rate of TSH secretion by the anterior pituitary is exposure of an animal to cold. Exposure of rats for several weeks sometimes increases the output of thyroid hormones more than 100 per cent and can increase the basal metabolic rate as much as 50 per cent. Indeed, even human beings moving to arctic regions have been known to develop basal metabolic rates 15 to 20 per cent above normal.

Various emotional reactions can also affect the output of TRH and TSH and can therefore indirectly affect the secretion of thyroid hormone.

Neither the emotional effects nor the effect of cold is observed when the hypophysial stalk is cut, illustrating that both these effects are mediated by way of the hypothalamus.

Inverse Feedback Effect of Thyroid Hormone on Anterior Pituitary Secretion of TSH — Feedback Regulation of Thyroid Secretion. Increased thyroid hormone in the body fluids decreases the secretion of TSH by the anterior pituitary. When the rate of thyroid hormone secretion rises to about 1.75 times normal, the rate of TSH secretion falls essentially to zero. Almost all this feedback depressant effect occurs even when the anterior pituitary has been completely separated from the hypothalamus. Therefore, as illustrated in Figure 50-5, it is probable that increased thyroid hormone inhibits anterior pituitary secretion of TSH mainly by a direct effect on the anterior pituitary itself, though perhaps secondarily by much weaker effects acting through the hypothalamus.

One mechanism that has been suggested for the feedback effect on the anterior pituitary gland is that thyroid hormone reduces the number of TRH receptors on the cells that secrete TSH. Therefore, the stimulating effect on these cells by TRH from the hypothalamus is greatly reduced.

Regardless of the mechanism of the feedback, its effect is to maintain an almost constant concentration of free thyroid hormones in the circulating body fluids.

DISEASES OF THE THYROID

Hyperthyroidism

Most effects of hyperthyroidism are obvious from the preceding discussion of the various physiologic effects of thyroid hormone. However, some specific effects should be mentioned especially in connection with the development and treatment of hyperthyroidism.

Causes of Hyperthyroidism (Toxic Goiter, Thyrotoxicosis, Graves's Disease). In most patients with hyperthyroidism, the thyroid gland is increased to two to three times normal size, with tremendous folding of the follicular cell lining into the follicles, so that the number of cells is increased several times as much as the size of the gland. Also, each cell increases its rate of secretion severalfold; radioactive iodine uptake studies indicate that these hyperplastic glands secrete thyroid hormone at a rate as great as 5 to 15 times normal.

These changes in the thyroid gland are similar to those caused by excessive thyroid-stimulating hormone. However, radioimmunoassay studies have shown the plasma TSH concentrations usually to be less than normal rather than enhanced, and often to be essentially zero. On the other hand, one or more globulin antibodies having actions similar to that of TSH are found in the blood of almost all these patients. These antibodies bind with the thyroid cell membranes, and it is believed that they bind with the same membrane receptors that bind TSH and that this induces continual activation of the cells, with resultant development of the hyperthyroidism. One of these antibodies, found in 50 to 80 per cent of thyrotoxic patients, is called *long-acting thyroid stimulator* (LATS).

The antibodies that cause hyperthyroidism almost certainly develop as the result of autoimmunity that has developed against thyroid tissue. Presumably, at some time in the history of the person an excess of thyroid cell antigens has been released from the thyroid cells, and this has resulted in the formation of antibodies against the thyroid gland itself.

Symptoms of Hyperthyroidism. The symptoms of hyperthyroidism are obvious from the preceding discussion of the physiology of the thyroid hormones: intolerance to heat, increased sweating, mild to extreme weight loss, varying degrees of diarrhea, muscular weakness, nervousness and other psychic disorders, extreme fatigue yet inability to sleep, and tremor of the hands.

Exophthalmos. Most, but not all, persons with hyperthyroidism develop some degree of protrusion of the eyeballs, as illustrated in Figure 50-6. This condition is called *exophthalmos.*

The cause of the protrusion is edematous swelling of the retro-orbital tissues and degenerative changes in the extraocular muscles. The factor or factors that initiate these changes are still in serious dispute. In most patients, antibodies that react with the retro-orbital tissues can be found in the blood. Therefore, there is much reason to believe that exophthalmos, like hyperthyroidism itself, is an autoimmune process. Usually, the exophthalmos greatly ameliorates with treatment of the hyperthyroidism.

Diagnostic Tests for Hyperthyroidism. In the usual patient with hyperthyroidism, the most accurate diagnostic test is direct measurement of the concentration of "free" thyroxine and triiodothyronine in the plasma using appropriate radioimmunoassay procedures.

Other tests that are frequently used are these:

1. The basal metabolic rate is usually increased to +30 to +60 in severe hyperthyroidism.
2. The rate of uptake of a standard injected dose of radioactive iodine by the normal thyroid gland, when measured by a calibrated radioactive detector placed over the neck, is about 4 per cent per hour. In the hyperthyroid person, this can rise to as high as 20 to 25 per cent per hour.

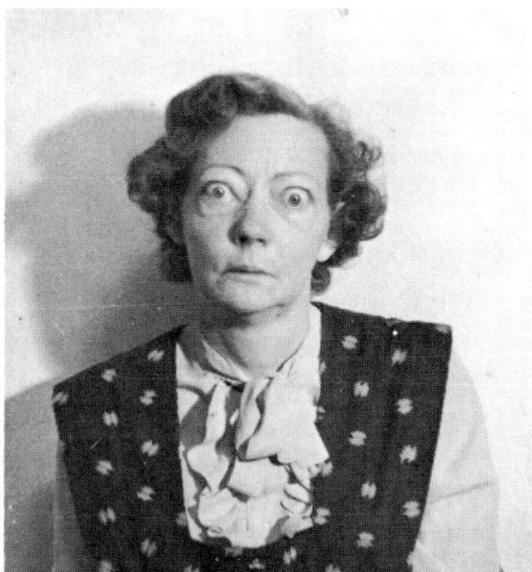

Figure 50-6. Patient with exophthalmic hyperthyroidism. Note protrusion of the eyes and retraction of the superior eyelids. The basal metabolic rate was +40. (Courtesy of Dr. Leonard Posey.)

Physiology of Treatment in Hyperthyroidism. The most direct treatment of hyperthyroidism is surgical removal of the thyroid gland. However, treatment of less severe cases can be achieved with antithyroid drugs such as propylthiouracil, a drug that blocks the formation of thyroid hormones in the thyroid cells.

Hypothyroidism

The effects of hypothyroidism, in general, are opposite to those of hyperthyroidism, but here again, a few physiological mechanisms peculiar to hypothyroidism are involved.

Endemic Colloid Goiter. The term *goiter* means a greatly enlarged thyroid gland. As was pointed out in the discussion of iodine metabolism, about 50 mg of iodine is needed each year for the formation of adequate quantities of thyroid hormone. In certain areas of the world, notably in the Swiss Alps and in the Great Lakes region of the United States, insufficient iodine is present in the soil for the foodstuffs to contain even this minute quantity of iodine. Therefore, prior to the introduction of iodized table salt, many persons living in these areas developed extremely large thyroid glands called *endemic goiters.*

The mechanism for development of the large endemic goiters is the following: Lack of iodine prevents production of thyroid hormone by the thyroid gland; as a result, no hormone is available to inhibit production of TSH by the anterior pituitary and this allows the pituitary to secrete excessively large quantities of TSH. The TSH then causes the thyroid cells to secrete tremendous amounts of thyroglobulin (colloid) into the follicles, and the gland grows larger and larger. But unfortunately, owing to lack of iodine, increased thyroxine and triiodothyronine production does not occur. The follicles become tremendous in size, and the thyroid gland may increase to as large as 300 to 500 grams or more, which is more than ten times the normal size.

Idiopathic Nontoxic Colloid Goiter. Enlarged thyroid glands almost identical with those of endemic colloid goiter frequently develop even when the affected persons receive sufficient quantities of iodine in their diets. These goitrous glands may secrete normal quantities of thyroid hormones, but more frequently the secretion of hormone is depressed, as in endemic colloid goiter.

The exact cause of the enlarged thyroid gland in patients with idiopathic colloid goiter is not known, but most of these patients show signs of mild thyroiditis; therefore, it has been suggested that thyroiditis causes slight hypothyroidism, which then leads to increased TSH secretion and progressive growth of the noninflamed portions of the gland. This could explain why these glands usually are very nodular, with some portions of the gland growing while other portions are being destroyed by thyroiditis.

In some persons with colloid goiter, the thyroid glands have abnormal enzyme systems, which leads to diminished thyroid hormone formation and resultant excess stimulation of the thyroid gland by TSH. And, finally, some foods contain *goitrogenic substances* that have an antithyroid activity, thus also leading to TSH-stimulated enlargement of the thyroid gland. Such goitrogenic substances are found in some varieties of turnips and cabbages.

Characteristics of Hypothyroidism. Whether hypothyroidism is due to endemic colloid goiter, idiopathic colloid goiter, destruction of the thyroid gland by irritation, surgical removal of the thyroid gland, or destruction of the thyroid gland by various other diseases, the physiological effects are the same. These include extreme somnolence with 14 to 16 hours of sleep a day; extreme muscular sluggishness; slowed heart rate; decreased cardiac output; decreased blood volume; increased weight; constipation; mental sluggishness; failure of many trophic functions in the body as evidenced by depressed growth of hair and scaliness of the skin; development of a frog-like husky voice; and, in severe cases, development of an edematous appearance throughout the body called myxedema.

Myxedema. The patient with almost total lack of thyroid function develops *myxedema.* Figure 50-7 shows such a patient with bagginess under the eyes and swelling of the face. In this condition, for reasons not yet explained, greatly increased quantities of proteoglycans, containing mainly hyaluronic acid, collect in the interstitial spaces and form an edema characterized by a myxomatous gel in the interstitial spaces.

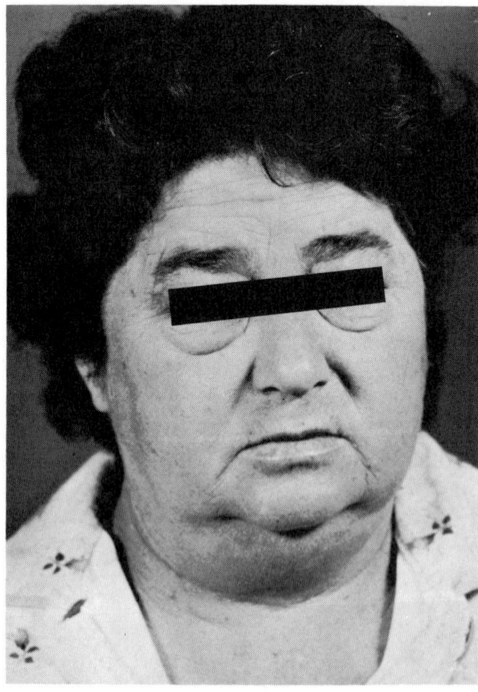

Figure 50-7. Patient with myxedema. (Courtesy of Dr. Herbert Langford.)

Arteriosclerosis in Hypothyroidism. Lack of thyroid hormone increases the quantity of blood lipids, with especially large amounts of cholesterol, and the increase in blood cholesterol is usually associated with atherosclerosis and arteriosclerosis. Therefore, many hypothyroid patients, particularly those with myxedema, develop severe arteriosclerosis, which results in peripheral vascular disease, deafness, and often extreme coronary sclerosis with consequent early demise.

Diagnostic Tests in Hypothyroidism. The tests already described for diagnosis of hyperthyroidism give the opposite results in hypothyroidism. The free thyroxine in the blood is low. The basal metabolic rate in myxedema ranges between −30 and −50. And the rate of radioactive iodine uptake by the thyroid gland (except in iodine deficiency hypothyroidism) measures less than 1 per cent per hour rather than the normal of approximately 4 per cent per hour. However, just as important for diagnosis as the various diagnostic tests are the characteristic symptoms of hypothyroidism just discussed.

Treatment of Hypothyroidism. Figure 50-4 shows the effect of thyroxine on the basal metabolic rate, illustrating that the hormone normally has a duration of action of more than 1 month. Consequently, it is easy to maintain a steady level of thyroid hormone activity in the body by daily oral ingestion of a tablet or so of desiccated thyroid gland or thyroxine. Furthermore, proper treatment of the hypothyroid patient results in such complete normality that formerly myxedematous patients properly treated have lived into their nineties after treatment for over 50 years.

Cretinism. Cretinism is the condition caused by extreme hypothyroidism during infancy and childhood, and it is characterized especially by failure of growth. Cretinism results from (a) congenital lack of a thyroid gland *(congenital cretinism),* (b) failure of the thyroid gland to produce thyroid hormone because of a genetic deficiency of the gland, or (c) iodine lack in the diet *(endemic cretinism).* The severity of endemic cretinism varies greatly, depending on the amount of iodine in the diet, and whole populations of an endemic area have occasionally had cretinoid tendencies.

A newborn baby without a thyroid gland may have absolutely normal appearance and function because it had been supplied with thyroid hormone by the mother while *in utero,* but a few weeks after birth its movements become sluggish, and both its physical and mental growth are greatly retarded. Treatment of the cretin at any time usually causes normal return to physical growth, but unless the cretin is treated within a few months after birth, its mental growth will be permanently retarded.

REFERENCES

Burrow, G. N., et al.: Thyroid Function and Disease. Philadelphia, W. B. Saunders Co., 1989.
Delange, F., et al. (eds.): Research in Congenital Hypothyroidism. New York, Plenum Publishing Corp., 1989.
DeLong, G. R., et al. (eds.): Iodine and the Brain. New York, Plenum Publishing Corp., 1989.
Dussault, J. H., and Ruel, J.: Thyroid hormones and brain development. Annu. Rev. Physiol., 49:321, 1987.
Felig, P., et al. (eds.): Endocrinology and Metabolism. 2nd ed. New York, McGraw-Hill Book Co., 1987.
Green, W. L. (ed.): The Thyroid. New York, Elsevier Science Publishing Co., 1987.
LiVolsi, V. A.: Pathology of the Thyroid. Philadelphia, W. B. Saunders Co., 1989.
Medeiros-Neto, G. A., and Gaitan, E. (eds.): Frontiers in Thyroidology. New York, Plenum Publishing Corp., 1987.
Pinchera, A., et al. (eds.): Thyroid Autoimmunity. New York, Plenum Publishing Corp., 1987.
Samuels, H. H., et al.: Regulation of gene expression by thyroid hormone. Annu. Rev. Physiol., 51:623, 1989.

QUESTIONS

1. Explain the anatomy of both secretion and absorption into the blood of the thyroid metabolic hormones.
2. What is the importance of *iodide trapping* for the formation of thyroid hormones?
3. Give the chemical steps required for the formation of thyroid hormone within the structure of *thyroglobulin.*
4. Explain the storage of thyroglobulin and the release of the thyroid metabolic hormones from the thyroglobulin into the circulating blood.
5. How are *thyroxine* and *triiodothyronine* transported to the tissues?
6. Explain the mechanism by which thyroid hormones cause increased protein synthesis in cells and tell how this affects the metabolic rate of the body.
7. What is the effect of the thyroid hormones on the cellular *enzyme systems,* especially on the enzyme systems of the *mitochondria?*
8. What is the effect of thyroid hormone on growth, especially in children?
9. Explain briefly the effects of thyroid hormone on carbohydrate metabolism, fat metabolism, body weight, function of the cardiovascular system, function of the gastrointestinal tract, function of the central nervous system, muscle tremor, and sleep.
10. What are the chemical compositions of TRH and TSH, and what are their respective functions in the control of thyroid hormone secretion?
11. What are the feedback mechanisms from the body tissues back to the hypothalamus, pituitary gland, and thyroid gland that play important roles in the regulation of thyroid hormone secretion?
12. Explain the causes and effects of *hyperthyroidism.*
13. What is *exophthalmos,* and what is its cause?
14. What is meant by *endemic colloid goiter,* and what is its cause?
15. What are the causes of *hypothyroidism,* and what are its effects on the body?
16. What is *myxedema,* and why does it develop in severe hypothyroidism?
17. What are the characteristics of *cretinism,* and how does the lack of thyroid hormones cause this abnormality?

51

The Adrenocortical Hormones

The two *adrenal glands,* each of which weighs about 4 grams, lie at the superior poles of the two kidneys. Each gland is composed of two distinct parts, the *adrenal medulla* and the *adrenal cortex.* The adrenal medulla, the central 20 per cent of the gland, is functionally related to the sympathetic nervous system; it secretes the hormones *epinephrine* and *norepinephrine* in response to sympathetic stimulation. In turn, these hormones cause almost the same effects as direct stimulation of the sympathetic nerves in all parts of the body. These hormones and their effects were discussed in detail in Chapter 41 in relation to the sympathetic nervous system.

The adrenal cortex secretes an entirely different group of hormones, called *corticosteroids.* These hormones are all synthesized from the steroid cholesterol, and they all have similar chemical formulas. However, very slight differences in their molecular structures give them several very different but very important functions.

Mineralocorticoids and Glucocorticoids. Two major types of adrenocortical hormones, the *mineralocorticoids* and the *glucocorticoids,* are secreted by the adrenal cortex. In addition to these, small amounts of sex hormones are secreted, especially *adrogenic hormones,* which exhibit approximately the same effects in the body as the male sex hormone testosterone. These are normally in such small amounts that they are of only slight importance, though in certain abnormalities of the adrenal cortices, extreme quantities can be secreted and can then result in masculinizing effects.

The *mineralocorticoids* have gained this name because they especially affect the electrolytes of the extracellular fluids — sodium and potassium, in particular. The *glucocorticoids* have gained their name because they exhibit an important effect in increasing blood glucose concentration. However, the glucocorticoids have additional effects on both protein and fat metabolism that likely are equally important if not more so to body function than are the effects on carbohydrate metabolism.

Over 30 different steroids have been isolated from the adrenal cortex, but only 2 of these are of major importance to the endocrine function of the human body — *aldosterone,* which is the principal mineralocorticoid, and *cortisol,* which is the principal glucocorticoid.

Chemistry of the Adrenocortical Hormones

Figure 51–1 illustrates the chemical formulas of aldosterone and cortisol. *Aldosterone* has an oxygen atom bound at the number 18 carbon of the cholesterol nucleus that is most important in providing the mineralocorticoid activity of aldosterone. The glucocorticoid activity of *cortisol* is provided principally by the presence of a keto-oxygen on carbon number 3 and the hydroxylation of carbon numbers 11 and 21.

In addition to aldosterone and cortisol, which respectively are the principal mineralocorticoid and glucocorticoid hormones, still other steroids having one or both of these activities are normally secreted in small amounts by the adrenal cortex. And several additional potent steroid hormones not normally formed in the adrenal glands have been synthesized and are used in various forms of therapy. The more important of these adrenocortical hormones are the following:

Mineralocorticoids

Aldosterone (very potent, accounts for 95 per cent or more of mineralocorticoid activity)

Desoxycorticosterone (one fifteenth as potent as aldosterone, very small quantities secreted)

Corticosterone (slight activity)

9α-Fludrocortisone (synthetic, slightly more potent than aldosterone)

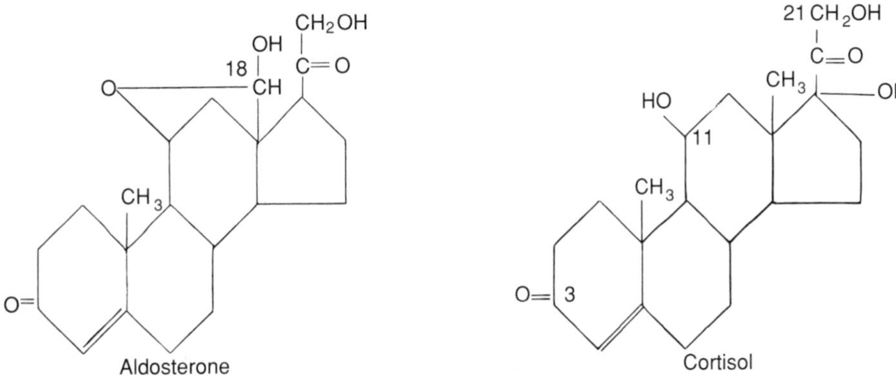

Figure 51-1. The two important corticosteroids.

Glucocorticoids

Cortisol (very potent, accounts for about 95 per cent of all glucocorticoid activity)

Corticosterone (about 4 per cent of total glucocorticoid activity, but much less potent than cortisol)

Cortisone (synthetic, almost as potent as cortisol)

Prednisone (synthetic, four times as potent as cortisol)

Dexamethasone (synthetic, 30 times as potent as cortisol)

FUNCTIONS OF THE MINERALOCORTICOIDS—ALDOSTERONE

Loss of adrenocortical secretion usually causes death within 3 days to 2 weeks unless the person receives extensive salt therapy or mineralocorticoid therapy. Without mineralocorticoids, the potassium ion concentration of the extracellular fluid rises markedly, the sodium and chloride concentrations decrease, and the total extracellular fluid volume and blood volume also become reduced. The person soon develops diminished cardiac output, which proceeds to a shocklike state followed by death. This entire sequence can be prevented by the administration of aldosterone or some other mineralocorticoid. Therefore, the mineralocorticoids are said to be the immediate "life-saving" portion of the adrenocortical hormones, whereas the glucocorticoids are of particular importance in helping a person resist different types of stresses, as discussed later in the chapter.

Aldosterone exerts at least 95 per cent of the mineralocorticoid activity of the adrenocortical secretion, but cortisol, the major glucocorticoid secreted by the adrenal cortex, also provides a small amount of mineralocorticoid activity.

Renal Effects of Aldosterone

By far the most important function of aldosterone is to cause transport of sodium and potassium through the renal tubular walls and, to a smaller extent, transport of hydrogen ions. The mechanisms of these effects were discussed in detail in Chapter 21. However, let us summarize briefly the renal and body fluid effects of aldosterone.

Effect on Tubular Reabsorption of Sodium and Tubular Secretion of Potassium. It will be recalled from Chapter 21 that aldosterone causes an exchange transport of sodium and potassium—that is, absorption of sodium and simultaneous excretion of potassium by the tubular epithelial cells—in the distal tubule, collecting tubule, and collecting duct. Therefore, aldosterone causes sodium to be conserved in the extracellular fluid while potassium is excreted into the urine.

A high concentration of aldosterone in the plasma can decrease the sodium loss into the urine to as little as a few milligrams a day. At the same time, potassium loss into the urine increases manyfold.

Conversely, total lack of aldosterone secretion can cause loss of as much as 20 grams of sodium in the urine a day, an amount equal to one fifth of all the sodium in the body. But, at the same time, potassium is conserved tenaciously.

Therefore, the net effect of excess aldosterone in the plasma is to increase the total quantity of sodium in the extracellular fluid while decreasing the potassium. In turn, the increase in tubular reabsorption of sodium causes water reabsorption as well, mainly because the absorbed sodium causes osmosis of water through the tubular epithelium. Thus, an excess of aldosterone can increase the extracellular fluid volume to as much as 10 to 15 per cent above normal, or the volume may decrease to as low as 20 to 25 per cent below normal in the absence of aldosterone.

Hypokalemia and Muscle Paralysis; Hyperkalemia and Cardiac Toxicity. The excessive loss of potassium ions from the extracellular fluid into the urine under the influence of aldosterone causes a serious decrease in the plasma potassium concentration, often from the normal value of 4.5 mEq/liter to as low as 1 to 2 mEq/liter. This condition is called *hypokalemia.* When the potassium ion concentration falls below approximately one half normal, muscle paralysis or at least severe muscle weakness often develops. This is caused by effects on the nerve and muscle fiber membranes (see Chapter 5), which prevent transmission of action potentials.

On the other hand, when aldosterone is deficient, the extracellular fluid potassium ion concentration can rise above normal, causing *hyperkalemia.* When it rises to 60 to 100 per cent above normal, serious cardiac toxicity, including weakness of contraction and arrhythmia, becomes evident: a still higher concentration of potassium leads inevitably to cardiac death.

Effect of Aldosterone on Increasing Tubular Hydrogen Ion Secretion, with Resultant Mild Alkalosis. Though aldosterone mainly causes potassium to be secreted into the tubules in exchange for sodium reabsorption, to a much smaller extent it also causes tubular secretion of hydrogen ions in exchange for sodium. The obvious effect is to decrease the hydrogen ion concentration in the extracellular fluid. However, this effect is not a strong one, usually causing only a mild degree of alkalosis.

Effect of Aldosterone on Circulatory Function. In the absence of aldosterone secretion, a decrease in extracellular fluid volume to 20 to 25 per cent below normal and a comparable decrease in plasma volume cause *circulatory shock* to develop rapidly. Indeed, in complete lack of aldosterone, a person not treated with extra intake of salt, administration of a mineralocorticoid drug, or both is likely to die of circulatory shock within as few as 4 to 8 days.

In the case of hypersecretion of aldosterone, not only is the extracellular fluid volume increased but blood volume and cardiac output are increased as well. Each of these can increase to as much as 15 to 25 per cent above normal in the first few days of excess aldosterone secretion, but after compensations occur, the volumes and the cardiac output usually return to no more than 5 to 10 per cent above normal. Nevertheless, over a prolonged period of time even these small increases are sufficient to cause moderate to severe hypertension, as we discuss later in the chapter in relation to primary aldosteronism.

Cellular Mechanism of Aldosterone Action

Although for many years we have known the overall effects of mineralocorticoids on the body, the basic action of aldosterone on the tubular cells to increase transport of sodium is still only partly understood. The sequence of events that leads to increased sodium reabsorption seems to be the following:

First, because of its lipid solubility in the cellular membranes, aldosterone diffuses to the interior of the tubular epithelial cells.

Second, in the cytoplasm of the tubular cells, aldosterone combines with a highly specific cytoplasmic *receptor protein,* a protein with a stereomolecular configuration that allows only aldosterone or extremely similar compounds to combine.

Third, the aldosterone-receptor complex diffuses into the nucleus, where it may undergo further alterations, and then it induces specific portions of the DNA to form one or more types of messenger RNA related to the process of sodium and potassium transport.

Fourth, the messenger RNA diffuses back into the cytoplasm, where in conjunction with the ribosomes, it causes protein formation. The protein formed is one or more enzymes, or carrier substances, required for sodium and potassium transport, probably a specific ATPase that catalyzes energy transfer from cytoplasmic ATP to the sodium-potassium transport mechanism of the cell membrane.

Thus, aldosterone does not have an immediate effect on sodium and potassium transport, but must await the sequence of events that leads to the formation of the specific intracellular substance or substances required for transport. Approximately 20 to 30 minutes are required before new RNA appears in the cells, and approximately 45 minutes are required before the rates of sodium and potassium transport begin to increase; the effect reaches maximum only after several hours.

Regulation of Aldosterone Secretion

The regulation of aldosterone secretion is so deeply intertwined with the regulation of extracellular fluid electrolyte concentrations, extracellular fluid volume, blood volume, arterial pressure, and many special aspects of renal function that it is not possible to discuss the regulation of aldosterone secretion independently of all these other factors. This subject has already been presented in Chapter 22, to which the reader is referred. However, it is important to list here, also, the most important factors that are presently known to play essential roles in the regulation of aldosterone secretion. In the probable order of their importance they are

1. Increased potassium ion concentration of the extracellular fluid increases secretion;
2. Increased renin-angiotensin system activation increases secretion;
3. Increased quantity of body sodium *decreases* secretion;
4. Adrenocorticotropic hormone (ACTH) from the anterior pituitary gland increases secretion.

This very potent effect of potassium ions is exceedingly important because it establishes a powerful feedback mechanism for control of extracellular fluid potassium ion concentration as follows: (1) An increase in potassium ion concentration causes increased secretion of aldosterone. (2) The aldosterone in turn potently affects the kidneys, causing enhanced excretion of potassium. (3) Therefore, the potassium ion concentration returns toward normal. This effect of potassium ions on aldosterone secretion results from a direct influence of the potassium ions on the adrenocortical cells themselves, though the intracellular mechanism is unknown.

When an animal or human being is placed on a sodium-deficient diet, after several days the rate of aldosterone secretion increases markedly even though the sodium ion concentration of the body fluids does not fall significantly. Suggestions as to the cause of this phenomenon have included the following:

1. The diminished sodium leads to diminished extracellular fluid volume, with resultant diminished cardiac output and renal blood flow. The reduced renal blood flow causes enhanced formation of angiotensin, and the angiotensin stimulates aldosterone secretion.
2. Lack of sodium causes retention of potassium by the kidneys. The elevated potassium could then also cause the increased aldosterone secretion.

Effect of the Renin-Angiotensin System on Aldosterone Secretion. Infusion of moderate amounts of angiotensin into an animal can cause acute increases in aldosterone secretion of as much as eightfold. However, if the angiotensin infusion is continued, the rate of aldosterone secretion falls in about 12 hours to only 50 to 100 per cent above normal. Yet, even so, in many clinical conditions the renin-angiotensin system is the cause of excessive aldosterone secretion because tremendous quantities of angiotensin are often formed.

FUNCTIONS OF THE GLUCOCORTICOIDS

Even though mineralocorticoids can save the life of an acutely adrenalectomized animal, the animal still is far from normal. Instead, its metabolic systems for utilization of carbohydrates, proteins, and fats are considerably deranged. Furthermore, without glucocorticoids the animal cannot resist different types of physical or even mental stress, and minor illnesses such as respiratory tract infections can lead to death. Therefore, the glucocorticoids have functions just as important to long-continued life of the animal as do the mineralocorticoids. These functions are explained in the following sections.

At least 95 per cent of the glucocorticoid activity of the adrenocortical secretions results from the secretion of *cortisol,* also known as *hydrocortisone.* In addition, a small amount of glucocorticoid activity is provided by *corticosterone* that is secreted in small amounts.

Effects of Cortisol on Carbohydrate Metabolism

Stimulation of Gluconeogenesis. By far the best-known metabolic effect of cortisol and other glucocorticoids on metabolism is their ability to stimulate gluconeogenesis (formation of glucose from proteins and some other substances) by the liver, often increasing the rate of gluconeogenesis as much as six- to tenfold. This results mainly from two different effects of cortisol:

First, all the enzymes required to convert amino acids into glucose are increased in the liver cells. This results from the effect of the glucocorticoids to activate DNA transcription in the liver cell nuclei in the same way that aldosterone functions in the renal tubular cells, with formation of messenger RNAs that in turn lead to the array of enzymes required for gluconeogenesis.

Second, cortisol causes mobilization of amino acids from the extrahepatic tissues, mainly from muscle. As a result, more amino acids become available in the plasma to enter into the gluconeogenesis process of the liver and thereby to promote the formation of glucose.

Decreased Glucose Utilization by the Cells. Cortisol also causes a moderate decrease in the rate of glucose utilization by the cells. Though the cause of this decrease is unknown, most physiologists believe that somewhere between the point of entry of glucose into the cells and its final degradation cortisol directly delays the rate of glucose utilization.

Elevated Blood Glucose Concentration, and Adrenal Diabetes. Both the increased rate of gluconeogenesis and the moderate reduction in rate of glucose utilization by the cells cause the blood glucose concentration to rise. The increased blood glucose concentration is occasionally great enough—50 per cent or more above normal—that the condition is called *adrenal diabetes* (meaning elevated blood glucose concentration); it has many similarities to pituitary diabetes, which was discussed in Chapter 49 but is quite different from the diabetes caused by insulin deficiency.

Effects of Cortisol on Protein Metabolism

Reduction in Cellular Protein. One of the principal effects of cortisol on the metabolic systems of the body is reduction of the protein stores in essentially all body cells except those of the liver. This reduction is caused both by decreased protein synthesis and increased catabolism of protein already in the cells. Both these effects may possibly result from decreased amino acid transport into extrahepatic tissues, discussed below, but this probably is not the only cause, since cortisol also depresses the formation of RNA in many extrahepatic tissues, including especially muscle and lymphoid tissue.

Increased Liver and Plasma Proteins Caused by Cortisol. Coincidently with the reduced proteins elsewhere in the body, the liver proteins become enhanced. Furthermore, the plasma proteins (which are produced by the liver and then released into the blood) are also increased. These are exceptions to the protein depletion that occurs elsewhere in the body. This difference is probably caused by enhancement of the liver enzymes required for protein synthesis.

Increased Blood Amino Acids, Diminished Transport of Amino Acids into Extrahepatic Cells, and Enhanced Transport into Hepatic Cells. Recent studies in isolated tissues have demonstrated that cortisol depresses amino acid transport into muscle cells and perhaps into other extrahepatic cells. But, in contrast, it enhances transport into liver cells.

The increased plasma concentration of amino acids, plus the fact that cortisol enhances transport of amino acids into the hepatic cells, could also account at least partly for expanded utilization of amino acids by the liver in the presence of cortisol — such effects as (1) increased rate of deamination of amino acids by the liver, (2) increased protein synthesis in the liver, (3) increased formation of plasma proteins by the liver, and (4) increased conversion of amino acids to glucose — that is, enhanced gluconeogenesis.

Thus, it is possible that many of the effects of cortisol on the metabolic systems of the body can be explained very simply from this ability of cortisol to mobilize amino acids.

Effects of Cortisol on Fat Metabolism

Mobilization of Fatty Acids. In much the same manner that cortisol promotes amino acid mobilization from muscle, it also promotes mobilization of fatty acids from adipose tissue. This in turn increases the concentration of free fatty acids in the plasma, which also increases their utilization for energy. Cortisol moderately enhances the oxidation of fatty acids in the cells as well, perhaps as a secondary result of the reduced availability of glycolytic products for metabolism.

The increased mobilization of fats, combined with their increased oxidation in the cells, is one of the factors that help to shift the metabolic systems of the cells from utilization of glucose for energy to utilization of fatty acids in times of starvation or other stresses. This cortisol mechanism, however, requires several hours to become fully developed — not nearly so rapid or powerful an effect as the similar shift elicited by a decrease in insulin, as discussed in the following chapter. Nevertheless, it is probably an important factor for long-term conservation of body glucose and glycogen.

Other Effects of Cortisol

Function of Cortisol in Different Types of Stress. It is amazing that almost any type of stress, whether physical or neurogenic, causes an immediate and marked increase in ACTH (adrenocorticotropic hormone) secretion by the anterior pituitary gland, followed within minutes by greatly increased secretion of cortisol by the adrenal gland. Some of the types of stress that increase cortisol release are the following:

1. Trauma of almost any type
2. Infection
3. Intense heat or cold
4. Injection of norepinephrine and other sympathomimetic drugs
5. Surgery
6. Injection of a necrotizing substance beneath the skin
7. Restraint of an animal that prevents movement
8. Almost any debilitating disease

Thus, a wide variety of nonspecific stimuli can cause marked increase in the rate of cortisol secretion by the adrenal cortex.

Yet even though we know that cortisol secretion often increases greatly in stressful situations, we still are not sure why this is of significant benefit to the animal. One guess, which is probably as good as any other, is that the glucocorticoids cause rapid mobilization of amino acids and fats from their cellular stores, making these available both for energy and for synthesis of other compounds needed by the different tissues of the body. Indeed, it is well known that when proteins are released from most of the tissue cells, the liver cells can use the mobilized amino acids to form both glucose and new proteins. It has also been shown that damaged tissues momentarily depleted of proteins can also utilize the newly available amino acids to form new proteins that are essential to the lives of the cells. Or perhaps the amino acids are used to synthesize such essential intracellular substances as purines, pyrimidines, and creatine phosphate, which are necessary for maintenance of cellular life.

Anti-Inflammatory Effects of Cortisol. When tissues are damaged by trauma, by infection with bacteria, or in almost any other way, they almost always become inflamed. In some conditions the inflammation is more damaging than the trauma or disease itself. Administration of large amounts of cortisol can usually block this inflammation or even reverse many of its effects once it has begun.

Basically, there are five main stages of inflammation: (1) release from the damaged tissue cells of chemical substances that activate the inflammation process — chemicals such as histamine, bradykinin, and proteolytic enzymes; (2) an increase in blood flow in the inflamed area caused by some of the released products from the tissues, a condition called *erythema;* (3) leakage of large quantities of almost pure plasma out of the capillaries into the damaged areas, followed by clotting of the tissue fluid, which causes a *nonpitting type of edema;* (4) infiltration of the area by leukocytes; and, finally, (5) tissue healing, which is often accomplished at least partially by ingrowth of fibrous tissue.

One of the most important anti-inflammatory effects of cortisol is its ability to cause *stabilization of the intracellular lysosomal membranes.* That is, cortisol makes it much more difficult than normal for the membranes of the lysosomes to rupture. Therefore, most of the proteolytic enzymes released by damaged cells that cause inflammation and that are mainly formed in the lysosomes are released in greatly decreased quantity.

Even after inflammation has become well established, administration of cortisol can often reduce inflammation within hours to several days. The immediate effect is to block most of the factors that are promoting the inflammation. Then the rate of healing is also increased. This probably results from those same factors that allow the body to resist many other types of physical stress when large quantities of cortisol are secreted; perhaps the enhancement of healing results from the mobilization of amino acids and their use to repair the damaged tissues; perhaps it results from increased amounts of glucose and fatty acids available for cellular energy; or perhaps it depends on some catalytic effect of cortisol to inactivate or remove inflammatory products.

Regardless of the precise mechanisms by which the anti-inflammatory effect occurs, this effect of cortisol can play a major role in combating certain types of diseases, such as rheumatoid arthritis, rheumatic fever, and acute glomerulonephritis. All of these are characterized by severe local inflammation, and the harmful effects to the body are caused mainly by the inflammation itself, not by other aspects of the disease. When cortisol or other glucocorticoids are administered to patients with these diseases, the inflammation almost invariably subsides within 24 to 48 hours. And even though the cortisol does not correct the basic disease condition but merely prevents the damaging effects of the inflammatory response, this alone can be a life-saving measure.

Regulation of Cortisol Secretion—Adrenocorticotropic Hormone (ACTH)

Control of Cortisol Secretion by ACTH. Unlike aldosterone secretion by the adrenal cortex, which is controlled mainly by potassium and angiotensin acting directly on the adrenocortical cells themselves, almost no stimuli have *direct* effects on the adrenal cells to control cortisol secretion. Instead, secretion of cortisol is controlled almost entirely by *adrenocorticotropic hormone* (ACTH) secreted by the anterior pituitary gland, as illustrated in Figure 51–2. This hormone, also called *corticotropin* or *adrenocorticotropin,* is *a large polypeptide chain* composed of 39 amino acids. It also enhances the production of adrenal androgens by the adrenal cortex. Small amounts of ACTH are required for aldosterone secretion, providing a permissive role that allows the other more important factors to exert their more powerful controls.

Control of ACTH Secretion by the Hypothalamus—Corticotropin-Releasing Factor (CRF). In the same way that other pituitary hormones are controlled by releasing hormones, or factors, from the hypothalamus, so also does an important releasing factor control ACTH secretion. This is called *corticotropin-releasing factor* (CRF). It is *a small peptide* that is secreted into the primary capillary plexus of the hypophysial portal system in the median eminence of the hypothalamus and then carried to the anterior pituitary gland, where it induces ACTH secretion.

The anterior pituitary gland can secrete only small

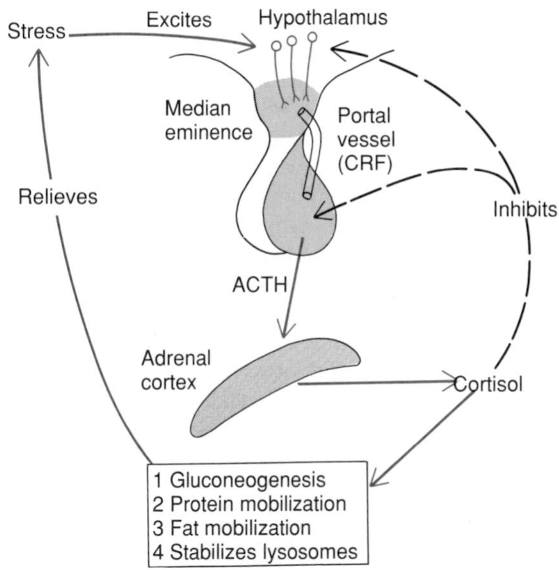

Figure 51–2. Mechanism for regulation of glucocorticoid secretion.

quantities of ACTH in the absence of CRF. Instead, most conditions that cause high ACTH secretory rates initiate this secretion by signals that begin in the hypothalamus and then are transmitted by CRF to the anterior pituitary gland.

Effect of Physiological Stress on ACTH Secretion. It was pointed out earlier in the chapter that almost any type of physical or mental stress can lead within minutes to greatly enhanced secretion of ACTH and consequently of cortisol as well, often increasing cortisol secretion as much as 20-fold. This effect is illustrated forcefully by the curves in Figure 51–3, which shows a manyfold increase in plasma

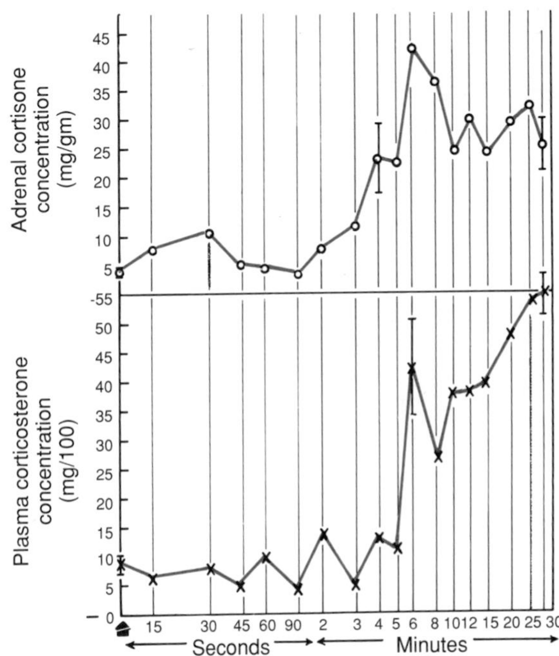

Figure 51–3. Rapid reaction of the adrenal cortex of a rat to stress caused by fracture of the tibia and fibula. (Courtesy of Drs. Guillemin, Dear, and Lipscomb.)

corticosterone concentration in a rat within minutes after tibia and fibula had been broken (corticosterone is the principal glucocorticoid secreted by the rat adrenal in place of cortisol). It is believed that pain stimuli caused by the stress are first transmitted upward through the brain stem to the perifornical area of the hypothalamus and from here into the paraventricular nucleus of the hypothalamus and eventually to the median eminence, as shown in Figure 51-2, where CRF is secreted into the hypophysial portal system. Within minutes the entire control sequence leads to large quantities of the glucocorticoids in the blood.

Inhibitory Effect of Cortisol on the Hypothalamus and the Anterior Pituitary—Decreased ACTH Secretion. Cortisol has direct negative feedback *effects* on (1) the hypothalamus, decreasing the formation of CRF, and (2) the anterior pituitary gland, decreasing the formation of ACTH. These feedbacks help regulate the plasma concentration of cortisol. That is, whenever the concentration becomes too great, these feedbacks automatically reduce this concentration back toward a normal control level.

Summary of the Control System. Figure 51-2 illustrates the overall system for control of cortisol secretion. The central key to this control is the excitation of the hypothalamus by different types of stress. These stresses activate the entire system to cause rapid release of cortisol, and the cortisol in turn initiates a series of metabolic effects directed toward relieving the damaging nature of the stressful state. In addition, there is also direct feedback of the cortisol to the hypothalamus and anterior pituitary gland to decrease the concentration of cortisol in the plasma at times when the body is not experiencing stress. However, the stress stimuli are the prepotent ones; they can always break through this direct inhibitory feedback control of cortisol.

Secretion of Melanocyte-Stimulating Hormone (MSH) Along with ACTH

When ACTH is secreted by the anterior pituitary gland, several other hormones with similar chemical structures are secreted simultaneously, including especially *melanocyte-stimulating hormone* (MSH). Under normal conditions, this hormone is not known to be secreted in enough quantity to have a significant effect on the body, but this may not be true when the rate of secretion of ACTH is very high, as occurs in Addison's disease, which will be discussed later.

MSH causes the *melanocytes,* which are located in abundance at the border between the dermis and the epidermis of the skin, to form the pigment *melanin* and to disperse it in the cells of the epidermis. Injection of melanocyte-stimulating hormone into a person over a period of 8 to 10 days can cause intense darkening of the skin. The effect is much greater in persons with genetically dark skins than in light-skinned persons.

In some lower animals, an intermediate "lobe" of the pituitary gland, called the *pars intermedia,* is highly developed, lying between the anterior and the posterior pituitary lobes. This lobe secretes an especially large amount of melanocyte-stimulating hormone. Furthermore, this secretion is independently controlled by the hypothalamus in response to the amount of light to which an animal is exposed or to other environmental factors. For instance, some arctic animals develop darkened fur in the summer yet have entirely white fur in the winter.

ACTH, because of its similarity to MSH, has about one thirtieth as much melanocyte-stimulating effect as MSH. Furthermore, because the quantities of MSH secreted in the human being are extremely small while those of ACTH are large, it is likely that ACTH is considerably more important normally than MSH in determining the amount of melanin in the skin.

ABNORMALITIES OF ADRENOCORTICAL SECRETION

Hypoadrenalism—Addison's Disease

Addison's disease results from failure of the adrenal cortices to produce adrenocortical hormones, and this failure in turn is most frequently caused by *primary atrophy* of the adrenal cortices, probably resulting from autoimmunity against the cortices, but also frequently caused by tuberculous destruction of the adrenal glands or invasion of the adrenal cortices by cancer. Basically, the disturbances in Addison's disease are these:

Mineralocorticoid Deficiency. Lack of aldosterone secretion greatly decreases sodium reabsorption and consequently allows sodium ions, chloride ions, and water to be lost into the urine in profusion. The net result is a greatly decreased extracellular fluid volume. Furthermore, the person develops hyperkalemia (excess potassium in the extracellular fluids) and acidosis because of failure of potassium and hydrogen ions to be secreted in exchange for sodium reabsorption.

As the volume of extracellular fluid becomes depleted, the plasma volume also falls, the red blood cell concentration rises markedly, the cardiac output decreases, and the patient dies in shock. Death usually occurs in the untreated patient 4 days to 2 weeks after complete cessation of mineralocorticoid secretion.

Glucocorticoid Deficiency. Loss of cortisol secretion makes it impossible for the person with Addison's disease to maintain normal blood glucose concentration between meals because of an inability to synthesize significant quantities of glucose by gluconeogenesis. Furthermore, lack of cortisol reduces the mobilization of both proteins and fats from the tissues, thereby depressing many other metabolic functions of the body. This sluggishness of energy mobilization when cortisol is not available is one of the major detrimental effects of glucocorticoid lack. However, even when excess quantities of glucose and other nutrients are available, the person's muscles are still weak, indicating that glucocorticoids are also needed to maintain other metabolic functions of the tissues besides simply energy metabolism.

Lack of adequate glucocorticoid secretion also makes the person with Addison's disease highly susceptible to the deteriorating effects of different types of stress, and even a mild respiratory infection can sometimes cause death.

Treatment of Persons with Addison's Disease. The untreated person with full-blown Addison's disease dies within a few days because of consuming weakness and eventual circulatory shock. Yet such a person can usually live for years if small quantities of mineralocorticoids and glucocorticoids are administered daily.

The Addisonian Crisis. As noted earlier in the chapter, great quantities of glucocorticoids are occasionally secreted in response to different types of physical or mental stress. In the person with Addison's disease, the output of glucocorticoids does not increase during stress. Yet whenever such a person is specifically subjected to different types of trauma, disease, or other stresses such as surgical operations, he or she is likely to develop an acute need for excessive amounts of glucocorticoids and must be given as much as ten or more times the normal quantities in order to prevent severe debility or even death.

This critical need for extra glucocorticoids and the associated severe debility in times of stress is called *addisonian crisis.*

Hyperadrenalism — Cushing's Disease

Hypersecretion of cortisol by the adrenal cortex causes a complex of hormonal effects called Cushing's disease, resulting from either a cortisol-secreting tumor of one adrenal cortex or general hyperplasia of both adrenal cortices. The hyperplasia in turn is usually caused by increased secretion of ACTH by the anterior pituitary. Most abnormalities of Cushing's disease are ascribable to abnormal amounts of cortisol, but increased secretion of androgens is often of significance as well.

A special characteristic of Cushing's disease is mobilization of fat from the lower part of the body, with concomitant extra deposition of fat in the thoracic region, giving rise to a so-called "buffalo" torso. The excess secretion of steroids also leads to an edematous appearance of the face, and the androgenic potency of some of the hormones causes acne and hirsutism (excess growth of facial hair). The total appearance of the face is frequently described as a "moon face," as illustrated to the left in Figure 51–4 in a patient with Cushing's disease prior to treatment.

Effects on Carbohydrate and Protein Metabolism. The abundance of glucocorticoids secreted in Cushing's disease causes increased blood glucose concentration, sometimes to values as high as 200 mg per 100 ml of blood after meals, which is called *adrenal diabetes.* This effect results mainly from enhanced gluconeogenesis.

The effects of glucocorticoids on protein catabolism in Cushing's disease are often profound, causing greatly decreased proteins almost everywhere in the body except for the liver and the plasma. The loss of

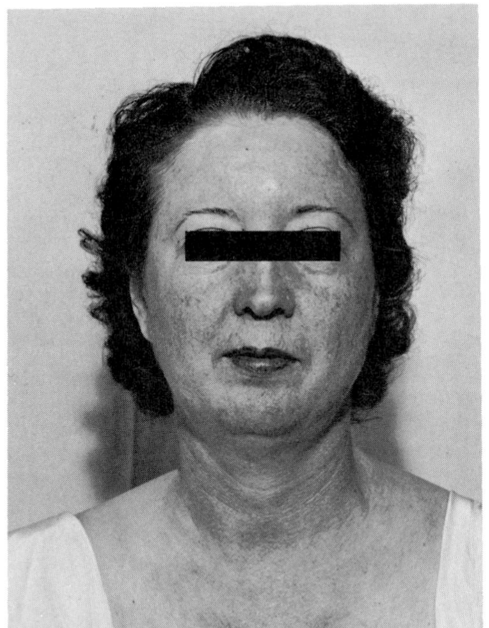

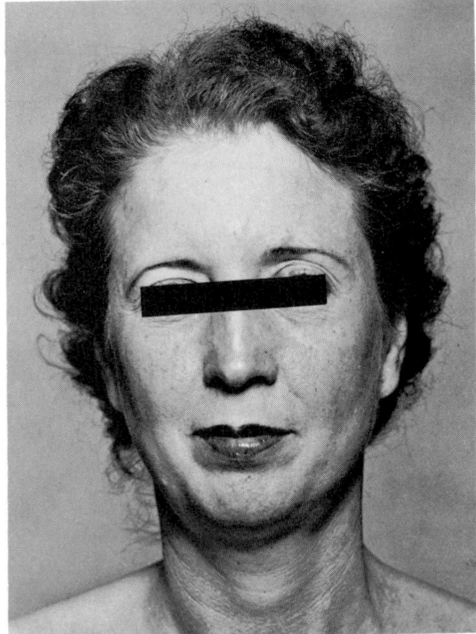

Figure 51–4. A person with Cushing's disease before subtotal adrenalectomy (left) and after subtotal adrenalectomy (right). (Courtesy of Dr. Leonard Posey.)

protein from the muscles in particular causes severe weakness. The loss of protein synthesis in the lymphoid tissues leads to a suppressed immune system, so that many of these patients die of infections. Even the collagen fibers in the subcutaneous tissue are diminished, so that the subcutaneous tissues tear easily, resulting in development of large *purplish striae;* these are actually scars where the subcutaneous tissues have torn apart. In addition, lack of protein deposition in the bones causes *osteoporosis* with consequent weakness of the bones.

Treatment of Cushing's Disease. Treatment in Cushing's disease consists of removing an adrenal tumor if this is the cause or of decreasing the secretion of ACTH if possible. Hypertrophied pituitary glands or even small tumors in the pituitary gland that oversecrete ACTH can be surgically or microsurgically removed or can be destroyed by radiation. If ACTH secretion cannot easily be decreased, the only satisfactory treatment usually is bilateral total or partial adrenalectomy followed by the administration of adrenal steroids to make up for any insufficiency that develops.

Primary Aldosteronism

Occasionally, a small tumor of the zona glomerulosa cells (cells located on the outer surface of the adrenal cortex) occurs and secretes large amounts of aldosterone. The effects of the excess aldosterone are those discussed earlier in the chapter. The most important effects are hypokalemia, slight increase in extracellular fluid volume and blood volume, very slight increase in plasma sodium concentration (usually not over a 2 to 3 per cent increase), and moderate hypertension. Especially interesting in primary aldosteronism are occasional periods of muscular paralysis caused by the hypokalemia. The paralysis is caused by a depressant effect of the hypokalemia on action potential transmission, as explained in Chapter 5.

Treatment of primary aldosteronism is usually surgical removal of the adrenal tumor.

REFERENCES

Burnstein, K. L., and Cidlowski, J. A.: Regulation of gene expression by glucocorticoids. Annu. Rev. Physiol., 51:683, 1989.

D'Agata, R., and Chrousos, G. P.: Recent Advances in Adrenal Regulation and Function. New York, Raven Press, 1987.

DeGroot, L. J. (ed.): Endocrinology. 2nd ed. Philadelphia, W. B. Saunders Co., 1989.

Funder, J. W.: Adrenal steroids: New answers, new questions. Science, 237:236, 1987.

Jones, M. T., and Gilham, B.: Factors involved in the regulation of adrenocorticotropic hormone/β-lipotropic hormone. Physiol. Rev., 68:743, 1988.

Kannan, C. R.: The Adrenal Gland. New York, Plenum Publishing Corp., 1988.

Moudgil, V. K. (ed.): Steroid Receptors in Health and Disease. New York, Plenum Publishing Corp., 1988.

Parker, L.: Adrenal Androgens in Clinical Medicine. San Diego, CA, Academic Press, 1988.

Quinn, S. J., and Williams, G. H.: Regulation of aldosterone secretion. Annu. Rev. Physiol., 50:409, 1988.

Schatzberg, A. F., and Nemeroff, C. B. (eds.): The Hypothalamic-Pituitary-Adrenal Axis. New York, Raven Press, 1988.

Seldin, D. W., and Giebisch, G.: The Regulation of Potassium Balance. New York, Raven Press, 1989.

Seldin, D. W., and Giebisch, G.: The Regulation of Sodium and Chloride Balance. New York, Raven Press, 1989.

QUESTIONS

1. What is the difference between the *adrenal medulla* and the *adrenal cortex?*
2. Describe, in general, the chemistry of the *adrenocortical hormones.*
3. Why are the adrenocortical hormones divided into *mineralocorticoids* and *glucocorticoids?*
4. What are the effects of *aldosterone* on sodium absorption and potassium secretion by the renal tubules?
5. How does *hypokalemia* cause muscle paralysis? On the other hand, how does *hyperkalemia* cause cardiac toxicity?
6. Explain the cellular mechanism for aldosterone action.
7. Review briefly the regulation of aldosterone secretion. What are the specific effects of potassium ions and angiotensin on aldosterone secretion?
8. What are the most important glucocorticoids secreted by the body?
9. What are the effects of *cortisol* on carbohydrate metabolism? How does cortisol increase *gluconeogenesis?*
10. What is the effect of cortisol on protein metabolism, especially on the *mobilization of amino acids* from the peripheral tissues, and what are its effects on liver proteins and plasma proteins?
11. What are the effects of cortisol on fat metabolism?
12. Explain what we know about the role of cortisol in protecting the body against different types of stress.
13. What is the role of cortisol in neutralizing the effects of inflammation, and why is this important?
14. What are the chemical characteristics of *CRF* and *ACTH,* and how do these function in the control of glucocorticoid secretion by the adrenal cortex?
15. What are the feedback effects from the body that help to control secretion of ACTH by the anterior pituitary gland and therefore control the secretion of glucocorticoids?
16. What is the relationship of ACTH to *melanocyte-stimulating hormone,* and what are the effects of both of these on body pigmentation?
17. What are the causes of *Addison's disease,* and what are the functional abnormalities of the body that it causes?
18. What are the causes of and the functional abnormalities caused by *Cushing's disease?*
19. What are the clinical characteristics of *primary aldosteronism,* and what are the physiological mechanisms of these effects?

52

Insulin, Glucagon, and Diabetes Mellitus

The pancreas, in addition to its digestive functions, secretes two important hormones, *insulin* and *glucagon.* The purpose of this chapter is to discuss the functions of these hormones in regulating glucose, lipid, and protein metabolism, also to discuss briefly the disease *diabetes mellitus,* which is caused by hyposecretion of insulin.

Physiological Anatomy of the Pancreas. The pancreas is composed of two major types of tissues, as shown in Figure 52–1: (1) the *acini,* which secrete digestive juices into the duodenum, and (2) the *islets of Langerhans,* which secrete insulin and glucagon directly into the blood. The digestive secretions of the pancreas were discussed in Chapter 43.

The islets of Langerhans of the human being contain three major types of cells, the *alpha, beta,* and *delta* cells, which are distinguished from one another by their structure and staining characteristics. The beta cells secrete insulin, the alpha cells secrete glucagon, and the delta cells secrete somatostatin, the important functions of which are still not entirely clear.

INSULIN

Insulin is a very large polypeptide (small protein) with a molecular weight of 5808 in the case of human insulin. It is composed of two amino acid chains connected to each other by disulfide linkages.

Before insulin can exert its function it must first bind with a large *receptor protein* in the cell membrane.

The Basic Function of Insulin: Activation of Target Cell Receptors by Insulin, and the Resulting Cellular Effects

To initiate its effects on target cells, insulin first binds with and activates a membrane receptor protein having a molecular weight of about 300,000. It is the activated receptor, not the insulin, that causes the subsequent effects.

The insulin receptor is a combination of four separate subunits held together by disulfide linkages, *two alpha subunits* that lie entirely outside the cell membrane and *two beta subunits* that penetrate through the membrane with an end of each of these protruding into the cell cytoplasm. The insulin binds with the alpha subunits on the outside of the cell; but because of the linkages with the beta subunits, the portions of the beta subunits protruding into the cell become autophosphorylated. This makes them become an activated enzyme, a local *protein kinase,* which in turn causes phosphorylation of multiple other cytosol enzymes. The net effect is to activate some of these enzymes while inactivating others. Thus, in this roundabout way, insulin directs the intracellular metabolic machinery to produce the desired effects. Unfortunately, from this point on, the molecular mechanisms are almost entirely unknown.

Nevertheless, the end effects of insulin stimulation are clear. These are basically the following:

1. Within seconds after insulin binds with its membrane receptors, the membranes of muscle cells, adipose cells, and many other types of cells in the body—constituting about 80 per cent of all cells—become highly permeable to glucose. This allows rapid entry of glucose into the cells. Inside the cell, the glucose is immediately phosphorylated and becomes a substrate for all the usual carbohydrate metabolic functions. The increased glucose transport is believed to result from opening of gates in a glucose transport protein, a membrane protein with a molecular weight of about 55,000.
2. In addition to increased membrane permeability for glucose, the cell membrane also becomes more permeable for many of the amino acids,

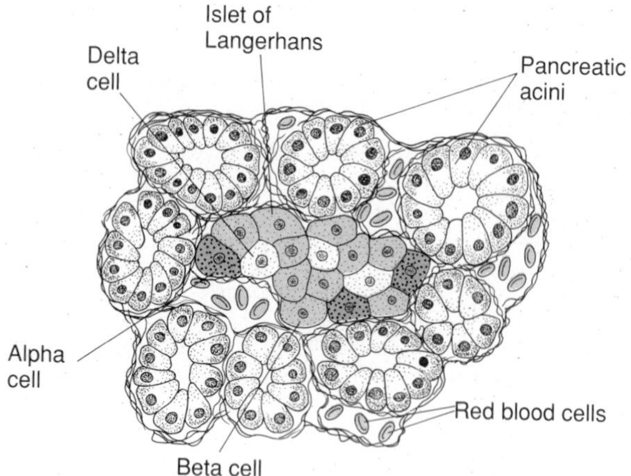

Figure 52–1. Physiologic anatomy of the pancreas.

potassium ions, magnesium ions, and phosphate ions.

3. Slower effects occur during the next 10 to 15 minutes to change the activity levels of still many more intracellular metabolic enzymes. These effects result mainly from the changed states of phosphorylation of the enzymes.
4. Still much slower effects continue to occur for hours and even for several days. These result from changed rates of translation of messenger RNAs at the ribosomes to form new proteins and still slower effects from changed rates of transcription of DNA in the cell nucleus. In this way, insulin remolds much of the cellular enzymatic machinery to achieve its metabolic goals.

Effect of Insulin on Carbohydrate Metabolism

Immediately after a high carbohydrate meal, the glucose that is absorbed into the blood causes rapid secretion of insulin. The insulin in turn causes rapid uptake, storage, and use of glucose by almost all tissues of the body, but especially by the muscles, adipose tissue, and liver.

Effect of Insulin in Promoting Glucose Metabolism in Muscle

During much of the day, muscle tissue depends not on glucose for its energy but instead on fatty acids. The principal reason for this is that the normal *resting muscle* membrane is only slightly permeable to glucose except when the muscle fiber is stimulated by insulin; and between meals, the amount of insulin that is secreted is too small to promote significant amounts of glucose entry into the muscle cells.

However, under two conditions the muscles do utilize large amounts of glucose. One of these is during periods of moderate to heavy exercise. This usage of glucose does not require large amounts of insulin because exercising muscle fibers, for reasons not understood, become highly permeable to glucose even in the absence of insulin because of the contraction process itself.

The second condition for muscle usage of large amounts of glucose is during the few hours after a meal. At this time the blood glucose concentration is high; also, the pancreas is secreting large quantities of insulin, and the extra insulin causes rapid transport of glucose into the muscle cells. This causes the muscle cell during this period of time to utilize carbohydrates, and to do so preferentially over fatty acids because the flow of fatty acids from the adipose tissue is strongly inhibited by insulin, as we discuss later.

Storage of Glycogen in Muscle. If the muscles are not exercising during the period following a meal and yet glucose is transported into the muscle cells in abundance, then most of the glucose is stored in the form of muscle glycogen instead of being used for energy, up to a limit of about 2 per cent concentration. The glycogen can later be used for energy by the muscle. It is especially useful for short periods of extreme energy use by the muscles and even to provide spurts of anaerobic energy for a few minutes at a time by glycolytic breakdown of the glycogen to lactic acid, which can occur even in the absence of oxygen.

Insulin Facilitation of Glucose Transport Through the Muscle Cell Membrane. Insulin has a direct effect on the muscle cell membrane to *facilitate glucose transport.* This is illustrated by the experimental results depicted in Figure 52–2. The lower curve labeled "control" shows the concentration of free glucose measured inside the cell when no insulin was present, illustrating that the glucose concentration remained almost exactly zero despite increased extracellular glucose concentration up to as high as 750 mg/dl. In contrast, the curve labeled "insulin" illustrates that the intracellular glucose concentration rose to as high as 400 milligrams when insulin was added. Thus, it is clear that insulin can increase the rate of transport of glucose into the resting muscle cell by at least 10- to 20-fold.

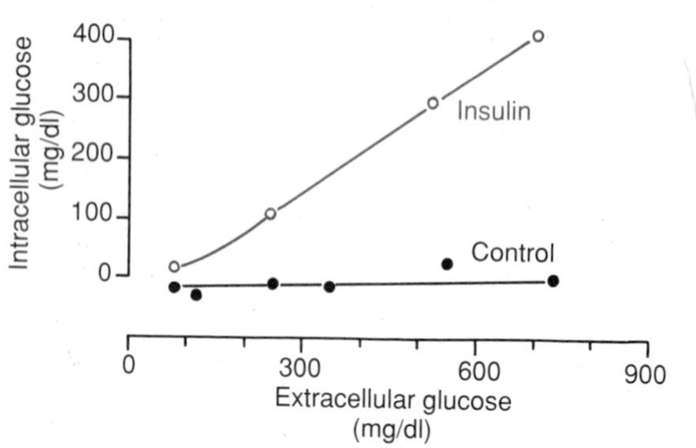

Figure 52–2. Effect of insulin in enhancing the concentration of glucose inside muscle cells. Note that in the absence of insulin (control) the intracellular glucose concentration remained near zero despite very high extracellular glucose concentrations of glucose. (From Park, Morgan, Kaji, and Smith, *in* Eisenstein [ed.]: The Biochemical Aspects of Hormone Action. Boston, Little, Brown & Company.)

Effect of Insulin on Promoting Liver Uptake, Storage, and Use of Glucose

One of the most important of all the effects of insulin is to cause most of the glucose absorbed after a meal to be stored almost immediately in the liver in the form of glycogen. Then, between meals, when food is not available and the blood glucose concentration begins to fall, the liver glycogen is split back into glucose, which is released back into the blood to keep the blood glucose concentration from falling too low.

The mechanism by which insulin causes glucose uptake and storage in the liver includes several almost simultaneous steps:

1. Insulin *inhibits liver phosphorylase,* the enzyme that causes liver glycogen to split into glucose. This obviously prevents breakdown of the glycogen that is already in the liver cells.
2. Insulin causes *enhanced uptake of glucose* from the blood by the liver cells. It does this by *increasing the activity of the enzyme glucokinase,* which is the enzyme that causes the initial phosphorylation of glucose after it diffuses into the liver cells. Once phosphorylated, the glucose is *temporarily* trapped inside the liver cells, because phosphorylated glucose cannot diffuse back through the cell membrane.
3. Insulin also increases the activities of the enzymes that promote glycogen synthesis.

The net effect of all these actions is to increase the amount of glycogen in the liver. The glycogen can increase to a total of about 5 to 6 per cent of the liver mass, which is equivalent to almost 100 grams of stored glycogen.

Release of Glucose from the Liver Between Meals. After the meal is over and the blood glucose level begins to fall to a low level, several events now transpire that cause the liver to release glucose back into the circulating blood:

1. The decreasing blood glucose causes the pancreas to decrease its insulin secretion.
2. The lack of insulin then reverses all the effects listed above for glycogen storage, essentially stopping further synthesis of glycogen in the liver and preventing further uptake of glucose by the liver from the blood.
3. The lack of insulin (along with increase of glucagon, which will be discussed later) activates the enzyme *phosphorylase,* which causes the splitting of glycogen into *glucose phosphate.*
4. The enzyme *glucose phosphatase,* which has been inhibited by insulin, now becomes activated by the insulin lack and causes the phosphate radical to split away from the glucose; and this allows the free glucose to diffuse back into the blood.

Thus, the liver removes glucose from the blood when it is present in excess after a meal and returns it to the blood when it is needed between meals. Ordinarily, about 60 per cent of the glucose in the meal is stored in this way in the liver and then returned later.

Other Effects of Insulin on Carbohydrate Metabolism in the Liver. When the quantity of glucose entering the liver cells is more than can be stored as glycogen, *insulin promotes the conversion of all of this excess glucose into fatty acids.* These fatty acids are subsequently packaged as triglycerides in very low density lipoproteins and transported to the adipose tissue and deposited as fat.

Insulin also *inhibits gluconeogenesis.* It does this mainly by decreasing the quantities and activities of the liver enzymes required for gluconeogenesis.

Lack of Effect of Insulin on Glucose Uptake and Usage by the Brain

The brain is quite different from most other tissues of the body in that insulin has either little or no effect on uptake or use of glucose. Instead, *the brain cells are permeable to glucose without the intermediation of insulin.*

The brain cells are also quite different from most other cells of the body in that they normally use only glucose for energy. Therefore, it is essential that the blood glucose level be maintained always above a critical level, which is one of the important functions of the blood glucose control system. When the blood glucose does fall too low, into the range of 20 to 50 mg/dl, symptoms of *hypoglycemic shock* develop, characterized by progressive nervous irritability that leads to fainting, convulsions, and even coma.

Effect of Insulin on Carbohydrate Metabolism in Other Cells

Insulin increases glucose transport into and glucose usage by most other cells of the body (with the exception of the brain cells, as noted) in the same way that it affects glucose transport through the muscle cell membrane. The transport of glucose into adipose cells is essential for providing the glycerol portion of the fat molecule for deposition of fat in these cells.

Effect of Insulin on Fat Metabolism

Though not quite as visible as the acute effects of insulin on carbohydrate metabolism, insulin also affects fat metabolism in ways that, in the long run, are equally as important. Especially dramatic is the long-term effect of insulin lack in causing extreme atherosclerosis, often leading to heart attacks, cerebral strokes, and other vascular accidents. But, first, let us discuss the acute effects of insulin on fat metabolism.

Effect of Insulin Excess on Fat Synthesis and Storage

Insulin has several different effects that lead to fat storage in adipose tissue. Insulin increases the utilization of glucose by most of the body's tissues, which automatically decreases the utilization of fat, thus functioning as a "fat sparer." However, insulin also promotes fatty acid synthesis. Almost all of this synthesis occurs in the liver cells, and the fatty acids are then transported in the lipoproteins to the adipose cells to be stored. However, a minute part of the synthesis occurs in the fat cells themselves.

Storage of Fat in the Adipose Cells. Insulin has two essential effects that are required for fat storage in adipose cells:

1. Insulin *inhibits the action of hormone-sensitive lipase.* This is the enzyme that causes hydrolysis of the triglycerides already stored in the fat cells. Therefore, the release of fatty acids into the circulating blood is inhibited.
2. Insulin *promotes glucose transport through the cell membrane into the fat cells* in exactly the same way that it promotes glucose transport into muscle cells. Some of this glucose is then utilized to synthesize small amounts of fatty acids; but, more important, it also forms large quantities of the substance *α-glycerophosphate.* This substance supplies the *glycerol* that combines with fatty acids to form the triglycerides that are the storage form of fat in adipose cells. Therefore, when insulin is not available, storage of the large amounts of fatty acids transported from the liver in the lipoproteins is almost totally blocked.

Increased Metabolic Use of Fat Caused by Insulin Lack

All aspects of fat breakdown and use for providing energy are greatly *enhanced in the absence of insulin.* This occurs even normally between meals when secretion of insulin is minimal, but it becomes extreme in diabetes mellitus when secretion of insulin is almost zero. The resulting effects are as follows:

Lipolysis of Storage Fat and Release of Free Fatty Acids During Insulin Lack. In the absence of insulin, all the aforementioned effects of insulin causing storage of fat are reversed. The most important effect is that the enzyme *hormone-sensitive lipase* in the fat cells becomes strongly activated. This causes hydrolysis of the stored triglycerides, releasing large quantities of fatty acids and glycerol into the circulating blood. Consequently, the plasma concentration of free fatty acids begins to rise within minutes. This free fatty acid then becomes the main energy substrate used by essentially all tissues of the body besides the brain. Figure 52–3 illustrates the approximate effects of insulin lack on the plasma concentration of free fatty acids, glucose, and acetoacetic acid. Note that immediately after removal of the pancreas the free fatty acid concentration in the plasma begins to rise, rising considerably more rapidly even than the concentration of glucose.

Effect of Insulin Lack on Plasma Cholesterol and Phospholipid Concentrations. The excess of fatty acids in the plasma also promotes liver conversion of some of the fatty acids into phospholipids and

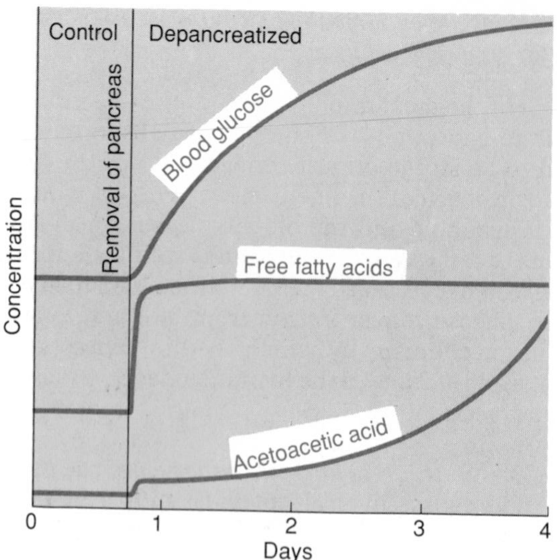

Figure 52–3. Effect of removing the pancreas on the concentrations of blood glucose, plasma free fatty acids, and acetoacetic acid.

cholesterol, two of the major products of fat metabolism. These two substances, along with excess triglycerides formed at the same time in the liver, are then discharged into the blood in the lipoproteins. Occasionally, the plasma lipoproteins increase as much as threefold in the absence of insulin, giving a total concentration of plasma lipids of several per cent rather than the normal 0.6 per cent. This high lipid concentration—especially the high concentration of cholesterol—leads to rapid development of atherosclerosis in persons with serious diabetes.

Acidotic Effects of Insulin Lack. Insulin lack also causes excessive amounts of *acetoacetic acid* to be formed from fatty acids in the liver cells. Therefore, so much acetoacetic acid is released from the liver that it cannot all be metabolized by the tissues. As illustrated in Figure 52–3, its concentration rises during the days following cessation of insulin secretion, sometimes reaching concentrations as high as 10 mEq/liter or more. We see later that in severe diabetes the acetoacetic acid can cause severe *acidosis* and *coma,* which often leads to death.

Effect of Insulin on Protein Metabolism and Growth

Effect of Insulin on Protein Synthesis and Storage. During the few hours following a meal when excess quantities of nutrients are available in the circulating blood, not only carbohydrates and fats but proteins as well are stored in the tissues; insulin is required for this to occur. The manner in which insulin causes protein storage is not as well understood as the mechanisms for both glucose and fat storage. Some of the facts follow:

1. Insulin causes active transport of many of the amino acids into the cells. Thus insulin shares with growth hormone the capability of increasing the uptake of amino acids into cells.

2. Insulin has a direct effect on the ribosomes in *increasing the translation of messenger RNA*, thus forming new proteins. In some unexplained way, insulin "turns on" the ribosomal machinery.
3. Over a longer period of time insulin also *increases the rate of transcription of selected DNA genetic sequences* in the cell nuclei, thus forming increased quantities of RNA and still more protein synthesis—especially promoting a vast array of enzymes for storage of carbohydrates, fats, and proteins.
4. Insulin also *inhibits the catabolism of proteins*, thus decreasing the rate of amino acid release from the cells, especially from the muscle cells.

In summary, insulin promotes protein formation and also prevents the degradation of proteins. Conversely, virtually all protein storage comes to a complete halt when insulin is not available.

Effect of Insulin on Growth—Its Synergistic Effect with Growth Hormone. Because insulin is required for the synthesis of proteins, it is equally as essential for growth of an animal as is growth hormone. This is illustrated in Figure 52-4, which shows that a depancreatized, hypophysectomized rat without therapy hardly grows at all. Furthermore, administration of either growth hormone or insulin one at a time causes almost no growth. Yet a combination of both these hormones does cause dramatic growth. Thus it appears that the two hormones function synergistically to promote growth, each performing a specific function that is separate from that of the other. Perhaps part of this necessity for both hormones results from the fact that each promotes cellular uptake of a different selection of amino acids, all of which are required if growth is to be achieved.

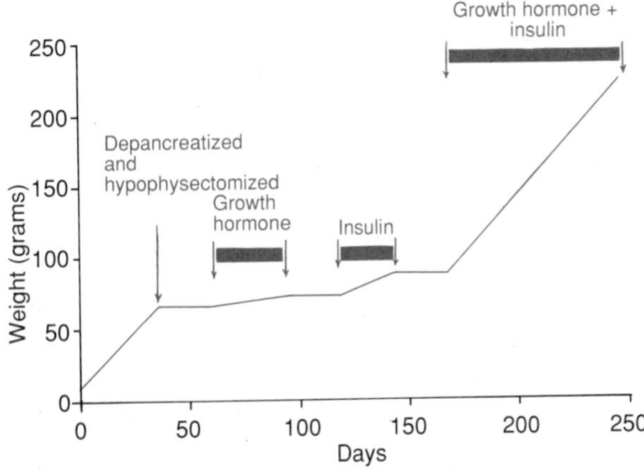

Figure 52-4. Effect of growth hormone, insulin, and growth hormone plus insulin on growth in a depancreatized and hypophysectomized rat.

Control of Insulin Secretion

Stimulation of Insulin Secretion by Blood Glucose

At the normal fasting level of blood glucose of 80 to 90 mg/dl, the rate of insulin secretion is minimal—on the order of 25 ng/min/kg of body weight. If the blood glucose concentration is suddenly increased to a level two to three times normal and is kept at this high level thereafter, insulin secretion increases markedly in two stages, as shown by the changes in plasma insulin concentration seen in Figure 52-5.

1. Plasma insulin concentration increases almost tenfold within 3 to 5 minutes after acute elevation of the blood glucose; this results from immediate dumping of performed insulin from the beta cells of the islets of Langerhans. However, the initial high rate of secretion is not maintained; instead, the insulin concentration decreases about halfway back toward normal in another 5 to 10 minutes.
2. After about 15 minutes, insulin secretion rises a second time and reaches a new plateau in 2 to 3 hours, this time usually at a rate of secretion even greater than that in the initial phase. This secretion results both from additional release of preformed insulin and from activation of the enzyme system that synthesizes and releases new insulin from the cells.

Feedback Relationship Between Blood Glucose Concentration and Insulin Secretion Rate. As the concentration of blood glucose rises above 100 mg/dl of blood, the rate of insulin secretion rises rapidly, reaching a peak some 10 to 25 times the basal level at blood glucose concentrations of between 400 and 600 mg/dl, as illustrated in Figure 52-6. Thus, the increase in insulin secretion under a glucose stimulus is dramatic both in its rapidity and in the tremendous level of secretion achieved. Furthermore, the turn-off of insulin secretion is almost equally as rapid, occurring within minutes after reduction in blood glucose concentration back to the fasting level.

This response of insulin secretion to an elevated blood glucose concentration provides an extremely important feedback mechanism for regulating blood glucose concentration. That is, any rise in blood glucose increases insulin secretion, and the insulin in

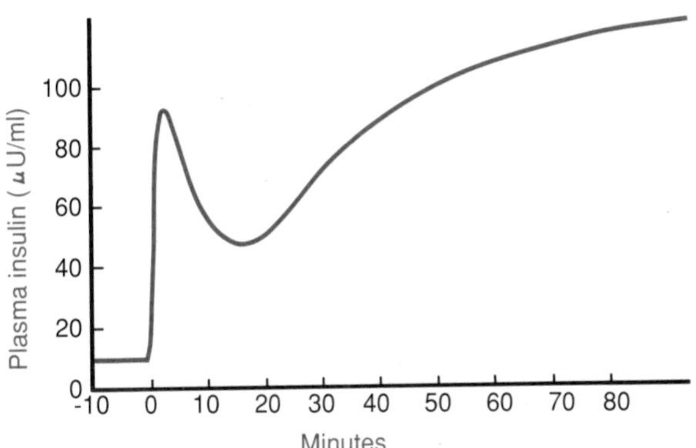

Figure 52-5. Increase in plasma insulin concentration following a sudden increase in blood glucose to two to three times the normal range. Note an initial rapid surge in insulin concentration and then a delayed but higher and continuing increase in concentration beginning 15 to 20 minutes later.

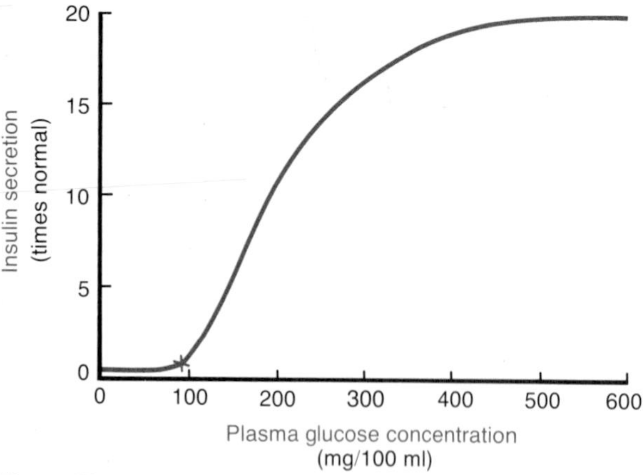

Figure 52–6. Approximate increase in insulin secretion at different plasma glucose levels.

turn causes transport of glucose into the liver, muscle, and other cells, thereby reducing the blood glucose concentration back toward the normal value.

Stimulation of Insulin Secretion by Some Amino Acids

In addition to excess glucose stimulating insulin secretion, many of the amino acids have a similar effect. The most potent of these are *arginine* and *lysine.* This stimulation of insulin secretion seems to be a purposeful response, because the insulin in turn promotes transport of the amino acids into the tissue cells and also promotes intracellular formation of protein. That is, the insulin is important for proper utilization of excess amino acids in the same way that it is important for the utilization of carbohydrates.

Role of Insulin in Switching Between Carbohydrate and Lipid Metabolism

From the preceding discussions it should be clear that insulin promotes the utilization of carbohydrates for energy and depresses the utilization of fats. Conversely, lack of insulin causes fat utilization mainly to the exclusion of glucose utilization, except by brain tissue. Furthermore, the signal that controls this rapid switching mechanism is principally the blood glucose concentration. When the glucose concentration is low, insulin secretion is suppressed, and fat is utilized almost exclusively for energy everywhere except in the brain; when the glucose concentration is high, insulin secretion is stimulated, and carbohydrate is utilized instead of fat until the excess blood glucose is stored. Therefore, one of the most important functional roles of insulin in the body is to control which of these two foods, from moment to moment, will be utilized by the cells for energy.

GLUCAGON AND ITS FUNCTIONS

Glucagon, a hormone secreted by the alpha cells of the islets of Langerhans, has several functions that are opposite to those of insulin. Most important of these is its effect in *increasing* the blood glucose concentration.

Like insulin, glucagon is a large polypeptide. It has a molecular weight of 3485 and is composed of a chain of 29 amino acids. On injection of purified glucagon into an animal, a profound *hyper*glycemic effect occurs. One microgram of glucagon per kilogram of body weight can elevate the blood glucose concentration approximately 20 mg/dl of blood in about 20 minutes. For this reason, glucagon is frequently called *hyperglycemic hormone.*

The two major effects of glucagon on glucose metabolism are (1) breakdown of liver glycogen *(glycogenolysis)* and (2) increased *gluconeogenesis.*

Glycogenolysis and Increased Blood Glucose Concentration Caused by Glucagon. The most dramatic effect of glucagon is its ability to cause glycogenolysis in the liver, which in turn increases the blood glucose concentration within minutes.

Glucagon does this by the following complex cascade of events:

1. It activates *adenyl cyclase* in the liver cell membrane,
2. which causes the formation of *cyclic AMP,*
3. which activates *protein kinase regulator protein,*
4. which activates *protein kinase,*
5. which activates *phosphorylase b kinase,*
6. which converts *phosphorylase b* into *phosphorylase a,*
7. which promotes the degradation of glycogen into glucose-1-phosphate,
8. which then is dephosphorylated and the glucose released from the liver cells.

This sequence of events is exceedingly important for several reasons. First, it is one of the most thoroughly studied of all the *second messenger* functions of cyclic AMP. Second, it illustrates a cascading system in which each succeeding product is produced in greater quantity than the preceding product; therefore the sequence represents a potent *amplifying* mechanism, which explains how only a few micrograms of glucagon can have the extreme effect of causing hyperglycemia.

Infusion of glucagon for about 4 hours can cause such intensive liver glycogenolysis that all of the liver stores of glycogen become totally depleted.

Gluconeogenesis Caused by Glucagon. Even after all the glycogen in the liver has been exhausted under the influence of glucagon, continued infusion of this hormone causes continued hyperglycemia. This results from an effect of glucagon that increases the rate of gluconeogenesis in the liver cells. It is achieved by activating multiple enzymes that are required for gluconeogenesis. Also, glucagon increases the extraction of amino acids from the blood by the liver cells, thus making a greater quantity of these available to be converted into glucose.

Glucagon-Like Effect of Epinephrine. Epinephrine (and to a slight extent norepinephrine as well) is also a potent promoter of liver glycogenolysis, having an effect almost exactly the same as that of glucagon, though not quite as strong.

Regulation of Glucagon Secretion

Inhibitory Effect of Blood Glucose. Changes in blood glucose concentration have exactly the opposite effect on glucagon secretion as on insulin secretion. That is, a *decrease* in blood glucose increases glucagon secretion. Especially when the blood glucose falls to as low as 70 mg/dl of blood, the pancreas secretes large quantities of glucagon. The glucagon rapidly mobilizes glucose from the liver; thus glucagon helps protect against hypoglycemia.

Excitatory Effect of Amino Acids. High concentrations of amino acids, as occur in the blood after a protein meal (especially the amino acids *alanine* and *arginine*), stimulate the secretion of glucagon. This is the same effect that amino acids have in stimulating insulin secretion. Thus, in this instance the glucagon and insulin responses are not opposites.

The importance of amino acid stimulation of glucagon secretion is that the glucagon then promotes rapid conversion of the amino acids to glucose, thus making even more glucose available to the tissues.

SUMMARY OF BLOOD GLUCOSE REGULATION

In the normal person the blood glucose concentration is very narrowly controlled, usually in a range between 80 and 90 mg/dl of blood in the fasting person each morning before breakfast. This concentration increases to 120 to 140 mg/dl during the first hour or so following a meal, but the feedback systems for control of blood glucose return the glucose concentration very rapidly back to the control level, usually within 2 hours after the last absorption of carbohydrates. Conversely, in starvation the gluconeogenesis function of the liver provides the glucose that is required to maintain the fasting blood glucose level.

The mechanisms for achieving this high degree of control have been presented in this chapter. However, let us summarize these briefly.

1. The liver functions as a very important *blood glucose-buffer system.* That is, when the blood glucose rises to a very high concentration following a meal and the rate of insulin secretion also increases, as much as two thirds of the glucose absorbed from the gut is almost immediately stored in the liver in the form of glycogen. Then during the succeeding hours, when both the blood glucose concentration and the rate of insulin secretion fall, the liver releases the glucose back into the blood.
2. It is very clear that both insulin and glucagon function as important and separate feedback control systems for maintaining a normal blood glucose concentration. When the concentration level rises too high, insulin is secreted; the insulin in turn causes the blood glucose concentration to decrease toward normal. Conversely, a decrease in blood glucose stimulates glucagon secretion; the glucagon then functions in the opposite direction to increase the glucose toward normal. Under most normal conditions, the insulin feedback mechanism is much more important than the glucagon mechanism.
3. Also, in hypoglycemia a direct effect of low blood glucose on the hypothalamus stimulates the sympathetic nervous system. In turn, epinephrine secreted by the adrenal glands causes still further release of glucose from the liver. This, too, helps protect against severe hypoglycemia.
4. And, finally, over a period of hours and days, both growth hormone and cortisol are secreted in response to prolonged hypoglycemia, and they both decrease the rate of glucose utilization by most cells of the body. This, too, helps return the blood glucose concentration toward normal.

Importance of Blood Glucose Regulation. One might ask, Why is it important to maintain a constant blood glucose concentration, particularly since most tissues can shift to utilization of fats and proteins for energy in the absence of glucose? The answer is that glucose is the *only* nutrient that normally can be utilized by the *brain, retina,* and *germinal epithelium of the gonads* in sufficient quantities to supply them with their required energy. Therefore, it is important to maintain a blood glucose concentration at a sufficiently high level to provide this necessary nutrition.

Most of the glucose formed by gluconeogenesis during the interdigestive period is used for metabolism in the brain. Indeed, it is important that the pancreas not secrete any insulin during this time, for otherwise the scant supplies of glucose that are available would all go into the muscles and other peripheral tissues, leaving the brain without its normal nutritive source.

DIABETES MELLITUS

In most instances, diabetes mellitus results from diminished secretion of insulin by the beta cells of the islets of Langerhans. Heredity usually plays a major role in determining in whom diabetes will develop and in whom it will not. Sometimes it does this by increasing the susceptibility of the beta cells to viruses, or by favoring the development of autoimmune antibodies against the beta cells, thus leading to their destruction. In other instances there appears to be a simple hereditary tendency for beta cell degeneration.

Obesity also plays a role in the development of diabetes. One reason is that in obesity the beta cells of the islets of Langerhans become less responsive to stimulation by increased blood glucose; therefore, the blood insulin levels do not increase when needed. Another reason is that obesity decreases the number of insulin receptors in the insulin target cells throughout the body, thus making the amount of insulin that is available even less effective in promoting its usual metabolic effects.

Pathological Physiology of Diabetes

Most of the pathological conditions in diabetes mellitus can be attributed to one of the following three major effects of insulin lack: (1) decreased utilization of glucose by the body cells, with a resultant increase in blood glucose concentration to as high as 300 to 1200 mg per dl; (2) markedly increased mobilization of fats from the fat storage areas, causing abnormal fat metabolism as well as deposition of lipids in the vascular walls, resulting in atherosclerosis; and (3) depletion of protein in the tissues of the body.

However, in addition, some special pathophysiological problems occur in diabetes mellitus that are not so readily apparent. These are the following:

Loss of Glucose and Water in the Urine of the Diabetic Person. When the quantity of glucose entering the kidney tubules in the glomerular filtrate rises too high, a significant proportion of the glucose begins to spill into the urine. Usually, glucose spillage will occur when the blood glucose level rises over 180 mg/dl. Consequently, it is frequently stated that the blood *threshold* for the appearance of glucose in the urine is approximately 180 mg/dl.

The loss of glucose in the urine causes *diuresis,* which means loss of an excessive amount of water in the urine, because of the osmotic effect of glucose in the tubules to prevent tubular reabsorption of water. The overall effect is dehydration of the extracellular space, which then causes dehydration of the intracellular spaces as well. Thus, one of the important features of diabetes is a tendency for extracellular and intracellular dehydration to develop, and these states are often associated with collapse of the circulation.

Acidosis in Diabetes. The shift from carbohydrate to fat metabolism in diabetes has already been discussed. When the body depends almost entirely on fat for energy, the level of acetoacetic acid (and β-hydroxybutyric acid, a derivative of acetoacetic acid) in the body fluids may rise from 1 mEq/liter to as high as 10 mEq/liter. This is obviously likely to result in acidosis.

Obviously, all the usual reactions that occur in metabolic acidosis take place in diabetic acidosis, including *rapid and deep breathing.* But, most important of all, the acidosis can lead to *coma* and death, as discussed later.

Treatment of Diabetes

The theory of treatment of diabetes mellitus is based on the administration of enough insulin to enable the patient's metabolism of carbohydrate, fat, and protein to be as nearly normal as possible. Optimal therapy can prevent most acute effects of diabetes and can greatly delay the chronic effects as well.

Ordinarily, the severely diabetic patient is given a single dose of a long-acting insulin (a preparation that releases insulin slowly) each day; this increases overall carbohydrate metabolism throughout the day. Then additional quantities of regular insulin (a short-acting preparation lasting only a few hours) are given at those times of the day when the blood glucose level tends to rise too high — meal times, for example. Thus each patient is established on an individualized routine of treatment.

Diet of the Diabetic. The insulin requirements of a diabetic are established with the patient on a standard diet containing normal, well-controlled amounts of carbohydrates, for any change in the quantity of carbohydrate intake changes the requirements for insulin. In a normal person, the pancreas has the ability to adjust the quantity of insulin produced to the intake of carbohydrate; but in the completely diabetic person, this control function has been totally lost.

In the obesity type of diabetes, the disease can often be controlled by weight reduction alone. The decreased fat reduces the insulin requirements, and the pancreas can then often supply the need.

Relationship of Treatment to Arteriosclerosis. Diabetic patients have an extremely strong tendency to develop atherosclerosis, arteriosclerosis, severe coronary heart disease, and multiple microcirculatory lesions. Indeed, those who have relatively poorly controlled diabetes throughout childhood are likely to die of heart disease in their twenties.

In the early days of treating diabetes, the tendency was to reduce drastically the carbohydrates in the diet so that the insulin requirements would be minimized. This procedure kept the blood sugar level down to normal values and prevented loss of glucose in the urine, but it did not prevent the abnormalities of fat metabolism, especially the atherosclerosis. Consequently, the tendency at present is to allow the patient an almost normal carbohydrate diet and then to give simultaneously large quantities of insulin to metabolize the carbohydrates. This depresses the rate of fat metabolism and also depresses the high level of blood cholesterol that occurs in diabetes as a result of abnormal fat metabolism.

Because the complications of diabetes — such as atherosclerosis, greatly increased susceptibility to infection, diabetic retinopathy, cataracts, hypertension, and chronic renal disease — are more closely associated with the level of the blood lipids than with the level of blood glucose, it is the object of many clinics treating diabetes to administer sufficient glucose and insulin to bring the concentrations of the blood lipids near to normal.

Diabetic Coma

If diabetes is not controlled satisfactorily, severe dehydration and acidosis may result; sometimes, even when the person is receiving treatment, sporadic changes in metabolic rates of the cells, such as might occur during bouts of fever, can also precipitate dehydration and acidosis.

If the pH of the body fluids falls below approximately 7.0, the diabetic person develops coma. Also, in addition to the acidosis, dehydration is believed to exacerbate the coma. Once the diabetic person reaches this stage, the outcome is usually fatal unless immediate treatment is provided. Indeed, instead of the 60 to 80 units of insulin per day usually necessary for control of severe diabetes, several times this much insulin must often be given the first day of treatment of coma.

Administration of insulin often will not by itself reverse the abnormal physiology in diabetic coma. In addition, it is usually necessary to correct both the dehydration and acidosis immediately. The dehydration is ordinarily corrected by rapidly administering large quantities of sodium chloride solution, and the acidosis is often corrected by administering sodium bicarbonate or sodium lactate solution.

REFERENCES

Baskin, D. G., et al.: Insulin in the brain. Annu. Rev. Physiol., 49:335, 1987.

Camerini-Davalos, R. A., and Cole, H. S.: Prediabetes. New York, Plenum Publishing Corp., 1988.

DeGroot, L. J. (ed.): Endocrinology. 2nd ed. Philadelphia, W. B. Saunders Co., 1989.

Felig, P., et al. (eds.): Endocrinology and Metabolism. 2nd ed. New York, McGraw-Hill Book Co., 1987.

Goren, H. J., et al.: Insulin Action and Diabetes. New York, Raven Press, 1988.

Krall, L. P., and Beaser, R.: Joslin Diabetes Manual. 12th ed. Philadelphia, Lea & Febiger, 1989.

Meisler, M. H., and Howard, G.: Effects of insulin on gene transcription. Annu. Rev. Physiol., 51:701, 1989.

Nishimoto, I., and Kojima, J.: Calcium signalling system triggered by insulin-like growth factor II. News Physiol. Sci., 4:94, 1989.

Prentki, M., and Matschinsky, F. M.: Ca^{2+}-cAMP, and phospholipid-derived messengers in coupling mechanisms of insulin secretion. Physiol. Rev., 67:1185, 1987.

Sonne, O.: Receptor-mediated endocytosis and degradation of insulin. Physiol. Rev., 68:1129, 1988.

Standaert, M. L., and Pollet, R. J.: Insulin-glycerolipid mediators and gene expression. FASEB J., 2:2453, 1988.

QUESTIONS

1. Give the physiologic anatomy of the pancreas for secreting the pancreatic hormones.
2. What is the chemical nature of *insulin?*
3. Explain the effect of insulin on glucose uptake by the liver and later release from the liver back into the blood.
4. Explain the role of insulin in increasing the utilization of glucose by muscle. How does insulin increase *membrane transport* of glucose?
5. What is the effect of insulin on glucose uptake by the brain?
6. Explain the effect of insulin on *storage of fat* in the adipose tissues.
7. Explain the effects of *lack of insulin* on the *release of fatty acids* from the fat tissues as well as on the *increase in plasma lipid concentrations.*
8. How does insulin promote *growth,* and why does *insulin lack* cause *protein depletion* in the cells and weakness of muscles?
9. Explain the control of insulin secretion by the blood glucose concentration.
10. What other factors help control insulin secretion?
11. Explain the important role of insulin for switching between carbohydrate and lipid metabolism.
12. Explain the *cascade method* by which extremely minute quantities of *glucagon* can cause marked release of glucose from the liver.
13. Explain the factors that control glucagon secretion.
14. Discuss the overall integration of the different hormonal and metabolic systems in the control of blood glucose concentration.
15. In *diabetes* what happens to the following factors: blood glucose concentration, rate of urine excretion, concentration of glucose in the urine, acid-base balance of the body fluids, blood concentration of cholesterol and other lipids, and state of body hydration?
16. What is the basic goal of current treatment of diabetes, and how is this achieved by the use of diet, *short-acting insulin,* and *long-acting insulin?*
17. What are the characteristics of *diabetic coma,* and what is the physiology of its treatment?

53

Parathyroid Hormone, Calcitonin, Calcium and Phosphate Metabolism, Vitamin D, Bone, and Teeth

The physiology of both parathyroid hormone and the hormone calcitonin is closely related to calcium and phosphate metabolism, the function of vitamin D, and the formation of bone and teeth. Therefore these are discussed together in the present chapter.

CALCIUM AND PHOSPHATE IN EXTRACELLULAR FLUID AND PLASMA —FUNCTION OF VITAMIN D

Absorption of Calcium and Phosphate

By far the major sources of calcium in the diet are milk and milk products, which are also major sources of phosphate, but phosphate is also present in many other dietary foods, including especially the meats.

Calcium is poorly absorbed from the intestinal tract because of the relative insolubility of many of its compounds and also because bivalent cations are poorly absorbed through the intestinal mucosa. On the other hand, phosphate is absorbed exceedingly well most of the time except when excess calcium is in the diet; the calcium tends to form almost insoluble calcium phosphate compounds in the intestines that fail to be absorbed but instead pass on through the bowels to be excreted in the feces. In other words, the major problem in the absorption of calcium and phosphate is actually a problem of calcium absorption alone, for if this is absorbed, phosphate will also be absorbed.

About seven eighths of the daily intake of calcium is not absorbed and therefore is excreted in the feces; the remaining one eighth is eventually excreted in the urine.

Vitamin D and Its Role in Calcium Absorption

Vitamin D has a potent effect in increasing calcium absorption from the intestinal tract; it also has important effects on both bone deposition and bone reabsorption, as will be discussed later in the chapter. However, vitamin D itself is not the active substance that actually causes these effects. Instead, the vitamin D must first be converted through a succession of reactions in the liver and the kidney to the final active product, *1,25-dihydroxycholecalciferol.* Figure 53–1 illustrates the succession of steps that leads to the formation of this substance from vitamin D. Some of the important features of this schema are the following:

The Vitamin D Compounds. Several different compounds derived from sterols belong to the vitamin D family, and they all perform more or less the same functions. The most important of them is *cholecalciferol,* called vitamin D_3. Most of this substance is formed in the skin as a result of irradiation of *7-dehydrocholesterol* by ultraviolet light from the sun. Consequently, appropriate exposure to the sun prevents vitamin D deficiency.

Conversion of Cholecalciferol to 25-Hydroxycholecalciferol in the Liver and Its Feedback Control. The first step in the activation of cholecalciferol is to convert it to 25-hydroxycholecal-

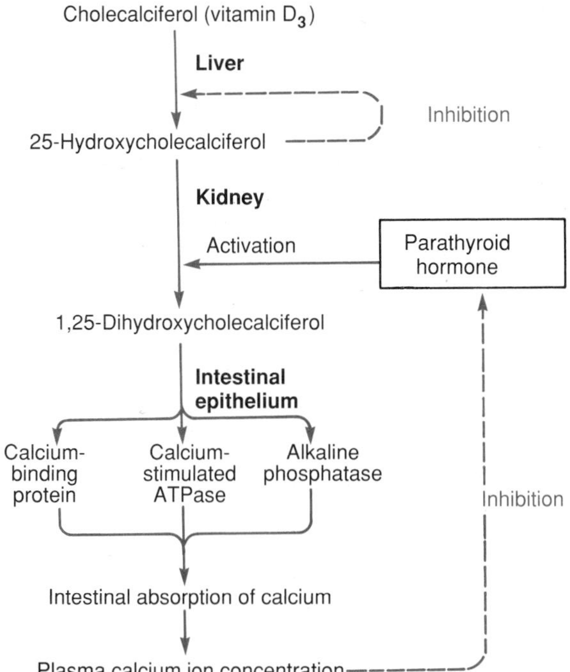

Figure 53-1. Activation of vitamin D_3 to form *1,25-dihydroxycholecalciferol;* and the role of vitamin D in controlling the plasma calcium concentration.

ciferol; this conversion occurs in the liver. The process, however, is a limited one, because the 25-hydroxycholecalciferol itself has a feedback inhibitory effect on the conversion reactions. This feedback effect is extremely important for two reasons.

First, the feedback mechanism regulates very precisely the concentration of 25-hydroxycholecalciferol in the plasma. The intake of vitamin D_3 can change as much as a hundredfold, and yet the concentration of 25-hydroxycholecalciferol still remains within a few percentage points of its normal mean value. Obviously, this high degree of feedback control prevents excessive action of vitamin D_3 when it is present in too high a concentration in the diet.

Second, this controlled conversion of vitamin D_3 to 25-hydroxycholecalciferol conserves the vitamin D_3 for future use, because once converted, it persists in the body for only a short time, whereas in the vitamin D_3 form it can be stored in the liver for as long as several months.

Formation of 1,25-Dihydroxycholecalciferol in the Kidneys and Its Control by Parathyroid Hormone. Figure 53-1 illustrates that 25-hydroxycholecalciferol is converted in the kidneys to 1,25-dihydroxycholecalciferol. This latter substance is the active form of vitamin D; none of the previous products in the schema of Figure 53-1 have very much vitamin D effect. Therefore in the absence of the kidneys, vitamin D is almost totally ineffective.

Note also in Figure 53-1 that the conversion of 25-hydroxycholecalciferol to 1,25-dihydroxycholecalciferol requires parathyroid hormone. In the absence of this hormone, either none or almost none of the 1,25-dihydroxycholecalciferol is formed. Therefore, parathyroid hormone exerts a potent effect in determining the functional effects of vitamin D in the body, specifically its effects on calcium absorption in the intestines and its effect on bone.

Hormonal Effect of 1,25-Dihydroxycholecalciferol on the Intestinal Epithelium in Promoting Calcium Absorption. 1,25-Dihydroxycholecalciferol has several effects on the intestinal epithelium in promoting intestinal absorption of calcium. Probably the most important of these effects is that it causes formation of a *calcium-binding protein* in the intestinal epithelial cells. The rate of calcium absorption seems to be directly proportional to the quantity of this calcium-binding protein. Furthermore, this protein remains in the cells for several weeks after the 1,25-dihydroxycholecalciferol has been removed from the body, thus causing a prolonged effect on calcium absorption.

Other effects of 1,25-dihydroxycholecalciferol that might play a role in promoting calcium absorption are (1) the formation of a calcium-stimulated ATPase in the brush border of the epithelial cells and (2) the formation of an alkaline phosphatase in the epithelial cells. Unfortunately, the precise details of calcium absorption are still unknown.

Feedback Effect of Calcium Ion Concentration on the Formation of 1,25-Dihydroxycholecalciferol. Later in the chapter we shall see that the rate of secretion of parathyroid hormone is controlled almost entirely and very potently by the plasma calcium ion concentration. When the calcium ion concentration rises, this immediately inhibits parathyroid hormone secretion; in the absence of this hormone, 1,25-dihydroxycholecalciferol cannot be formed in the kidneys. Thus, this is a *negative* feedback mechanism for control of the plasma concentration of 1,25-dihydroxycholecalciferol and also of the plasma calcium ion concentration. That is, an increase in the calcium ion concentration decreases parathyroid secretion, which decreases 1,25-dihydroxycholecalciferol, which decreases the absorption of calcium from the intestinal tract, and thus returns the calcium ion concentration to its normal value.

Calcium in Plasma and Interstitial Fluid

The concentration of calcium in plasma is approximately 9.4 mg/dl, normally varying between 9.0 and 10.0 mg/dl; this is equivalent to approximately 2.4 millimoles per liter. It is apparent from these limits that the calcium level in the plasma is regulated within narrow limits, and mainly by parathyroid hormone, as discussed later in the chapter.

The calcium in the plasma is present in three different forms, as shown in Figure 53-2. (1) Approximately 40 per cent of the calcium is combined with the plasma proteins and consequently is not diffusible through the capillary membrane. (2) Approximately 10 per cent of the calcium (0.2 mmol per liter) is diffusible through the capillary membrane but is combined with other substances of the plasma and interstitial

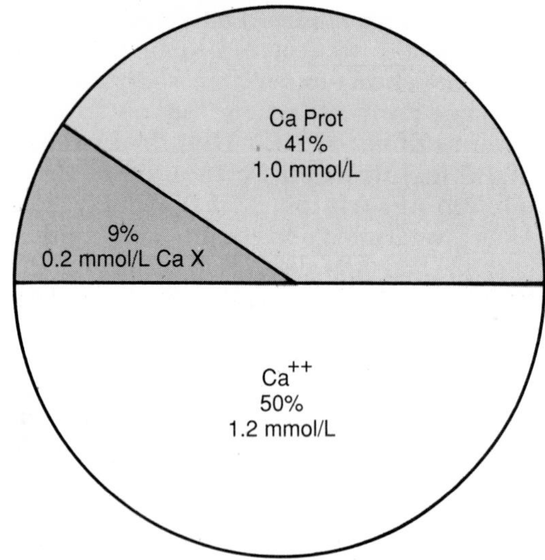

Figure 53-2. Distribution of ionic calcium *(Ca^{--})*, diffusible but un-ionized calcium *(Ca X)*, and nondiffusible calcium proteinate *(Ca Prot)* in blood plasma.

fluids (citrate and phosphate, for instance) in such a manner that it is not ionized. (3) The remaining 50 per cent of the calcium in the plasma is both diffusible through the capillary membrane and ionized. Thus, the plasma and interstitial fluids have a normal *calcium ion concentration of approximately 1.2 mmol per liter.* This ionic calcium is important for most functions of calcium in the body, including its effect on the heart, on the nervous system, and on bone formation.

Inorganic Phosphate in Extracellular Fluids

Inorganic phosphate in the plasma is mainly in two forms: HPO_4^{--} and $H_2PO_4^-$. The concentration of both of these together is approximately 1.3 mmol per liter. Because it is difficult to determine chemically the exact ratio of HPO_4^{--} to $H_2PO_4^-$ in the blood, ordinarily the total quantity of phosphate is expressed in terms of milligrams of *phosphorus* per dl of blood. The average total quantity of inorganic phosphorus represented by both phosphate ions is about 4 mg per dl.

Effects of Abnormal Calcium Concentration in the Body Fluids

Tetany Resulting from Hypocalcemia. When the extracellular fluid concentration of calcium ions falls below normal, the nervous system becomes progressively more excitable because of increased neuronal membrane permeability. Especially, the peripheral nerve fibers become so excitable that they begin to discharge spontaneously, initiating nerve impulses that pass to the peripheral skeletal muscles, where they elicit tetanic contraction. Consequently, hypocalcemia causes tetany.

Figure 53-3 illustrates tetany in the hand, which usually occurs before generalized tetany all over the body develops. This is called *carpopedal spasm.*

Acute hypocalcemia in the human being ordinarily causes essentially no other significant effects besides tetany, because tetany kills the patient before other effects can develop. Tetany ordinarily occurs when the blood concentration of calcium falls from its normal level of 9.4 mg to approximately 6 mg per dl, which is only 35 per cent below the normal calcium concentration, and it is usually lethal at about 4 mg per dl.

In experimental animals, in which the level of calcium can be reduced beyond the normal lethal stage, extreme hypocalcemia can cause marked dilatation of the heart, changes in cellular enzyme activities, increased cell membrane permeability in other cells besides nerve cells, and impaired blood clotting.

Hypercalcemia. When the level of calcium in the body fluids rises above normal, the nervous system is depressed, and reflex activities of the central nervous system becomes sluggish. Also, increased calcium ion concentration causes constipation and lack of appetite, probably because of depressed contractility of the muscular walls of the gastrointestinal tract. The depressive effects of an increased calcium level begin to appear when the blood level of calcium rises above approximately 12 mg per dl, and they can become marked as the calcium level rises above 15 mg per dl. When the level of calcium rises above approximately 17 mg per dl in the body fluids, calcium phosphate is likely to precipitate throughout the blood and soft tissues, an effect that can be rapidly lethal.

BONE AND ITS RELATIONSHIPS WITH EXTRACELLULAR CALCIUM AND PHOSPHATES

Bone is composed of a tough *organic matrix* that is greatly strengthened by deposits of *calcium salts.* Average *compact bone* contains by weight approximately 30 per cent matrix and 70 per cent salts. How-

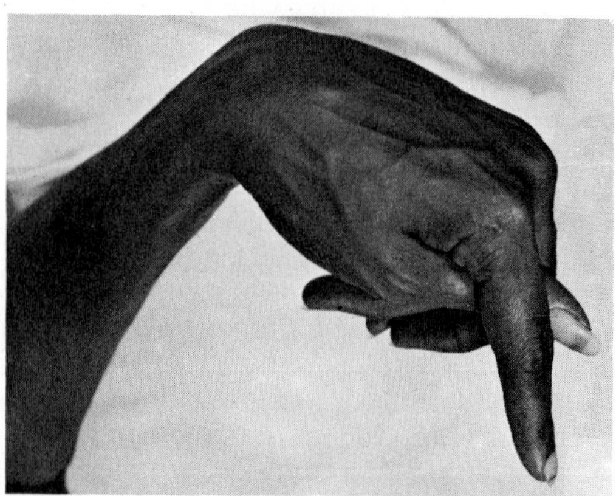

Figure 53-3. Hypocalcemic tetany in the hand, called "carpopedal spasm." (Courtesy of Dr. Herbert Langford.)

ever, *newly formed bone* may have a considerably higher percentage of matrix in relation to salts.

The Organic Matrix of Bone. The organic matrix of bone is 90 to 95 per cent *collagen fibers,* and the remainder is a homogeneous medium called *ground substance.* The collagen fibers extend primarily along the lines of tensional force. These fibers give bone its great tensile strength.

The ground substance is composed of extracellular fluid plus *proteoglycans,* especially *chondroitin sulfate* and *hyaluronic acid.* The precise function of these is not known, though perhaps they help to control the deposition of calcium salts.

The Bone Salts. The crystalline salts deposited in the organic matrix of bone are composed principally of *calcium* and *phosphate,* and the formula for the major crystalline salt, known as *hydroxyapatite,* is $Ca_{10}(PO_4)_6(OH)_2$. Each crystal—about 400 angstroms long, 10 to 30 angstroms thick, and 100 angstroms wide—is shaped like a long, flat plate. The relative ratio of calcium to phosphorus can vary markedly under different nutritional conditions, the Ca/P ratio on a weight basis varying between 1.3 and 2.0.

Magnesium, sodium, potassium, and *carbonate* ions are also present among the bone salts, though x-ray diffraction studies fail to show definite crystals formed by them. Therefore, they are believed to be adsorbed to the surfaces of the hydroxyapatite crystals rather than organized into distinct crystals of their own. This ability of many different types of ions to adsorb to bone crystals extends to many ions normally foreign to bone, such as *strontium, uranium, plutonium* and the *other transuranic elements, lead, gold, other heavy metals,* and *at least 9 of 14 of the major radioactive products released by explosion of the hydrogen bomb.* Deposition of radioactive substances in bone can cause prolonged irradiation of the bone tissues, and if a sufficient amount is deposited, an osteogenic cancer almost invariably eventually develops.

Tensile and Compressional Strength of Bone. Each collagen fiber of bone is composed of repeating periodic segments every 640 angstroms along its length; hydroxyapatite crystals lie adjacent to each segment of the fiber bound tightly to it. This intimate bonding prevents the crystals and collagen fibers from slipping out of place, which is essential in providing strength to the bone. In addition, the segments of adjacent collagen fibers overlap each other, also causing the hydroxyapatite crystals to be overlapped like bricks keyed to each other in a brick wall.

The collagen fibers of bone, like those of tendons, have great tensile strength, while the calcium salts, which are similar in physical properties to marble, have great compressional strength. These combined properties, plus the degree of bondage between the collagen fibers and the crystals, provide a bony structure that has both extreme tensile and compressional strength. Thus, bones are constructed in exactly the same way that reinforced concrete is constructed. The steel of reinforced concrete provides the tensile strength, while the cement, sand, and rock provide the compressional strength. Indeed, the compressional strength of bone is greater than, and the tensile strength approaches, that of reinforced concrete.

PRECIPITATION AND ABSORPTION OF CALCIUM AND PHOSPHATE IN BONE —EQUILIBRIUM WITH THE EXTRACELLULAR FLUIDS

Supersaturated State of Calcium and Phosphate Ions in Extracellular Fluids with Respect to Hydroxyapatite. The concentrations of calcium and phosphate ions in extracellular fluid are considerably greater than those required to cause precipitation of hydroxyapatite. However, because of the large number of ions required to form a single molecule of hydroxyapatite, it is very difficult for all of these ions to come together simultaneously. Therefore, hydroxyapatite crystals fail to precipitate in tissues other than bone, despite the state of supersaturation of the ions.

Mechanism of Bone Calcification. The initial stage of bone production is the secretion of collagen and ground substance by the *osteoblasts.* The collagen polymerizes rapidly to form collagen fibers, and the resultant tissue becomes *osteoid,* a cartilage-like material but differing from cartilage in that calcium salts precipitate in it. As the osteoid is formed, some osteoblasts become entrapped in it, and these are called *osteocytes.*

Within a few days after the osteoid is formed, calcium salts begin to precipitate on the surfaces of the collagen fibers. The precipitates appear at periodic intervals along each collagen fiber, forming minute nidi that gradually over a period of days and weeks grow into the finished product, *hydroxyapatite crystals.*

The initial calcium salts to be deposited are not hydroxyapatite crystals but amorphous compounds (noncrystalline), probably a mixture of such salts as $CaHPO_4 \cdot 2H_2O$, $Ca_3(PO_4)_2 \cdot 3H_2O$, and others. Then by a process of substitution and addition of atoms, these salts are reshaped into the hydroxyapatite crystals.

It is still not known what causes calcium salts to be deposited in osteoid. One theory holds that at the time of formation the collagen fibers are specially constituted in advance for causing precipitation of calcium salts. It is also believed that the osteoblasts secrete a substance into the osteoid to neutralize an inhibitor that normally prevents hydroxyapatite crystallization. Once the inhibitor has been neutralized, the natural affinity of the collagen fibers for calcium salts supposedly causes the precipitation. In support of this theory is the fact that properly prepared collagen fibers from other tissues of the body as well as bone will also cause precipitation of hydroxyapatite crystals from plasma.

Exchangeable Calcium

If soluble calcium salts are injected intravenously, the calcium ion concentration can be made to increase immediately to very high levels. However, within 30 minutes to an hour or so, the calcium ion concentration returns to normal. Likewise, if large quantities of calcium ions are removed from the circulating body fluids, the calcium ion concentration again returns to normal within 30 minutes to an hour or so. These effects result from the fact that the bone and other body tissues contain a type of *exchangeable* calcium that is always in equilibrium with the calcium ions in the extracellular fluids. Most of this exchangeable calcium is in the bone, and it normally amounts to about 0.4 to 1.0 per cent of the total bone calcium. Most of this calcium is probably readily mobilizable salts such as $CaHPO_4$ and the other amorphous salts.

The importance of exchangeable calcium to the body is that it provides a rapid buffering mechanism to keep the calcium ion concentration in the extracellular fluids from rising to excessive levels or falling to very low levels under transient conditions of excess or diminished availability of calcium.

Deposition and Absorption of Bone—Remodeling of Bone

Deposition of Bone by the Osteoblasts. Bone is continually being deposited by *osteoblasts,* and it is continually being absorbed where *osteoclasts* are active. Osteoblasts are found on the outer surfaces of the bones and in the bone cavities, as illustrated in Figure 53-4. A small amount of osteoblastic activity occurs continually in all living bones (on about 4 per cent of all surfaces in adult bone), so that at least some new bone is being formed constantly.

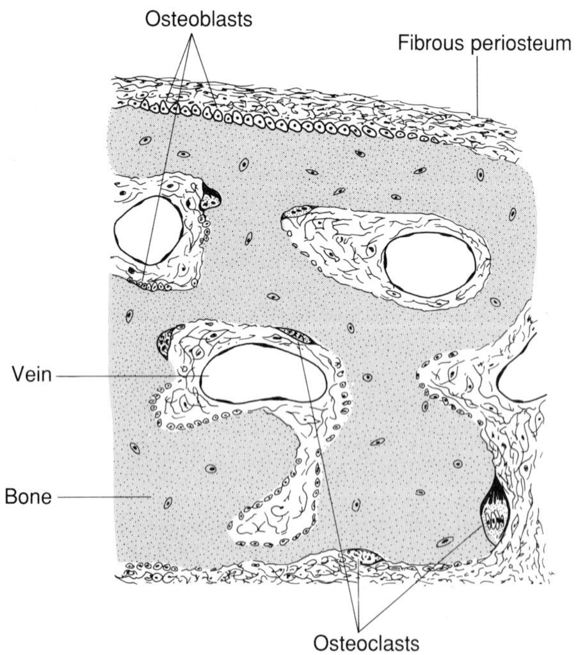

Figure 53-4. Osteoblastic and osteoclastic activity in the same bone.

Absorption of Bone—Function of the Osteoclasts. Bone is also being continually absorbed in the presence of osteoclasts, which are normally active at any one time on about 1 per cent of the bone surfaces. Later in this chapter we will see that parathyroid hormone controls the bone absorptive activity of osteoclasts.

Histologically, bone absorption occurs immediately adjacent to the osteoclasts, as illustrated in Figure 53-4. The mechanism of this absorption is believed to be the following: The osteoclasts send out villus-like projections toward the bone and from these "villi" secrete two types of substances: (1) proteolytic enzymes, released from the lysosomes of the osteoclasts, and (2) several acids, including citric acid and lactic acid. The enzymes presumably digest or dissolute the organic matrix of the bone, while the acids cause solution of the bone salts.

Equilibrium Between Bone Deposition and Absorption. Normally, except in growing bones, the rates of bone deposition and absorption are equal to each other, so that the total mass of bone remains constant. Usually, osteoclasts exist in small masses, and once a mass of osteoclasts begins to develop, it usually eats away at the bone for about 3 weeks, eating out a tunnel that may be as great as 1 mm in diameter and several mm in length. At the end of this time, the osteoclasts disappear, and the tunnel is invaded by osteoblasts instead. Bone deposition then occurs for several months, the new bone being laid down in successive layers on the inner surfaces of the cavity until the tunnel is filled. Deposition of new bone ceases when the bone begins to encroach on the blood vessels supplying the area. The canal through which these vessels run, called the *haversian canal,* therefore, is all that remains of the original cavity. Each new area of bone deposited in this way is called an *osteon,* shown in Figure 53-5.

Value of Continual Remodeling of Bone. The continual deposition and absorption of bone have a number of physiologically important functions. First, bone ordinarily adjusts its strength in proportion to the degree of bone stress. Consequently, bones thicken when subjected to heavy loads. Second, even the shape of the bone can be rearranged for proper support of mechanical forces by deposition and absorption of bone in accordance with stress patterns. Third, new organic matrix is needed as the old organic matrix degenerates. In this manner the normal toughness of bone is maintained. Indeed, the bones of children, in whom the rate of deposition and absorption is rapid, show little brittleness in comparison with the bones of old age, at which time the rates of deposition and absorption are slow.

Control of the Rate of Bone Deposition by Bone Stress. Bone is deposited in proportion to the compressional load that the bone must carry. For instance, the bones of athletes become considerably heavier than those of nonathletes. Also, if a person has one leg in a cast but continues to walk on the

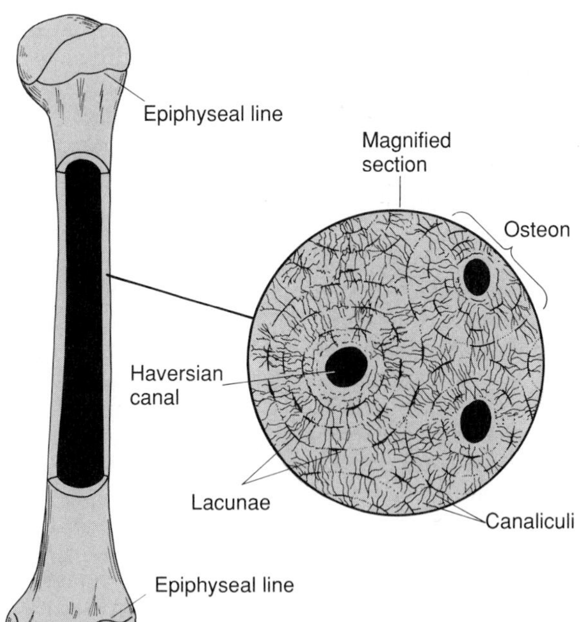

Figure 53-5. The structure of bone.

opposite leg, the bone of the leg in the cast becomes thin and decalcified, while the opposite bone remains thick and normally calcified. Therefore, continual physical stress stimulates osteoblastic deposition of bone.

The deposition of bone at points of compressional stress has been suggested to be caused by a *piezo-electric* effect, as follows: Compression of bone causes a negative potential at the compressed site and a position potential elsewhere in the bone. It has been shown that minute quantities of current flowing in bone cause osteoblastic activity at the negative end of the current flow, which could explain the increased bone deposition at compression sites.

Repair of a Fracture. A fracture of a bone in some way maximally activates all the periosteal and intraosseous osteoblasts involved in the break. Immense numbers of new osteoblasts are formed almost immediately from *osteoprogenitor cells,* which are bone stem cells. Therefore, within a short time a large bulge of osteoblastic tissue and new organic bone matrix, followed shortly by the deposition of calcium salts, develops between the two broken ends of the bone. This is called a *callus.* It is reshaped into an appropriate structural bone during the ensuing months.

PARATHYROID HORMONE

For many years it has been known that increased activity of the parathyroid gland causes rapid absorption of calcium salts from the bones with resultant hypercalcemia in the extracellular fluid; conversely, hypofunction of the parathyroid glands causes hypocalcemia, often with resultant tetany, as described earlier in the chapter. Also, parathyroid hormone is important in phosphate metabolism as well as in calcium metabolism.

Physiological Anatomy of the Parathyroid Glands. Normally there are four parathyroid glands in the human being; these are located immediately behind the thyroid gland—one behind each of the upper and each of the lower poles of the thyroid. Each parathyroid gland is approximately 6 mm long, 3 mm wide, and 2 mm thick and has a macroscopic appearance of dark brown fat; for this reason the parathyroid glands are difficult to locate.

Removal of half the parathyroid glands usually causes little physiological abnormality. However, removal of three of four normal glands usually causes transient hypoparathyroidism. But even a small quantity of remaining parathyroid tissue is usually capable of enough hypertrophy to perform the function of all the glands.

The parathyroid gland of the adult human being, illustrated in Figure 53-6, contains mainly *chief cells* and *oxyphil cells,* but oxyphil cells are absent in many animals and in young humans. The chief cells secrete most of the parathyroid hormone. The function of the oxyphil cells is not certain; they are believed to be aged chief cells that no longer secrete hormone.

Chemistry of Parathyroid Hormone. Parathyroid hormone has been isolated in a pure form. It is a small protein with a molecular weight of approximately 9500 and is composed of a polypeptide chain of 84 amino acids.

Effect of Parathyroid Hormone on Calcium and Phosphate Concentrations in Extracellular Fluid

Figure 53-7 illustrates the effects on blood calcium and phosphate concentrations caused by suddenly beginning to infuse parathyroid hormone into an animal and continuing the infusion for an indefinite period of time. Note that at the onset of infusion the calcium ion concentration begins to rise and reaches a plateau level in about 4 hours. On the other hand, the phosphate concentration falls and reaches a depressed plateau level within an hour or two. The rise in calcium concentration is caused principally by (1) a direct effect of parathyroid hormone in causing cal-

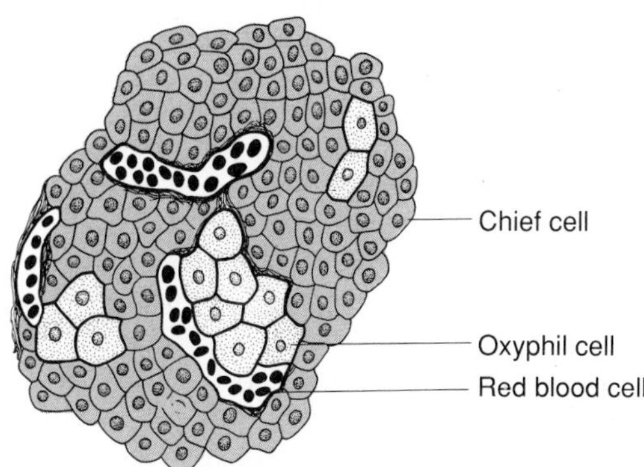

Figure 53-6. Histological structure of a parathyroid gland.

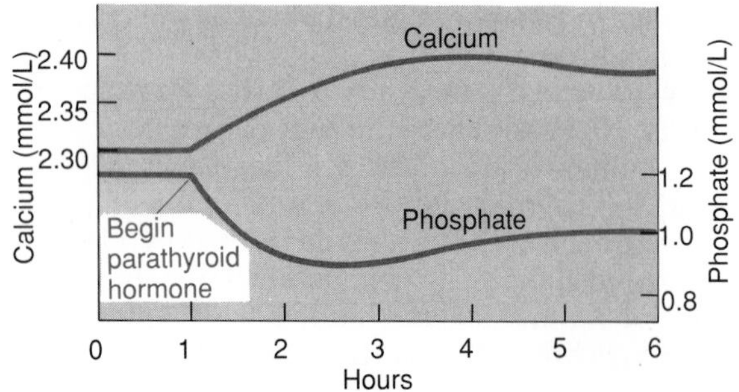

Figure 53-7. Approximate changes in calcium and phosphate concentrations during the first 5 hours of parathyroid hormone infusion at a moderate rate.

cium and phosphate absorption from the bone and (2) an effect on the kidneys to decrease the excretion of calcium in the urine. The decline in phosphate concentration, on the other hand, is caused by a very strong effect of parathyroid hormone on the kidney, resulting in excessive renal phosphate excretion that is usually great enough to override the increased phosphate absorption from the bone.

Calcium and Phosphate Absorption from Bone Caused by Parathyroid Hormone

Parathyroid hormone seems to have two separate effects on bone in causing absorption of calcium and phosphate. One effect, very rapid, takes place in minutes and probably results from activation of the already existing bone cells to promote the calcium and phosphate absorption. The second phase is a much slower one, requiring several days or even weeks to become fully developed, and it results from the proliferation of osteoclasts, followed by greatly increased osteoclastic reabsorption of the bone itself, not merely absorption of calcium phosphate salts from the bone.

The Rapid Phase of Calcium and Phosphate Absorption—Osteolysis. When large quantities of parathyroid hormone are injected, the calcium ion concentration in the blood begins to rise within minutes, long before any new bone cells can be developed. Histological studies have shown that the parathyroid hormone causes removal of bone salts from the bone matrix in the vicinity of the osteocytes lying within the bone itself and also in the vicinity of the osteoblasts along the bone surface. Yet, strangely enough, one does not usually think of either osteoblasts or osteocytes functioning to cause bone salt absorption, because both these types of cells are osteoblastic in nature and are normally associated with bone deposition and its calcification. However, recent studies have shown that the osteoblasts and osteocytes form a system of interconnected cells that spreads over all the bone surfaces except the small surface areas that are adjacent to the osteoclasts. Also, long filmy processes extend from osteocyte to osteocyte throughout the bone structure, and these processes also connect with the surface osteocytes and osteoblasts. This extensive system is called the *osteocytic membrane system,* and it is believed to provide a membrane that separates the bone itself from the extracellular fluid. Between the osteocytic membrane and the bone is a small amount of fluid called simply *bone fluid.* Indirect experiments suggest that the osteocytic membrane pumps calcium ions from the bone fluid into the extracellular fluid, creating a calcium ion concentration in the bone fluid only one third of that in the extracellular fluid. When the osteocytic pump becomes excessively activated, the bone fluid calcium concentration falls even lower, and calcium phosphate salts are then absorbed from the bone. This effect is called *osteolysis,* and it occurs without absorption of the bone matrix. When the pump is inactivated, the bone fluid calcium concentration rises to a higher level, and calcium phosphate salts are then redeposited in the matrix.

But where does parathyroid hormone fit into this picture? It seems that parathyroid hormone can strongly activate the calcium pump, thereby causing rapid removal of calcium phosphate salts from the amorphous bone crystals that lie near the osteocytic membrane. The parathyroid hormone is believed to stimulate calcium absorption by increasing the calcium permeability of the bone fluid side of the osteocytic membrane, thus allowing calcium ions to diffuse into the cells from the bone fluid. Then the calcium pump on the other side of the cell membrane transfers the calcium ions the rest of the way into the extracellular fluid.

The Slow Phase of Bone Absorption and Calcium Phosphate Release—Activation of the Osteoclasts. A much better-known effect of parathyroid hormone is activation of the osteoclasts. These in turn set about their usual task of gobbling up the bone.

Activation of the osteoclastic system occurs in two stages: (1) immediate activation of the osteoclasts that are already formed and (2) formation of new osteoclasts. Usually, several days of excess parathyroid hormone cause the osteoclastic system to become well developed, but it can continue to grow for literally months under the influence of very strong parathyroid hormone stimulation.

Bone contains such great amounts of calcium in comparison with the total amount in all the extracellular fluids (about 1000 times as much) that even when parathyroid hormone causes a great rise in calcium concentration in the fluids, it is impossible to discern any immediate effect at all on the bones. Yet prolonged administration or secretion of parathyroid hormone finally results in evident absorption in all the bones with development of large cavities filled with very large, multinucleated osteoclasts.

Effect of Parathyroid Hormone on Phosphate and Calcium Excretion by the Kidneys

Administration of parathyroid hormone causes immediate and rapid loss of phosphate in the urine. This effect is caused by diminished renal tubular reabsorption of phosphate ions.

Parathyroid hormone also causes renal tubular *reabsorption* of calcium at the same time that it diminishes phosphate reabsorption. Were it not for this effect of parathyroid hormone on the kidneys to increase calcium reabsorption, the continual loss of calcium into the urine would eventually deplete the bones of this mineral.

Effect of Vitamin D on Bone and Its Relation to Parathyroid Activity

Vitamin D plays important roles in both bone absorption and bone deposition. Administration of extreme quantities of vitamin D causes absorption of bone in much the same way that administration of parathyroid hormone does. Also, in the absence of vitamin D, the effect of parathyroid hormone in causing bone absorption is greatly reduced or even prevented. Therefore, it is possible, if not likely, that parathyroid hormone functions in bone the same way that it functions in the kidneys and intestines—that is, by causing the conversion of vitamin D to 1,25-dihydroxycholecalciferol, which in turn acts to cause the bone absorption.

Vitamin D in much smaller amounts promotes bone calcification. Obviously, one of the ways in which it does so is to increase calcium and phosphate absorption from the intestines. However, even in the absence of such increase, it still enhances the mineralization of bone. Here again, the mechanism of the effect is unknown, but it probably results from the ability of 1,25-dihydroxycholecalciferol to cause transport of calcium ions through cell membranes—perhaps through the osteoblastic or osteocytic cell membranes.

Control of Parathyroid Secretion by Calcium Ion Concentration

Even the slightest decrease in calcium ion concentration in the extracellular fluid causes the parathyroid glands to increase their rate of secretion and eventually to hypertrophy. For instance, the parathyroid glands become greatly enlarged in *rickets,* in which the level of calcium is usually depressed only a few per cent; they also become greatly enlarged in pregnancy, even though the decrease in calcium ion concentration in the mother's extracellular fluid is hardly measurable; and they are greatly enlarged during lactation because calcium is used for milk formation.

On the other hand, any condition that increases the calcium ion concentration causes decreased activity and reduced size of the parathyroid glands. Such conditions include (1) excess quantities of calcium in the diet, (2) increased vitamin D in the diet, and (3) bone absorption caused by factors other than parathyroid hormone (for example, bone absorption caused by disuse of the bones).

Figure 53–8 illustrates quantitatively the relationship between plasma calcium concentration and plasma parathyroid hormone concentration. The solid curve shows the acute relationship when the calcium concentration is changed over a period of a few hours. This shows that a decrease in calcium concentration from 9.4 to 8.4 mg/dl doubles or triples the plasma parathyroid hormone. On the other hand, the approximate chronic relationship that one finds when the calcium ion concentration changes over a period of many weeks, thus allowing time for the glands to hypertrophy, is illustrated by the dashed line; this illustrates that chronically, approximately a 1 per cent decrease in calcium can give as much as a 100 per cent increase in parathyroid hormone. Obviously, this is the basis of the body's extremely potent feedback system for control of plasma calcium ion concentration.

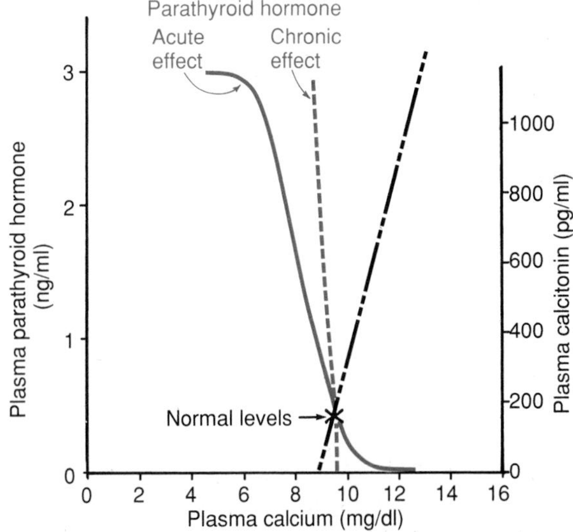

Figure 53–8. Approximate effect of plasma calcium concentration on the plasma concentrations of parathyroid hormone and calcitonin. Note especially that long-term, chronic changes of only a small percentage in calcium concentration can cause as much as 100 per cent change in parathyroid hormone concentration.

CALCITONIN

About 30 years ago, a new hormone that has *weak* effects on blood calcium opposite to those of parathyroid hormone was discovered. This hormone is named *calcitonin,* because it reduces the blood calcium ion concentration. In the human being, it is secreted not by the parathyroid glands but instead by the thyroid gland, by *parafollicular cells,* or C cells, in the interstitium between the thyroid follicles.

Calcitonin is a large polypeptide with a molecular weight of approximately 3400; it has a chain of 32 amino acids.

Effect of Calcitonin in Decreasing Plasma Calcium Concentration. In young animals, calcitonin decreases blood calcium ion concentration very rapidly, beginning within minutes after injection of the calcitonin. Thus the effect of calcitonin on blood calcium ion concentration is exactly opposite that of parathyroid hormone, and it occurs several times as rapidly.

Calcitonin reduces plasma calcium concentration in at least two separate ways:

1. The immediate effect is to decrease the absorptive activities of the osteoclasts and probably also the osteolytic effect of the osteocytic membrane throughout the bone, thus shifting the balance in favor of deposition of calcium in the rapidly exchangeable pool of bone calcium salts.
2. The second and more prolonged effect is to prevent formation of new osteoclasts.

Calcitonin has only a weak effect on plasma calcium concentration in the adult human being. The reason for this is simply that the daily rates of bone absorption and deposition of calcium are small, and the stimulatory effect of calcitonin cannot alter the rates enough to make much difference.

Effect of Plasma Calcium Concentration on the Secretion of Calcitonin

An increase in plasma calcium concentration of about 10 per cent causes an immediate three- to sixfold increase in the rate of secretion of calcitonin, which is illustrated by the dot-dash line of Figure 53-8. This provides a second hormonal feedback mechanism for controlling the plasma calcium ion concentration, but one that works exactly opposite to the parathyroid hormone system. That is, an increase in calcium concentration causes increased calcitonin secretion, and the increased calcitonin in turn reduces the plasma calcium concentration back toward normal.

However, there are two major differences between the calcitonin and the parathyroid feedback systems. First, the calcitonin mechanism operates more rapidly, reaching peak activity in less than an hour, in contrast with the 3 to 4 hours required for peak activity to be attained following the onset of parathyroid secretion.

The second difference is that the calcitonin mechanism acts mainly as a short-term regulator and has little long-term effect, month in and month out, on calcium ion concentration — contrary to the powerful long-term effect of the parathyroid hormone system. As was pointed out above, the calcitonin mechanism is a very weak one in the normal human adult, anyway. Therefore, over a prolonged period of time it is almost entirely the parathyroid system that sets the long-term level of calcium ions in the extracellular fluid.

PHYSIOLOGY OF PARATHYROID AND BONE DISEASES

Hypoparathyroidism

When the parathyroid glands do not secrete sufficient parathyroid hormone, the osteoclasts of the bone become almost totally inactive. As a result, bone reabsorption is so depressed that the level of calcium in the body fluids decreases.

If the parathyroid glands are suddenly removed, the calcium level in the blood falls from the normal of 9.4 mg/dl to 6 to 7 mg/dl within 2 to 3 days. When this level is reached, the usual signs of tetany develop. Among the muscles of the body that are especially sensitive to tetanic spasm are the laryngeal muscles. Laryngeal spasm obstructs respiration, which is a usual cause of death in tetany unless appropriate treatment is applied.

Treatment of Hypoparathyroidism

Parathyroid Hormone (Parathormone). Parathyroid hormone is occasionally used for treating hypoparathyroidism. However, because of the expense of this hormone, because its effect lasts only a few hours, and because the tendency of the body to develop immune bodies against it makes it progressively less active in the body, treatment of hypoparathyroidism with parathyroid hormone is rare in present-day therapy.

Vitamin D and Calcium Therapy. In most patients administration of extremely large quantities of vitamin D, as high as 100,000 units per day, along with 1 to 2 grams of calcium, will suffice to keep the calcium ion concentration in a normal range. At times it may be necessary to administer 1,25-dihydroxycholecalciferol instead of the nonactivated form of vitamin D because of its much more potent and rapid action, but this can also cause unwanted effects, because it is sometimes difficult to prevent overactivity by this activated form of vitamin D.

Hyperparathyroidism

The cause of hyperparathyroidism is most often a tumor in one of the parathyroid glands.

In hyperparathyroidism, extreme osteoclastic activity occurs in the bones, and this elevates the calcium ion concentration in the extracellular fluid while usually (but not always) depressing the concentration of phosphate ions because of increased renal excretion of phosphate.

In severe hyperparathyroidism, the osteoclastic absorption of bone soon far outstrips osteoblastic deposition, and the bone may be eaten away almost entirely. Indeed, often the reason a hyperparathyroid person comes to the doctor is a broken bone. X-ray films of the bones show extensive decalcification, and occasionally, large punched-out cystic areas of the bones, that are filled with osteoclasts in the form of so-called *giant cell tumors.* Obviously, multiple fractures of the weakened bones result from only slight trauma.

The obvious treatment of hyperparathyroidism is surgical removal of the parathyroid tumor, but this is a difficult procedure because these tumors are often only a few millimeters in size and are difficult to find at operation.

Rickets

Rickets occurs mainly in children as a result of calcium or phosphate deficiency *in the extracellular fluid.* Yet, ordinarily, rickets is not due to lack of calcium or phosphate in the diet but instead to a deficiency of vitamin D. However, if the child is properly exposed to sunlight, the ultraviolet rays will form enough vitamin D_3 in the skin to prevent rickets by promoting calcium and phosphate absorption from the intestines, as discussed earlier in the chapter.

Children who remain indoors through the winter generally do not receive adequate quantities of vitamin D without some supplementary therapy in the diet. Rickets tends to occur especially in the spring months because vitamin D formed during the preceding summer can be stored for several months in the liver, and also, calcium and phosphorus absorption from the bones must take place for several months before clinical signs of rickets become apparent.

Effects of Rickets on Bone. During prolonged deficiency of calcium and phosphate in the body fluids, increased parathyroid hormone secretion protects the body against hypocalcemia by causing osteoclastic absorption of the bone; this in turn causes the bone to become progressively weaker and imposes marked physical stress on the bone, resulting in rapid osteoblastic activity. The osteoblasts lay down large quantities of organic bone matrix, osteoid, which does not become calcified because the calcium and phosphate concentrations are insufficient to cause calcification. Consequently, the newly formed, uncalcified osteoid gradually takes the place of other bone that is being reabsorbed.

Obviously, hyperplasia of the parathyroid glands is marked in rickets because of the decreased blood calcium level.

Tetany in Rickets. In the early stages of rickets, tetany almost never occurs, because the parathyroid glands continually stimulate osteoclastic absorption of bone and therefore maintain an almost normal level of calcium in the body fluids. However, when the bones become exhausted of calcium, the level of calcium may fall rapidly. As the blood level of calcium falls below 7 mg/dl, the usual signs of tetany develop, and the child may die of tetanic laryngeal spasm unless intravenous calcium is administered, which relieves the tetany immediately.

Treatment of Rickets. The treatment of rickets depends on supplying adequate calcium and phosphate in the diet and also on administering vitamin D.

Osteoporosis

Osteoporosis is the most common of all bone diseases in adults, especially in old age. It is a different disease from osteomalacia and rickets, for it results from diminished organic bone matrix rather than abnormal bone calcification. Usually, in osteoporosis the osteoblastic activity in the bone is less than normal, and consequently the rate of bone ostoid deposition is depressed. But occasionally, as in hyperparathyroidism, the cause of the diminished bone is excess osteoclastic activity.

Among common causes of osteoporosis are (1) lack of physical stress on the bones because of inactivity; (2) malnutrition to the extent that sufficient protein matrix cannot be formed; (3) postmenopausal lack of estrogen secretion, for estrogens have an osteoblast-stimulating activity; and (4) old age, in which growth hormone and other growth factors diminish greatly, plus the fact that many of the protein anabolic functions are poor anyway, so that bone matrix cannot be deposited satisfactorily.

PHYSIOLOGY OF THE TEETH

The teeth cut, grind, and mix the food. To perform these functions, the jaws have powerful muscles capable of providing an occlusive force of as much as 50 to 100 pounds between the front teeth and as much as 150 to 200 pounds for the jaw teeth. Also, the upper and lower teeth are provided with projections and facets that interdigitate, so that each set of teeth fits with the other. This fitting is called *occlusion,* and it allows even small particles of food to be caught and ground between the tooth surfaces.

Functions of the Different Parts of the Teeth

Figure 53–9 illustrates a sagittal section of a tooth, showing its major functional parts: the *enamel, dentine, cementum,* and *pulp.* The tooth can also be divided into the *crown,* which is the portion that protrudes out of the gum into the mouth, and the *root,*

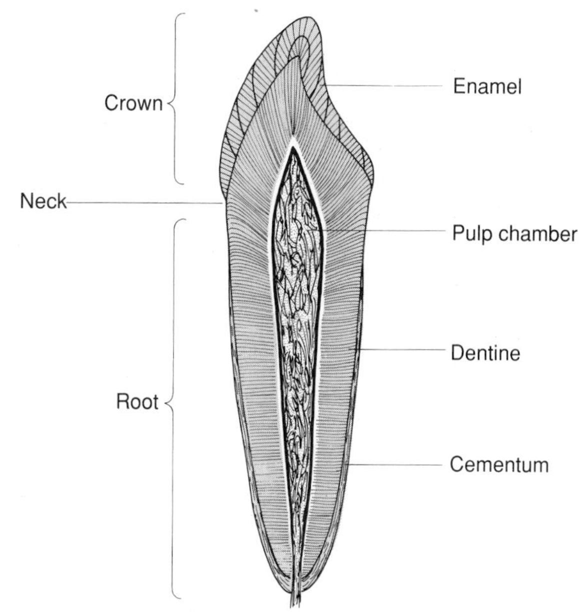

Figure 53–9. Functional parts of a tooth.

which is the portion that protrudes into the bony socket of the jaw. The collar between the crown and the root where the tooth is surrounded by gum is called the *neck.*

Dentine. The main body of the tooth is composed of dentine, which has a strong, bony structure. Dentine is made up principally of hydroxyapatite crystals similar to those in bone but much denser. These are embedded in a strong meshwork of collagen fibers. In other words, the principal constituents of dentine are very much the same as those of bone. The major difference is its histological organization, for dentine does not contain any osteoblasts, osteoclasts, or spaces for blood vessels or nerves. Instead, it is deposited and nourished by a layer of cells called *odontoblasts,* which line the wall of the pulp cavity.

The calcium salts in dentine make it extremely resistant to compressional forces, while the collagen fibers make it tough and resistant to tensional forces that might result when the teeth are struck by solid objects.

Enamel. The outer surface of the tooth is covered by a layer of enamel that is formed prior to eruption of the tooth by special epithelial cells called *ameloblasts.* Once the tooth has erupted, no more enamel is formed. Enamel is composed of very large and extremely dense crystals of hydroxyapatite with adsorbed carbonate, magnesium, sodium, potassium, and other ions embedded in a meshwork of very strong and almost completely insoluble protein fibers that are similar to (but not identical with) the keratin of hair. The dense crystalline structure of the salts makes the enamel extremely hard, much harder than the dentine. Also, the special protein fiber meshwork makes enamel very resistant to acids, enzymes, and other corrosive agents, because this protein is one of the most insoluble and resistant proteins known.

Cementum. Cementum is a bony substance secreted by cells of the *periodontal membrane,* which lines the tooth socket. Many collagen fibers pass directly from the bone of the jaw, through the periodontal membrane, and then into the cementum. These collagen fibers and the cementum hold the tooth in place. When the teeth are exposed to excessive strain, the layer of cementum becomes thicker and stronger. Also, it increases in thickness and strength with age, causing the teeth to become progressively more firmly seated in the jaws.

Pulp. The inside of each tooth is filled with pulp, which in turn is composed of connective tissue with an abundant supply of nerves, blood vessels, and lymphatics. The cells lining the surface of the pulp cavity are the odontoblasts, which, during the formative years of the tooth, lay down the dentine but at the same time encroach more and more on the pulp cavity, making it smaller. In later life the dentine stops growing, and the pulp cavity thereafter remains essentially constant in size. However, the odontoblasts are still viable and send projections into small *dentinal tubules* that penetrate all the way through the dentine; they are of importance for providing nutrition and for exchange of calcium, phosphate, and other minerals.

Dentition

All human beings and most other mammals develop two sets of teeth during a lifetime. The first teeth are called the *deciduous teeth,* or *milk teeth,* and they number 20 in the human being. These erupt between the seventh month and second year of life, and they last until the sixth to the thirteenth year. After each deciduous tooth is lost, a permanent tooth replaces it, and an additional 8 to 12 molars appear posteriorly in the jaw, making the total number of permanent teeth 28 to 32, depending on whether the four *wisdom teeth* finally appear, which does not occur in everyone.

Formation of the Teeth. Figure 53–10 illustrates the formation and eruption of teeth. Figure 53–10A shows invagination of the oral epithelium into the *dental lamina;* this is followed by the development of a tooth-producing organ. The outer epithelial cells form ameloblasts, which form the enamel on the outside of the tooth. The inner epithelial cells invaginate upward to form a pulp cavity and also to form the odon-

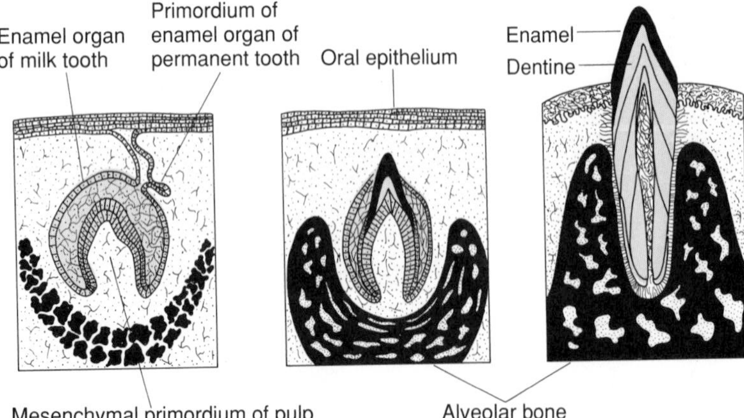

Figure 53–10. *A,* Primordial tooth organ. *B,* the developing tooth. *C,* The erupting tooth.

toblasts that secrete dentine. Thus, enamel is formed on the outside of the tooth, and dentine is formed on the inside, giving rise to an early tooth as illustrated in Figure 53–10B.

Eruption of Teeth. During early childhood, the teeth begin to protrude from the jaw bone through the oral epithelium into the mouth. The cause of eruption is unknown, though several theories have been offered in an attempt to explain this phenomenon. The most likely theory is that growth of the tooth root as well as the bone underneath the tooth progressively shoves the tooth forward.

Development of the Permanent Teeth. During embryonic life, a tooth-forming organ also develops in the dental lamina for each permanent tooth that will be needed after the deciduous teeth are gone. These tooth-producing organs slowly form the permanent teeth throughout the first 6 to 20 years of life. When each permanent tooth becomes fully formed, it, like the deciduous tooth, pushes upward through the bone of the jaw. In so doing it erodes the root of the deciduous tooth and eventually causes it to loosen and fall out. Soon thereafter, the permanent tooth erupts to take the place of the original one.

Metabolic Factors in Development of the Teeth. The rate of development and the speed of eruption of teeth can be accelerated by both thyroid and growth hormones. Also, the deposition of salts in the early forming teeth is affected considerably by various factors of metabolism, such as the availability of calcium and phosphate in the diet, the amount of vitamin D present, and the rate of parathyroid hormone secretion. When all these factors are normal, the dentine and enamel will be correspondingly healthy, but when they are deficient, the calcification of the teeth also may be defective so that the teeth will be abnormal throughout life.

Mineral Exchange in Teeth

The salts of teeth, like those of bone, are composed basically of hydroxyapatite with adsorbed carbonates and various cations bound together in a hard crystalline substance. Also, new salts are constantly being deposited while old salts are being reabsorbed from the teeth, as also occurs in bone. However, experiments indicate that deposition and reabsorption occur mainly in the dentine and cementum, while very little occurs in the enamel. Most of what does occur in the enamel is by exchange of minerals with the saliva rather than the fluids of the pulp cavity. The rate of absorption and deposition of minerals in the cementum is approximately equal to that in the surrounding bone in the jaw, while the rate of deposition and absorption of minerals in the dentine is only one third that of bone. The cementum has characteristics almost identical with those of usual bone, including the presence of osteoblasts and osteoclasts, while dentine does not have these characteristics, as explained above; this difference undoubtedly accounts for the varying rates of mineral exchange.

The mechanism by which minerals are deposited and reabsorbed from the dentine is not clear. It is probable that the small processes of the odontoblasts that protrude into the tubules of the dentine are capable of absorbing salts and then of providing new salts to take the place of the old.

In summary, rapid mineral exchange occurs in the dentine and cementum of teeth, though the mechanism of this exchange in dentine is unknown. On the other hand, enamel exhibits extremely slow mineral exchange so that it maintains most of its original mineral complement throughout life.

Dental Abnormalities

The two most common dental abnormalities are *caries* and *malocclusion.* Caries means erosions of the teeth, whereas malocclusion means failure of the projections of the upper and lower teeth to interdigitate properly.

Caries and the Role of Fluorine. It is generally agreed by research investigators that dental caries results from the action of bacteria on the teeth, the most common of which is *Streptococcus mutans.* The first event in the development of caries is the deposit of *plaque,* a film of precipitated products of saliva and food, on the teeth. Large numbers of bacteria inhabit this plaque and are readily available to cause caries. However, these bacteria depend to a great extent on carbohydrates for their food. When carbohydrates are available, their metabolic systems are strongly activated and they also multiply. In addition, they form acids, particularly lactic acid, and proteolytic enzymes. The acids are the major culprit in the causation of caries, because the calcium salts of teeth are slowly dissolved in a highly acid medium. And once the salts have been absorbed, the remaining organic matrix is rapidly digested by the proteolytic enzymes.

Enamel is far more resistant to demineralization by acids than is dentine, primarily because the crystals of enamel are very dense and also are about 200 times as large as the dentine crystals. Therefore, the enamel of the tooth is the primary barrier to the development of caries. Once the carious process has penetrated through the enamel to the dentine, it then proceeds many times as rapidly because of the high degree of solubility of the dentine salts.

Because of the dependence of the caries causing bacteria on carbohydrates, it is frequently taught that a diet high in carbohydrate content will lead to excessive development of caries. However, it is not the quantity of carbohydrate ingested but instead the frequency with which it is eaten that is important. If eaten in many small portions throughout the day, as in the form of candy, the bacteria are supplied with their preferential metabolic substrate for many hours of the day, and the development of caries is extreme. If the carbohydrates, even though in large amounts, are eaten only at mealtimes, the extensiveness of the caries is greatly reduced.

The teeth of some people are more resistant to

caries than those of others. Studies show that teeth of children who drink water containing small amounts of fluorine develop enamel that is more resistant to caries than the enamel in children who drink water not containing fluorine. Fluorine does not make the enamel harder than usual, but instead it displaces hydroxyl ions in the hydroxyapatite crystals, which in turn makes the enamel several times less soluble. It is also believed that the fluorine might be toxic to some of the bacteria as well. Finally, when small pits do develop in the enamel, fluorine is believed to promote deposition of calcium phosphate to "heal" the enamel surface. Regardless of the precise means by which fluorine protects the teeth, it is known that small amounts of fluorine deposited in enamel make teeth about three times as resistant to caries as are teeth without fluorine.

Malocclusion. Malocclusion is usually caused by a hereditary abnormality that causes the teeth of one jaw to grow to an abnormal position. In malocclusion, the teeth cannot perform their normal grinding or cutting action adequately. Occasionally malocclusion also results in abnormal displacement of the lower jaw in relation to the upper jaw, causing such undesirable effects as pain in the mandibular joint or deterioration of the teeth.

The orthodontist can often correct malocclusion by applying prolonged gentle pressure against the teeth with appropriate braces. The gentle pressure causes absorption of alveolar jaw bone on the compressed side of the tooth socket and deposition of new bone on the tensional side of the socket. In this way the tooth gradually moves to a new position as directed by the applied pressure.

REFERENCES

Avioli, L., and Krane, S. M.: Metabolic Bone Disease. 2nd ed. Philadelphia, W. B. Saunders Co., 1989.

Canalis, E.: Bone-related growth factors. Triangle, 27:11, 1988.

Carney, S. L., and Muir, H.: The structure and function of cartilage proteoglycans. Physiol. Rev., 68:858, 1988.

Chambers, T. J.: The effect of calcitonin on the osteoclast. Triangle, 27:53, 1988.

DeLuca, H. F.: The vitamin D story: A collaborative effort of basic science and clinical medicine. FASEB J., 2:224, 1988.

Einhorn, T. A.: Biomechanical properties of bone. Triangle, 27:27, 1988.

Fiskum, G. (ed.): Cell Calcium Metabolism. New York, Plenum Publishing Corp., 1989.

Grossman, L. I., et al: Endodontic Practice. 11th ed. Philadelphia, Lea & Febiger, 1988.

Martin, R. B., and Burr, D. B.: Structure, Function, and Adaptation of Compact Bone, New York, Raven Press, 1989.

Minghetti, P. P., and Norman, A. W.: 1,25(OH)$_2$-vitamin D$_3$ receptors: Gene regulation and genetic circuitry. FASEB J., 2:3043, 1988.

Provenza, D. V.: Fundamentals of Oral Histology and Embryology. 2nd ed. Philadelphia, Lea & Febiger, 1988.

Riggs, B. L., and Melton, L. J., III: Osteoporosis: Etiology, Diagnosis, and Management. New York, Raven Press, 1988.

Tam, C. S., et al. (eds.): Metabolic Bone Disease: Cellular and Tissue Mechanisms. Boca Raton, Fla., CRC Press, Inc., 1988.

Wozney, J. M., et al.: Novel regulators of bone formation: Molecular clones and activities. Science, 242:1528, 1988.

QUESTIONS

1. Explain the steps by which *vitamin D* is converted into *1,25-dihydroxycholecalciferol.* What is the role of parathyroid hormone in this conversion?
2. What is the feedback mechanism in the conversion process of the above question that keeps the concentration of 1,25-dihydroxycholecalciferol at a reasonably constant level?
3. How does 1,25-dihydroxycholecalciferol function to control the absorption of calcium from the intestinal tract?
4. What proportion of the calcium in the plasma is in ionic form?
5. What are the effects on the body of *hypocalcemia* and *hypercalcemia?*
6. Describe the way in which the organic matrix of bone and the bone salts are structured to provide both compressional strength and tensional strength of the bone.
7. What is the composition of *hydroxyapatite?*
8. During bone calcification, what salts are first laid down in the bone, and how are these converted to hydroxyapatite?
9. What is meant by *exchangeable calcium,* and how does it function to buffer the calcium concentration of the extracellular fluid?
10. Explain the histological mechanisms by which bone is continually being remodeled. What is the value of continual remodeling of bone?
11. What is the chemical composition of *parathyroid hormone?*
12. What is the effect of parathyroid hormone on plasma calcium and plasma phosphate concentrations? How does parathyroid hormone act on the bone to cause calcium removal? What is the difference between the rapid phase and the slow phase of calcium and phosphate absorption?
13. What is the effect of parathyroid hormone on calcium and phosphate excretion by the kidneys?
14. Describe the effect of plasma calcium ion concentration on the rate of parathyroid hormone secretion. How does this function as a means for negative feedback control of the calcium ion concentration?
15. What is the chemical composition of *calcitonin,* and where is it formed in the body?
16. How do the functions of calcitonin differ from those of parathyroid hormone?
17. In *hypoparathyroidism,* what causes tetany?
18. In *hyperparathyroidism,* why is it that the first symptom of the disease is often a broken bone?
19. In *rickets,* why is it that *tetany* and symptoms of *bone weakness* and *lack of bone growth* occur in the spring months of the year? Describe the effects of rickets on bones.
20. Describe the functional parts of the *teeth.*
21. What are the special characteristics of enamel that make it highly resistant to the development of caries?
22. How does *mineral exchange* occur in the different parts of teeth?
23. Describe the cause and development of *caries.* What is the role of *fluorine* in preventing caries?

54

Male Reproductive Functions, the Male Sex Hormones, and the Pineal Gland

Male reproductive functions can be divided into three major subdivisions: first, spermatogenesis, which means simply the formation of sperm; second, performance of the male sexual act; and third, regulation of male sexual functions by the various hormones. Associated with these reproductive functions are the effects of the male sex hormones on the accessory sexual organs, on cellular metabolism, on growth, and on other functions of the body.

Physiological Anatomy of the Male Sexual Organs. Figure 54–1 illustrates the various portions of the male reproductive system. The testis is composed of about 900 coiled *seminiferous tubules,* each over half a meter long, in which the sperm are formed. The sperm then empty into the *epididymis,* another coiled tube approximately 6 meters long. The epididymis leads into the *vas deferens,* which enlarges into the *ampulla of the vas deferens* immediately before the vas enters the body of the *prostate gland.* A *seminal vesicle,* one located on each side of the prostate, empties into the prostatic end of the ampulla, and the contents from both the ampulla and the seminal vesicle pass into an *ejaculatory duct* leading through the body of the prostate gland to empty into the *internal urethra. Prostate ducts* in turn empty from the prostate gland into the ejaculatory duct. Finally, the *urethra* is the last connecting link from the testis to the exterior. The urethra is supplied with mucus derived from a large number of minute *urethral glands* located along its entire extent and even more so from bilateral *bulbourethral glands* located near the origin of the urethra.

SPERMATOGENESIS

Spermatogenesis occurs in all the seminiferous tubules during active sexual life, beginning at an average age of 13 years as the result of stimulation by anterior pituitary gonadotropic hormones and continuing throughout the remainder of life.

The Steps of Spermatogenesis

The seminiferous tubules, one of which is illustrated in Figure 54–2A, contain a large number of small to medium-sized germinal epithelial cells called *spermatogonia,* which are located in two to three layers along the outer border of the tubular epithelium. These continually proliferate to replenish themselves, and a portion of them differentiate through definite stages of development to form sperm, as shown in Figure 54–2B.

In spermatogenesis, some of the spermatogonia grow continually to form considerably enlarged cells called *spermatocytes.* Then the spermatocyte divides in two stages by the process of *meiosis* (in which there is no formation of new chromosomes, only separation of the chromosomal pairs) to form four *spermatids,* each containing 23 chromosomes. The spermatids do not divide again but instead mature for almost 2 months to become spermatozoa.

The Sex Chromosomes. In each spermatogonium one of the 23 pairs of chromosomes carries the genetic information that determines the sex of the

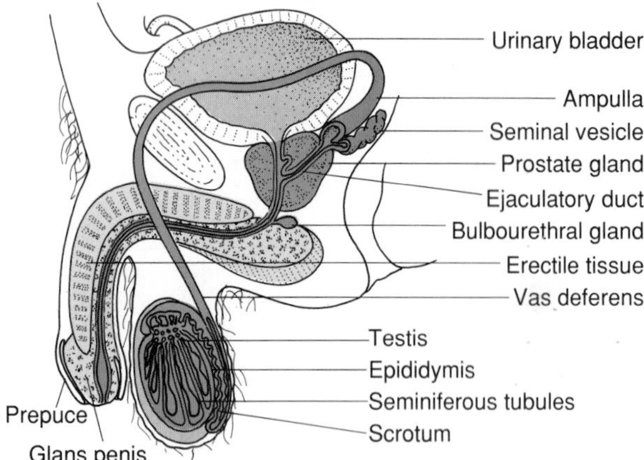

Figure 54-1. The male reproductive system. (Modified from Fawcett: Bloom and Fawcett: A Textbook of Histology. 10th ed. Philadelphia, W. B. Saunders Company, 1985.)

eventual offspring. This pair is composed of one X chromosome, which is called the *female chromosome,* and one Y chromosome, the *male chromosome.* During meiotic division the sex-determining chromosomes are separated between the spermatids, so that half the sperm become *male sperm* containing the Y chromosome and the other half *female sperm* containing the X chromosome. The sex of the offspring is determined by which of these two types of sperm fertilizes the ovum. This will be discussed further in Chapter 56.

Formation of Sperm. When the spermatids are first formed, they still have the usual characteristics of epithelioid cells, but during their maturation most of the cytoplasm disappears, and each spermatid begins to elongate into a spermatozoon, illustrated in Figure 54-3, composed of a *head, neck, body,* and *tail.* To form the head, the nuclear material is condensed into a compact mass, and the cell membrane contracts around the nucleus. It is this nuclear material that fertilizes the ovum.

At the top of the sperm head is a cap called the *acrosome,* which is formed from the Golgi apparatus and contains hyaluronidase and proteases that play important roles in the entry of the sperm into the ovum.

The *centrioles* are aggregated in the neck of the sperm, and the *mitochondria* are arranged in a spiral in the body.

Extending beyond the body is a long tail, which is mainly an outgrowth of one of the centrioles. This has almost the same structure as a cilium, which was described in detail in Chapter 2. The tail contains two paired microtubules down the center and nine double microtubules arranged around the border. This whole structure is called the *axoneme.*

To and fro movement of the tail (flagellar movement) provides motility for the sperm. This movement results from a to-and-fro longitudinal sliding motion between the anterior and posterior tubules that make up the axoneme. Normal sperm move in a straight line at a velocity of 1 to 4 mm per minute.

Function of the Sertoli Cells. The Sertoli cells of the germinal epithelium, known as the *sustentacular*

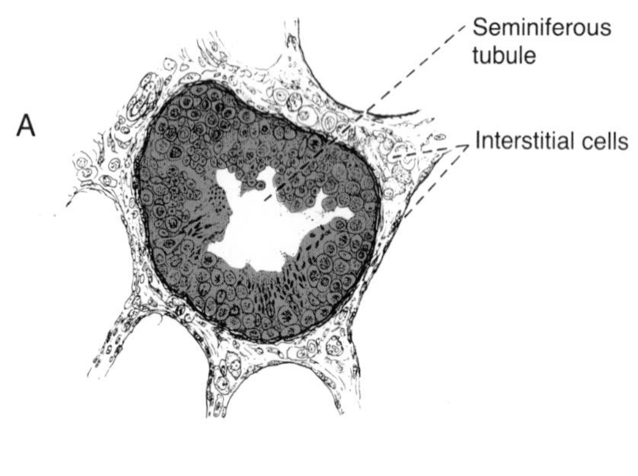

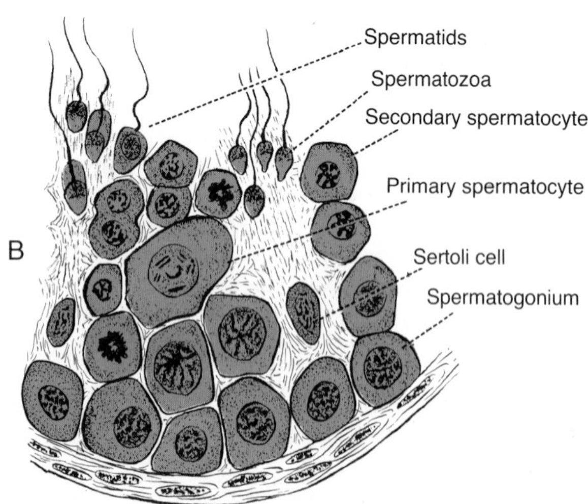

Figure 54-2. *A,* Cross-section of a seminiferous tubule. *B,* Spermatogenesis.

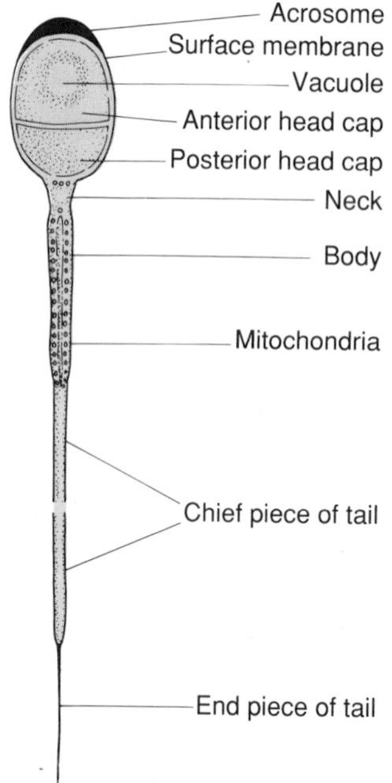

Figure 54-3. Structure of the human spermatozoon.

cells, are illustrated in Figure 54–2B. These cells are large, extending from the base of the seminiferous epithelium all the way to the lumen of the tubule. The spermatids attach themselves to the Sertoli cells, and a specific relationship exists between the two cells that causes the spermatids to change into spermatozoa. The Sertoli cells provide nutrient material, hormones, and enzymes that are necessary for causing appropriate changes in the spermatids. The Sertoli cells also remove the excess cytoplasm as the spermatids are converted to spermatozoa, a process called *spermiation.*

Maturation of Sperm in the Epididymis. Following formation in the seminiferous tubules, the sperm pass into the *epididymis.* Sperm removed from the seminiferous tubules are completely nonmotile, and they cannot fertilize an ovum. However, after the sperm have been in the epididymis for some 18 to 24 hours, they develop the capability of motility, even though inhibitory proteins in the epididymal fluid still prevent motility until after ejaculation. The sperm also become capable of fertilizing the ovum, a process called *maturation.* The epididymis secretes a copious quantity of fluid containing hormones, enzymes, and special nutrients that are essential for sperm maturation.

Storage of Sperm. A small quantity of sperm can be stored in the epididymis, but most sperm are stored in the vas deferens and ampulla of the vas deferens. They can remain stored, maintaining their fertility, in these areas for at least a month, though during normal sexual activity storage ordinarily is no longer than a few days.

Physiology of the Mature Sperm. The usual motile and fertile sperm are capable of flagellated movement through the fluid media at a rate of approximately 1 to 4 mm per minute. Furthermore, *normal* sperm travel in a straight line rather than in circles. The activity of sperm is greatly enhanced in neutral and slightly alkaline media such as exist in the ejaculated semen, but it is greatly depressed in mildly acid media, and strong acid media can cause rapid death of sperm. Though sperm can live for many weeks in the genital ducts of the testes, the life of sperm in the female genital tract is only 1 to 2 days.

Function of the Seminal Vesicles

The seminal vesicles are secretory glands lined with an epithelium that secretes a mucoid material containing an abundance of *fructose* and other nutrient substances, as well as large quantities of *prostaglandins* and *fibrinogen.* During the process of ejaculation, each seminal vesicle empties its contents into the ejaculatory duct shortly after the vas deferens empties the sperm. This adds greatly to the bulk of the ejaculated semen, and the fructose and other substances in the seminal fluid are of considerable nutrient value for the ejaculated sperm until one of them fertilizes the ovum. The prostaglandins are believed to aid fertilization in two ways: (1) by acting on the cervical mucus to make it more receptive to sperm and (2) possibly causing reverse peristaltic contractions in the uterus and fallopian tubes to move the sperm toward the ovaries (a few sperm reach the upper end of the fallopian tubes within 5 minutes).

Function of the Prostate Gland

The prostate gland secretes a thin, milky, alkaline fluid containing citric acid, calcium, and several other substances. During emission, the capsule of the prostate gland contracts simultaneously with the contractions of the vas deferens, so that the thin, milky fluid adds to the bulk of the semen. The alkaline characteristic of the prostatic fluid may be quite important for successful fertilization of the ovum, because the fluid of the vas deferens is relatively acidic owing to the presence of metabolic end-products of the sperm and consequently inhibits sperm motility and fertility. Also, the vaginal secretions of the female are acidic (pH of 3.5 to 4.0). Sperm do not become optimally motile until the pH of the surrounding fluids rises to approximately 6 to 6.5. Consequently, it is probable that prostatic fluid neutralizes the acidity of these other fluids after ejaculation and greatly enhances the motility and fertility of the sperm.

Semen

Semen, which is ejaculated during the male sexual act, is composed of the fluids from the vas deferens, the seminal vesicles, the prostate gland, and the mucous glands, especially the bulbourethral glands. The major bulk of the semen is seminal vesicle fluid (about 60 per cent), which is the last to be ejaculated and serves to wash the sperm out of the ejaculatory duct and urethra. The average pH of the combined semen is approximately 7.5, the alkaline prostatic fluid having neutralized the mild acidity of the other portions of the semen. The prostatic fluid gives the semen a milky appearance, while fluid from the seminal vesicle and from the mucous glands gives the semen a mucoid consistency. Indeed, a clotting enzyme of the prostatic fluid causes the fibrinogen of the seminal vesicle fluid to form a weak coagulum, which then dissolves during the next 15 to 30 minutes because of lysis by a fibrinolysin formed from a prostatic profibrinolysin. In the early minutes after ejaculation, the sperm remain relatively immobile, possibly because of the viscosity of the coagulum. However, after the coagulum dissolutes, the sperm simultaneously become highly motile.

Though sperm can live for many weeks in the male genital ducts, once they are ejaculated in the semen, their maximal life span is only 24 to 48 hours at body temperature. At lowered temperatures, however, semen may be stored for several weeks, and when frozen at temperatures below −100°C, sperm have been preserved for years.

Effect of Sperm Count on Fertility. The usual quantity of semen ejaculated at each coitus averages approximately 3.5 ml, and in each milliliter of semen is an average of approximately 120 million sperm, though even in normal persons this number can vary from 35 million to 200 million. Therefore, an average of 400 million sperm are usually present in each ejaculate. When the number of sperm in each milliliter falls below approximately 20,000,000, the person is likely to be infertile. Thus, even though only a single sperm is necessary to fertilize the ovum, the ejaculate must contain a tremendous number of sperm for at least one to fertilize the ovum. A possible reason for this requirement is the need for enzymes from many sperm to allow penetration of one through the protective coating of the ovum.

The Acrosome Enzymes, the "Acrosome Reaction," and Penetration of the Ovum

When the ovum is expelled from the ovarian follicle into the abdominal cavity and fallopian tube, it carries with it multiple layers of granulosal cells. Before a sperm can fertilize the ovum, it must first pass through the granulosa cell layer, and then it must penetrate through the thick covering of the ovum itself, the *zona pellucida.* Fortunately, the acrosome begins to release its enzymes. It is believed that the hyaluronidase among these enzymes is especially important in opening pathways between the granulosa cells so that the sperm can reach the ovum.

On reaching the zona pellucida of the ovum, the anterior membrane of the sperm binds specifically with a receptor protein in the zona pellucida. Then, rapidly, the entire anterior membrane of the acrosome dissolves, and all the acrosomal enzymes are immediately released. Within minutes, these open a penetrating pathway for passage of the sperm head through the zona pellucida, and the sperm genetic material enters the oocyte to cause fertilization; then the embryo begins to develop, as discussed in Chapter 56.

THE MALE SEXUAL ACT

Neuronal Stimulus for Performance of the Male Sexual Act

The most important nerve signals for initiating the male sexual act originate in the glans penis, for the glans contains a highly organized sensory end-organ system that transmits into the central nervous system a special modality of sensation called *sexual sensation.* The massaging action of intercourse on the glans stimulates the sensory end-organs, and the sexual sensations in turn pass through the pudendal nerve, thence through the sacral plexus into the sacral portion of the spinal cord, and finally up the cord to undefined areas of the cerebrum. Impulses may also enter the spinal cord from areas adjacent to the penis to aid in stimulating the sexual act. For instance, stimulation of the scrotum and perineal structures in general can send impulses into the cord which add to the sexual sensation. Sexual sensations can even originate in internal structures, such as irritated areas of the urethra, the bladder, the prostate, the seminal vesicles, the testes, and the vas deferens. Indeed, one of the causes of "sexual drive" is probably overfilling of the sexual organs with secretions. Infection and inflammation of these sexual organs sometimes cause almost continual sexual desire, and aphrodisiac drugs, such as cantharides, increase the sexual desire by irritating the bladder and urethral mucosa.

The Psychic Element of Male Sexual Stimulation. Appropriate psychic stimuli can greatly enhance the ability of a person to perform the sexual act. Simply thinking sexual thoughts or even dreaming that the act of intercourse is being performed can cause the male sexual act to occur and to culminate in ejaculation. Indeed, *nocturnal emissions* during dreams occur in many men during some stages of sexual life, especially during the teens.

Integration of the Male Sexual Act in the Spinal Cord. Though psychic factors usually play an important part in the male sexual act and can actually initiate it, the cerebrum is probably not absolutely necessary for its performance, for appropriate genital stimulation can cause ejaculation in some animals and in an occasional human being after their spinal cords have been cut above the lumbar region. Therefore, the male sexual act results from inherent reflex mechanisms integrated in the sacral and lumbar spinal cord, and these mechanisms can be activated by either psychic or direct sexual stimulation or both.

Stages of the Male Sexual Act

Erection; Role of the Parasympathetic Nerves. Erection is the first effect of male sexual stimulation, and the degree of erection is proportional to the degree of stimulation, whether this be psychic or physical.

Erection is caused by parasympathetic impulses that pass from the sacral portion of the spinal cord to the penis. These parasympathetic impulses dilate the arteries of the penis, thus allowing arterial blood to flow under high pressure into the *erectile tissue* of the penis, illustrated in Figure 54–4. This erectile tissue is composed of large, cavernous venous sinusoids, which are normally relatively empty but become dilated tremendously when arterial blood flows into them under pressure. Also, these erectile bodies are surrounded by strong fibrous coats; therefore, high pressure within the sinusoids causes ballooning of the erectile tissue to such an extent that the penis becomes hard and elongated.

Lubrication, Another Parasympathetic Function. During sexual stimulation, parasympa-

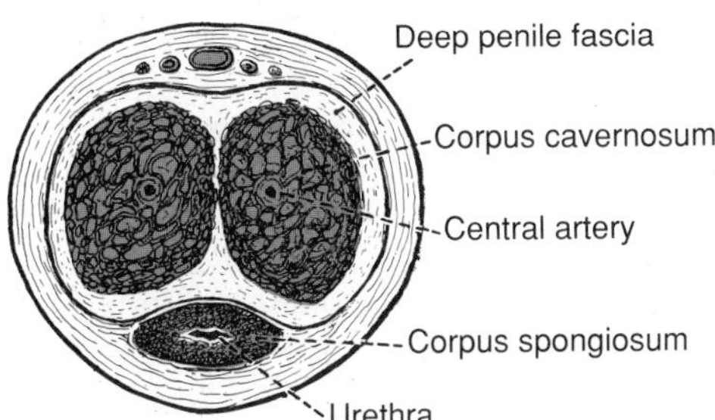

Figure 54-4. Erectile tissue of the penis.

thetic impulses, in addition to promoting erection, cause the urethral glands and the bulbourethral glands to secrete mucus. This mucus flows through the urethra during intercourse to aid in the lubrication of coitus. However, most of the lubrication of coitus is provided by the female sexual organs rather than by the male. Without satisfactory lubrication, the male sexual act is rarely successful because unlubricated intercourse causes pain impulses that inhibit rather than excite sexual sensations.

Emission and Ejaculation; A Sympathetic Nervous Function. Emission and ejaculation are the culmination of the male sexual act. When the sexual stimulus becomes extremely intense, the reflex centers of the spinal cord begin to emit *sympathetic impulses* that leave the cord at L-1 and L-2 and pass to the genital organs to initiate *emission,* the forerunner of ejaculation.

Emission begins with contraction of the vas deferens and the ampulla to cause expulsion of sperm into the internal urethra. Then, contractions in the seminal vesicles and the muscular coat of the prostate gland expel seminal fluid and prostatic fluid, forcing the sperm forward. All these fluids mix with the mucus already secreted by the bulbourethral glands to form the semen. The process to this point is *emission.*

The filling of the internal urethra then elicits signals that are transmitted to the sacral regions of the cord. In turn, signals from the sacral cord further excite the rhythmic contraction of the internal genital organs and also cause contraction of the ischiocavernosus and bulbocavernosus skeletal muscles that compress the bases of the penile erectile tissue. These effects together cause rhythmic, wavelike increases in pressure in the genital ducts and urethra, which project the semen from the urethra to the exterior. This process is called *ejaculation.* At the same time, rhythmic contractions of the pelvic muscles and even of some of the muscles of the body trunk cause thrusting movements of the pelvis and penis, which also help propel the semen into the deepest recesses of the vagina and perhaps even through the cervix into the uterus.

This entire period of emission and ejaculation is called the *male orgasm.* At its termination, the male sexual excitement disappears almost entirely within 1 to 2 minutes and erection ceases, a process called *resolution.*

TESTOSTERONE AND OTHER MALE SEX HORMONES

Secretion of Testosterone by the Interstitial Cells of the Testes. The testes secrete several male sex hormones, which are collectively called *androgens.* However, one of these, *testosterone,* is so much more abundant and potent than the others that it can be considered to be the significant hormone responsible for the male hormonal effects.

Testosterone is formed by the *interstitial cells of Leydig,* which lie in the interstices between the seminiferous tubules, as illustrated in Figure 54-5, and constitute about 20 per cent of the mass of the adult testes. Interstitial cells in the testes are not numerous in a child, but they *are* numerous in a newborn male infant and also in the adult male any time after puberty; at both these times the testes secrete large quantities of testosterone.

Secretion of Androgens Elsewhere in the Body. The term *androgen* is used synonymously with the term male sex hormone, but it also includes male sex hormones produced elsewhere in the body besides the testes. For instance, the adrenal gland secretes at least five different androgens, though the total masculinizing activity of all these is normally so slight that they do not cause significant masculine characteristics even in women. But when an adrenal tumor of the androgen-producing cells occurs, the quantity of androgenic hormones may become great enough to cause all the usual male secondary sexual characteristics.

Chemistry of Testosterone. All androgens are steroid compounds, as illustrated by the formula in Figure 54-6 for *testosterone* and its closely related hormone, *dihydrotestosterone,* also secreted in small quantities by the testes. Both in the testes and in the

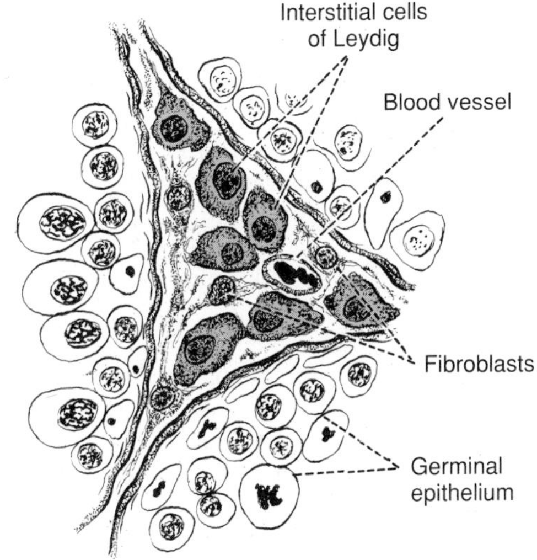

Figure 54-5. Interstitial cells of Leydig located in the interstices between the seminiferous tubules.

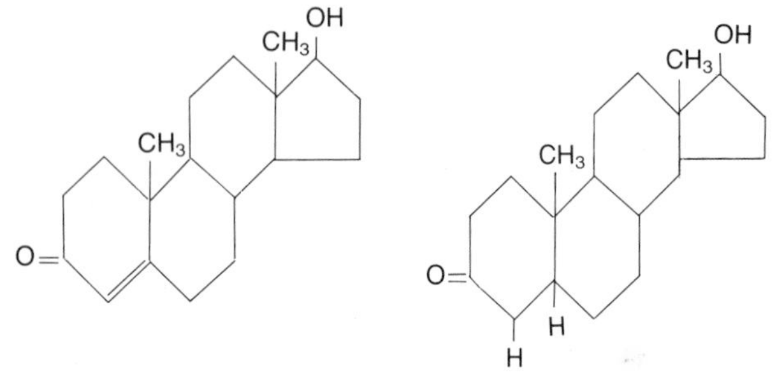

Figure 54-6. Testosterone and dihydrotestosterone.

adrenals, the androgens can be synthesized either from cholesterol or directly from acetyl coenzyme A.

Metabolism of Testosterone. After secretion by the testes, testosterone, most of it loosely bound with plasma protein, circulates in blood for about 30 minutes to an hour before it either becomes fixed to the tissues or is degraded into inactive products that are subsequently excreted.

Much of the testosterone that becomes fixed to the tissues is converted within the cells to dihydrotestosterone, which is also shown in Figure 54-6; it is in this form that testosterone performs many of its intracellular functions.

Degradation and Excretion of Testosterone. The testosterone that does not become fixed to the tissues is rapidly converted, mainly by the liver, into *androsterone* and *dehydroepiandrosterone* and is simultaneously conjugated either as glucuronides or sulfates. These are excreted either in the bile into the intestinal tract or into the urine.

Functions of Testosterone

In general, testosterone is responsible for the distinguishing characteristics of the masculine body. Even during fetal life, the testes are stimulated by chorionic gonadotropin from the placenta to produce a small quantity of testosterone, but essentially no testosterone is produced during childhood until approximately the age of 10 to 13 years. Then testosterone production increases rapidly at the onset of puberty and lasts throughout most of the remainder of life, dwindling rapidly beyond the age of 40 years to perhaps one third the peak value by the age of 80 years.

Functions of Testosterone During Fetal Development. Testosterone begins to be elaborated by the male at about the second month of embryonic life. Injection of large quantities of male sex hormone into gravid animals causes development of male sexual organs in the fetus even when the fetus is female. Also, removal of the fetal testes in a male fetus causes development of female sexual organs. Therefore, the presence or absence of testosterone in the fetus is the determining factor in the development of male or female genital organs and characteristics. That is, testosterone secreted by the genital ridges and the subsequently developing testes is responsible for the development of the male sex characteristics, including the growth of a penis and a scrotum rather than the formation of a clitoris and a vagina. Also, it causes development of the prostate gland, the seminal vesicles, and the male genital ducts, while at the same time suppressing the formation of female genital organs.

Effect on the Descent of the Testes. The testes usually descend into the scrotum during the last two months of pregnancy, when the testes are secreting adequate quantities of testosterone. If a male child is born with undescended testes, administration of testosterone will often cause the testes to descend in the usual manner if the inguinal canals are large enough to allow the testes to pass. Or administration of gonadotropic hormones, which stimulate the interstitial cells of the testes to produce testosterone, can also cause the testes to descend. Thus, the stimulus for descent of the testes is testosterone, indicating again that testosterone is an important hormone for male sexual development during fetal life.

Effect of Testosterone on Development of Adult Primary and Secondary Sexual Characteristics. Testosterone secretion after puberty causes the penis, the scrotum, and the testes all to enlarge about eightfold until about the age of 20 years. In addition, testosterone causes the secondary sexual characteristics of the male to develop at the same time, beginning at puberty and ending at maturity. These secondary sexual characteristics, in addition to the sexual organs themselves, distinguish the male from the female as follows:

Distribution of Body Hair. Testosterone causes growth of hair (1) over the pubis, (2) on the face, (3) usually on the chest, and (4) less often on other regions of the body, such as the back. It also causes the hair on most other portions of the body to become more prolific.

Baldness. Testosterone in some men decreases the growth of hair on the top of the head; a man who does not have functional testes does not become bald. However, many virile men never become bald, for baldness is a result of two factors: first, a *genetic background* for the development of baldness and, second, superimposed on this genetic background, *large quantities of androgenic hormones.* A woman who has the appropriate genetic background and who develops a long-sustained androgenic tumor becomes bald in the same manner as a man.

Effect on the Voice. Testosterone secreted by the testes or injected into the body causes hypertrophy of the laryngeal mucosa and enlargement of the larynx. These effects cause at first a relatively discordant, "cracking" voice, but this gradually changes into the typical masculine bass voice.

Effect on the Skin. Testosterone increases the thickness of the skin over the entire body and increases the ruggedness of the subcutaneous tissues.

Effect on Protein Formation and Muscular Development. One of the most important male characteristics is the development of increasing musculature following puberty; men average about a 50 per cent increase in muscle mass over that in women. This is associated with increased protein in other parts of the body as well. Many of the changes in the skin are due to deposition of proteins in the skin, and the changes in the voice even result, at least partly, from the protein anabolic function of testosterone.

Because of the very great effect that testosterone has on the body musculature, it (or more usually a synthetic androgen instead) is widely used by athletes to improve their muscular performance. This practice is to be severely deprecated because of prolonged harmful effects of excess testosterone, as we shall discuss in Chapter 57 in relation to sports physiology. Testosterone is also sometimes used in old age as a "youth hormone" to improve muscle strength and vigor.

Effect on Bone Growth and Calcium Retention. Following puberty or following prolonged injection of testosterone, the bones grow considerably in thickness and also deposit substantial amounts of calcium salts. Thus, testosterone increases the total quantity of bone matrix, and this also causes calcium retention. The increase in bone matrix is believed to result from the general protein anabolic function of testosterone.

When great quantities of testosterone (or any other androgen) are secreted in the still-growing child, the rate of bone growth increases markedly, causing a spurt in total body growth as well. However, the testosterone also causes the epiphyses of the long bones to unite with the shafts of the bones at an early age in life. Therefore, despite the rapidity of growth, the early uniting of the epiphyses prevents the person from growing as tall as he would grow were testosterone not secreted at all. Even in normal men the final adult height is slightly less than that which would have been attained had the person been castrated prior to puberty.

Effect on the Red Blood Cells. The average man has about 700,000 more red blood cells per cubic millimeter than the average woman. However, this difference may be due partly to increased metabolic rate following testosterone administration rather than to a direct effect of testosterone on red blood cell production.

Basic Intracellular Mechanism of Action of Testosterone

Probably all or almost all the effects just listed result from increased rate of protein formation in the target cells. This has been studied extensively in the prostate gland, one of the organs that is most affected by testosterone. In this gland, testosterone enters the cells within a few minutes after secretion, is there converted to *dihydrotestosterone,* and binds with a cytoplasmic receptor protein. This combination then migrates to the nucleus, where it binds with a nuclear protein and induces the DNA-RNA transcription process. Within 30 minutes RNA polymerase has become activated, and the concentration of RNA begins to increase in the cells; this is followed by progressive increase in cellular protein. After several days the quantity of DNA in the gland has also increased, and there has been a simultaneous increase in the number of prostatic cells.

Therefore, it is assumed that testosterone greatly stimulates production of proteins in general, though increasing more specifically those proteins in target organs or tissues responsible for the development of male sexual characteristics.

Control of Male Sexual Functions by the Anterior Pituitary Gland Gonadotropic Hormones—FSH and LH

The anterior pituitary gland secretes two major gonadotropic hormones: (1) *follicle-stimulating hormone* (FSH) and (2) *luteinizing hormone* (LH). Both of these play major roles in the control of male sexual function.

Regulation of Testosterone Production by LH. Testosterone is produced by the interstitial cells of Leydig when the testes are stimulated by LH from the pituitary gland, and the quantity of testosterone secreted varies approximately in proportion to the amount of LH available.

Injection of purified LH into a child causes cells that look like fibroblasts in the interstitial areas of the testes to develop into interstitial cells of Leydig, though mature Leydig cells are not normally found in the child's testes until after the age of approximately 10 years.

Effect of Human Chorionic Gonadotropin on the Fetal Testes. During gestation the placenta secretes large quantities of *human chorionic gonadotropin,* a hormone that has almost the same properties as LH. This hormone stimulates the formation of interstitial cells in the testes of the fetus and causes testosterone secretion. As pointed out earlier in the chapter, the secretion of testosterone during fetal life is necessary for promoting formation of male sexual organs.

Regulation of Spermatogenesis by FSH and Testosterone. The conversion of spermatogonia into spermatocytes in the seminiferous tubules is stimulated by FSH from the anterior pituitary gland. This results from the effect of FSH to stimulate the Sertoli cells, which are responsible for converting the spermatids into sperm, a process called *spermiation.*

However, FSH cannot by itself cause complete formation of spermatozoa. For spermatogenesis to proceed to completion, testosterone must be secreted simultaneously by the interstitial cells. Thus testosterone diffusing from the interstitial cells into the seminiferous tubules apparently is necessary for final maturation of the spermatozoa. Because testosterone is secreted by the interstitial cells under the influence of LH, both FSH and LH must be secreted by the anterior pituitary gland if spermatogenesis is to occur.

Regulation of Pituitary Secretion of LH and FSH by the Hypothalamus — Gonadotropin-Releasing Hormone

The gonadotropins, like corticotropin and thyrotropin, are secreted by the anterior pituitary gland mainly in response to nervous activity in the hypothalamus. For instance, psychic stimuli can affect fertility of the male animal, as exemplified by the fact that transporting a bull under uncomfortable conditions can often cause almost complete temporary sterility. In the human being, too, it is known that various psychic stimuli feeding into the hypothalamus can cause marked excitatory or inhibitory effects on gonadotropin secretion, in this way sometimes greatly altering the degree of fertility.

Gonadotropin-Releasing Hormone (GnRH), the Hypothalamic Hormone That Stimulates Gonadotropin Secretion. In both men and women, the hypothalamus controls gonadotropin secretion by way of the hypothalamic-hypophysial portal system, as discussed in Chapter 49. Though there are two different gonadotropic hormones, luteinizing hormone and follicle-stimulating hormone, only one hypothalamic releasing hormone has been discovered; this is called *gonadotropin-releasing hormone (GnRH).* Because this hormone has an especially strong effect on inducing luteinizing hormone secretion by the anterior pituitary gland, it is often also called *luteinizing hormone-releasing hormone* (LHRH).

Reciprocal Inhibition of Hypothalamic–Anterior Pituitary Secretion of Gonadotropic Hormones by Testicular Hormones. *Feedback Control of Testosterone Secretion.* The following negative feedback control system operates continuously to control very precisely the rate of testosterone secretion:

1. The hypothalamus secretes *gonadotropin-releasing hormone,* which stimulates the anterior pituitary gland to secrete *luteinizing hormone.*
2. Luteinizing hormone in turn stimulates *hyperplasia of the Leydig cells* of the testes and also stimulates production of *testosterone* by these cells.
3. The testosterone in turn feeds back *negatively* to the hypothalamus, inhibiting production of gonadotropin-releasing hormone. This obviously limits the rate at which testosterone will be produced. On the other hand, when testosterone production is too low, lack of inhibition of the hypothalamus leads to return of testosterone secretion to the normal level.

Feedback Control of Spermatogenesis—Role of Inhibin. It is known, too, that spermatogenesis by the testes inhibits the secretion of FSH. It is believed that the Sertoli cells secrete a hormone that has a direct inhibitory effect mainly on the anterior pituitary gland (but perhaps slightly on the hypothalamus as well) to inhibit the secretion of FSH. A glycoprotein hormone having a molecular weight between 10,000 and 30,000 and called *inhibin* has been isolated from cultured Sertoli cells and is probably responsible for most of the feedback control of FSH secretion and of spermatogenesis. This feedback cycle is the following:

1. Follicle-stimulating hormone stimulates the Sertoli cells that provide nutrition for the developing spermatozoa.
2. The Sertoli cells release inhibin that in turn feeds back negatively to the anterior pituitary gland to inhibit the production of FSH. Thus, this feedback cycle maintains a constant rate of spermatogenesis, without underproduction or overproduction, that is required for male reproductive function.

Puberty and Regulation of Its Onset. During the first 10 years of life, the male child secretes almost no gonadotropins and consequently almost no testosterone. Then, at the age of about 10 years, the anterior pituitary gland begins to secrete progressively increasing quantities of gonadotropins, and this is followed by a corresponding increase in testicular function. By approximately the age of 13 years, the male child reaches full adult sexual capability. This period of change is called *puberty.*

The cause of the onset of puberty is the following: *During childhood, the hypothalamus simply does not secrete significant amounts of gonadotropin-releasing hormone.* Then, for reasons not understood, some maturation process in the brain causes the hypothalamus to begin secreting GnRH at the time of puberty. This secretion will not occur if the neuronal connections between the hypothalamus and other parts of the brain are not intact. Therefore, the present belief is that the maturation process probably occurs elsewhere in the brain instead of in the hypothalamus. One suggested locus is the amygdala.

ABNORMALITIES OF MALE SEXUAL FUNCTION

The Prostate Gland and Its Abnormalities

The prostate gland remains relatively small throughout childhood but begins to grow at puberty under the stimulus of testosterone. This gland reaches an almost stationary size by the age of 20 years and remains this size up to the age of approximately 50 years. At that time in some men, it begins to degenerate along with the decreased production of testosterone by the testes. A benign fibroadenoma frequently develops in the prostate in older men and causes urinary obstruction. This hypertrophy is not caused by testosterone.

Cancer of the prostate gland is an extremely common cause of death, resulting in approximately 2 to 3 per cent of all male deaths.

Once cancer of the prostate gland does occur, the cancerous cells are usually stimulated to more rapid growth by testosterone and are inhibited by removal of the testes so that testosterone cannot be formed. Also, prostatic cancer can usually be inhibited by administration of estrogens. Some patients who have prostatic cancer that has already metastasized to almost all the bones of the body can be successfully treated for a few months to years by removal of the testes, by estrogen therapy, or by both; following this therapy the metastases degenerate and the bones heal. This treatment does not completely stop the cancer but does slow it down and greatly diminishes the severe bone pain.

Testicular Tumors and Hypergonadism in the Male

An *interstitial cell tumor* on rare occasions develops in a testis, but when one does develop it sometimes produces as much as 100 times the normal quantity of testosterone. When such tumors develop in young children, they cause rapid growth of the musculature and bones but also early uniting of the epiphyses, so that the eventual adult height actually is less than that which would have been achieved otherwise. Obviously, such interstitial cell tumors cause excessive development of the sexual organs and of the secondary sexual characteristics. In the adult male, small interstitial cell tumors are difficult to diagnose because masculine features are already present.

Much more common than the interstitial cell tumors are tumors of the germinal epithelium. Because germinal cells are capable of differentiating into almost any type of cell, many of these tumors contain multiple types of tissue, such as placental tissue, hair, teeth, bone, and skin, all found together in the same tumorous mass called a *teratoma.* Often these tumors secrete no hormones, but if a significant quantity of placental tissue develops in the tumor, it may secrete large quantities of human chorionic gonadotropin that has functions very similar to those of LH. Also, estrogenic hormones are frequently secreted by these tumors and cause the condition called *gynecomastia,* which means overgrowth of the breasts.

THE PINEAL GLAND—ITS FUNCTION IN CONTROLLING SEASONAL FERTILITY

The pineal gland is a small nervous tissue-glandular body protruding from the midbrain above and behind the superior colliculi. Some physiologists have claimed for many years that the pineal gland plays important roles in the control of sexual activities and reproduction, functions that still others have said were nothing more than the zealous imaginings of physiologists preoccupied with sexual delusions.

But now, after years of turmoil and dispute, it looks as though the sex advocates have at last won. For, in some lower animals in which the pineal gland has been removed or in which the nervous circuits to the pineal gland have been sectioned, the normal annual periods of seasonal fertility are lost. To these animals such seasonal fertility is very important because it allows birth of the offspring in the spring and summer months when survival is most likely. The mechanism of this effect is still not entirely clear, but it seems to be the following:

First, the pineal gland is controlled by nerve signals elicited by the amount of light seen by the eyes each day. For instance, in the hamster, more than 13 hours of darkness each day activates the pineal gland, while less than that amount of darkness fails to activate it.

Second, the pineal gland secretes *melatonin* and several other similar substances. Either melatonin or one of the other substances then passes either by way of the blood or through the fluid of the third ventricle to the anterior pituitary gland to *inhibit* gonadotropic hormone secretion, and the gonads become inhibited and even involuted. This is what occurs during the early winter months. But after about 4 months of dysfunction, the gonadotropic hormone secretion breaks through the inhibitory effect of the pineal gland, and the gonads become functional once more, ready for a full springtime of activity.

But does the pineal gland have a similar function in controlling reproduction in human beings? The answer to this is still far from known. However, tumors in the region of the pineal gland are often associated with serious hypo- or hypergonadal dysfunction. So perhaps the pineal gland does play at least some role in controlling sexual drive and reproduction in humans.

REFERENCES

Cooke, B. A., and Sharpe, R. M.: The Molecular and Cellular Endocrinology of the Testis. New York, Raven Press, 1988.

DeGroot, L. J., et al. (eds.): Endocrinology. 2nd ed. Philadelphia, W. B. Saunders Co., 1989.

Hinton, B. T., and Turner, T. T.: Is the epididymis a kidney analogue? News Physiol. Sci., 3:28, 1988.

Knobil, E., et al. (eds.): The Physiology of Reproduction. New York, Raven Press, 1988.

Leung, P. C. K., et al. (eds.): Endocrinology and Physiology of Reproduction. New York, Plenum Publishing Corp., 1987.

Mahesh, V. B., et al. (eds.): Regulation of Ovarian and Testicular Function. New York, Plenum Publishing Corp., 1987.

Marx, J. L.: Sexual responses are—almost—all in the brain. Science, 241:903, 1988.

Negro-Vilar, A., et al.: Andrology and Human Reproduction. New York, Raven Press, 1988.

Reppert, S. M., et al.: Putative melatonin receptors in a human biological clock. Science, 242:78, 1988.

Soules, M. R.: Problems in Reproductive Endocrinology and Infertility. New York, Elsevier Science Publishing Co., 1989.

Spark, R. F.: The Infertile Male. New York, Plenum Publishing Corp., 1988.

Wassarman, P. M.: Eggs, sperm, and sugar: A recipe for fertilization. News Physiol. Sci., 3:120, 1988.

QUESTIONS

1. Describe the physiological anatomy of the *testes* and the other male sex organs.
2. Give the steps of *spermatogenesis.*
3. What determines the sex of a *sperm?*
4. Give the characteristics of the mature sperm.
5. What is the function of the *Sertoli cells* during the formation of sperm?
6. What is the role of the *epididymis* during the maturation of the sperm?
7. What are the respective roles of the *seminal vesicles* and the *prostate gland* in the formation of *semen?*
8. What is the composition of semen?
9. What is the relationship of *sperm count* to *fertility,* and what possible role does the secretion by sperm of *hyaluronidase* and *proteinases* play in this effect?
10. What are the types of stimuli that can lead to sexual sensations and culmination of the sexual act?
11. What are the roles of the parasympathetic and the sympathetic nerves in *erection, lubrication,* and *emission* and *ejaculation?*
12. What is the chemistry of *testosterone,* and by what cells is it formed?
13. What are the functions of testosterone during fetal development?
14. What are the effects of testosterone on the male sexual organs during adolescence?
15. What are the effects of testosterone on body hair, baldness, the voice, the skin, muscle development, bone growth, and the red blood cells?
16. What is the basic intracellular mechanism by which testosterone performs most or all of its functions?
17. Explain the control of *testosterone secretion* by GnRH and LH. Give the feedback control mechanism that maintains a relatively constant rate of testosterone secretion.
18. Explain the effects of GnRH, FSH, LH, and testosterone in the control of *spermatogenesis.*
19. What is the feedback mechanism for control of spermatogenesis? How does the hormone *inhibin* enter into this?
20. What causes the onset of *puberty?*
21. Why are tumors of the germinal epithelium frequently of the *teratoma* type in which multiple types of body tissues are found, such as hair, teeth, skin, and so forth?
22. Explain how the *pineal gland* might control seasonal fertility in animals.

55

Female Physiology Before Pregnancy and the Female Hormones

The sexual and reproductive functions in the female can be divided into two major phases: first, preparation of the body for conception, and second, the period of gestation. The present chapter is concerned with the preparation of the body for gestation, and the following chapter presents the physiology of pregnancy.

PHYSIOLOGICAL ANATOMY OF THE FEMALE SEXUAL ORGANS

Figure 55–1 illustrates the principal organs of the human female reproductive tract, including the *ovaries*, the *fallopian tubes*, the *uterus*, and the *vagina*. Reproduction begins with the development of ova in the ovaries. A single ovum is expelled from an ovarian follicle into the abdominal cavity in the middle of each monthly sexual cycle. This ovum then passes through one of the fallopian tubes into the uterus, and if it has been fertilized by a sperm, it implants in the uterus, where it develops into a fetus, a placenta, and fetal membranes.

At puberty, the two ovaries contain 300,000 to 400,000 ova. Each ovum surrounded by a single layer of *granulosa cells* is called a *primordial follicle*. During all the reproductive years of a woman, only about 400 of these follicles develop enough to expel their ova; the remainder degenerate. At the end of reproductive capability, which is called *menopause*, only a few primordial follicles remain in the ovaries, and even these degenerate soon thereafter.

THE FEMALE HORMONAL SYSTEM

The female hormonal system, like that of the male, consists of three different hierarchies of hormones:

1. A hypothalamic releasing hormone: *gonadotropin-releasing hormone* (GnRH).
2. The anterior pituitary hormones: *follicle-stimulating hormone* (FSH) and *luteinizing hormone* (LH), both of which are secreted in response to the same releasing hormone from the hypothalamus.
3. The ovarian hormones: *estrogen* and *progesterone*, which are secreted by the ovaries in response to the two hormones from the anterior pituitary gland.

The various hormones are not secreted in constant, steady amounts but at drastically differing rates during different parts of the female sexual month, as will be explained later in the chapter.

Before it is possible to discuss the interplay between these different hormones, it is first necessary to describe some of their specific functions and their relationships to the function of the ovaries.

FUNCTION OF THE ANTERIOR PITUITARY GONADOTROPIC HORMONES IN CONTROLLING THE MONTHLY OVARIAN CYCLE

The normal reproductive years of a woman are characterized by monthly rhythmical changes in the

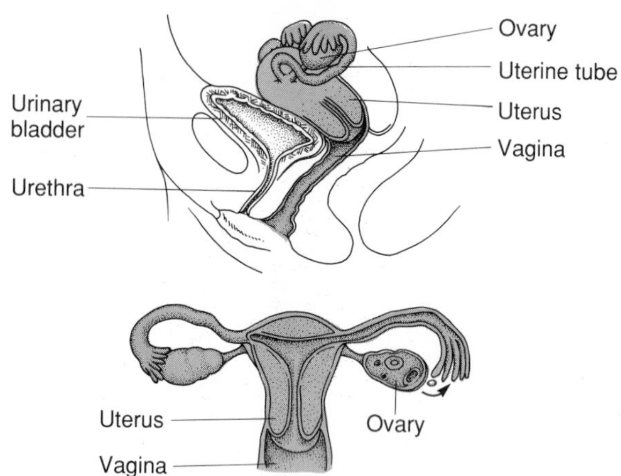

Figure 55-1. The female reproductive organs.

rates of secretion of the female hormones and corresponding changes in the sexual organs themselves. This rhythmical pattern is called the *female sexual cycle* (or less accurately, the *menstrual cycle*). The duration of the cycle averages 28 days. It may be as short as 20 days or as long as 45 days even in completely normal women, though abnormal cycle length is often associated with decreased fertility.

The two significant results of the female sexual cycle are: First, only a *single* mature ovum is normally released from the ovaries each month, so that only a single fetus can begin to grow at a time. Second, the uterine endometrium is prepared for implantation of the fertilized ovum at the required time of the month.

The Anterior Pituitary Gonadotropic Hormones. The ovarian changes during the sexual cycle are completely dependent on gonadotropic hormones secreted by the anterior pituitary gland. Ovaries that are not stimulated by these gonadotropic hormones remain completely inactive, which is essentially the case throughout childhood, when almost no gonadotropic hormones are secreted. However, at the age of about 8 years, the pituitary begins secreting progressively more and more gonadotropic hormones, which culminates in the initiation of monthly sexual cycles between the ages of 11 and 15 years; this culmination is called *menarche,* and this period of life in the girl is called *puberty.*

The anterior pituitary secretes two different hormones that are known to be essential for function of the ovaries: (1) *follicle-stimulating hormone* (FSH), and (2) *luteinizing hormone* (LH). Both these are small glycoproteins having molecular weights of about 30,000.

During each month of the female sexual cycle, there is a cyclic increase and decrease of FSH and LH, as illustrated in the lower half of Figure 55-2. These cyclic variations in turn cause cyclic ovarian changes, which are explained in the following sections.

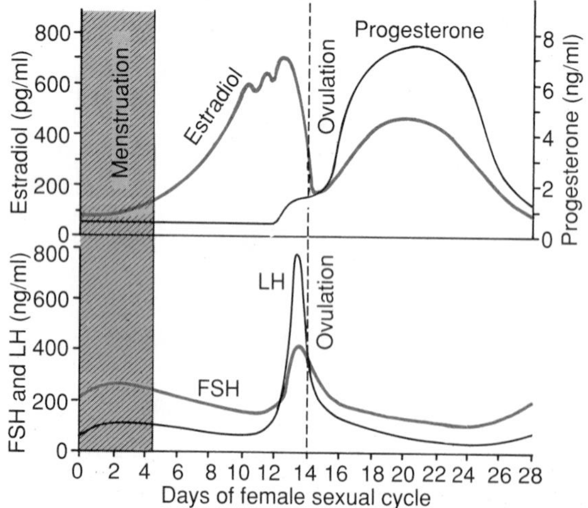

Figure 55-2. Approximate plasma concentrations of the gonadotropins and ovarian hormones during the normal female sexual cycle.

Follicular Growth—Function of FSH

Figure 55-3 depicts the various stages of follicular growth in the ovaries, illustrating, first, the primordial follicle. Throughout childhood the primordial follicles do not grow, but at puberty, when FSH and LH from the anterior pituitary gland begin to be secreted in large quantities, the entire ovaries and especially many of the follicles within them begin to grow. The first stage of follicular growth is enlargement of the ovum itself and growth of additional layers of granulosa cells; the follicle is then known as the *primary follicle.* Then, a few weeks before ovulation still many more layers of granulosa cells develop, as well as several layers of *theca cells* around the granulosa cells. The theca cells originate from the stroma of the ovary and soon take on epithelioid characteristics. It is then the combination of the granulosa and theca cells that secrete the ovarian hormones estrogens and progesterone.

The Vesicular Follicles. At the beginning of each

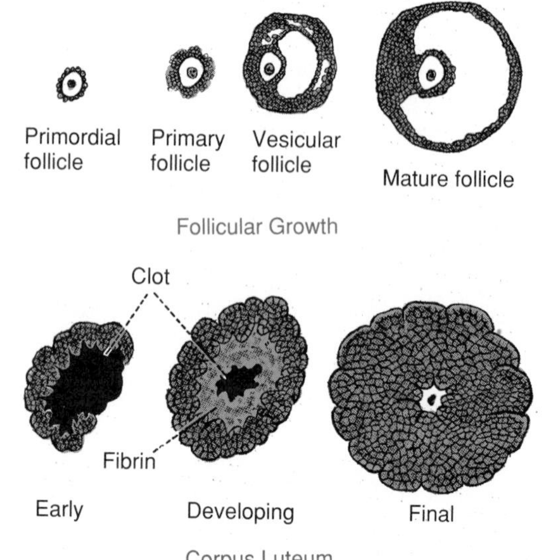

Figure 55-3. Stages of follicular growth in the ovary, showing also formation of the corpus luteum. (Modified from Arey: Developmental Anatomy. 7th ed. Philadelphia, W. B. Saunders Company, 1974.)

month of the female sexual cycle, at the time of menstruation, the concentrations of the pituitary hormones FSH and LH increase. These hormones then cause accelerated growth of the theca and granulosa cells in about 20 of the ovarian follicles each month. These cells in turn secrete a *follicular fluid* that contains a high concentration of estrogen, one of the important female sex hormones discussed later. The accumulation of this fluid in the follicle causes an *antrum* to appear within the mass of theca and granulosa cells, as illustrated at the third stage in Figure 55-3.

After the antrum is formed, the theca and granulosa cells continue to proliferate, the rate of secretion accelerates, and each of the growing follicles is now called a *vesicular follicle.*

As the vesicular follicle enlarges, the theca and granulosa cells now develop mainly at one pole of the follicle. It is in this mass that the ovum is located.

Maturation of Only One Follicle, Atresia of the Remainder. After a week or more of growth—but before ovulation occurs—one of the follicles begins to outgrow all the others; the remainder begin to involute (a process called *atresia*), and these follicles are said to become *atretic.* The cause of the atresia is unknown, but it has been postulated to be the following: The one follicle that becomes more highly developed than the others also secretes more estrogen than the others. Furthermore, this estrogen causes a *positive* feedback effect in that single local follicle, because the extra estrogen causes increasing numbers of both FSH and LH receptors on the granulosa cells and thecal cells, thus promoting an explosive increase in the rate of secretion of fluid and hormones into this one rapidly developing follicle. Yet, at the same time, the large amounts of estrogen from this follicle act on the hypothalamus to depress secretion of FSH and LH by the anterior pituitary gland; it is believed in this way to block further growth of the less well developed follicles that have not yet initiated their own intrinsic positive feedback stimulation. Therefore, the largest follicle continues to grow because of its intrinsic positive feedback effects while all the other follicles stop growing and, indeed, involute.

This process of atresia obviously is important in that it allows only one of the follicles to grow large enough to ovulate. This single follicle reaches a size of approximately 1 to 1.5 cm at the time of ovulation.

Ovulation

Ovulation in a woman with a normal 28-day female sexual cycle occurs 14 days after the onset of menstruation.

Shortly before ovulation the protruding outer wall of the follicle swells rapidly, and a small area in the center of the capsule, called the *stigma,* protrudes like a nipple. In another half hour or so, fluid begins to ooze from the follicle through the stigma. About 2 minutes later, the stigma ruptures widely, and a more viscous fluid that has occupied the central portion of the follicle is evaginated outward into the abdomen. This viscous fluid carries with it the ovum surrounded by several thousand granulosa cells called the *corona radiata.*

Need for LH to Cause Ovulation—Preovulatory Surge of LH. Luteinizing hormone is necessary for final follicular growth and ovulation. Without this hormone, even though large quantities of FSH are available, the follicle will not progress to the stage of ovulation.

Approximately 2 days before ovulation, for reasons that are not completely known at present but that are discussed in more detail later in the chapter, the rate of secretion of LH by the anterior pituitary gland increases markedly, rising sixfold to tenfold and peaking about 16 hours before ovulation. FSH also increases about twofold at the same time, and these two hormones act synergistically to cause the extremely rapid swelling of the follicle that culminates in ovulation.

The Corpus Luteum—The Luteal Phase of the Ovarian Cycle

During the last day before ovulation and continuing for a day or so after ovulation, the granulosa cells, under the stimulation of luteinizing hormone, undergo rapid physical and chemical change, a process called *luteinization.* Thus, the mass of granulosa cells still remaining in the ovary at the site of the ruptured follicle becomes the *corpus luteum,* as illustrated in the lower half of Figure 55-3; this then secretes large quantities of the hormones progesterone and estrogen. These cells become greatly enlarged and develop lipid inclusions that give the cells a distinctive yellowish color, from which is derived the term *luteum,* which means *yellow.*

In the normal woman, the corpus luteum grows to approximately 1.5 cm, reaching this stage of development approximately 7 or 8 days following ovulation. After this, it begins to involute and loses its secretory function as well as its lipid characteristics approximately 12 days following ovulation, becoming then the so-called *corpus albicans,* which during the ensuing few weeks is replaced by connective tissue.

The Role of LH. The conversion of the granulosa cells into the *lutein cells* in the corpus luteum requires the presence of luteinizing hormone (LH). Indeed, this is the reason for its name. Also, in the continued presence of LH the degree of growth of the corpus luteum is enhanced, its secretion is greater, and its life is extended.

Termination of the Ovarian Cycle and Onset of the Next Cycle. After several days of the luteal phase of the ovarian cycle, the large amounts of estrogen and progesterone secreted by the corpus luteum cause a feedback effect to the hypothalamus to decrease the secretion of both FSH and LH. Therefore, during this period no new follicles begin to grow in the ovary. However, when the corpus luteum degenerates completely at the end of 12 days of its life (approximately on the 26th day of the female sexual cycle), the loss of feedback suppression now allows the anterior pituitary gland once again to begin secreting increased quantities of FSH and LH. The FSH and LH initiate growth of new follicles to begin a new ovarian cycle. At the same time, the paucity of secretion of progesterone and estrogen leads to menstruation by the uterus, as explained later.

Summary

Approximately each 28 days, the gonadotropic hormones FSH and LH from the anterior pituitary gland cause new follicles to begin to grow in the ovaries, one of which finally ovulates at the 14th day of the cycle. During all this early growth of the follicles, estrogen is secreted.

Following ovulation, the secretory cells of the follicle develop into a corpus luteum, which secretes large quantities of both of the female hormones progesterone and estrogen. In another 2 weeks the corpus luteum degenerates, whereupon the ovarian hormones estrogen and progesterone decrease greatly and menstruation begins. A new ovarian cycle then follows.

FUNCTIONS OF THE OVARIAN HORMONES—ESTRADIOL AND PROGESTERONE

The two types of ovarian sex hormones are the *estrogens* and the *progestins.* By far the most important of the estrogens is the hormone *estradiol,* and by far the most important progestin is *progesterone.* The estrogens mainly promote proliferation and growth of specific sex-related cells in the body and are responsible for development of most secondary sexual characteristics of the female. On the other hand, the progestins are concerned almost entirely with final preparation of the uterus for pregnancy and the breasts for lactation.

Chemistry of the Sex Hormones

The Estrogens. In the normal nonpregnant woman, estrogens are secreted in major quantities only by the ovaries, though minute amounts are also secreted by the adrenal cortices. In pregnancy, tremendous quantities are also secreted by the placenta, as we shall discuss in the following chapter.

Only three estrogens are present in significant quantities in the plasma of the human female: *β-estradiol, estrone,* and *estriol,* the formulas for which are illustrated in Figure 55–4. The principal estrogen secreted by the ovaries is β-estradiol. Small amounts of estrone are also secreted, and estriol is a very weak estrogenic oxidative product derived from both estradiol and estrone, the conversion occurring mainly in the liver.

The estrogenic potency of β-estradiol is 12 times that of estrone and 80 times that of estriol. Considering these relative potencies, the total estrogenic effect of β-estradiol is usually many times that of the other two together. For this reason β-estradiol is considered to be the major estrogen, though the estrogenic effects of estrone are far from negligible.

The Progestins. By far the most important of the progestins is progesterone. However, small amounts of another progestin, *17-α-hydroxyprogesterone* also are secreted along with progesterone, and it has essentially the same effects. Yet for practical purposes, it is usually proper to consider progesterone to be the single important progestin.

In the normal nonpregnant female, progesterone is secreted in significant amounts only during the latter half of each ovarian cycle when it is secreted by the corpus luteum.

Synthesis of the Estrogens and Progestins. Note from the chemical formulas of the estrogens and progesterone in Figure 55–4 that all these are steroids. They are synthesized in the ovaries mainly from cholesterol derived from the blood but to a slight extent also from acetyl coenzyme A, multiple molecules of which can combine to form the appropriate steroid nucleus.

Functions of the Estrogens—Effects on the Primary and Secondary Sexual Characteristics

The principal function of the estrogens is to cause cellular proliferation and growth of the tissues of the sexual organs and of other tissues related to reproduction.

Effect on the Sexual Organs. During childhood, estrogens are secreted only in small quantities, but following puberty the quantity of estrogens secreted under the influence of the pituitary gonadotropic hormones increases some 20-fold or more. At this time the female sexual organs change from those of a child to those of an adult. The fallopian tubes, uterus, and vagina all increase in size. Also, the external genitalia enlarge, with deposition of fat in the mons pubis and labia majora and with enlargement of the labia minora.

In addition, estrogens change the vaginal epithelium from a cuboidal into a stratified type, which is considerably more resistant to trauma and infection than is the prepubertal epithelium. More important, however, are the changes that take place in the endometrium under the influence of estrogens, for estrogens cause marked proliferation of the endometrium and development of the endometrial glands that will later be used to aid in nutrition of the implanting ovum. These effects are discussed later in the chapter in connection with the endometrial cycle.

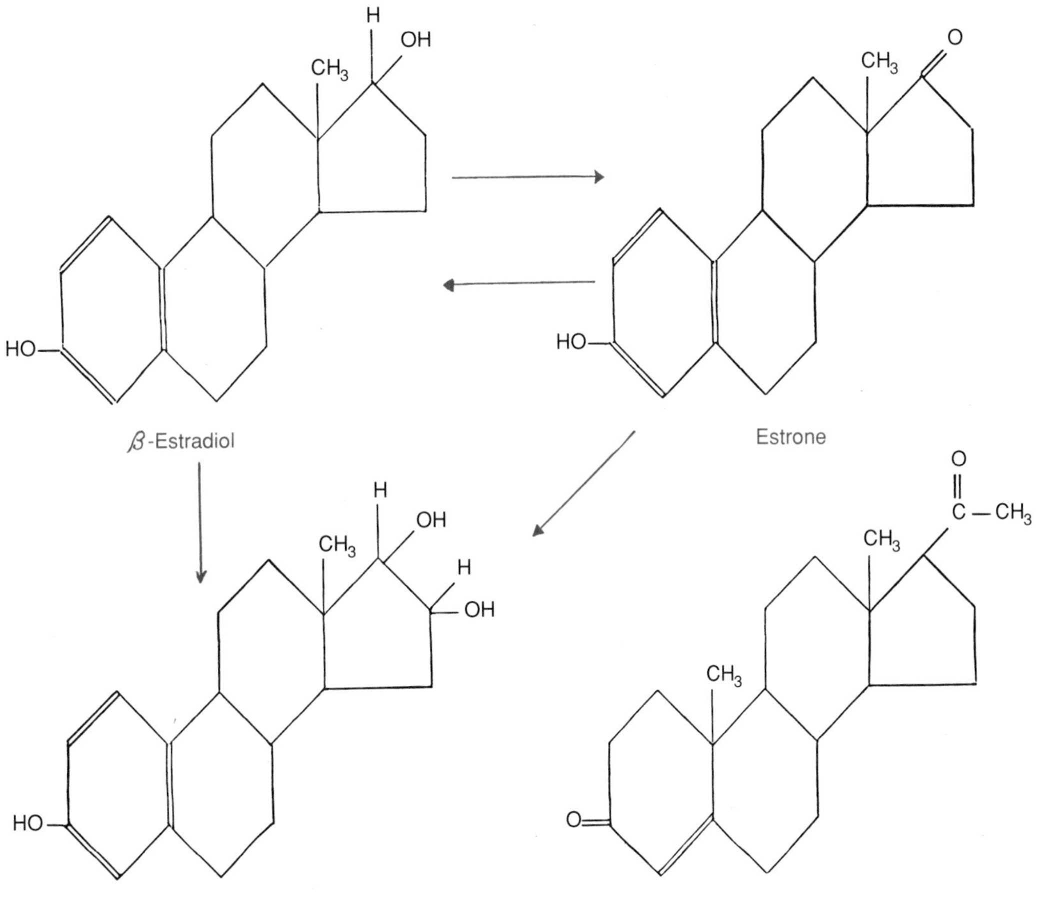

β-Estradiol

Estrone

Estriol

Progesterone

Figure 55-4. Chemical formulas of the principal female hormones.

Effect on the Breasts. Estrogens cause fat deposition in the breasts, development of the stromal tissues of the breasts, and growth of an extensive ductile system. The lobules and alveoli of the breast develop to a slight extent, but it is progesterone and prolactin that cause the determinative growth and function of these structures. In summary, the estrogens initiate growth of the breasts and the breasts' milk-producing apparatus, and they are also responsible for the characteristic external appearance of the mature female breast, but they do not complete the conversion of the breasts into milk-producing organs, a subject discussed in the following chapter.

Effect on the Skeleton. Estrogens cause increased osteoblastic activity. Therefore, at puberty, when the female enters her reproductive years, her height increases rapidly for several years. However, estrogens have another potent effect on skeletal growth that eventually stops the increasing height: that is, the estrogens cause early uniting of the epiphyses with the shafts of the long bones. This effect is much stronger in the female than is a similar effect of testosterone in the male. As a result, growth of the female usually ceases several years earlier than growth of the male. The female eunuch who is completely devoid of estrogen production usually grows several inches taller than the normal mature female because her epiphyses do not unite early.

Effect on Fat Deposition. Estrogens cause deposition of increased quantities of fat in the subcutaneous tissues. As a result, the overall specific gravity of the female body, as judged by flotation in water, is considerably less than that of the male body, which contains more protein and less fat. In addition to deposition of fat in the breasts and subcutaneous tissues, estrogens cause especially marked deposition of fat in the buttocks and thighs, causing the broadening of the hips that is characteristic of the feminine figure.

Effect on the Skin. Estrogens cause the skin to become more vascular than normal; this effect often results in greater bleeding of cut surfaces than is observed in men.

The Basic Intracellular Functions of Estrogens

Thus far we have discussed the gross effects of estrogens on the body. The cellular mechanism behind these effects is: Estrogens circulate in the blood for only a few minutes before they are delivered to the target cells. On entry into these cells, they combine within 10 to 15 seconds with "receptor" protein molecules and then, in combination with this protein, interact with specific portions of the chromosomal DNA in the cell nucleus. This immediately initiates the process of transcription; therefore, RNA begins to be produced within a few minutes. In addition, over many hours new DNA may also be produced, resulting eventually in division of the cell. The RNA diffuses to the cytoplasm, where it causes greatly increased protein formation and subsequently altered cellular function.

One of the principal differences between the protein anabolic effect of the estrogens and that of testosterone is that estrogen causes its effect almost exclusively in a few specific target organs, such as the uterus, the breasts, the skeleton, and certain fatty areas of the body, whereas testosterone has a more generalized effect throughout the body.

Functions of Progesterone

Effect on the Uterus. By far the most important function of progesterone is *to promote secretory changes in the endometrium,* thus preparing the uterus for implantation of the fertilized ovum. This function is discussed later in connection with the endometrial cycle of the uterus.

Effect on the Fallopian Tubes. Progesterone also promotes secretory changes in the mucosal lining of the fallopian tubes. These secretions are important for nutrition of the fertilized, dividing ovum during the several days while it traverses the fallopian tube prior to implantation in the uterus.

Effect on the Breasts. Progesterone promotes development of the lobules and alveoli of the breasts, causing the alveolar cells to proliferate, to enlarge, and to become secretory in nature. However, progesterone does not cause the alveoli actually to secrete milk, for, as discussed in the following chapter, milk is secreted only after the prepared breast is further stimulated by prolactin from the anterior pituitary.

Progesterone also causes the breasts to swell. Part of this swelling is due to the secretory development in the lobules and alveoli, but part also results somewhat from increased fluid in the subcutaneous tissue itself.

The Endometrial Cycle and Menstruation

Associated with the cyclic production of estrogens and progesterone by the ovaries is an endometrial cycle operating through the following stages: first, proliferation of the uterine endometrium; second, secretory changes in the endometrium; and third, desquamation of the endometrium, which is known as *menstruation.* The various phases of the endometrial cycle are illustrated in Figure 55–5.

Proliferative Phase (Estrogen Phase) of the Endometrial Cycle. At the beginning of each menstrual cycle, most of the endometrium is desquamated by the process of menstruation. After menstruation, only a thin layer of endometrial stroma remains at the base of the original endometrium, and the only epithelial cells left are those located in the remaining deep portions of the glands and crypts of the endometrium. *Under the influence of estrogens,* secreted in increasing quantities by the vesicular follicles of the ovary during the first part of the ovarian cycle, the stromal cells and the epithelial cells proliferate rapidly. The endometrial surface is re-epithelialized within 4 to 7 days after the beginning of menstruation. For the first 2 weeks of the sexual cycle—that is, until ovulation—the endometrium increases greatly in thickness, owing to increasing numbers of stromal cells and to progressive growth of the endometrial glands, as well as ingrowth of blood vessels into the endometrium, all of which effects are promoted by the estrogens. At the time of ovulation the endometrium is approximately 2 to 3 mm thick.

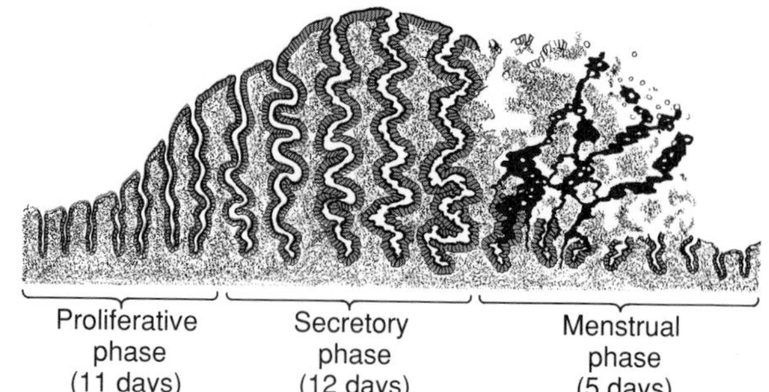

Figure 55–5. Phases of endometrial growth and menstruation during each monthly female sexual cycle.

Secretory Phase (Progestational Phase) of the Endometrial Cycle. During the latter half of the sexual cycle, progesterone as well as estrogens is secreted in large quantity by the corpus luteum. The estrogens cause slight additional cellular proliferation, and progesterone causes considerable swelling and secretory development of the endometrium. The glands increase in tortuosity, secretory substances accumulate in the glandular epithelial cells, and the glands secrete small quantities of endometrial fluid. Also, the cytoplasm of the stromal cells increases, lipid and glycogen deposits increase greatly in these cells, and the blood supply to the endometrium further increases in proportion to the developing secretory activity. The thickness of the endometrium approximately doubles during the secretory phase, so that toward the end of the monthly cycle the endometrium has a thickness of 5 to 6 mm.

The whole purpose of all these endometrial changes is to produce a highly secretory endometrium containing large amounts of stored nutrients that can provide appropriate conditions for implantation of a fertilized ovum during the latter half of the monthly cycle.

Menstruation. Approximately 2 days before the end of the monthly cycle, the ovarian hormones estrogens and progesterone decrease sharply to low levels of secretion, as was illustrated in Figure 55–2, and menstruation follows. Menstruation is caused by this sudden reduction in both progesterone and estrogens at the end of the monthly ovarian cycle. The first effect is decreased stimulation of the endometrial cells by these two hormones, followed rapidly by involution of the endometrium itself to about 65 per cent of its previous thickness. During the 24 hours preceding the onset of menstruation, the blood vessels leading to the mucosal layers of the endometrium become vasospastic, presumably because of some effect of the involution, such as release of a vasoconstrictor material. The vasospasm and loss of hormonal stimulation cause beginning necrosis in the endometrium. As a result, blood seeps into the tissues of the vascular layer of the endometrium, the hemorrhagic areas growing over a period of 24 to 36 hours. Gradually, the necrotic outer layers of the endometrium separate from the uterus at the site of the hemorrhages, until, at approximately 48 hours following the onset of menstruation, all the superficial layers of the endometrium have desquamated. The desquamated tissue and blood in the uterine vault initiate uterine contractions that expel the uterine contents.

During normal menstruation, approximately 40 ml of blood and an additional 35 ml of serous fluid are lost. This menstrual fluid is normally nonclotting, because a *fibrinolysin* is released along with the necrotic endometrial material.

Within 4 to 7 days after menstruation starts, the loss of blood ceases, for by this time the endometrium has become completely re-epithelialized.

REGULATION OF THE FEMALE MONTHLY RHYTHM: INTERPLAY BETWEEN THE OVARIAN AND THE HYPOTHALAMIC-PITUITARY HORMONES

Now that we have presented the major cyclic changes that occur during the female sexual cycle, we can attempt to explain the basic rhythmical mechanism that causes these cyclic variations.

Function of the Hypothalamus in the Regulation of Gonadotropin Secretion — Gonadotropin-Releasing Hormone

As pointed out in Chapter 49, secretion of most of the anterior pituitary hormones is controlled by releasing hormones formed in the hypothalamus and then transported to the anterior pituitary gland by way of the hypothalamic-hypophysial portal system. In the case of the gonadotropins, at least one releasing hormone, *gonadotropin-releasing hormone (GnRH),* is important. This has been purified and has been found to be a decapeptide having the following formula:

Glu-His-Trp-Ser-Tyr-Gly-Leu-Arg-
Pro-Gly-NH_2

Intermittent, Pulsatile Secretion of GnRH by the Hypothalamus — and Pulsatile Release of LH From the Anterior Pituitary. The hypothalamus does not secrete GnRA continuously, but instead secretes it in pulses lasting several minutes that occur every 1 to 3 hours. Furthermore, when GnRH is infused continuously so that it is available all of the time rather than in these pulses, its effects in causing release of LH and FSH by the anterior pituitary gland are completely lost. Therefore, for reasons unknown, the pulsatile nature of GnRH release is absolutely essential to its function.

The pulsatile release of GnRH also causes pulsatile output of LH.

To a slight extent, the secretion of FSH rises and falls with the hypothalamic pulses of GnRH, but there is a more important prolonged effect on FSH secretion that persists for many hours rather than changing pulse to pulse.

Hypothalamic Centers for Release of GnRH. The neuronal activity that causes pulsatile release of GnRH occurs primarily in the mediobasal hypothalamus. In turn, multiple neuronal centers in the brain's limbic system transmit signals into the hypothalamus to modify both the intensity of GnRH release and the frequency of the pulses, thus providing a possible explanation of why psychic factors very often modify female sexual function.

Negative Feedback Effect of Estrogen, Progesterone, and Inhibin on Secretion of Follicle-Stimulating Hormone and Luteinizing Hormone

Estrogen in small amounts and progesterone in large amounts inhibit the production of FSH and LH. These feedback effects mainly operate directly on the anterior pituitary gland but to a lesser extent on the hypothalamus to decrease secretion of GnRH, especially by altering the frequency of the GnRH pulses.

In addition to the feedback effects of estrogen and progesterone, still another hormone is involved. This is *inhibin,* which is secreted along with the steroid sex hormones by the corpus luteum. This inhibin inhibits the secretion of FSH by the anterior pituitary gland and LH to a lesser extent as well. Therefore, it is believed that inhibin might be especially important in causing the decrease in secretion of FSH and LH toward the end of the female sexual month.

Positive Feedback Effect of Estrogen Before Ovulation — The Preovulatory Luteinizing Hormone Surge

For reasons not completely understood, the anterior pituitary gland secretes greatly increased amounts of LH for a period of 1 to 2 days beginning 24 to 48 hours before ovulation. This effect is illustrated in Figure 55-2, and the figure shows a much smaller preovulatory surge of FSH as well.

Experiments have shown that infusion of estrogen into a female above a critical rate for a period of 2 to 3 days during the first half of the ovarian cycle will cause rapidly accelerating growth of the follicles and also rapidly accelerating secretion of ovarian estrogens. During this period the secretion of both FSH and LH by the anterior pituitary gland is at first suppressed slightly. Then abruptly the secretion of LH increases six-to eightfold, and the secretion of FSH increases about twofold. The cause of this abrupt increase in secretion of the gonadotropins is not known. However, several possible causes are as follows: (1) It has been suggested that estrogen at this point in the cycle has a peculiar *positive feedback effect* to stimulate pituitary secretion of the gonadotropins; this is in sharp contrast to its normal negative feedback effect that occurs during the remainder of the female monthly cycle. (2) The granulosa cells of the follicles begin to secrete small but increasing quantities of progesterone a day or so prior to the preovulatory LH surge, and it has been suggested that this might be the factor that stimulates the excess LH secretion.

Regardless of its cause, without this normal preovulatory surge of LH, ovulation will not occur.

Feedback Oscillation of the Hypothalamic-Pituitary-Ovarian System

Now, after discussing much of the known information about the interrelationships of the different components of the female hormonal system, we can digress from the area of proven fact into the realm of speculation and attempt to explain the feedback oscillation that controls the rhythm of the female sexual cycle. It seems to operate in approximately the following sequence of three successive events:

1. The Postovulatory Secretion of the Ovarian Hormones and Depression of Gonadotropins. The easiest part of the cycle to explain is the events that occur during the postovulatory phase—between ovulation and the beginning of menstruation. During this time the corpus luteum secretes large quantities of both progesterone and estrogen and probably the additional hormone inhibin as well. All these hormones together have a combined negative feedback effect on the anterior pituitary gland and the hypothalamus to cause suppression of both FSH and LH, decreasing these to their lowest levels at about 3 to 4 days before the onset of menstruation. These effects are illustrated in Figure 55–2.

2. The Follicular Growth Phase. Two to three days before menstruation the corpus luteum involutes, and the secretion of estrogen, progesterone, and inhibin decreases to a low ebb. This releases the hypothalamus and anterior pituitary from the feedback effect of these hormones; and a day or so later, at about the time that menstruation begins, FSH increases as much as twofold; then several days after menstruation begins, LH secretion increases as much as twofold as well. These hormones initiate new follicular growth and progressive increase in the secretion of estrogen, reaching a peak estrogen secretion at about 12.5 to 13 days after the onset of menstruation. During the first 11 to 12 days of this follicular growth the rates of secretion of the gonadotropins FSH and LH decrease slightly because of the negative feedback effect mainly of estrogen on the anterior pituitary gland. Then comes a sudden increase in secretion of both of these hormones, leading to the preovulatory surge of LH, followed by ovulation.

3. Preovulatory Surge of LH and FSH; Ovulation. At approximately 11.5 to 12 days after the onset of menstruation, the decline in secretion of FSH and LH comes to an abrupt halt. It is believed that the high level of estrogens at this time (or the beginning secretion of progesterone by the follicles) causes a positive feedback effect principally on the anterior pituitary, as explained earlier, which leads to a terrific surge of secretion of LH and to a lesser extent of FSH. Whatever the cause of this preovulatory LH and FSH surge, the LH leads to both ovulation and subsequent secretion by the corpus luteum. Thus, the hormonal system begins a new round of the cycle until the next ovulation.

Puberty

Puberty means the onset of adult sexual life, and as pointed out earlier in the chapter, it is caused by a gradual increase in gonadotropic hormone secretion by the pituitary, beginning approximately in the eighth year of life.

In the female, as in the male, the infantile pituitary gland and ovaries are capable of full function if appropriately stimulated. However, as is also true in the male and for reasons not yet understood, the hypothalamus does not secrete significant quantities of gonadotropin-releasing hormone during childhood. Experiments have shown that the hypothalamus itself is perfectly capable of secreting this hormone, but there is lack of the appropriate signal from some other brain area to cause the secretion. Therefore, it is now believed that the onset of puberty is initiated by some maturation process occurring elsewhere in the brain than the hypothalamus, perhaps somewhere in the limbic system.

The Menopause

At an age of 40 to 50 years, women's sexual cycles usually become irregular, and ovulation fails to occur during many of these cycles. After a few months to a few years, the cycles cease altogether. This cessation of the cycles is called the *menopause.*

The cause of the menopause is "burning out" of the ovaries. In other words, throughout a woman's sexual life many of the primordial follicles grow into vesicular follicles with each sexual cycle, and eventually almost all the ova either are ovulated (about 0.1 per cent of the total) or degenerate. Therefore at the age of about 45 years, only a few primordial follicles still remain to be stimulated by FSH and LH; the production of estrogens by the ovaries also decreases as the number of primordial follicles approaches zero. When estrogen production falls below a critical value, the estrogens can no longer inhibit the production of FSH and LH sufficiently to cause oscillatory cycles. Consequently, FSH and LH (mainly FSH) are produced thereafter in large and continuous quantities. Estrogens continue to be produced in subcritical quantities for a short time after the menopause, but over a few years, as the final remaining primordial follicles become atretic, the production of estrogens by the ovaries falls almost to zero.

ABNORMALITIES OF SECRETION BY THE OVARIES

Hypogonadism. Less than normal secretion by the ovaries can result from poorly formed ovaries or lack of ovaries. When ovaries are absent from birth or when they never become functional, *female eunuchism* occurs. In this condition the usual secondary sexual characteristics do not appear, and the sexual organs remain infantile. Especially characteristic of this condition is excessive growth of the long bones because the epiphyses do not unite with the shafts of these bones as early as in the normal adolescent woman. Consequently, the female eunuch is as tall as her male counterpart of similar genetic background, or perhaps even slightly taller.

When the ovaries of a fully developed woman are removed, the sexual organs regress to some extent, so that the uterus becomes almost infantile in size, the vagina becomes smaller, and the vaginal epithelium becomes thin and easily damaged. The breasts atrophy and become pendulous, and the pubic hair becomes considerably thinner. These same changes occur in the woman after the menopause.

Irregularity of Menses and Amenorrhea Due to Hypogonadism. The quantity of estrogens produced by the ovaries must rise above a critical value if they are to be capable of inhibiting the production of follicle-stimulating hormone sufficiently to cause an oscillatory sexual cycle. Consequently, in hypogonadism or when the gonads are secreting small quantities of estrogens as a result of other factors, the ovarian cycle likely will not occur normally. Instead, several months may elapse between menstrual periods, or menstruation may cease altogether (amenorrhea). Characteristically, ovulation often fails to occur in these prolonged ovarian cycles, presumably due to insufficient secretion of luteinizing hormone, which is necessary for ovulation.

Hypersecretion by the Ovaries. Extreme hypersecretion of hormones by the ovaries is a rare clinical entity, for excessive secretion of estrogens automatically decreases the production of gonadotropins by the pituitary, and this in turn limits the production of the ovarian hormones. Consequently, hypersecretion of feminizing hormones is recognized clinically only when a feminizing tumor develops.

Rarely, a granulosa cell tumor develops in an ovary, more often after menopause than before. Such a tumor secretes large quantities of estrogens, which exert the usual estrogenic effects, including hypertrophy of the uterine endometrium and irregular bleeding from it. In fact, bleeding is often the first indication that such a tumor exists.

THE FEMALE SEXUAL ACT

Stimulation of the Female Sexual Act. As is true in the male sexual act, successful performance of the female sexual act depends on both psychic stimulation and local sexual stimulation.

Also, as in men, the thinking of erotic thoughts can lead to female sexual desire, and this aids greatly in the performance of the female sexual act. Such desire is probably based as much on one's background training as on physiological drive, though sexual drive does increase in proportion to the level of secretion of the sex hormones. Desire also changes during the sexual month, reaching a peak near the time of ovulation, probably because of the high levels of estrogen secretion during the preovulatory period.

Local sexual stimulation in women occurs in more or less the same manner as in men, for massage, irritation, or other types of stimulation of the perineal region, sexual organs, and urinary tract create sexual sensations. The glans of the *clitoris* is especially sensitive for initiating sexual sensations. As in men, the sexual sensory signals are mediated to the sacral segments of the spinal cord through the pudendal nerve and sacral plexus. Once these signals have entered the spinal cord, they are transmitted thence to the cerebrum. Also, local reflexes integrated in the sacral and lumbar spinal cord are at least partially responsible for female sexual reactions.

Female Erection and Lubrication. Located around the introitus and extending into the clitoris is erectile tissue almost identical with the erectile tissue of the penis. This erectile tissue, like that of the penis, is controlled by the parasympathetic nerves that pass through the pelvic nerves to the external genitalia. In the early phases of sexual stimulation, the parasympathetics dilate the arteries allowing rapid accumulation of blood in the erectile tissue, so that the introitus tightens around the penis; this aids the male greatly in his attainment of sufficient sexual stimulation for ejaculation to occur.

Parasympathetic signals also pass to the bilateral Bartholin's glands located beneath the labia minora to cause secretion of mucus immediately inside the introitus. This mucus is responsible for much of the lubrication during sexual intercourse, though much is also provided by mucus secreted by the vaginal epithelium and a small amount secreted from the male urethral glands. The lubrication in turn is necessary for establishing during intercourse a satisfactory massaging rather than an irritative sensation, which may be provoked by a dry vagina. Massaging constitutes the optimal type of sensation for evoking the appropriate reflexes that culminate in both the male and female climaxes.

The Female Orgasm. When local sexual stimulation reaches maximum intensity, and especially when the local sensations are supported by appropriate psychic conditioning signals from the cerebrum, reflexes are initiated that cause the female orgasm, also called the *female climax.* The female orgasm is analogous to emission and ejaculation in the male, and it perhaps helps promote fertilization of the ovum. Indeed, the human female is known to be somewhat more fertile when inseminated by normal sexual intercourse rather than by artificial methods, thus indicating an important function of the female orgasm. Possible effects that could result in greater fertility are:

First, during the orgasm the perineal muscles of the female contract rhythmically, which results from spinal cord reflexes similar to those that cause ejaculation in the male. It is possible, also, that reflexes involving the sympathetic nervous system increase uterine and fallopian tube motility during the orgasm, thus helping transport the sperm toward the ovum, but the information on this subject is scanty.

Second, in many lower animals, copulation causes the posterior pituitary gland to secrete oxytocin; this effect is probably mediated through the amygdaloid nuclei and then through the hypothalamus to the pituitary. The oxytocin in turn causes increased rhythmic contractility of the uterus, which has been postulated to cause rapid transport of the sperm. Sperm have been shown to traverse the entire length of the fallopian tube in the cow in approximately 5 minutes, a rate at least ten times as fast as that which the swimming motions of the sperm themselves could achieve. Whether or not this occurs in the human female is unknown.

In addition to the possible effects of the orgasm on fertilization, the intense sexual sensations that develop during the orgasm also pass to the cerebrum and cause intense muscle tension throughout the body. But after culmination of the sexual act, this gives way during the succeeding minutes to a sense of satisfaction characterized by relaxed peacefulness, an effect called *resolution.*

FEMALE FERTILITY

The Fertile Period of Each Sexual Cycle. The ovum remains viable and capable of being fertilized for probably no longer than 24 hours after it is expelled from the ovary. Therefore, sperm must be available soon after ovulation if fertilization is to take place. On the other hand, a few sperm can remain viable in the female reproductive tract for up to 72 hours, though most of them for not more than 24 hours. Therefore, for fertilization to take place, intercourse usually must occur some time between one day prior to ovulation and one day after ovulation.

The Rhythm Method of Contraception. A method of contraception often practiced is to avoid intercourse near the time of ovulation. The difficulty with this method is the impossibility of predicting the exact time of ovulation. Yet the interval between ovulation and the next succeeding onset of menstruation is almost always between 13 and 15 days. In other words, if the periodicity of the menstrual cycle is 28 days, ovulation usually occurs within one day of the 14th day of the cycle. If, on the other hand, the periodicity of the cycle is 40 days, ovulation usually occurs within one day of the 26th day of the cycle. Finally, if the periodicity of the cycle is 21 days, ovulation usually occurs within one day of the 7th day of the cycle. Therefore, it is usually stated that avoidance of intercourse for 4 days prior to the calculated day of ovulation and 3 days afterward prevents conception. But such a method of contraception can be used only when the periodicity of the menstrual cycle is regular.

Hormonal Suppression of Fertility—"The Pill." It has long been known that administration of either estrogen or progesterone, if given in appropriate quantity during the first half of the monthly female cycle, can inhibit ovulation. The reason for this is that administration of either of these can prevent the preovulatory surge of LH secretion by the pituitary gland, which, it will be recalled, is essential in causing ovulation.

The reason the administration of estrogen or progesterone prevents the preovulatory surge of LH secretion is not fully understood. However, experimental work has suggested that immediately before the surge occurs there is probably a sudden depression of estrogen secretion by the ovarian follicles, and that this might be the necessary signal for causing the feedback effect that leads to the surge. Obviously, administration of the sex hormones could prevent the initial hormonal depression that might be the initiating signal for ovulation.

The problem in devising methods for hormonal suppression of ovulation has been to develop appropriate combinations of estrogens and progestins that will suppress ovulation but that will not cause unwanted effects of these two hormones. For instance, too much of either of the hormones can cause abnormal menstrual bleeding patterns. However, use of certain synthetic progestins in place of progesterone, especially the 19-norsteroids, along with small amounts of estrogens will usually prevent ovulation and yet also allow almost a normal pattern of menstruation. Therefore, almost all "pills" used for control of fertility consist of some combination of synthetic estrogens and synthetic progestins. The main reason for using synthetic estrogens and synthetic progestins is that the *natural* hormones are almost entirely destroyed by the liver within a short time after they are absorbed from the gastrointestinal tract into the portal circulation. However, many of the *synthetic* hormones can resist this destructive propensity of the liver, thus allowing oral administration.

The medication is usually begun in the early stages of the monthly cycle and continued beyond the time that ovulation normally would have occurred. Then the medication is stopped, allowing menstruation to occur and a new cycle to begin.

Anovulation and Female Sterility. Approximately one of every six to eight marriages is infertile; in about 60 per cent of these, the infertility is due to female sterility.

Occasionally, no abnormality whatsoever can be discovered in the female genital organs, in which case it must be assumed that the infertility is due either to abnormal physiological function of the genital system or to abnormal development of the ova themselves.

However, one of the most common causes of female sterility is failure to ovulate. This can result from either hyposecretion of gonadotropic hormones, in which case the intensity of the hormonal stimuli simply is not sufficient to cause ovulation, or from abnormal ovaries that will not allow ovulation. For instance, thick capsules occasionally exist on the outside of the ovaries and prevent ovulation.

Lack of ovulation caused by hyposecretion of the pituitary gonadotropic hormones can usually be treated by administration of *human chorionic gonadotropin,* a hormone that will be discussed in the following chapter and that is extracted from the human placenta. This hormone, though secreted by the placenta, has almost exactly the same effects as luteinizing hormone and therefore is a powerful stimulator of ovulation. However, excess use of this hormone can cause ovulation from many follicles simultaneously; and multiple births result. As many as seven babies have been born to mothers treated for infertility with this hormone.

REFERENCES

DeGroot, L. J., et al. (eds.): Endocrinology. 2nd ed. Philadelphia, W. B. Saunders Co., 1989.

DeJong, F. H.: Inhibin. Physiol. Rev., 68:555, 1988.

Dicztausy, E., and Bygdeman, M.: Fertility Regulation Today and Tomorrow. New York, Raven Press, 1987.

Dufau, M. L.: Endocrine regulation and communicating functions of the Leydig cell. Annu. Rev. Physiol., 50:483, 1988.

Gruhn, J. G., and Kazer, R. R.: Hormonal Regulation of the Menstrual Cycle. New York, Plenum Publishing Corp., 1989.

Keyes, P. L., and Wiltbank, M. C.: Endocrine regulation of the corpus luteum. Annu. Rev. Physiol., 50:465, 1988.

Knobil, E., et al. (eds.): The Physiology of Reproduction. New York, Raven Press, 1988.

Richards, J. S., and Hedin, L.: Molecular aspects of hormone action in ovarian follicular development, ovulation, and luteinization. Annu. Rev. Physiol., 50:441, 1988.

Rories, C., and Spelsberg, T. C.: Ovarian steroid action on gene expression: Mechanisms and models. Annu. Rev. Physiol., 51:653, 1989.

Soules, M. F.: Problems in Reproductive Endocrinology and Infertility. New York, Elsevier Science Publishing Co., 1989.

Wassarman, P. M.: Eggs, sperm, and sugar: A recipe for fertilization. News Physiol. Sci., 3:120, 1988.

Wynn, R. M., and Jollie, W. (eds.): The Biology of the Uterus. 2nd ed. New York, Plenum Publishing Corp., 1989.

QUESTIONS

1. Describe the physiological anatomy of the female sexual organs.
2. Describe the monthly changes in the ovaries and control of the ovarian cycle by the anterior pituitary *gonadotropic hormones.*
3. What are the characteristics of the *vesicular follicles,* what do they secrete, and what is their fate?
4. Describe *ovulation.* What are the roles of *FSH* and *LH* leading up to ovulation, and what is the role of the *preovulatory surge of LH?*
5. Describe the formation of the *corpus luteum,* its secretion of *progesterone* and *estrogen* and its control by LH.
6. Describe, in general, the chemistry of the estrogens and progesterone.
7. What are the effects of the estrogens on the female sex organs, the breasts, and the skin?
8. How do the estrogens function intracellularly to cause their hormonal effects?
9. What are the functional effects of progesterone on the uterus, the fallopian tubes, and the breast?
10. Describe the monthly changes in the *uterine endometrium.* What are the roles of estrogen and progesterone in controlling the endometrial cycle?
11. Describe the sequential changes in the endometrium that cause menstruation and the hormonal effects that lead to menstruation.
12. Explain the role of the *hypothalamus* in secreting *GnRH* and the effect of this secretion in controlling the secretion of FSH and LH by the anterior pituitary gland. What is the cause of the preovulatory surge of luteinizing hormone?
13. Explain the sequential changes in secretory rates of GnRH, the anterior pituitary hormones, and the ovarian hormones that are responsible for the monthly *female sexual cycle.*
14. What leads to *puberty?*
15. What is the cause of the *menopause?*
16. What are the clinical characteristics of *hypogonadism?*
17. What are the clinical characteristics of *hypersecretion by the ovaries?*
18. Describe the sexual sensory signals that lead to female excitement during the sexual act.
19. What is the role of the parasympathetic nervous system in female *erection* and *lubrication,* and what is the possible role of the sympathetic nervous system in the female *orgasm?*
20. How can one calculate with reasonable accuracy the few days of the female sexual cycle when the female will be fertile?
21. What is the physiological basis of hormonal *suppression of fertility?*
22. How can female sterility caused by *anovulation* frequently be treated with hormones?

56

Pregnancy, Lactation, and Fetal and Neonatal Physiology

In the preceding two chapters, the sexual functions of men and women were described to the point of fertilization of the ovum. If the ovum becomes fertilized, a completely new sequence of events called *gestation,* or *pregnancy,* takes place, and the fertilized ovum eventually develops into a full-term fetus. This chapter discusses these events.

Maturation of the Ovum

Shortly before the ovum is released from the follicle, each of the 23 pairs of chromosomes loses one of its partners, so that 23 *unpaired* chromosomes remain in the mature ovum. It is at this point that ovulation occurs, and soon thereafter, usually after the ovum enters the tip of the fallopian tube, fertilization occurs.

Fertilization of the Ovum

After coitus, the first sperm are transported through the uterus to the ovarian end of the fallopian tubes within 5 to 10 minutes. This is many times more rapid than the motility of the sperm themselves can account for, which indicates that propulsive movements of the uterus and fallopian tubes might be responsible for much of the sperm movement. Yet, even with this aid, of the nearly one half billion sperm deposited in the vagina, only 1000 to 3000 succeed in traversing the fallopian tubes to reach the proximity of the ovum.

Only one sperm is required for fertilization of the ovum, the process of which is illustrated in Figure 56-1. Furthermore, almost never does more than one sperm enter the ovum for the following reason: The zona pellucida of the ovum has a lattice-type structure, and once this is punctured, some substance (perhaps one of the proteolytic enzymes of the sperm acrosome) diffuses throughout the lattice to prevent penetration by additional sperm. Indeed, many sperm do attempt to penetrate the zona pellucida but become inactivated after traveling only part way through.

Once a sperm enters the ovum, its head swells rapidly to form a *male pronucleus,* which is also illustrated in Figure 56-1. Later, the 23 chromosomes of the male pronucleus and the 23 of the *female pronucleus* align themselves to re-form a complete complement of 46 chromosomes (23 pairs) in the fertilized ovum.

Sex Determination. The sex of a child is determined by the type of sperm that fertilizes the ovum — that is, whether it is a male or a female sperm. It will be recalled from Chapter 54 that a male sperm carries a *Y sex chromosome and 22 autosomal chromosomes,* while a female sperm carries the same 22 autosomal chromosomes but an *X sex chromosome.* On the other hand, the ovum has an X sex chromosome, not a Y chromosome. After recombination of the male and female pronuclei during fertilization, the fertilized ovum then contains 44 autosomal chromosomes and either 2 X chromosomes, which causes a female child to develop, or an X and a Y chromosome, which causes a male child to develop.

Transport and Implantation of the Developing Ovum

Entry of the Ovum into the Fallopian Tube. When ovulation occurs, the ovum along with its at-

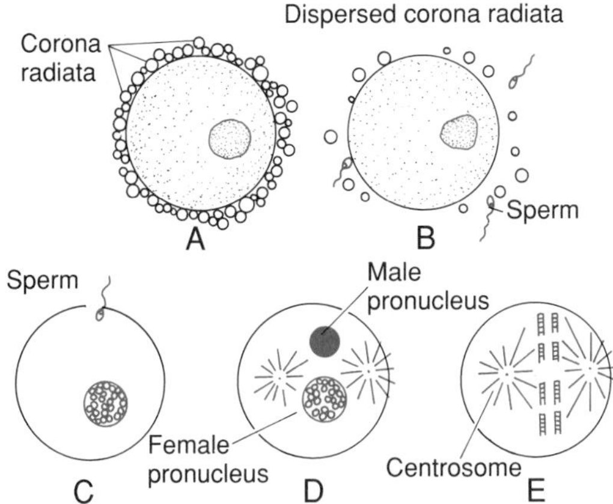

Figure 56–1. Fertilization of the ovum, showing *A*, the mature ovum surrounded by the corona radiata; *B*, dispersal of the corona radiata; *C*, entry of the sperm; *D*, formation of the male and female pronuclei; and *E*, reorganization of a full complement of chromosomes and beginning division of the ovum. (Modified from Arey: Developmental Anatomy. 7th ed. Philadelphia, W. B. Saunders Company, 1974.)

tached granulosa cells, the *corona radiata,* is expelled directly into the peritoneal cavity and must then enter one of the fallopian tubes. The fimbriated end of each fallopian tube falls naturally around the ovaries, and the inner surfaces of the fimbriated tentacles are lined with ciliated epithelium, the *cilia* of which continuously beat toward the *ostium* of the fallopian tube. One can actually see a slow fluid current flowing toward the ostium. By this means the ovum enters one or the other fallopian tube.

Transport of the Ovum Through the Fallopian Tube. Fertilization of the ovum normally takes place soon after the ovum enters the fallopian tube. After fertilization has occurred, 3 to 4 days are normally required for transport of the ovum through the tube into the cavity of the uterus. This transport is effected mainly by a feeble fluid current in the fallopian tube resulting from action of the ciliated epithelium that lines the tube, the cilia always beating toward the uterus. It is possible also that weak contractions of the fallopian tube aid in the passage of the ovum.

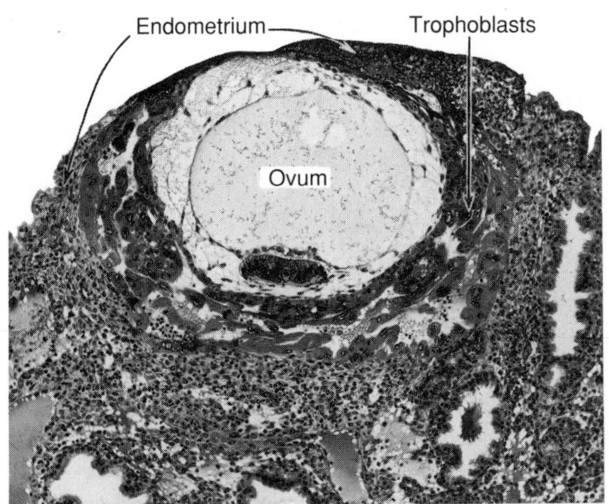

Figure 56–2. Implantation of the early human embryo, showing trophoblastic digestion and invasion of the endometrium. (Courtesy of Dr. Arthur Hertig.)

This delayed transport of the ovum through the fallopian tube allows several stages of division to occur, and the ovum develops first to a mass of cells called the *morula* and then to the stage of a *blastocyst* soon after it enters the uterus. During this time, large quantities of secretions are formed by secretory cells that line the fallopian tube. These secretions are for nutrition of the developing ovum.

Implantation of the Blastocyst in the Uterus. After reaching the uterus, the developing morula and then blastocyst usually remains in the uterine cavity an additional 2 to 5 days before it implants in the endometrium, which means that implantation ordinarily occurs on the seventh or eighth day following ovulation. During this time the developing mass of cells obtains its nutrition from the endometrial secretions, called uterine milk. Figure 56–2 shows a very early stage of implantation, illustrating that the blastocyst has a cavity with the embryo, shown in color, beginning to develop along one wall of the cavity.

Implantation results from the action of *trophoblastic cells* that develop over the surface of the blastocyst. These cells secrete proteolytic enzymes that digest and liquefy the cells of the endometrium. Simultaneously, much of the fluid and nutrients thus released is actively absorbed into the blastocyst as a result of phagocytosis by the trophoblastic cells; these absorbed substances provide the sustenance for further growth. Also, at the same time, additional trophoblastic cells form cords of cells that extend into the deeper layers of the endometrium and attach to them. Thus, the blastocyst eats a hole in the endometrium and attaches to it at the same time.

Once implantation has taken place, the trophoblastic and underlying blastocyst cells proliferate rapidly; and they, along with cells from the mother's endometrium, form the placenta and the various membranes of pregnancy.

Early Intrauterine Nutrition of the Embryo. As the trophoblastic cells invade the endometrium, digesting and imbibing it, the stored nutrients in the large endometrial cells, called *decidual cells,* are used by the embryo for appropriate growth and development. During the first week after implantation, this is the only means by which the embryo can obtain any nutrients, and the embryo continues to obtain a large measure of its total nutrition in this way for at least 8 weeks, though the placenta also begins to provide slight amounts of nutrients after approximately the sixteenth day beyond fertilization (a little over a week after implantation).

FUNCTION OF THE PLACENTA

The structure of the placenta is illustrated in Figure 56–3. Note that the fetus's blood flows through two *umbilical arteries* to the capillaries of the villi, and thence back through the *umbilical vein* into the fetus.

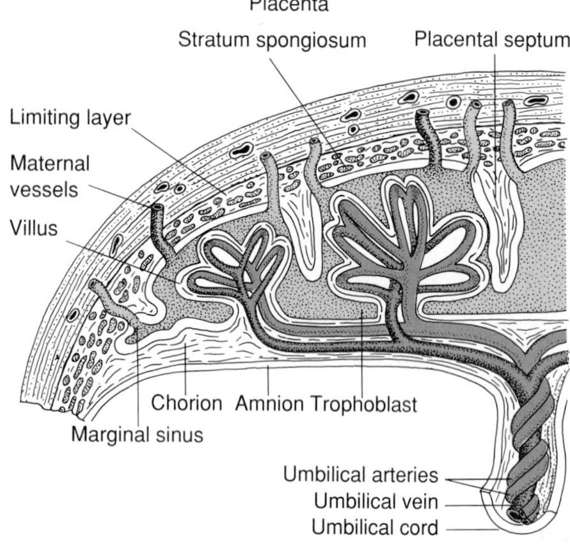

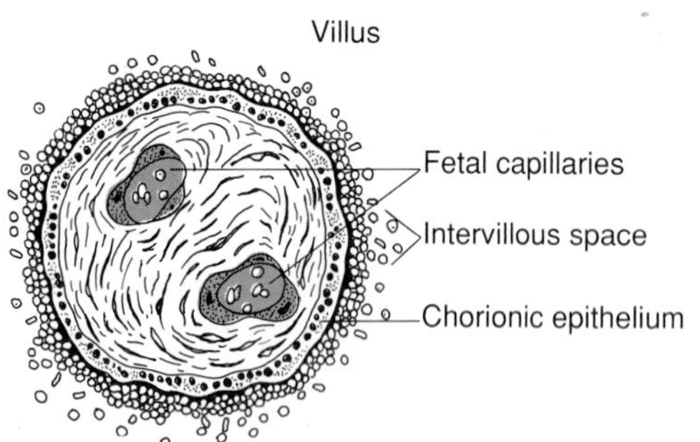

Figure 56-3. *Above,* Organization of the mature placenta. *Below,* Relationship of the fetal blood in the villus capillaries to the mother's blood in the intervillous spaces. (Modified from Gray and Goss: Anatomy of the Human Body. Philadelphia, Lea & Febiger; and from Arey: Developmental Anatomy. 7th ed. Philadelphia, W. B. Saunders Company, 1974.)

On the other hand, the mother's blood flows from the *uterine arteries* into large *blood sinuses* surrounding the villi and then back into the *uterine veins* of the mother.

The lower part of Figure 56-3 illustrates the fetal blood in the capillaries of the villus that protrudes into the blood sinuses of the placenta. The capillaries of the villus are lined with an extremely thin endothelium and are surrounded by a layer of *mesenchymal tissue* that is covered on the outside of the villus by a layer of *trophoblast cells.*

Diffusion Through the Placental Membrane

The major function of the placenta is to allow *diffusion* of foodstuffs from the mother's blood into the fetus's blood and diffusion of excretory products from the fetus back into the mother.

In the early months of development, placental permeability is relatively slight because the villar membranes have not yet been reduced to their minimum thickness. However, as the placenta becomes older, the permeability increases progressively until the last month or so of pregnancy.

Diffusion of Oxygen Through the Placental Membrane. Almost exactly the same principles are applicable for the diffusion of oxygen through the placental membrane as through the pulmonary membrane; these principles were discussed in Chapter 28. The dissolved oxygen in the blood of the large placental sinuses simply passes through the villar membrane into the fetal blood because of a pressure gradient of oxygen from the mother's blood to the fetus's blood. The mean Po_2 in the mother's blood in the placental sinuses is approximately 50 mm Hg toward the end of pregnancy, and the mean Po_2 in the blood leaving the villi and returning to the fetus after it has been oxygenated is about 30 mm Hg. Therefore, the mean pressure gradient for diffusion of oxygen through the placental membrane is about 20 mm Hg.

One might wonder how it is possible for a fetus to obtain sufficient oxygen when the fetal blood leaving the placenta has a Po_2 of only 30 mm Hg. However, most of the hemoglobin of the fetus is *fetal hemoglobin,* a type of hemoglobin synthesized in the fetus prior to birth. At low Po_2s, fetal hemoglobin can carry as much as 20 to 30 per cent more oxygen than can maternal hemoglobin.

Also, the *hemoglobin concentration of the fetal blood is about 50 per cent greater than that of the mother,* which is also an important factor in enhancing the amount of oxygen transported to the fetal tissues.

Diffusion of Carbon Dioxide Through the Placental Membrane. Carbon dioxide is continuously formed in the tissues of the fetus in the same way that it is formed in maternal tissues. The only means for excreting the carbon dioxide is through the placenta. The Pco_2 builds up in the fetal blood until it is about 48 mm Hg, in contrast with 40 to 45 mm Hg in maternal blood. Thus, a small pressure gradient for carbon dioxide develops across the placental membrane, but this is sufficient to allow adequate diffusion of carbon dioxide from the fetal blood into the maternal blood, because the extreme solubility of carbon dioxide in the water of the placental membrane allows carbon dioxide to diffuse about 20 times as rapidly as oxygen.

Diffusion of Foodstuffs Through the Placental Membrane. Other metabolic substrates needed by the fetus diffuse into the fetal blood in the same manner as oxygen. For instance, the glucose level in the fetal blood ordinarily is approximately 20 to 30 per cent lower than the glucose level in the maternal blood, for glucose is metabolized rapidly by the fetus. This in turn causes rapid diffusion of additional glucose from the maternal blood into the fetal blood.

Because of the high solubility of fatty acids in cell membranes, these too diffuse from the maternal blood into the fetal blood. Also, such substances as potassium, sodium, and chloride ions diffuse from the maternal blood into the fetal blood.

Active Absorption by the Placental Membrane. The cells that line the outer surfaces of the villi can also actively absorb certain nutrients from the maternal blood in the placenta during the first half of pregnancy at least and perhaps even throughout the entire pregnancy. For instance, the measured *amino acid* concentration of fetal blood is greater than that of maternal blood, and *calcium* and *inorganic phosphate* occur in greater concentration in fetal blood than in maternal blood. These effects indicate that the placental membrane has the ability to absorb actively at least small amounts of certain substances even during the latter part of pregnancy.

Excretion Through the Placental Membrane. In the same manner that carbon dioxide diffuses from the fetal blood into the maternal blood, other excretory products formed in the fetus diffuse into the maternal blood and then are excreted by the mother's kidneys along with her own excretory products. These include especially waste products such as *urea, uric acid,* and *creatinine.* For instance, the level of urea in the fetal blood is only slightly greater than in maternal blood, because urea diffuses through the placental membrane with considerable ease.

HORMONAL FACTORS IN PREGNANCY

In pregnancy, the placenta forms large quantities of *human chorionic gonadotropin, estrogens, progesterone,* and *human chorionic somatomammotropin,* the first three of which, and perhaps the fourth as well, are essential to the continuance of pregnancy.

Human Chorionic Gonadotropin and Its Effects—Persistence of the Corpus Luteum and Prevention of Menstruation

Menstruation normally occurs approximately 14 days after ovulation, at which time most of the secretory endometrium of the uterus sloughs away from the uterine wall and is expelled to the exterior. If this were to happen after implantation of an ovum, the pregnancy would terminate. However, this is prevented by the secretion of human chorionic gonadotropin in the following manner:

Coincidently with the development of the trophoblast cells from the early dividing ovum, the hormone *human chorionic gonadotropin* is secreted into the fluids of the mother. As illustrated in Figure 56–4, the secretion of this hormone can first be measured 8 days after ovulation, just as the ovum is first implanting in the endometrium. Then the rate of secretion rises rapidly to reach a maximum approximately 8 weeks after ovulation, and decreases to a relatively low value by 16 to 20 weeks after ovulation.

Function of Human Chorionic Gonadotropin. Human chorionic gonadotropin is a glycoprotein having a molecular weight of 39,000 and very much the same molecular structure and function as luteinizing hormone secreted by the pituitary. By far its most important function is to prevent the normal involution of the corpus luteum at the end of the female sexual cycle. Instead, it causes the corpus luteum to secrete even larger quantities of its usual hormones, progesterone and estrogens. These excess hormones cause the endometrium to continue growing and to store large amounts of additional nutrients rather than to be passed in the menstruum.

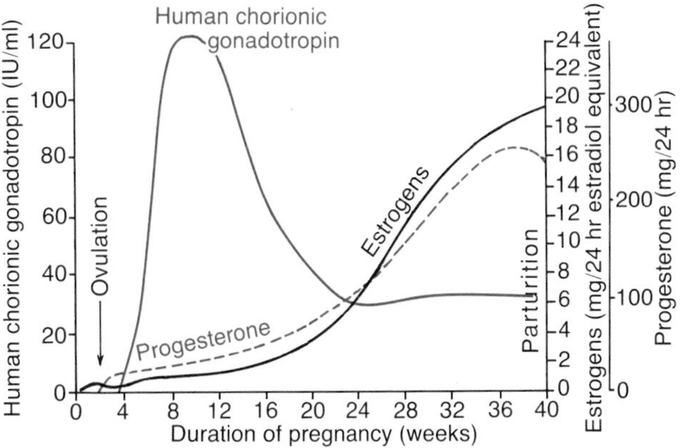

Figure 56–4. Rates of secretion of estrogens, progesterone, and chorionic gonadotropin at different stages of pregnancy.

If the corpus luteum is removed before approximately the seventh to eleventh week of pregnancy, spontaneous abortion usually occurs, but after this time the placenta itself secretes sufficient quantities of progesterone and estrogens to maintain pregnancy.

Effect of Human Chorionic Gonadotropin on the Fetal Testes. Human chorionic gonadotropin also exerts an *interstitial cell-stimulating effect* on the testes, thus resulting in the production of testosterone in male fetuses. This small secretion of testosterone during gestation is the factor that causes the fetus to grow male sex organs. Near the end of pregnancy, the testosterone secreted by the fetal testes also causes the testicles to descend into the scrotum.

Secretion of Estrogens by the Placenta

The placenta, like the corpus luteum, secretes both estrogens and progesterone. Figure 56–4 shows that the daily production of placental estrogens increases markedly to about 30 times normal toward the end of pregnancy.

Function of Estrogens in Pregnancy. In the discussions of estrogens in the preceding chapter it was pointed out that these hormones exert mainly a proliferative function on certain reproductive and associated organs. During pregnancy, the extreme quantities of estrogens cause (1) enlargement of the uterus, (2) enlargement of the breasts and growth of the breast glandular tissue, and (3) enlargement of the female external genitalia.

The estrogens also relax the various pelvic ligaments, so that the sacroiliac joints become relatively limber and the symphysis pubis becomes elastic. These changes facilitate easy passage of the fetus through the birth canal.

There is much reason to believe that estrogens also affect the development of the fetus during pregnancy, for example, by affecting the rate of cell reproduction in the early embryo.

Secretion of Progesterone by the Placenta

Progesterone is also a hormone essential for pregnancy. In addition to being secreted in moderate quantities by the corpus luteum at the beginning of pregnancy, it is secreted in tremendous quantities by the placenta, averaging about one quarter gram per day toward the end of pregnancy. Indeed, the rate of progesterone secretion increases by as much as tenfold during the course of pregnancy, as illustrated in Figure 56-4.

The special effects of progesterone that are essential for normal progression of pregnancy are the following:

1. As pointed out earlier, progesterone causes decidual cells to develop in the uterine endometrium, and these cells then play an important role in the nutrition of the early embryo.
2. Progesterone has a special effect in decreasing the contractility of the gravid uterus, thus preventing uterine contractions from causing spontaneous abortion.
3. Progesterone also contributes to the development of the ovum even prior to implantation, for it specifically increases the secretions of the fallopian tubes and uterus to provide appropriate nutritive matter for the developing *morula* and *blastocyst.* There are some reasons to believe, too, that progesterone even affects cell cleavage in the early developing embryo.
4. The progesterone secreted during pregnancy also helps to prepare the breasts for lactation, as discussed later in the chapter.

Human Chorionic Somatomammotropin

Recently, a new hormone called *human chorionic somatomammotropin* has been discovered. This is a protein having a molecular weight of about 38,000 that begins to be secreted about the fifth week of pregnancy and increases progressively throughout the remainder of pregnancy. Human chorionic somatomammotropin has several important effects:

First, when administered to several different types of lower animals, human chorionic somatomammotropin causes at least partial development of the breasts.

Second, this hormone has weak actions similar to those of growth hormone, causing deposition of protein tissues in the same way that growth hormone does.

Third, human chorionic somatomammotropin has recently been found to have important actions on both glucose metabolism and fat metabolism in the mother, effects that perhaps are important for nutrition of the fetus. The hormone causes decreased utilization of glucose by the mother, thereby making larger quantities of glucose available to the fetus. Furthermore, the hormone promotes release of free fatty acids from the fat stores of the mother, thus providing an alternative source of energy for her metabolism.

Therefore, it is beginning to appear that human chorionic somatomammotropin is a general metabolic hormone that has specific nutritional implications for both the mother and fetus.

RESPONSE OF THE MOTHER TO PREGNANCY

The presence of a growing fetus in the uterus adds an extra physiological load on the mother, and much of the response of the mother to pregnancy is due to this increased load. However, special effects include the following:

Blood Flow Through the Placenta; Cardiac Output. About 625 ml of blood flows through the maternal circulation of the placenta each minute during the latter stages of gestation. This flow increases the cardiac output of the mother in the same manner that arteriovenous shunts increase the output. This factor, plus a general increase in the mother's metabolism, increases her cardiac output to 30 to 40 per cent above normal.

Blood Volume of the Mother. The maternal blood volume shortly before birth of the baby is approximately 30 per cent above normal. This increase occurs at least partly because of increased secretion during pregnancy of aldosterone and estrogens, both of which cause increased fluid retention by the kidneys.

At the time of birth of the baby, the mother has approximately 1 to 2 liters of extra blood in her circulatory system. Only about one fourth of this amount is normally lost during delivery of the baby, thereby allowing a considerable safety factor for the mother.

Nutrition During Pregnancy. The growing fetus assumes priority for many of the nutritional elements in the mother's body, and many portions of the fetus continue to grow even if the mother does not eat a sufficiently nourishing diet.

By far the greatest growth of the fetus occurs during the last trimester of pregnancy; the weight of the child almost doubles during the last two months of pregnancy. Ordinarily, the mother does not absorb sufficient protein, calcium, phosphorus, and iron from the gastrointestinal tract during the last month of pregnancy to supply the fetus. However, from the beginning of pregnancy the mother's body has been storing these substances to be used during the latter months of pregnancy. Some of this storage is in the placenta, but most of it is in the normal storage depots of the mother.

If appropriate nutritional elements are not present in the mother's diet, a number of maternal deficiencies can occur during pregnancy. Such deficiencies often occur for calcium, phosphates, iron, and the vitamins. For example, approximately 375 mg of iron is needed by the fetus to form its blood, and an additional 600 mg is needed by the mother to form her own extra blood. The normal store of nonhemoglobin iron in the mother at the outset of pregnancy is often only 100 mg or so. Therefore, in general, the obstetrician supplements the diet of the mother with the needed substances. It is especially important that the mother receive large quantities of vitamin D, for although the total quantity of calcium utilized by the fetus is small, calcium even normally is poorly absorbed by the gastrointestinal tract. Finally, shortly before birth of the baby vitamin K is often added to the mother's diet so that the baby will have sufficient prothrombin to prevent postnatal hemorrhage.

The Amniotic Fluid and Its Formation. Normally, the volume of amniotic fluid (the fluid that surrounds the fetus in the uterus) is between 500 ml and 1 liter. Studies with isotopes of the rate of formation of amniotic fluid show that on the average the water in amniotic fluid is completely replaced once every 3 hours, and the electrolytes sodium and potassium are replaced once every 15 hours. Yet, strangely enough, the sources of the fluid and the points of reabsorption are mainly unknown. A portion of the fluid is derived from renal excretion by the fetus, and a small amount of absorption occurs by way of the fetal gastrointestinal tract. But about one half of the fluid turnover is believed to occur through the amniotic membranes.

Preeclampsia and Eclampsia

Approximately 4 per cent of all pregnant women develop a rapid rise in arterial blood pressure associated with loss of large amounts of protein in the urine at some time during the latter 4 months of pregnancy. This condition, called *preeclampsia,* is often also characterized by salt and water retention by the kidneys, weight gain, and development of edema. In addition, arterial spasm occurs in many parts of the body, most significantly in the kidneys, brain, and liver. Both the renal blood flow and the glomerular filtration rate are decreased, which is exactly opposite to the changes that occur in the normal pregnant woman. The renal effects are caused at least partly by thickened glomerular tufts that contain a protein deposit in the basement membranes.

Various attempts have been made to prove that preeclampsia is caused by excessive secretion of placental or adrenal hormones, but proof of a hormonal basis is still lacking. Another plausible theory is that preeclampsia results from some type of autoimmunity or allergy resulting from the presence of the fetus. Indeed, the acute symptoms disappear within a few days after birth of the baby.

Eclampsia is a severe degree of preeclampsia characterized by extreme vascular spasticity throughout the body, clonic convulsions followed by coma, greatly decreased kidney output, malfunction of the liver, often extreme hypertension, and a generalized toxic condition of the body. Usually, it occurs shortly before parturition. Without treatment, a very high percentage of eclamptic patients die. However, with optimal and immediate use of rapidly acting vasodilating drugs to reduce the arterial pressure to normal, followed by immediate termination of pregnancy—by cesarean operation if necessary—the mortality has been reduced to 1 per cent or less.

PARTURITION

Increased Uterine Contractility Near Term

Parturition simply means the process by which the baby is born. At the termination of pregnancy, the uterus becomes progressively more excitable until finally it begins strong rhythmic contractions with such force that the baby is expelled. The exact cause of the increased activity of the uterus is not known, but at least two major categories of effects lead up to the culminating contractions responsible for parturition; these are, first, progressive hormonal changes that cause increased excitability of the uterine musculature and, second, progressive mechanical changes caused by enlargement of the baby.

Hormonal Factors That Cause Increased Uterine Contractility

Ratio of Estrogens to Progesterone. Progesterone inhibits uterine contractility during pregnancy, thereby helping to prevent expulsion of the fetus. On the other hand, estrogens have a definite tendency to increase the degree of uterine contractility. Both these hormones are secreted in progressively greater quantities throughout pregnancy, but from the seventh month onward, estrogen secretion increases more than progesterone secretion. Therefore, it has been postulated that the *estrogen to progesterone ratio* increases sufficiently toward the end of pregnancy to be at least partly responsible for the increased contractility of the uterus.

Effect of Oxytocin on the Uterus. Oxytocin is a hormone secreted by the posterior pituitary gland that specifically causes uterine contraction (see Chapter 49). Experiments in animals have shown that irritation or stretching of the uterine cervix, such as that occurring at the end of pregnancy, causes a neurogenic reflex to the posterior pituitary gland that increases the rate of oxytocin secretion. Therefore this hormone probably helps considerably to increase uterine contractions.

Mechanical Factors That Increase the Contractility of the Uterus

Stretch of the Uterine Musculature. Simply stretching smooth muscle organs usually increases their contractility. Furthermore, intermittent stretch, like that occurring repetitively in the uterus because of movements of the fetus, can also elicit smooth muscle contraction.

Note especially that twins are born on the average *19 days* earlier than a single child, which emphasizes the importance of mechanical stretch in promoting parturition.

Stretch or Irritation of the Cervix. There is much reason to believe that stretch or irritation of the uterine cervix is particularly important in directly eliciting uterine contractions. The mechanism of this effect is probably transmission of action potentials through the muscle of the uterus itself from the cervix to the body of the uterus.

Onset of Labor — A Positive Feedback Theory for its Initiation

During most of the months of pregnancy, the uterus undergoes periodic episodes of weak and slow rhythmic contractions called *Braxton Hicks's contractions.* These become progressively stronger toward the end of pregnancy; and they eventually change rather suddenly, within hours, to exceptionally strong contractions that start stretching the cervix and, later, forcing the baby through the birth canal. This process is called *labor,* and the strong contractions that result in final parturition are called *labor contractions.*

On the basis of our new understanding of control systems in the past few years, a theory has been proposed for explaining the onset of labor based on positive feedback. This theory suggests that stretch of the cervix by the fetus's head finally becomes great enough to elicit a reflex increase in contractility of the uterine body. This pushes the baby forward, which stretches the cervix some more and initiates a new cycle. Thus, the process continues again and again until the baby is expelled. This theory is illustrated in Figure 56–5. We know at least two positive feedbacks that could lead to birth of the baby, as follows:

(1) Stretch of the cervix causes the entire body of the uterus to contract, and this stretches the cervix still more because of the downward thrust of the baby's head. (2) Cervical stretch also causes the pituitary gland to secrete oxytocin, which is still another cause of increased uterine contractility.

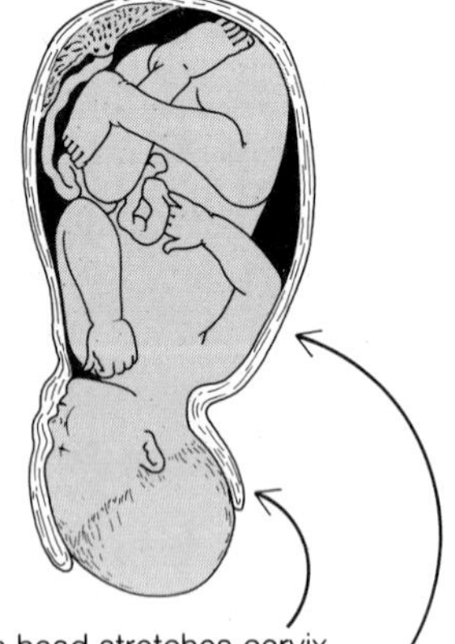

Figure 56–5. Theory for the onset of intensely strong contractions during labor.

To summarize the theory, we can assume that multiple factors increase the contractility of the uterus toward the end of pregnancy. Eventually, a uterine contraction becomes strong enough to irritate the uterus enough to increase its contractility still more because of positive feedback, and to result in a second contraction stronger than the first, a third stronger than the second, and so forth. Once these contractions become strong enough to cause this type of increasing feedback, with each contraction greater than the one preceding, the process proceeds to completion.

Abdominal Muscle Contractions During Labor

Once labor contractions become strong and painful, neurogenic reflexes, mainly from the birth canal to the spinal cord and thence back to the abdominal muscles, cause intense abdominal muscle contractions along with the uterine contractions. These abdominal contractions add greatly to the positive feedback forces that cause expulsion of the baby.

Mechanics of Parturition

At the beginning of labor, strong contractions might occur only once every 30 minutes. As labor progresses, the contractions finally appear as often as once every 1 to 3 minutes, and the intensity of contraction increases greatly with only a short period of relaxation between contractions.

The combined contractions of the uterine and abdominal musculature during delivery of the baby cause a downward force on the fetus of approximately 25 pounds during each strong contraction. It is fortunate that the contractions of labor occur intermittently, because strong contractions impede or sometimes even stop blood flow through the placenta and would cause death of the fetus were the contractions continuous.

In 19 of 20 births the head is the first part of the baby to be expelled; in most of the remaining instances the buttocks are presented first. The head acts as a wedge to open the structures of the birth canal as the fetus is forced downward from above.

The first major obstruction to expulsion of the fetus is the uterine cervix. Toward the end of pregnancy the cervix becomes soft, which allows it to stretch when labor pains cause the body of the uterus to contract. The so-called *first stage of labor* is the period of progressive cervical dilatation, which continues until the cervical opening is as large as the head of the fetus. This stage usually lasts 8 to 24 hours in the first pregnancy but often only a few minutes if the mother has had many pregnancies.

Once the cervix has dilated fully, the fetal membranes usually rupture, and the amniotic fluid is lost through the vagina. Then the fetus's head moves rapidly into the birth canal and, with additional force from above, continues to wedge its way through the canal until delivery is effected. This is called the *second stage of labor;* it may last from as little as a minute after many pregnancies up to half an hour or more in the first pregnancy.

Separation and Delivery of the Placenta

During the succeeding 10 to 45 minutes after birth of the baby, the uterus contracts to a very small size, which causes a *shearing* effect between the walls of the uterus and the placenta and consequent separation of the placenta from its implantation site. Separation of the placenta opens the placental sinuses and causes bleeding. However, the amount of bleeding is limited to an average of 350 ml by the following mechanism: The smooth muscle fibers of the uterine musculature are arranged in figure of eights around the blood vessels as they pass through the uterine wall. Therefore, contraction of the uterus following delivery of the baby constricts the vessels that had previously supplied blood to the placenta.

Labor Pains

With each uterine contraction, the mother experiences considerable pain. The pain in early labor is probably caused mainly by hypoxia of the uterine muscle resulting from compression of the blood vessels to the uterus. This contraction pain is greatly reduced when the sympathetic *hypogastric nerves,* which carry the sensory fibers leading from the uterus, have been sectioned. However, during the second stage of labor, when the fetus is being expelled through the birth canal, much more severe pain is caused by cervical stretch, perineal stretch, and stretch or tearing of structures in the vaginal canal itself. This pain is conducted by somatic nerves instead of by the hypogastric nerves.

Involution of the Uterus

During the first 4 to 5 weeks following parturition, the uterus involutes. Its weight becomes less than one half its immediate postpartum weight within a week, and in 4 weeks the uterus may be as small as it had been prior to pregnancy. During early involution of the uterus the placental site on the endometrial surface autolyzes, causing a vaginal discharge known as *lochia,* which is first bloody and then serous, and continues for approximately a week and a half in all. After this time, the endometrial surface will have become re-epithelialized and ready for normal, nongravid sex life again.

LACTATION

Development of the Breasts

The breasts begin to develop at puberty; this development is stimulated by the estrogens of the monthly sexual cycles that stimulate growth of the stroma and ductile system plus deposition of fat to give mass to the breasts. However, much additional growth occurs during pregnancy, and the glandular tissue only then becomes completely developed for actual production of milk.

All through pregnancy, the tremendous quantities of estrogens secreted by the placenta—plus additional quantities of growth hormone, prolactin, and several other hormones—cause the ductile system of the breasts to grow and to branch. Simultaneously, the stroma of the breasts also increases, and large quantities of fat are laid down in the stroma.

Then the action of progesterone causes growth of the lobules, budding of alveoli, and development of secretory characteristics in the cells of the alveoli, most of which occurs in response to the very large amount of progesterone secreted by the placenta during pregnancy.

Initiation of Lactation—Function of Prolactin

Though estrogen and progestrone are essential for the physical development of the breasts during pregnancy, both of these hormones also have a specific effect to inhibit the actual secretion of milk. On the other hand, the hormone *prolactin* has exactly the opposite effect, promotion of the secretion of milk. This hormone is secreted by the mother's anterior pituitary gland, and its concentration in her blood rises steadily from the fifth week of pregnancy until birth of the baby, at which time it has risen to very high levels, usually about ten times the normal nonpregnant level. This is illustrated in Figure 56-6. In addition, the placenta secretes large quantities of *human chorionic somatomammotropin,* which also has mild lactogenic properties, thus supporting the prolactin from the mother's pituitary. Even so, because of suppression by estrogens and progesterone, only a few milliliters of fluid are secreted each day until after the baby is born. This fluid is called *colostrum;* it contains essentially the same concentrations of proteins and lactose as milk but almost no fat, and its maximum rate of production is about 1/100 the subsequent rate of milk production.

Immediately after the baby is born, the sudden loss of both estrogen and progesterone secretion by the placenta allows the lactogenic effect of the prolactin from the mother's pituitary gland to assume its natural milk-promoting role, and within 2 or 3 days, the breasts begin to secrete copious quantities of milk instead of colostrum.

Following birth of the baby, the *basal level* of pro-

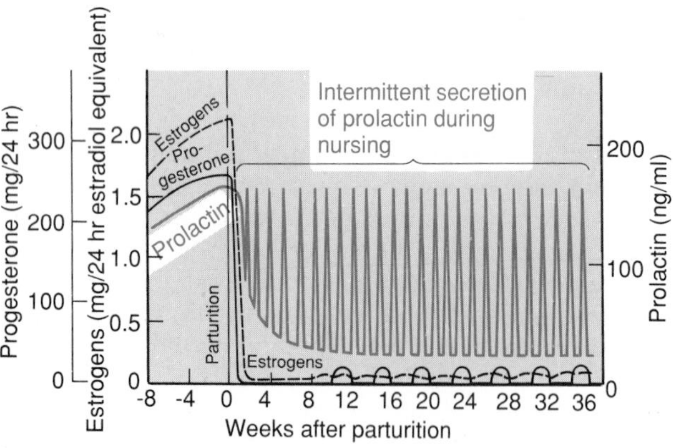

Figure 56-6. Changes in rates of secretion of estrogens, progesterone, and prolactin for 8 weeks prior to parturition and for 36 weeks thereafter. Note especially the decrease of prolactin secretion back to basal levels within a few weeks, but also the intermittent periods of marked prolactin secretion (for about 1 hour at a time) during and after periods of nursing.

lactin secretion returns during the next few weeks to the nonpregnant level, as shown in Figure 56-6. However, each time the mother nurses her baby, nervous signals from the nipples to the hypothalamus cause approximately a tenfold to twentyfold surge in prolactin secretion lasting about 1 hour, which is also shown in the figure. The prolactin in turn acts on the breasts to provide the milk for the next nursing period. If this prolactin surge is absent, if it is blocked as a result of hypothalamic or pituitary damage, or if nursing does not continue, the breasts lose their ability to produce milk within a few days. However, milk production can continue for several years if the child continues to suckle, but the rate of milk formation normally decreases considerably within 7 to 9 months.

Hypothalamic Control of Prolactin Secretion. Though secretion of most of the anterior pituitary hormones is enhanced by neurosecretory releasing factors transmitted from the hypothalamus to the anterior pituitary gland through the hypothalamic-hypophysial portal system, the secretion of prolactin is normally controlled by an exactly opposite effect. That is, the hypothalamus synthesizes a *prolactin inhibitory hormone* (PIH). This hormone is probably the small amine *dopamine*. Under normal conditions, large amounts of PIH are continuously transmitted to the anterior pituitary gland so that the normal rate of prolactin secretion is slight. However, it is believed that during lactation the formation of a *prolactin releasing factor* (PRF) may be formed intermittently at the time of nursing, causing the surges in prolactin secretion that occur at that time.

The Ejection (or "Let-Down") Process in Milk Secretion—Function of Oxytocin

Milk is secreted continuously into the alveoli of the breasts, but milk does not flow easily from the alveoli into the ductile system and therefore does not continually leak from the breast nipples. Instead, the milk must be ejected, or "let-down" from the alveoli to the ducts before the baby can obtain it. This process is caused by a combined neurogenic and hormonal reflex involving the hormone *oxytocin* as follows:

When the baby suckles the breast, sensory signals are transmitted through somatic nerves to the spinal cord and then to the hypothalamus, there causing *oxytocin* secretion. This hormone flows in the blood to the breasts, where it causes *myoepithelial cells* that surround the outer walls of the alveoli to contract, thereby expressing the milk from the alveoli into the ducts. Thus, within 30 seconds to a minute after a baby begins to suckle the breast, milk begins to flow. This process is called *milk ejection,* or *milk let-down.*

Suckling on one breast causes milk flow not only in that breast but also in the opposite breast. Also, it is especially interesting that the sound of the baby crying is often enough of a signal to cause milk ejection.

The Composition of Milk and the Metabolic Drain on the Mother Caused by Lactation

Table 56-1 gives the contents of human milk and cow's milk.

At the height of lactation, 1.5 liters of milk may be formed each day. With this amount of lactation, great quantities of metabolic substrates are drained from the mother. For instance, approximately 50 grams of fat enter the milk each day, and approximately 100 grams of lactose, which must be derived from the mother's glucose. Also, some 2 to 3 grams of calcium phosphate may be lost each day, and unless the mother is drinking large quantities of milk and has an adequate intake of vitamin D, the output of calcium and phosphate by the lactating mammae will be much greater than the intake of these substances. To supply the excess calcium and phosphate, the parathyroid glands enlarge greatly, and the bones become progressively decalcified. The problem of decalcification is usually not very great during pregnancy, but it can be a distinct problem during lactation.

GROWTH AND FUNCTIONAL DEVELOPMENT OF THE FETUS

During the first 2 to 3 weeks of gestation, the fetus remains almost microscopic in size, but thereafter its

Table 56-1 PERCENTAGE COMPOSITION OF MILK

	Human Milk	Cow's Milk
Water	88.5	87.0
Fat	3.3	3.5
Lactose	6.8	4.8
Casein	0.9	2.7
Lactalbumin and other protein	0.4	0.7
Ash	0.2	0.7

dimensions increase almost in proportion to age. At 12 weeks the length of the fetus is approximately 10 cm; at 20 weeks, approximately 25 cm, and at term (40 weeks), approximately 53 cm (about 21 inches). Because the weight of the fetus is proportional to the cube of the length, the weight increases approximately in proportion to the cube of the age of the fetus. Therefore, the weight of the fetus remains almost nothing during the first months and reaches only 1 pound at 5.5 months of gestation. Then during the last trimester of pregnancy, the fetus gains tremendously, so that 2 months prior to birth the weight averages 3 pounds; at 1 month prior to birth, 4.5 pounds; and at birth, 7 pounds.

Development of the Fetal Organ Systems

Within 1 month after fertilization of the ovum, all the different organs of the fetus are already at least partly formed, and during the next 2 to 3 months, the minute details of the different organs are established. Beyond the fourth month, the organs of the fetus are grossly the same as those of the newborn child, even including most of the smaller structures of the organs. However, cellular development of these structures is usually far from complete and requires the entire remaining 5 months of pregnancy for full maturation. Even at birth the cells of certain structures, particularly those of the nervous system, the kidneys, and the liver, still lack full development, as is discussed in more detail later in the chapter.

The Circulatory System. The human heart begins beating during the fourth week following fertilization, contracting at the rate of about 65 beats per minute. The rate increases steadily as the fetus grows and reaches approximately 140 per minute immediately before birth.

Formation of Blood Cells. Nucleated red blood cells begin to be formed in the yolk sac and mesothelial layers of the placenta at about the third week of fetal development. This is followed a week later by the formation of non-nucleated red blood cells by the fetal mesenchyme and by the endothelium of the fetal blood vessels. Then at approximately 6 weeks, the liver begins to form blood cells, and in the third month the spleen and other lymphoid tissues of the body also begin forming blood cells. Finally, from approximately the third month on, the bone marrow forms more and more red and white blood cells while the other structures completely lose their ability to form blood cells, except for lymphocytes.

The Respiratory System. Obviously, respiration cannot occur during fetal life. However, respiratory movements do take place beginning at the end of the first trimester of pregnancy. Tactile stimuli or fetal asphyxia especially cause respiratory movements.

The Nervous System. Most of the peripheral reflexes of the fetus are well developed by the third to fourth month of pregnancy. However, some of the more important higher functions of the central nervous system are still undeveloped even at birth. Indeed, myelinization of some major tracts of the central nervous system becomes complete only after approximately a year of postnatal life.

The Gastrointestinal Tract. Even in midpregnancy the fetus ingests and absorbs large quantities of amniotic fluid, and during the latter 2 to 3 months, gastrointestinal function approaches that of the normal newborn infant. Small quantities of *meconium* are continually formed in the gastrointestinal tract and excreted from the bowels into the amniotic fluid. Meconium is composed partly of unabsorbed residue of amniotic fluid and partly of excretory products from the gastrointestinal mucosa and glands.

The Kidneys. The fetal kidneys are capable of excreting urine during at least the latter half of pregnancy, and urination occurs normally *in utero.* However, the renal control systems for regulation of extracellular fluid electrolyte balances and acid-base balance are almost nonexistent until after midfetal life and do not reach full development until about a month after birth.

ADJUSTMENTS OF THE INFANT TO EXTRAUTERINE LIFE

Onset of Breathing

The most obvious effect of birth on the baby is loss of the placental connection with the mother and therefore loss of this means for metabolic support. And by far the most important immediate adjustment required of the infant is to begin breathing.

Cause of Breathing at Birth. Following completely normal delivery from a mother who has not been depressed by anesthetics, the child ordinarily begins to breathe immediately and has a completely normal respiratory rhythm from the outset. The promptness with which the fetus begins to breathe indicates that breathing is initiated by sudden exposure to the exterior world, probably resulting from a slightly asphyxiated state incident to the birth process but also from sensory impulses originating in the suddenly cooled skin. However, if the infant does not breathe immediately, its body becomes progressively more hypoxic and hypercapnic, which provides additional stimulus to the respiratory center and usually causes breathing within a few seconds to a few minutes after birth.

Delayed and Abnormal Breathing at Birth—Danger of Hypoxia. If the mother has been depressed by a general anesthetic during delivery, which at least partially anesthetizes the child as well, respiration is likely to be delayed for several minutes, which illustrates the importance of using as little obstetrical anesthesia as feasible. Also, many infants who have had head trauma during delivery are slow to breathe or sometimes will not breathe at all. This can result from two possible effects: First, in a few infants, intracranial hemorrhage or brain contusion causes a concussion syndrome with a greatly depressed respiratory center. Second, and probably much more important, prolonged fetal hypoxia during delivery causes serious depression of the respiratory center. Hypoxia frequently occurs during delivery because of (1) compression of the umbilical cord, (2) premature separation of the placenta, (3) excessive contraction of the uterus, which cuts off blood flow to the placenta, or (4) excessive anesthesia of the mother.

Degree of Hypoxia That an Infant Can Tolerate. In the adult, failure to breathe for only 4 minutes often causes death, but a newborn infant often survives as long as 10 to 15 minutes of failure to breathe after birth. Unfortunately, though, permanent brain impairment often ensues if breathing is delayed more than 8 to 10 minutes. Indeed, actual lesions develop, mainly in brain stem areas, thus affecting many motor functions of the body. This is believed to be one of the causes of *cerebral palsy.*

Expansion of the Lungs at Birth. At birth, the walls of the alveoli are held together by the surface tension of the viscid fluid that fills them. More than 25 mm Hg of negative pressure is required to oppose the effects of this surface tension and therefore to open the alveoli for the first time. But once the alveoli are open, further respiration can be effected with relatively weak respiratory movements. Fortunately, the first inspirations of the newborn infant are extremely powerful, usually capable of creating as much as 50 mm Hg negative pressure in the intrapleural space.

Figure 56-7 illustrates the tremendous forces required to open the lungs at the onset of breathing. To the left is shown the pressure-volume curve (compliance curve) for the first breath after birth. Observe first the lowermost curve, which shows that the lungs do not expand at all until the negative pressure has reached −40 cm water (−30 mm Hg). Then as the negative pressure increases to −60 cm water, only about 40 ml of air enters the lungs. Then, to deflate the lungs, considerable positive pressure is required, probably because of the resistance offered by the viscid fluid in the bronchioles.

Note that the second breath is much easier. However, breathing does not become completely normal until about 40 minutes after birth, as shown by the third compliance curve, the shape of which compares favorably with that of the normal adult.

Respiratory Distress Syndrome. A few infants, especially premature infants, develop severe respiratory distress during the few hours to several days following birth and frequently succumb within the next day or so. The alveoli of these infants at death contain large quantities of proteinaceous fluid, almost as if pure plasma had leaked out of the capillaries into the alveoli.

One of the most characteristic findings in these infants is failure to secrete adequate quantities of *surfactant,* a substance normally secreted into the alveoli that decreases the surface tension of the alveolar fluid, therefore allowing the alveoli to open easily. The surfactant secreting cells (the type II alveolar epithelial cells) do not begin to secrete surfactant until the last 1 to 3 months of gestation. Therefore, many premature babies and some full-term babies are born without the capability of secreting surfactant, which therefore causes both a tendency of the lungs to collapse and to develop pulmonary edema. The role of surfactant in preventing these effects was discussed in Chapter 27.

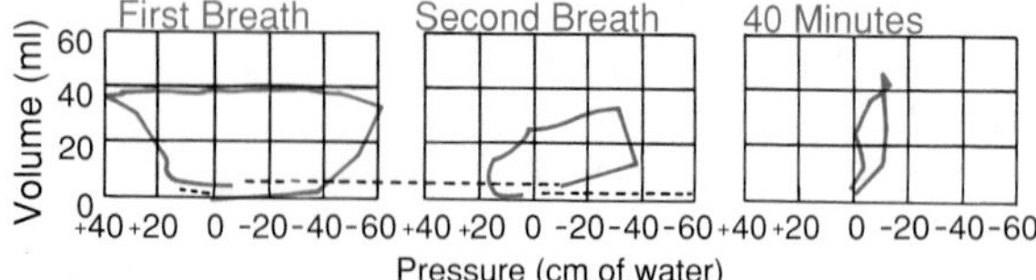

Figure 56-7. Pressure-volume curves of the lungs (compliance curves) of a newborn baby immediately after birth, showing *(a)* the extreme forces required for breathing during the first two breaths of life and *(b)* development of a nearly normal compliance within 40 minutes after birth. (From Smith: *Sci. Am., 209:32.* © 1963 by Scientific American, Inc. All rights reserved.)

Circulatory Readjustments at Birth

Almost as important as the onset of breathing at birth are the immediate circulatory adjustments that allow adequate blood flow through the lungs. Because the lungs are mainly nonfunctional during fetal life, it is not necessary for the fetal heart to pump much blood through the lungs. On the other hand, the fetal heart must pump large quantities of blood through the placenta. As illustrated in Figure 56-8, most of the blood entering the right atrium from the inferior vena cava is directed in a straight pathway across the posterior aspect of the right atrium and thence through the *foramen ovale* directly into the left atrium. Thus, the well-oxygenated blood from the placenta enters the left side of the heart without going through the right ventricle and lungs. Instead, it is pumped by the left ventricle mainly into the vessels of the head and forelimbs.

The blood entering the right atrium from the superior vena cava is directed downward through the tricuspid valve into the right ventricle. This blood is mainly deoxygenated blood from the head region of the fetus, and it is pumped by the right ventricle into the pulmonary artery. Then almost all of the blood passes through the *ductus arteriosus* into the descending aorta and through the two umbilical arteries into the placenta, where this deoxygenated blood becomes oxygenated.

Changes in the Fetal Circulation at Birth. The basic changes in the fetal circulation at birth were discussed in Chapter 18 in relation to congenital anomalies of the ductus arteriosus and foramen ovale that persist throughout life. Briefly, these are as follows:

First, the tremendous blood flow through the placenta ceases, which *approximately doubles the systemic vascular resistance at birth.* This obviously *increases the aortic pressure* as well as the pressures in the left ventricle and left atrium.

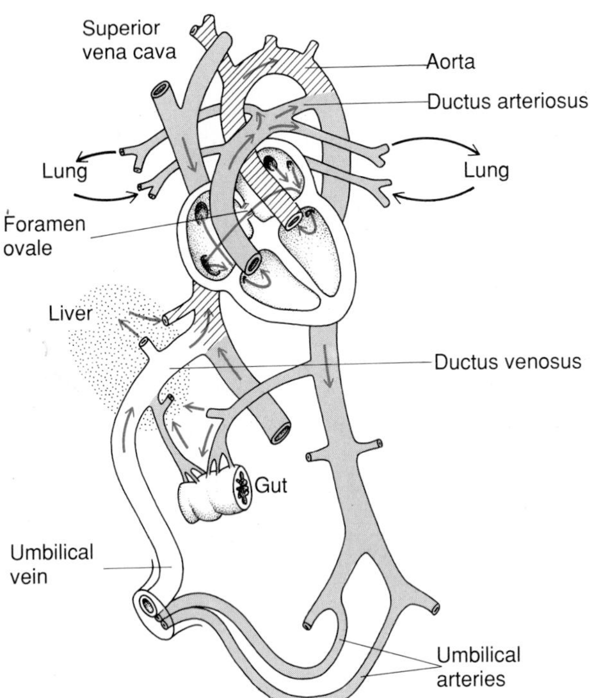

Figure 56-8. Organization of the fetal circulation. (Modified from Arey: Developmental Anatomy. 7th ed. Philadelphia, W. B. Saunders Company, 1974.)

Second, the *pulmonary vascular resistance decreases greatly* as a result of expansion of the lungs. In the unexpanded fetal lungs, the blood vessels are compressed because of the small volume of the lungs. Immediately upon expansion these vessels are no longer compressed, and the resistance to blood flow decreases severalfold. Also, in fetal life the hypoxia of the lungs causes considerable tonic vasoconstriction of the lung blood vessels, but vasodilation takes place when aeration of the lungs eliminates the hypoxia. These changes reduce the resistance of blood flow through the lungs as much as fivefold, which obviously *reduces the pulmonary arterial pressure, the right ventricular pressure, and the right atrial pressure.*

Closure of the Foramen Ovale. The *low right atrial pressure* and the *high left atrial pressure* that occur secondary to the changes in pulmonary and systemic resistance at birth cause a tendency for blood to flow backward from the left atrium into the right atrium rather than the other direction, as occurred during fetal life. Consequently, the small valve that lies over the foramen ovale on the left side of the atrial septum closes over this opening, thereby preventing further flow.

Closure of the Ductus Arteriosus. Similar effects occur in relation to the ductus arteriosus, for the increased systemic resistance *elevates the aortic pressure* while the decreased pulmonary resistance *reduces the pulmonary arterial pressure.* As a consequence, immediately after birth, blood begins to flow backward from the aorta into the pulmonary artery rather than in the other direction as in fetal life. However, after only a few hours the muscular wall of the ductus arteriosus constricts markedly, and within 1 to 8 days the constriction is sufficient to stop all blood flow. This is called *functional closure* of the ductus arteriosus. Then sometime during the next 1 to 4 months, the ductus arteriosus ordinarily becomes anatomically *occluded* by growth of fibrous tissue into its lumen.

Ductus closure almost certainly results from the increased oxygenation of the blood flowing through the ductus. In fetal life the Po_2 of the ductus blood is only 15 to 20 mm Hg, but it increases to about 100 mm Hg within a few hours after birth. Furthermore, many experiments have shown that the degree of contraction of the smooth muscle in the ductus wall is closely related to the availability of oxygen.

In addition, for reasons unknown the level of prostaglandins in the circulating blood decreases, and this, too, helps close the ductus.

In one of several thousand infants, the ductus fails to close, resulting in a *patent ductus arteriosus,* the consequences of which were discussed in Chapter 18.

SPECIAL FUNCTIONAL PROBLEMS IN THE NEONATAL INFANT

The most important characteristic of the newborn infant is instability of the various hormonal and neurogenic control systems. This results partly from the immature development of the different organs of the body and partly from the fact that the control systems simply have not become adjusted to the completely new way of life.

Cardiac Output. The cardiac output of the newborn infant averages 550 ml per minute, which is about two times as much in relation to body weight as in the adult. Occasionally, a child is born with an especially low cardiac output caused by hemorrhage through the placental membrane into the mother's blood prior to birth.

Arterial Pressure. The arterial pressure during the first day after birth averages about 70/50; it increases slowly during the next several months to approximately 90/60. Then there is a much slower rise during the subsequent years until the adult pressure of 115/70 is attained at adolescence.

Fluid Balance, Acid-Base Balance, and Renal Function. The rate of fluid intake and fluid excretion in the infant is seven times as great in relation to weight as in the adult, which means that even a slight alteration of fluid balance can cause rapidly developing abnormalities. Also, the rate of metabolism in the infant is two times as great in relation to body mass as in the adult, which means that two times as much acid is normally formed, leading to a tendency toward acidosis in the infant. Finally, functional development of the kidneys is not complete until approximately the end of the first month of life. For instance, the kidneys of the newborn can concentrate urine to only one and a half times the osmolality of the plasma instead of the normal three- to fourfold in the adult.

Therefore, considering the immaturity of the kidneys together with the marked fluid turnover and rapid formation of acid in the infant, one can readily understand that among the most important problems of infancy are acidosis and dehydration.

Liver Function. During the first few days of life, liver function may be quite deficient, as evidenced by the following effects:

1. The liver of the newborn conjugates bilirubin with glucuronic acid poorly and therefore excretes bilirubin only slightly during the first few days of life.
2. The liver of the newborn is deficient in forming plasma proteins, so that the plasma protein concentration falls in the first few weeks of life to 1 g/100 ml less than that for older children. Occasionally, the protein concentration falls so low that the infant actually develops hypoproteinemic edema.
3. The gluconeogenesis function of the liver is particularly deficient. As a result, the blood glucose level of the unfed newborn infant falls to about 30 to 40 mg/100 ml, and the infant must depend on its stored fats for energy until feeding can occur.
4. The liver of the newborn often also forms too little of the factors needed for normal blood coagulation.

Digestion, Absorption, and Metabolism of Energy Foods. In general, the ability of the newborn infant to digest, absorb, and metabolize foods is not different from that of the older child, with the following three exceptions:

First, secretion of pancreatic amylase in the newborn infant is deficient, so that the infant utilizes starches less adequately than do older children. However, the infant readily assimilates disaccharides and monosaccharides.

Second, absorption of fats from the gastrointestinal tract is somewhat less than in the older child. Consequently, milk with a high fat content, such as some varieties of cow's milk, is frequently inadequately utilized.

Third, because the liver functions are imperfect during at least the first week of life, the glucose concentration in the blood is unstable and often low.

Metabolic Rate and Body Temperature. The normal metabolic rate of the newborn in relation to body weight is about two times that of the adult, which accounts also for the two times as great cardiac output and two times as great minute respiratory volume in the infant.

However, since the body surface area is very large in relation to the body mass, heat is readily lost from the body. As a result, the body temperature of the newborn infant, particularly of the premature infant, falls. Figure 56–9 shows that the body temperature of even the normal infant falls several degrees during the first few hours after birth but returns to normal in 7 to 8 hours. Still, the body temperature regulatory mechanisms remain poor during the early days of life,

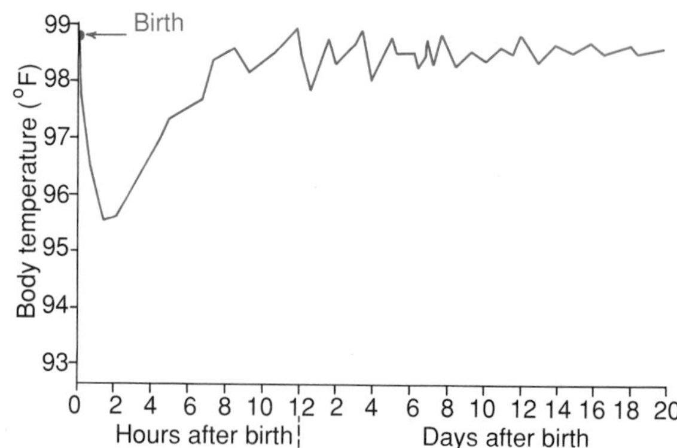

Figure 56–9. Fall in body temperature of the infant immediately after birth and instability of body temperature during the first few days of life.

at first allowing marked deviations in temperature, which are also illustrated in Figure 56–9.

Nutritional Needs During the Early Weeks of Life. Three specific problems occur in the early nutrition of the infant, as follows:

Need for Calcium. In the newborn infant rapid ossification of the bones has only begun at birth, so that a ready supply of calcium is needed throughout infancy.

Need for Iron. If the mother has had adequate amounts of iron in her diet, the liver of the infant usually has stored enough iron to keep forming blood cells for 4 to 6 months after birth. But if the mother has had insufficient iron in her diet, anemia is likely to supervene in the infant after about 3 months of life. Therefore, administration of iron in some form is desirable by the second or third month of life.

Vitamin C Deficiency. Ascorbic acid (vitamin C) is not stored in significant quantities in the fetal tissues; yet it is required for proper formation of cartilage, bone, and other intercellular structures of the infant. Furthermore, milk, especially cow's milk, has poor supplies of ascorbic acid. For this reason, orange juice or other sources of ascorbic acid are usually prescribed by the third week of life.

Immunity. Fortunately, the newborn infant inherits much immunity from its mother because many antibodies diffuse from the mother's blood through the placenta into the fetus. However, the neonate itself does not form antibodies to a significant extent. By the end of the first month, the blood gamma globulins, which contain the antibodies, have decreased to less than one half the original level, with a corresponding decrease in immunity. Therefore, the baby's own immunization processes begin to form antibodies, and the gamma globulin concentration returns essentially to normal by the age of 6 to 20 months.

Endocrine Problems. Ordinarily, the endocrine system of the infant is highly developed at birth, and the infant rarely exhibits any immediate endocrine abnormalities. However, there are special instances in which endocrinology of infancy is important.

1. If a pregnant mother bearing a *female child* is treated with an androgenic hormone or if she develops an androgenic tumor during pregnancy, the child will be born with a high degree of

masculinization of its sexual organs, thus resulting in a type of *hermaphroditism.*

2. An infant born of a diabetic mother will have considerable hypertrophy and hyperfunction of its islets of Langerhans. As a consequence, the infant's blood glucose concentration may fall to as low as 20 mg per 100 ml or even lower shortly after birth. Fortunately, the newborn infant, unlike the adult, only rarely develops insulin shock or coma from this low level of blood glucose concentration.

   Because of metabolic deficits in the diabetic mother, the fetus is often stunted in growth, and growth of the newborn infant and tissue maturation are often impaired. Also, there is a high rate of intrauterine mortality, and of those fetuses that do come to live birth, there is still a high mortality rate. Two thirds of the infants who die succumb to the respiratory distress syndrome, which was described earlier in the chapter.
3. Occasionally, a child is born with hypofunctional adrenal cortices, perhaps resulting from *agenesis* of the glands or *exhaustion atrophy,* which can occur when the adrenal glands have been overstimulated.

Special Problems of Prematurity

All the problems just noted for neonatal life are especially exacerbated in prematurity. These can be categorized under the following two headings: (1) immaturity of certain organ systems and (2) instability of the different homeostatic control systems. Because of these effects, a premature baby rarely lives if it is born more than 2.5 to 3 months prior to term.

The respiratory system is especially likely to be underdeveloped in the premature infant. The vital capacity and the functional residual capacity of the lungs are unusually small in relation to the size of the infant. Also, surfactant secretion is seriously depressed. As a consequence, respiratory distress is a common cause of death. Also, the low functional residual capacity in the premature infant is often associated with periodic breathing of the Cheyne-Stokes type.

Another major problem of the premature infant is its inability to ingest and absorb adequate food. If the infant is more than 2 months premature, the digestive and absorptive systems are almost always inadequate. The absorption of fat is so poor that the premature infant must have a low fat diet. Furthermore, the premature infant has unusual difficulty in absorbing calcium and therefore can develop severe rickets before the difficulty is recognized. For this reason, special attention must be paid to adequate calcium and vitamin D intake.

Immaturity of the different organ systems in the premature infant creates a high degree of instability in the homeostatic systems of the body. For instance, the acid-base balance can vary tremendously, particularly when the food intake varies from time to time. And one of the particular problems of the premature infant is inability to maintain normal body temperature. Its temperature tends to approach that of its surroundings. At normal room temperature the baby's temperature may stabilize in the low 90s or even in the 80s. Statistical studies show that a body temperature maintained below 35.5° C (96° F) is associated with a particularly high incidence of death, which explains the common use of the incubator in the treatment of prematurity.

REFERENCES

Reproduction and Lactation

Ben-Jonathan, N., et al.: Suckling-induced rise in prolactin: Mediation by prolactin-releasing factor from posterior pituitary. News Physiol. Sci., 3:172, 1988.

DeGroot, L. J., et al. (eds.): Endocrinology. 2nd ed. Philadelphia, W. B. Saunders Co., 1989.

Hanson, L. A.: Biology of Human Milk. New York, Raven Press, 1988.

Kaufmann, P., and Miller, R. K. (eds.): Placental Vascularization and Blood Flow. New York, Plenum Publishing Corp., 1988.

Knobil, E., et al. (eds.): The Physiology of Reproduction. New York, Raven Press, 1988.

Leung, P. C. K., et al. (eds.): Endocrinology and Physiology of Reproduction. New York, Plenum Publishing Corp., 1987.

Stern, L., et al.: Physiologic Foundations of Perinatal Care. New York, Elsevier Science Publishing Co., 1989.

Vonderhaar, B. K., and Ziska, S. E.: Hormonal regulation of milk protein gene expression. Annu. Rev. Physiol., 51:641, 1989.

Wolf, D. P., et al. (eds.): In Vitro Fertilization and Embryo Transfer. New York, Plenum Publishing Corp., 1988.

Fetal and Neonatal Physiology

Cooke, J.: The early embryo and the formation of body pattern. Am. Sci., 76:35, 1988.

Gold, J. J., and Josimovich, J. B. (eds.): Gynecologic Endocrinology. 4th ed. New York, Plenum Publishing Corp., 1987.

Jones, C. T., and Rolph, T. P.: Metabolism during fetal life: A functional assessment of metabolic development. Physiol. Rev., 65:357, 1985.

Knobil, E., et al. (eds.): The Physiology of Reproduction. New York, Raven Press, 1988.

Lumbers, E. R.: Renal function during intrauterine life. News Physiol. Sci., 2:220, 1987.

Mortola, J. P.: Dynamics of breathing in newborn mammals. Physiol. Rev., 67:187, 1987.

Naeye, R. L.: Diseases of the Fetus and Newborn: Clinical Correlations and Medical-Legal Considerations. St. Louis, C. V. Mosby Co., 1989.

Rories, C., and Spelsberg, T. C.: Ovarian steroid action on gene expression: Mechanisms and models. Annu. Rev. Physiol., 51:653, 1989.

QUESTIONS

1. Describe the *fertilization* of the ovum.
2. Describe the *transport* and *implantation* of the developing morula and blastocyst.
3. How do the early-developing morula and blastocyst derive their *nutrition* from the uterus?
4. In what ways is *diffusion* through the placental mem-

brane similar to diffusion through the respiratory membrane?

5. Describe the diffusion of oxygen, carbon dioxide, and the various food substances through the placental membrane.
6. Explain the role of *human chorionic gonadotropin* in the maintenance of pregnancy during the first few weeks after fertilization.
7. What are the functions of the *estrogens* and the *progesterone* secreted by the placenta?
8. How does the mother respond to pregnancy in relation to each of the following factors: placental blood flow and cardiac output, mother's blood volume, mother's nutrition during pregnancy, and formation of amniotic fluid?
9. What are the characteristics of *preeclampsia* and *eclampsia?*
10. Discuss the factors that increase *uterine contractility* toward the end of pregnancy. How does increased contractility lead to a possible positive feedback cycle that culminates in labor and birth of the baby?
11. Describe the mechanics of *parturition.* What specific feedback mechanisms at the time of labor probably play major roles in enhancing the *labor contractions* and causing parturition to go to completion?
12. Discuss the factors that cause growth and development of the breasts and their glandular apparatus.
13. Explain the hormonal mechanisms that prevent *lactation* before birth but cause it to begin immediately after birth. What is the role of *prolactin* in maintaining the capability of the breasts to secrete milk for many months if the baby continues to suckle?
14. Explain the function of *oxytocin* in *milk ejection.*
15. What are some of the metabolic drains on the mother during lactation?
16. Which organs of the fetus are not fully developed at the time of birth?
17. Describe the onset of breathing. Why is *surfactant* important in this?
18. Explain the changes in pressure in different parts of the circulatory system immediately after birth that cause the immediate closure of the *foramen ovale* and the closure over a period of hours of the *ductus arteriosus.*
19. What are some of the special nutritional needs of the newborn infant?
20. Explain what happens to the fetus when the mother is given an androgenic hormone or when she has diabetes during pregnancy.
21. What are some of the special problems of prematurity, especially problems related to the respiratory system and to the maintenance of body temperature?

XIV

SPORTS PHYSIOLOGY

57

Sports Physiology

No other normal stresses to which the body is exposed even nearly approach the extreme stresses of heavy exercise. In fact, if some of the extremes of exercise were continued for even slightly prolonged periods of time, they might easily be lethal. Therefore, in the main, sports physiology is a discussion of the ultimate limits to which most of the bodily mechanisms can be stressed. To give one simple example: In a person who has extremely high fever, approaching the level of lethality, the body metabolism increases to about 100 per cent above normal. By comparison, the metabolism of the body during a marathon race increases to 2000 per cent above normal.

The Female and the Male Athlete

Most of the quantitative data that will be given in this chapter will be for the young male adult, not because it is desirable to know only these values but because it is only in this class of athletes that relatively complete measurements have been made. However, for those measurements that have been made in women, almost identically the same basic physiological principles apply equally as to men except for quantitative differences caused by differences in body size, body composition, and the presence or absence of the male sex hormone testosterone. In general, most quantitative values for women — such as muscle strength, pulmonary ventilation, and cardiac output, all of which are related mainly to the muscle mass — will vary between two thirds and three quarters of the values recorded in men. On the other hand, when measured in terms of strength per square centimeter of cross-sectional area, the female muscle can achieve almost exactly the same maximum force of contraction as that of the male — between 3 and 4 kg/cm^2. Therefore, much of the difference in total muscle performance lies in the extra percentage of the male body that is muscle, caused by endocrine differences that we shall discuss later.

A good indication of the relative performance capabilities of the female versus the male athlete comes from the relative times required for running the marathon race. In a recent comparison, the top female performer had a running time about 12 per cent less than that of the top male performer. On the other hand, for some endurance events, women have at times held the records over men — for instance, for the two-way swim across the English Channel, where the availability of extra fat might be an advantage.

The hormonal differences between women and men certainly account for a large part if not most of the differences in athletic performance. *Testosterone* secreted by the male testicles has a powerful *anabolic effect* in causing greatly increased deposition of protein everywhere in the body, especially in the muscles. In fact, even the man who participates in very little sports activity but who nevertheless is well-endowed with testosterone will have muscles that grow to sizes 40 per cent or more greater than those of his female counterpart and with a corresponding increase in strength.

The female sex hormone *estrogen* probably also accounts for some of the difference between female and male performance, though not nearly so much as testosterone. Estrogen is known to increase the deposition of fat in the female, especially in certain tissues, such as the breasts, the hips, and the subcutaneous tissue. At least partly for this reason, the average nonathletic female has about 27 per cent body fat composition in contrast to the nonathletic male, who has about 15 per cent. This obviously is a detriment to the highest levels of athletic performance in those events in which performance depends upon speed or bodily strength; on the other hand, it could be an aid in grueling endurance athletic events that require the fat for energy.

Finally, one cannot neglect the effect of the sex hormones on temperament. There is no doubt that testosterone promotes aggressiveness and that estrogen is associated with a more mild temperament. Certainly a large part of competitive sports is the aggressive spirit that drives a person to maximal effort, often at the expense of judicious restraint.

THE MUSCLES IN EXERCISE

Strength, Power, and Endurance of Muscles

The final common denominator in athletic events is what the muscles can do for you — what strength they can give when it is needed, what power they can achieve in the performance of work, and how long they can continue in their activity.

The strength of a muscle is determined mainly by its size, with a *maximum contractile force of between 3 and 4 kilograms per square centimeter* of muscle cross-sectional area. Thus, the man who is well laced with testosterone and therefore has correspondingly enlarged muscles will be much stronger than those persons without the testosterone advantage. Also, the athlete who has enlarged his muscles through an exercise training program likewise will have increased muscle strength.

To give an example of muscle strength, a world-class weight lifter might have a quadriceps muscle with a cross-sectional area as great as 150 square centimeters. This would translate into a maximal contractile strength of 525 kilograms (or 1155 pounds), with all this force applied to the patellar tendon. Therefore, one can readily understand how it is possible for this tendon to be ruptured or actually to be avulsed from its insertion into the tibia below the knee. Also, when such forces occur in tendons that span a joint, similar forces are applied as well to the surfaces of the joints, or sometimes to ligaments spanning the joints, thus accounting for such happenings as displaced cartilages, compression fractures about the joint, or torn ligaments.

The *holding strength* of muscles is about 40 per cent greater than the contractile strength. That is, if a muscle is already contracted and a force then attempts to stretch out the muscle, as occurs when landing after a jump, this requires about 40 per cent more force than can be achieved by a shortening contraction. Therefore, the force of 525 kilograms calculated previously for the patellar tendon becomes 735 kilograms (1617 pounds). This obviously further compounds the problems of the tendons, joints, and ligaments. It can also lead to internal tearing in the muscle itself. In fact, stretching out of a maximally contracted muscle is one of the best ways to insure the highest degree of muscle soreness.

The *power* of muscle contraction is different from muscle strength, for power is a measure of the total amount of work that the muscle can perform in a given period of time. This is determined not only by the strength of muscle contraction but also by its *distance of contraction* and the *number of times that it contracts each minute.* Muscle power is generally measured in *kilogram meters (kg-m) per minute.* That is, a muscle that can lift a kilogram weight to a height of 1 meter or that can move some object laterally against a force of 1 kilogram for a distance of a meter in 1 minute is said to have a power of 1 kg-m/min. The maximum power achievable by all the muscles in the body of a highly trained athlete with all the muscles working together is approximately the following:

	kg-m/min
First 8 to 10 seconds	7000
Next 1 minute	4000
Next half hour	1700

Thus, it is clear that a person has the capability of an extreme power surge for a short period of time, such as during a 100 meter dash that can be completed entirely within the first 10 seconds, whereas for long-term endurance events the power output of the muscles is only one fourth as great as during the initial power surge.

Yet this does not mean that one's athletic performance is four times as great during the initial power surge as it is for the next half hour, because the efficiency for translation of muscle power output into athletic performance is often much less during rapid activity than during less rapid but sustained activity. Thus, the velocity of the hundred meter dash is only 1.75 times as great as the velocity of the 30 minute race despite the fourfold difference in short-term versus long-term muscle power capability.

The final measure of muscle performance is *endurance.* This, to a great extent, depends on the nutritive support for the muscle — more than anything else on the amount of glycogen that has been stored in the muscle prior to the period of exercise. A person on a high carbohydrate diet stores far more glycogen in muscles than a person on either a mixed diet or a high fat diet. Therefore, endurance is greatly enhanced by a high carbohydrate diet. When athletes run at speeds typical for the marathon race, their endurance as measured by the time that they can sustain the race until complete exhaustion is approximately the following:

	minutes
High carbohydrate diet	240
Mixed diet	120
High fat diet	85

The corresponding amounts of glycogen stored in the muscle are approximately the following:

	gm/kg muscle
High carbohydrate diet	40
Mixed diet	20
High fat diet	6

The Muscle Metabolic Systems in Exercise

The same basic metabolic systems are present in muscle as in all other parts of the body; these were discussed in detail in Chapters 45 through 48. However, special quantitative measures of the activities of three metabolic systems are exceedingly important in understanding the limits of physical activity. These are (1) the *phosphagen system,* (2) the *glycogen-lactic acid system,* and (3) the *aerobic system.*

The Phosphagen System

Adenosine Triphosphate. The basic source of energy for muscle contraction is adenosine triphosphate (ATP), which has the following basic formula:

$$\text{Adenosine}-PO_3 \sim PO_3 \sim PO_3^-$$

The bonds attaching the last two phosphate radicals to the molecule, designated by the symbol ~, are *high-energy phosphate bonds.* Each of these bonds stores 7300 calories of energy per mole of ATP under standard conditions (and as much as 12,000 calories under the physical conditions in the body, which was discussed in detail in Chapter 45). Therefore, when one phosphate radical is removed from the molecule, 7300 calories of energy that can be used to energize the muscle contractile process is released. Then, when the second phosphate radical is removed, still another 7300 calories becomes available. Removal of the first phosphate converts the ATP into *adenosine diphosphate* (ADP), and removal of the second converts this ADP into *adenosine monophosphate* (AMP).

Unfortunately, the amount of ATP present in the muscles, even in the well-trained athlete, is sufficient to sustain maximal muscle power for only about 3 seconds, maybe enough for half of a 50 meter dash. Therefore, except for a few seconds at a time, it is essential that new adenosine triphosphate be formed continuously, even during the performance of athletic events. Figure 57-1 illustrates the overall metabolic system, showing the breakdown of ATP first to ADP and then to AMP, with the release of energy to the muscles for contraction. To the left-hand side of the figure are illustrated the three different metabolic mechanisms that are responsible for reconstituting a continuous supply of adenosine triphosphate in the muscle fibers. These are the following:

Release of Energy from Phosphocreatine. Phosphocreatine (also called *creatine phosphate*) is another chemical compound that has a high energy phosphate bond, with the following formula:

$$\text{Creatine} \sim PO_3^-$$

This can decompose to *creatine* and *phosphate ion,* as illustrated to the left in Figure 57-1, and in doing so releases large amounts of energy. In fact, the high-energy phosphate bond of phosphocreatine has more energy than the bond of ATP—10,300 calories per mole, in comparison with 7300. Therefore, the phosphocreatine can easily provide enough energy to reconstitute the high energy bonds of the ATP. Furthermore, most muscle cells have two to four times as much phosphocreatine as ATP.

A special characteristic of energy transfer from phosphocreatine to ATP is that it occurs within a small fraction of a second. Therefore, in effect, all the energy stored in the muscle phosphocreatine is instantaneously available for muscle contraction, just as is the energy stored in ATP.

The cell phosphocreatine plus its ATP are called the *phosphagen energy system.* These together can provide maximal muscle power for a period of 8 to 10 seconds, almost enough for the 100 meter run. Thus, the energy from the phosphagen system is used for maximal short bursts of muscle power.

The Glycogen-Lactic Acid System

The stored glycogen in muscle can be split into glucose and the glucose then utilized for energy. The initial stage of this process, called *glycolysis,* occurs entirely without use of oxygen and therefore is said to be *anaerobic metabolism* (see Chapter 45). During glycolysis, each glucose molecule is split into two *pyruvic acid molecules,* and energy is released to form several ATP molecules. Ordinarily the pyruvic acid then enters the mitochondria of the muscle cells and reacts with oxygen to form still many more ATP molecules. However, when there is insufficient oxygen for this second stage (the oxidative stage) of glucose metabolism to occur, most of the pyruvic acid is converted into *lactic acid,* which then diffuses out of the muscle cells into the interstitial fluid and blood. Therefore, in effect, much of the muscle glycogen becomes lactic acid, but in doing so considerable amounts of adeno-

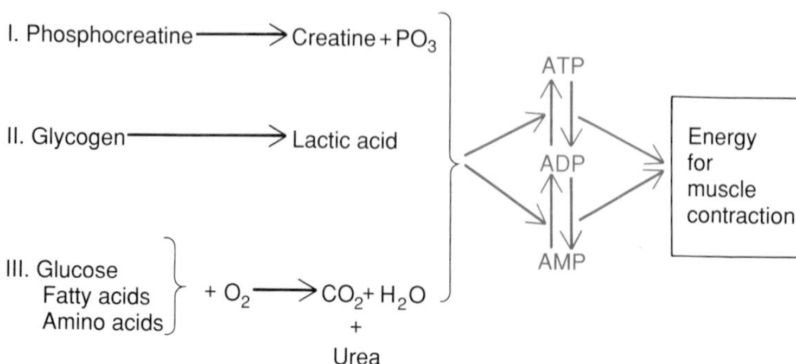

Figure 57-1. The three important metabolic systems that supply energy for muscle contraction.

sine triphosphate are formed entirely without the consumption of oxygen.

Another characteristic of the glycogen-lactic acid system is that it can form ATP molecules about 2.5 times as rapidly as can the oxidative mechanism of the mitochondria. Therefore, when large amounts of adenosine triphosphate are required for short to moderate periods of muscle contraction, this anaerobic glycolysis mechanism can be used as a rapid source of energy. It is not as rapid as the phosphagen system, but about half as rapid.

Under optimal conditions the glycogen-lactic acid system can provide 1.3 to 1.6 minutes of maximal muscle activity in addition to the 8 to 10 seconds provided by the phosphagen system.

The Aerobic System

The aerobic system means the oxidation of foodstuffs in the mitochondria to provide energy. That is, as illustrated to the left in Figure 57-1, glucose, fatty acids, and amino acids from the foods—after some intermediate processing—combine with oxygen to release tremendous amounts of energy that are used to convert AMP and ADP into ATP, as was discussed in Chapter 45.

In comparing this aerobic mechanism of energy supply with the glycogen-lactic acid system and the phosphagen system, the relative *maximal rates of power generation* in terms of ATP utilization are the following:

	M of ATP/min
Aerobic system	1
Glycogen-lactic acid system	2.5
Phosphagen system	4

On the other hand, when comparing the systems for endurance, the relative values are the following:

	Time
Phosphagen system	8 to 10 seconds
Glycogen-lactic acid system	1.3 to 1.6 minutes
Aerobic system	unlimited time (as long as nutrients last)

Thus, one can readily see that the phosphagen system is the one utilized by the muscle for power surges of a few seconds, and the aerobic system is required for prolonged athletic activity. In between is the glycogen-lactic acid system, which is especially important for giving extra power during such intermediate races as the 200- to 800-meter runs.

What Types of Sports Utilize Which Energy Systems?

By considering the vigor of a sports activity and its duration, one can estimate very closely which of the energy systems are used for each activity. Various approximations are presented in Table 57-1.

Table 57-1 ENERGY SYSTEMS USED IN VARIOUS SPORTS

Phosphagen system, almost entirely
100-meter dash
Jumping
Weight lifting
Diving
Football dashes
Phosphagen and glycogen-lactic acid systems
200-meter dash
Basketball
Baseball home run
Ice hockey dashes
Glycogen-lactic acid system, mainly
400-meter dash
100-meter swim
Tennis
Soccer
Glycogen-lactic acid and aerobic systems
800-meter dash
200-meter swim
1500-meter skating
Boxing
2000-meter rowing
1500-meter run
1 mile run
400-meter swim
Aerobic system
10,000-meter skating
Cross-country skiing
Marathon run (26.2 miles, 42.2 km)
Jogging

Recovery of the Muscle Metabolic Systems After Exercise

In the same way that the energy from phosphocreatine can be used to reconstitute adenosine triphosphate, so also can energy from the glycogen-lactic acid system be used to reconstitute both phosphocreatine and ATP. And then energy from the oxidative metabolism of the aerobic system can be used to reconstitute all the other systems—the ATP, the phosphocreatine, and also the glycogen-lactic acid system.

Reconstitution of the lactic acid system means mainly the removal of the excess lactic acid that has accumulated in all the fluids of the body. This is especially important because *lactic acid causes extreme fatigue.* When adequate amounts of energy are available from oxidative metabolism, removal of lactic acid is achieved in two ways: First, a small portion of it is converted back into pyruvic acid and then metabolized oxidatively by all of the body tissues. Second, the remaining lactic acid is reconverted into glucose mainly in the liver; and the glucose in turn is used to replenish the glycogen stores of the muscles.

Recovery of the Aerobic System After Exercise. During the early stages of heavy exercise even a portion of one's aerobic energy capability is depleted. This results from two effects: (1) the so-called *oxygen debt* and (2) *depletion of the glycogen stores* of the muscles.

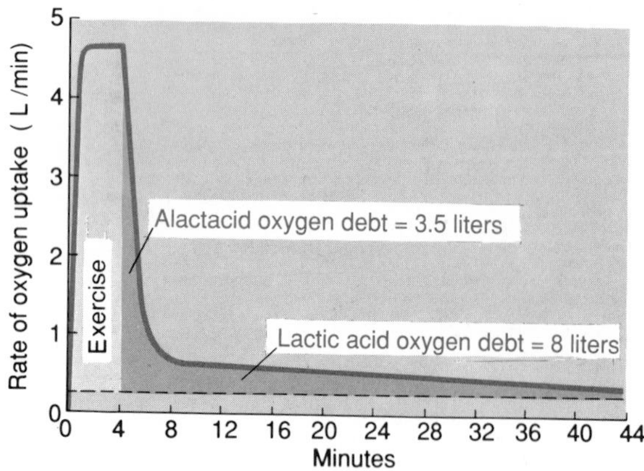

Figure 57-2. Rate of oxygen uptake by the lungs during maximal exercise for 4 minutes and then for almost 1 hour after the exercise is over. This figure demonstrates the principle of *oxygen debt*.

The Oxygen Debt. The body normally contains about 2 liters of stored oxygen that can be used for aerobic metabolism even without breathing any new oxygen. This stored oxygen consists of the following: (1) 0.5 liter in the air of the lungs; (2) 0.25 liter dissolved in the body fluids; (3) 1 liter combined with the hemoglobin of the blood; and (4) 0.3 liter stored in the muscle fibers themselves, combined with myoglobin, an oxygen binding chemical similar to hemoglobin.

In heavy exercise, almost all of this stored oxygen is used within a minute or so for aerobic metabolism. Then, after the exercise is over, this stored oxygen must be replenished by breathing extra amounts of oxygen over and above the normal requirements. In addition, about 9 liters more of oxygen must be consumed to provide for reconstituting both the phosphagen system and the lactic acid system. All of this extra oxygen that must be "repaid," about 11.5 liters, is called the oxygen debt.

Figure 57-2 illustrates this principle of oxygen debt. During the first 4 minutes of the figure, the person exercises very heavily, and the rate of oxygen uptake increases about 15-fold. Then, even after the exercise is over, the oxygen uptake still remains above normal, at first very high while the body is reconstituting the phosphagen system and also repaying the stored oxygen portion of the oxygen debt, then for another hour at a lower level while the lactic acid is removed. The early portion of the oxygen debt is called the *alactacid oxygen debt* and amounts to about 3.5 liters. The latter portion is called the *lactic acid oxygen debt* and amounts to about 8 liters.

Recovery of Muscle Glycogen. Recovery from exhaustive muscle glycogen depletion is not a simple matter. This often requires days, rather than the seconds, minutes, or hours required for recovery of the phosphagen and lactic acid metabolic systems. Figure 57-3 illustrates this recovery process under three different conditions: first in persons on a high carbohydrate diet; second, in persons on a high fat/high protein diet; and third, in persons with no food. Note that on a high carbohydrate diet, full recovery occurs in approximately 2 days. On the other hand, persons on a high fat/high protein diet or on no food at all show extremely little recovery even after as long as 5 days. The messages of this comparison are (1) that it is important for an athlete to have a high carbohydrate diet before a grueling athletic event and (2) not to participate in exhaustive exercise during the 48 hours preceding the event.

Nutrients Used During Muscle Activity

Although we have emphasized the importance of a high carbohydrate diet and large stores of muscle glycogen for maximal athletic performance, this does not mean that only carbohydrates are used for muscle energy—it means simply that carbohydrates are used by preference. Actually, the muscles use large amounts of fat for energy in the form of *fatty acids* and *acetoacetic acid* (see Chapter 46) and also use to a much less extent proteins in the form of *amino acids*.

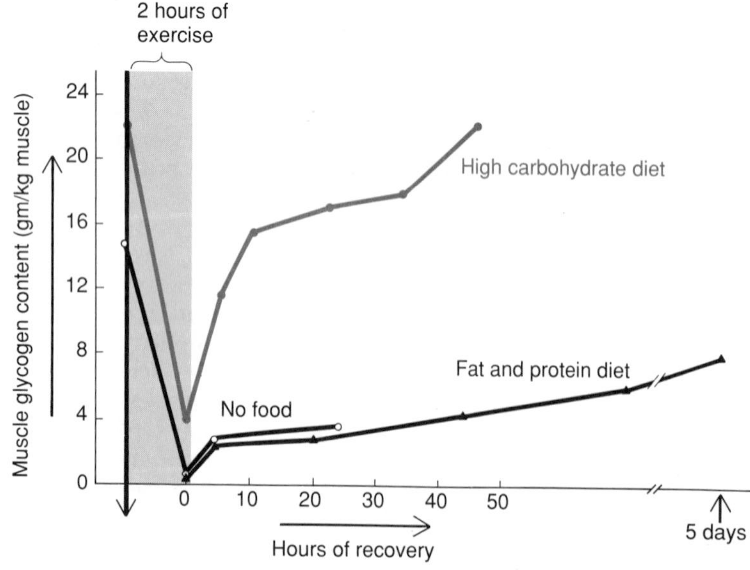

Figure 57-3. Effect of diet on the rate of muscle glycogen replenishment following prolonged exercise. (From Fox: Sports Physiology. Philadelphia, Saunders College Publishing, 1979.)

In fact, even under the best conditions, in those endurance athletic events that last longer than 4 to 5 hours, the glycogen stores of the muscle become depleted and are then of little further use for energizing muscle contraction. Instead, the muscle now depends upon energy from other sources, mainly from fats.

Figure 57–4 illustrates the approximate relative usage of carbohydrates and fat for energy during prolonged exhaustive exercise under three different dietary conditions: high carbohydrate diet, mixed diet, and high fat diet. Note that most of the energy is derived from carbohydrate during the first few seconds or minutes of the exercise, but at the time of exhaustion, as much as 60 to 85 per cent of the energy is being derived from fats, rather than carbohydrates.

Not all the energy from carbohydrates comes from the stored muscle glycogen. In many persons almost as much glycogen is stored in the liver as in the muscles; and this can be released into the blood in the form of glucose, then taken up by the muscles as an energy source. In addition, glucose solutions given to an athlete to drink during the course of an athletic event (in optimal concentrations of 2 to 2.5 per cent) can provide as much as 30 to 40 per cent of the energy required during prolonged events such as marathon races.

In essence, then, if muscle glycogen and blood glucose are available, these are the energy nutrients of choice for intense muscle activity. Even so, for a real endurance event one can expect fat to supply more than 50 per cent of the required energy after about the first 3 to 4 hours.

Effect of Athletic Training on Muscles and Muscle Performance

Importance of Maximal Resistance Training. One of the cardinal principles of muscle development during athletic training is the following: Muscles that function under no load, even if they are exercised for hours upon end, increase little in strength. At the other extreme, muscles that contract at or near their maximal force of contraction will develop strength very rapidly even if the contractions are performed only a few times each day. Utilizing this principle, experiments on muscle building have shown that 6 maximal or nearly maximal muscle contractions performed in three separate sets 3 days a week give approximately optimal increase in muscle strength and without producing chronic muscle fatigue. The upper curve in Figure 57–5 illustrates the approximate percentage increase in strength that can be achieved in the previously untrained person by this optimal resistive training program, showing that the muscle strength increases about 30 per cent during the first 6 to 8 weeks but almost plateaus after that time. Along with this increase in strength is an approximately equal percentage increase in muscle mass, which is called *muscle hypertrophy.*

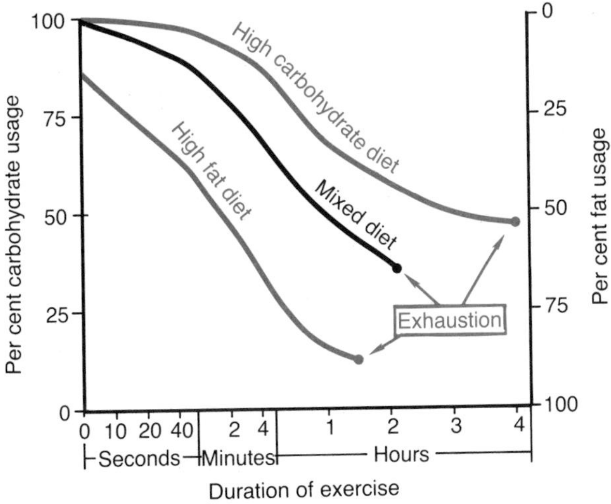

Figure 57–4. Effect of duration of exercise as well as type of diet on relative percentages of carbohydrate or fat used for energy by muscles. (Based partly on data in Fox: Sports Physiology. Philadelphia, Saunders College Publishing, 1979.)

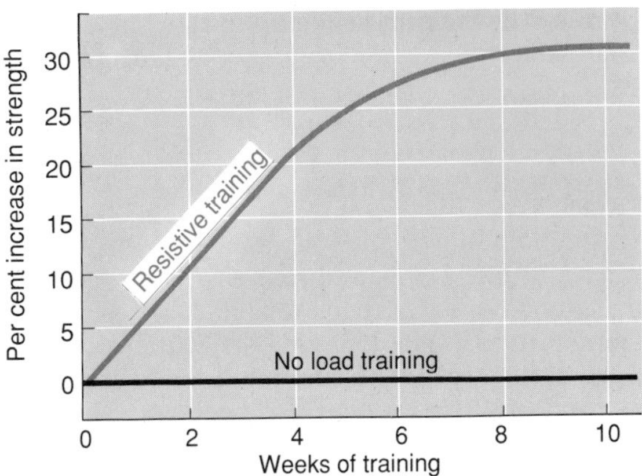

Figure 57–5. Approximate effect of optimal resistive exercise training on increase in muscle strength over a training period of 10 weeks.

Muscle Hypertrophy. The basic size of a person's muscles is determined mainly by heredity plus the level of testosterone secretion, which, in men, causes considerably larger muscles than in women. However, with training, the muscles can become hypertrophied perhaps an additional 30 to 60 per cent. Most of this hypertrophy results from increased diameter of the muscle fibers; but this is not entirely true, because a very few greatly enlarged muscle fibers are believed to split down the middle along their entire length to form entirely new fibers, thus increasing the numbers of fibers slightly.

The changes that occur inside the hypertrophied muscle fibers themselves include (1) increased numbers of myofibrils, proportionate to the degree of hypertrophy; (2) up to 120 per cent increase in mitochondrial enzymes; (3) as much as 60 to 80 per cent increase in the components of the phosphagen metabolic system, including both ATP and phosphocreatine; (4) as much as 50 per cent increase in stored glycogen; and (5) as much as 75 to 100 per cent increase in stored triglyceride (fat). Because of all these changes, the capabilities of both the anaerobic and the aerobic metabolic systems are increased, increasing especially the maximum oxidation rate and efficiency of the oxidative metabolic system as much as 45 per cent.

Fast Twitch and Slow Twitch Muscle Fibers

In the human being, all muscles have varying percentages of *fast twitch* and *slow twitch muscle fibers.* For instance, the gastrocnemius muscle has a higher preponderance of fast twitch fibers, which gives it the capability of very forceful and rapid contraction of the type used in jumping. On the other hand, the soleus muscle has a higher preponderance of slow twitch muscle fibers and therefore is used to a greater extent for prolonged lower leg muscle activity.

The basic differences between the fast twitch and the slow twitch fibers are the following:

1. Fast twitch fibers are about two times as large in diameter.
2. The enzymes that promote rapid release of energy from the phosphagen and glycogen–lactic acid energy systems are two to three times as active in fast twitch fibers as in slow twitch fibers, thus making the maximal power that can be achieved by fast twitch fibers as great as two times that of slow twitch fibers.
3. Slow twitch fibers are mainly organized for endurance, especially for generation of aerobic energy. They have far more mitochondria than the fast twitch fibers. In addition, they contain considerably more myoglobin, a hemoglobin-like protein that combines with oxygen within the muscle fiber; and even more important, myoglobin increases the rate of diffusion of oxygen throughout the fiber by shuttling oxygen from one molecule of myoglobin to the next. In addition, the enzymes of the aerobic metabolic system are considerably more active in slow twitch fibers than in fast twitch fibers.
4. The number of capillaries per mass of fibers is greater in the vicinity of slow twitch fibers than in the vicinity of fast twitch fibers.

In summary, fast twitch fibers can deliver extreme amounts of power for a few seconds to a minute or so. On the other hand, slow twitch fibers provide endurance, delivering prolonged strength of contraction over many minutes to hours.

Hereditary Differences Among Athletes for Fast Twitch Versus Slow Twitch Muscle Fibers. Some persons have considerably more fast twitch than slow twitch fibers, and others have more slow twitch fibers; this obviously could determine to some extent the athletic capabilities of different individuals. Unfortunately, athletic training has not been shown to change the relative proportions of fast twitch and slow twitch fibers however much an athlete might wish to develop one type of athletic prowess over another. Instead, this is determined almost entirely by genetic inheritance, and this in turn helps determine which area of athletics is most suited to each person: some people are born to be marathoners; others are born to be sprinters and jumpers. For example, the following are recorded percentages of fast twitch versus slow twitch fiber in the quadriceps muscles of different types of athletes:

	Fast Twitch	*Slow Twitch*
Marathoners	18	82
Swimmers	26	74
Average man	55	45
Weight lifters	55	45
Sprinters	63	37
Jumpers	63	37

RESPIRATION IN EXERCISE

Although one's respiratory ability is of relatively little concern in the performance of sprint types of athletics, it is critical for maximal performance in endurance athletics.

Oxygen Consumption and Pulmonary Ventilation in Exercise. Normal oxygen consumption for a young adult man at rest is about 250 ml/min. However, under maximal conditions this can be increased to approximately the following average levels:

	ml/min
Untrained average man	3600
Athletically trained average man	4000
Male marathon runners	5100

Figure 57–6 illustrates the relationship between oxygen consumption at different degrees of exercise and *pulmonary ventilation.* It is clear from this figure, as would be expected, that there is a linear relationship. In round numbers, both oxygen consumption and pulmonary ventilation increase about 20-fold between the resting state and maximum intensity of exercise.

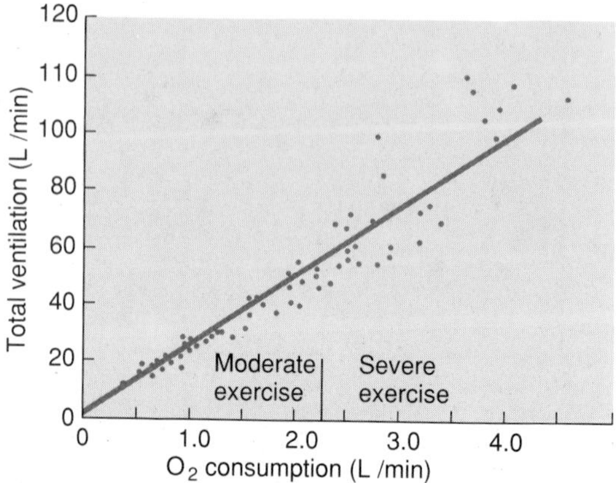

Figure 57–6. Effect of exercise on oxygen consumption and ventilatory rate. (From Gray: Pulmonary Ventilation and Its Physiological Regulation. Springfield, Ill., Charles C Thomas.)

The Limits of Pulmonary Ventilation. How severely do we stress our respiratory systems during exercise? This can be answered by the following comparison for the normal man:

	liters/min
Pulmonary ventilation at maximal exercise	100 to 110
Maximal breathing capacity	150 to 170

Thus, the maximal breathing capacity is about 50 per cent greater than the actual pulmonary ventilation during maximal exercise. This obviously provides an element of safety for athletes, giving them extra ventilation that can be called on in such conditions as (1) exercise at high altitudes, (2) exercise under very hot conditions, and (3) abnormalities in the respiratory system.

The important point is that the respiratory system is not normally the most limiting factor in the delivery of oxygen to the muscles during maximal muscle aerobic metabolism. We shall see shortly that the ability of the heart to pump blood to the muscles is usually a greater limiting factor.

Effect of Training on $\dot{V}O_2$ Max. The abbreviation for the rate of oxygen usage under maximal aerobic metabolism is $\dot{V}O_2$ Max. Figure 57–7 illustrates the progressive effect of athletic training on $\dot{V}O_2$ Max recorded in a group of subjects beginning at the level of no training and then pursuing the training program for 7 to 13 weeks. In this study, it is surprising that the $\dot{V}O_2$ Max increased only about 10 per cent. Furthermore, the frequency of training, whether two times or five times per week, had little effect on the increase in $\dot{V}O_2$ Max. Yet, as was pointed out earlier, the $\dot{V}O_2$ Max of marathoners is about 45 per cent greater than that of the untrained person. Part of this greater $\dot{V}O_2$ Max of the marathoner is genetically determined; that is, those persons who have greater chest sizes in relation to body size and stronger respiratory muscles select themselves to become marathoners. However, it is also very likely that the very prolonged training of the marathoner does increase the $\dot{V}O_2$ Max by values considerably greater than the 10 per cent that has been recorded in short-term experiments such as that in Figure 57–7.

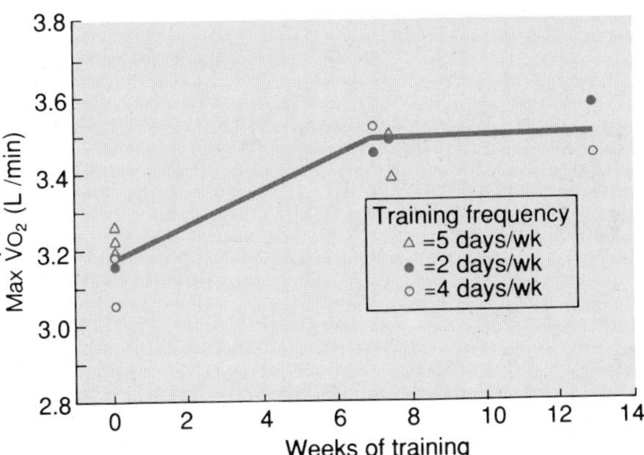

Figure 57–7. Increase in $\dot{V}O_2$ Max over a period of 7 to 13 weeks of athletic training. (From Fox: Sports Physiology. Philadelphia, Saunders College Publishing, 1979.)

The O_2 Diffusing Capacity of Athletes. The O_2 *diffusing capacity* is a measure of the rate at which oxygen can diffuse from the alveoli into the blood. This is expressed in terms of *milliliters of oxygen that will diffuse for each millimeter of mercury difference between alveolar partial pressure of oxygen and pulmonary blood oxygen pressure.* That is, if the partial pressure of oxygen in the alveoli is 91 mm Hg while the pressure in the blood is 90 mm Hg, the amount of oxygen that diffuses through the respiratory membrane each minute is the diffusing capacity. The following are measured values for different diffusing capacities:

	ml/min
Nonathlete at rest	23
Nonathlete during maximal exercise	48
Speed skaters during maximal exercise	64
Swimmers during maximal exercise	71
Oarsmen during maximal exercise	80

The most startling fact about these results is the almost threefold increase in diffusing capacity between the resting state and the state of maximal exercise. This results mainly from the fact that blood flow through many of the pulmonary capillaries is very sluggish or even dormant in the resting state, whereas in exercise increased blood flow through the lungs causes all the pulmonary capillaries to be perfused at their maximal level, thus providing far greater surface area through which oxygen can diffuse into the pulmonary capillary blood.

It is also clear from these values that those athletes who require greater amounts of oxygen per minute have higher diffusing capacities. Is this because persons with naturally greater diffusing capacities choose these types of sports, or is it because something about the training procedures increases the diffusing capacity? The answer is not known; but one must believe that training does play some role, particularly endurance training.

The Blood Gases During Exercise. Because of the great usage of oxygen by the muscles in exercise, one would expect the oxygen pressure of the arterial blood to decrease markedly during strenuous athletics and the carbon dioxide pressure of the venous blood to increase far above normal. However, this normally is not the case. Both of these values remain nearly normal, illustrating the extreme ability of the respiratory system to provide very adequate aeration of the blood even in heavy exercise, which illustrates another very important point. The blood gases do not have to become abnormal for respiration to be stimulated in exercise. Instead, respiration is stimulated mainly by neurogenic mechanisms in exercise, as discussed in Chapter 29. Part of this stimulation results from direct stimulation of the respiratory center by the same nervous signals that are transmitted from the brain to the muscles to cause the exercise. Part is believed to result from sensory signals transmitted into the respiratory center from the contracting muscles and moving joints. All this nervous stimulation of respiration is normally sufficient to provide almost exactly the proper increase in pulmonary ventilation to keep the blood respiratory gases — the oxygen and the carbon dioxide — almost normal.

Effect of Smoking on Pulmonary Ventilation in Exercise. It is widely stated that smoking can decrease an athlete's "wind." This is true for many reasons. First, one effect of nicotine is constriction of the terminal bronchioles of the lungs, which increases the resistance of air flow into and out of the lungs. Second, the irritating effects of smoke cause increased fluid secretion in the bronchial tree, as well as some swelling of the epithelial linings. Third, nicotine paralyzes the cilia on the surfaces of the respiratory epithelial cells that normally beat continuously to remove excess fluids and foreign particles from the respiratory tract. As a result, much debris accumulates in the respiratory passageways and adds further to the difficulty of breathing. Putting all these factors together, even the light smoker will feel respiratory strain during maximal exercise, and the level of performance obviously may be reduced.

Much more severe are the effects of chronic smoking. There are very few chronic smokers in whom some degree of emphysema does not develop. In this disease, the following occur: (1) chronic bronchitis, (2) obstruction of many of the terminal bronchioles, and (3) destruction of many alveolar walls. In severe emphysema, as much as four fifths of the respiratory membrane can be destroyed; then even the slightest exercise can cause respiratory distress. In fact, many such patients cannot even perform the athletic feat of walking across the floor of a single room without gasping for breath. Such is the indictment of smoking.

THE CARDIOVASCULAR SYSTEM IN EXERCISE

Muscle Blood Flow. The final common denominator of cardiovascular function in exercise is to deliver oxygen and other nutrients to the muscles. For this purpose, the muscle blood flow increases drastically during exercise. Figure 57–8 illustrates a recording of muscle blood flow in the calf of a person for a period of 6 minutes during strong intermittent contraction. Note not only the great increase in flow — about 13-fold — but also that the flow decreased during each muscle contraction. Two points can be made from this study: (1) The actual contractile process itself temporarily decreases muscle blood flow because the contracting muscle compresses the intramuscular blood vessels; therefore, strong tonic contractions can cause rapid muscle fatigue because of lack of delivery of enough oxygen and nutrients during the continuous contraction. (2) The blood flow to

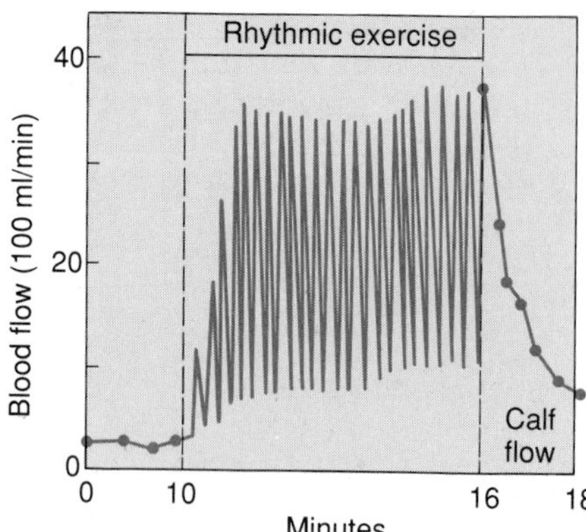

Figure 57–8. Effects of muscle exercise on blood flow in the calf of a leg during strong rhythmical contraction. The blood flow was much less during contraction than between contractions. (From Barcroft and Dornhorst: *J. Physiol., 109:*402, 1949.)

muscles during exercise can increase markedly. The following comparison illustrates the maximal increase in blood flow that can occur in the well-trained athlete.

	ml/100 gm muscle/min
Resting blood flow	3.6
Blood flow during maximal exercise	90

Thus, muscle blood flow can increase a maximum of about 25-fold during the most strenuous exercise. About half this increase in flow results from intramuscular vasodilation caused by the direct effects of increased muscle metabolism, as was explained in Chapter 14. The other half results from multiple factors, the most important of which is probably the moderate increase in arterial blood pressure that occurs in exercise, usually about a 30 per cent increase. The increase in pressure not only forces more blood through the blood vessels but also stretches the walls of the arterioles and further reduces the vascular

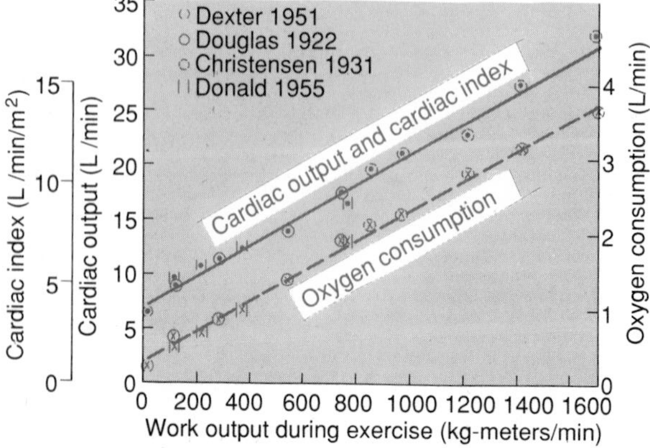

Figure 57–9. Relationship between cardiac output and work output (solid line) and between oxygen consumption and work output (dashed line) during different levels of exercise. (From Guyton, Jones, and Coleman: Circulatory Physiology: Cardiac Output and Its Regulation. Philadelphia, W. B. Saunders Company, 1973.)

resistance. Therefore, a 30 per cent increase in blood pressure can often more than double the blood flow; this is added to the great increase in flow already caused by the metabolic vasodilation.

Work Output, Oxygen Consumption, and Cardiac Output During Exercise. Figure 57–9 illustrates the interrelationships among work output, oxygen consumption, and cardiac output during exercise. It is not surprising that all these are directly related to each other, as shown by the linear functions, because the muscle work output increases oxygen consumption, and oxygen consumption in turn dilates the muscle blood vessels, thus increasing venous return and cardiac output. Typical cardiac outputs at several levels of exercise are the following:

	liters/min
Average young man at rest	5.5
Maximal output during exercise in young untrained man	23
Maximal output during exercise in male marathoner	30

Thus, the normal untrained person can increase cardiac output a little over fourfold, and the well-trained athlete can increase output about sixfold. Individual marathoners have been clocked at cardiac outputs as great as 35 to 40 liters/min.

Effect of Training on Heart Hypertrophy and on Cardiac Output. From the foregoing data, it is clear that marathoners can achieve maximal cardiac outputs about 40 per cent greater than that achieved by the untrained person. This results mainly from the fact that the heart chambers of marathoners enlarge about 40 per cent; along with enlargement of the chambers, the heart mass increases 40 per cent or more as well. Therefore, not only do the skeletal muscles hypertrophy during athletic training but the heart does also. However, heart enlargement and increased pumping capacity occur only in the endurance types, not in the sprint types, of athletic training.

Even though the heart of the marathoner is considerably larger than that of the normal person, resting cardiac output is almost exactly the same as that in the normal person. However, this normal cardiac output is achieved by a large stroke volume at a reduced heart rate. Table 57–2 compares stroke volume and heart rate in the untrained person and the marathoner.

Table 57–2 COMPARISON OF CARDIAC OUTPUT BETWEEN MARATHONER AND NONATHLETE

	Stroke Volume (ml)	Heart Rate (beats/min)
Resting		
Nonathlete	75	75
Marathoner	105	50
Maximum		
Nonathlete	110	195
Marathoner	162	185

Thus, the heart-pumping effectiveness of each heart beat is 40 to 50 per cent greater in the highly trained athlete than in the untrained person, but there is a corresponding decrease in heart rate at rest.

Role of Stroke Volume and Heart Rate in Increasing the Cardiac Output. Figure 57–10 illustrates the approximate changes in stroke volume and heart rate as the cardiac output increases from its resting level of about 5.5 liters/min to 30 liters/min in the marathon runner. The *stroke volume* increases from 105 to 162 milliliters, an increase of about 50 per cent; whereas the heart rate increases from 50 to 185 beats per minute, an increase of 270 per cent. Therefore, the heart rate increase accounts by far for a greater proportion of the increase in cardiac output than does the increase in stroke volume during strenuous exercise. The stroke volume normally reaches its maximum by the time the cardiac output has increased only halfway to its maximum. Any further increase in cardiac output must occur by increasing the heart rate.

Relationship of Cardiovascular Performance to $\dot{V}O_2$ Max. During maximal exercise, both the heart rate and the stroke volume are increased to about 95 per cent of their maximal levels. Since the cardiac output is equal to stroke volume *times* heart rate, one finds that the cardiac output is about 90 per cent of the maximum that the person can achieve. This is in contrast to about 65 per cent of maximum for pulmonary ventilation. Therefore, one can readily see that the cardiovascular system is normally much more limiting on $\dot{V}O_2$ Max than is the respiratory system. For this reason, it is frequently stated that the performance that can be achieved by the marathoner mainly depends on his or her heart, for this is the most limiting link in the delivery of adequate oxygen to the exercising muscles. Therefore, the 40 per cent advantage in maximal cardiac output that the marathoner has over the average untrained male is probably the single most important physiological benefit of the marathoner's training program.

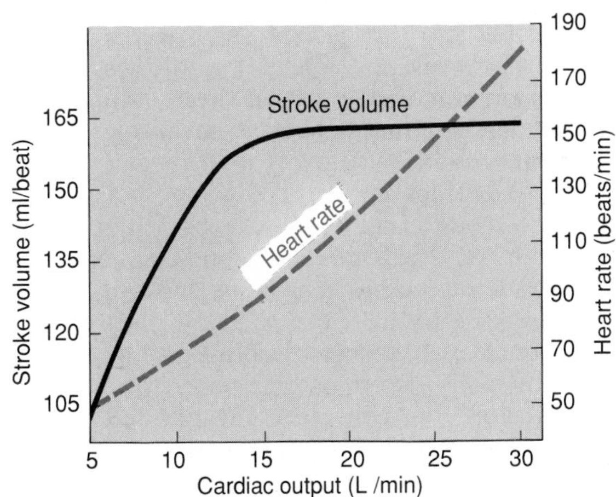

Figure 57–10. Approximate stroke volume output and heart rate at different levels of cardiac output in a marathon athlete.

Effect of Heart Disease and Old Age on Athletic Performance. Because of the critical limitation that the cardiovascular system places on maximal performance in endurance athletics, one can readily understand that any type of heart disease that reduces the maximum cardiac output will cause an almost corresponding decrease in achievable muscle power. Therefore, a person with congestive heart failure frequently has difficulty achieving even the muscle power required to climb out of bed, much less to walk across the floor.

The maximal cardiac output of older persons also decreases considerably — there is as much as a 50 per cent decrease between the teens and the age of 80 years. Again, one finds that the maximal achievable muscle power is greatly reduced.

BODY HEAT IN EXERCISE

Almost all the energy released by the body's metabolism of nutrients is eventually converted into body heat. This applies even to the energy that causes muscle contraction, for the following reasons: First, the maximal efficiency for conversion of nutrient energy into muscle work, even under the best of conditions, is only 20 to 25 per cent; the remainder of the nutrient energy is converted into heat during the course of the intracellular chemical reactions. Second, almost all the energy that does go into creating muscle work still becomes body heat because all but a small portion of this energy is used for (1) overcoming viscous resistance to the movement of the muscles and joints, (2) overcoming the friction of the blood flowing through the blood vessels, and (3) other similar effects — all of which convert the muscle contractile energy into heat.

Now, recognizing that the oxygen consumption by the body can increase as much as 20-fold in the well-trained athlete and that the amount of heat liberated in the body is directly proportional to the oxygen consumption (as discussed in Chapter 47), one quickly realizes that tremendous amounts of heat are injected into the internal body tissues during endurance athletic events.

Next, with a vast rate of heat flow into the body on a very hot and humid day, so that the sweating mechanism cannot eliminate the heat, an intolerable and even lethal condition called *heat stroke* can easily develop in the athlete.

Heat Stroke. During endurance athletics, even under normal environmental conditions the body temperature often rises from its normal level of 37°C to 40°C (98.6°F to 102°F to 103°F). With very hot and humid conditions or excess clothing, the body temperature can easily rise to as high as 41.1°C to 42.5°C (106°F to 108°F). At this level the elevated temperature itself becomes destructive to tissue cells, especially destructive to brain cells. When this happens, multiple symptoms begin to appear, including extreme weakness, exhaustion, headache, dizziness, nausea, profuse sweating, confusion, staggering gait, collapse, and unconsciousness.

This whole complex is called heat stroke, and failure to treat it immediately can lead to death. In fact, even though the person has stopped exercising, the temperature does not easily decrease by itself. One of the reasons for this is that at these high temperatures the temperature-regulating mechanism itself often fails (see Chapter 47). A second reason is that the high temperature approximately doubles the rates of all intracellular chemical reactions, thus liberating still far more heat.

The treatment of heat stroke is to reduce the body temperature as rapidly as possible. The most practical way to do this is to remove all clothing, maintain a spray of water on all surfaces of the body or continually sponge the body, and blow air over the body with a strong fan. Experiments have shown that this treatment can reduce the temperature either as rapidly or almost as rapidly as any other procedure, though some physicians prefer total immersion of the body in ice water containing a mush of crushed ice if available.

BODY FLUIDS AND SALT IN EXERCISE

As much as a 5 to 10 pound weight loss has been recorded in athletes in a period of 1 hour during endurance athletic events under hot and humid conditions. Essentially all of this weight loss results from loss of sweat. Loss of enough sweat to decrease body weight only 3 per cent can significantly diminish a person's performance, and a 5 to 10 per cent rapid decrease in weight can often be very serious, leading to muscle cramps, nausea, and other effects. Therefore, it is essential to replace fluid as it is lost.

Replacement of Salt and Potassium. Sweat contains a large amount of salt, for which reason it has long been stated that all athletes should take salt (sodium chloride) tablets when performing exercise on hot and humid days. Unfortunately, overuse of salt tablets has often done more harm than good. Furthermore, if an athlete becomes acclimatized to the heat by progressive increase in athletic exposure over a period of 1 to 2 weeks rather than performing maximal athletic feats on the first day, the sweat glands also become acclimatized, so that the amount of salt lost in the sweat is only a small fraction of that prior to acclimatization. This sweat gland acclimatization results mainly from increased aldosterone secretion by the adrenal cortex. The aldosterone in turn has a direct effect on the sweat glands, increasing the reabsorption of sodium chloride from the sweat before it issues forth from the sweat gland tubules onto the surface of the skin. Once the athlete is acclimatized, only rarely do salt supplements need to be considered during athletic events.

On the other hand, recent experience by military units suddenly exposed to heavy exercise in the desert has demonstrated still another electrolyte problem —

the problem of potassium loss. Potassium loss results partly from the increased secretion of aldosterone during heat acclimatization, which increases the loss of potassium in the urine as well as in the sweat. As a consequence of these new findings, some of the newer supplemental fluids for athletics are beginning to contain properly proportioned amounts of potassium and sodium, usually in the form of fruit juices.

DRUGS AND ATHLETES

Without belaboring this issue, let us list some of the effects of drugs in athletics:

First, *caffeine* can increase athletic performance. In one experiment on a marathon runner, his running time for the marathon was reduced by 7 per cent by judicious use of caffeine in amounts similar to those found in one to three cups of coffee.

Second, use of *male sex hormones (androgens)* to increase muscle strength undoubtedly can increase athletic performance under some conditions, especially in women and in men who are poorly endowed with normal testosterone secretion. Unfortunately, some of the synthetic testosterone analog preparations can cause liver damage and even liver cancer. In men, any type of male sex hormone preparation also leads to decreased testicular function, including both decreased formation of sperm and decreased secretion of the person's own natural testosterone, with residual effects lasting at least for many months and perhaps indefinitely. In a woman, even more dire effects can occur because she is not normally adapted to the male sex hormone—hair on the face, a bass voice, ruddy skin, cessation of menses.

Other drugs, such as *amphetamines* and *cocaine,* have been reputed to increase one's athletic performance. However, it is equally true that overuse of these drugs can lead to deterioration of performance. Furthermore, experiments have failed to prove the value of these drugs except as a psychic stimulant. Some athletes have been known to die during athletic events because of interaction between such drugs and the norepinephrine and epinephrine released by the sympathetic nervous system during exercise. One of the causes of death under these conditions is overexcitability of the heart, leading to ventricular fibrillation, which is lethal within seconds.

REFERENCES

Barrow, H. M., and Brown, J. D.: Man and Movement: Principles of Physical Education, 4th ed. Philadelphia, Lea & Febiger, 1988.

Fisher, A. G., and Jensen, C. R.: Scientific Basis of Athletic Conditioning. 3rd ed. Philadelphia, Lea & Febiger, 1989.

Franklin, B. A., et al. (eds.): Exercise in Modern Medicine. Baltimore, Williams & Wilkins, 1988.

Friedman, M. J., and Ferkel, R. D. (eds.): Prosthetic Ligament Reconstruction of the Knee. Philadelphia, W. B. Saunders Co., 1988.

Gowitzke, B. A., and Milner, M.: Scientific Bases of Human Movement. 3rd ed. Baltimore, Williams & Wilkins, 1988.

Jones, N. L.: Clinical Exercise Testing. 3rd ed. Philadelphia, W. B. Saunders Co., 1988.

Nordin, M., and Frankel, V. H. (eds.): Basic Biomechanics of the Musculoskeletal System. 2nd ed. Philadelphia, Lea & Febiger, 1989.

Rasch, P. J. (ed.): Kinesiology and Applied Anatomy. 7th ed. Philadelphia, Lea & Febiger, 1989.

Smith, N. J., and Stanitski, C. L.: Sports Medicine: A Practical Guide. Philadelphia, W. B. Saunders Co., 1987.

Strauss, R. H.: Drugs and Performance in Sports. Philadelphia, W. B. Saunders Co., 1987.

Stray-Gundersen, J.: Unethical alterations of oxygen-carrying capacity in endurance athletes. News Physiol. Sci., 3:241, 1988.

Thomas, J. A. (ed.): Drugs, Athletes, and Physical Performance. New York, Plenum Publishing Corp., 1988.

Wagner, P. D.: The lungs during exercise. News Physiol. Sci., 2:6, 1987.

QUESTIONS

1. Discuss the differences between the female and the *male* athlete.
2. What is the relationship between *muscle cross-sectional area* and *muscle strength*?
3. How does *muscle power* differ from *muscle strength*?
4. Characterize the three important metabolic systems that supply energy in exercise.
5. Explain the mechanisms for recovery of each of the above three metabolic systems after they are depleted.
6. How do the different nutrients contribute to muscle energy during endurance athletics?
7. Explain the principles of *muscle building* and the changes in the muscle fibers during *muscle hypertrophy.*
8. What are the differences between *fast twitch* and *slow twitch* fibers?
9. Approximately how much can the untrained person and the trained person increase their rates of *oxygen consumption* above the resting level during *maximal exercise*?
10. What are the effects of maximal exercise on *blood oxygen* and *carbon dioxide concentrations*? Why do these effects occur?
11. How much can *muscle blood flow* increase during *maximal exercise*? What are the causes of this increase?
12. Explain the relationship between *work output, oxygen consumption,* and *cardiac output* during exercise.
13. What are the relationships of both respiratory and cardiovascular performance to $\dot{V}O_2$ *Max*?
14. Discuss the perils of excess *body heat* during exercise.
15. Discuss the problems of *fluid and electrolyte loss* during exercise. Discuss their replacement.

Index

Note: Page numbers in *italics* refer to illustrations; page numbers followed by (t) refer to tables.